THE ILLUSTRATED ENCYCLOPEDIA OF Natural Remedies

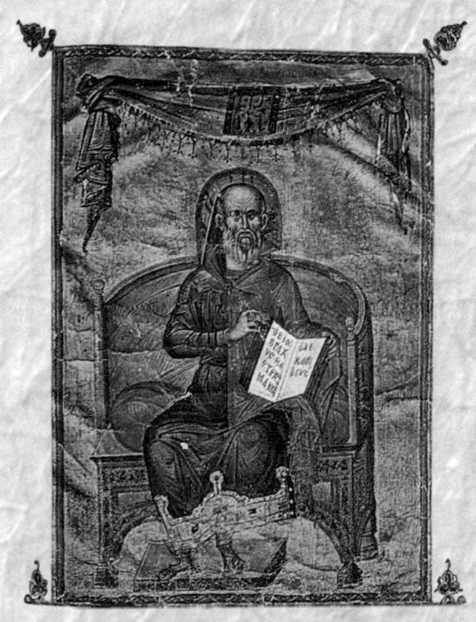

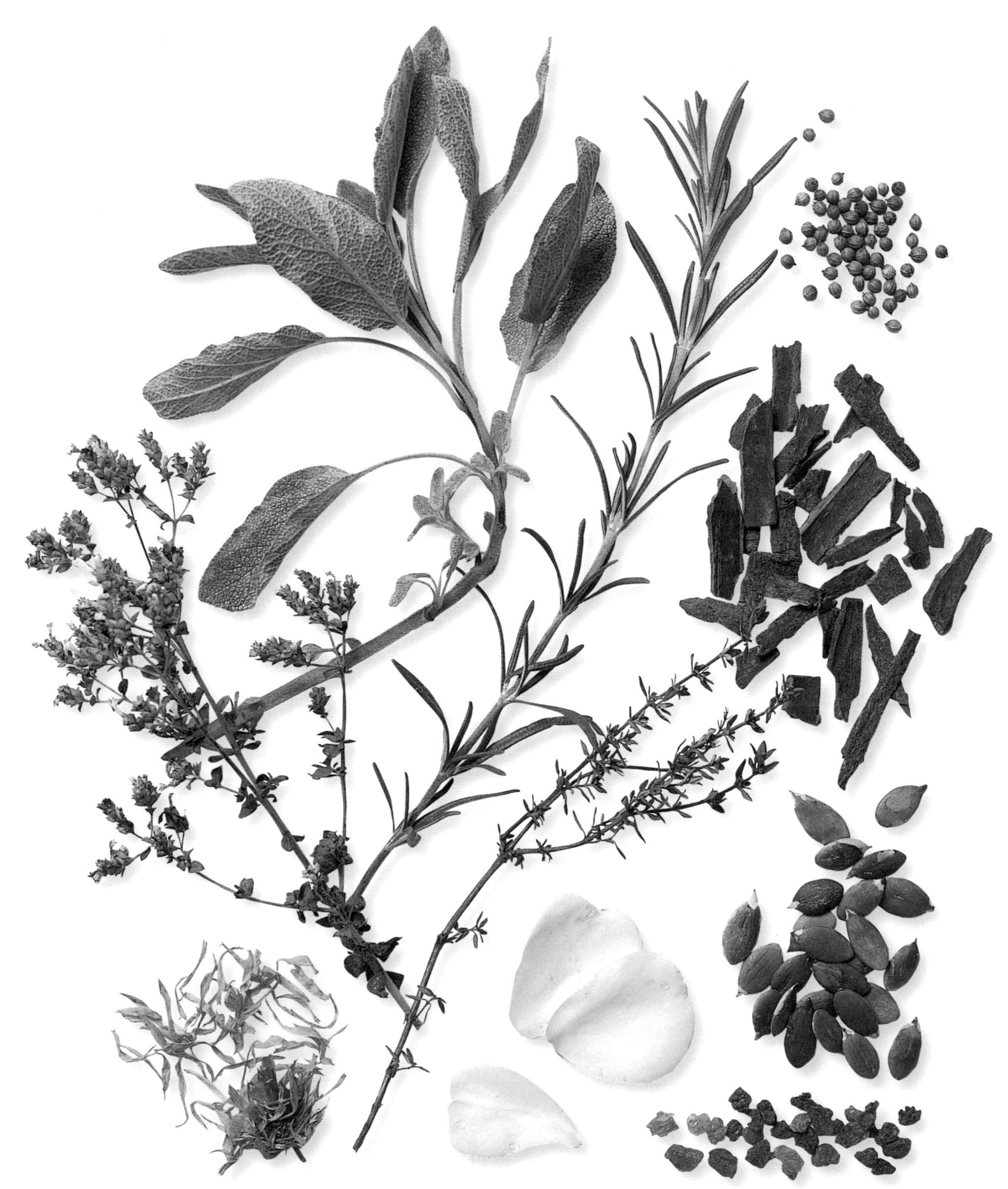

THE ILLUSTRATED ENCYCLOPEDIA OF

Natural Remedies

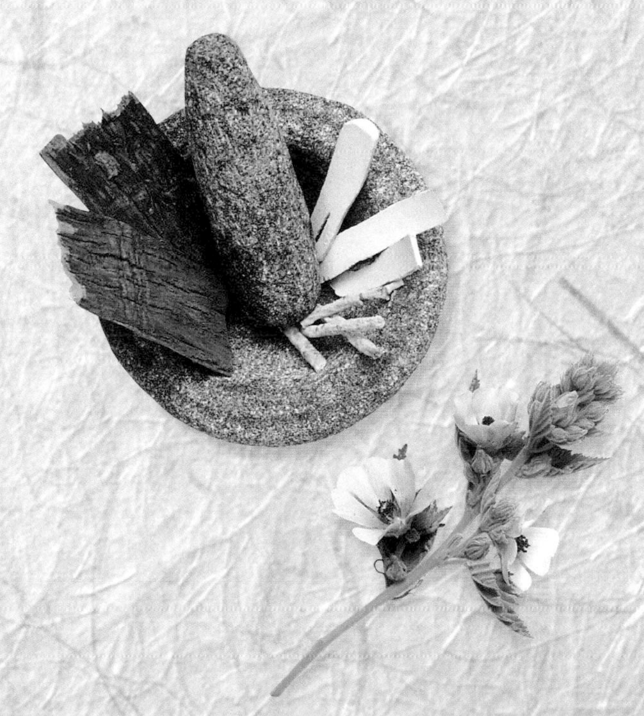

C. NORMAN SHEALY

M.D., Ph.D.

ELEMENT

Shaftesbury, Dorset • Boston, Massachusetts • Melbourne, Victoria

First published in Great Britain in 1998 by
ELEMENT BOOKS LIMITED
Shaftesbury, Dorset, SP7 8BP

Published in the USA in 1998 by
ELEMENT BOOKS INC
160 North Washington Street, Boston, MA 02114

Published in Australia in 1998 by
ELEMENT BOOKS
and distributed by Penguin Australia Ltd
487 Maroondah Highway, Ringwood, Victoria 3134

NOTE FROM THE PUBLISHER
Any information given in this book is not intended to be taken as a replacement for medical advice. Any person with a condition requiring medical attention should consult a qualified practitioner or therapist.

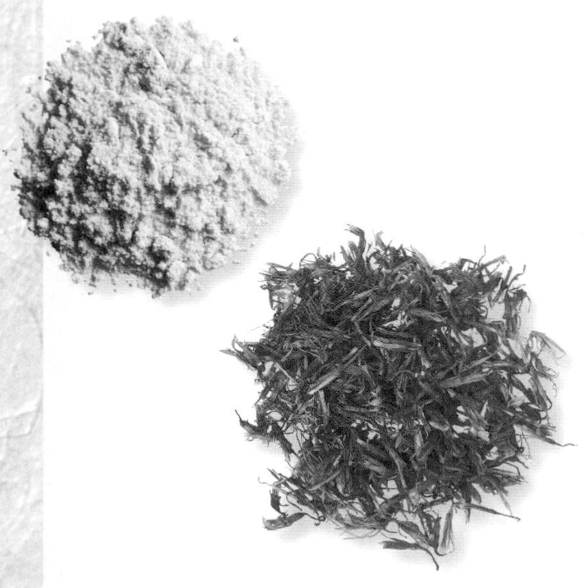

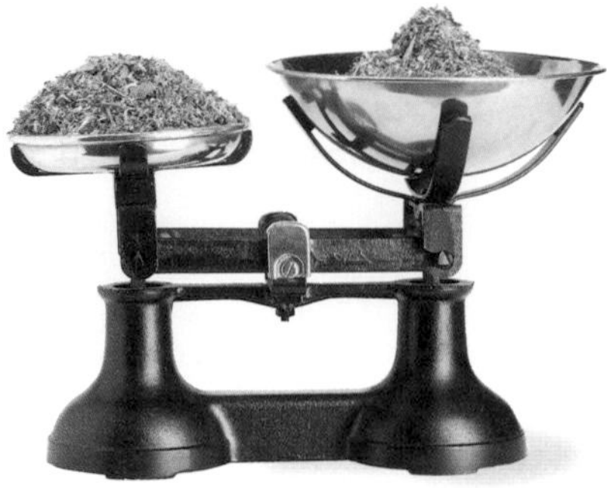

Editor in Chief **C. Norman Shealy** M.D., Ph.D.
General Editor **Karen Sullivan**

Designed and created with
The Bridgewater Book Company Limited

ELEMENT BOOKS LIMITED
Editorial Director Julia McCutchen
Managing Editor Miranda Spicer
Editor Katie Worrall
Production Director Roger Lane
Production Sarah Golden

THE BRIDGEWATER BOOK COMPANY
Art Director Terry Jeavons
Designers Jane Lanaway, Glyn Bridgewater
Page layout John Christopher, Richard Constable, Chris Lanaway, Andrew Lawes, Angela Neal, Michael Whitehead, and Ginny Zeal
Managing Editor Anne Townley
Editor Fiona Corbridge
Picture research Vanessa Fletcher
Three dimensional models Mark Jamieson
Studio photography Guy Ryecart, Ian Parsons
Illustrations Michael Courtney, Lorraine Harrison, Ivan Hissey, Mainline Design

Printed and bound in Great Britain by
Butler & Tanner Limited, Frome and London

Library of Congress Cataloging in Publication data available

ISBN 1 86204 186 5 PB
ISBN 1 86204 409 0 HB

ACKNOWLEDGMENTS

The publishers wish to thank the following for the use of pictures:

A–Z BOTANICAL pp. 28T, 32BR, 33TR, 79TR, 92TL, 97C, 116CL, 132BR, 183TR, 184TR, 203BL, 229TL, 229TR, 230CL, 232TR, 239TL, 239TR, 240TL, 241T

AUSTRALIAN BUSH ESSENCES pp. 230BL, 230TR, 231TR. 238TL. 240BL

C. W. DANIEL PUBLISHERS pp. 141CR, 141BR

BRIDGEMAN ART LIBRARY pp. 2, 78

e.t.archive pp. 18–19

GARDEN PICTURE LIBRARY pp. 41CL, 107TL, 153CR, 16TL, 185CR, 197TR, 213B, 218BL, 222TL, 22BR, 225TR, 233TL

HARRY SMITH pp. 33C, 152CL

HOUSES AND INTERIORS p. 93CR

HUTCHISON PICTURE LIBRARY pp. 68BL, 70B, 105BR, 189B, 190BL

IMAGE BANK pp. 18TL, 18BL, 80BL, 291TR

NATURAL HISTORY PHOTOGRAPHIC AGENCY: pp. 99BR, 199L, 216B

OXFORD SCIENTIFIC FILMS pp. 188TL, 176T

SCIENCE PHOTO LIBRARY pp. 75L, 184B, 196CR, 277BR, 390TL, 341BR, 398TL, 424, 448TR

WELEDA UK LTD, manufacturers of homeopathic remedies pp. 174TL, 174CL, 174BL,

ZEFA pp. 10BL, 10/11, 11TR, 18CL, 34BL, 40TL, 45CB, 47BL, 50T, 51BL, 58TL, 69T, 74C, 75R 77B, 78/79, 88T, 95BL, 105TL, 105BC, 108CL, 141TR, 155TL, 168BR, 174TR, 193TL, 197BL, 201TR, 207C, 210/211, 212BL, 214T, 215CR, 228BR, 237TL, 237TR, 242TR, 242BR, 244/245, 261T, 266CR, 267T, 276TL, 287T, 307, 324L, 330TR, 335BR, 391, 417TR, 427, 439

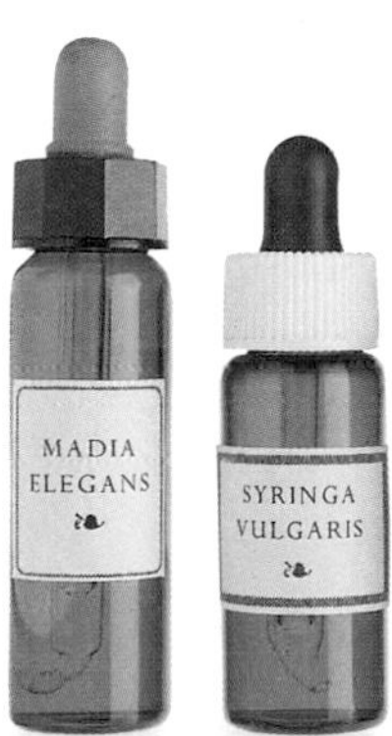

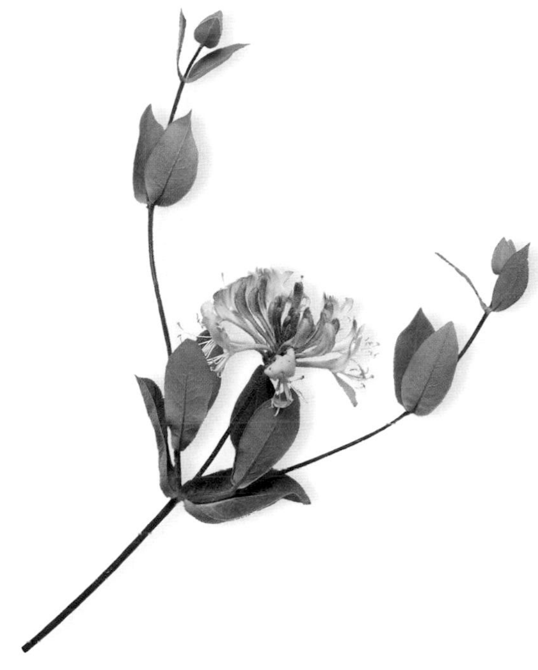

SPECIAL THANKS TO

Maria Anderson, Philip Auchinvole, Tony Bannister, Jan Boyle, Glyn Bridgewater, Stephanie Brotherstone, Deena Bunn, Kimberley Bunn, Adam Carne, Rob Chappell, Judith Cox, Naomi Denny, Juliette Denny, Nina Downey, Rebecca Drury, Cathy Glendinning, Paul Golding, Rachel Gould, Paul Harley, Deborah Heath, Julia Holden, Simon Holden, Natalie Jerome, Carolyn Jikeimi-Roberts, Mette Lauritzen, Jan Lewington, Kay Macmullan, Jack Martin, Jim McClean, Norma McClean, Henry Milne, Helen Omand, Elin Osmond, Wendy Oxberry, Sunny Pitcher, Caron Riley, Vincent Riley, Warren Saunders, Michelle Sawyer, Stephen Sparshatt, Sarah Stanley, Andrew Stemp, Neil Strowger, Jenny Sullivan, Bethany Sword, Lauren Sword, Sheila Sword, Gav Tuffnell, Mary Watson, Derek Watts, Louise Williams, Robert Williams.

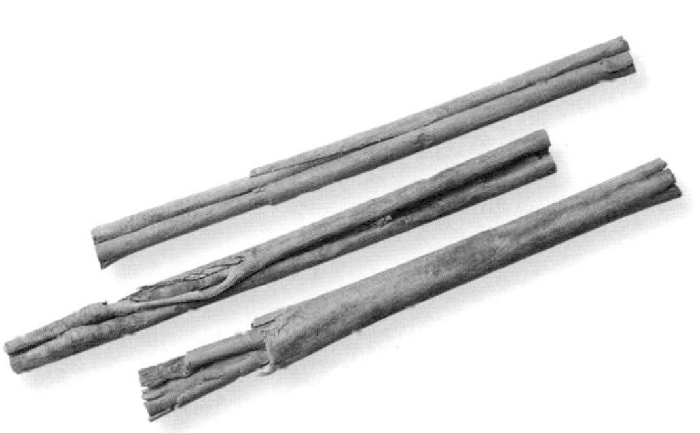

CONTENTS

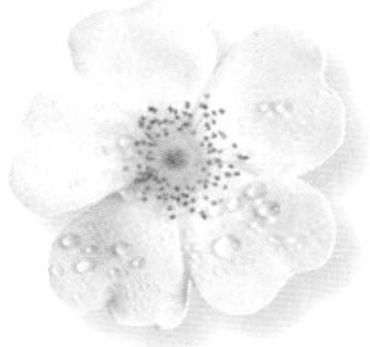

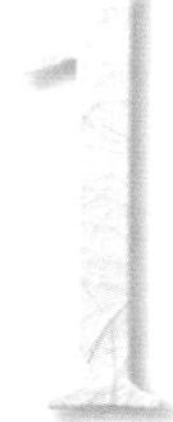

PART ONE

THERAPIES AND HEALING REMEDY SOURCES

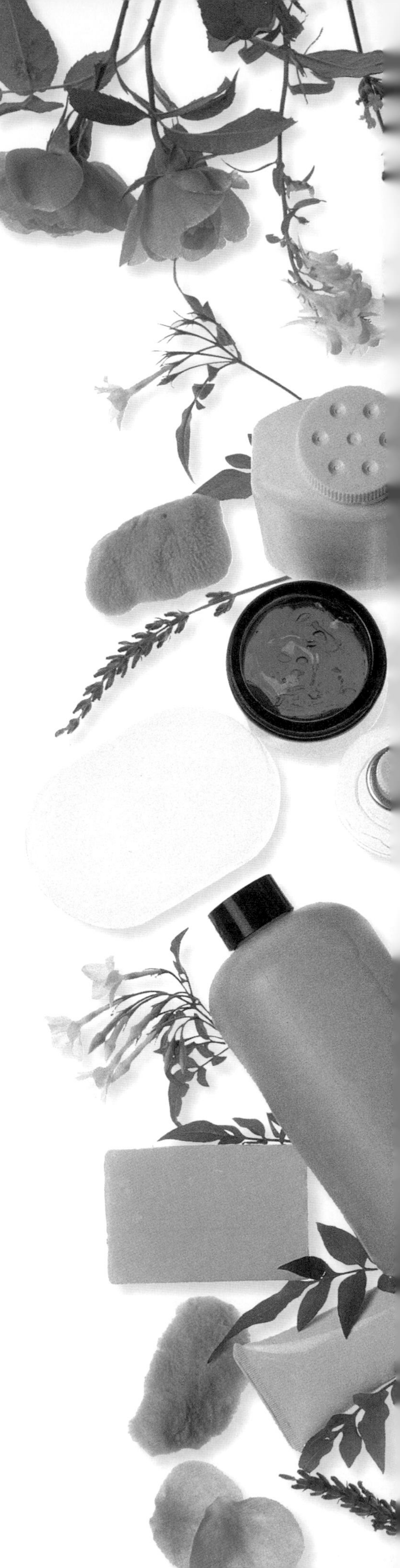

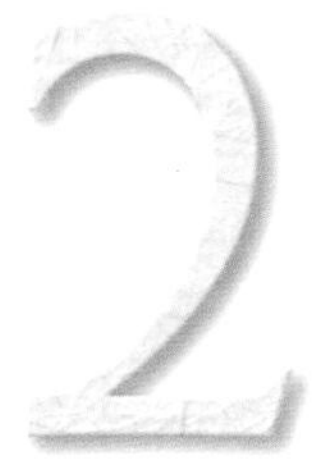

PART TWO

TREATING COMMON AILMENTS

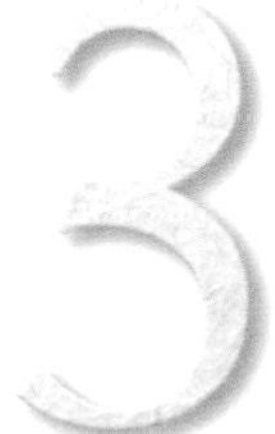

PART THREE

REFERENCE SECTION

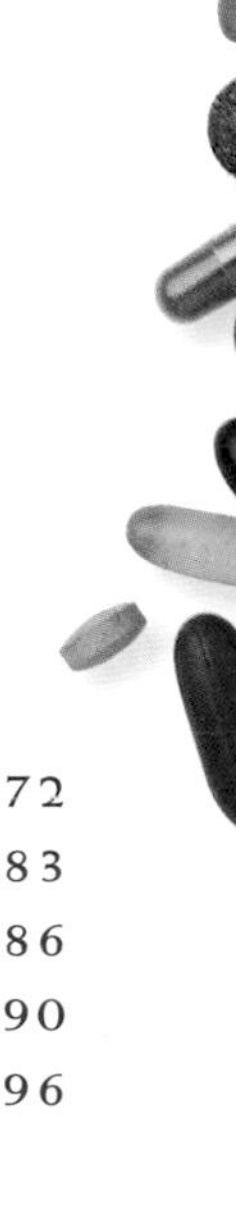

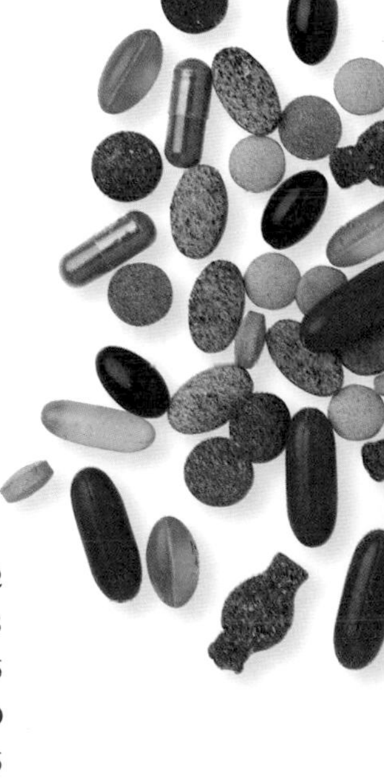

FOREWORD

THE "FATHER OF MEDICINE" *is generally considered to be Hippocrates who was born around 460 B.C.E. on the island of Cos, and died around 370 B.C.E. The body of work that is attributed to Hippocrates consists of 79 books and 59 treatises on which modern medicine is said to be founded. It is particularly interesting that a great deal of his writing addresses the role model of the physician – he should look healthy and well-nourished, wear decent clothes, and have a degree of friendliness. Other than that, the most consistent commentary is on attention to anatomical detail, and precautions about the limitations of therapy, especially surgery.*

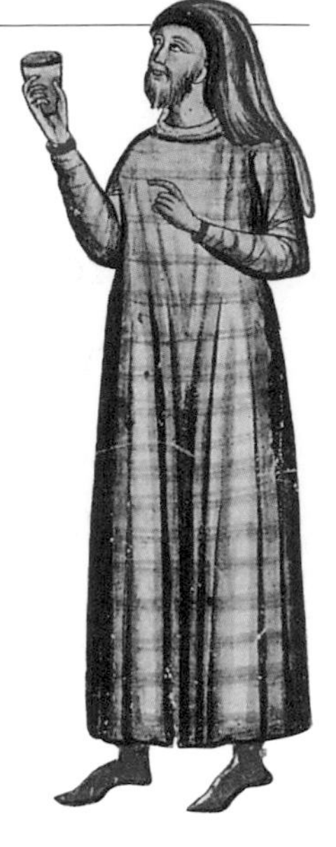

ABOVE *The role of the physician was central to the work of Hippocrates who is considered to be the founder of modern medicine.*

In terms of theory, modern medicine dates from the work of Hippocrates, although the history of natural therapy extends back to long before his time. From those early days in Greece, two major schools of thought have dominated Western medicine – on the one hand rationalism, and on the other empiricism. Essentially the rationalists believe that science can ultimately know all the answers about life, and even create it. The "success" of recent experiments into cloning has certainly appeared to give credence to this view. In contrast, empiricists, or naturalists, believe in the ineffable quality of the universe, the natural order of life, and a concept of the divine, or vital force. Interestingly, empiricism has been embraced to a greater extent by the general public and rationalism by the Western medical society. Individuals seem to feel much more at home with a way of understanding health and disease that relies on sensory input and personal experience.

ABOVE *Eastern philosophy is based on a belief in wholeness which is at odds with much of Western thinking about medicine.*

The dramatic increase in popularity of Ayurveda and Chinese Medicine in the West can be seen as a return to what is in essence a naturalist or empiricist approach, although both these therapies have developed into organized

RIGHT *Holistic therapies address both the spiritual and physical aspects of illness and disease.*

systems. Homeopathy was developed very much later, at a time when Western medicine was in a remarkably non-scientific pit of superstition and useless therapy which was often worse than no therapy at all. It is a very subtle approach to healing, perhaps ultimately dealing at an anatomic level in the "vital force" of the universe, and its popularity is also increasing. These therapies, and the others covered in this book, put the reader back in touch with empirical approaches to health, giving him or her the opportunity to grasp and use insights which Western physicians have largely ignored. The idea is to choose remedies from this book according to intuition, with the introductory chapters as a guide, and judge their results according to your own sensory perception.

ABOVE Attention to diet is an important part of almost every natural therapy.

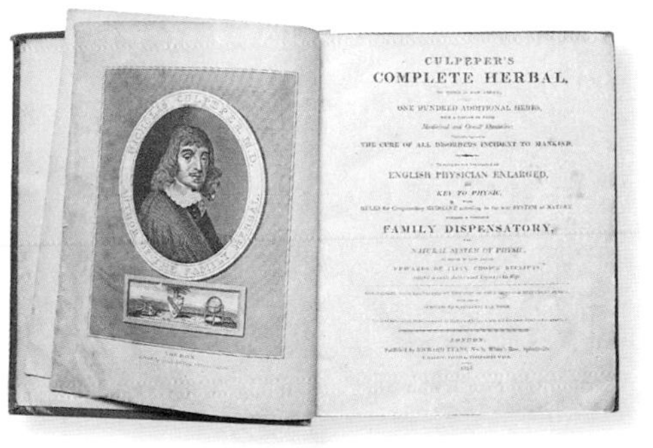

ABOVE There is a wealth of medical knowledge enshrined in old texts that is now being rediscovered by new generations.

When I asked my Professor of Medicine, Eugene A. Stead Jr., M.D., in 1978 what he considered to be the role of a physician, he answered that it is to be a triage officer. "Triage" is a term which is often used in connection with battle or disaster victims, and means the allocation of treatment to patients according to the principle of maximizing the number of survivors. A triage officer would stand at the door when a patient was significantly ill and advise when medicine or surgery was truly needed to save life or function. Dr. Stead advised that when life and function are not at risk, as in the vast majority of symptomatic illnesses, the patient should "go into the department stores and choose that which most appeals."

In this wonderful and comprehensive book, you have a remarkable department store of choices. May your browsing be healing.

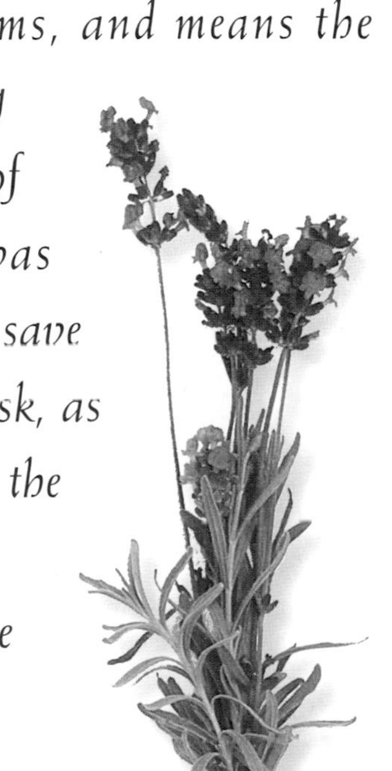

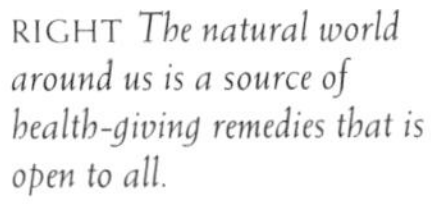
RIGHT The natural world around us is a source of health-giving remedies that is open to all.

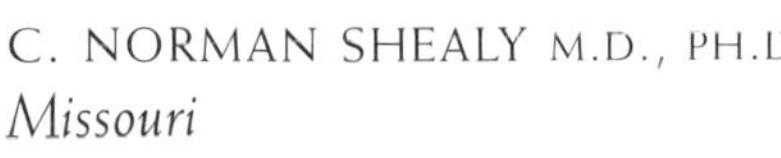
C. NORMAN SHEALY M.D., PH.D
Missouri

INTRODUCTION

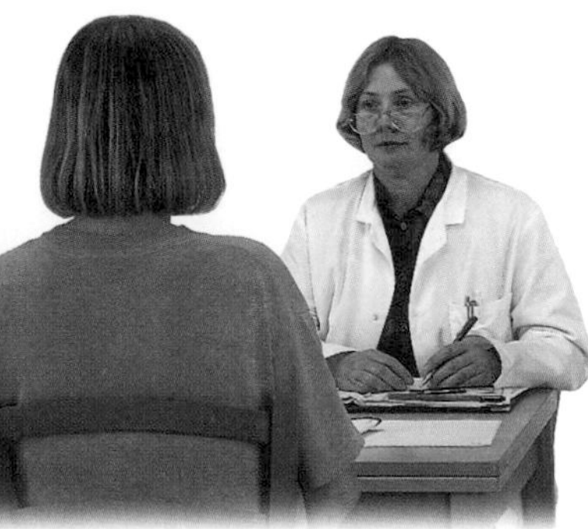

ABOVE *The claims of conventional medicine are today being questioned by increasing numbers of people.*

The increased use of natural medicines and remedies over the past decade has prompted one of the most exciting developments in healthcare in our time. Many of the tenets of modern medicine have been challenged, and the crisis that conventional healthcare is now facing is the result of its own philosophy. The main premise of conventional medicine is that curing disease will lead to good health. This ignores the fundamental concept that pathology is individual to the sufferer, and that prevention is ultimately more important than treatment for the population at large.

This idea is borne out by the fact that modern medicine is simply not as efficient or effective as we have been led to believe; indeed, evidence suggests that it may cause and create more fatal diseases than it cures, and despite the huge sums of money invested, the populations of the U.K., Australia, the U.S. and most of Europe do not live as long or as healthily as people from other cultures, where healthcare investment is substantially lower.

Adverse drug reactions and side-effects are one of the 10 most common reasons for hospitalization in the U.S., and a 1997 survey indicates that avoidable deaths from unnecessary surgery total nearly 100,000 per year. The information provided to doctors and physicians throughout the course of their careers is largely funded by the pharmaceutical industry which earns billions each year from sales of prescription and over-the-counter medicines. As a result, we, in the West, have been encouraged to adopt a "pill-popping" approach to health – taking an average of 26.5 million pills per hour. Sleeping tablets, analgesics (painkillers), antihistamines, sedatives, and antidepressants rank among the top 20 drugs prescribed by physicians, and more than 52 million aspirin or paracetamol tablets are taken each day in the U.S.

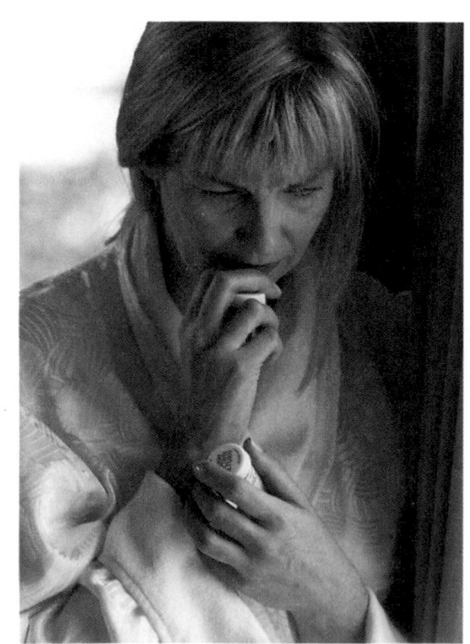

BELOW *The quick fix, pill-dispensing option of much modern medicine neglects underlying causes of ill-health.*

Perhaps the most alarming result of this over–dependence upon drugs is the fact that we have stopped taking responsibility for our own health. When we have a headache, we take a painkiller; when we have a cold, we might take an antihistamine. We suppress the symptoms of health conditions because we want to feel better; we no longer accept the logic that pain or discomfort is a message from our body that something is wrong. We have become used to the idea that someone or something else can deal with our health problems. By taking a pill or conventional medicine in some form, we do experience a relief from symptoms, but what is important to

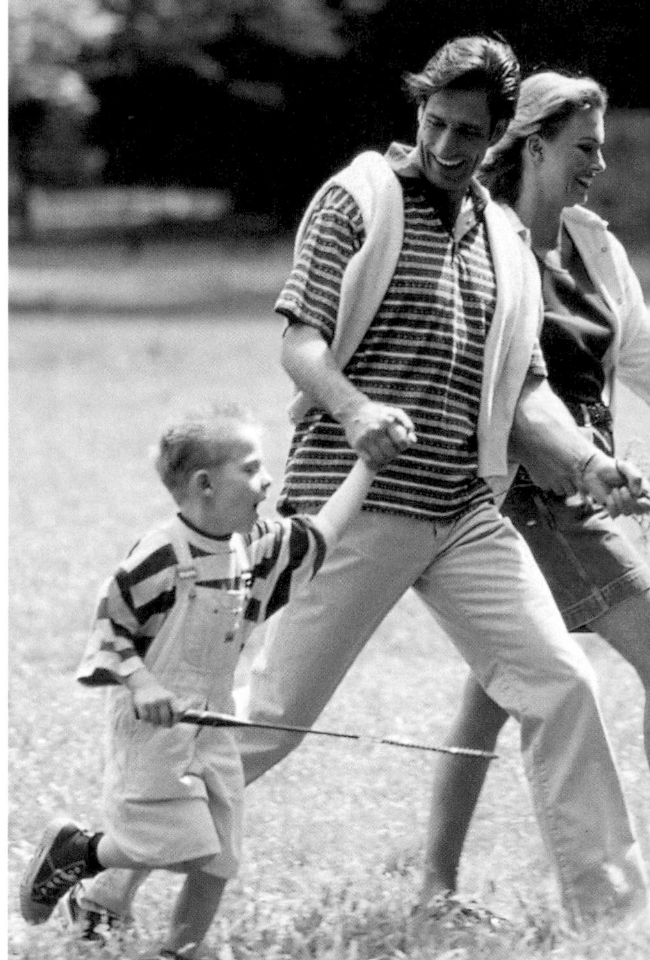

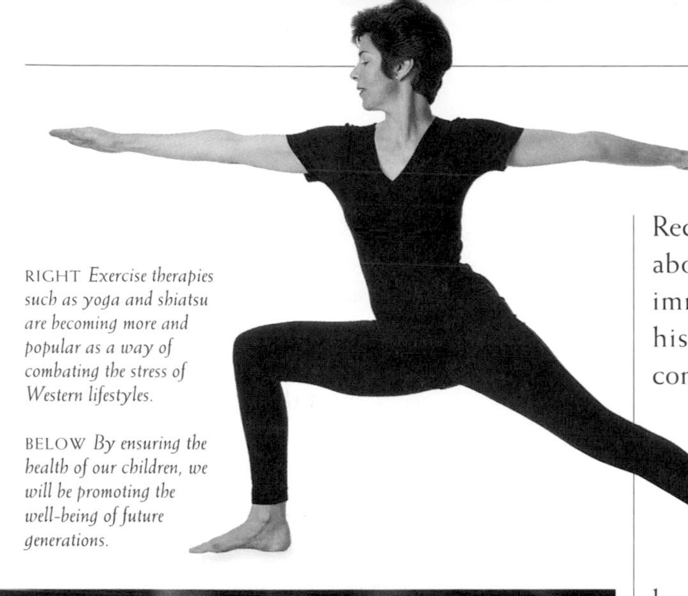

RIGHT *Exercise therapies such as yoga and shiatsu are becoming more and popular as a way of combating the stress of Western lifestyles.*

BELOW *By ensuring the health of our children, we will be promoting the well-being of future generations.*

remember is that the cause of the pain or illness remains. By treating the symptoms, or suppressing them, we are doing nothing to treat the root cause. Eczema sufferers apply ointments and creams to the surface of the skin; they make take anti-inflammatories or antihistamines to ease the itching, but the cause of the eczema is still there and the body's reaction has been masked by drugs. They have not been cured, their illness has merely been controlled.

Recently, this trend has begun to change. Scares about the side-effects and long-term effects of immunization, abuse of painkillers, anti-histamines, and antibiotics have proved that conventional medicine, despite its many miracles, has been overused and we have become far too dependent on it. Many of us are no longer happy to accept the risks of prescription drugs, and are realizing that there are natural, healthy alternatives. With the increased interest in diet, emotional health and well-being, and exercise, we are becoming more in tune with our bodies and are choosing to listen to the messages they give. Even more importantly, we are taking steps to prevent illness rather than simply treat it when it does arise, and for this reason we are willing to try natural substances that not only treat health conditions, at cause level, but work with the body to keep it well. Natural remedies are more likely to make you feel better, more vital and more alert; they have fewer side-effects and because they work actively to prevent illness, they are, perhaps, the answer to the healthcare crisis that has been spiralling out of control.

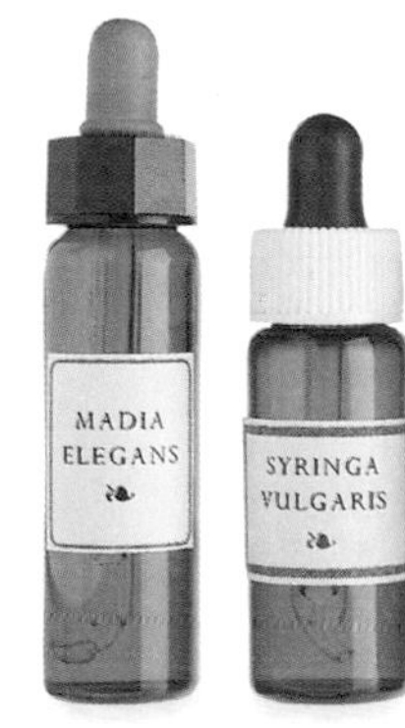

Our understanding of how different cultures approach healthcare is blossoming, and figures show that many of the most common Western illnesses, such as eczema, asthma, cancer, chronic fatigue syndrome, and digestive problems simply do not exist to the same degree in other countries. We have a cornucopia of information at our fingertips, and a greater understanding of how disease can be prevented and cured using herbs, oils, homeopathic remedies, food, vitamins and nutritional supplements, and other substances that encourage our bodies to work at their optimum level.

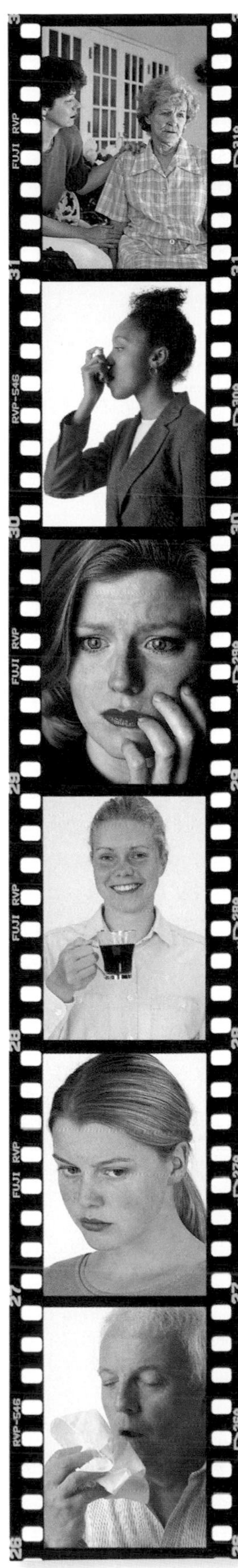

ABOVE RIGHT *The time may be approaching when remedies derived from natural sources will supplant the synthetic medicines of Western healthcare.*

RIGHT *A wide range of ailments can be alleviated by holistic therapies, from life-threatening diseases like cancer to minor disorders like the common cold.*

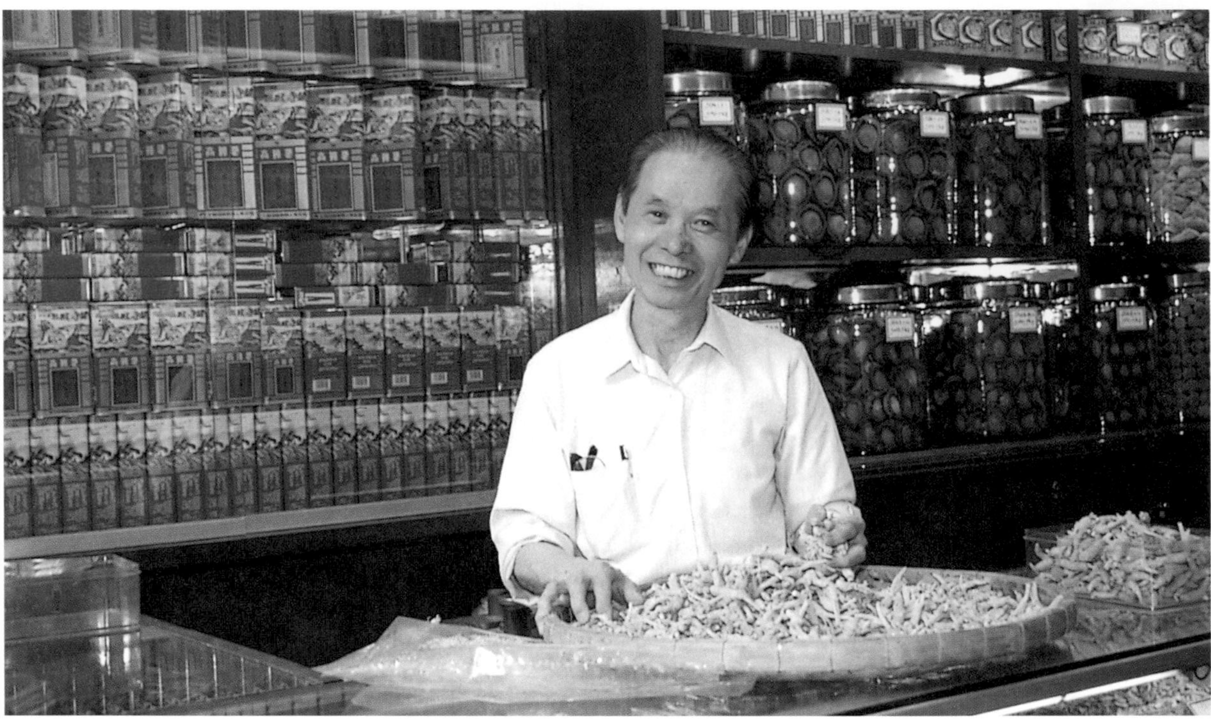

LEFT *Traditional Chinese Medicine is one of the most popular natural therapies.*

A HEALTHY MIND IN A HEALTHY BODY

The modern clinical emphasis on separating different aspects of our physical, mental, and spiritual health has resulted in a dehumanizing of medicine. By treating the whole person, holistic therapies can restore the proper balance and promote a sense of complete well-being, inside and out.

The sale of natural products has increased by over 200 percent over the last five years, and more than 20 percent of the U.S. population has consulted a natural health practitioner over the last year. Our approach to our health is changing dramatically, and this increased interest is being fed by a broad range of products from around the world that are now available in our local shops and stores.

Our growing understanding of holistic treatment has encouraged us to examine the healing practices of cultures from around the world, and from each we can gather invaluable information about diet, lifestyle, illness, health and well-being.

ABOVE *Ayurveda, the traditional medicine of India, uses herbal treatments to restore the body's natural balance.*

This book concentrates on the remedies that form the basis of eight international therapeutic disciplines: homeopathy, aromatherapy, Chinese herbal medicine, herbalism, Ayurveda, flower essences, folk or traditional medicine (also called home remedies), and nutrition. These remedies can be used to encourage and enhance good health and to treat and prevent illnesses, both chronic and acute. Many of these remedies are derived from plants, which have a wide variety of therapeutic uses; indeed, up to 140 conventional drugs in use today are based on plants and herbs.

A large percentage of these remedies have been in use for thousands of years, and it was the practice of herbalism and other disciplines that made it possible for so many of our conventional drugs to be created. However, in practice, pharmaceutical companies isolate and often synthesize the active ingredient of a plant or herb, and many practitioners believe that this causes side-effects and other problems, that do not occur when the substance is taken in its whole, natural form.

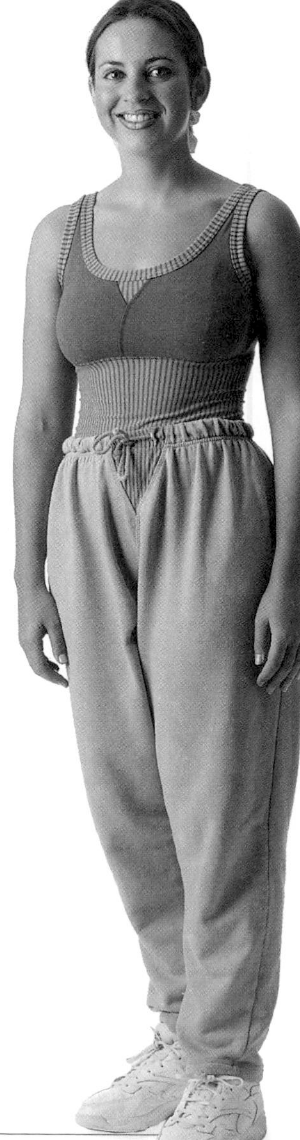

RIGHT *Natural healing therapies treat the whole person.*

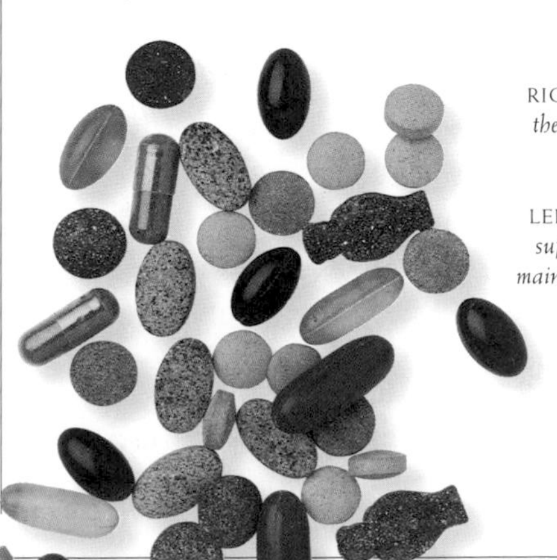

LEFT *Dietary and other supplements can help to maintain our constitutional harmony.*

REMEDY SOURCES

Natural medicine uses many different kinds of substances as the basis for healing remedies.

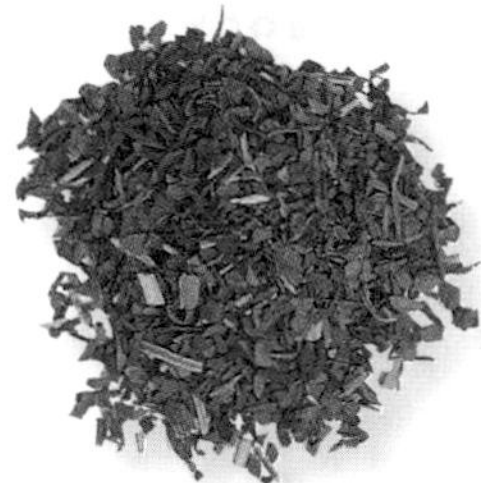

AYURVEDA
Ayurvedic tea is a simple form of healing remedy.

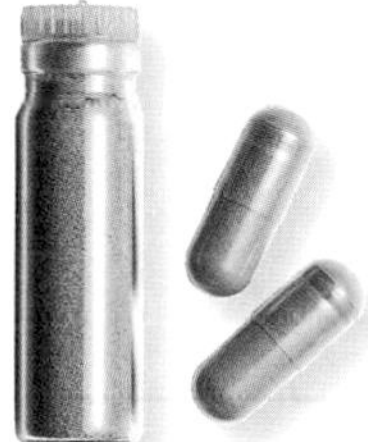

CHINESE HERBS
Chinese herbal remedies come in various forms including lozenges and powders.

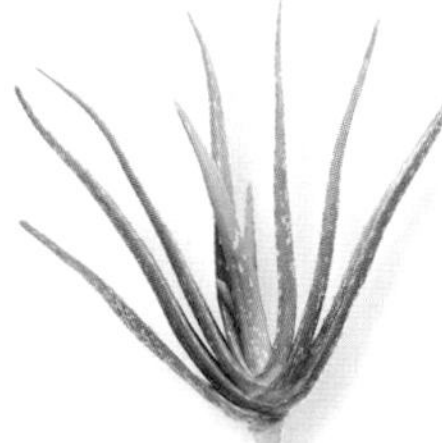

HERBS AND PLANTS
The leaves, shoots, seeds, and even roots of many plants have therapeutic qualities.

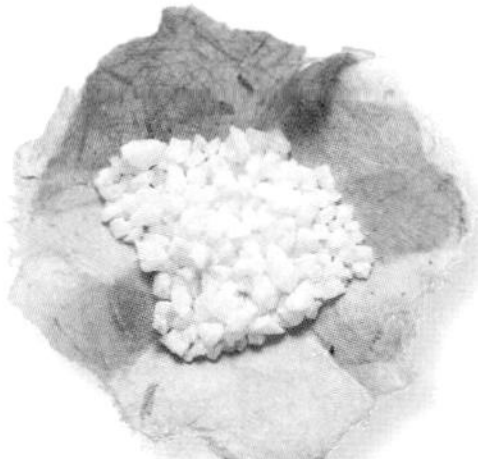

HOMEOPATHY
Homeopathic remedies most often are given in the form of tablets.

Isolating the active ingredients of plants produces powerful, often toxic, drugs, while medical herbalism offers a gentler, safer, and less disruptive effect, allowing the body to undertake its own natural healing process.

There are over 1000 remedies outlined in this book, many of which you can grow in your own garden or on the windowsill, or purchase from a reputable health shop. Others will be items from your larder or store cupboard – everyday goods with healing and therapeutic properties that may surprise you. Each of the remedy sources has a data file of features, cautions, and other useful information, and there are often recipes for practical applications. Each of the main eight disciplines is also introduced, which helps you to understand how, for instance, the use of something like cinnamon or ginseng differs between Western and Chinese herbalism, and between folk medicine and Ayurveda. You'll learn how a rose aromatherapy oil is different from a rose flower essence, how vitamin C and healthy bacteria can encourage good health, and how Belladonna, a poisonous substance, can be taken in tiny dilutions to relieve fevers and other problems. You'll discover natural alternatives to caffeine and sleeping pills, laxatives, and antacids, in remedies that strengthen your mind and body, lift your mood, calm your nerves, and enhance your resistance to infection and illness.

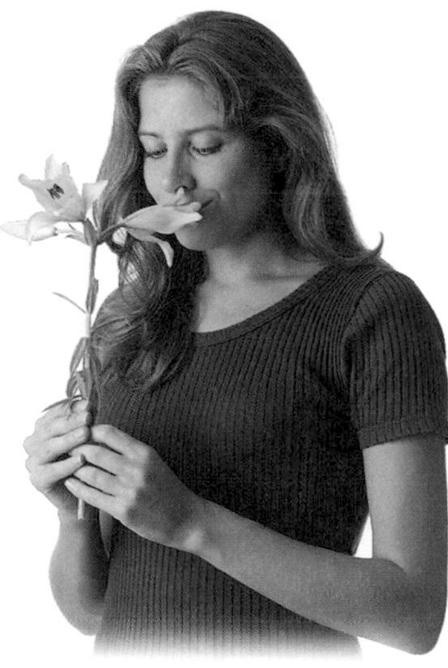

ABOVE *The restoration of the body's natural rhythms is an important aspect of holistic therapy.*

BELOW *A well-stocked herb garden, used with care and skill, will be of more therapeutic benefit than any number of proprietary medicines.*

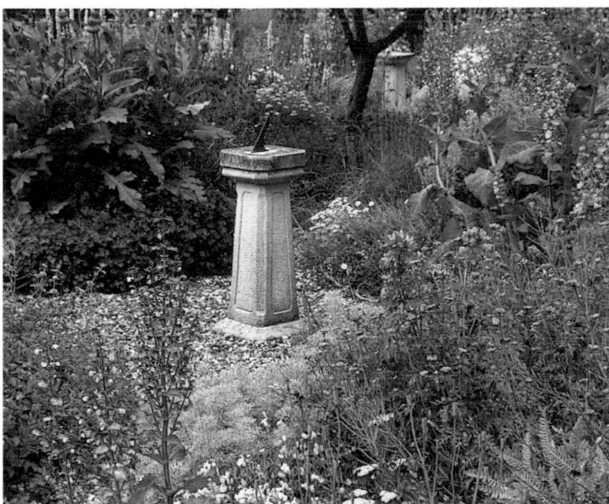

Over 200 common ailments are also discussed in detail, with practical examples of how you can use the remedies from around the world to cure or prevent them. There are also suggestions for stocking a complete home medicine chest, so you can have on hand all the essential remedies to keep you healthy.

We are on the brink of an exciting new era in healthcare, and with the benefit of these remedies, presented in easy-to-follow files, grouped by the discipline in which they are most often used, you and your family can experiment with safe substitutes to conventional medicines by following the comprehensive instructions. The remedies in this book form the basis of a "stay-well" philosophy, with substances to boost immunity, help prevent cancer and heart disease, encourage emotional well-being and relaxation, enhance your strength, and keep your body's systems functioning the way they should. These remedies are the medicine of the future, and this is the essential guide for anyone who wants to take responsibility for their own health. By using only a few of these remedies, you can live longer and with a better quality of life. These are the secrets of good health from around the world; experiment with care and you'll be amazed at the results.

KAREN SULLIVAN
London

ABOVE *A simple plant like Meadowsweet is a treasure store of healing properties waiting to be unlocked.*

HOW TO USE THIS BOOK

This exhaustive and gloriously illustrated reference work is dedicated to the whole spectrum of alternative healing remedies. Aimed at the general reader, this comprehensive book covers the origins, methods, principles and remedies of eight alternative therapies - Ayurveda, Aromatherapy, Flower Remedies, Chinese Herbal Medicine, Herbalism, Homeopathy, Vitamins and Minerals, and Traditional Home and Folk Remedies.

PART ONE: **Therapies and Healing Remedy Sources.** Eight chapters cover the different therapies. In each case, the background and history of the therapy are covered together with how it works, information on visiting a practitioner and extensive guidelines for self-help. Following the introduction to the therapy, the major remedies and remedy sources are covered with details on how the substance is obtained or made, what they treat and how they should be taken. "Therapy Connections" highlight the remedy sources which are common to more than one therapy giving a full picture of the properties and various uses of one particular remedy source.

PART TWO: **Treating Common Ailments.** 185 pages of common ailments and the relevant remedies with which they can be treated. In many cases, information on how the remedies should be prepared will be accompanied by step-by-step photographic sequences. Caution boxes will make clear the situations in which the remedies are not suitable. Cross-referencing directs the reader back to Part One where the source of the remedy, its properties and uses are outlined in detail. A final chapter is devoted to the best remedies to be kept in your Home Remedy Chest.

PART THREE: **Reference Section.** Consists of a full glossary of terms, a list of useful addresses and books for further reading.

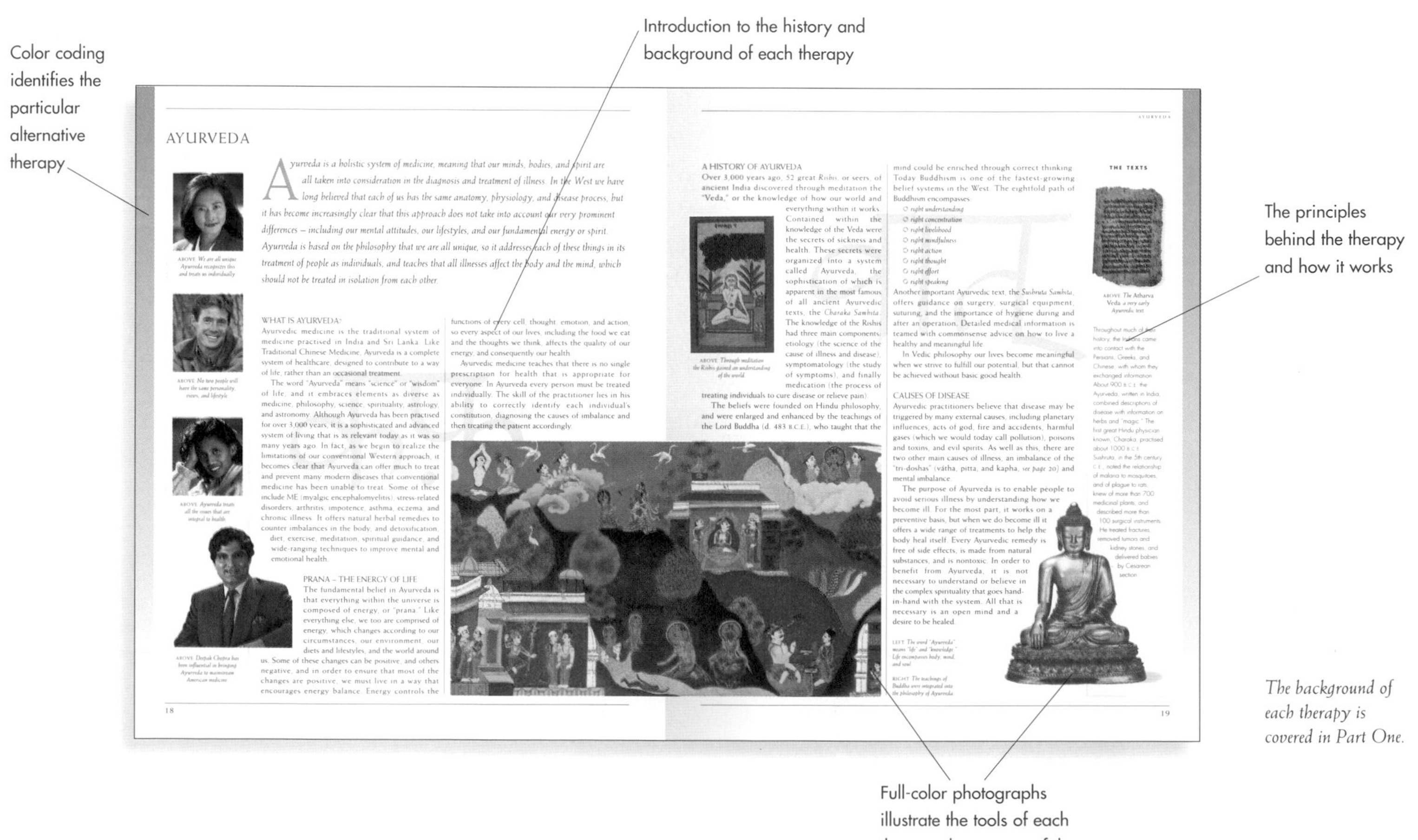

The remedy source is described and illustrated

"Therapy Connections" refer you to other therapies which use the same remedy source

The remedy sources are listed in Part One.

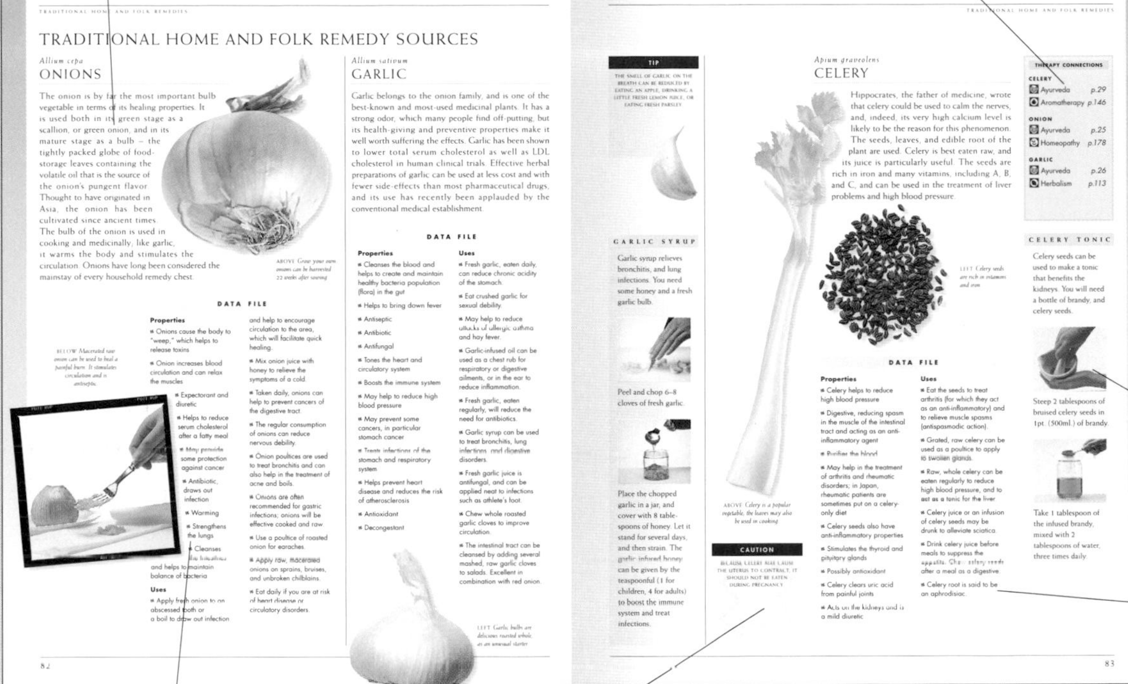

Step-by-step photographs demonstrate how to prepare the remedy

How to use the remedy source in particular treatments

Bullet points highlight the properties of the remedy source

Cautions warn when it is inadvisable to use a particular remedy

Ailments, grouped according to the body system affected, each have a descriptive introduction

The different remedies for the ailment in question are listed with cross-references to its detailed entry in the therapy chapter in Part One

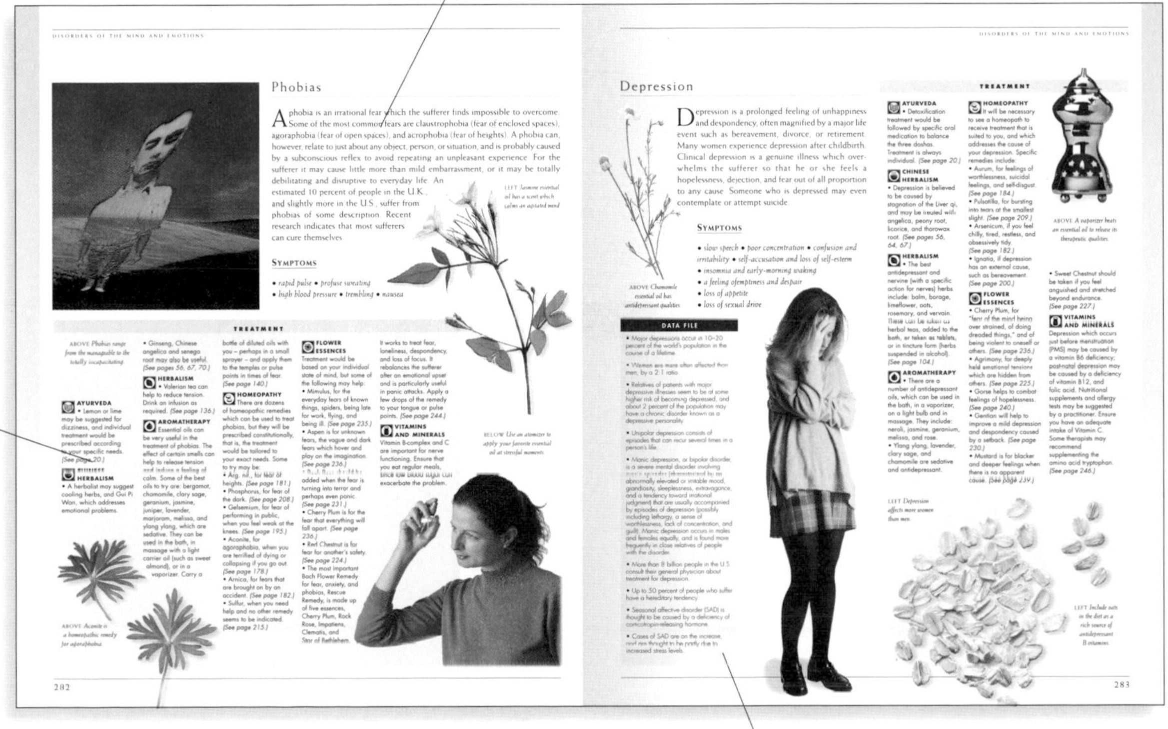

Specific illnesses appear in Part Two, Treating Common Ailments.

A "Data File" gives the latest facts and figures about this ailment

1

PART ONE

THERAPIES AND HEALING REMEDY SOURCES

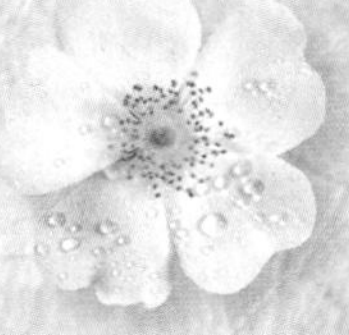

AYURVEDA

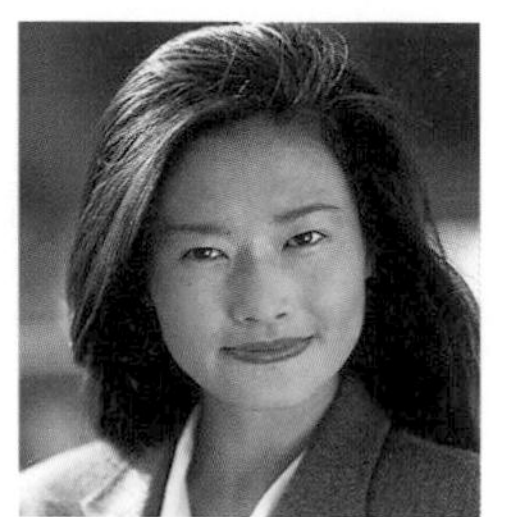

ABOVE *We are all unique. Ayurveda recognizes this and treats us individually.*

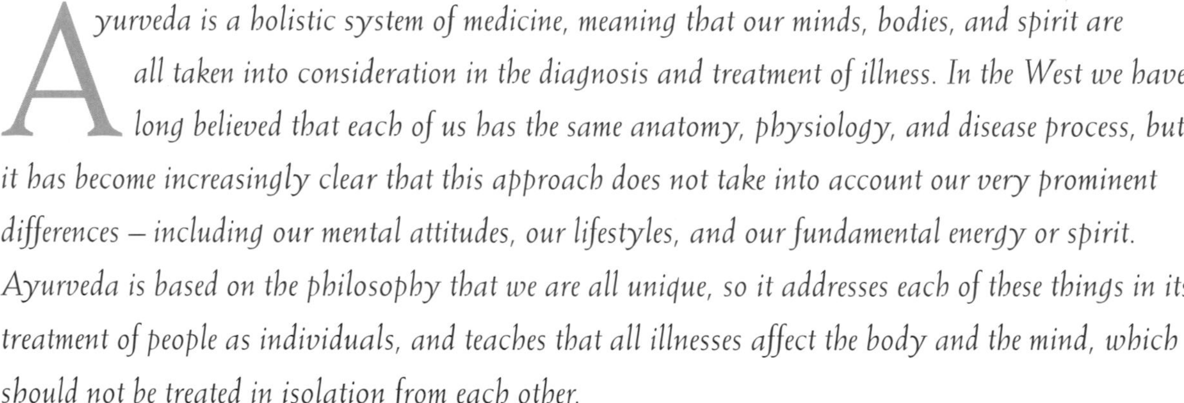

Ayurveda is a holistic system of medicine, meaning that our minds, bodies, and spirit are all taken into consideration in the diagnosis and treatment of illness. In the West we have long believed that each of us has the same anatomy, physiology, and disease process, but it has become increasingly clear that this approach does not take into account our very prominent differences – including our mental attitudes, our lifestyles, and our fundamental energy or spirit. Ayurveda is based on the philosophy that we are all unique, so it addresses each of these things in its treatment of people as individuals, and teaches that all illnesses affect the body and the mind, which should not be treated in isolation from each other.

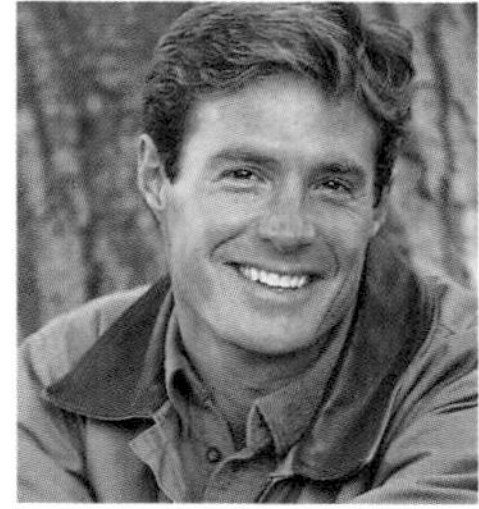

ABOVE *No two people will have the same personality, views, and lifestyle.*

WHAT IS AYURVEDA?

Ayurvedic medicine is the traditional system of medicine practised in India and Sri Lanka. Like Traditional Chinese Medicine, Ayurveda is a complete system of healthcare, designed to contribute to a way of life, rather than an occasional treatment.

The word "Ayurveda" means "science" or "wisdom" of life, and it embraces elements as diverse as medicine, philosophy, science, spirituality, astrology, and astronomy. Although Ayurveda has been practised for over 3,000 years, it is a sophisticated and advanced system of living that is as relevant today as it was so many years ago. In fact, as we begin to realize the limitations of our conventional Western approach, it becomes clear that Ayurveda can offer much to treat and prevent many modern diseases that conventional medicine has been unable to treat. Some of these include ME (myalgic encephalomyelitis), stress-related disorders, arthritis, impotence, asthma, eczema, and chronic illness. It offers natural herbal remedies to counter imbalances in the body, and detoxification, diet, exercise, meditation, spiritual guidance, and wide-ranging techniques to improve mental and emotional health.

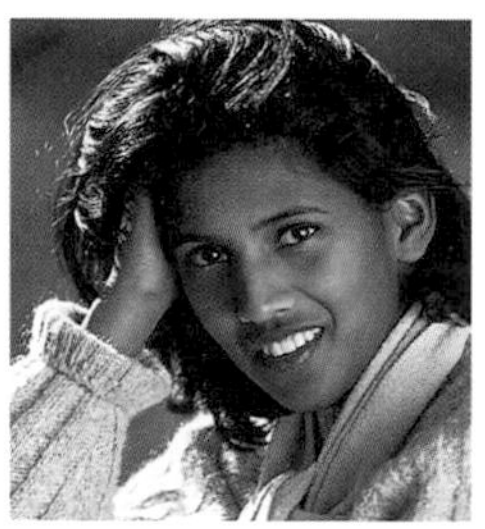

ABOVE *Ayurveda treats all the issues that are integral to health.*

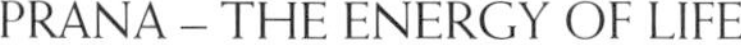

PRANA – THE ENERGY OF LIFE

The fundamental belief in Ayurveda is that everything within the universe is composed of energy, or "prana." Like everything else, we too are comprised of energy, which changes according to our circumstances, our environment, our diets and lifestyles, and the world around us. Some of these changes can be positive, and others negative, and in order to ensure that most of the changes are positive, we must live in a way that encourages energy balance. Energy controls the functions of every cell, thought, emotion, and action, so every aspect of our lives, including the food we eat and the thoughts we think, affects the quality of our energy, and consequently our health.

ABOVE *Deepak Chopra has been influential in bringing Ayurveda to mainstream American medicine.*

Ayurvedic medicine teaches that there is no single prescription for health that is appropriate for everyone. In Ayurveda every person must be treated individually. The skill of the practitioner lies in his ability to correctly identify each individual's constitution, diagnosing the causes of imbalance and then treating the patient accordingly.

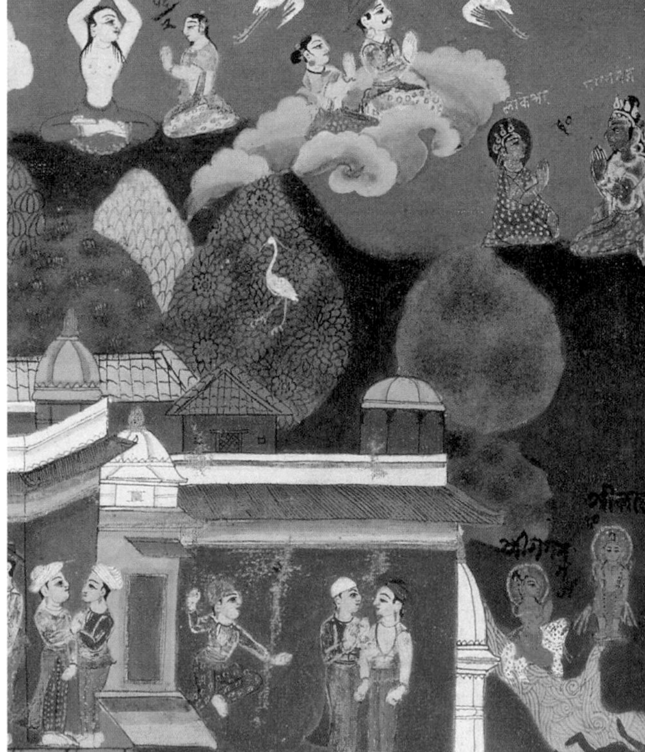

A HISTORY OF AYURVEDA

Over 3,000 years ago, 52 great *Rishis*, or seers, of ancient India discovered through meditation the "Veda," or the knowledge of how our world and everything within it works. Contained within the knowledge of the Veda were the secrets of sickness and health. These secrets were organized into a system called Ayurveda, the sophistication of which is apparent in the most famous of all ancient Ayurvedic texts, the *Charaka Samhita*. The knowledge of the Rishis had three main components: etiology (the science of the cause of illness and disease), symptomatology (the study of symptoms), and finally medication (the process of treating individuals to cure disease or relieve pain).

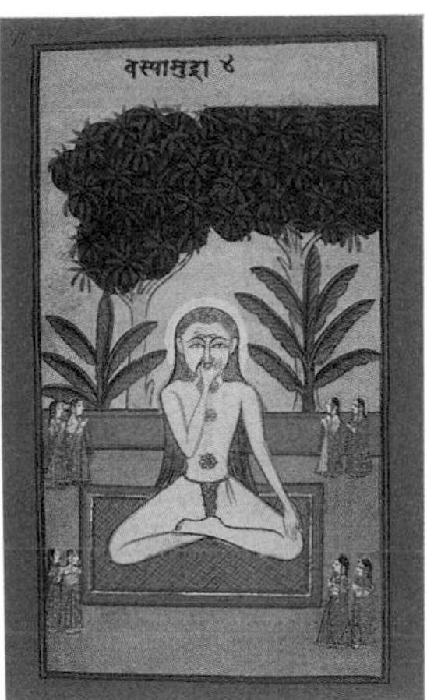

ABOVE *Through meditation the Rishis gained an understanding of the world.*

The beliefs were founded on Hindu philosophy, and were enlarged and enhanced by the teachings of the Lord Buddha (d. 483 B.C.E.), who taught that the mind could be enriched through correct thinking. Today Buddhism is one of the fastest-growing belief systems in the West. The eightfold path of Buddhism encompasses:

- *right understanding*
- *right concentration*
- *right livelihood*
- *right mindfulness*
- *right action*
- *right thought*
- *right effort*
- *right speaking*

Another important Ayurvedic text, the *Sushruta Samhita*, offers guidance on surgery, surgical equipment, suturing, and the importance of hygiene during and after an operation. Detailed medical information is teamed with commonsense advice on how to live a healthy and meaningful life.

In Vedic philosophy our lives become meaningful when we strive to fulfill our potential, but that cannot be achieved without basic good health.

CAUSES OF DISEASE

Ayurvedic practitioners believe that disease may be triggered by many external causes, including planetary influences, acts of god, fire and accidents, harmful gases (which we would today call pollution), poisons and toxins, and evil spirits. As well as this, there are two other main causes of illness, an imbalance of the "tri-doshas" (vátha, pitta, and kapha, *see page* 20) and mental imbalance.

The purpose of Ayurveda is to enable people to avoid serious illness by understanding how we become ill. For the most part, it works on a preventive basis, but when we do become ill it offers a wide range of treatments to help the body heal itself. Every Ayurvedic remedy is free of side effects, is made from natural substances, and is nontoxic. In order to benefit from Ayurveda, it is not necessary to understand or believe in the complex spirituality that goes hand-in-hand with the system. All that is necessary is an open mind and a desire to be healed.

LEFT *The word "Ayurveda" means "life" and "knowledge." Life encompasses body, mind, and soul.*

RIGHT *The teachings of Buddha were integrated into the philosophy of Ayurveda.*

THE TEXTS

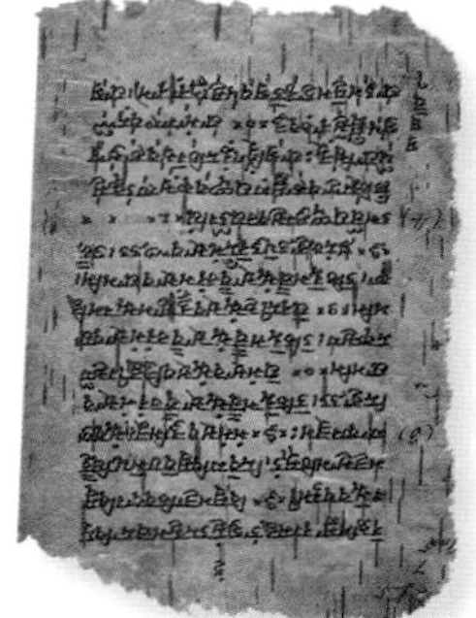

ABOVE *The* Atharva Veda: *a very early Ayurvedic text.*

Throughout much of their history, the Indians came into contact with the Persians, Greeks, and Chinese, with whom they exchanged information. About 900 B.C.E. the Ayurveda, written in India, combined descriptions of disease with information on herbs and "magic." The first great Hindu physician known, Charaka, practised about 1000 B.C.E. Sushruta, in the 5th century C.E., noted the relationship of malaria to mosquitoes, and of plague to rats, knew of more than 700 medicinal plants, and described more than 100 surgical instruments. He treated fractures, removed tumors and kidney stones, and delivered babies by Cesarean section.

HOW DOES IT WORK?

THE FIVE ELEMENTS

The universe consists of five elements, Ether (space), Air, Earth, Fire, and Water. Our bodies consist of a combination of these elements. All five elements exist in all things, including ourselves.

- **ETHER** corresponds to the spaces in the body: the mouth, nostrils, thorax, abdomen, respiratory tract, and cells.
- **AIR** is the element of movement so it represents muscular movement, pulsation, expansion and contraction of the lungs and intestines, even the movement in every cell.
- **FIRE** controls enzyme functioning. It shows itself as intelligence, fuels the digestive system, and regulates metabolism.
- **WATER** is in plasma, blood, saliva, digestive juices, mucous membranes, and cytoplasm, the liquid inside cells.
- **EARTH** manifests in the solid structures of the body: the bones, nails, teeth, muscles, cartilage, tendons, skin, and hair.

The five elements also relate to our senses: sound is transmitted through Ether; Air is related to touch; Fire is related to sight; Water is related to taste; and Earth is connected to smell.

Ayurveda teaches that all organic matter is formed from the Earth element, which "gave birth" to other matter. All five elements may be present in all matter: Water, when it is frozen, becomes solid like Earth; Fire melts it back to Water; Fire can turn Water to steam, which is dispersed within the Air and the Ether.

Our constitutions are very important in Ayurveda, and each of us is individual, according to our specific energies. We inherit many aspects of our constitution, and we can live a healthy and happy life if we strive to attain a good quality of spirit (with no envy, hatred, anger, or ego), and maintain a healthy diet and lifestyle.

Your constitution is determined by the state of your parents' doshas at the time of your conception, and each individual is born in the "prakruthi" state, which means that you are born with levels of the three doshas that are right for you. But, as we go through life, diet, environment, stress, trauma, and injury cause the doshas to become imbalanced, a state known as the "vikruthi" state. When levels of imbalance are excessively high or low it can lead to ill health. Ayurvedic practitioners work to restore individuals to their "prakruthi" state.

THE THREE DOSHAS

There are three further bio-energies, called doshas, which exist in everything in the universe, and which are composed of different combinations of the five elements. The three doshas affect all body functions, on both a mental and a physical level. Good health is achieved when all three doshas work in balance. Each one has its role to play in the body.

- VÁTHA is the driving force; it relates mainly to the nervous system and the body's energy.
- PITTA is Fire; it relates to the metabolism, digestion, enzymes, acid, and bile.
- KAPHA is related to Water in the mucous membranes, phlegm, moisture, fat, and lymphatics.

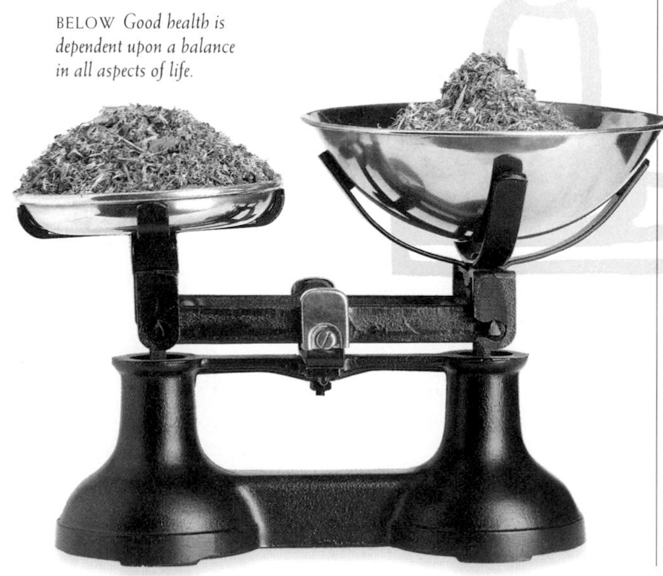

BELOW *Good health is dependent upon a balance in all aspects of life.*

VÁTHA

VÁTHA is a combination of the elements Air and Ether, with Air being the most dominant. Its qualities are light, cold, dry, rough, subtle, mobile, clear, dispersing, erratic, and astringent. Vátha is the lightest of the three doshas, portrayed by the color blue. Predominantly vátha people are thin with dry, rough, or dark skin; large, crooked or protruding teeth; a small, thin mouth, and dull, dark eyes.

Characteristics:

- Often constipated
- Frequent but sparse urine and little perspiration
- Highly original and creative mind
- Poor long-term memory
- Rapid speech
- Tendency to anxiety and depression
- High sex drive (or none at all)
- Love of travel
- Dislike of cold weather

RIGHT *Vátha people tend to be thin, with light bones.*

The balance of the three doshas depends on a variety of factors, principally correct diet and exercise, maintaining good digestion, healthy elimination of body wastes, and ensuring balanced emotional and spiritual health.

We will be made up of a combination of two or all three types of dosha, although we may tend to be predominantly one. Some sub-groups include vátha-pitta, vátha–kapha or pitta–kapha.

THE FUNDAMENTAL QUALITIES

The principle of qualities in Ayurveda is similar to the Chinese concept of yin and yang, in that every quality has its opposite, and good health depends on finding a balance between the two extremes of qualities such as slow and fast, wet and dry, cloudy and clear. For example, hot and cold exist together as a pair of qualities, and everything in between is composed of levels of heat and cold. Heat relates to pitta, an imbalance of which can cause problems such as fevers, heartburn, or emotional disturbances such as anger or jealousy. If you have an excess of pitta you need to reduce your heat quality by eating fewer pitta foods, such as onions, garlic, and beef, and introduce more "cooling" foods, such as eggs, cheese, and lentils.

PITTA

PITTA is mostly Fire with some Water. Its qualities are light, hot, oily, sharp, liquid, sour, and pungent. Pitta is "medium" and portrayed by the color red. Pitta types seem to conform to a happy medium, and are of medium height and build, with soft, fair, freckled, or bright skin; soft, fair, light brown, or reddish hair that goes prematurely gray; small, yellowish teeth, and an average-sized mouth.

Characteristics:

- Speaks clearly, but often sharply
- Enjoys light but uninterrupted sleep
- Intelligent
- Clear memory
- Jealous
- Ambitious
- Passionately sexual
- Interested in politics
- Dislikes heat
- Loves luxury
- Loose stools and a tendency to diarrhea
- Strong appetite
- Great thirst

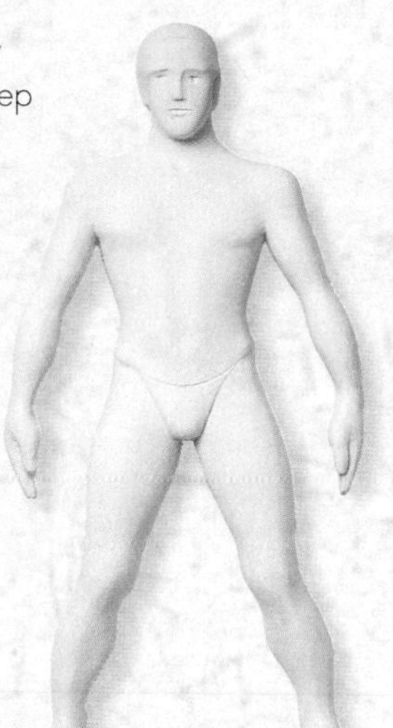

RIGHT *Pitta people are of medium build, and fair-skinned.*

KAPHA

KAPHA is a combination of mostly Water and some Earth. Its qualities are heavy, cold, oily, slow, slimy, dense, soft, static, and sweet. Kapha is the heaviest of the doshas, and is portrayed by yellow. Kapha people tend to be large-framed and often overweight, with thick, pale, cool, and oily skin; thick, wavy and oily hair, either very dark or very light; strong white teeth, and a large mouth with full lips.

Characteristics:

- Speaks slowly and monotonously, and needs plenty of deep sleep
- Sluggish or slow but steady appetite
- Heavy sweating
- Large soft stools
- Business-like
- Good memory
- Passive, bordering on lethargic
- Dislikes cold and damp
- Delights in good food and familiar places

RIGHT *Kapha people are often large and overweight.*

AGNI AND DIGESTION

In Ayurveda good digestion is the key to good health. Poor digestion produces "ama," a toxic substance that is believed to be the cause of illness. Ama is seen in the body as a white coating on the tongue, but it can also line the colon and clog blood vessels. Ama occurs when the metabolism is impaired as a result of an imbalance of "agni." Agni is the Fire which, when it is working effectively, maintains normality in all the functions of the body. Uneven agni is caused by imbalances in the doshas, and such factors as eating and drinking too much of the wrong foods, smoking, and repressing emotions.

MALAS

Malas represent the effective elimination of waste products and there are three main types:

- *Sharkrit or pureesha (feces)*
- *Mootra (urine)*
- *Sweda (sweat)*

Ama is a fourth type of waste, which cannot be eliminated, and an accumulation of which causes disease. Comprised of toxic materials, a build-up of ama is the result of an unhealthy diet and lifestyle, and the ingestion of toxins.

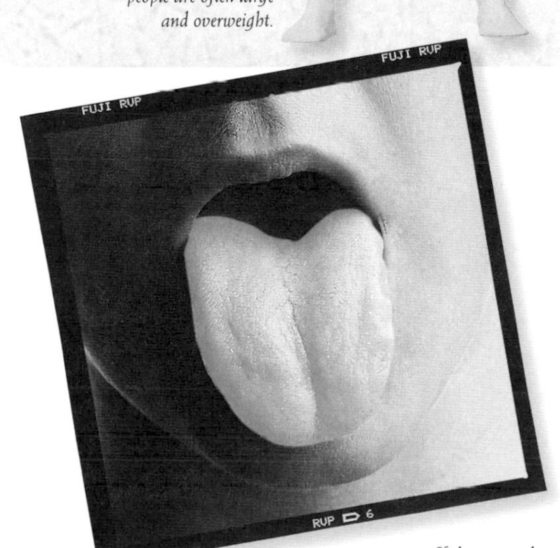

ABOVE *If the tongue has a white coating, it indicates that the body is out of balance.*

THE SEVEN TISSUES

Imbalance in the doshas also causes imbalance in the seven body tissues, or "dhatus." These are: plasma (rasa), blood (raktha), muscle (mamsa), fat (madas), bone (asthi), marrow and nerves (majja), and reproductive tissues (shukra). The dhatus support and derive energy from each other, so when one is affected the others also suffer.

THE THREE DOSHAS

The three doshas, or tridoshas, come from the five basic eternal substances, the pancha-mahabhutas. Each is made up of different elements.

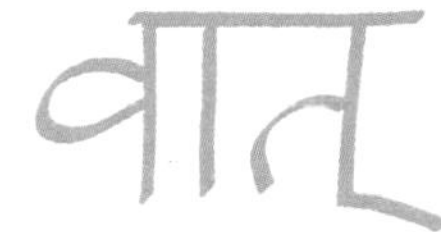

ABOVE *Vátha Sanskrit symbol and icon. Vátha consists of vayu (air) and akasha (space).*

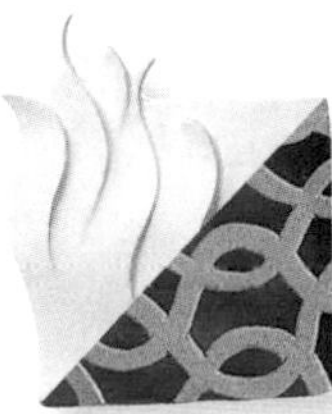

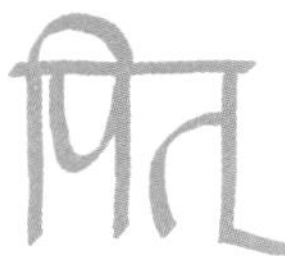

ABOVE *Pitta Sanskrit symbol and icon. Pitta consists of tejas (fire) and jala (water).*

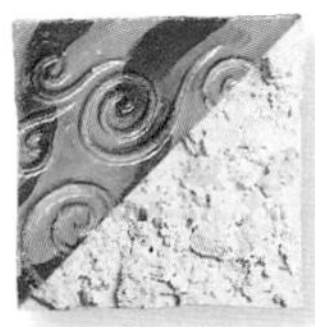

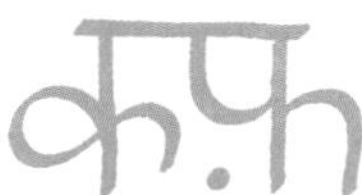

ABOVE *Kapha Sanskrit symbol and icon. Kapha consists of jala (water) and prthvi (earth).*

AYURVEDIC TREATMENT

WHAT CAN AYURVEDA TREAT?

- Allergies
- Anxiety
- Arthritis
- Back pain
- Bronchitis
- Circulation problems
- Colds
- Digestive complaints such as irritable bowel syndrome, constipation, indigestion
- Dyslexia
- Eczema
- Headaches
- High blood pressure
- Insomnia
- Irritability and emotional stress
- Obesity
- Skin problems
- Water retention

Ayurveda will keep the immune system strong and capable of fighting off infection, and able to address chronic disorders from within.

SHODANA

In Ayurvedic medicine it is essential to detoxify the body before prescribing restorative treatment. Shodana is used to eliminate disease, blockages in the digestive system, or any causes of imbalance in the doshas. Where shodana is required the practitioner can use "panchakarma" therapy, and sometimes a preparatory therapy called "purwakarma." Purwakarma breaks down into two types of preparatory treatment, known as "snehana" and "swedana":

- **Snehana** involves massaging herbal oils into the skin to encourage elimination of toxins. Blended oils are used to treat specific disorders, such as stress, anxiety, insomnia, arthritis, or circulation problems. Oils can also be massaged into the scalp for depression, insomnia, and memory problems. Snehana can sometimes involve lying in an oil bath, which is thought to be even more effective at allowing you to absorb the properties from herbal oils.
- **Swedana** means sweating. It is sometimes used in conjunction with the oil treatment, but on a separate day. Steam baths are used to encourage the elimination of toxins through the pores, and, together with the oil treatments, they make the detoxification process much more effective.

PANCHAKARMA

This is a profound detoxification. It is traditionally a fivefold therapy, but all five aspects are used only in very rare cases. You may need only two or three of the following treatments:

- **Nirhua vasti** (*oil enema therapy*). The oil is passed through a tube to the rectum, using gravity, rather than pressure, so that it does not cause damage. Oil enemas are often used to eliminate váthа or pitta-oriented problems, such as in the treatment of constipation, irritable bowel syndrome, diarrhea, indigestion, and fungal infections.
- **Ánuvasana vasti** (*herbal enema*). The practitioner makes a herbal decoction and passes it through the tube. The selection of a herbal enema rather than an oil one depends on the patient's problem and the contraindications.
- **Vireka** (*herbal laxative therapy*). Vireka is used as a normal part of any detoxification therapy, and is also used to treat pitta-oriented disease, such as gastrointestinal problems, and vátha problems, such as constipation and irritable bowel syndrome. It also helps with inflammatory skin complaints, fluid retention, liver problems, and energy problems.
- **Vamana** (*therapeutic vomiting*). This is a traditional treatment for respiratory and catarrhal problems such as bronchitis, sinusitis, and asthma, but it is rarely used today.
- **Nasya** (*herbal inhalation therapy*). This treatment involves inhaling the vapor from medicinal herbs infused in boiling water. It is used mostly to eliminate Kapha-oriented problems, ear, eyes, nose and throat disorders, headaches, migraine, neuralgia, sinusitis, catarrh, and bronchitis.

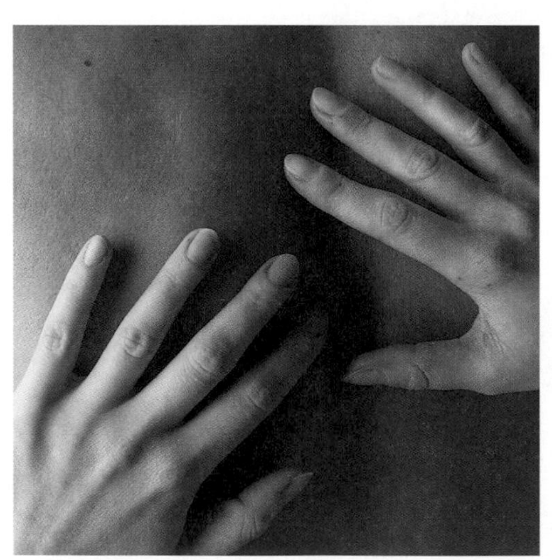

ABOVE *Snehana uses herbal oils to help eliminate toxins from the body.*

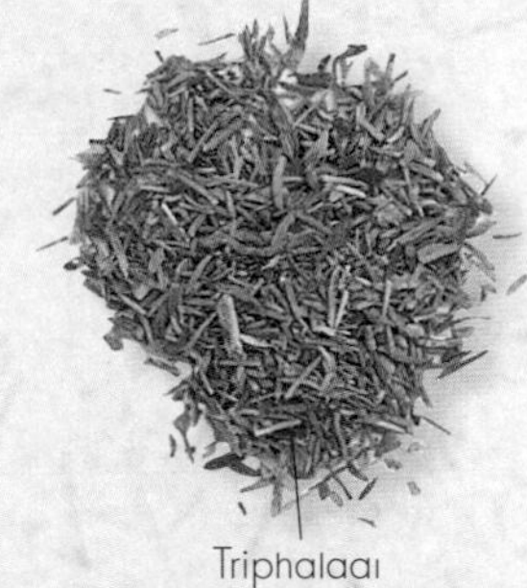

Guggul

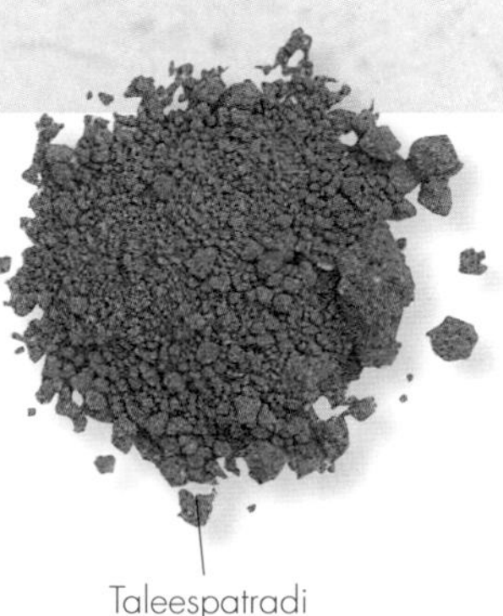

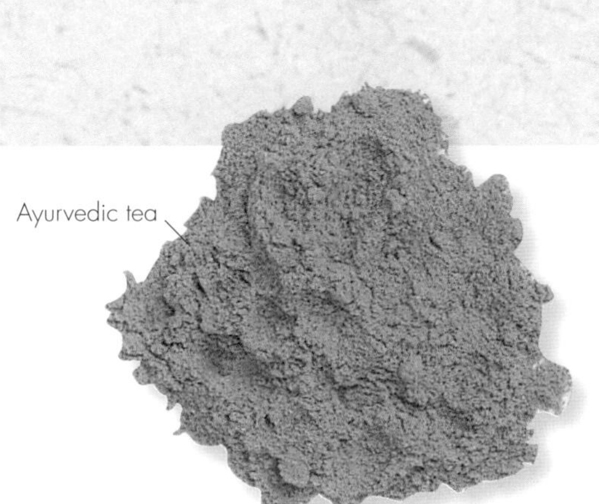

SAMANA

After the detoxification process the practitioner may prescribe herbal or mineral remedies to correct imbalances in the doshas. These are to stimulate agni and restore balance in the doshas. They are not prescribed to eradicate disease, because the disease is just a symptom of doshic imbalance. Herbal remedies are usually prescribed in liquid form or as dried herbs, although they can also come in powder or tablet form. The ingredients are pre-prepared, but the blends are prescribed for the individual. Each ingredient is classified by the effect it has on lowering or increasing the levels of the doshas.

Prescriptions are usually made up of groups of herbs, to which you add eight cups of water and boil until the liquid is reduced to one cup. You may have to take the remedy two or three times a day.

Your practitioner will also advise on lifestyle, food, and exercise. There is no single healthy diet in Ayurveda, just a diet that is best for you. It is important to eat to suit your constitution, and the practitioner may prepare a diet sheet for you to use.

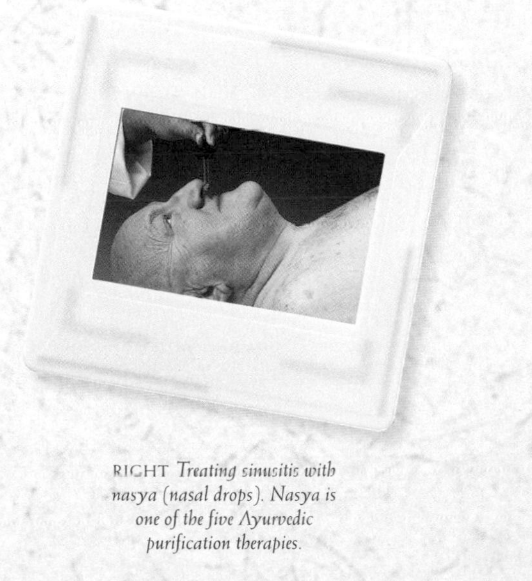

RIGHT *Treating sinusitis with nasya (nasal drops). Nasya is one of the five Ayurvedic purification therapies.*

PLANT POWER

In many cases the whole plant is used in an Ayurvedic treatment; in others, only part. All plants are associated with the following properties and effects:

- THE THREE DOSHAS. Plants can be used to increase or decrease an influence as required.
- SHAD RASA (the tastes). Every plant contains one or more of the six basic tastes, which are sweet, acidic, salty, pungent, bitter, and astringent.
- GUNAS (the properties). The gunas are distinctive characteristics that can be related to matter, thoughts, and ideas. There is a belief that everything in the universe is made up of complementary opposites (*see yin and yang, in Chinese Herbal Medicine, page 48*). There are 20 gunas: hot and cold, hard and soft, oily and dry, light and heavy, dull and sharp, subtle and gross, slimy and rough, unmoving and mobile, turbid and transparent, solid and liquid. The properties of each guna are related to the doshas, and specific substances, which are characterized by specific gunas, can increase or decrease dosha influence throughout the body. The properties of each guna can affect the doshas.

LEFT *Yoga harmonizes mind and body, and can thus be regarded as an Ayurvedic treatment.*

Many herbs are used in Ayurvedic preparations, and are sold as essences, pills, powders, pastes, and potencized remedies. Often they are herbs that are known and used in the West, although they are used differently in Ayurvedic medicine.

Herbs can have many effects on the body, including purifying the blood, binding stools, aiding digestion, expelling worms, improving coagulation, healing fractures, increasing appetite, lowering fever, reducing toxins, balancing the tridoshas (or increasing or decreasing the three doshas), strengthening the heart, among others.

It is usually safe to combine taking Ayurvedic herbal remedies and orthodox medicines. However, you should inform your Ayurvedic practitioner of any medication you are currently taking or have taken in the past.

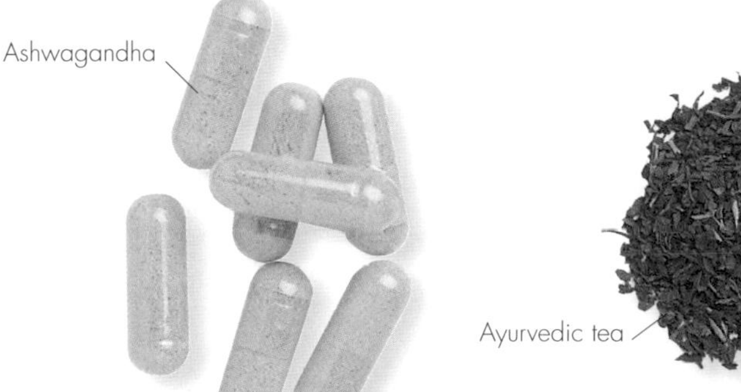

LEFT *Ayurvedic remedies come in many forms, some ready to use: liquid herbal remedies, dried herbs, powders, capsules, tablets.*

OTHER USEFUL AYURVEDIC TREATMENTS INCLUDE:

- Meditation
- Breathing exercises
- Marma puncture (rather like acupuncture; adjusting energy levels in the body by stimulating energy points in the body, which can stimulate some of its functions and maintain health
- Marma therapy, applying pressure or massage to marma points
- Yoga
- Unblocking chakras, which are centres of energy located along the mid-line of the body which distribute energy to the 107 marma points on the body
- Rejuvenation therapy, or rasayana, which helps to promote and preserve health and longevity in the healthy, and to cure disease in the sick
- Psychotherapy or counseling

AYURVEDIC REMEDY SOURCES

Achillea millefolium

YARROW *GANDANA*

Yarrow is a sacred plant to many cultures. In China, yarrow stalks were used to cast the I Ching, to read the future for the emperor. Ayurvedics use the herb as a "heal-all" because it has so many uses – allowing you to keep your head in the heavens and your feet on the ground. Yarrow balances emotional upsets, and is a frequent addition to treatments during the menopause.

LEFT *Yarrow flowers in early summer. Gather it at this time.*

CAUTION

DO NOT ADMINISTER YARROW TO CHILDREN UNDER TWO YEARS OLD.

THOSE WITH SENSITIVE SKIN MAY BE IRRITATED WHEN EXPOSED TO THE SUN WHILE USING YARROW.

IT SHOULD NOT BE USED IN CASES OF HIGH VÁTHA.

DATA FILE

Properties

Yarrow is bitter, pungent, astringent, cooling, and drying. It acts as a diaphoretic, antispasmodic, anti-inflammatory, antiphlogistic, antiseptic, and tonic. Yarrow is carminative, alterative, sedative, vulnerary, and emmenagogic.

Part of Plant Used

The leaves, stalks, flowers, and fruits.

Conditions Treated

Used for hemorrhages, ulcers, measles, colds, fever, nosebleeds, abscesses, vaginitis, varicose veins, headache, menopause, hemorrhoids, gout, cellulite, acne, sunburn, smallpox, and chicken pox. Yarrow has healing effects on mucous membranes, eases diarrhea, and improves blood clotting.

Form Taken

Skin patches, lotion, bath, compress, massage oil.

Used With Other Herbs?

Angelica, cedarwood, cinnamon, clove, lavender, lemon, licorice, myrrh, myrtle, sarsaparilla, St. John's wort, turmeric.

HOW TO USE

❧ Yarrow reduces pitta and kapha; it increases vátha with its cooling, drying properties. ❧ **Legend has it that Achilles used yarrow to staunch his soldiers' wounds during the Trojan war.** ❧ For wound treatment, simply press fresh leaves and flower tops into cuts and scrapes on the way to washing and bandaging them. ❧ **As an infusion to relieve menstrual cramps or hot flushes, steep 2 teaspoons of the dried herb in a cup of boiling water for about 10 minutes. Add honey to taste, and drink warm.**

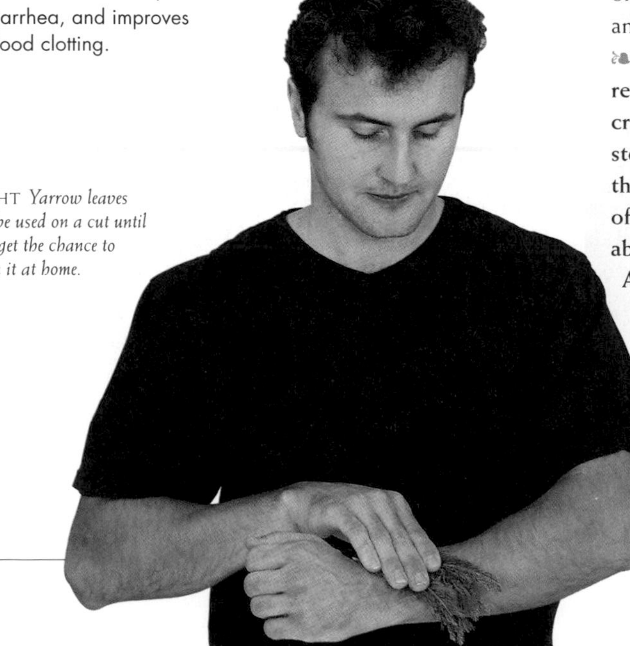

RIGHT *Yarrow leaves can be used on a cut until you get the chance to clean it at home.*

Acorus calamus

CALAMUS ROOT *VACHA*

Also known as sweet flag or myrtle flag, this rhizome is a reddish, hairy root, known throughout Asia for its medicinal properties. The word "vacha" means speech in Sanskrit, and calamus root is traditionally used as a brain tonic and to improve the capacity for speech.

DATA FILE

Properties

This herb is pungent and bitter, with astringent qualities. It is a stimulant, a heating/drying agent which warms vátha and decreases kapha states. It can be used as a decongestant and expectorant. Calamus root is emetic and anticonvulsive; it is a bronchio-dilator, increases circulation to the brain, and so can reduce brain toxins.

Part of Plant Used

The root.

Conditions Treated

Calamus strengthens the adrenals, improves muscle tissue, helps circulation and is useful in periods of weakness. It has a beneficial effect on gingivitis (gum disease), and a massage with calamus oil will stimulate lymphatic drainage. The herb increases endurance and stamina, and has been used for the treatment of arthritis, shock, coughs, and nagging sinus headaches.

Form Taken

Use the herb externally in a compress or as massage oil.

Used With Other Herbs?

Calamus mixes well with ginger, yarrow, lemon, orange, cinnamon, and also with cedar.

HOW TO USE

❧ Calamus reduces kapha and vátha, and increases pitta. ❧ **Calamus root is often used to improve the memory.** ❧ A simple formula for boosting your brain power: mix ¼ of a teaspoon of the powdered root with a ½ teaspoon of honey. Take internally every morning and evening. Use any time you are experiencing mental stress and overstimulation. A great help at exam time!

LEFT *Calamus leaves and young rhizome (rootstock). Rhizomes are thick horizontal underground stems.*

CAUTION

CALAMUS CAN CAUSE BLEEDING DISORDERS, SUCH AS NOSEBLEEDS AND HEMORRHOIDS, IF USED IN EXCESS.

USE ONLY THE RECOMMENDED DOSE.

CALAMUS CAN HAVE A VERY STRONG AND LONG-LASTING ODOR. IT MAY BE APPROPRIATE TO USE IT IN CONJUNCTION WITH ROSEMARY, LAVENDER, OR A SWEET-SMELLING HERB.

THERAPY CONNECTIONS

YARROW

Herbalism p.112

ONION

Traditional and Folk Remedies p.82

Homeopathy p.178

VÁTHA

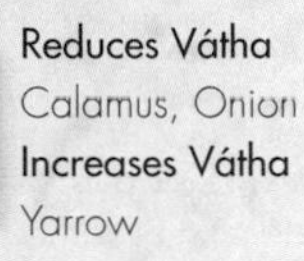

Reduces Vátha
Calamus, Onion
Increases Vátha
Yarrow

PITTA

Reduces Pitta
Yarrow
Increases Pitta
Calamus, Onion

KAPHA

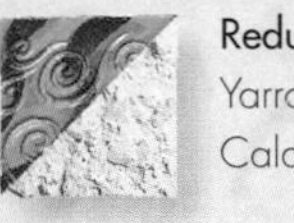

Reduces Kapha
Yarrow,
Calamus, Onion

Allium cepa

ONION *DUNGRI*

Onion and its relative garlic are members of the lily family. They are some of the oldest known medicinal plants, rich in trace elements, minerals, and sulfur. Remedies using onion date back to 3000 B.C.E. Ayurvedic practitioners prescribed onion for cancer and leprosy. Onion stimulates the production of saliva and digestive juices, as well as the flow of tears!

RIGHT *Slices of raw onion can be placed directly on a burn to soothe the pain.*

DATA FILE

Properties

Onion is a pungent, sweet bulb with heating and drying qualities. It is an excellent stimulant, carminative, and expectorant. The juice is disinfectant, rejuvenative, and antispasmodic. Onion has a rejuvenating effect on all tissues and body systems: the digestive, respiratory, nervous, reproductive, and circulatory systems.

Part of Plant Used

The bulb.

Conditions Treated

Onion has been used to treat a broad spectrum of ailments, including but not limited to nerve rejuvenation, colds, skin disease, parasites, bronchial disorders, asthma, joint problems and arthritis, cysts and growths, fluid retention. Onion helps eliminate lead and other heavy metals from the body, and is beneficial for diabetics and patients with cancer.

Form Taken

Onion can be peeled and eaten raw, cooked, powdered, juiced, taken as a tea, decoction, infusion, in food, and as an oil.

Used With Other Herbs?

Combines well with ginger, black pepper, cumin, coriander, eucalyptus.

HOW TO USE

❧ Onion reduces kapha and vátha, and increases pitta. Its stimulating effects aid in the secretion of digestive juices. ❧ **Onion juice has been used to treat infected wounds, amebic dysentery, and, at one time, juice applied to the ear was said to cure deafness!** ❧ Onion may be used directly on the skin for natural relief from burns. Simply place slices of raw onion on the burned skin, or apply a homemade lotion of onion juice mixed with salt. This preparation is also effective for insect bites and stings. ❧ **For an antibiotic treatment, peel and eat (raw or cooked) one-quarter of one sweet white onion, two to four times a day. The onion must be chewed, crushed, chopped, or bruised to access its antibiotic properties.**

BELOW *Include onion in food as often as possible for its health-enhancing properties.*

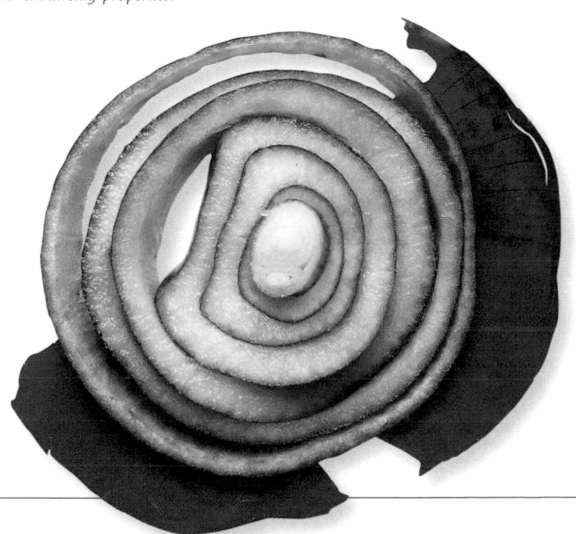

CAUTION

NURSING MOTHERS BEWARE: ONION IN YOUR BREAST MILK MAY CAUSE COLIC IN YOUR INFANT.

SOME PEOPLE HAVE ALLERGIES TO ONION AND MAY DEVELOP A SKIN RASH. IF ONE APPEARS, DISCONTINUE USE.

CONSULT A PHYSICIAN BEFORE CONSUMING LARGE QUANTITIES OF ONION FOR MEDICINAL PURPOSES.

SOME PEOPLE HAVE TROUBLE DIGESTING RAW ONION. IF THIS IS THE CASE, STEAM OR BLANCH THE ONION BEFORE EATING.

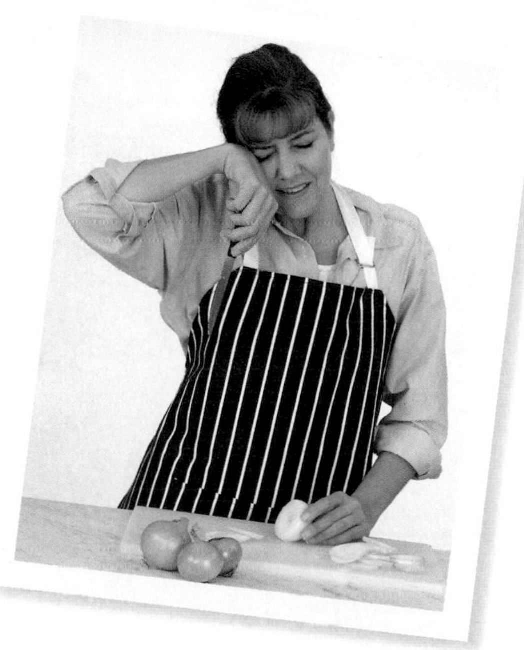

ABOVE *Tears – a well-known side-effect of chopping onions. Onions also stimulate the secretion of digestive juices.*

THERAPY CONNECTIONS

GARLIC
Traditional and Folk Remedies p.82
Herbalism p.113

ALOE VERA
Herbalism p.114

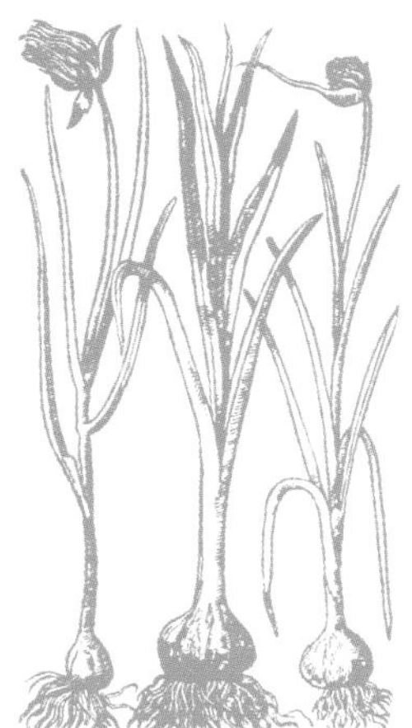
GARLIC
Allium sativum.

Allium sativum

GARLIC *LASHUNA*

Garlic is one of the oldest known medicinal plants. A remedy using garlic was found on a Sumerian clay tablet which dated back to 3000 B.C.E. Ayurvedic practitioners prescribed garlic liberally for cancer and leprosy. When the British came to India, leprosy became known as "peelgarlic," because of the frequent sight of lepers peeling and eating garlic cloves.

CAUTION

NURSING MOTHERS BEWARE: GARLIC IN YOUR BREAST MILK MAY CAUSE COLIC IN YOUR INFANT.

SOME PEOPLE HAVE ALLERGIES TO GARLIC AND MAY DEVELOP A SKIN RASH. IF ONE APPEARS, DISCONTINUE GARLIC USE.

CONSULT A PHYSICIAN BEFORE CONSUMING LARGE QUANTITIES OF GARLIC FOR MEDICINAL PURPOSES.

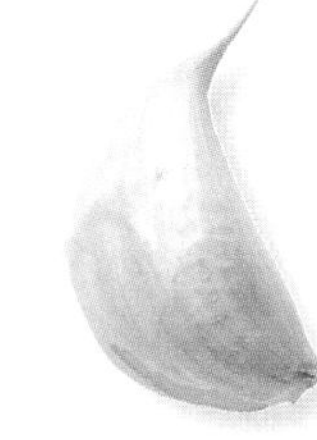
ABOVE *Grow your own garlic by planting individual cloves in the fall.*

DATA FILE

Properties

Garlic is a pungent, sweet bulb with heating and drying qualities. It is an excellent stimulant, carminative, and expectorant. The juice is disinfectant, rejuvenative, and antispasmodic. Garlic has a rejuvenating effect on all tissues and systems: digestive, respiratory, nervous, reproductive, and circulatory.

Part of Plant Used

The bulb.

Conditions Treated

Garlic has been used to treat a broad spectrum of ailments, including but not limited to nerve rejuvenation, colds, skin disease, parasites, joint problems and arthritis, cysts and growths, fluid retention. Like onion, garlic helps eliminate lead and other heavy metals from the body. It is beneficial to diabetics and cancer patients.

Form Taken

Garlic cloves can be chewed, cooked, powdered, taken as a tea, decoction, infusion, in food, and as an infused oil.

Used With Other Herbs?

Ginger, black pepper, cumin, coriander, eucalyptus.

VÁTHA

Reduces Vátha
Garlic
Balances Vátha
Aloe Vera

PITTA

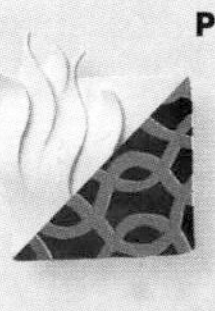
Increases Pitta
Garlic
Balances Pitta
Aloe Vera

KAPHA

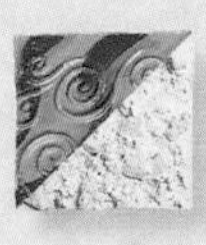
Reduces Kapha
Garlic
Balances Kapha
Aloe Vera

HOW TO USE

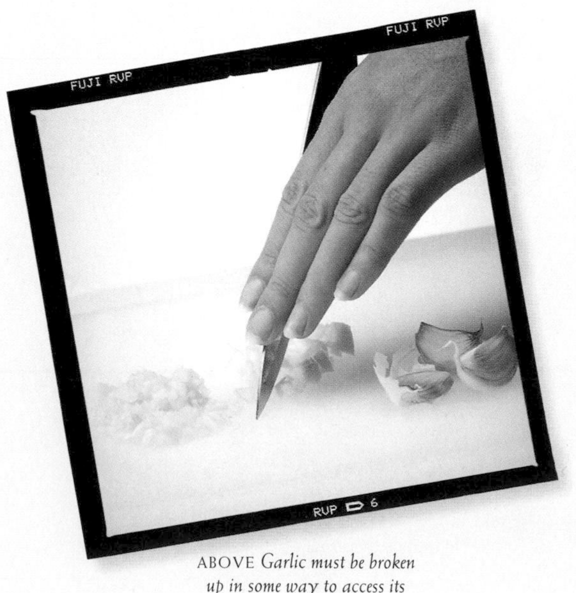

ABOVE *Garlic must be broken up in some way to access its healing properties.*

❧ Garlic reduces kapha and vátha, and increases pitta. ❧ **Its stimulating effect aids in the secretion of digestive juices.** ❧ Garlic juice has been used to treat infected wounds and amebic dysentery. ❧ **Garlic may be used as a natural antibiotic, and as a blood pressure and cholesterol reducer.** ❧ To obtain antibiotic effects, 6–12 cloves of garlic a day are recommended. Peel and chew three cloves of garlic at a time, two to four times a day. ❧ **The garlic must be chewed, crushed, chopped, or bruised to access its antibiotic properties.**

Aloe vera

ALOE VERA *KUMARI*

Aloe can be grown anywhere, and is often grown as a houseplant on the kitchen windowsill. Its fame as a treatment for burns and scalds goes back to Alexander the Great, who used an island off Somalia for the sole purpose of obtaining the "amazing wound-healing" plant. Another part of the aloe – the latex – is a powerful laxative, and is obtained in fresh aloe juice.

DATA FILE

Properties

Aloe vera has bitter, cooling, sweet qualities. It is astringent, and an excellent blood cleanser. Aloe vera alleviates all three doshas, and specifically reduces pitta (cooling pitta rashes, burns, and ulcers). Aloe vera works on the thyroid, the pituitary gland, and the ovaries.

Part of Plant Used

The leaf, the gel, the juice.

Conditions Treated

Aloe vera relieves inflammation, soothes muscle spasm, purifies the blood, and cleanses the liver. Fresh aloe gel scooped or expressed from the spongy leaves of the plant can be spread on the skin to heal burns, scalds, scrapes, sunburn, and wounds. Apply the gel directly to the outer eyelid for conjunctivitis. For cosmetic purposes, the gel can give skin a healthy glow – but use the fresh gel. Commercially packaged products use stabilized aloe, which has none of the fresh herb's healing properties.

Form Taken

Drink aloe juice for internal conditions, apply the gel externally. To soothe wounds, clean the wound with soap and water. Cut several inches off an older leaf, slice it lengthwise, and apply the gel to the wound. Allow it to dry. You can leave the gel on the wound for several hours, or if it is painful, wash it off and reapply later.

Used With Other Herbs?

Barberry, cinnamon, cloves, licorice, St. John's wort.

HOW TO USE

Aloe Vera is good for all doshas; it will bring balance equally to kapha, pitta, and vátha.

You can make your own aloe vera medicated oil by slicing up the leaves of the aloe vera plant, and placing them in a glass jar.

Cover the leaves with vegetable oil. Any vegetable oil can be used as the base. Allow the mixture to soak for 60 days, then strain. Keep the oil in a dark glass container. Label the container, as the scent is subtle, and will not be easy to identify. The oil will keep indefinitely.

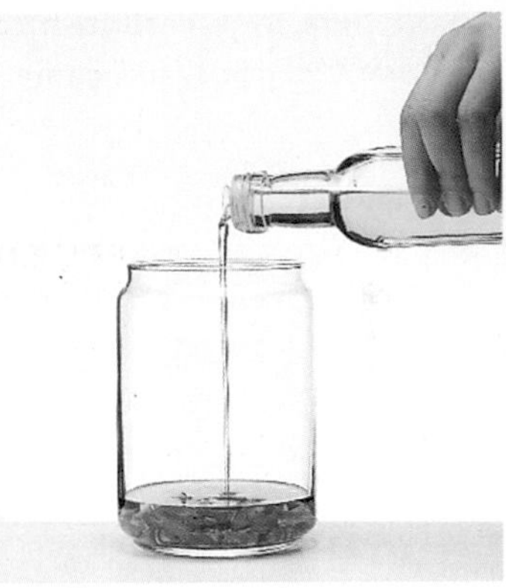

BELOW *Aloe vera gel helps to relieve the inflammation of conjunctivitis.*

Rub gel on outer eyelid

Aloe vera gel

LEFT *Aloe vera is a succulent requiring a minimum temperature of 10°C (50°F).*

CAUTION

ALOE VERA GEL CAN CAUSE SKIN IRRITATION IN SOME PEOPLE. IF IRRITATION OCCURS, DISCONTINUE USE.

ALOE VERA CONTAINS A POWERFUL LAXATIVE – ANTHRAQUINONE – WHICH CAN CAUSE DIARRHEA AND INTESTINAL CRAMPS. IF YOU USE ALOE JUICE OR SUPPLEMENTS AS A LAXATIVE, USE UNDER THE GUIDANCE OF A PHYSICIAN, AND NEVER EXCEED THE RECOMMENDED DOSAGE.

Angelica

ANGELICA *CHORAKA*

In the West, angelica has been associated with magic and sorcery for centuries. Necklaces of angelica leaf were thought to be protection against spells and illness, and its presence in a garden or cupboard was a defense against charges of witchcraft. Chinese angelica, or dong quai, has been used in Asia for thousands of years, and is enjoying renewed popularity as a gynecological aid. Ayurvedic practitioners prescribe the herb for menstrual problems, as well as arthritis, abdominal pains, and flu.

HOW TO USE

- In general, angelica balances all three doshas. If used in excess, or in high pitta states, it will increase pitta.
- **It is a wonderful expectorant and digestive aid.**
- You can prepare the leaves and seeds as an infusion for a mild treatment, or use the root in a decoction for a stronger effect. For an infusion, use 1 teaspoon of the powdered leaves or seeds in a cup or teapot. Add 1 cup of boiling water. Steep for 10–15 minutes, then strain.
- **For a decoction, take 3 teaspoons of the powdered root. Add 3 cups of water, and bring to a boil. Cover and simmer for 5 minutes. Remove from the heat and let stand for 15 minutes. Drink up to 2 cups a day. Sweeten with honey or anise if necessary.**

LEFT *Most of the angelica plant is useful: collect the root, leaves and seeds. The plant is a biennial.*

THERAPY CONNECTIONS

ANGELICA

Chinese Herbal Medicine p.55
Herbalism p.115
Aromatherapy p.146

CELERY SEED

Traditional Home and Folk Remedies p.83
Aromatherapy p.146

DATA FILE

Properties

Angelica is pungent, sweet, heating, and moisturizing. It is stimulant, expectorant, tonic, emmenagogue, carminative, and diaphoretic. Angelica has antibacterial properties, and has been used to induce menstruation and abortion.

Part of Plant Used

The roots, leaves, and seeds.

Conditions Treated

Amenorrhea, menstrual cramps, PMS, anemia, headaches, colds, flu, hiccups, arthritis, rheumatism, poor circulation, adrenal excess, digestive disorders, heartburn, bronchitis, poor blood clotting, also poor liver function.

Form Taken

As an inhalant, nose drops, in a vaporizer, tea, tincture, massage oil.

Used With Other Herbs?

Rose, St. John's wort, yarrow, vetiver, fennel, cumin, chamomile.

VÁTHA

Reduces Vátha
Celery seed
Balances Vátha
Angelica
Neutralizes Vátha
Barberry

PITTA

Increases Pitta
Celery seed, Barberry
Balances Pitta
Angelica

KAPHA

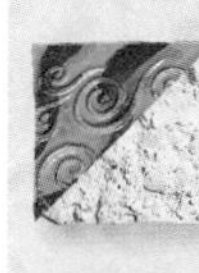

Reduces Kapha
Celery seed
Balances Kapha
Angelica, Barberry

CAUTION

FRESH ANGELICA ROOTS ARE POISONOUS. DRYING ELIMINATES ALL DANGER.

DO NOT USE WITH HYPERTENSION, HEART DISEASE, OR HIGH PITTA CONDITIONS.

ANGELICA CAN INCREASE PHOTOSENSITIVITY; USE A SUNSCREEN IF SPENDING TIME OUTDOORS.

PREGNANT WOMEN SHOULD AVOID ANGELICA BECAUSE OF ITS HISTORY AS AN ABORTIFACIENT.

Cramping pains

LEFT *Use angelica to treat painful menstrual cramps. Drink a cup of angelica decoction twice a day.*

Apium graveolens

CELERY SEED *AJWAN*

Celery seed, or *ajwan*, grows wild in India all year round. Traditional Ayurvedic practitioners prescribe celery seed to reduce high vátha states – indigestion, nervous stomach, and ungrounded emotions. In aromatherapy, celery seed oil can be used to counteract jet lag and exposure to smog and toxic environments. Celery seed is a strong diuretic, so you may want to drink extra water when taking this herb.

HOW TO USE

Celery seed reduces kapha and vátha, and increases pitta. **It is most commonly used as a diuretic, since fluid retention aggravates high blood pressure, congestive heart conditions, premenstrual syndrome, arthritis, and gout.** For a mildly diuretic infusion, or to bring on menstruation, crush 1½ teaspoons of celery seeds. Add 1 cup of boiling water. Cover and let steep for 15–20 minutes. You may drink up to 3 cups of the infusion a day.

LEFT *Celery seed contains several oils, including apiol, a valuable curative.*

DATA FILE

Properties

Celery seed has pungent, salty qualities, and a heating/moisturizing effect. It is used as a stimulant and expectorant, an antispasmodic and lithotrophic (dispels stones). Celery seed is a strong diuretic. It also contains chemicals – phthalides – which have a sedative effect and can ease insomnia.

Part of Plant Used

The juice, roots, and seeds.

Conditions Treated

The common cold, coughs, sinus congestion, respiratory infections, bronchitis, laryngitis, arthritis, digestive problems, high blood pressure, insomnia, diseases of the liver and spleen, and irregular menstruation.

Form Taken

As a food, a tea or infusion, a steam, a powder, massage oil, or a gargle.

Used With Other Herbs?

Basil, black pepper, camphor, eucalyptus, sandalwood.

ABOVE RIGHT *Celery seed tea before bed lessens the risk of insomnia.*

CAUTION

CELERY SEED MAY CAUSE MINOR DISCOMFORT IN SOME PEOPLE. IF YOU ARE EXPERIENCING A STOMACH UPSET OR DIARRHEA WHILE TAKING CELERY SEED, DISCONTINUE USE.

PREGNANT WOMEN SHOULD NOT TAKE CELERY SEED WITHOUT A PHYSICIAN'S APPROVAL BECAUSE OF ITS STRONG DIURETIC PROPERTIES.

DO NOT GIVE CELERY SEED TO CHILDREN UNDER TWO YEARS OLD.

Berberis vulgaris

BARBERRY

Barberry has been in use as a healing herb for thousands of years. The Egyptians used it to prevent plagues – a testimony to its antibiotic properties. The Ayurvedics were more likely to prescribe it for dysentery, mouth ulcers, sore throats, and skin infections. Barberry has been proven to be a more powerful antibiotic and antibacterial agent than many current pharmaceutical products.

CAUTION

BARBERRY MAY STIMULATE THE UTERUS AND SHOULD NOT BE TAKEN BY PREGNANT WOMEN.

BARBERRY IS A VERY POWERFUL HERB, AND SHOULD BE USED IN SMALL DOSES AND UNDER THE SUPERVISION OF A PHYSICIAN OR ALTERNATIVE HEALTHCARE PRACTITIONER.

IF THE DOSAGE IS TOO HIGH, BARBERRY CAN CAUSE NAUSEA, VOMITING, HAZARDOUS DROPS IN BLOOD PRESSURE, AND DIZZINESS.

DATA FILE

Properties

Barberry is a stimulant, a respiratory aid, and is antibiotic, antibacterial, and antifungal. It decreases heart rate, shrinks tumors, stimulates intestinal movement, reduces bronchial constriction, and enlarges blood vessels.

Part of Plant Used

The berries, roots, and the ground bark.

Conditions Treated

Skin infections, urinary tract infections, diarrhea, dysentery, cholera, arthritis, conjunctivitis, high blood pressure, throat infections, mouth ulcers, abnormal uterine bleeding.

Form Taken

Tea or infusion, gargle, eyewash, douche, compress, and powder.

Used With Other Herbs?

Garlic, ginger, saffron, wild sunflower.

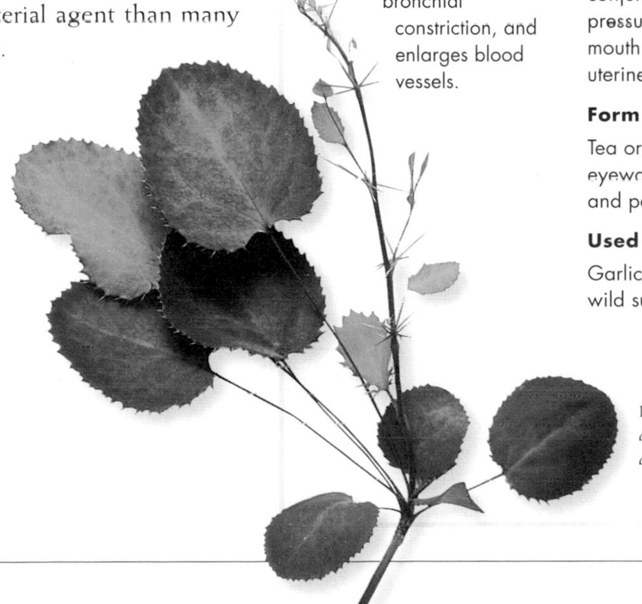

LEFT *Barberry makes a bitter tonic with strong antibiotic effects.*

HOW TO USE

Barberry can be used to treat a variety of symptoms in its decoction form. Take 1 teaspoon of powdered root bark in a small enamel pan. Add 2 cups of water. Cover and boil for 15–30 minutes, with as little liquid loss as possible. Allow to cool. The taste will be quite bitter. Sweeten with honey to taste. Drink up to one cup a day. **For a compress to treat conjunctivitis, soak a clean cloth in the decoction (before you add any honey). Place over the eye.**

Brassica nigra

MUSTARD *RAI*

Mustard is an annual plant cultivated as a spice all over the world. It has been used for centuries as a pungent condiment and healing herb by the Chinese, the Greeks, and the Ayurvedics. Mustard is peculiar in that its strong taste develops only after the seeds are crushed and come into contact with water or saliva.

ABOVE *Ready-powdered mustard seeds can be mixed with warm water to form a thick paste. Spread on a piece of cloth to form a poultice.*

DATA FILE

Properties

Antiseptic, warming, carminative, antibacterial, antiseptic, and antiviral. Mustard aids digestion and eases gastric distention. It is an emetic, rubefacient, and a laxative. It acts as an irritant, encouraging blood flow toward the surface of the skin in cases of rheumatism, sciatica, peritonitis, and neuralgia, and for various muscle aches and pains.

Part of Plant Used

Seed, pods.

Conditions Treated

For centuries, mustard plasters have been used to treat chest colds and coughs. Mustard is also beneficial for backache, joint pain, digestive upsets, hiccups, and as a laxative. Mustard eases constipation, minor aches and pains, and muscle stiffness.

Form Taken

As a spice or oil, in compresses and poultices.

Used With Other Herbs?

Aloe vera, ginger, garlic, and onion.

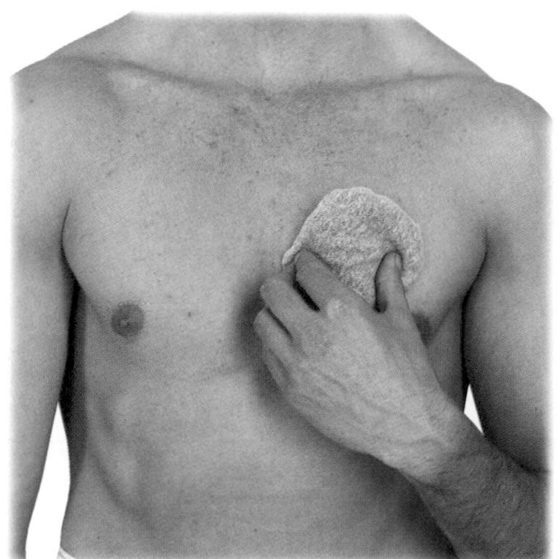

ABOVE *A mustard poultice, or plaster, helps to relieve the symptoms of a chest cold.*

HOW TO USE

❧ Mustard reduces pitta and kapha, and has a neutral effect on vátha. ❧ **Mustard oil can be rectified with alcohol (1 part oil to 40 parts alcohol) and used as a lotion for joint pains, arthritis, and sluggish circulation.** ❧ A mustard foot bath will clear blood congestion in the head, warm up cold feet, and lower a fever in the early stages of illness. Put one-quarter of a cup of mustard seed in a small cloth bag or a large tea strainer. Steep in hot water for 5 minutes. Soak the feet until the water cools off.

CAUTION

LARGE AMOUNTS OF MUSTARD CAN CAUSE IRRITATION AND INFLAMMATION. DO NOT LET UNDILUTED MUSTARD OIL COME IN CONTACT WITH THE SKIN.

DO NOT USE MUSTARD PLASTERS FOR MORE THAN 10–15 MINUTES AT A TIME, OR BLISTERING AND IRRITATION CAN OCCUR.

Carum carvi

CARAWAY *SUSHAVI*

This perennial plant is found in the wild in North America, Europe, and Asia. Caraway is best known in Europe in the making of rye bread, where the addition of caraway seeds aids in the digestion of starch. It is also a favorite addition to laxative herbs, tempering their violent effects. Caraway seeds, infused and allowed to cool, soothe colicky children and can be added to desserts to speed digestion after a rich meal.

DATA FILE

Properties

Caraway is a pungent, heating/drying agent, known for its stimulant and carminative properties. As an antispasmodic, caraway will soothe the muscles in the digestive process. It can also relax uterine tissue and is therefore beneficial for menstrual cramps.

Part of Plant Used

Seed.

Conditions Treated

Caraway aids the digestive process, both internally and in external application. It soothes indigestion, gas, colic, flatulence, and accumulation of toxins and fluids. It is also beneficial as a scalp treatment. The oil can be used as an enema for intestinal parasites. A stomach massage with a very small amount of the oil will reduce flatulence. Caraway seeds can be added to any laxative to temper its strength and to soothe the colon.

Form Taken

Teas, as an oil for stomach massage, in an inhaler, and as a spice to aid the digestion of starches.

Used With Other Herbs?

Caraway blends well with dill, fennel, anise, basil, cardamom, and jasmine.

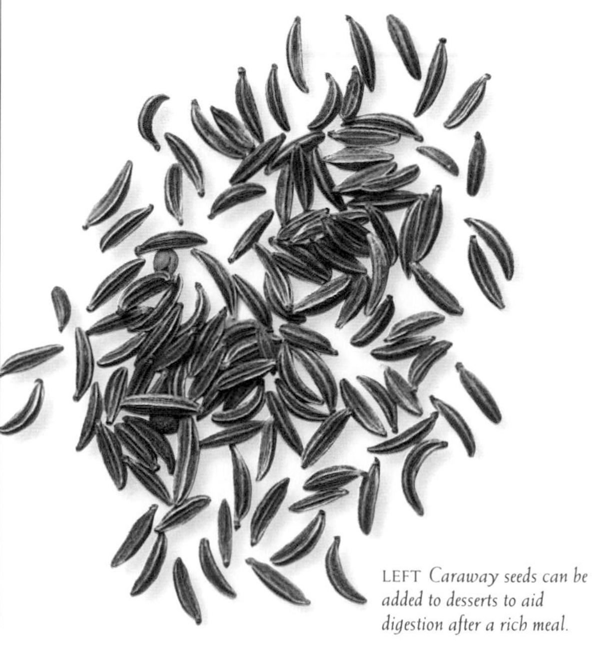

LEFT *Caraway seeds can be added to desserts to aid digestion after a rich meal.*

HOW TO USE

❧ Caraway reduces vátha and kapha, and increases pitta. It clears kapha mucus build-up and soothes vátha emotion. Caraway increases pitta digestive fire. ❧ **Eat a teaspoonful of the seeds to aid digestion, or make an infusion.**

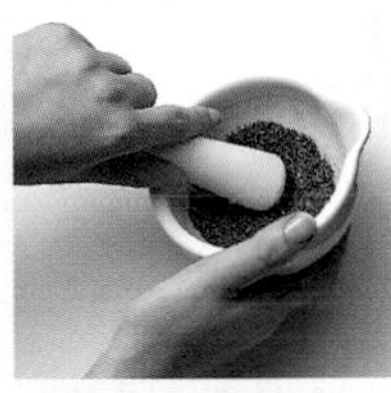

❧ Finely crush 9 teaspoonsful of seeds using a pestle and mortar.

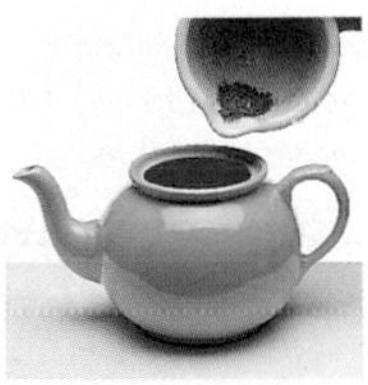

❧ Place the seeds in a pot and add boiling water.

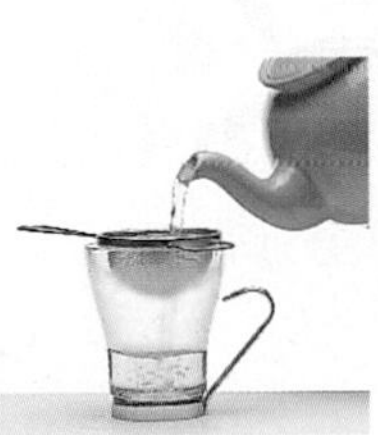

❧ Allow the infusion to stand for 20 minutes, then strain and drink as needed, up to 3 cups a day.

THERAPY CONNECTIONS

MUSTARD

Traditional and Folk Remedies *p.98*

Flower Remedies *p.239*

CAYENNE PEPPER

Herbalism *p.118*

VÁTHA

Reduces Vátha
Caraway, Cayenne Pepper
Neutralizes Vátha
Mustard

PITTA

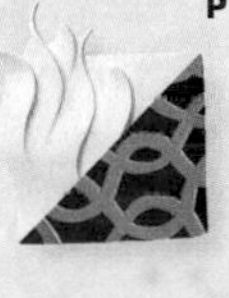

Reduces Pitta
Mustard
Increases Pitta
Caraway, Cayenne pepper

KAPHA

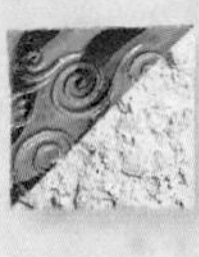

Reduces Kapha
Caraway, Mustard, Cayenne pepper

Capsicum annuum

CAYENNE PEPPER *MERCHI*

This fiery red pepper, used the world over in cooking, is known to many Westerners by its Caribbean name, cayenne. Ironically, only a tiny amount of the world's red pepper supply comes from the Caribbean – India and Africa are the main producers. One traditional cayenne prescription is to put the powder into socks to warm cold feet!

ABOVE *Add a teaspoonful of cayenne pepper to a cup of boiling water to make an infusion. Drink a tablespoonful in hot water.*

DATA FILE

Properties

Cayenne pepper assists digestion by stimulating the flow of saliva and stomach secretions. It is analgesic and warming, increasing circulation. It has strong digestive, carminative, and emetic properties. Cayenne acts as a decongestant and an expectorant.

Part of Plant Used

The pod.

Conditions Treated

Cayenne alleviates colds, gastrointestinal and bowel problems, and is used as a digestive aid. Externally, cayenne treats arthritis and muscle soreness. Creams containing cayenne are frequently used in the treatment of shingles.

Form Taken

Raw, powdered, as a spice, oil, tea, or plaster.

Used With Other Herbs?

Garlic, onion, coriander, lemon, ginger.

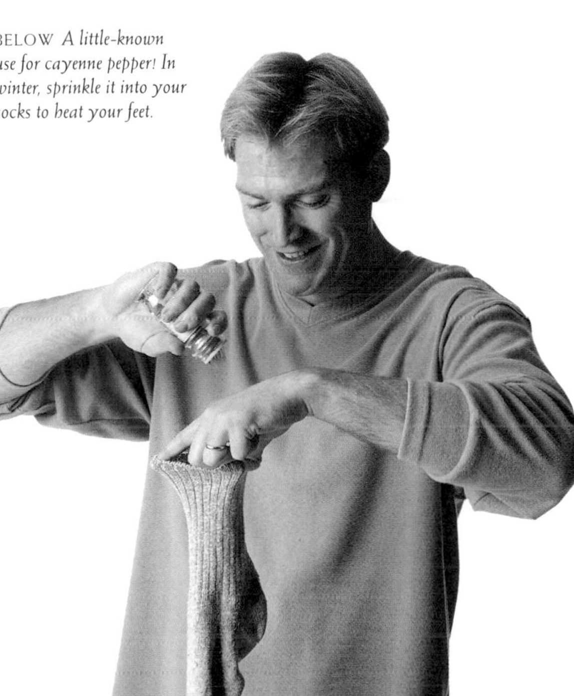

BELOW *A little-known use for cayenne pepper! In winter, sprinkle it into your socks to heat your feet.*

HOW TO USE

❧ Cayenne, with its warming and mucus-relieving qualities, increases pitta and reduces kapha and vátha. Externally, cayenne can be used for arthritis and muscle soreness, and internally as a digestive aid and a treatment for colds, fever, toothache, diarrhea, and constipation. For a pain-relieving muscle rub, mix a half-teaspoon of cayenne powder or puréed fresh cayenne to 1 cup of warm vegetable oil.

CAUTION

DO NOT GIVE TO CHILDREN UNDER TWO YEARS OLD.

USE RUBBER GLOVES WHEN CHOPPING CAYENNE PEPPERS, AS THEY MAY BURN. IF BURNING DOES OCCUR, WASH WITH VINEGAR SEVERAL TIMES, RINSING CAREFULLY.

PEPPER OIL WILL CAUSE SEVERE PAIN ON CONTACT WITH SENSITIVE TISSUES, SUCH AS EYES OR GENITALS.

Cassia angustifolia
SENNA

The Chinese name for this herb is *Fan-Hsieh-Yeh*, or "foreign-country laxative herb." Senna has a very strong laxative effect on the body. Indian senna (*C. angustifolia*) is a close relative of North African and American senna, but its properties are much milder. Still a powerful laxative, it is gentler on the body. The seed pods can be used instead of the leaves for a still milder treatment.

DATA FILE

Properties
Bitter, pungent, cooling, and purging. It is cathartic, antiseptic, antispasmodic, cholagogue, and cleansing. Senna acts mostly on the lower half of the body.

Part of Plant Used
The leaves and the whole seed pods.

Conditions Treated
Senna is the most powerful herbal treatment for constipation, especially when it is chronic. Do not use if you suffer from hemorrhoids. Senna has sometimes been used to reduce fevers, and is an ingredient in sore throat remedies.

Form Taken
Used as a powder, a tea, or a supplement.

Used With Other Herbs?
Anise, cardamom, cinnamon, coriander, fennel, ginger, nutmeg, and orange.

BELOW *Only use North American and African senna with other herbs.*

HOW TO USE

❧ Senna reduces kapha and vátha, and increases pitta. ❧ **A senna infusion will give you the benefits of senna's laxative power. Steep 3½ oz. (80g.) of senna leaves, ½ teaspoon of coriander, and ½ teaspoon of ginger in 1 quart (1l.) of hot water for 15 minutes. Take 1–4 tablespoons at a time. The infusion is more palatable cold than hot.** ❧ For children or the elderly, senna pods have a more gentle laxative effect. Steep 3–4 pods in 4–5 tablespoons of cold water. Take 1 or 2 tablespoons at a time. ❧ **For adults, use 6–12 pods for the same amount of water.**

Cedrus deodara
CEDAR *DEVADARU*

The wood we know of for its insect repellent qualities (the cedar chest which protects woolens from moths) is also, according to the Ayurvedics, an excellent treatment for dandruff. Considered a soothing tonic to the skin, cedar is often used in men's perfumes and toiletries, particularly aftershave lotions.

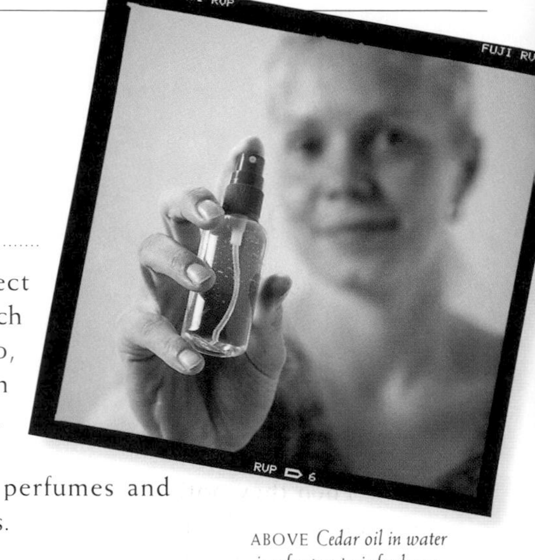

ABOVE *Cedar oil in water is a fragrant air freshener. Put it in an atomizer and spray your rooms.*

DATA FILE

Properties
Cedar is bitter and pungent, with antiseptic, diuretic qualities. It is useful as a nervine and expectorant. Cedar has a heating, drying effect on the body. The astringent, tonic qualities in cedar make it an excellent antidote to oily skin, oily scalp, and dandruff.

Part of Plant Used
The wood and bark.

Conditions Treated
Bronchitis, urinary infections, fear and nervous tension, oily hair, hair loss, oily skin, dandruff, sensitive skin, as a rub for sore joints and muscles, and to provoke sluggish menstrual cycles.

Form Taken
Oil for massage and inhalation; made into a tea or an infusion.

Used With Other Herbs?
Blends well with camphor, sandalwood, and vetiver.

VÁTHA

Reduces Vátha
Senna, Camphor
Balances Vátha
Gotu Kola
Increases Vátha
Cedar

PITTA

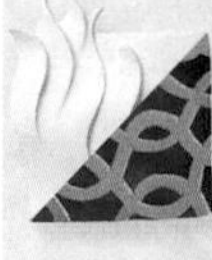

Reduces Pitta
Cedar
Balances Pitta
Gotu Kola
Increases Pitta
Senna, Camphor

KAPHA

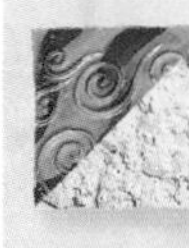

Reduces Kapha
Senna, Camphor, Cedar
Balances Kapha
Gotu Kola

HOW TO USE

❧ Cedar will reduce pitta and kapha, while increasing vátha.
❧ **Cedar is an excellent air freshener, deodorizer, and insect repellent – add oil of cedar to water in an atomizer and spray the room, or add ten drops to a tablespoon of vegetable oil and rub it on to skin.**

CAUTION

CEDAR SHOULD NOT BE TAKEN BY PREGNANT WOMEN, AS IT WILL STIMULATE THE MENSTRUAL CYCLE, AND ACTS AS A POSSIBLE ABORTIFACIENT.

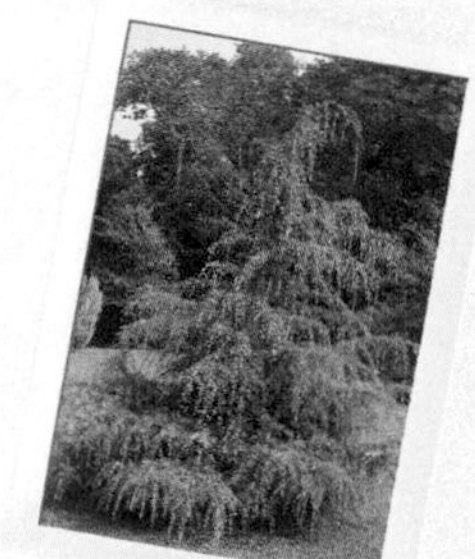

RIGHT Cedrus deodara *grows quickly to reach a maximum height of 80ft. (25m.).*

Centella asiatica

GOTU KOLA *BRAHMI*

According to tradition, the natives of Sri Lanka were the first people to use gotu kola. They noticed that elephants, animals renowned for their longevity, loved to eat the rounded gotu kola leaves. Hence the proverb "Two leaves a day keeps old age away." The Ayurvedics used gotu kola like ginseng, as a tonic for longevity. Then they noticed it was beneficial for many skin diseases, including leprosy. Today it is used to aid a variety of conditions.

DATA FILE

Properties

Bitter, stimulating, cooling, and moistening. Gotu kola neutralizes blood acids and may lower body temperature. It acts as a nervine, a diuretic, and a rejuvenating tonic. It is excellent for hair growth and as a treatment for baldness.

Part of Plant Used

The seeds, nuts, and roots.

Conditions Treated

Gotu kola stimulates the central nervous system. It aids in the elimination of fluids, shrinks tissues, decreases fatigue and depression, and stimulates sexual appetite. Gotu kola is recommended for rheumatism, blood disease, mental disorder, high blood pressure, a sore throat, tonsillitis, cystitis, venereal disease, insomnia, and to relieve stress.

Form Taken

Used as a massage oil, shampoo, poultice, tea, and skin cream.

Used With Other Herbs?

Sandalwood, lemon.

HOW TO USE

❧ Gotu kola has a balancing effect on all three doshas. ❧ **Gotu kola infusions, taken as a beverage, will improve circulation in the legs and treat varicose veins.**
❧ They will also act as a soporific in cases of insomnia. ❧ **Used as a compress, the infusion will relieve psoriasis.**
❧ To make an infusion, pour 2 cups of boiling water over 1 teaspoon of the herb. Let steep for 10 minutes. Drink up to 2 cups a day, adding lemon or honey to taste if desired.
❧ **If the results of a compress are disappointing, try strengthening the infusion used.**

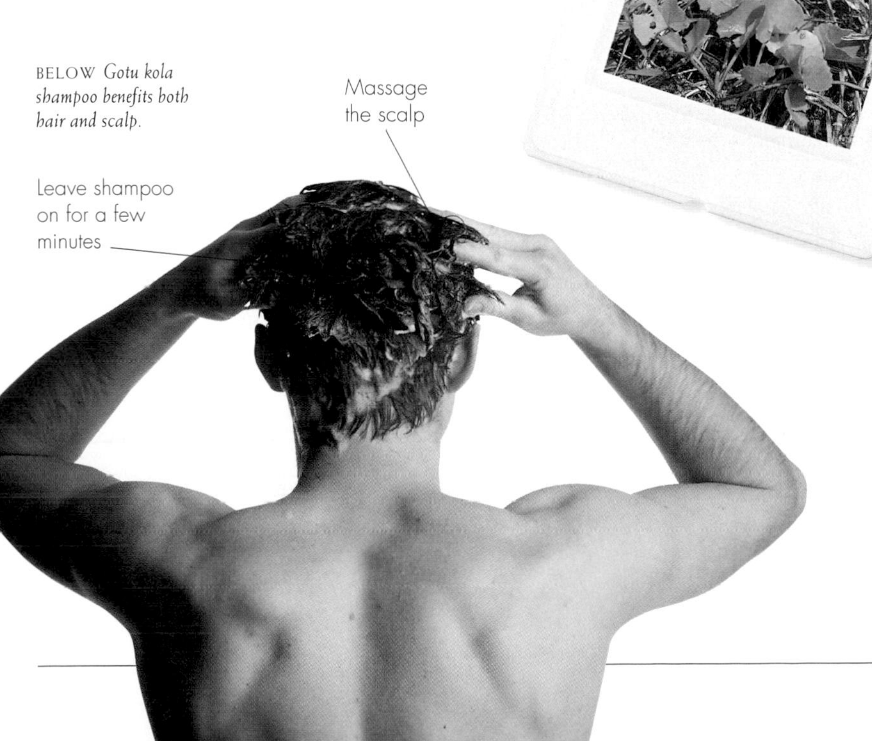

RIGHT *Gotu kola is reputed to prolong life, and acts as a general tonic.*

BELOW *Gotu kola shampoo benefits both hair and scalp.*

Cinnamomum camphora

CAMPHOR *KARPURA*

When camphor is steam-distilled, it is fractionalized into blue, brown, and white camphors. Blue camphor is the heaviest and weakest, and it is used mostly in perfume distillation. Brown camphor contains strong carcinogens and should be avoided. White camphor has medicinal qualities and is the most readily available.

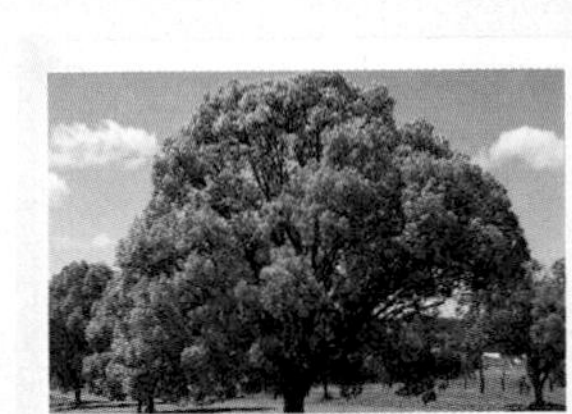

RIGHT *The camphor tree is a large evergreen grown in warm regions.*

HOW TO USE

❧ Camphor reduces kapha and vátha, and it increases pitta when used in excess. ❧ **For bronchitis and colds, try a camphor inhalation. Half-fill an enamel pan or heat-proof dish with just-boiled water. Add 7 drops of oil of camphor. Use a towel to form a "tent" over the bowl. Inhale deeply for several minutes. Stop if you feel dizzy or if the steam is too hot for your skin.**

DATA FILE

Properties

Camphor is a pungent, sour, heating substance. It has moisturizing properties which recommend it for use as an expectorant, decongestant, and bronchial dilator. Camphor is frequently employed for its twin analgesic and antiseptic qualities.

Part of Plant Used

The twigs and the leaves. Both have a strong camphor smell. Make sure that you purchase camphor which has been steam-distilled from natural sources.

Conditions Treated

Camphor clears the mind and eases headaches. It alleviates joint and muscle pain. It acts on the nervous system and tissues, as well as the respiratory system. Camphor is indicated for bronchitis, asthma, coughs, arthritis, rheumatism, and gout. It also helps nasal and sinus congestion.

Form Taken

Use as a massage oil, compress, salve, steam inhalation, and in lotions.

Used With Other Herbs?

Use camphor in small doses only. Blends with rosemary, eucalyptus, and juniper.

Cinnamomum zeylanicum

CINNAMON *TWAK, TAJ*

Cinnamon originally grew in southern Asia. Ancient Ayurvedic practitioners used it as a treatment for fevers, diarrhea, and to mask unpleasant flavors in other healing herbs. The Greeks used cinnamon to treat bronchitis, but the Europeans championed the use of cinnamon in baking. Do not confuse cinnamon with cassia, or Chinese cinnamon, a more pungent herb which is frequently added to spiced meats.

DATA FILE

Properties

Cinnamon is a pungent, sweet astringent, with stimulating, heating qualities. It acts as a diaphoretic, parasiticide, antispasmodic, aphrodisiac, analgesic, and diuretic. Cinnamon's antiseptic, antibacterial, and antifungal qualities have frequently been utilized in toothpastes and as a treatment for gum disease. As an anti-yeast agent, cinnamon has been used to treat Candida and other yeast infections.

Part of Plant Used

The bark and the leaf.

Conditions Treated

Cinnamon is recommended for respiratory ailments such as colds, sinus congestion, and bronchitis. As a digestive aid, it relieves dyspepsia, intestinal infections, and parasites. It aids circulation and helps to alleviate anemia. Cinnamon is useful for the treatment of scabies and lice. Its benefits as an aid to circulation are especially powerful during the menopause, and cinnamon's properties will increase the appetite – both sexual and gastronomic.

Form Taken

As a tea, spice, inhalant, massage oil, or powder.

Used With Other Herbs?

Cardamom, orange, nutmeg, and licorice.

HOW TO USE

❧ Cinnamon reduces vátha and kapha, and increases pitta.

❧ **Because of its strong antibacterial effect, cinnamon can be used to treat minor scrapes and cuts.**

❧ Cinnamon contains the natural anesthetic oil eugenol, which will help relieve the pain of minor wounds. To treat cuts and scrapes, wash the affected area thoroughly. Pat dry. Sprinkle powdered cinnamon lightly over the area, then bind or bandage. Repeat treatment as needed until the area is healed.

CAUTION

DO NOT USE CINNAMON IN CASES OF HIGH PITTA.

CINNAMON WILL AGGRAVATE BLEEDING, AND CAN BE A SKIN IRRITANT AND A CONVULSIVE IN HIGH DOSES.

CINNAMON BARK OIL IN PARTICULAR CAN BE AN IRRITANT AND IS NOT RECOMMENDED FOR USE ON THE SKIN.

CINNAMON INFUSIONS SHOULD NOT BE GIVEN TO CHILDREN UNDER TWO.

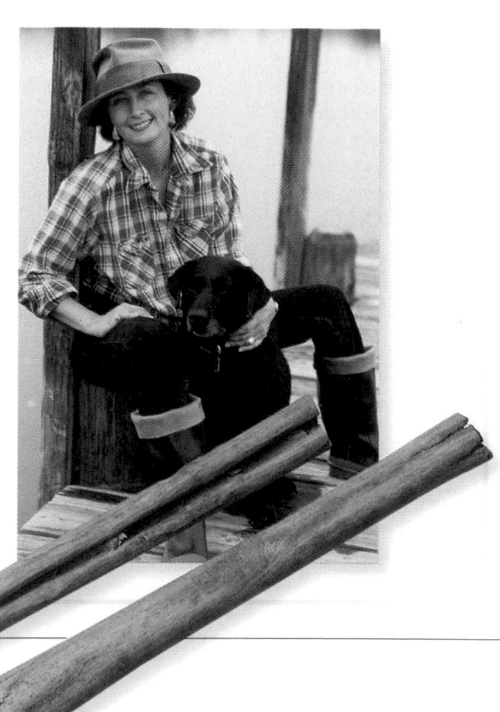

ABOVE LEFT *Cinnamon has powerful circulatory benefits during the menopause.*

BELOW LEFT *Cinnamon sticks are the dried inner bark of the shoots.*

Comiphora mukul

MYRRH *BOLA*

ABOVE *Myrrh resin was used by the ancient Egyptians for embalming.*

Myrrh is the gum from a shrub native to northeastern Africa and southwestern Asia. The shrub can grow to 30ft. (9m.) tall. Myrrh exudes from natural cracks or man-made incisions in the bark. It leaves the tree as a pale yellow liquid, which hardens into a yellowish-red or reddish-brown substance which is collected for use. This resin or gum has been used for thousands of years for its healing properties. In the Bible, myrrh is one of the gifts the wise men brought to the Christ child.

DATA FILE

Properties

Myrrh is an alterative. It is analgesic, emmenagogic, rejuvenative, astringent, expectorant, antispasmodic, and antiseptic. Its tonic effects benefit all tissues of the body.

Part of Plant Used

The sap or gum.

Conditions Treated

Myrrh is a treatment for amenorrhea, dysmenorrhea, menopause, coughs, asthma, bronchitis, arthritis, rheumatism, traumatic injuries, ulcerated surfaces, anemia, pyorrhea, excessive weight, halitosis, gum disease, sore throat, canker sores, and mouth ulcers. Myrrh is used for embalming, to clean wounds, as a douche, to stimulate menstrual flow, to promote lung drainage, and to treat hemorrhoids.

Form Taken

As a lotion or salve, a massage oil, a gargle, an incense, plaster, or infusion.

Used With Other Herbs?

Frankincense, juniper, cypress, geranium, aloe, and pine.

HOW TO USE

❧ Myrrh reduces kapha and vátha, while increasing pitta. ❧ **Its antiseptic and antifungal properties recommend it for sore throats, swollen gums, and cold sores. Myrrh oil can be used directly on sore gums, or to make a gargle.**

❧ A gargle: mix 1 teaspoon of myrrh and 1 teaspoon of boric acid in 1pt. (500ml.) of boiling water. Stand for 30 minutes, then strain. Reheat and gargle. Do not swallow. Add 1 teaspoon of golden seal to cure bad breath.

CAUTION

DO NOT USE MYRRH IN CASES OF HIGH PITTA.

Coriandrum sativum

CORIANDER

DHANYAKA, DHANIA

By all accounts, coriander, or dhanyaka, originated in India. Two thousand years ago, it was imported to China. The herb was said to "stimulate arousal and confer immortality." A popular ingredient in curry spice blends, coriander retains its aphrodisiac status – but immortality has yet to be demonstrated!

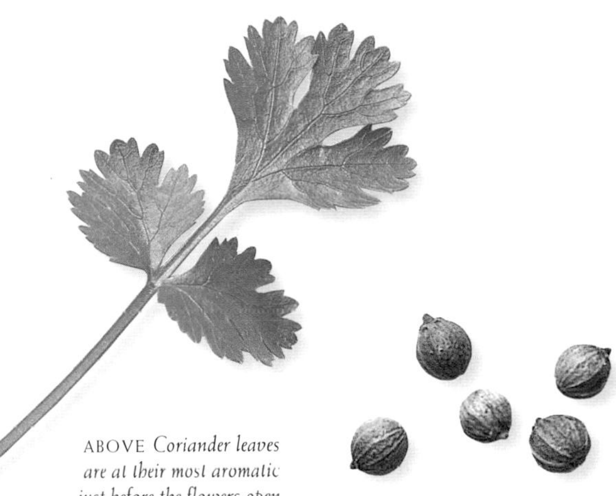

ABOVE *Coriander leaves are at their most aromatic just before the flowers open.*

DATA FILE

Properties

Coriander is a bitter, pungent herb, with a sweet, pleasant taste. Its energy is cooling and moisturizing. It has strong stimulant and alterative properties. Coriander acts as a diuretic and diaphoretic. Coriander stimulates the plasma, blood, and muscles. It is thought to be an aphrodisiac because of its phyto-estrogen content.

Part of Plant Used

The seeds and the leaves.

Conditions Treated

Coriander alleviates urinary infections, cystitis, rashes, hives, burns, digestive disorders such as gas pains, vomiting, and indigestion. Coriander is beneficial for respiratory problems – it eases allergies and hay fever. It purifies the blood, decongests the liver, and reduces heat and fever in the body. As an anti-inflammatory, coriander benefits arthritis. Coriander is typically an ingredient in eyewashes for blindness, and has been indicated as a remedy for measles.

Form Taken

As a spice, a tea or infusion, a compress, douche, shampoo, and massage oil.

Used With Other Herbs?

Used with lemon, cajeput, lavender, cardamom, clove, nutmeg, jasmine, sandalwood, and cypress.

THERAPY CONNECTIONS

CINNAMON

Chinese Herbal Medicine *p.59*

Aromatherapy *p.150*

MYRRH

Aromatherapy *p.155*

CORIANDER

Aromatherapy *p.156*

HOW TO USE

Coriander reduces all three doshas. **Its antifungal, antibacterial properties were noted by the Romans, who used coriander to preserve meats.** Like cinnamon, coriander powder can be sprinkled on cuts and scrapes to prevent infection. **The infusion makes an excellent digestive aid.** Bruise 1 teaspoon of the seeds (or use ½ teaspoon of the powder). Place in a cup, and add 1 cup boiling water. Let steep for 5 minutes. Drink up to 3 cups a day after meals. This same infusion, at half-strength, may be given, with caution, to children under two years of age for colic.

Drink up to 3 cups a day, after meals

RIGHT *Drinking coriander infusion helps with digestive problems.*

CAUTION

IN HIGH DOSES, CORIANDER MAY CAUSE KIDNEY IRRITATION.

DURING PREGNANCY, USE ONLY UNDER RECOMMENDATION FROM YOUR PHYSICIAN.

VÁTHA

Reduces Vátha
Cinnamon, Myrrh, Coriander

PITTA

Increases Pitta
Cinnamon, Myrrh, Coriander

KAPHA

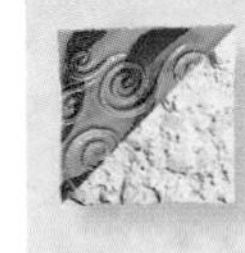

Reduces Kapha
Cinnamon, Myrrh, Coriander

Crocus sativus

SAFFRON *KESAR, NAGAKESHARA*

Saffron is a small, perennial crocus with purple flowers cultivated in Spain, France, Sicily, Iran, and India. The young plant does not flower for the first few years. When it matures, it produces flowers with golden stigmas which are quite expensive to harvest. The stigmas, or threads, are highly valued for their medicinal and aphrodisiac properties, as well as their delicious flavor.

DATA FILE

Properties

Saffron is warming, digestive, stimulant, and rejuvenating. It has anodyne, antispasmodic properties;
it is frequently used as an emmenagogue and expectorant. Saffron has been highly valued in Ayurvedic tradition for its aphrodisiac properties, especially its sweet, heavy aroma and taste.

Part of Plant Used

The stigmas or threads.

Conditions Treated

Aids digestion and improves appetite. Benefits menstrual pain and irregularity, menopause, impotence, infertility, anemia, enlarged liver, hysteria, depression, insomnia, neuralgia, lumbago, rheumatism, cough, asthma, gastro-intestinal complaints, colic, and chronic diarrhea.

Form Taken

Whole threads as a spice, in oils, infusions, and food. The oil can be used as a massage oil, a perfume, or a bath.

Used With Other Herbs?

Cedarwood, champa, lavender, rosewood, sandalwood.

HOW TO USE

❧ Saffron can be used to balance all three doshas.
❧ **A saffron infusion can be helpful for irregular menstruation and menstrual pains.** ❧ **Steep 6–10 stigmas in ½ cup of boiling water. Take 1 cup a day, unsweetened.** ❧ Saffron is prized for its aphrodisiac qualities. Try it to inspire your romantic encounters!

CAUTION

DO NOT USE DURING PREGNANCY, AS THE HERB CAN PROMOTE MISCARRIAGE.

SAFFRON CAN BE NARCOTIC IN LARGE DOSES – DO NOT EXCEED THE MEDICINAL AMOUNT INDICATED. A DOSE OF ⅓OZ. (10–12G.) CAN BE FATAL FOR HUMANS.

BELOW *Saffron threads. Saffron comes from the iris family, and is used both as a spice and a yellow dye.*

Cuminum cyminum

CUMIN *JEERA*

Cumin seeds are pungent and savory brown seeds with a flavor common to Indian and Middle Eastern cooking. Heating the seeds, by cooking or infusing, aids the digestive power of the cumin. Cumin is very rich in vitamins and minerals, and is an antidote to weakness and fatigue.

CAUTION

AN EXCESS OF CUMIN MAY CAUSE NAUSEA.

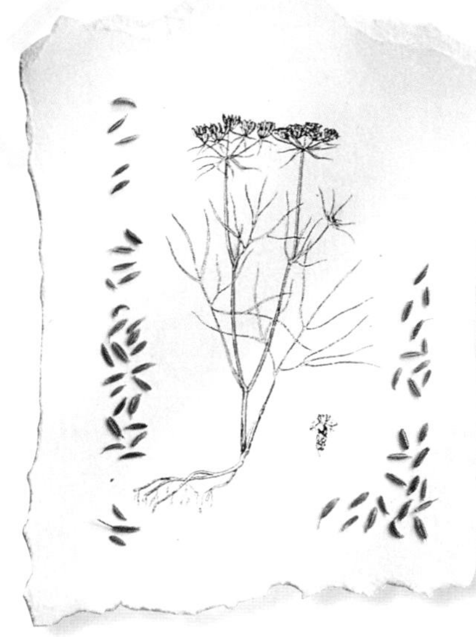

RIGHT *Cumin is an aromatic spice much used in Indian cooking to aid digestion.*

DATA FILE

Properties

Cumin has a pungent, bitter effect, with neutral to cooling properties. It acts as a blood cleanser, a carminative, aiding in the absorption of nutrients to the system. Cumin is a physical and sexual stimulant. It is antispasmodic, alterative, and acts as a lactagogue and immune builder.

Part of Plant Used

The seed.

Conditions Treated

Digestive disorders and gas pains, anemia, migraine, allergies, nervous conditions, low breast milk, and lack of sexual drive. Cumin builds up the immune system of people who suffer severe allergies.

Form Taken

In a compress, as a spice and infusion, in massage oil, and as an inhalation.

Used With Other Herbs?

Because of its overpowering smell, use cumin in small amounts when mixing with other herbs. Cumin is frequently used with lemon, black pepper, coriander, lavender, and rosemary.

HOW TO USE

❧ Cumin reduces kapha and pitta, and increases vátha.

❧ To relieve abdominal pain, add the seeds to food.

❧ Abdominal pain can also be treated with a cumin seed poultice. First, soak 2 table-spoons of cumin seeds in hot water for two hours.

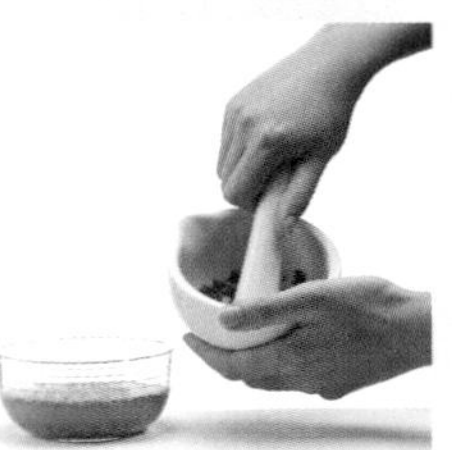

❧ Strain, dry, then crush the seeds with a heavy object (a clean stone, rolling pin, or hammer).

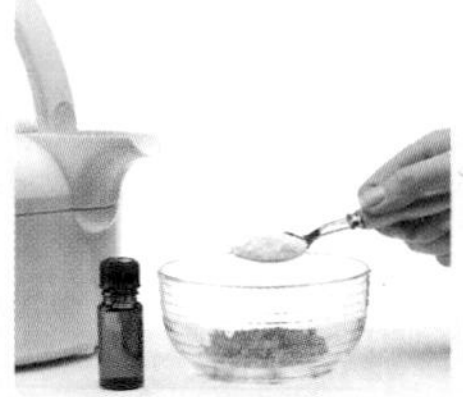

❧ Add several drops of peppermint oil, a little flour and some hot water – just enough to make a paste. Mix well. Spread this mixture on a piece of muslin or thin cloth, and apply over the abdomen to relieve liver, stomach, and gall bladder pains.

Curcuma longa

TURMERIC *HARIDRA, HALDI*

Turmeric holds a place of honor in Ayurvedic medicine. It is a symbol of prosperity, and was believed to be a cleanser for all the systems in the body. Turmeric was prescribed as a digestive aid, a treatment for fever, infections, dysentery, arthritis, jaundice, and it has been used as a basic ingredient in curries for thousands of years.

RIGHT *The leaves of the turmeric plant. Turmeric originates from south Asia.*

DATA FILE

Properties

Antiseptic, warming, pungent, bitter, and astringent. Turmeric acts as a stimulant, an alterative, and carminative, with vulnerary, antibacterial properties. Turmeric has a bright yellow color, and is sometimes used as a dye and a food coloring.

Part of Plant Used

The roots.

Conditions Treated

Indigestion, poor circulation, cough, amenorrhea, pharyngitis, skin disorders, diabetes, arthritis, anemia, wounds, bruises, and all immune system deficiencies. Because of its energizing effect on the immune system, turmeric is being studied for use in the treatment of HIV and AIDS.

Form Taken

As a massage oil, in facial creams and lotions, in compresses, or as a food or spice.

Used With Other Herbs?

Ginger, musk, wild sunflower.

VÁTHA

Reduces Vátha
Turmeric
Increases Vátha
Cumin
Balances Vátha
Saffron

PITTA

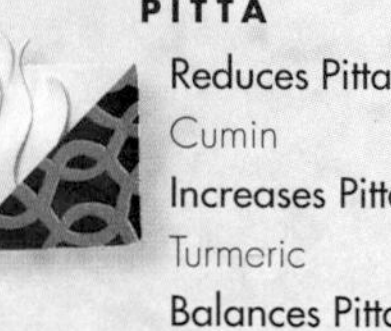

Reduces Pitta
Cumin
Increases Pitta
Turmeric
Balances Pitta
Saffron

KAPHA

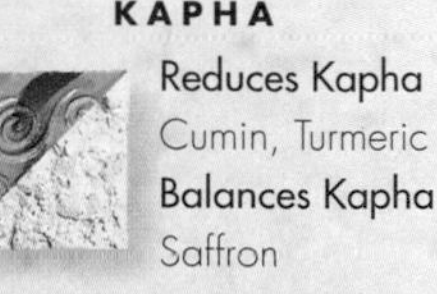

Reduces Kapha
Cumin, Turmeric
Balances Kapha
Saffron

CAUTION

DO NOT USE IN CASES OF HEPATITIS, EXTREMELY HIGH PITTA, OR PREGNANCY.

TURMERIC IS SAID TO REDUCE FERTILITY, AND WOULD NOT BE RECOMMENDED FOR SOMEONE TRYING TO CONCEIVE.

HOW TO USE

❧ Reduces kapha and vátha, and increases pitta. ❧ **Reduces fat, purifies blood, and aids circulation.** ❧ It benefits digestion, and can help rid the body of intestinal parasites. ❧ **A turmeric infusion will benefit all these conditions, and reduce arthritis pain.** ❧ Warm 1 cup of milk and remove it from the heat before it boils. Stir in 1 teaspoon of turmeric powder. Drink up to 3 cups of this a day.

LEFT *Turmeric rhizomes are ground to make the familiar yellow powder.*

BELOW *Using turmeric face cream to improve problem skin.*

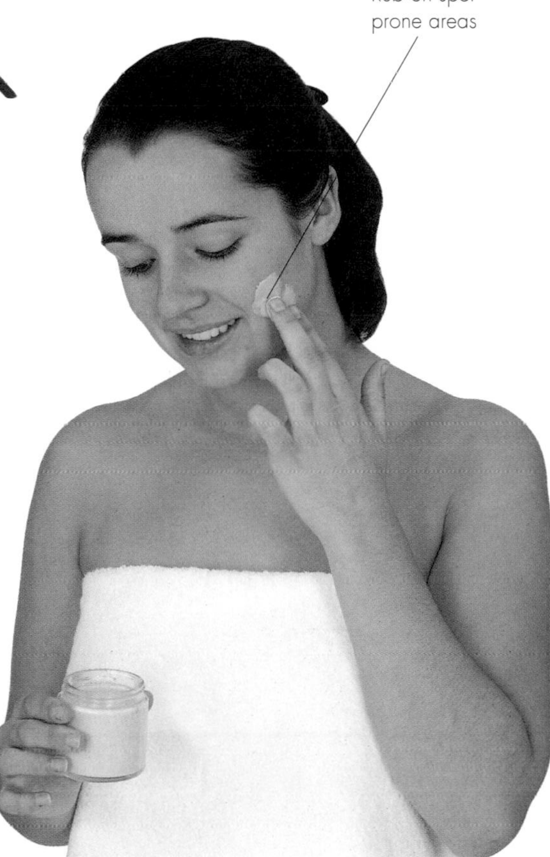

Elettaria cardamomum

CARDAMOM *ELAICHI*

Cardamom is a stimulating plant which eases the brain, the respiratory and the digestive systems. Its sweet, warming energy brings joy and clarity to the mind, and is particularly good for opening the flow of prana, or vital energy, through the body. Added to milk, cardamom will neutralize mucus-forming properties; added to coffee, it detoxifies caffeine.

LEFT *and* BELOW *Cardamom leaves and seeds. The main cardamom producers are Sri Lanka and India.*

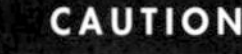

CAUTION

DO NOT USE WITH ULCERS, OR IN HIGH PITTA STATES.

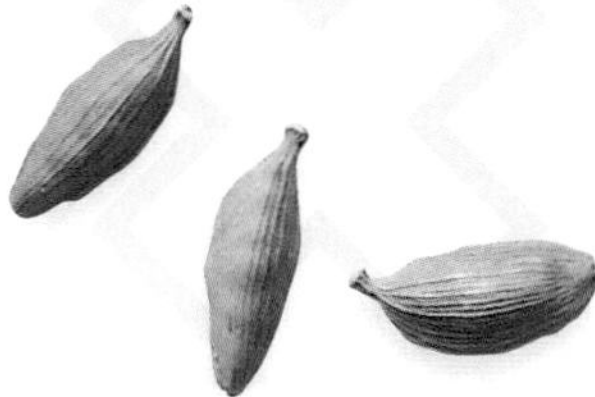

DATA FILE

Properties

Cardamom is a stimulant, an expectorant, a diaphoretic, and has aphrodisiac properties. Its qualities are pungent and sweet, with heating/moisturizing effects on the doshas. Cardamom aids in the digestion of fats and starches, stimulates the spleen, and calms acid stomach and acid regurgitation. Cardamom suppresses vomiting when eaten with a banana.

Part of Plant Used

The seeds and root.

Conditions Treated

Cardamom aids respiratory problems such as coughs, colds, bronchitis, asthma, and loss of voice. It also benefits the digestive system in cases of vomiting, belching, and indigestion. Cardamom's stimulating effects bring mental clarity and good humor.

Form Taken

Tea, as an additive to milk and food, as a bath, inhalation, or massage oil.

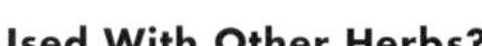

Used With Other Herbs?

Cardamom blends well with orange, anise, caraway, ginger, and coriander.

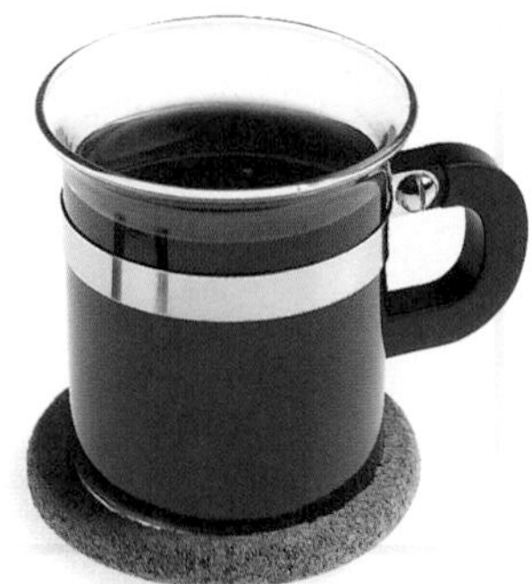

LEFT *Cardamom can be added to coffee to neutralize the caffeine.*

HOW TO USE

❧ Cardamom reduces kapha and vátha, and stimulates pitta. ❧ **Because of its soothing nervine properties, it will calm a fluttery high vátha state by kindling agni (fire).** ❧ Cardamom removes excess kapha mucus from the stomach and lungs. ❧ **Basundi, a milk-based digestive aid, is also a delicious dessert. To make this, take 2 cups of full cream milk, 2 teaspoons of cardamom powder, 2 tablespoons of ground almonds and pistachio, a pinch of saffron powder, and add honey to taste. Bring the milk to the boil and simmer until it thickens. Stir frequently to prevent burning. Add cardamom, chopped nuts, and a little honey. Continue to stir, and cook for another minute or two. Remove from heat, and add honey to taste. Let the mixture cool before eating. Serves two or three people.**

Eugenia carophyllata

CLOVES *LAVANGA*

Clove is the bud of a tropical evergreen tree. Now common as a kitchen spice, clove was a rare, prized substance for thousands of years. The demand for cloves and other Asian herbs spurred explorers like Magellan (who brought cloves to Spain) to circle the globe. Its sweetening, deodorizing properties have long been used externally in potpourris, incense, and air fresheners. Clove can also be used as an internal deodorizer, freshening the breath and reducing body odor.

ABOVE *Cloves: the dried flower buds of* Eugenia carophyllata *which originated in Indonesia.*

DATA FILE

Properties

Clove has pungent and heating properties. It functions as an analgesic, expectorant, stimulant, and carminative. Clove has antifungal properties useful for treating athlete's foot, and it deodorizes the mouth and breath. As an anesthetic it has been used in treating toothache.

Part of Plant Used

Dried flower buds (either whole or powdered).

Conditions Treated

Clove is recommended for colds, coughs, asthma, laryngitis, pharyngitis, toothache, indigestion, vomiting, hiccups, low blood pressure, and impotence. Clove tones muscles, and expectant mothers are recommended to eat cloves in the last month of pregnancy to strengthen the uterus.

Form Taken

As an oil, a compress, inhalation, massage oil, lotion, spice, and tea.

Used With Other Herbs?

Cardamom, cinnamon, lavender, ginger, orange, bay leaf.

HOW TO USE

❧ Cloves reduce kapha and vátha, and increase pitta. ❧ **Clove has long been used to fight bacteria, tooth decay, and anesthetize dental pain.** ❧ For temporary relief of toothache prior to visiting your dentist, clean your teeth gently and thoroughly. Dip a Q-tip in pure clove oil. Apply it to the affected tooth and surrounding gum area.

CAUTION

CLOVE SHOULD NOT BE GIVEN TO CHILDREN UNDER TWO, NURSING MOTHERS, AND SHOULD BE USED WITH CARE BY PREGNANT WOMEN.

EXTERNAL USE OF THE OIL MAY CAUSE A RASH.

Glycyrrhiza glabra

LICORICE *MULATHI*

Licorice is one of the most popular healing herbs in Ayurvedic medicine. It has been used for ulcers and malaria, to treat throat and respiratory problems, and to soothe rashes and infections. Due to its strong, sweet taste, the herb is sometimes used in recipes to mask the unpleasant taste of another herb.

RIGHT *Licorice root is sweet-tasting and used in confectionery and medicine.*

CAUTION

LICORICE MAY INCREASE BLOOD PRESSURE SLIGHTLY AND CAN CAUSE MILD ADRENAL STIMULATION.

IN PREGNANT AND NURSING WOMEN, CASES OF HIGH BLOOD PRESSURE OR HIGH ADRENAL FUNCTION, IT SHOULD BE USED ONLY ON THE ADVICE OF A PHYSICIAN.

DATA FILE

Properties

Licorice is sweet and astringent. It is a demulcent, expectorant, and germicide, with laxative and alterative properties. It has been used with muscle problems because of its anti-inflammatory, antiarthritic properties. Licorice is antibacterial and antiviral.

Part of Plant Used

The root and the bark.

Conditions Treated

Strengthens the nerves, promotes the memory, treats asthma, bronchitis, throat problems, digestive disorders, disorders of the spleen, liver disease, Addison's disease, inflamed gallbladder, colds, coughs, constipation, ulcers, and gastritis. Licorice powder has also been used externally to treat genital herpes and cold sores.

Form Taken

As a powder, a tea or infusion, a food, or an oil.

Used With Other Herbs?

Black pepper, clove, fenugreek, ginger, long pepper, sage, turmeric.

THERAPY CONNECTIONS

CARDAMOM
Chinese Herbal Medicine p.55
Aromatherapy p.158

CLOVES
Traditional Home and Folk Remedies p.90

LICORICE
Traditional Home and Folk Remedies p.91
Herbalism p.122
Chinese Herbal Medicine p.64

VÁTHA

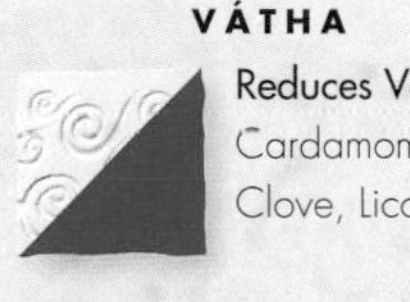

Reduces Vátha
Cardamom, Clove, Licorice

PITTA

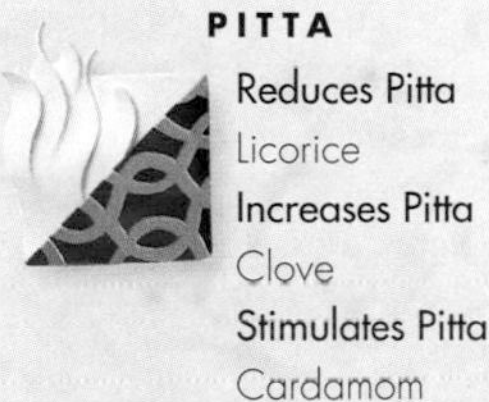

Reduces Pitta
Licorice
Increases Pitta
Clove
Stimulates Pitta
Cardamom

KAPHA

Reduces Kapha
Cardamom, Clove

RIGHT *Licorice is a perennial growing to 4ft. (1.2m.) high with purple and white flowers.*

HOW TO USE

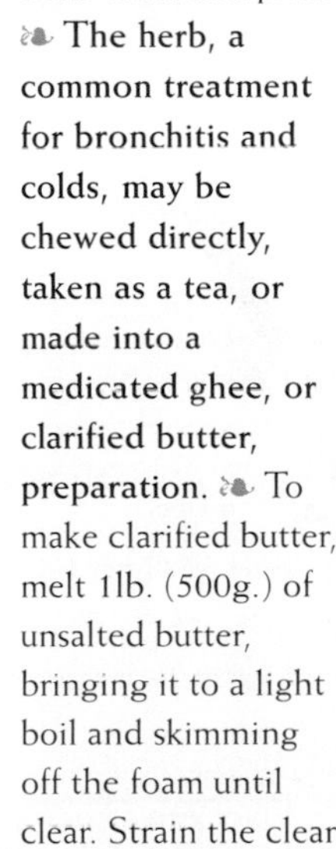

❧ Licorice reduces both vátha and pitta. ❧ **The herb, a common treatment for bronchitis and colds, may be chewed directly, taken as a tea, or made into a medicated ghee, or clarified butter, preparation.** ❧ To make clarified butter, melt 1lb. (500g.) of unsalted butter, bringing it to a light boil and skimming off the foam until clear. Strain the clear butter through cheesecloth, and let it cool.

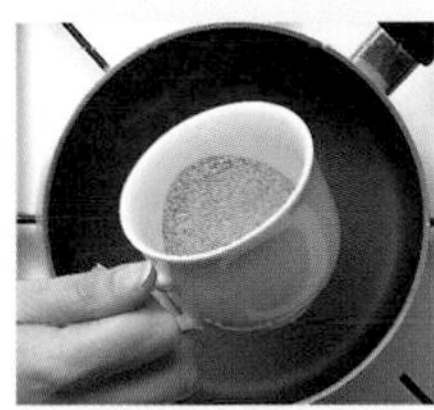

❧ **For licorice medicated ghee, you will need 2 cups of water, ¼ cup of licorice powder, and 2 tablespoons of pure ghee. Boil the water, add the licorice powder, then boil the mixture for 12 minutes.**

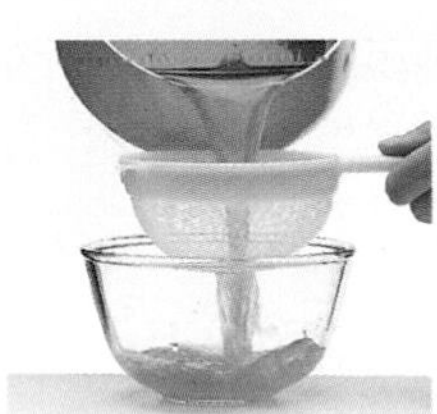

❧ **Remove from the heat and strain with a fine sieve.**

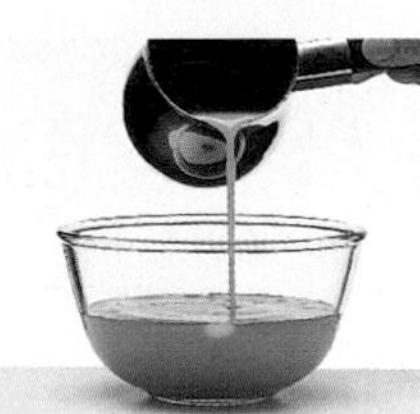

❧ **Add ghee to the remaining liquid, let it stand for 10 minutes, then administer externally or add it to food while it is still warm.**

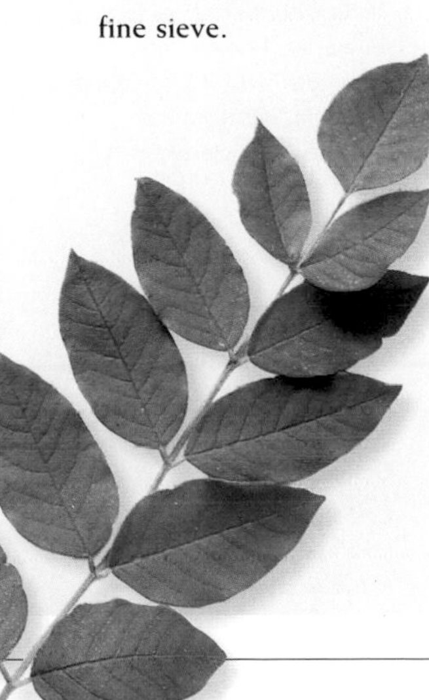

Inula helenium

WILD SUNFLOWER

ELECAMPANE, SURIA-MUKHI

Traditional Ayurvedic and Chinese herbalists have long used the dried root of the wild sunflower, or elecampane, to treat bronchial infections, asthma, and whooping cough. The Greeks were convinced of the healing properties of the herb for intestinal disorders such as dysentery, pinworm, and parasites. Today, elecampane is used to treat the respiratory and digestive systems, menstrual problems, and to aid kidney function.

ABOVE *The root of the wild sunflower is dug up in the fall and dried.*

CAUTION

TRADITIONALLY USED TO STIMULATE THE UTERUS SO SHOULD BE AVOIDED BY PREGNANT WOMEN.

SOME PEOPLE DEVELOP A RASH WHEN IN CONTACT WITH THE HERB OR ITS OIL. IF SO, DISCONTINUE USE.

DO NOT GIVE WILD SUNFLOWER TO CHILDREN UNDER TWO YEARS OF AGE.

HOW TO USE

❧ Elecampane increases pitta, and reduces kapha and vátha with its warming, drying qualities. A decoction treats both respiratory and digestive upsets. Put 3 cups of water and 2 teaspoons of powdered root into an enamel pan. Cover and boil gently for 30 minutes. Allow to cool. The taste will be bitter. Sweeten with honey if desired. Take 2 tablespoons at a time, up to 2 cups a day. Store the mixture in a refrigerator.

DATA FILE

Properties

Wild sunflower is a sweet, bitter, pungent herb with warming, drying qualities. It acts as an expectorant, a tonic for the nervous system, a rejuvenative, and a galactagogue (induces milk secretion). Elecampane's antibacterial and antifungal qualities support its use in the effective expulsion of intestinal parasites.

Part of Plant Used

The roots.

Conditions Treated

Colds, bronchial infections, coughs, lung congestion and infection. It aids digestive disorders such as amebic dysentery, pinworms, hookworms, and giardiasis. It stimulates the brain, kidneys, stomach, and uterus, and eases sciatica. Wild sunflower has been used to treat menstrual cramps.

Form Taken

Inhalations, massage oils, and lotions.

Used With Other Herbs?

Cedarwood, cinnamon, lavender, frankincense, musk, and tuberose.

CAUTION

USE OF THE HERB MAY CAUSE PHOTOSENSITIVITY IN SOME PEOPLE.

Hypericum perforatum

ST. JOHN'S WORT

St. John's wort is a bushy, flowering shrub found the world over. The leaves and flowers have long been used for their diuretic, emmenagogic and anti-depressant qualities. The Ancient Greek scholar, Galen, describes the herb as the antidote to intestinal worms. Scientists have recently discovered that the herb is a source of hypercin, which may counter the HIV virus.

HOW TO USE

❧ St. John's wort reduces pitta and kapha, and increases váthа. An oil extract of St. John's wort can be used internally for stomachache, colic, or intestinal disorders. Externally, the oil will soothe wounds, burns, and treat skin cancer. Put the fresh leaves and flowers in a glass jar, and fill it with olive oil. Close the jar and leave it for six to seven weeks, shaking it often. The oil will turn red. Strain the oil through a cloth. If a watery layer appears when the oil has stood for a while, decant or siphon it off. Stored in a dark container, the oil will keep for up to two years. Use the oil externally or take internally, 10–15 drops in water.

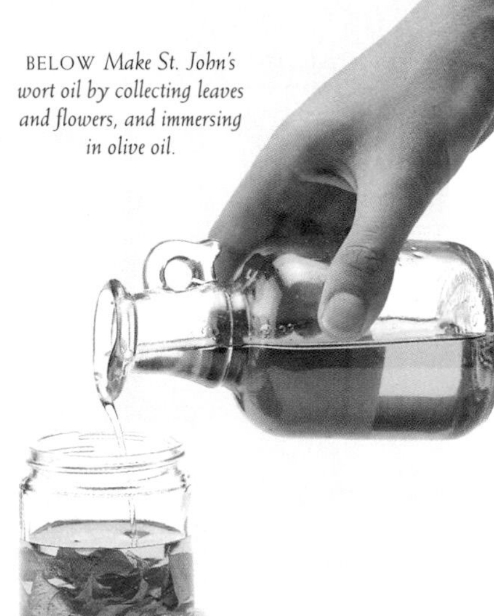

BELOW *Make St. John's wort oil by collecting leaves and flowers, and immersing in olive oil.*

BELOW *St. John's wort should be gathered when the plant is in flower.*

DATA FILE

Properties

Bitter, astringent, sweet, and cooling. St. John's wort has moisturizing, vulnerary, antispasmodic, anti-inflammatory properties. It is an expectorant, a nutritive tonic, and a ervine.

Part of Plant Used

The leaves and the flowers.

Conditions Treated

Spinal problems, skin problems, joint pain, problems associated with aging, trauma, and eczema. St. 'ohn's wort has been indicated for stomachache, colic, congestion in the lungs, insomnia, anemia, headache, jaundice, catarrh, burns, wounds, and sores. It can be used to treat carcinoma, bedwetting, melancholy, depression, uterine cramping, and menstrual problems.

Form Taken

As a massage lotion, compress, or salve; as a tea, tincture, or infusion.

Used With Other Herbs?

Angelica, chamomile, rosewood, yarrow.

THERAPY CONNECTIONS

ST. JOHN'S WORT

Herbalism p.124

Homeopathy p.199

Medicago sativa

ALFALFA

Alfalfa is grown the world over, primarily as food for livestock. The ancient Chinese, noticing their cattle preferred grazing in alfalfa, started to sprout alfalfa shoots to use as a vegetable. Ancient Arabs fed it to their horses to increase speed and endurance. They called it al-fac-facah, "father of every food," and introduced it to the Spanish, who changed the name to alfalfa. Ayurvedics have used alfalfa to cleanse the liver, detoxify the blood, treat ulcers, arthritis, and fluid retention.

RIGHT *Alfalfa has deep roots and so is resistant to drought. It has mauve flowers in summer.*

DATA FILE

Properties

Alfalfa is bitter and astringent, with cooling properties. It is high in chlorophyll and nutrients. It alkalizes and detoxifies the body, aids the liver, and is good for anemia, ulcers, diabetes, hemorrhaging, and arthritis. Alfalfa promotes pituitary gland function and contains antifungal agents.

Part of Plant Used

The leaves, petals, flowers, and sprouts.

Conditions Treated

Ayurvedic medicine notes alfalfa's ability to soothe ulcers, as well as reduce arthritis and fluid retention. Alfalfa leaves help to reduce blood cholesterol levels and clean plaque deposits from arterial walls. The sprouts produce a similar but lesser effect; however, the sprouts help neutralize carcinogens in the colon, binding them and speeding their elimination from the body. Alfalfa has been used to treat anemia, colitis, sciatica, and rheumatism. Sip the infusion for a natural breath freshener.

Form Taken

Take as a tea, a supplement, or in sprouts.

Used With Other Herbs?

Fenugreek, garlic, ginger, saffron, turmeric.

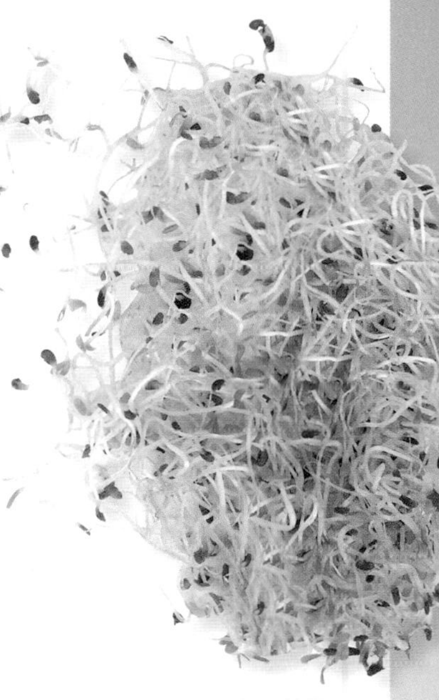

ABOVE *Originally from southwest Asia, alfalfa is now grown all over the world.*

VÁTHA

Reduces Vátha
Alfalfa
Increases Vátha
St. John's wort

PITTA

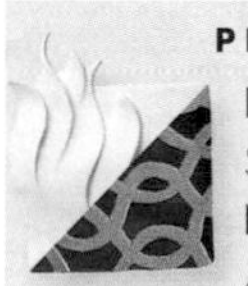

Reduces Pitta
St. John's wort
Neutralizes Pitta
Alfalfa

KAPHA

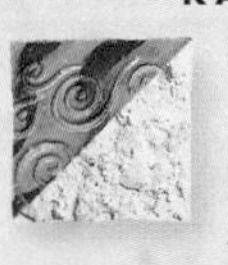

Reduces Kapha
St. John's wort
Increases Kapha
Alfalfa

HOW TO USE

❧ Alfalfa reduces both kapha and vátha, and has a neutral effect on pitta. ❧ **It is a great detoxifier and can be used on a regular basis to cleanse the system and provide refreshing chlorophyll.** ❧ The tea can be used to reduce cholesterol. Use 2 teaspoons of the herb to 1 cup of boiling water. Let it steep for 15 minutes. Drink up to 3 cups of the tea a day.

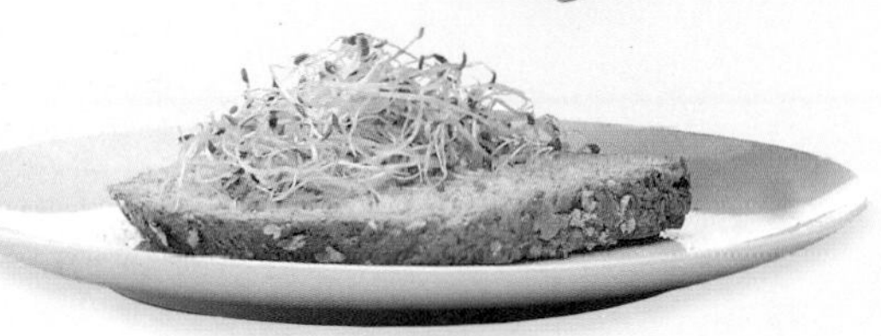

LEFT *Add alfalfa sprouts to a sandwich for a nutritious, tasty snack.*

CAUTION

NEVER EAT ALFALFA SEEDS BECAUSE THEY CONTAIN HIGH LEVELS OF THE TOXIC AMINO ACID CANAVANINE. OVER TIME, EATING THE SEEDS COULD RESULT IN IMPAIRED FUNCTIONING OF THE PLATELETS AND WHITE BLOOD CELLS.

THE ALFALFA PLANT ALSO CONTAINS SAPONINS, CHEMICALS WHICH MAY AFFECT RED BLOOD CELLS. IN RECOMMENDED DOSES, ALFALFA IS CONSIDERED COMPLETELY SAFE.

PREGNANT AND NURSING WOMEN SHOULD CONSULT A PHYSICIAN BEFORE USE.

Myristica fragrans

NUTMEG *JAIPHALA*

Nutmeg is a tropical evergreen tree native to Indonesia. The brown, wrinkled fruit contains a kernel which is covered by a bright red membrane. The membrane produces the spice mace. The 2–4in. (5–10cm.) kernel provides us with nutmeg. Many healing remedies use mace and nutmeg together.

CAUTION

CAN BE VERY TOXIC. EATING AS FEW AS TWO NUTMEG KERNELS CAN CAUSE DEATH. USE ONLY IN THE MEDICINAL AMOUNT. CONSULT A PHYSICIAN BEFORE USING NUTMEG MEDICINALLY.

PREGNANT WOMEN AND PEOPLE IN HIGH PITTA CONDITION SHOULD AVOID NUTMEG.

NUTMEG HAS HALLUCINOGENIC PROPERTIES.

DATA FILE

Properties

Warming, stimulant, rejuvenating. Nutmeg improves appetite and digestion. It is highly aromatic, carminative, and has strong hallucinogenic properties when ingested in large quantities. However, nutmeg is also highly toxic when ingested in large doses, and is only recommended for use in small doses of 1 teaspoonful or less.

Part of Plant Used

The kernel of the seed.

Conditions Treated

Nutmeg is calming and sleep-inducing, making it an excellent remedy for insomnia and other sleep disorders. It has been used to treat diarrhea and vomiting. Nutmeg strengthens the heart and eases menstruation. In small quantities, it acts on the stomach, improving digestion and appetite, while dispelling flatulence or acid stomach. Nutmeg has been used to ease kidney trouble.

Form Taken

Whole or as a powder, as a tea, a spice, a massage oil, or an inhalation.

Used With Other Herbs?

Balsam, bay, cinnamon, cumin, lavender.

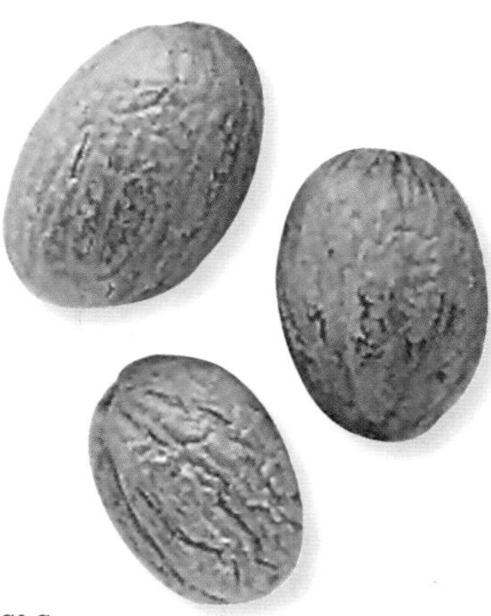

ABOVE *Whole nutmegs. The spice mace, also comes from the* Myristica *plant.*

BELOW *Nutmeg helps to thwart insomnia. Drink nutmeg tea before going to bed.*

HOW TO USE

❧ Nutmeg increases kapha and vátha, and has a neutral effect on pitta.

❧ **A nutmeg stomach tonic will relieve gas, nausea, and indigestion. Take 1½ teaspoons of powdered slippery elm bark, ½ teaspoon of nutmeg, and 1½ teaspoons of mace. Mix thoroughly and add a little cold water to make a smooth paste with no lumps. Bring 1pt. (500ml.) of light cream or ½pt. (250ml.) each of cream and water to the boiling point, remove from the heat, and quickly add the paste. Stir with a wooden spoon for 1 minute or until the powder is completely dissolved. Let cool until lukewarm. Drink ½ cup. You may take ½ cup up to three times daily, always warm, to help heal stomach problems.**

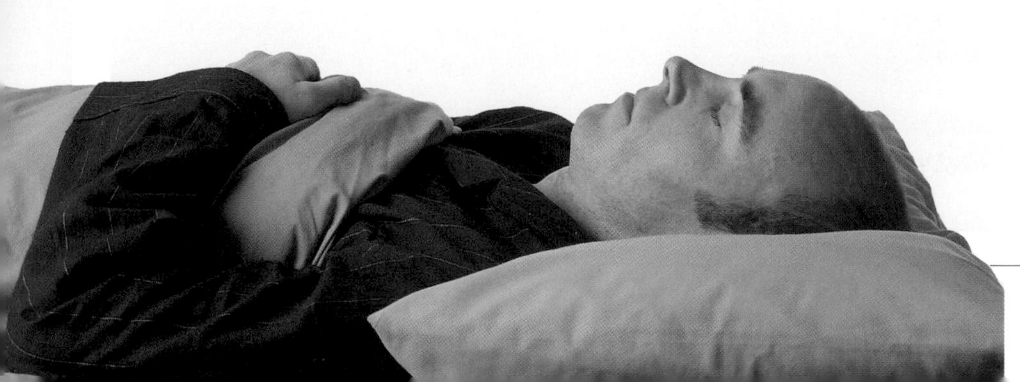

Ocymum basilicum

BASIL *TULSI*

There are many different varieties of basil. The Indian variety is also known as basil krishna, because it is said that Krishna wore garlands of this herb around his neck to increase his detachment and his faith. The faithful continue this practice, believing basil to be a protector in life and after death. Ayurvedics have used basil to treat stomach, kidney, and blood ailments.

ABOVE *Basil can be grown on a window-ledge if kept in a sunny position.*

HOW TO USE

❧ Basil reduces kapha and vátha, and increases pitta. ❧ **It has a strong effect on the emotions, and can ease fear or sadness.** ❧ Use a homemade infusion as an acne remedy. Steep 3 teaspoons of dried leaves in 1 cup of boiling water. Steep for 20 minutes. Apply with a cotton ball to freshly washed skin, or drink up to 3 cups of the tea per day as an internal antibacterial treatment.

CAUTION

AVOID USE WHEN IN A HIGH PITTA CONDITION, BECAUSE BASIL INCREASES PITTA.

USE WITH CARE DURING PREGNANCY, AS BASIL HAS BEEN USED AS A MENSTRUATION PROMOTER AND LABOR INDUCER.

DATA FILE

Properties

Basil acts as a diaphoretic, a febrifuge (a fever reducer), and a nervine. Basil is antibacterial, antiseptic, antifungal, and antispasmodic. Basil stimulates the immune system by increasing the production of antibodies.

Part of Plant Used

The leaves, the oil.

Conditions Treated

Basil can provide relief for colds, coughs, asthma, sinus congestion, headaches, arthritis, rheumatism, and fevers. Basil oil kills intestinal parasites, and as such is recommended for abdominal conditions, parasites, and stomachache. A basil poultice can be used to treat ringworm infections.

Form Taken

Basil can be drunk as a tea or juice, cooked into medicated ghee, used as an inhalation, massaged as a therapeutic oil, or made into a compress or poultice.

Used With Other Herbs?

Basil is wonderful when used in conjunction with camphor, rosemary, juniper, lemon, eucalyptus, myrtle, lavender, bergamot, lime, and clary sage. Great fragrances!

Piper longum

LONG PEPPER *PIPPALI*

Native to India and Java, these peppers are gathered and stored to ripen for use, in order to preserve the greatest heat potency. Long pepper, or pippali, is the primary ingredient in Ayurvedic medicine to treat kapha disorders. Together with ginger and black pepper, long pepper is used as a component in the Ayurvedic blend Trikatu.

CAUTION

LONG PEPPER SHOULD NOT BE GIVEN TO CHILDREN UNDER TWO YEARS OLD.

USE RUBBER GLOVES WHEN CHOPPING PEPPERS, AS IT MAY BURN THE FINGERTIPS. IF BURNING SHOULD OCCUR, WASH WITH VINEGAR SEVERAL TIMES, RINSING CAREFULLY.

PEPPER OIL CAN LINGER FOR SEVERAL HOURS, AND WILL CAUSE SEVERE PAIN IF IT COMES IN CONTACT WITH SENSITIVE TISSUES, SUCH AS EYES OR GENITALS.

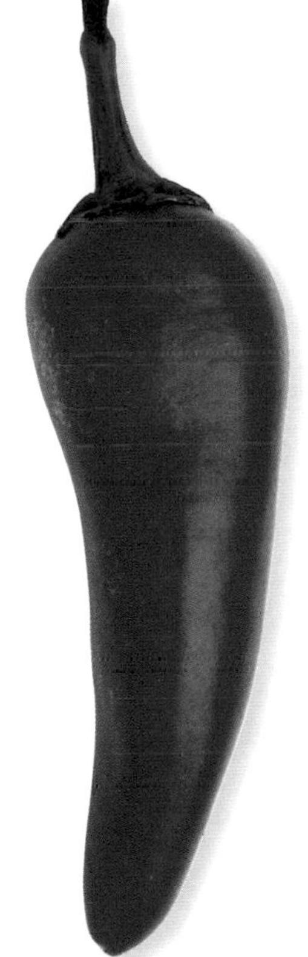

RIGHT *Long pepper obviously gets its name from its shape.*

HOW TO USE

❧ Long pepper restores kapha and vátha to balance, invigorating sluggish kapha, and warming vátha's coolness. ❧ **Its warming action increases pitta.** ❧ Use a pippali and rock salt tea to clear sore throats, sinus congestion, coughs, and hiccups. ❧ **To a large mug, add 1½ cups of boiling water, ½ teaspoon of long pepper powder, and ½ teaspoon of rock salt. Cover and let steep for 15 minutes. Pour the tea into another cup, leaving the sediment behind. Drink while warm.**

DATA FILE

Properties

Long pepper is a pungent, heating stimulant. It has strong digestive, carminative, and emetic properties. Long pepper acts as a decongestant and expectorant. It is analgesic and warming, and increases the circulation.

Part of Plant Used

The fruit (pepper).

Conditions Treated

Asthma, bronchitis, throat problems, digestive disorders, disorders of the spleen. Externally, long pepper can be used for arthritis and muscle soreness. Taken internally, it is useful as a digestive aid and a treatment for colds, fever, toothache, diarrhea, and constipation.

Form Taken

As a powder, a tea or infusion, a food, or an oil.

Used With Other Herbs?

Black pepper, fenugreek, ginger, turmeric.

BELOW *Pepper-infused oil's warming action benefits rheumatism and arthritis.*

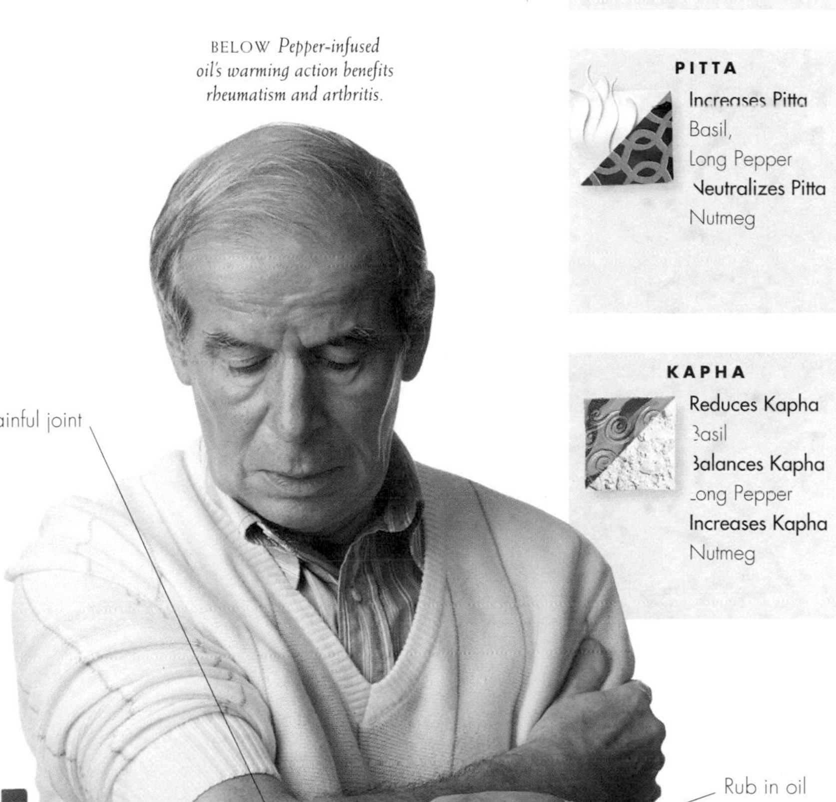

THERAPY CONNECTIONS

BASIL

Aromatherapy *p.164*

VÁTHA

Reduces Vátha
Basil
Balances Vátha
Long Pepper
Increases Vátha
Nutmeg

PITTA

Increases Pitta
Basil,
Long Pepper
Neutralizes Pitta
Nutmeg

KAPHA

Reduces Kapha
Basil
Balances Kapha
Long Pepper
Increases Kapha
Nutmeg

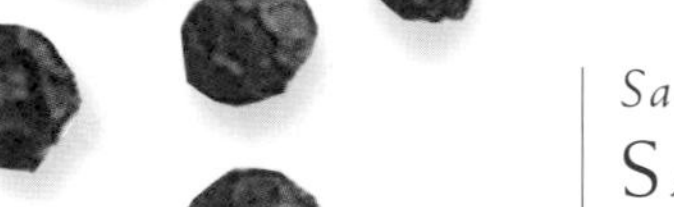

Piper nigrum

BLACK PEPPER

MARICH, MARI

In Ayurvedic traditions, black pepper or marich is named after the Sanskrit word for the sun. Black pepper contains very potent solar energy, and is a powerful digestive stimulant. Black pepper is rajasic, or energy-producing, in nature. The plant is native to South India, where the white-flowered shrub grows wild. The yellow berries, which are dried for peppercorns, turn red when they mature and are ready for harvesting.

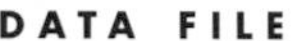

ABOVE *Peppercorns are dried, unripe berries which are crushed to produce the oil.*

CAUTION

DO NOT USE IN HIGH PITTA STATE OR IN CASES OF INFLAMMATION OF THE DIGESTIVE ORGANS.

OVERUSE OF STIMULANT HERBS CAN IMPAIR YOUR BODY'S NATURAL BALANCING SYSTEMS.

IF YOU FIND YOU ARE ATTRACTED TO ADDING PEPPER TO MOST OF YOUR FOOD, THEN START CUTTING BACK.

DATA FILE

Properties

Black pepper has a heating and drying effect. The taste is pungent and bitter, both properties good for balancing an overabundance of kapha.

Part of Plant Used

The pepper kernel and the oil made from it.

Conditions Treated

Black pepper stimulates the plasma and the blood, the nervous system, the spleen, and reduces fat. It is beneficial for chronic indigestion, toxins in the colon, sinus congestion, and can stimulate the circulation to help warm cold hands and feet.

Form Taken

Take as a spice, as an oil, a tea, or a compress.

Used With Other Herbs?

Black pepper combines well with orange, ginger, cypress, anise, sandalwood, lemon, and basil.

HOW TO USE

❧ Reduces kapha, increases pitta and vátha. ❧ **Use in cooking as a stimulant – black pepper's qualities are enhanced by heating.** ❧ The oil can be used to clear sinus congestion and stimulate fat reduction. To assist weight loss, blend 10 drops lavender oil, 10 drops black pepper oil, 5 drops sandalwood oil, 5 drops frankincense oil, and mix into 3fl. oz. (100ml.) almond oil. Store in a dark glass container. Clearly label the mixture to show it is for weight reduction use, and massage into areas where you want to lose weight.

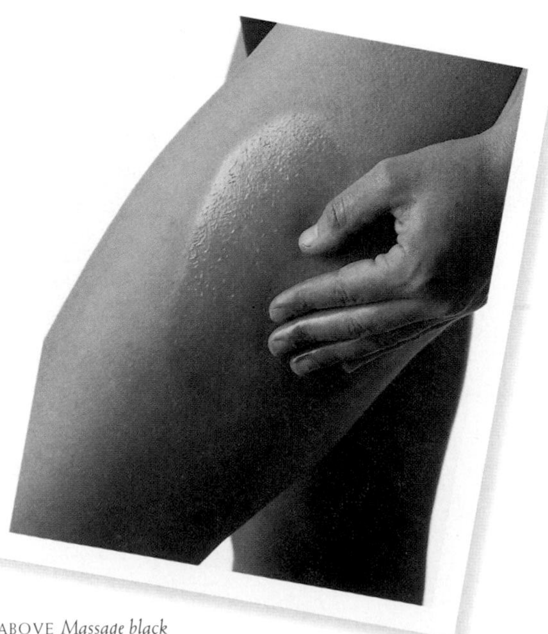

ABOVE *Massage black pepper oil into fat-prone areas to help weight loss.*

Santalum album

SANDALWOOD *CHANDANA*

Sandalwood is a small tree which grows primarily in India. While the aromatic wood is used to make scented carvings, the medicinal properties are in the oil, which can be pressed from the wood, or extracted with alcohol or water.

HOW TO USE

❧ Reduces pitta and vátha, and has a neutral effect on kapha. ❧ **A sandalwood decoction will reduce fever if taken internally; externally it can be used to treat acne and other skin problems.** ❧ To make a decoction, boil 1 heaped teaspoon of sandalwood in 1 cup of water. Cover and boil for several minutes. Strain and cool. Drink 1 or 2 cups a day, a tablespoon at a time. For external use, apply to freshly washed skin, and let dry. Repeat three times a day or as needed.

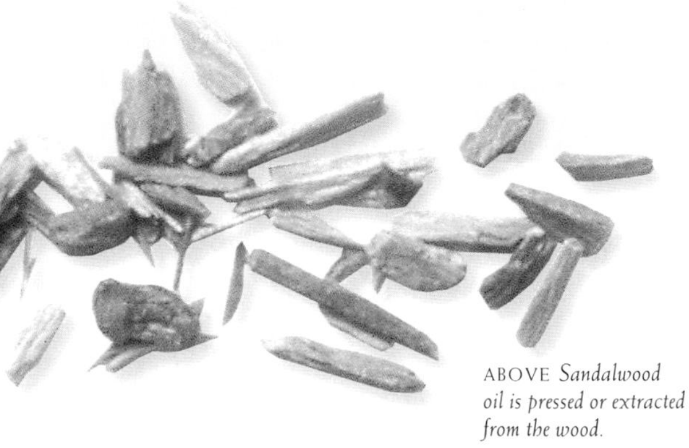

ABOVE *Sandalwood oil is pressed or extracted from the wood.*

DATA FILE

Properties

Bitter, sweet, astringent, cooling, moisturizing. Sandalwood is alterative, hemostatic, antipyretic, antiseptic, antibacterial, carminative, sedative, antispasmodic, and aphrodisiac. It works as a nervine, an expectorant, a diuretic, a disinfectant, and a moisturizer. It also helps to regenerate tissues.

Part of Plant Used

The wood.

Conditions Treated

Sandalwood has been used to treat cystitis, urethritis, vaginitis, acute dermatitis, herpes, bronchitis, palpitations, gonorrhea, sunstroke, dry skin, acne, laryngitis, nausea, tuberculosis, depression, insomnia, prostatitis, nervousness, anxiety, and impotence. Sandalwood can cure skin problems that are bacterial in origin.

Form Taken

In perfumes and massage oils; as a gargle, lotion, bath, inhalation, compress, or douche.

Used With Other Herbs?

Clove, geranium, musk, myrrh, tuberose, vetiver.

Trigonella foenum-graecum

FENUGREEK *METHICA*

Fenugreek is another healing herb whose qualities were brought to the attention of humans by animals. Farmers noticed that sick cattle would eat fenugreek plants even when they would not eat anything else. So fenugreek began to be used as a digestive aid and laxative. Fenugreek seeds contain a lot of bulk and mucilage, and, when mixed with water or saliva, become gelatinous and ease sluggish bowels.

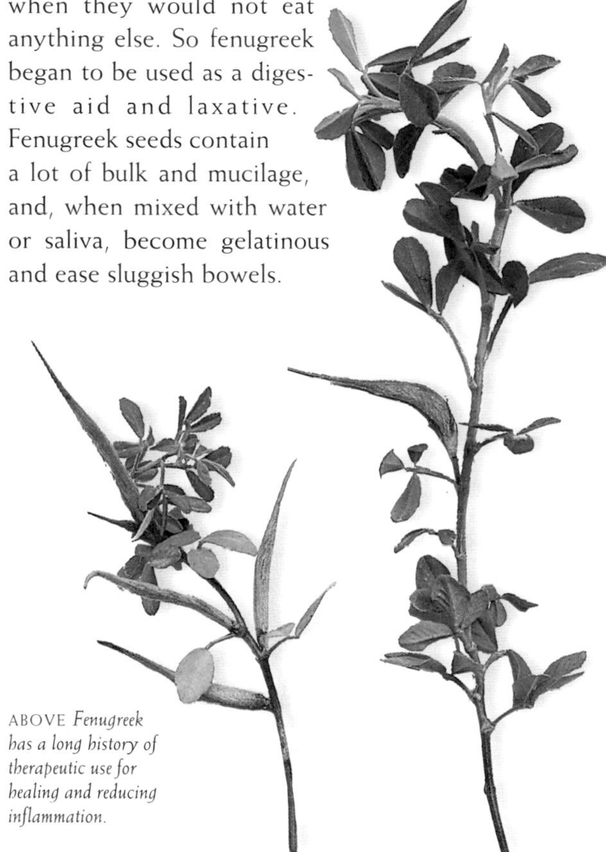

ABOVE *Fenugreek has a long history of therapeutic use for healing and reducing inflammation.*

CAUTION

FENUGREEK SEEDS MAY CAUSE WATER RETENTION AND WEIGHT GAIN.

BECAUSE OF ITS USE AS A UTERINE STIMULANT, FENUGREEK SHOULD NOT BE TAKEN BY PREGNANT WOMEN.

DO NOT GIVE FENUGREEK TO CHILDREN UNDER TWO YEARS.

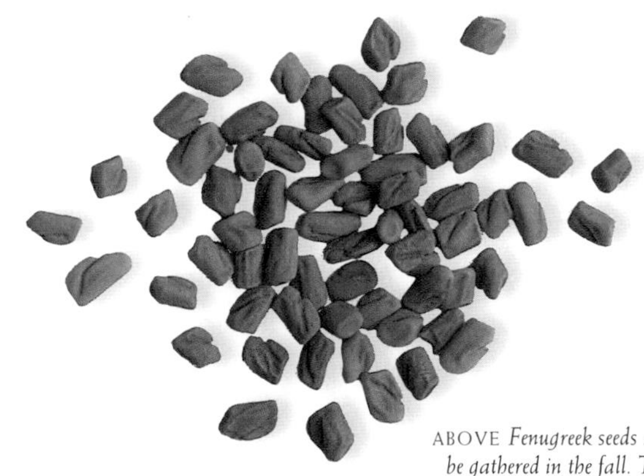

ABOVE *Fenugreek seeds should be gathered in the fall. Their bitterness soothes indigestion.*

DATA FILE

Properties

Antiseptic and warming. Fenugreek has expectorant qualities. It is anti-inflammatory, antiseptic, and soothing. The soothing expectorant qualities aid in promoting menstruation, as well as easing coughs, sore throats, and digestion (encouraging flow in the body).

Part of Plant Used

The seeds.

Conditions Treated

Constipation, digestive disorders, bronchitis, inflamed lungs, fevers, high cholesterol, eyestrain, sore throats, wounds, boils, rashes. It stimulates the uterus, promotes water retention and weight gain, reduces blood sugar levels, and lowers cholesterol.

Form Taken

As a spice, a tea, a massage oil, an inhalant, a poultice, or plaster.

Used With Other Herbs?

Peppermint, lemon, anise.

THERAPY CONNECTIONS

BLACK PEPPER
Traditional Home and Folk Remedies *p.97*
Aromatherapy *p.167*

SANDALWOOD
Aromatherapy *p.169*

VÁTHA

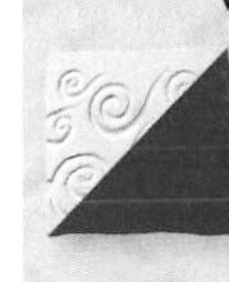

Reduces Vátha
Sandalwood, Fenugreek
Increases Vátha
Black pepper

PITTA

Reduces Pitta
Sandalwood
Increases Pitta
Black pepper, Fenugreek

KAPHA

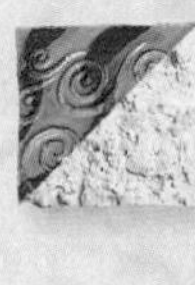

Reduces Kapha
Black pepper
Fenugreek
Neutralizes Kapha
Sandalwood

HOW TO USE

❧ Fenugreek reduces kapha and vátha, and increases pitta. ❧ **Fenugreek helps asthma and sinus problems by reducing mucus.** ❧ The seeds can be eaten by nursing mothers to increase milk production. ❧ **A fenugreek poultice can be used to treat boils and rashes.** ❧ Gargling a fenugreek decoction will soothe sore throats. ❧ **Fenugreek decoctions have many healing uses: to treat arthritis and aching joints, to bring on menstruation, to lower cholesterol, or to ease sore throats and laryngitis.** ❧ To make a decoction, bruise 2 tablespoons of fenugreek seeds. Add 4 cups of water. Bring to a boil, then cover and simmer for 10 minutes. Drink up to 3 cups a day. Add honey, lemon, or licorice to sweeten.

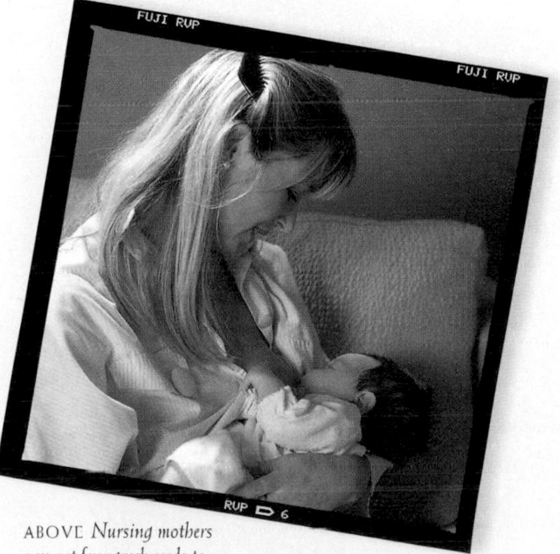

ABOVE *Nursing mothers can eat fenugreek seeds to increase their milk.*

Vattiveria zizanoiodes

VETIVER

Vetiver is a grassy plant known for its grounding, centering properties. In India, it is sown wherever there is soil erosion, to hold down the earth and prevent further damage to the land. Modern herbalists use it to enable an individual to connect to the earth and feel his or her purpose. It is helpful during emotionally stressful times and has been used as a tonic for women suffering PMS.

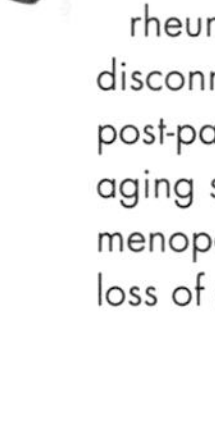

ABOVE *Vetiver has aromatic roots which yield a fragrant oil used in perfumes.*

DATA FILE

Properties

Warming, sweet, and bitter. Vetiver is an antiseptic tonic, grounding, regenerating, and strengthening. It is an aphrodisiac, and can be used to repel moths.

Part of Plant Used

The leaves and roots.

Form Taken

As a lotion, bath, massage oil, in patches and perfumes.

Used With Other Herbs?

Angelica, citrus, cinnamon, lavender, sandalwood, sage, yarrow.

Conditions Treated

Arthritis, root chakra blockage, nervousness, insomnia, rheumatism, stress, disconnectedness, anorexia, post-partum depression, aging skin, fatigue, menopause, loss of appetite.

VÁTHA

Reduces Vátha
Vetiver, Ginger

PITTA

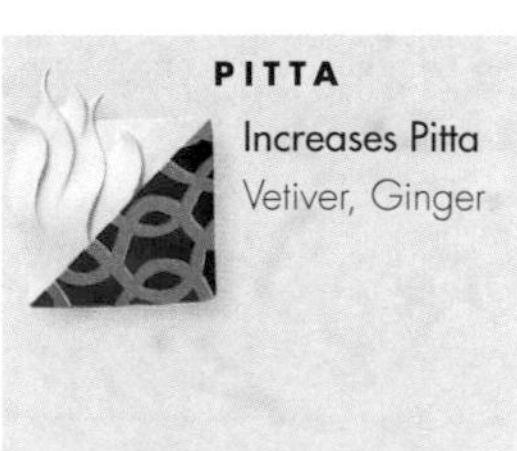

Increases Pitta
Vetiver, Ginger

KAPHA

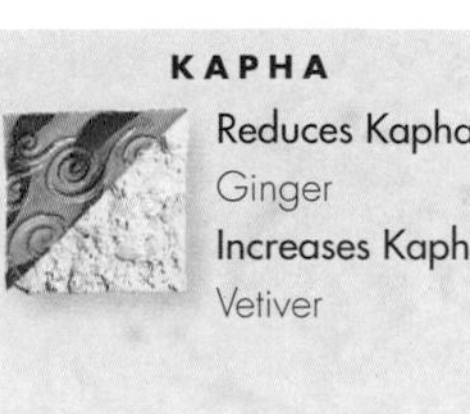

Reduces Kapha
Ginger
Increases Kapha
Vetiver

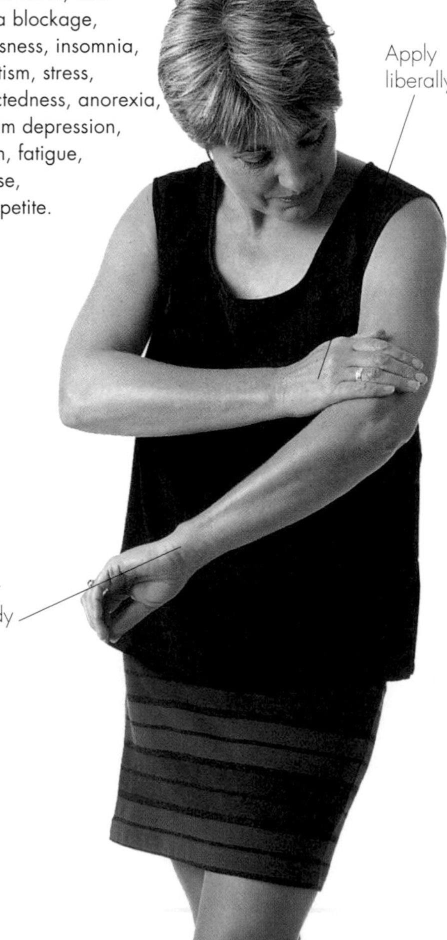

LEFT *Massage vetiver travel oil blend into your skin to help the body cope with a journey.*

HOW TO USE

❧ Vetiver reduces vátha, and increases both kapha and pitta. ❧ **Vetiver oil is particularly useful for jet lag, and for grounding and clarity while traveling.**

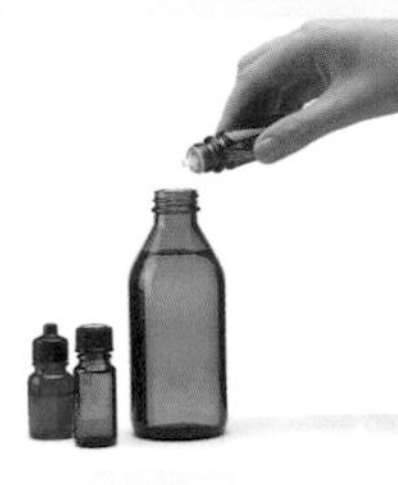

ABOVE *Add the essential oils to the base oil.*

❧ Use as a base 2fl. oz. (60ml.) apricot kernel oil. Add 5 drops vetiver oil, 5 drops geranium oil, and 2 drops juniper or grapefruit oils. Apply this mixture liberally all over your skin before travel. ❧ **Once traveling, reapply to as much of your body as possible every four or five hours.**

❧ You may also carry a damp washcloth to which the oils have been added. If you are flying, the flight attendant may heat the washcloth in the microwave for you. Shower or bathe upon arrival, and reapply the oils. Enjoy your trip!

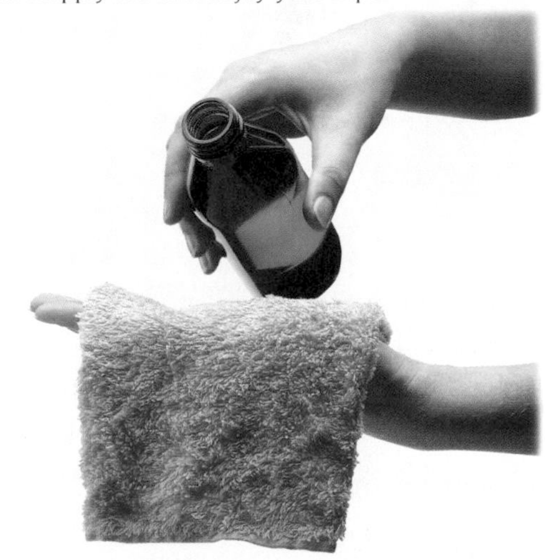

ABOVE *Apply the blend to a damp washcloth to pack and use during your journey.*

CAUTION

VETIVER HAS A VERY STRONG SMELL. DO NOT ALLOW IT TO OVERPOWER ANY BLEND YOU ARE MAKING WITH IT.

THERAPY CONNECTIONS

VETIVER
Aromatherapy *p.171*

GINGER
Aromatherapy *p.171*
Chinese Herbal Medicine *p.57*

ABOVE *Children will enjoy making gingerbread – and eating the results of their handiwork!*

Zingiber officinalis

GINGER *ARDRAKA*

Ginger is native to India, where the ancient Ayurvedics used it to preserve food, as a digestive aid, and as a spiritual and physical cleanser. Garlic was shunned on the days leading up to religious festivities, but plenty of ginger would be consumed in order to be sweet-smelling and purified for the gods. The Greeks wrapped the root in a piece of bread and ate it after a heavy meal to prevent indigestion – this is the origin of gingerbread.

RIGHT *The fresh root of the ginger plant may be dried and powdered for convenience.*

CAUTION

DO NOT USE IN CASES OF HIGH FEVER, BLEEDING, WITH INFLAMMATORY SKIN CONDITIONS, OR IF ULCERS ARE PRESENT.

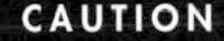

GINGER IN LARGE DOSES CAN BRING ON MENSTRUATION.

PREGNANT WOMEN WITH A HISTORY OF MISCARRIAGE SHOULD EXERCISE CAUTION AND CONSULT THEIR PHYSICIAN BEFORE USE.

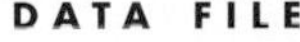

DATA FILE

Properties

Ginger is a pungent, sweet herb with warming/drying qualities. It acts as a stimulant, diaphoretic, antidepressant, and expectorant. Ginger stimulates all tissues of the body, and is highly recommended in cases where the illness is due to poor assimilation.

Part of Plant Used

The root.

Conditions Treated

Ginger is recommended for colds, coughs, flu, indigestion, vomiting, belching, abdominal pain, motion sickness, laryngitis, arthritis, hemorrhoids, headaches, impotence, diarrhea, heart disease, and memory loss.

Form Taken

As a food, a tea, a gargle, and a compress. Also used as a massage oil.

Used With Other Herbs?

Black pepper, eucalyptus, juniper, cedar, coriander, and all citrus.

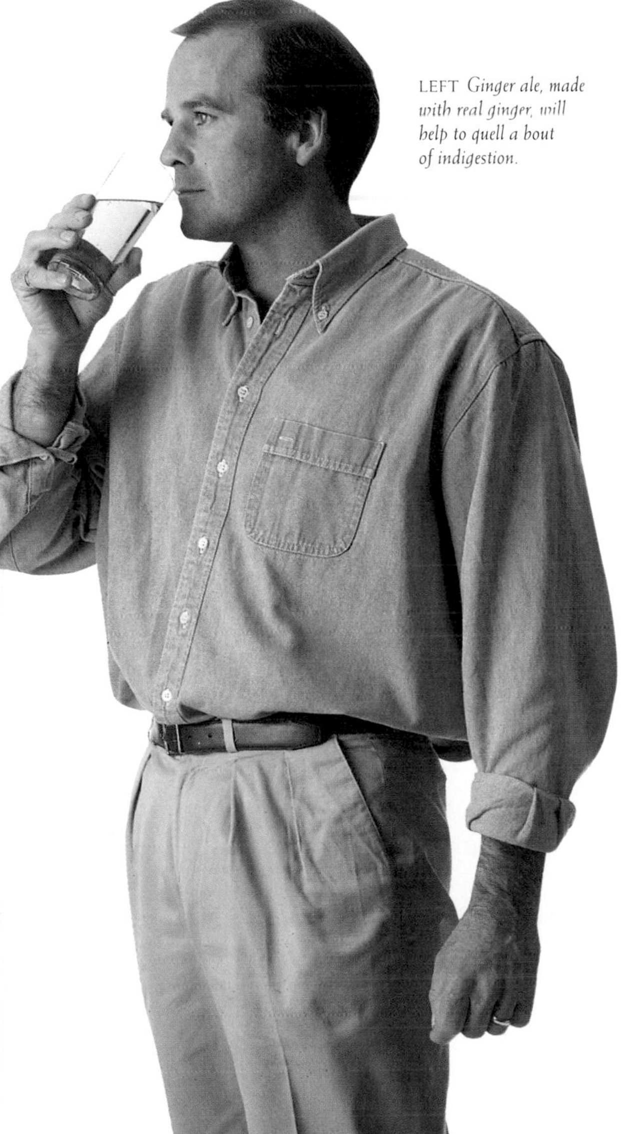

LEFT *Ginger ale, made with real ginger, will help to quell a bout of indigestion.*

HOW TO USE

ABOVE *Motion sickness responds well to remedies made with ginger.*

Ginger increases pitta in the body, reducing both kapha and vátha. **Its muscle-relaxant, heating pitta qualities can warm uterine walls, soothing menstrual cramps.** It is also frequently used as an antidote to travel sickness. **For motion sickness (on land, sea, or in the air), use a few drops of ginger oil on a small bandage and place behind the ear.** Alternatively, you may take ginger capsules, or make a ginger tea with 2 teaspoons of the grated root to 1 cup of boiling water. Let it steep for 5 minutes. Of course, you could also sip a glass of ginger ale (provided it is made from real, not synthetic, ginger).

CHINESE HERBAL MEDICINE

Chinese medicine is an ancient system of healing – acupuncture and Chinese herbal medicine grew up in tandem over 2,000 years. It is based on the philosophy of a very different civilization from our own, a civilization that perceived people as either "in harmony" or "out of harmony" with themselves and their surroundings. Traditional Chinese Medicine (TCM) sees disease in terms of patterns of disharmony, and so attempts to restore the balance in the person who is sick. Energy is believed to flow through channels called meridians, through which disease may be treated.

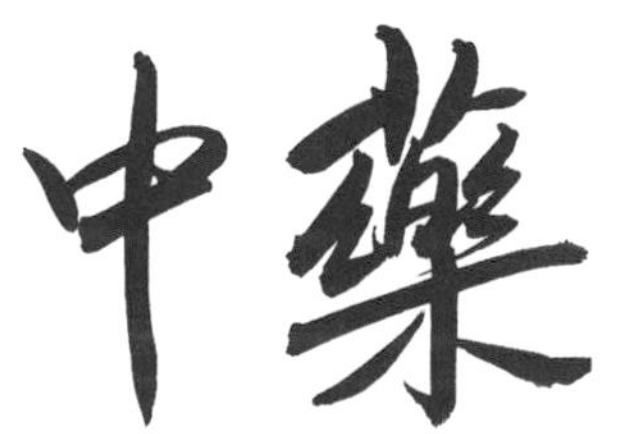

THE CHARACTERS FOR CHINESE MEDICINE

WHAT IS CHINESE HERBAL MEDICINE?

TCM uses terminology that sounds strange to most Westerners. Instead of talking about rheumatic diseases or neurological diseases it classifies diseases as being caused by Wind, Heat, Dampness, or Cold. Instead of talking about rheumatism in the knee joint, it may classify it as Cold–Damp in the Stomach meridian (*see page 50*). Western medicine focuses on a specific cause for a specific disease, and when it isolates that cause or agent it tries to control or destroy it. Chinese medicine is also concerned with the cause, but it focuses on the patient's response to that disease entity, both physiological and psychological. All the relevant information, including symptoms that may not seem related to the patient's main complaint, is collected together to enable the practitioner to discover the pattern of disharmony within that person, which can then be addressed by Chinese medicine. For instance, two patients coming with asthma may have completely different diagnoses according to Chinese medicine. The one with a pale face, prone to catching colds (Lung Qi Deficiency) will be given a completely different herbal formula to the patient who has a dry cough, thirst, and breathlessness on exertion (Lung Yin Deficiency). TCM does treat the same diseases – to a large extent people have the same problems the world over – it just perceives them in an entirely different way.

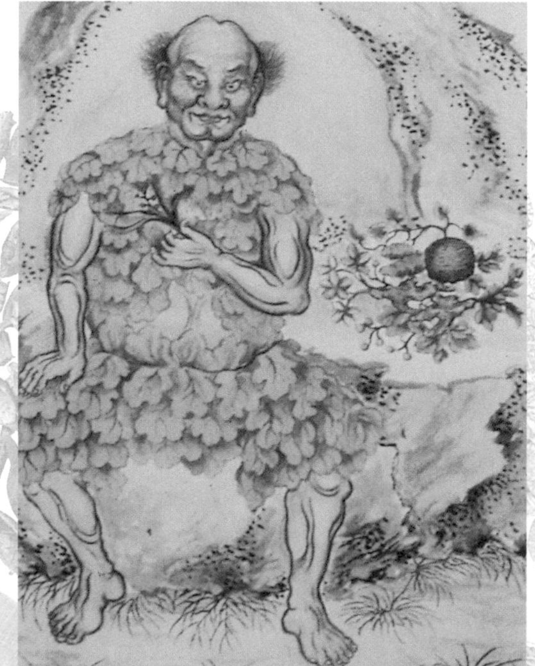

ABOVE *The Chinese god of medicine. Chinese medicine has an ancient heritage.*

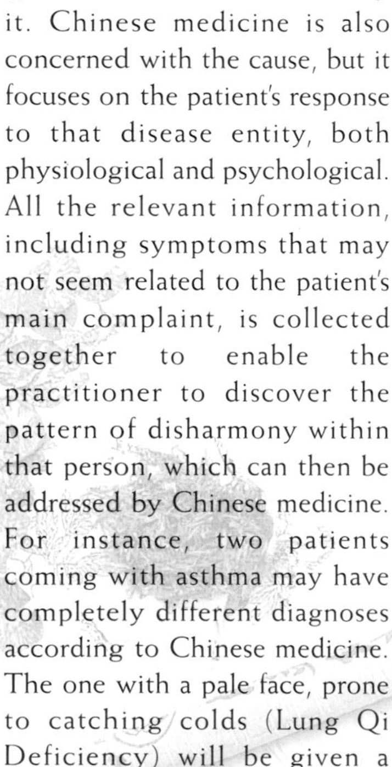

YIN AND YANG

Chinese medicine is based on the philosophy of yin and yang. These are the dual forces in the universe, seen both within nature and in human beings. They are used to explain the ongoing process of natural changes – yang is more prevalent during the day, while yin forces are more prevalent at night. There is no absolute yin or yang in living things – a cold yin-type illness may have aspects of yang, such as sharp, forceful contractions. Yin and yang both depend on each other and keep each other under control. However, it is when they go seriously out of balance and do not correct themselves that there is disease.

Everything has a yin and a yang aspect – for instance:

ITEM	YIN	YANG
Time	Night	Day
Season	Fall/Winter	Spring/Summer
Energy	Passivity/Stillness	Activity/Movement
Body	Front/Lower/Inside	Back/Upper/Outside
Breath	Inhalation	Exhalation
Temperature	Cold	Hot
Moisture	Wet/Damp	Dry
Direction	Downward	Upward

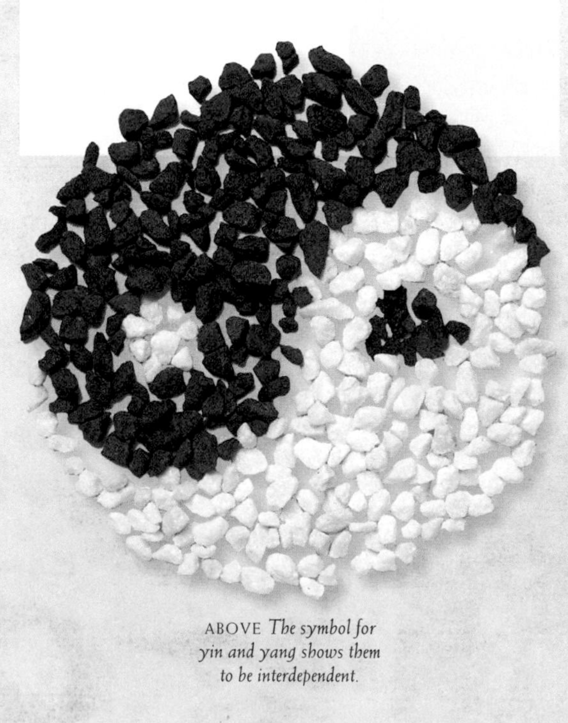

ABOVE *The symbol for yin and yang shows them to be interdependent.*

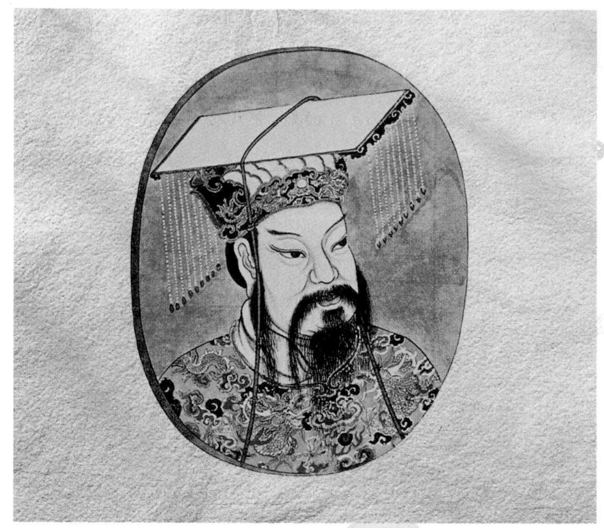

ABOVE *The* Inner Classic *takes the form of a dialog between the legendary* Yellow Emperor *and his minister* Qi Bo *on the topic of medicine.*

A SHORT HISTORY

The earliest herbal formulas in China were found to have been written down in the 3rd century B.C.E. In fact, the main book of the theory of Chinese medicine – the *Yellow Emperor's Inner Classic* – was compiled in the 1st century C.E., and is still taught in schools of TCM. Over the centuries, leading physicians have written down both herbal and acupuncture formulas, which explains the vast bulk of Chinese medicine reference books. The *Imperial Grace Formulary* of the Tai Pang Era (around 985 C.E.) for example, contains 16,834 entries, many of which are still commonly referred to today.

The early herbal formulas were very simple and elegant, while the later ones are much more complicated. Either type can be useful, depending on the patient and the physician's preferred manner of working. A practitioner of TCM, or someone practising Chinese herbal medicine specifically, will diagnose the patient's pattern of disharmony, find the tried and tested prescription which is closest to that patient's pattern, and add or subtract herbs to make it more suitable for that individual. Herbs are seldom used singly; they are usually combined in prescriptions containing 4–16 substances.

THE CHINESE THEORY OF LIFE

The Chinese believe that every living being is sustained by a basic Life Force, called "qi" (pronounced "chee"). Human beings receive their qi from a mixture of the influences of both Heaven and Earth. Therefore, we do have an element of the divine in us, which separates us from the animals. Chinese medicine works with the qi that we have to make us better. It may unblock the flow of qi in the body if it is stuck, or it may nourish qi if it is deficient.

We are born with a fixed amount of qi inherited from our parents (Yuan Qi – source or genetic qi). This is used both as our "reserve tank" and as a catalyst in most of the chemical processes of the body. We can nourish our Yuan Qi, though we cannot add to it. We may, however, deplete it through bad living practices – long-term lack of sleep or good food, drugs, drink, or years of excessive sex. The Chinese believe that this source qi is stored in the Kidneys (where its substance is called Jing or essence), and its functions include the control of sexual and reproductive activity in the body. We get our day-to-day qi from the air we breathe (Gong Qi) and the food we eat (Gu Qi).

Qi permeates the entire body; it directs the blood, nerve, and lymphatic systems (Ying Qi). It protects us from catching viruses and so on (Wei Qi), and fights them if they get into the body. It transforms the food we eat into bodily substances – blood, tears, sweat, and urine – keeps organs in their proper place, and prevents excessive loss of sweat. qi keeps the body warm and is naturally the source of movement and growth, as it has all these functions. We also use it in TCM to describe the functions of any Organ – for instance, Lung qi may be "weak" or Liver qi "blocked."

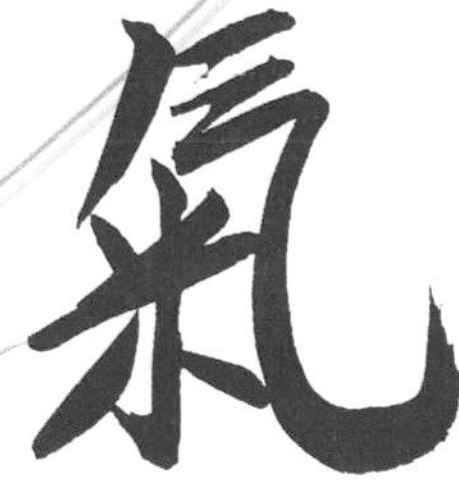

ABOVE *The Chinese character for qi. Qi is pronounced "chee," and often written as "chi."*

Gong Qi from the air

Gu Qi from food

Ying Qi runs the blood, nerve and lymphatic systems

Wei Qi protects against viruses

Yuan Qi stored in kidneys as Jing

RIGHT *The sources of qi: the air, food, and inherited genetic qi (Yuan Qi).*

MERIDIANS AND ORGANS

Although qi is everywhere in the body, it does have main pathways along which it flows, nourishing and warming the organs and body parts, and harmonizing their activity. These channels are called the meridian system (Jing-Luo). Most acupuncture points are sited along these channels, and most herbs a practitioner of Chinese medicine prescribes enter one or more of the meridian pathways. There are 12 main meridians, and these correspond to the 12 main organs in the body, such as the Liver, Heart, Stomach, Kidneys, Spleen, and so on. These meridians are bilateral – there is an identical pair on each side of the body. Some are more yin meridians, with functions more to do with storing the vital essences of the body. These are the Kidneys, Liver, Spleen, Heart, Lungs, and Pericardium. The other six are more yang meridians, with functions more to do with transportation of fluids and food. These are the Bladder, Gallbladder, Stomach, Small Intestine, Large Intestine, and the Triple Burner (a mechanism which regulates the overall body temperature and the Upper, Middle, and Lower parts (Jiaos) of the body). There are also six Extra meridians, one of which runs up the front center line of the body – the Ren Mai or Conception Vessel, and one of which runs up the spine – the Du Mai or Governor Vessel.

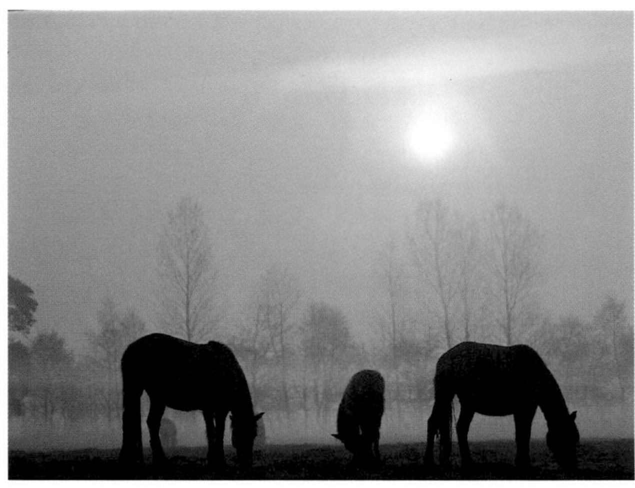

ABOVE *Chinese medicine sees harmony with nature and within ourselves as crucial for health.*

When a practitioner of Chinese medicine talks about an organ being out of balance, he or she usually refers to the meridian related to that organ, not necessarily the physical organ itself. For instance, the Liver meridian runs from the big toe, up the inside of the leg, through the genitals, and then deep into the Liver organ itself. There can be problems along the course of the meridian, and there is also a sphere of influence which each organ has within the body. The Liver controls the free flow of qi generally in the body, including the evenness of emotions, digestion, and menstruation. It also stores the blood, rules circulation in the tendons, has the major influence on the eyes, and manifests in the nails. It is therefore possible to see how diseases in these areas of the body may be treated via the Liver meridian.

In illness, different meridians exhibit different tendencies of disharmony – for instance, the Spleen has a tendency to deficiency causing Damp. This creates symptoms such as diarrhea or lassitude (tiredness). The Liver, on the other hand, has a tendency toward Rising yang, creating red sore eyes, migraines, and high blood pressure. It is these disharmonies that Chinese herbal medicine can address.

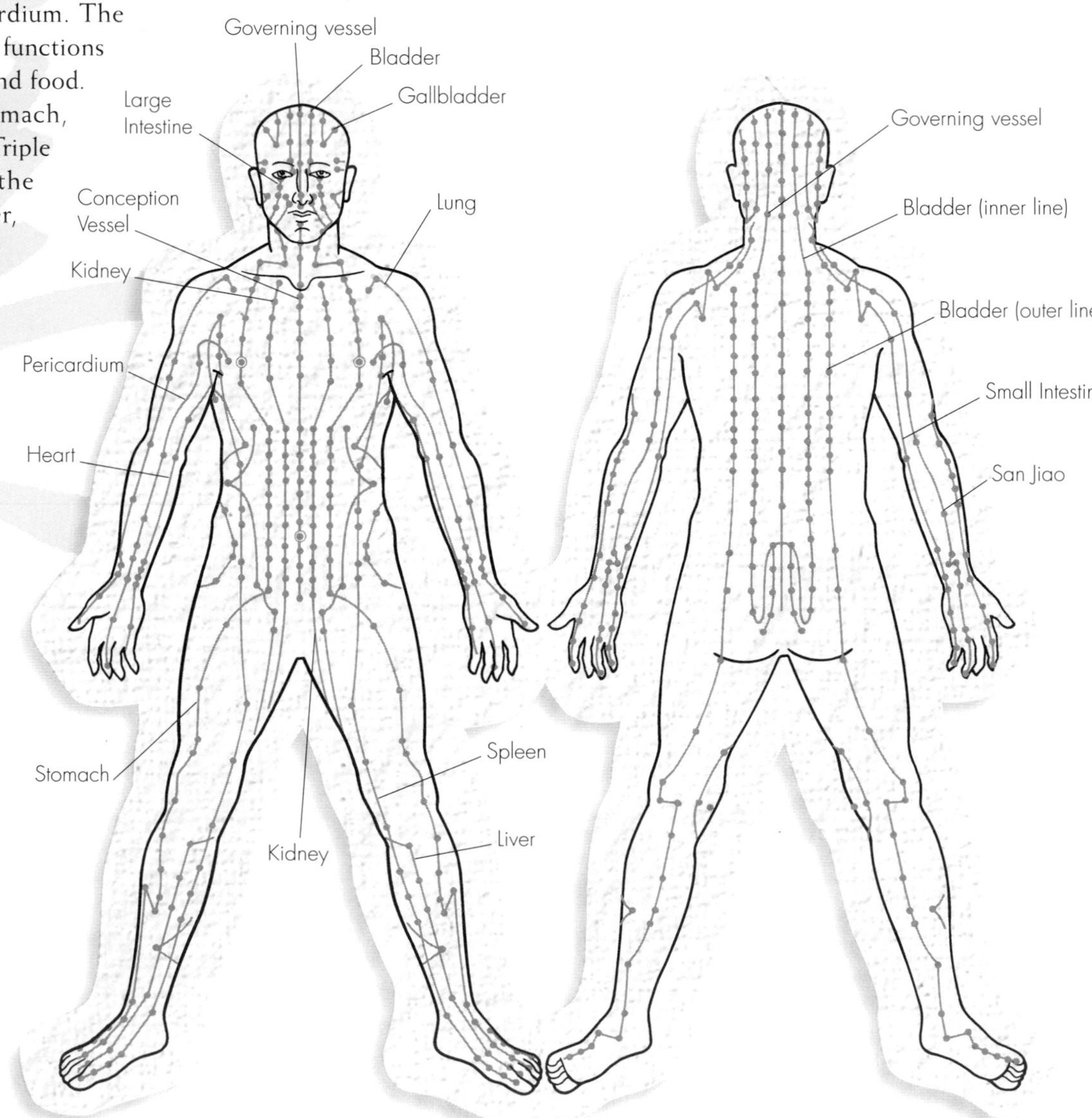

RIGHT *The 12 main meridians (energy channels) along which qi flows in the body.*

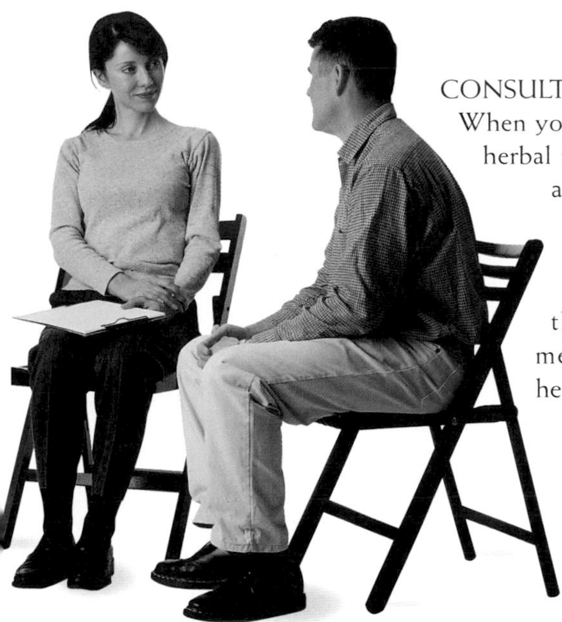

ABOVE *Find a registered practitioner from the national professional organization.*

CONSULTING A CHINESE HERBALIST

When you consult a practitioner of Chinese herbal medicine, he or she will first of all ask you in detail about your presenting condition – when it first appeared, your symptoms, what makes it worse or better. You will then be asked about your past medical history and your general health, for example:

- your appetite, diet, digestion, stools, and urination
- your sleep patterns, any pain – headaches, backache – ear, nose, and throat (ENT) problems
- intake of drugs, alcohol, nicotine
- body temperature (more hot or cold), circulation, and perspiration
- energy levels, mental, and emotional states
- gynecology – menstruation, pregnancies, menopause

Finally, your practitioner will take both radial (wrist) pulses and look at your tongue, in order to help him or her to make a diagnosis according to Chinese medicine. The practitioner may search through some books to check on the herbal prescription most suited to your condition, and will then write down a prescription. This will include anything from 4 to 20 herbs, and their dosages in grams or in *qian* (Chinese measurements). The names of the herbs will be in English, Latin, Pin-Yin (anglicized Chinese), or in Chinese characters. Your practitioner will then make up the prescription for you or refer you to a herbal supplier to have it made up elsewhere.

BELOW *A ginseng shop in Hong Kong. Ginseng is a useful but expensive herb.*

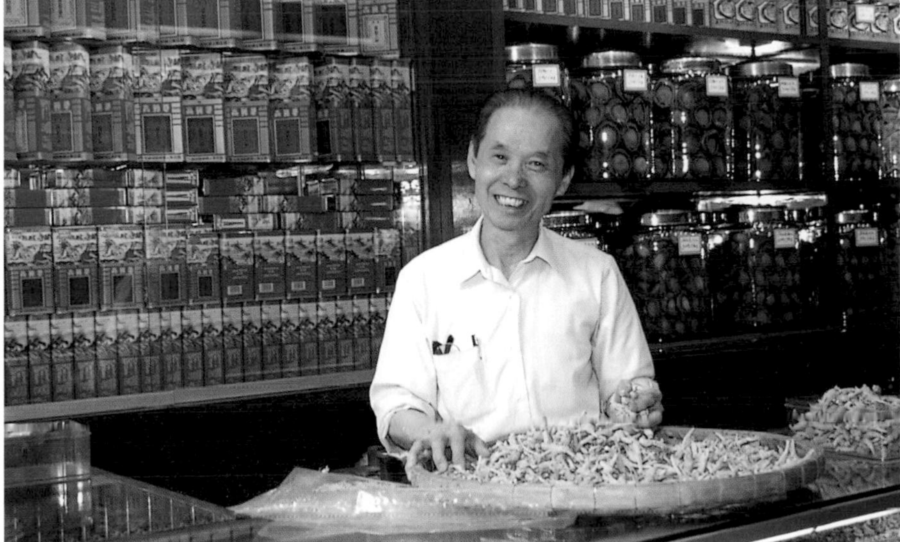

PREPARATIONS AND TREATMENT

There are many different ways of taking herbs. Individual herbs can be added to foods or taken as a tea, but Chinese herbs are rarely taken singly – they are much more effective when made into a composite prescription.

- **Decoctions** Packets of dried herbs are boiled for around 30 minutes, down to 2 cups, and then often boiled again to last two days. They smell worse than they taste!
- **Powders** One teaspoonful of cooked, freeze-dried herbs is taken two or three times a day, mixed with a little cold water to a paste; then a little boiling water is added. This is somewhat unpalatable but easy and effective.
- **Tinctures** One teaspoon of liquid taken two or three times a day. These are more palatable but not as strong as decoctions or powders.

Decoctions

- **Pills and capsules** These are used for patent remedies (prescriptions which have not been changed to suit the individual). They are easy to swallow, but you have to take a lot more than with Western drugs – sometimes eight tablets at a time.
- **Syrups** These are patent remedies, mainly good for coughs or children's tonics.
- **Plasters** These are used for rheumatic ailments (Wind–Damp); they are very effective for relieving local pain and stiffness. Treatment generally means taking herbs two or three times a day until the problem is gone.

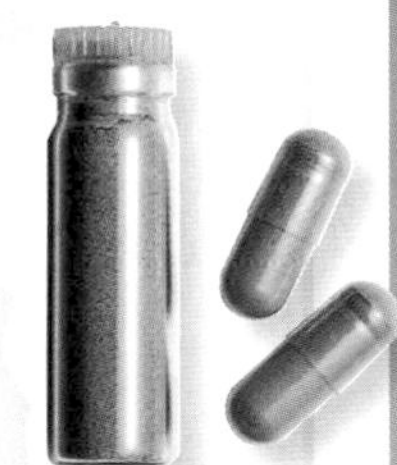

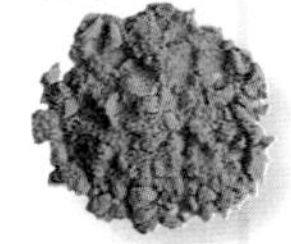

Powders and capsules

At first you will need to see your practitioner every one or two weeks so that he or she can alter the prescription as your symptoms improve. You may experience slight nausea, diarrhea, or digestive upset as your system becomes used to the herbs. In this case, you will need to halve your dosage and build it up again slowly; your practitioner may add more digestive herbs in order that you may tolerate it better. After that, you may be able to see or even telephone your practitioner once a month in order to report on progress, and so that the prescription can be changed accordingly. Herbal medicines should not be taken without review for more than 30 days.

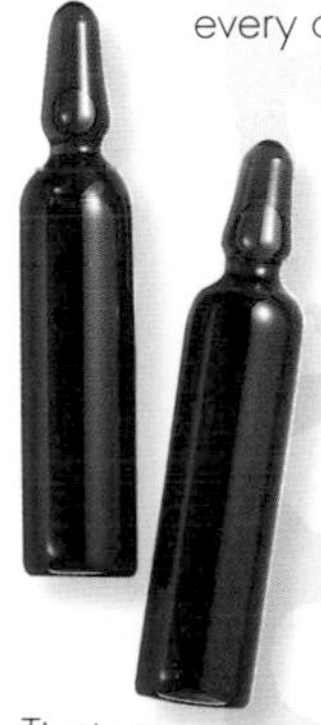

Tinctures

ABOVE *Chinese herbal preparations come in various forms, from raw and powdered herbs, to tinctures.*

THE HERBS USED

PLANTS

The medicinal use of herbs in China is believed to date back to about 2000 B.C.E., when Emperor Chi'en Nung wrote a book called the *Pen Tsao*, which listed the medicinal properties of over 300 plants. The Chinese word for herbalism, "Ben Cao," dates from about 500 B.C.E. "Ben" means a plant with a rigid stalk, and "Cao" means a grass-like plant. Herbalism developed to include the use of mineral and animal ingredients.

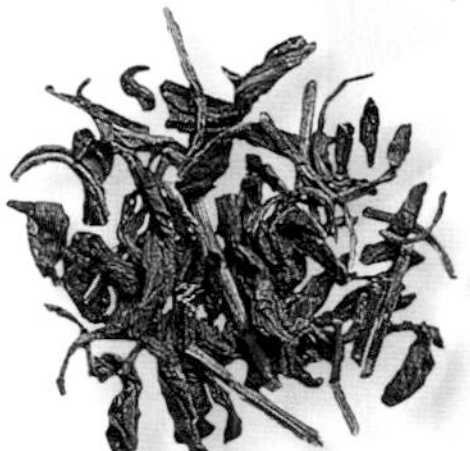

LEAF
Ren Shen (ginseng) leaf is sometimes used, but the root is more common.

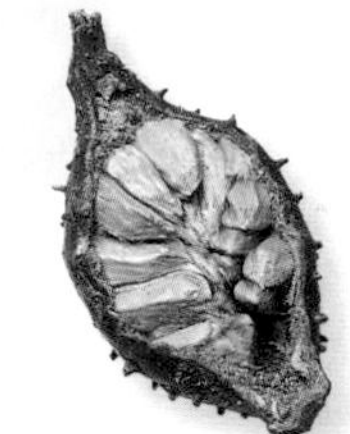

FLOWER
Jin Ying (rosehip) is an example of a flower that is used therapeutically.

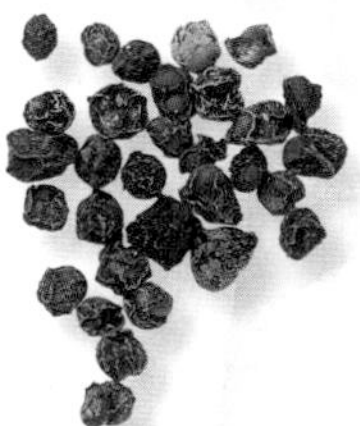

FRUIT
Wu Wei Zi (schisandra fruit) is sour and relieves sweating.

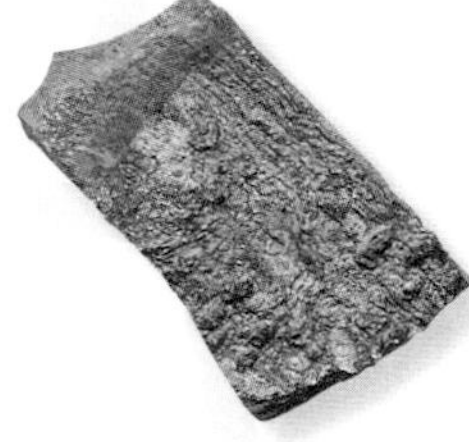

BARK
Rou Gui (cinnamon bark) is a warm herb and relieves Cold.

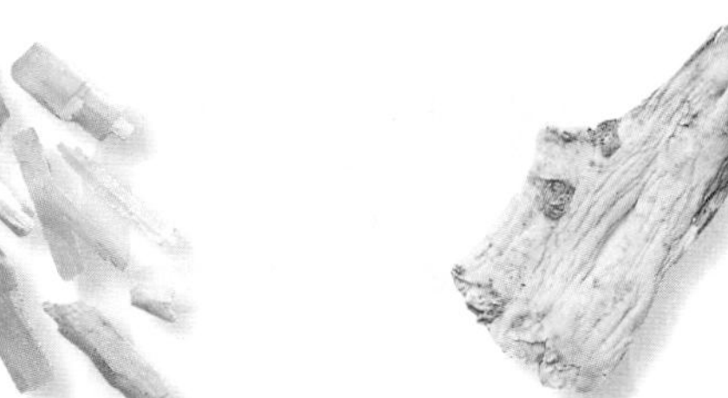

MINERAL
Shi Gao (gypsum) treats problems caused by excessive Heat.

ROOT
Jie Geng (platycodon root) moves Lung Qi.

ABOVE *A prescription may contain an assortment of herbs.*

Chinese herbs are mostly made of plant parts – leaves, flowers, fruit, or fruit peel, twigs, roots, bark, or fungus. There are some minerals, such as gypsum, but these are less commonly used. There are also animal parts in Traditional Chinese Herbal Medicine, such as snake, mammal bones, or deer horn. However, their importation has now been forbidden, and herbal practitioners find alternatives to prescribe.

PATENT HERBAL PREPARATIONS

These are sold as over-the-counter remedies for colds and flu, coughs and phlegm, even strep throat infections; also for rheumatic ailments, pain, and bruising from trauma. Patent remedies used for anything else must be diagnosed by a herbal practitioner, even tonics; for instance, do you need to tonify the qi, blood, yin, or yang? It is important to consult a herbal practitioner if you intend to use a patent remedy over a long period of time, such as a long-term tonic for an elderly person. Tonics should not be taken during an episode of cold or flu (Wind Invasion), as they tend to drive Wind deeper into the body.

ABOVE *Patent medicines are useful for common problems.*

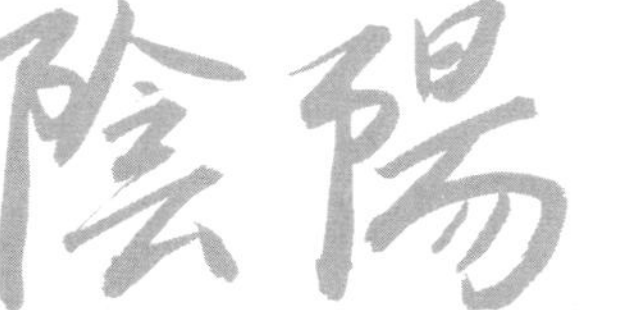

ABOVE *The Chinese characters for yin (left) and yang (right).*

SAFETY NOTE

IF PRESCRIBING HERBS OVER A LONG PERIOD OF TIME, IT IS IMPORTANT THAT THE PRACTITIONER PAYS PARTICULAR ATTENTION TO ANY LIVER OR KIDNEY SYMPTOMS WHICH MAY ARISE DURING THE COURSE OF TREATMENT. TOXIC HERBS ARE ILLEGAL IN THIS COUNTRY, BUT A VERY FEW INDIVIDUALS MAY EXPERIENCE IDIOSYNCRATIC REACTIONS TO HERBS – THESE ARE USUALLY DUE TO GENETIC ABNORMALITIES AND THE HERBS WOULD NOT CAUSE A REACTION IN MOST OTHER INDIVIDUALS. REGULAR LIVER FUNCTION TESTS ARE SOMETIMES ADVISED BY PRACTITIONERS, BUT THEIR VALUE IN THESE CASES IS STILL A MATTER OF DEBATE.

CAUTION

SOME PATENT REMEDIES CONTAINING ANIMAL PRODUCTS MAY STILL BE SOLD. THEY ARE NOW ILLEGAL IN THIS COUNTRY, SO PLEASE CHECK WITH THE PHARMACY FIRST. ALWAYS GO TO A REPUTABLE PRACTITIONER (CONSULT THE *REGISTER OF CHINESE HERBAL MEDICINE* [U.K.] OR YOUR STATE'S CHINESE MEDICINE ASSOCIATION [*SEE PAGE 478*]). SOME HERBAL PATENTS FOR INSOMNIA AND MENTAL DISTURBANCE CONTAIN MINERAL SUBSTANCES SUCH AS OYSTER SHELL OR MAGNETITE. IN EXCESS, THESE CAN CAUSE INDIGESTION, SO USE THEM FOR A LIMITED AMOUNT OF TIME AND FIND ALTERNATIVE PRESCRIPTIONS.

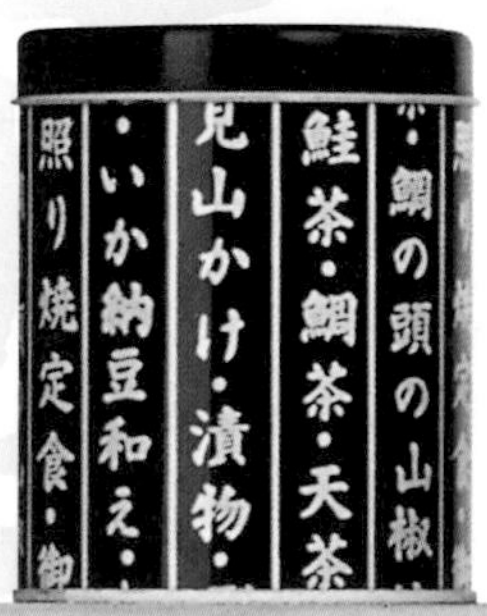

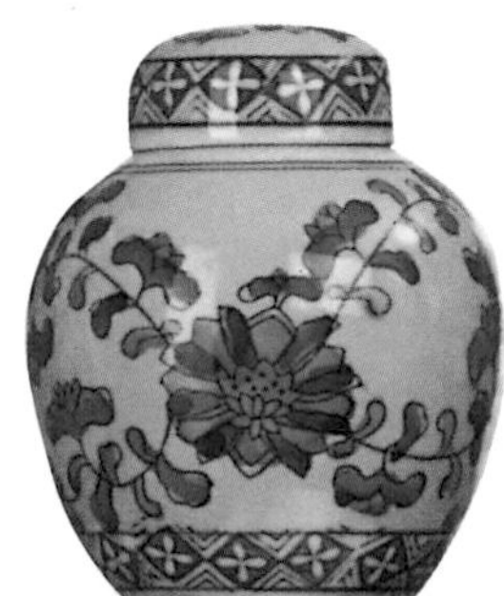

RIGHT *Herb storage jars. Herbs are kept separately to retain their individual properties.*

NOTES

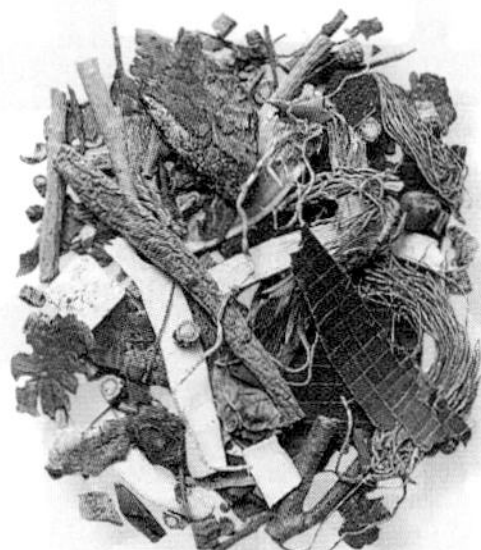

ABOVE *Herbal formulae have been developed over centuries, through experiment and observation.*

- Mention of organs, functions, or causes of disease (e.g. Spleen, harmonize, Dampness) refer to particular Chinese concepts. *(See Glossary, page 472.)*

- Chinese herbs are hardly ever used singly – they are used mainly in combination with other herbs to make a balanced prescription. Some of the most commonly used herbs involved in those prescriptions follow in the next section. Each herb also has a particular range of dosages assigned to it – when comparing it to other herbs in a prescription, one can see whether it is used in an average dose, or whether one would use a smaller or larger dose in that prescription. Both these features mean that it is important to consult a qualified herbalist before using the herbs, either in a herbal pharmacy or privately through the Register of Chinese Herbal Medicine Practitioners (U.K.) or your state's Chinese Medicine Association.

HERB TASTES AND FUNCTIONS

A Brief Note About Tastes

In the next section, we will mention the taste of each herb. In TCM, taste partly determines therapeutic function, so it is important to know what it signifies:

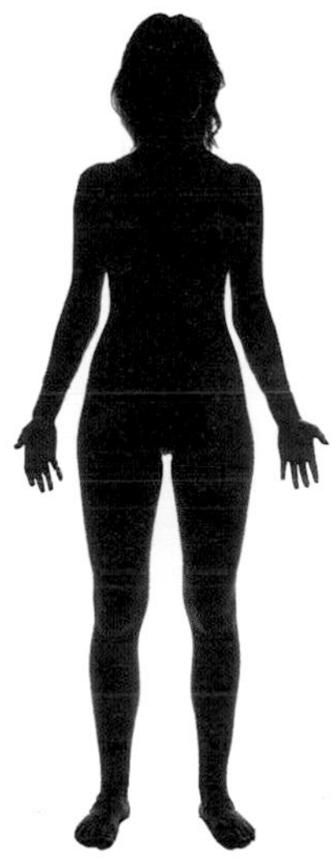

ABOVE *The taste of a herb relates to its action on qi in the body.*

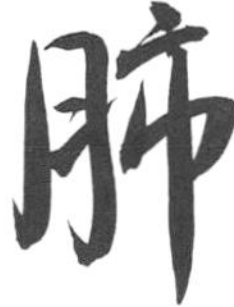

ACRID

- ACRID – Pungent or acrid substances disperse and move qi (energy).
- Acrid herbs mainly affect the Lung functions.

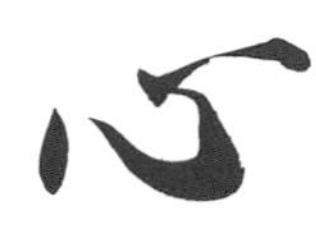

BITTER

- BITTER – These herbs reduce excess qi, drain and dry excess moisture.
- Bitter herbs mainly affect the Heart organ.

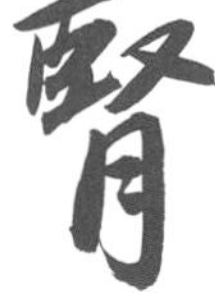

SALTY

- SALTY – these herbs purge (drain through the bowels) and soften.
- Salty herbs mainly affect the Kidney organ.

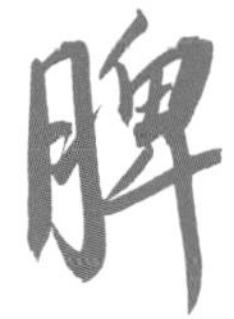

SWEET

- SWEET – Sweet substances tonify, harmonize, and strengthen qi, and may sometimes moisten.
- Sweet herbs mainly affect the Spleen organ.

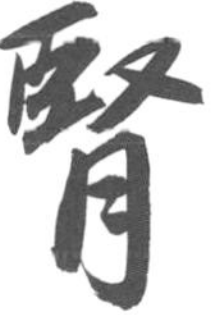

SOUR

- SOUR – Sour substances are astringent and prevent or reverse the abnormal leakage of fluids and energy.
- Sour herbs mainly affect the Kidney organ.

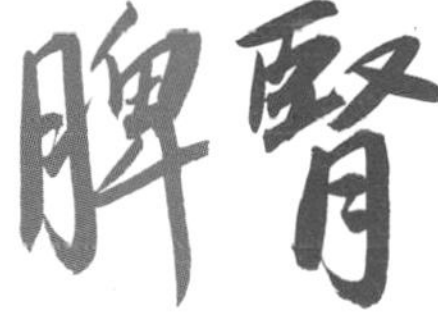

BLAND

- BLAND – Bland substances have none of these tastes, primarily leech out Dampness and promote urination.
- This helps both the Spleen and the Kidneys.

CHILDREN AND BABIES

Chinese herbal medicine can be very effective for children and babies. Children's dosages are usually half or a quarter of those given for adults. There are ways of encouraging children to take the herbs, either by involving them in the preparation of the prescription, or by sweetening it with honey, or by offering a cookie afterward! There are certain herbal powders especially formulated for babies.

PREGNANCY

Many herbs are expressly forbidden in pregnancy, whilst some are especially good for pregnant women. There are several which may help to prevent miscarriage. Only take herbs prescribed by a qualified practitioner when pregnant.

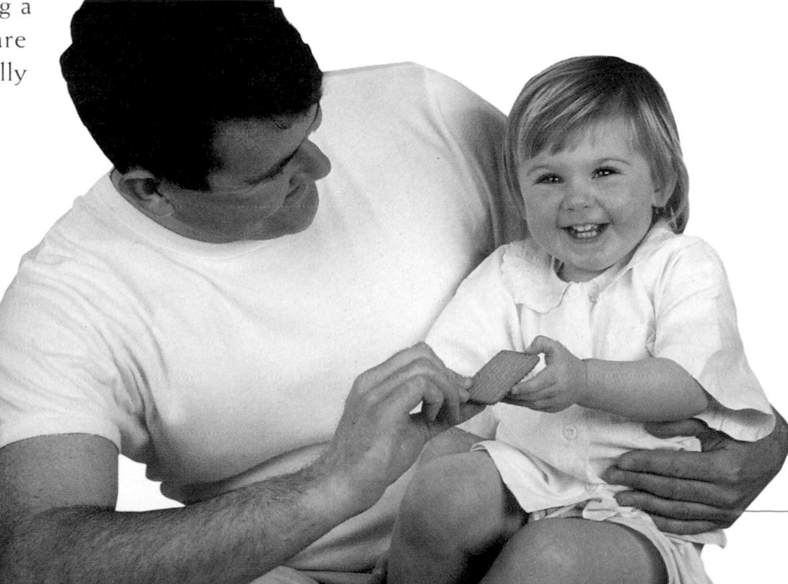

RIGHT *It can be difficult to persuade young children to take some Chinese remedies, due to their unfamiliar tastes. A reward will help!*

CHINESE HERBAL REMEDY SOURCES

Acanthopanax gracilistylus

WU JIA PI

This herb dispels Wind Dampness from the muscles, joints, and bones. Wind Dampness causes rheumatic and arthritic ailments. Wu Jia Pi also treats Damp Cold conditions where the circulation is obstructed, as in the swelling of the legs or stiff knee joints. The dried herb, or a decoction, can be taken in wine.

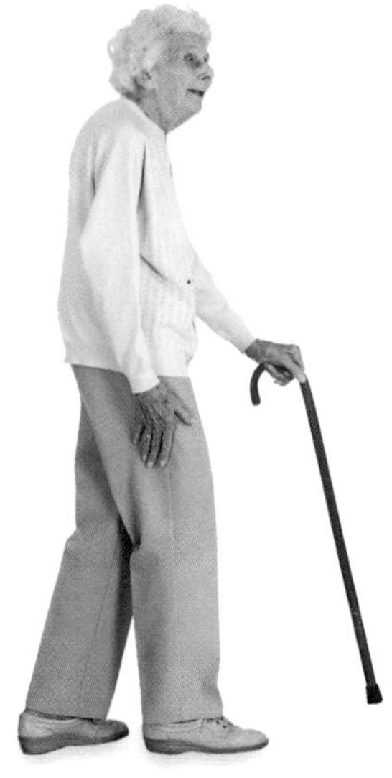

ABOVE *Arthritis, from Wind, Cold, and Damp, is treated through the Liver and Kidney meridians.*

HOW TO USE

Wu Jia Pi is a warm drying (acrid) herb which tonifies the Liver and Kidneys. These meridians decline as we get older, so it is especially useful in treating rheumatism, arthritis, or stiffness in the elderly or those suffering from long-term illness. It is particularly useful when the smooth flow of qi and blood is obstructed. It is also good for developmental delays in the motor functions of children. It is also used for difficulties with urination, and edema.

CAUTION

USE WITH CAUTION IN YIN DEFICIENCY WITH HEAT SIGNS, AS IT DRIES AND HEATS FURTHER.

DATA FILE

Properties

Acrid, Warm

Channels

Liver, Kidney

Functions and Uses

- Dispels Wind Dampness, and strengthens the sinews and bones: use for chronic Wind Cold Damp Painful Obstruction (Bi syndrome) when deficiency of the Liver and Kidneys causes weak sinews and bones.
- Transforms Dampness and reduces swelling: use for water retention.

THERAPY CONNECTIONS

HYSSOP

Aromatherapy *p.160*

CARDAMOM

Ayurveda *p.38*

Aromatherapy *p.158*

ANGELICA

Ayurveda *p.28*

Herbalism *p.115*

Aromatherapy *p.146*

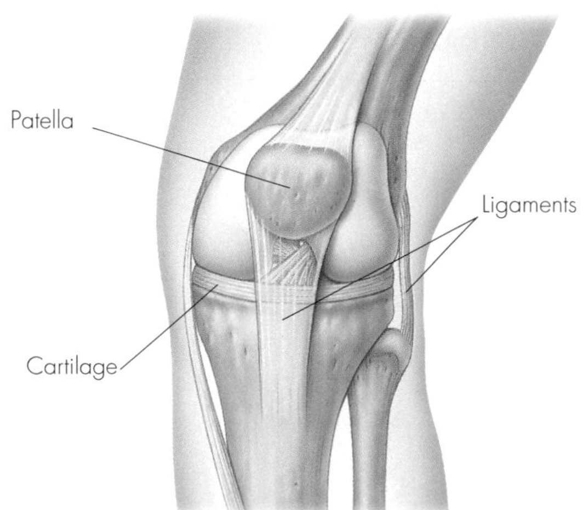

ABOVE *Wu Jia Pi has warming and drying qualities, and treats Damp conditions such as swollen or stiff joints.*

Agastache rugosa, wrinkled giant hyssop, patchouli

HUO XIANG

This herb transforms Dampness, a "pathogenic influence" which creates stagnation in the Middle Burner (Spleen and Stomach), with various digestive or fluid-retaining effects. Huo Xiang helps the Spleen to recover its function of transporting and transforming food in the body.

HOW TO USE

Huo Xiang is used specifically for stuck digestion, leading to bloating either above or below the navel, nausea, fatigue, lack of appetite, and a moist white coating on the tongue. It is the main herb in the patent formula Huo Xiang Zheng Qi Wan, which is used for gastric flu.

DATA FILE

Properties

Acrid, slightly Warm

Channels

Lung, Spleen, Stomach

Functions and Uses

- Fragrantly transforms Dampness: this means that it tonifies the Spleen so that it transforms the Dampness obstructing the middle area, which is interfering with the Spleen's normal digestive functions.
- Harmonizes the Middle Burner and stops vomiting; also used for morning sickness.
- Releases the exterior and expels Dampness, as in gastric flu.

CAUTION

NO HERBS USED FOR GETTING RID OF DAMP (SHOWN BY A THICK TONGUE COATING OR BY THE PRESENCE OF PHLEGM) MAY BE USED IN DEFICIENT YIN WITH HEAT SIGNS (SHOWN BY A PEELED TONGUE) – THEY WILL FURTHER DRY THE PATIENT UP AND MAKE THE CONDITION WORSE.

BELOW *Huo Xiang comes from wrinkled giant hyssop, a summer-flowering perennial.*

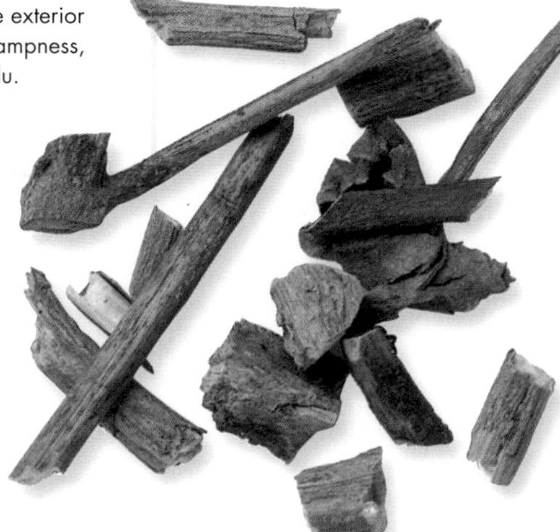

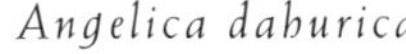

Alpinia oxyphylla, black cardamom

YI ZHI REN

This herb warms Internal Cold. Yi Zhi Ren is a cardamom, and all cardamoms warm the Middle area. Yi Zhi Ren also warms the Kidneys and controls fluids coming from that area – which makes it good for urinary incontinence, or frequency and enuresis (bed-wetting) from Cold-Deficient Spleen and Kidneys.

DATA FILE

Properties
Acrid, Warm

Channels
Kidney, Spleen

Functions and Uses

- Warms the Kidneys, firms the Jing-essence and holds in urine: this herb is used when the yang aspect of the Kidneys is Deficient and cannot hold sperm or urine in place.
- Warms the Spleen and stops diarrhea: Cold, Deficient Spleen or Stomach patterns causing diarrhea and other digestive symptoms.

CAUTION

CONTRAINDICATED FOR SPERMATORRHEA, FREQUENT URINATION, OR VAGINAL DISCHARGE DUE TO HEAT.

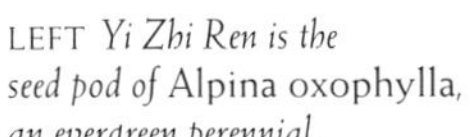

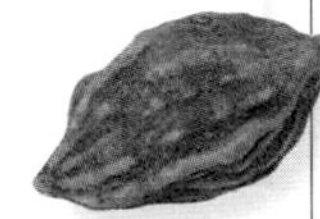

LEFT *Yi Zhi Ren is the seed pod of* Alpina oxophylla, *an evergreen perennial.*

HOW TO USE

Yi Zhi Ren is helpful in spermatorrhea, when men cannot hold the sperm or when it leaks out. When the Spleen yang is weak and Cold it does not transform the feces properly, leading to diarrhea. **There may also be vomiting, Cold abdominal pain (better with warmth), excessive saliva, and a thick unpleasant taste in the mouth.** It is very good for drooling. **Yi Zhi Ren is a valuable herb for warming the system, from infancy to old age.**

Angelica dahurica

BAI ZHI

Bai Zhi belongs to a group of warm, acrid herbs that release exterior conditions; that is, superficial illnesses caused by viruses, with symptoms in the skin or muscle layers. The herbs mainly affect the sweating mechanism, either causing the body to sweat, or if necessary stopping it from sweating.

ABOVE *Bai Zhi treats disorders via the Lung and Stomach meridians in the body.*

HOW TO USE

Bai Zhi is used mainly for sudden headaches (Wind-caused headaches), especially those along the Stomach channel, i.e. the front of the head, the forehead. **It is particularly good for headaches caused by sinusitis, and to help the sinusitis itself.** It is very good for ulcerated boils in cases where the pus is not yet discharged – use it with Jie Geng. **It is often added to prescriptions for vaginal discharge, especially for a white (Cold) discharge rather than a yellow, smelly one (Hot type). However, with the right combinations, one could use Bai Zhi for other types of headaches or discharges.**

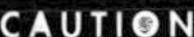

CAUTION

CONTRAINDICATED IN DEFICIENT BLOOD OR DEFICIENT YIN PATTERNS BECAUSE IT IS VERY DRYING. USE CAUTIOUSLY IF SORES HAVE ALREADY BURST.

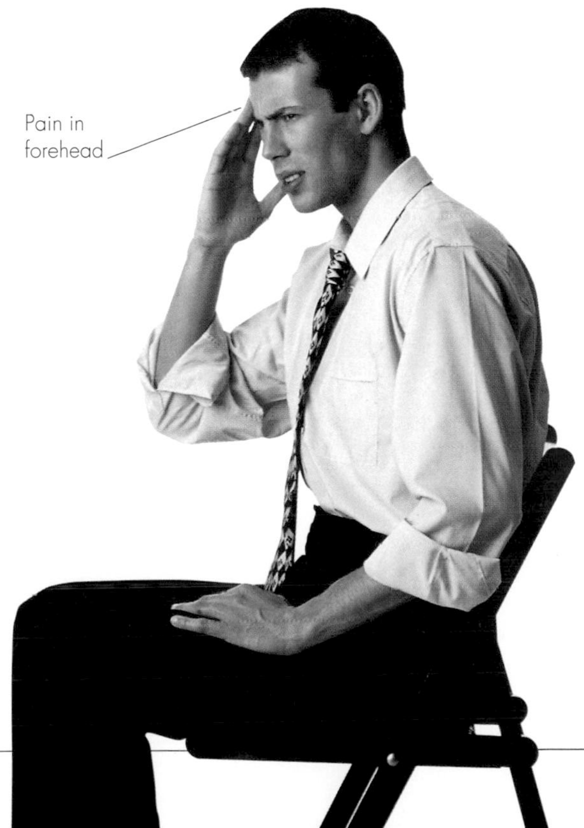

BELOW *A sudden headache will respond to treatment with Bai Zhi.*

DATA FILE

Properties
Acrid, Warm

Channels
Lung, Stomach

Functions and Uses

- Expels Wind and alleviates pain: use for externally contracted Wind Cold patterns, especially those with head symptoms.
- Reduces swelling and expels pus: use in the early stages of a sore in order to reduce swelling.
- Expels Dampness and alleviates discharge. It is used for treating leukorrhea (vaginal discharge) from Damp Cold in the lower abdominal area.
- Helps to open up the nasal passages.

Angelica sinensis, Chinese angelica

DANG GUI

Dang Gui is such a widely used herb that it has entered the Western herbal pharmacy. In TCM it is used to treat patterns of Blood Deficiency, and therefore affects mostly the Heart and Liver, which direct and store the Blood, respectively.

HOW TO USE

Dan Gui is unusual amongst Blood-tonifying herbs in that it both nourishes and invigorates blood circulation, and is therefore not cloying, as Shu di Huang can be. It is good for Blood-Deficient symptoms such as pale complexion, tinnitus, blurred vision, and palpitations, and is commonly used for all menstrual disorders, such as irregular menstruation, amenorrhea, or dysmenorrhea (painful menstruation). It is essential for pain in general as it moves the Blood – abdominal pain, traumatic injury, and even arthritic pain associated with Blood Deficiency (pain according to TCM may be caused by Stagnant Blood). It is useful for dry stools and helps heal sores.

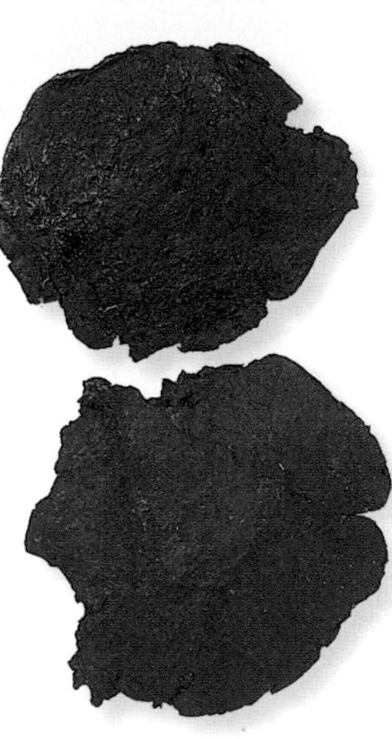

ABOVE *Dang Gui is recommended for all menstrual disorders.*

DATA FILE

Properties

Sweet, Acrid, Bitter, Warm

Channels

Heart, Liver, Spleen

Functions and Uses

- Tonifies the Blood and regulates the menses.
- Invigorates the Blood and disperses Cold: an important herb for stopping pain due to Blood stasis.
- Moistens the intestines and unblocks the bowels: like all tonifying herbs, Dang Gui is moistening – in this case it is also directed to the intestines.
- Reduces swelling, expels pus, generates new flesh, and alleviates pain: use for sores and abscesses.

CAUTION

USE WITH CAUTION FOR DIARRHEA OR ABDOMINAL SWELLING DUE TO DAMPNESS.

CONTRAINDICATED FOR YIN DEFICIENCY WITH HEAT SIGNS, AS IT IS WARMING.

Atractylodes macrocephala, atractylodes rhizome

BAI ZHU

This herb is one of a group that treat Qi Deficiency, and as we replenish our day-to-day energy from air and food, the two main organs involved are Lungs and Spleen.

CAUTION

CONTRAINDICATED IN CASES OF YIN DEFICIENCY WITH HEAT SIGNS, OR INJURED FLUIDS.

ABOVE *Bai Zhu gives qi a boost when fatigue is experienced.*

HOW TO USE

Bai Zhu is a major tonifying qi herb in cases of diarrhea, vomiting, fatigue, lack of appetite, lack of strength in the limbs, and is one of the herbs in the seminal tonifying prescription of the Four Gentlemen (Si Jun Zi Wan). It also helps Damp disorders such as edema and reduced urination, and is used in the Jade Screen prescription for spontaneous sweating due to Qi Deficiency. It is used for any type of threatened miscarriage when combined with other appropriate herbs.

DATA FILE

Properties

Sweet, Bitter, Warm

Channels

Spleen, Stomach

Functions and Uses

- Tonifies the Spleen and benefits the qi: use Bai Zhu to treat Spleen and Stomach Deficiency.
- Strengthens the Spleen and dries Dampness: use for digestive disorders, water retention and even for treating Damp Painful Obstruction (rheumatic ailments).
- Firms the exterior and stops sweating.
- Strengthens the Spleen and calms the fetus: for restless fetus when due to Spleen Deficiency not holding the fetus in.

LEFT *Bai Zhu may be used to help women who run the risk of miscarriage.*

Astragalus membranaceus, milk-vetch root

HUANG QI

This herb treats Qi Deficiency, and as we replenish our day-to-day energy from air and food, the two main organs involved are Lungs and Spleen (the main digestive organ in TCM).

HOW TO USE

Huang Qi is for Spleen-Deficient symptoms such as lack of appetite, fatigue, and diarrhea. Its action is also upward and outward, so it helps prolapsed uterus or uterine bleeding, but is also used in prescriptions to help the immune system fight viruses. It is used for frequent colds and helps excessive sweating. It is good for edema and pus-filled sores that have not yet discharged, and is also used in post-partum fever from severe loss of blood.

ABOVE *Huang Qi is an ascending herb: it tends to move upward and outward.*

DATA FILE

Properties

Sweet, slightly Warm

Channels

Lung, Spleen

Functions and Uses

- Tonifies the Spleen and benefits the qi: use for all Deficient Spleen patterns.
- Raises the yang qi of the Spleen and Stomach: use for prolapse – it makes things go up.
- Tonifies the Protective Qi (Wei Qi) and firms the exterior: goes to the outside of the body, and regulates the opening and closing of the pores.
- Benefits Water and reduces swelling.
- Tonifies the qi and Blood: particularly for severe loss of blood.

CAUTION

CONTRAINDICATED FOR FULL HEAT CONDITIONS OR YIN DEFICIENCY WITH FIRE – IT HEATS TOO MUCH.

DATA FILE

Properties

Acrid, slightly Bitter, Warm

Channels

Gall Bladder, Large Intestine, Spleen, Stomach

Functions and Uses

- Promotes the movement of qi and alleviates pain: use for Spleen, Stomach, Liver, or Gallbladder Stagnant Qi (pain is always a result of Stagnant Qi or Blood).
- Regulates Stagnant Qi in the Intestines.
- Strengthens the Spleen and prevents Stagnation: use Huang Qi with tonifying herbs to prevent their cloying side-effects.

CAUTION

CONTRAINDICATED IN CASES OF YIN DEFICIENCY OR DEPLETED FLUIDS.

Aucklandia lappa, costus root, saussurea

MU XIANG

Mu Xiang regulates and invigorates the qi when it becomes stuck or "stagnant," optimizing the function of the gastrointestinal tract and helping stop pain.

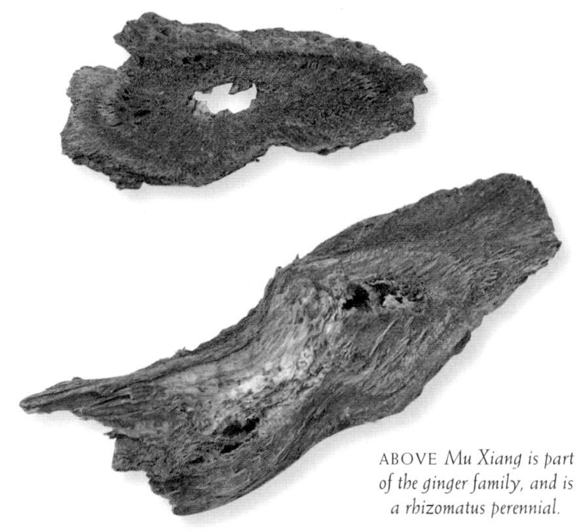

ABOVE *Mu Xiang is part of the ginger family, and is a rhizomatus perennial.*

HOW TO USE

Mu Xiang primarily helps digestive symptoms and pain. It is for Spleen or Stomach Stagnation symptoms such as lack of appetite, epigastric (above the navel) or abdominal pain or swelling, nausea, and vomiting. It is also used for Liver and Gallbladder Stagnation symptoms such as pain, swelling, or soreness in the flanks (sides). It is very good for diarrhea, dysentery, and tenesmus (a spasm of the rectum where one feels the need to defecate without being able to) due to Stagnation of qi in the Intestines rather than Deficiency. However, it also helps a Deficient Spleen regain its normal functions of transportation and transformation.

RIGHT *Mu Xiang helps to deal with lack of appetite, a symptom of Stomach Stagnation.*

THERAPY CONNECTIONS

GINGER

Ayurveda p.47

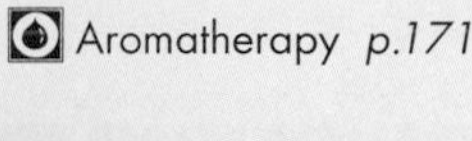

Aromatherapy p.171

Cannabis sativa, hemp, cannabis seeds

HUO MA REN

Huo Ma Ren comes into the category of Descending Downward: it facilitates the expulsion of the stool in cases of constipation. Huo Ma Ren is ungerminated cannabis seeds, but does not have the effects that smoking cannabis leaves or resin has.

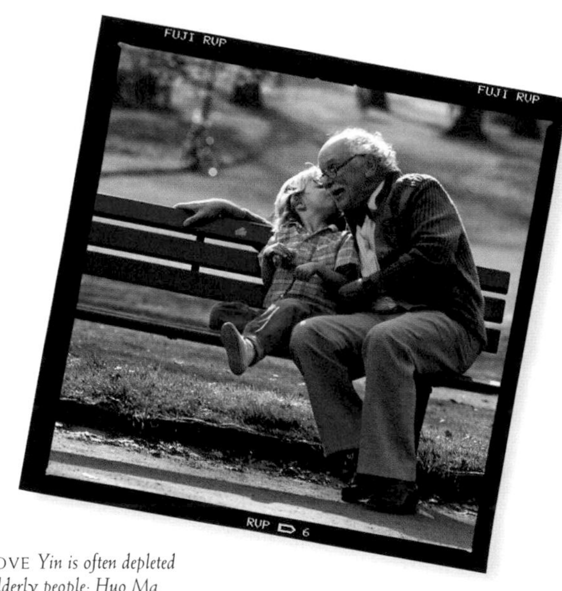

ABOVE *Yin is often depleted in elderly people: Huo Ma Ren helps to restore it.*

HOW TO USE

Huo Ma Ren is a moist laxative and therefore works gently by lubricating the Intestines. As it is mild in nature it is suitable for debilitated patients, the elderly, and those who are weakened by a febrile (feverish) disease or after childbirth. Also, as it is moistening, it is good for Blood Deficiency and general lack of fluids. One would often add Blood-nourishing herbs, such as Shu di Huang and Dang Gui for constipation due to Blood Deficiency, as in the elderly.

CAUTION

LONG-TERM USE MAY POSSIBLY RESULT IN VAGINAL DISCHARGE.

OVERDOSE MAY LEAD TO NAUSEA, VOMITING, AND DIARRHEA.

RIGHT *A cannabis plant. Huo Ma Ren is the ungerminated seeds of the plant.*

DATA FILE

Properties

Sweet, Neutral

Channels

Large Intestine, Spleen, Stomach

Functions and Uses

- Nourishes and moistens the Intestines: as it does not have a harsh effect, it is most suitable for constipation in the weak and elderly.
- Nourishes the yin: it mildly tonifies the yin and can be used in cases of Yin Deficiency with constipation. The yin is often depleted during a long illness like ME (or post-viral syndrome); also commonly in the elderly.
- Clears Heat and promotes healing of sores: use as an auxiliary herb for sores and ulcerations, taken orally or applied topically (locally).

Note: these seeds have been processed and therefore cannot germinate, so they cannot be considered an illegal drug.

Carthamus tinctorius, safflower flower

HONG HUA

This herb invigorates (or "regulates") the Blood, treating problems associated with Blood stasis. In TCM, these problems include pain and internal masses or growths.

HOW TO USE

Hong Hua is used for any Blood stasis patterns. These may include such gynecological problems as amenorrhea, post-partum dizziness, or fibroids. It may also include other tumors if they are caused by congealed blood, and many skin diseases, such as Kaposi's sarcoma, and scarlet fever. As it helps stuck Blood pain it is good for wounds or painful sores. It helps to bring out a measles' rash fully, and is useful for pain in the limbs. It also helps joint pain in arthritis.

DATA FILE

Properties

Acrid, Warm

Channels

Heart, Liver

Functions and Uses

- Invigorates the Blood and unblocks menstruation: it expels congealed Blood in the meridians and is not just for menstrual problems.
- Dispels Blood stasis and alleviates pain: it enters the Blood level of the channels (as opposed to qi or organ level).

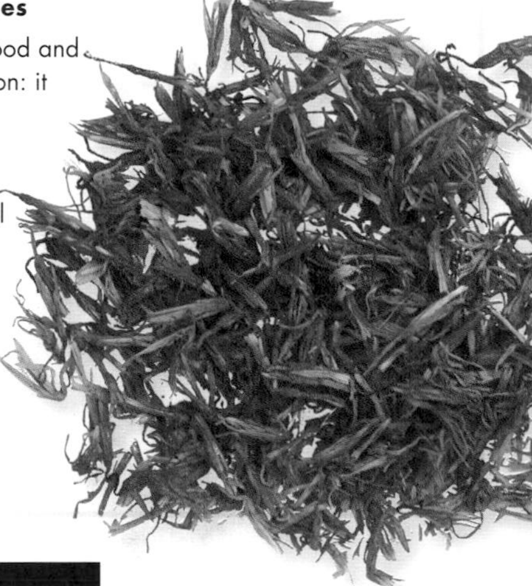

CAUTION

AS WITH MANY BLOOD-MOVING HERBS, DO NOT TAKE THIS DURING PREGNANCY.

ABOVE *Hong Hua is a pungent herb which helps move and invigorate the Blood.*

Cinnamomum cassia, cinnamon twigs

GUI ZHI

Gui Zhi belongs to a group of warm, acrid herbs that release exterior conditions; that is, superficial illnesses caused by viruses, with symptoms in the skin or muscle layers. These mainly cause sweating, or stop sweating where necessary.

HOW TO USE

Gui Zhi is used mainly for colds and flu, and commonly in combination with Bai Shao when there is too much sweating in a cold condition and the patient is becoming weak. It is often added to prescriptions for rheumatic complaints in the joints and limbs, especially the shoulders, caused by Cold Obstruction causing pain, where it sends warmth through the channels. Use for edema, where it sends warm yang energy through the meridians to move and transform the settled fluid. It is often used with licorice (Gan Cao) for palpitations and shortness of breath due to Deficient Heart yang. It can be used for menstrual cramps or irregular menstruation caused by Cold.

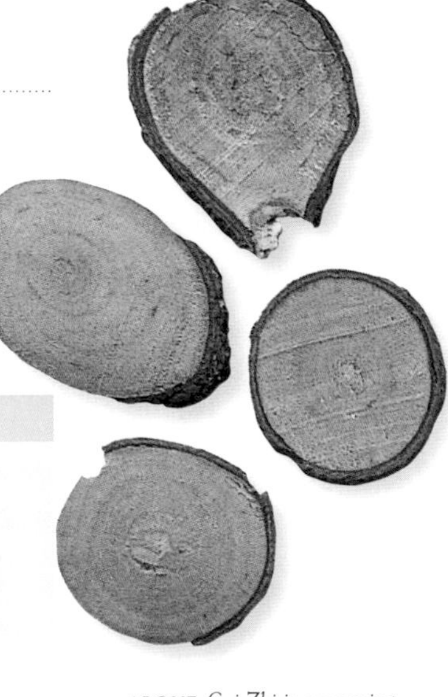

ABOVE *Gui Zhi is a warming herb, and is good for treating rheumatic complaints.*

CAUTION

CONTRAINDICATED IN WARM DISEASES, EITHER FROM FEVER, DEFICIENT YIN WITH HEAT SIGNS OR HEAT IN THE BLOOD WITH VOMITING.

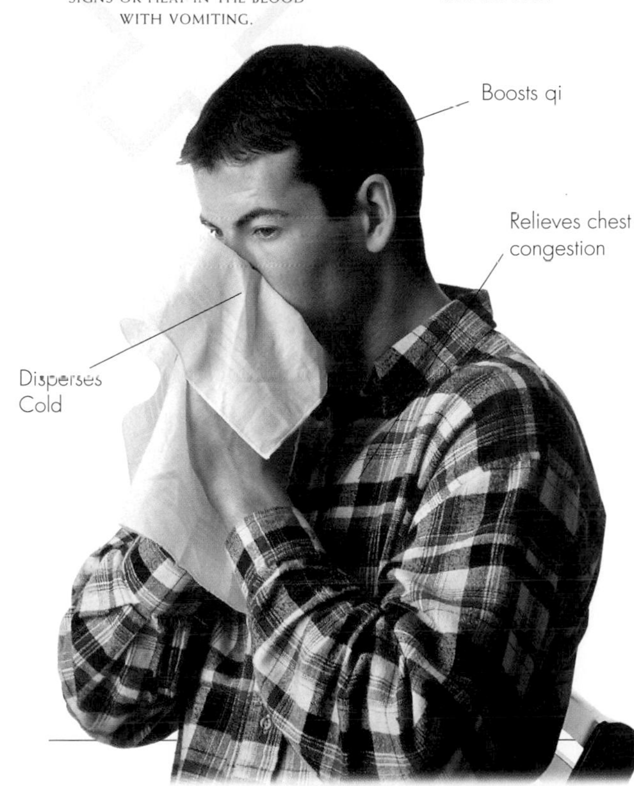

BELOW *Gui Zhi is a good treatment for colds and flu, often combined with Bai Shao.*

DATA FILE

Properties

Sweet and warm

Channels:

Lung, Bladder

Functions and Uses

- Adjusts the body's sweating in externally caused Cold conditions.
- Warms the meridians and disperses Cold: use for rheumatic ailments; also for gynecological problems caused by Cold obstructing the Blood.
- Moves the yang and transforms qi: use for water retention (edema) from Cold, where poor circulation of yang qi has failed to move the fluids in the body.
- Strengthens the Heart yang: use for palpitations when the active functioning of the Heart is weak.

Citrus reticulata, tangerine peel

CHEN PI

This herb regulates and invigorates the qi when it becomes stuck or "stagnant," optimizing the function of the gastrointestinal tract and helping stop pain.

HOW TO USE

Chen Pi is a very important herb as it "awakens the Spleen." It is for stagnant qi patterns with symptoms like epigastric (above the navel) or abdominal bloating, fullness, belching, nausea, and vomiting. It is very good for a lot of sticky sputum and other Phlegm Damp symptoms such as loss of appetite, fatigue, loose stools, and a thick, greasy tongue coating. It is therefore used for disorders affecting both the Spleen and the Lungs. It is particularly important for putting into tonifying prescriptions to make them more digestible.

DATA FILE

Properties

Acrid, Bitter, Warm, Fragrant

Channels

Spleen, Stomach, Lung

Functions and Uses

- Regulates the qi and strengthens the transportation function of the Spleen: it promotes the movement of qi in general, while directing it down.
- Dries Dampness and transforms Phlegm: use for a stuffy feeling in the chest and diaphragm.
- Helps prevent stagnation.

ABOVE *Chen Pi moves qi when it is stagnant, as revealed by Stomach disorders.*

CAUTION

CONTRAINDICATED IN DRY COUGH DUE TO YIN OR QI DEFICIENCY, AS IT IS DRYING (FRAGRANT) AND WARM.

USE WITH CAUTION WITH A RED TONGUE OR YELLOW PHLEGM (SYMPTOMS OF HEAT).

THERAPY CONNECTIONS

CINNAMON
Ayurveda p.34
Aromatherapy p.150

Codonopsis pilosula, codonopsis root

DANG SHEN

This herb is similar to Ren Shen: it treats Qi Deficiency, affecting primarily the Lungs and Spleen (the main digestive organ in TCM). It is less expensive than Ren Shen.

HOW TO USE

❧ Dang Shen does basically the same work as Ren Shen, but is not as strong. In prescriptions it is used in place of Ginseng to tonify the qi of the Spleen and Lungs, while ginseng is preferred for more serious situations, such as a patient who is barely conscious.

❧ It is used for lack of appetite, fatigue, tired limbs, diarrhea, vomiting, and prolapse – all symptoms of Spleen Qi Deficiency. It is also used for Lung Deficiency with chronic cough, shortness of breath, or copious sputum due to Spleen Deficiency. As it tonifies fluids, it is used in diabetes and the aftermath of febrile illnesses. It is the main herb in the seminal qi tonic prescription Si Jun Zi Wan ("Four Gentlemen"). Like all the qi tonics, it is sweet and cloying, and must therefore be combined with qi-moving herbs.

CAUTION

CONTRAINDICATED FOR PAINFUL URINATION OR DAMP–HEAT.

BELOW *Dang Shen enters all the channels, but especially the Lung and Spleen.*

DATA FILE

Properties

Sweet, Neutral

Channels

Lung, Spleen

Functions and Uses

- Tonifies the Middle area, benefits the qi and strengthens the Stomach and Spleen: use for all Deficient Qi patterns.
- Tonifies the Lungs.
- Strengthens the qi and nourishes fluids.

Coix lachryma jobi, seeds of Job's tears

YI YI REN

This is one of the Chinese herbs that transform Dampness, but it is more active on the Lower Burner than the Middle Burner.

HOW TO USE

❧ Like Fu Ling, Yi Yi Ren clears Dampness by promoting urination, but its Spleen-strengthening function is not as strong, and it works more on the Lower Burner (Kidneys) than on the Middle Burner (Spleen and Stomach). Use with Spleen-tonifying herbs to get rid of water retention; it may be used for Lung or Intestinal abscesses to help get rid of pus.

CAUTION

USE WITH CAUTION DURING PREGNANCY.

DATA FILE

Properties

Sweet, Bland, slightly Cold

Channels

Spleen, Lung, Kidney

Functions and Uses

- Promotes urination and leeches out Dampness: for edema or water retention in the legs.
- Clears Wind Dampness: this means Painful Obstruction syndrome, such as arthritic conditions.
- Clears Heat and expels pus: use when sores have become full of pus; pushes pus out.
- Strengthens Spleen and stops diarrhea: use when the Spleen is deficient, causing Damp diarrhea.
- Clears Damp Heat: for any digestive problems with a greasy yellow tongue coating.

Cornus officinalis, cornelian cherry fruit, dogwood fruit

SHAN ZHU YU

Shan Zhu Yu stabilizes and binds. It is sour and astringent, and helps keep in bodily substances which may leak, such as urine.

HOW TO USE

❧ Shan Zhu Yu is used for leakage of fluids due to weak Jing-essence, with symptoms such as excessive urination, incontinence, spermatorrhea, and premature ejaculation. In shock, it helps Liver and Kidney Deficiency, with such symptoms as lightheadedness, dizziness, sore and weak low back and knees, or impotence. It is useful for excessive uterine bleeding when the cause is Deficiency. It is one of the six herbs in the basic yin-tonifying prescription Liu Wei di Huang Wan (Six Flavor prescription), so if carefully combined it may tonify yin or yang.

DATA FILE

Properties

Sour, slightly Warm

Channels

Kidney, Liver

Functions and Uses

- Firms the Kidneys and retains the Jing-essence.
- Absorbs sweating and supports collapse: use for devastated yang and qi, as in shock.
- Tonifies and builds the Liver and Kidneys.
- Stabilizes the menses and stops bleeding.

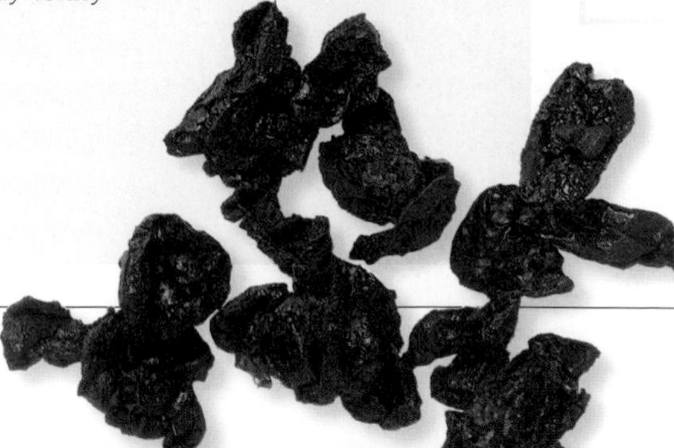

LEFT *Shan Zhu Yu is the fruit of the dogwood. It enters the Kidneys, where Jing is stored.*

BELOW *Huang Lian is used to treat halitosis caused by Stomach problems.*

Coptis chinensis, coptis rhizome, golden thread

HUANG LIAN

This herb clears Heat: this includes febrile conditions and any illnesses with Heat signs. It is one of the "Three Yellows," which are often used together for severe infections.

HOW TO USE

❧ Huang Lian deals with Damp Heat in the Middle Burner (digestive organs), and also the Heart and Pericardium. This latter leads to symptoms such as very high fever with delirium and disorientation. It can also be used to treat painful, red eyes and sore throat. It is very good with the infectious diseases still prevalent in the developing world. It is used for violent diarrhea and acid regurgitation from Stomach Heat. A decoction may be placed on sore, red eyes, boils, anal fissures, conjunctivitis, and used locally it is very good for treating trichomoniasis, a protozoan infection of the vagina.

DATA FILE

Properties

Bitter, Cold

Channels

Heart, Liver, Stomach, Large Intestine

Functions and Uses

- Clears Heat and detoxifies Fire Poison.
- Clears Heat and drains Dampness, especially in the Stomach and Intestines – dysentery, vomiting.
- Clears Heart Fire: symptoms such as irritability and insomnia.
- Stops Hot bleeding.
- Drains Stomach Fire: digestive dysfunction leading to bad breath and belching.
- Clears Heat topically: use for red mouth ulcers, boils, and abscesses.

CAUTION

DO NOT USE FOR DEFICIENT YIN PATTERNS, WHERE THE FLUID MAY BE DEFICIENT ANYWAY – HUANG LIAN WOULD DRY IT OUT MORE. LIKE ALL THE CLEARING HEAT HERBS IT IS COLD IN ENERGY, SO IT IS CONTRAINDICATED IN ANY DISEASES CAUSED BY COLD.

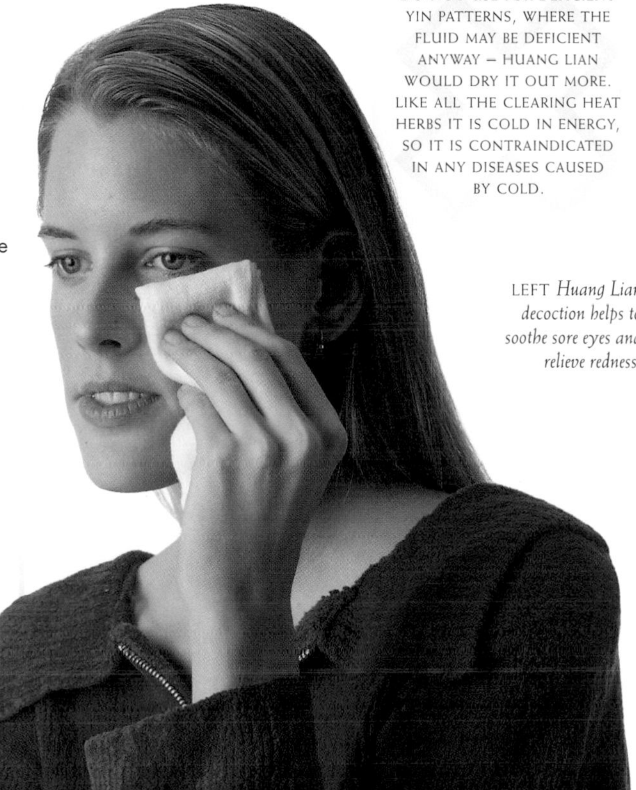

LEFT *Huang Lian decoction helps to soothe sore eyes and relieve redness.*

Crataegus pinnatifida, hawthorn fruit, crataegus

SHAN ZHA

This herb relieves digestive problems resulting from over-indulgence in greasy foods, and helps to promote efficient digestion by increasing gastrointestinal secretions and enzymatic functions.

RIGHT *Shan Zha deals with problems caused by an accumulation of greasy foods.*

DATA FILE

Properties

Sour, Sweet, slightly Warm

Channels

Liver, Spleen, Stomach

Functions and Uses

- Reduces and guides out food stagnation: for obstruction due to meat or greasy foods.
- Transforms Blood stasis and dissipates knottedness: enters the Blood level and is used for treating Blood stagnation disorders.
- Stops diarrhea: when the herb is slightly charred, it has an astringent effect.

THERAPY CONNECTIONS

HAWTHORN

Herbalism p.119

HOW TO USE

❧ Shan Zha is used for abdominal distention, belching, pain, and reduced appetite. It is also used for children who fail to thrive. It is especially useful if the symptoms are accompanied by diarrhea or chronic dysentery. It is particularly indicated for post-partum abdominal pain and menstrual pain when the cause is congealed Blood, and hernias with testicular pain and swelling. Recently it has also been used for hypertension (high blood pressure), coronary artery disease, and high cholesterol.

CAUTION

USE WITH CAUTION IN CASES OF SPLEEN AND STOMACH DEFICIENCY WITHOUT FOOD STAGNATION, AND IN DISEASES WITH ACID REGURGITATION.

Cuscuta chinensis, Chinese dodder seeds

TU SU ZI

This herb tonifies the yang, and as they are the basis of all the body's yang, it mainly affects the Kidneys. In TCM the Kidneys house the body's reserves, and the Kidney yang is also responsible for sexual and endocrine disorders.

HOW TO USE

Tu Su Zi helps the Jing-essence so is good for impotence, nocturnal emissions, and premature ejaculation, as well as such Kidney yang Deficient symptoms as sore lower back and knees, frequent urination, incontinence, and vaginal discharge. It is used for such Liver and Kidney Deficient symptoms as tinnitus (ringing in the ears), dizziness, blurred vision, or spots in front of the eyes. It stops leaking, so it is good for diarrhea or loose stools from Deficiency, and it also helps prevent threatened or habitual miscarriage. It is added to Kidney yang Deficient prescriptions to moisten the preparation.

DATA FILE

Properties

Acrid, Sweet, Neutral

Channels

Kidney, Liver

Functions and Uses

- Tonifies the Kidneys and benefits the Jing-essence: unlike most Kidney yang herbs, which are heating and therefore drying, Tu Su Zi is also moistening, so helps preserve the yin fluid.
- Tonifies the Liver and Kidneys and improves vision: use for patterns of Deficient Liver and Kidney yin and yang.
- Benefits the Spleen and Kidneys and stops persistent diarrhea.
- Calms the fetus.

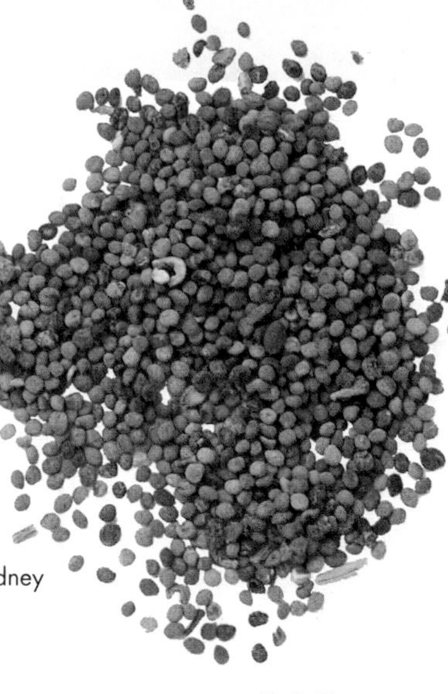

ABOVE *Tu Su Zi – Chinese dodder seed – is a moistening herb.*

CAUTION

ALTHOUGH THIS IS A NEUTRAL HERB, IT LEANS MORE TOWARD TONIFYING THE YANG AND SHOULD THEREFORE NOT BE USED FOR FIRE FROM YIN DEFICIENCY.

Cyperus rotundus, nut-grass rhizome

XIANG FU

This herb regulates and invigorates the qi when it becomes stuck or "stagnant," optimizing the function of the gastrointestinal tract and helping stop pain in various parts of the body, particularly menstrual and digestive pain.

LEFT *Xiang Fu is useful for treating gynecological disorders.*

HOW TO USE

Xiang Fu is a very widely used herb, as it has the ability to disperse stuck qi and to harmonize the energy, both in digestive and in gynecological disorders. It is particularly suitable for pain in the sides, fullness in the epigastrium (above the navel), pain and stuffiness in the chest, lack of appetite, wind and indigestion, as well as vomiting and diarrhea due to Liver qi invading the Spleen. It is also for swollen, tender breasts (due to PMS), and is an important herb for breast lumps. It is essential in prescriptions for dysmenorrhea (menstrual cramps) or irregular menstruation, and can be used in pregnancy for treating Liver qi stagnation patterns.

CAUTION

CONTRAINDICATED IN QI DEFICIENCY WITHOUT STAGNATION, AND IN YIN DEFICIENCY OR HEAT IN THE BLOOD.

DATA FILE

Properties

Acrid, slightly Bitter, slightly Sweet, Neutral

Channels

Liver, Triple Burner

Functions and Uses

- Moves qi and regulates Liver qi: in pathology, the Liver energy has a tendency to become "constrained," resulting in pain above the navel and around the ribs.
- Regulates menstruation and alleviates pain: according to TCM, the Liver is one of the main organs involved in gynecology, and the cause of menstrual pain is frequently due to "constrained Liver qi."

Gastrodia elata, gastrodia rhizome

TIAN MA

This herb has a sinking action – that is to say it takes qi down strongly.

HOW TO USE

Tian Ma is a very important herb for treating internal Liver Wind, with symptoms such as childhood convulsions or tantrums, epilepsy, spasms, or seizures. It is used for headaches, dizziness, and migraines caused by Wind Phlegm patterns, as well as Wind Stroke (stroke) with hemiplegia and numbness in the extremities. It is also good for rheumatic ailments in the lower back and limbs.

CAUTION

MAY BE TOXIC IN LARGE DOSES.

RIGHT *Tian Ma is a sweet herb which tonifies qi and treats the Liver.*

DATA FILE

Properties

Sweet, Neutral

Channels

Liver

Functions and Uses

- Calms the Liver, extinguishes Wind, and controls tremors. There are two kinds of Wind in TCM, external – which brings in cold or flu, or arthritic symptoms, and internal – which is generated by dysfunction of the Liver. This herb treats the second.
- Extinguishes Wind and alleviates pain: especially Wind Mucus head pain.
- Disperses painful obstruction caused by Wind Damp.

Eucommia ulmoides, eucommia bark

DU ZHONG

This herb belongs to a group that tonify the yang, and as the Kidneys are the basis of all the body's yang, it mainly affects the Kidneys. In TCM the Kidneys house the body's reserves, and the Kidney yang is also responsible for sexual and endocrine disorders.

BELOW *Du Zhong is the bark of* Eucommia ulmoides, *a 40ft. (12m.) deciduous, wide-spreading tree.*

DATA FILE

Properties

Sweet, slightly Acrid, Warm

Channels

Kidney, Liver

Functions and Uses

- Tonifies the Liver and Kidneys, strengthens the tendons and bones.
- Aids the smooth flow of qi and Blood: use to promote circulation.
- Calms the fetus: use for Cold (lack of yang) Deficient Kidney patterns during pregnancy.

HOW TO USE

Du Zhong is an expensive herb – it is necessary to kill the tree in order to get the bark. The Liver rules the sinews, the Kidneys rule the bones, so it is used for weak, sore, or painful lower back and knees, chronic fatigue, spermatorrhea (leaking of sperm), and frequent urination. Yang Deficient symptoms are always accompanied by Cold. It is the main herb for lower back pain caused by qi and Blood stagnation. It helps prevent miscarriage with bleeding during pregnancy, or when the fetus is restless, and it has recently been used for dizziness and lightheadedness due to hypertension from rising Liver yang.

CAUTION

CONTRAINDICATED FOR HEAT FROM YIN DEFICIENCY.

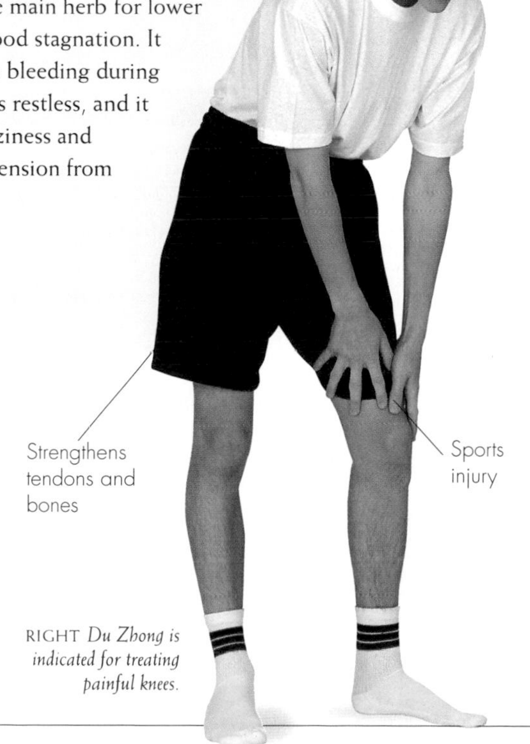

RIGHT *Du Zhong is indicated for treating painful knees.*

Fritillaria thunbergii, fritillaria bulb

ZHE BEI MU

Like Ban Xia, this herb transforms Phlegm, which in TCM is the accumulation of thick fluid mainly in the respiratory and digestive tracts, but which may occur in the muscles and other body tissues.

HOW TO USE

Zhe Bei Mu is a Cold herb which treats Phlegm Heat (as opposed to Ban Xia, which is warming), characterized by yellow sputum or sputum which is difficult to bring up. It is also indicated for Phlegm Fire coagulating and causing lumps in the breast or neck, and for Lung abscesses. Chuan Bei Mu is another form of this herb which is milder and not so cooling, and may be used for many types of cough, including dry yin deficient ones.

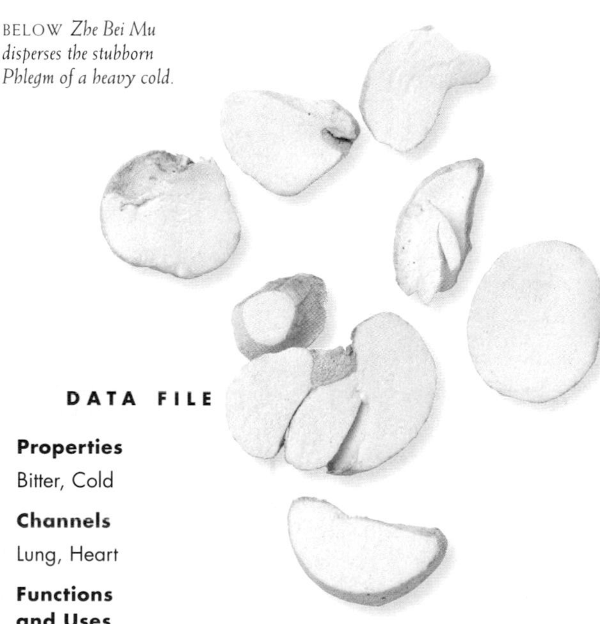

BELOW *Zhe Bei Mu disperses the stubborn Phlegm of a heavy cold.*

DATA FILE

Properties

Bitter, Cold

Channels

Lung, Heart

Functions and Uses

- Clears and transforms Phlegm Heat: use for acute Lung Heat patterns with productive yellow sputum.
- Clears Heat and dissipates nodules: use for Phlegm Fire which congeals and causes neck swellings.

CAUTION

INEFFECTIVE IN COUGHS DUE TO PHLEGM COLD.

Glycyrrhiza uralensis, licorice root

GAN CAO

This herb is one of a group that treat qi Deficiency and tonifies the Spleen. As we replenish our day-to-day energy levels by breathing in air and eating food, the two main organs involved are Lungs and Spleen (the main digestive organ in TCM).

CAUTION

CONTRAINDICATED FOR CASES OF EXCESS DAMPNESS, NAUSEA, OR VOMITING.

MAY CAUSE HIGH BLOOD PRESSURE OR EDEMA IF TAKEN FOR AN EXTENDED PERIOD OF TIME.

HOW TO USE

Gan Cao is a very useful herb, primarily because it is sweet and mild, so that it moderates the violent properties of other herbs in a prescription and makes them more digestible. Furthermore, it enters all 12 channels, so it can lead other herbs into those channels. It is used for Spleen Deficiency with shortness of breath, tiredness, and loose stools, and for Blood Deficiency with an irregular pulse and palpitations. It is used for any coughing and wheezing, and is good for spasms or cramps in the abdomen or legs. It is also useful for strep throat infections.

ABOVE *Gan Cao is useful for regulating the pulse.*

DATA FILE

Properties

Sweet, Neutral (raw), Warm (toasted)

Channels

All 12 channels

Functions and Uses

- Tonifies the Spleen and benefits the qi.
- Moistens the Lungs and stops coughing: because it is neutral it can be used to treat either Heat or Cold in the Lungs.
- Clears Heat and detoxifies Fire-Poison: use Gan Cao for sores or sore throats with pus.
- Moderates spasms and alleviates pain.
- Antidote for toxic substances, applied either internally or externally.
- Moderates and harmonizes the effects of other herbs.

Moderates spasms

Moistens the Lungs

RIGHT *Gan Cao stops coughing and soothes a sore throat.*

THERAPY CONNECTIONS

LICORICE

Ayurveda p.39

Traditional Home and Folk Remedies p.91

Herbalism p.122

Ledebouriella sesloides

FANG FENG

Fang Feng belongs to a group of warm, acrid herbs that release exterior conditions; that is, superficial illnesses caused by viruses, with symptoms in the skin or muscle layers. These herbs mainly cause sweating, or stop sweating where necessary.

HOW TO USE

Fang Feng means in English "guard against wind," so it is used particularly in ailments where Wind is predominant, according to TCM. This means it causes sweating (Acrid quality) in colds and flu. It is also useful in arthritis where the pain moves about from joint to joint (Wind type of arthritis). It treats numbness and trembling caused by Wind and Phlegm blocking the channels – for instance in convulsions associated with rabies or, more commonly, Parkinson's disease.

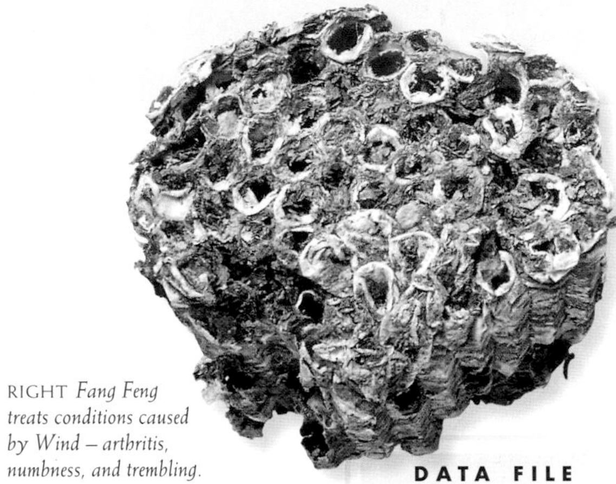

RIGHT *Fang Feng treats conditions caused by Wind – arthritis, numbness, and trembling.*

CAUTION

CONTRAINDICATED IN CASES OF DEFICIENT BLOOD WITH SPASMS – IT DOES NOT TONIFY THE BLOOD AND PRODUCES SWEATING, SO ONE WOULD HAVE TO ADD TONIFYING BLOOD HERBS TO STOP IT DEPLETING THE BLOOD FURTHER.

CONTRAINDICATED FOR CASES OF DEFICIENT YIN WITH HEAT SIGNS. YIN IS THE FLUID IN THE BODY AND IT KEEPS THE BODY COOL, SO DEFICIENT YIN CAN PRODUCE A "FALSE HEAT" SUCH AS IN MENOPAUSAL SWEATS. AS FANG FENG PRODUCES MORE SWEAT IT WOULD DEPLETE THE YIN FLUID EVEN FURTHER – IT NEEDS TO BE CAREFULLY COMBINED.

DATA FILE

Properties

Acrid, Sweet, slightly Warm

Channels

Bladder, Liver, Spleen

Functions and Uses

- Releases the Exterior and expels Wind: use for headaches, chills, and body aches from externally contracted Wind Cold.
- Expels Wind Dampness and alleviates pain: use for Exterior Wind Damp Painful Obstruction (rheumatic ailments).
- Expels Wind: Fang Feng alleviates trembling of the hands and feet.

Ligusticum chuanxiong, Szechuan lovage root, cnidium

CHUAN XIONG

This herb invigorates (or "regulates") the Blood, treating disorders associated with Blood stasis. In TCM these problems include pain and internal masses or growths.

DATA FILE

Properties

Acrid, Warm

Channels

Liver, Gallbladder, Pericardium

Functions and Uses

- Invigorates the Blood and promotes the circulation of qi: use for any Blood stasis patterns, especially in gynecology.
- Expels Wind and alleviates pain: it goes to the top and exterior parts of the body.

Itching caused by Wind

Enters Liver, Gallbladder and Pericardium

ABOVE *Itchy skin problems can be improved by taking Chuan Xiong.*

CAUTION

CONTRAINDICATED IN YIN DEFICIENCY WITH HEAT SIGNS (IT IS WARMING), HEADACHES DUE TO RISING LIVER YANG (UNLESS COMBINED CAREFULLY), QI DEFICIENCY (IT DOES NOT TONIFY), OR EXCESSIVE MENSTRUAL BLEEDING (IT MOVES BLOOD FURTHER).

HOW TO USE

Chuan Xiong is an important herb for gynecology, as many gynecological problems are caused by stagnant Blood circulation – problems such as dysmenorrhea (menstrual cramps), amenorrhea (lack of menstruation), difficult labor, or retained placenta. It is also used for chest, flank, and hypochondriac (above the navel) pain caused by Stagnant Qi and Blood. It is a leading herb for externally caught Wind disorders (viruses) with symptoms such as headaches, migraines, and dizziness. It is useful for arthritis and a variety of skin problems caused by Wind, including itching. As it moves the qi upward it is an essential herb used in combinations for treating all types of headaches.

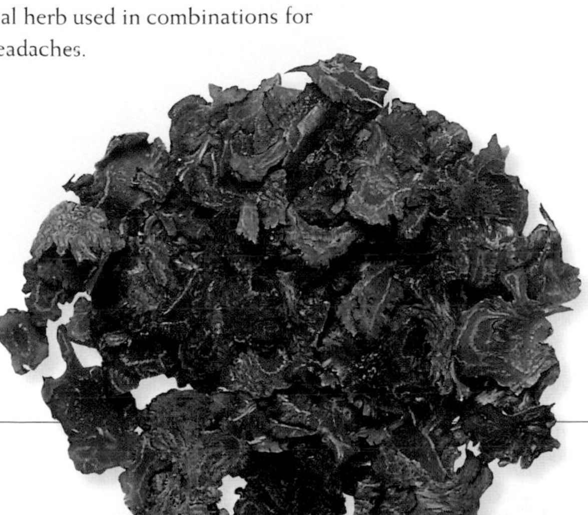

RIGHT *Chuan Xiong moves Stagnant Blood, and therefore eases painful periods.*

Lonicera japonica, honeysuckle flower, "Gold Silver flower"

JIN YIN HUA

Jin Yin Hua is one of a group of herbs that clear Heat: this includes febrile conditions and any illnesses with Heat signs, such as fever, inflammation, red eyes, aversion to heat, and hot skin eruptions.

HOW TO USE

Jin Yin Hua has a strong effect against many pathogenic bacteria. It is especially useful against Salmonella (food poisoning), and is effective against many streptococcus or staphylococcus infections. It is good for painful, hot swellings, particularly of the breast (mastitis), throat (viral or bacterial tonsillitis), or eyes (conjunctivitis). It is also used in "summer-heat diseases," where the hot weather produces fevers, sweating, and thirst. It is used for bad dysentery and bacterial urinary tract infections.

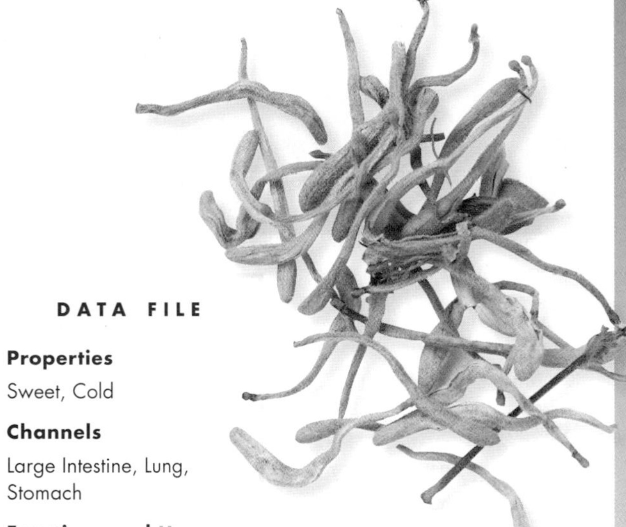

ABOVE *Jin Yin Hua is useful against food poisoning and throat infections.*

DATA FILE

Properties

Sweet, Cold

Channels

Large Intestine, Lung, Stomach

Functions and Uses

- Clears Heat and relieves toxicity: use Jin Yin Hua for hot, painful sores.
- Expels External Wind Heat: use for the early stages of febrile illnesses.
- Clears Damp Heat from Lower Burner: use for dysentery or cystitis.

CAUTION

CONTRAINDICATED IN CASES OF DIARRHEA DUE TO SPLEEN AND STOMACH DEFICIENCY – IT IS FOR STRONG INFECTIONS AND DOES NOT TONIFY WEAKNESS.

CONTRAINDICATED IN SORES WHICH DO NOT HAVE INFECTED PUS, BUT CLEAR LIQUID INSIDE.

Lycium barbarum, Chinese wolfberry fruit, matrimony vine fruit

GOU QI ZI

This herb treats patterns of Blood Deficiency, and in TCM the two organs most affected by this disorder are the Heart and Liver, which direct and store the Blood, respectively.

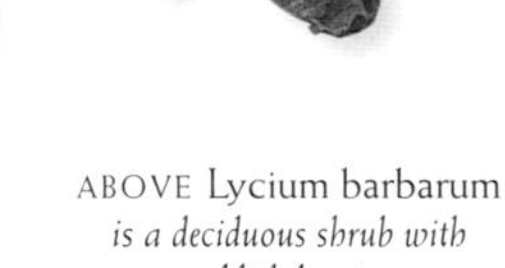

ABOVE Lycium barbarum *is a deciduous shrub with reddish berries.*

HOW TO USE

Gou Qi Zi is used for such Liver and Kidney Deficient symptoms as sore back and weak knees, impotence, leaking of sperm, and diabetes, particularly in the elderly, when the yin is in decline. It is used for Liver and Kidney Deficiency which leads to Blood and essence failing to nourish the eyes, so is good for failing or blurred vision, dizziness, dry, or sore eyes. As it enriches the yin of the Lungs, it is good for consumptive coughs.

CAUTION

CONTRAINDICATED IN FULL HEAT DISORDERS, ESPECIALLY EXTERNAL (VIRUSES), AND IN CASES OF SPLEEN DEFICIENCY WITH LOOSE STOOLS.

DATA FILE

Properties

Sweet, Neutral

Channels

Liver, Lung, Kidney

Functions and Uses

- Nourishes and tonifies the Liver and Kidneys: because this herb is neither Hot nor Cold, it is commonly used in treating Liver and Kidney Deficiency with patterns of Yin and Blood Deficiency.
- Benefits the Jing-essence and brightens the eyes: Jing (ancestral qi) is held in the Kidneys, while the Liver meridian goes to the eyes.
- Moistens the Lungs.

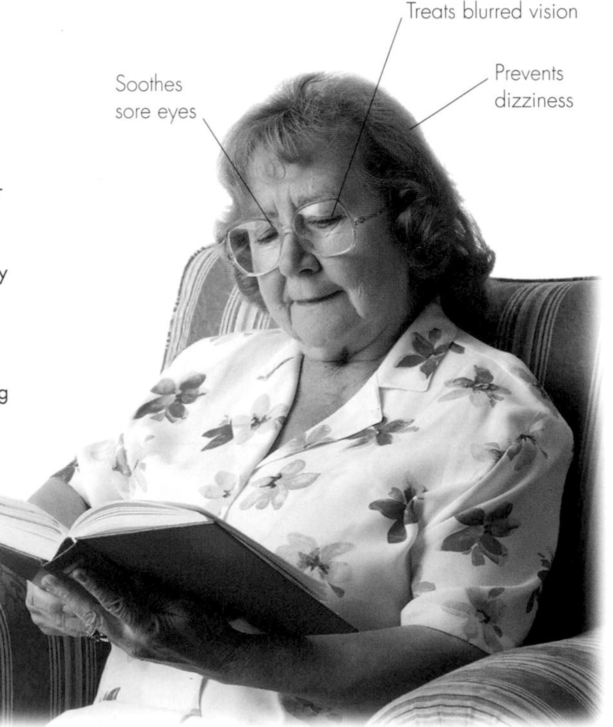

BELOW *Gou Qi Zi helps treat conditions in the elderly caused by depleted yin.*

Ophiopogon japonicus, ophiopogon tuber

MAI MEN DONG

This herb tonifies the yin, and it therefore moistens and nourishes fluid. Any of the major organs may suffer from a yin Deficiency, so Mai Men Dong is an important herb for their revitalization.

HOW TO USE

Mai Men Dong particularly strengthens the yin in the Upper part of the body, so it is good after febrile illness when the mouth is parched, and there is severe thirst or recurring fever. It is used for an irregular pulse and palpitations from the same causes of injury to the fluids or Blood. It is particularly for a dry cough, with or without mucus, and for Stomach Yin Deficiency, which includes stomachaches, "dry" vomiting, and a shiny tongue with little coating. It is also for diabetes, as well as being used to brighten the vision and strengthen the lower back. Like Tu Su Zi, it is added to prescriptions to moisten, but only in yin deficient patterns.

DATA FILE

Properties

Sweet, Bitter, slightly Cold

Channels

Lung, Stomach, Heart

Functions and Uses

- Moistens the Lungs and stops coughing.
- Tonifies the Stomach yin and generates fluid.

CAUTION

CONTRAINDICATED IN CASES OF DEFICIENCY WITHOUT HEAT SIGNS.

LIKE ALL TONIFYING YIN HERBS, IT AIDS DAMPNESS AND SHOULD THEREFORE NOT BE USED FOR COLD PHLEGMY COUGHING OR DEFICIENT SPLEEN WITH LOOSE STOOLS OR A THICK, GREASY TONGUE COATING.

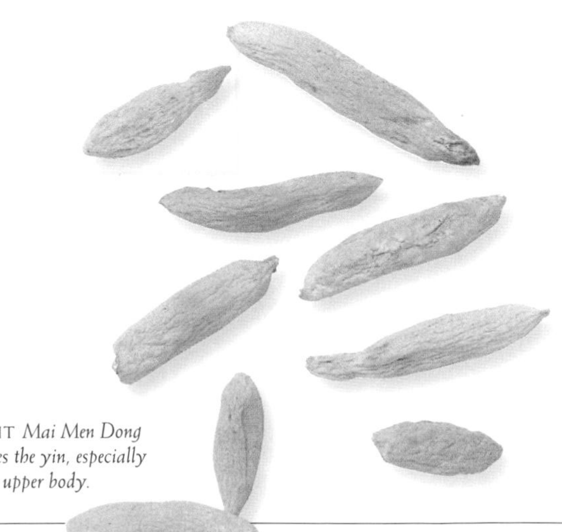

RIGHT *Mai Men Dong tonifies the yin, especially in the upper body.*

Paeonia lactiflora, white peony root

BAI SHAO

Bai Shao is a cooling herb with a sinking action – which means it takes qi down strongly. It is useful when the Liver is not fulfilling its function of making the Blood and qi flow smoothly.

HOW TO USE

Bai Shao has many uses and is an important herb. It treats headaches and dizziness due to rising Liver yang, and flank, chest, and abdominal pain from constrained (stuck) Liver Qi, or disharmony between the Liver and Spleen, which normally have a close relationship in the upper abdomen. Generally, this herb "softens" the Liver, treating spasms in the abdomen, or cramps in the hands or feet. It is good for menstrual irregularity or pain, or uterine bleeding, and, as it preserves the yin fluids, treats vaginal discharge and leaking of sperm. It treats excessive sweating in an external illness, or night sweating in Yin Deficiency.

DATA FILE

Properties

Bitter, Sour, Cool

Channels

Liver, Spleen

Functions and Uses

- Pacifies the Liver yang and alleviates pain: use for patterns of Liver yang rising, constrained Liver Qi or disharmonies between the Liver and the Spleen.
- Nourishes the Blood and regulates the menses.
- Preserves the yin.
- Adjusts the Ying and Wei: this refers to the balance between the inner and outer qi levels, which control the opening and closing of the pores.

CAUTION

EXERCISE CAUTION WITH DIARRHEA DUE TO COLD FROM DEFICIENCY, AS IT IS A COLD HERB.

BELOW *Bai Shao harmonizes the functions of the Liver and preserves the yin.*

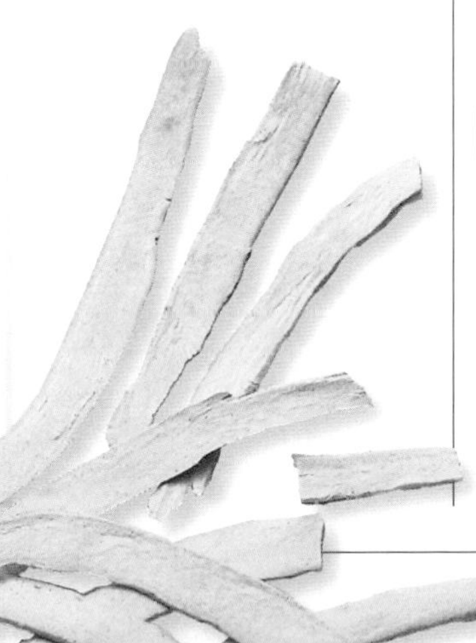

Panax ginseng, ginseng root, "man root"

REN SHEN

Ren Shen is an expensive herb as it takes six or seven years to cultivate. It is calming and has a proven effect on stress.

HOW TO USE

Ren Shen is invaluable because it tonifies both the qi (lack of energy) and the yin (lack of fluid). It is used after shock, with shallow respiration, shortness of breath, cold limbs, profuse sweating, and a weak pulse. It is good for Lung problems such as labored breathing and wheezing, and Spleen qi deficient problems such as lethargy, lack of appetite, bloating, and diarrhea, or, more severely, prolapse of the stomach, uterus, or rectum. It calms the Heart when there are palpitations, and in cases of anxiety, insomnia, or forgetfulness. As it is so expensive, it is usually substituted by Dang Shen in prescriptions.

ABOVE *Ren Shen calms anxiety and works on Heart Qi.*

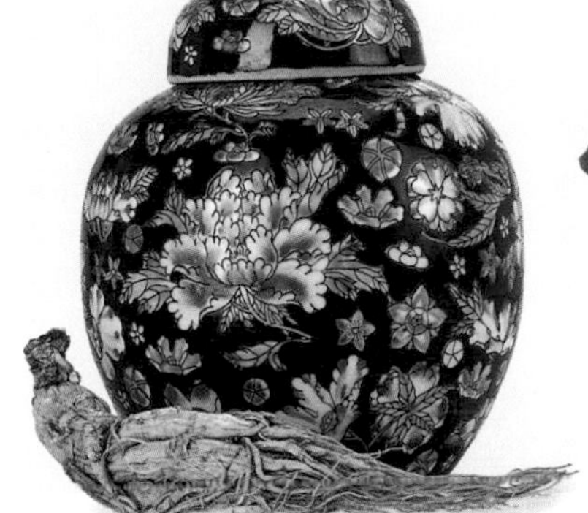

ABOVE *Ginseng should not be taken over an extended period.*

THERAPY CONNECTIONS

GINSENG
Herbalism p.126

CAUTION

CONTRAINDICATED FOR YIN DEFICIENCY WITH HEAT SIGNS (IT IS SLIGHTLY WARMING), HEAT EXCESS OR NO SIGNIFICANT QI DEFICIENCY.

OVERDOSE CAN LEAD TO HEADACHE, INSOMNIA, AND A RISE IN BLOOD PRESSURE.

DATA FILE

Properties

Sweet, slightly Bitter, slightly Warm

Channels

Lung, Spleen

Functions and Uses

- Strong tonifier of Root Qi: helps to revive an unconscious person.
- Tonifies the Lungs and benefits the qi.
- Strengthens the Spleen and tonifies the Stomach.
- Ren Shen generates fluid and stops thirst: use for diabetes when the qi and Blood have been injured by high fever and sweating.
- Benefits the Heart Qi and calms the spirit.

Panax notoginseng, notoginseng root, pseudoginseng root

SAN QI

This herb is used for bleeding or hemorrhage. Generally this herb is not used alone, but with other herbs that treat the cause of the bleeding, such as Hot Blood, Yin Deficiency, Spleen Deficiency, or stasis of the Blood.

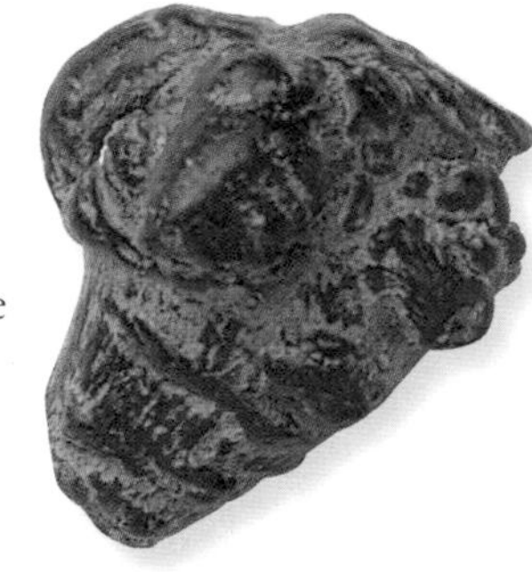

LEFT *San Qi treats pain in both the chest and the abdomen.*

HOW TO USE

San Qi has long been used in battle – soldiers carried this black powder with them to stem wounds. It is very expensive, and may be taken on its own or in a prescription. It is used for all kinds of internal and external bleeding, such as vomiting blood, nosebleed, blood in the urine or stool, uterine bleeding, or trauma-induced bleeding. It is good for chest and abdominal pain, as well as joint pain caused by congealed Blood. It can also be used after heart attacks to get rid of debris in the coronary artery, and is very useful after injuries, for swelling and pain due to falls, fractures, bruises, and sprains.

BELOW *Soldiers used to carry San Qi to stop bleeding.*

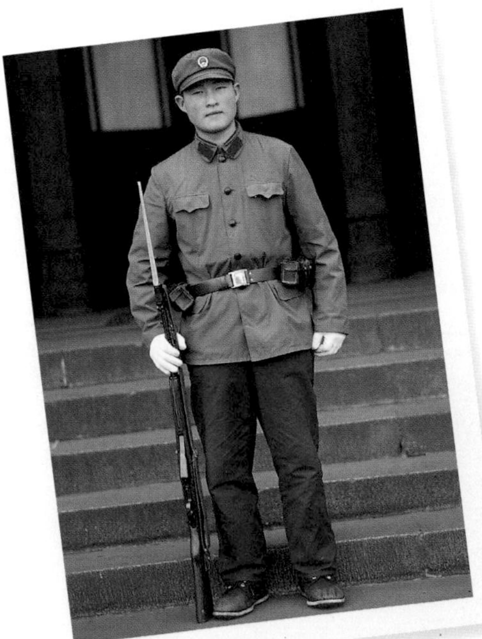

DATA FILE

Properties

Sweet, slightly Bitter, Warm

Channels

Liver, Stomach, Large Intestine

Functions and Uses

- Stops bleeding and transforms Blood stasis: because this herb can stop bleeding without causing Blood stasis, it is very widely used.
- Reduces swelling and alleviates pain: San Qi is a first choice for traumatic injuries.

CAUTION

CONTRAINDICATED DURING PREGNANCY.

USE WITH CAUTION IN PATIENTS WITH BLOOD OR YIN DEFICIENCY.

Phellodendron amurense, amur cork-tree bark, Cypress Rotundis, "Yellow Fir"

HUANG BAI, HUANG BO

This herb is one that clears Heat: this includes febrile conditions and any illnesses with Heat signs. It is one of the "Three Yellows," which are often used together for severe infections.

HOW TO USE

Huang Bai is particularly good for Damp Heat symptoms in the bottom third of the body, such as yellow, smelly vaginal discharge, foul-smelling diarrhea or dysentery. It is also used for red, swollen, and painful legs, and Damp Heat jaundice. It can be used for menopausal symptoms of hot sweats, or for afternoon fevers at the end of a long illness or when withdrawing from illicit drugs. It is good for leg ulcers which require antibiotics. It is a weaker (and cheaper) version of Huang Lian in its antimicrobial effects.

CAUTION

CONTRAINDICATED IN CASES OF SPLEEN DEFICIENCY, WITH OR WITHOUT DIARRHEA (SPLEEN DEFICIENCY MUST BE DIAGNOSED BY A QUALIFIED TCM PRACTITIONER).

DATA FILE

Properties

Bitter, Cold

Channels

Kidney, Bladder

Functions and Uses

- Drains Damp Heat, particularly in the Lower Burner: use Huang Bai for Damp Heat leukorrhea (vaginal discharge).
- Drains Kidney Fire: Ascending Kidney Fire with deficient yin signs, such as night sweating and a feeling of Heat in the patient's bones.
- Detoxifies Fire Poison, i.e. toxic sores with pus in them.

BELOW Phellodendron amurense *has dark, cork-like bark when the tree is old.*

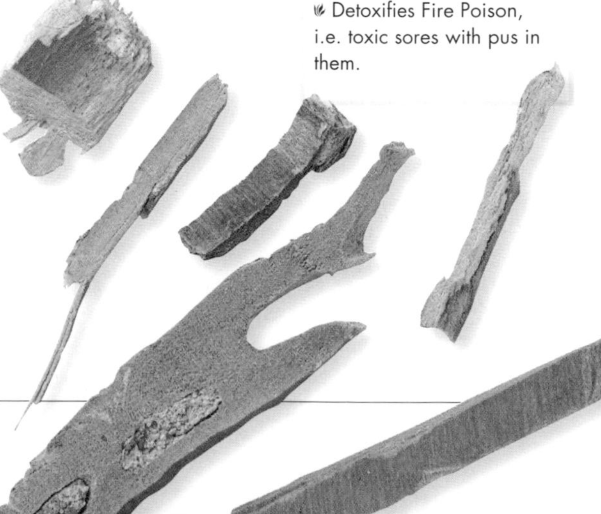

Pinellia ternata, pinellia rhizome

BAN XIA

This herb is one that transforms Phlegm, which in TCM is the accumulation of thick fluid mainly in the respiratory and digestive tracts, but which may occur in the muscles and other body tissues.

HOW TO USE

Ban Xia is one of the main herbs for drying Damp, and is used for abdominal and epigastric (upper abdominal) bloating and nausea, or for a stifling feeling in the chest due to Phlegm Damp – it is often used with Chen Pi. It can be added to prescriptions to avoid nausea from other herbs. It reduces any lumps or obstructions caused by Phlegm in the body.

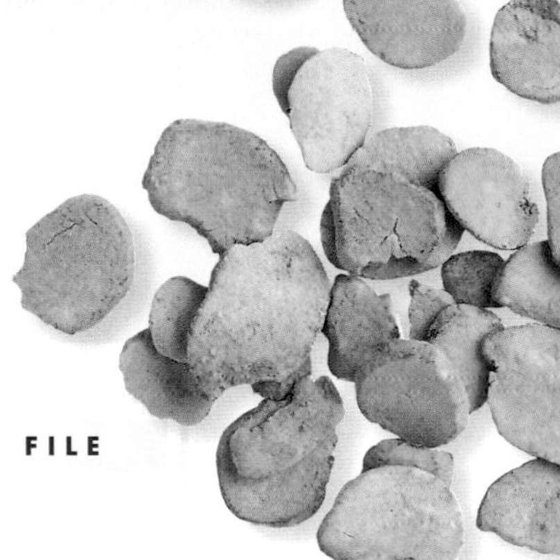

ABOVE *Ban Xia is used to treat an enlarged thyroid gland.*

DATA FILE

Properties

Acrid, Warm

Channels

Lung, Spleen, Stomach

Functions and Uses

- Dries Dampness, transforms Phlegm, and helps rebellious qi to descend: it is one of the main herbs for coughs with sputum. It helps the Spleen to dry out and so produce less mucus.
- Harmonizes the Stomach and stops vomiting: it takes qi down so helps Phlegm Dampness in the Stomach that rebels upward and causes vomiting.
- Dissipates nodules and reduces lumps: use for nodules caused by Phlegm lingering, such as goiter or lumps in the breast.

CAUTION

CONTRAINDICATED IN BLEEDING, COUGHS DUE TO YIN DEFICIENCY (DRY COUGHS) OR DEPLETED FLUIDS – IT IS VERY DRYING.

USE WITH CAUTION IN HEAT CASES.

IN VERY LARGE AMOUNTS, IT IS SOMEWHAT TOXIC (CAUSING NAUSEA), BUT CAN BE CURED BY GINGER.

Platycodon grandiflorum, balloon flower root

JIE GENG

This herb relieves coughing and wheezing. Like other cough remedies it treats the manifestation (presenting symptoms) of the problem, and therefore needs to be combined with other herbs that treat the root cause.

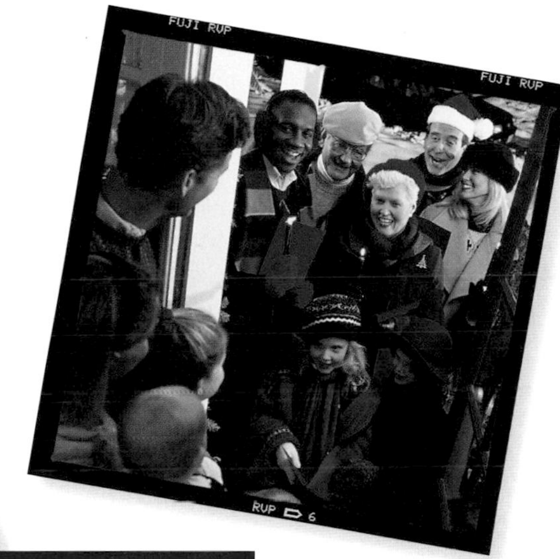

ABOVE *Carol singers in full voice. Jie Geng opens the voice and benefits the throat.*

CAUTION

CONTRAINDICATED IN COUGHING BLOOD (HEMOPTYSIS), AS IT MAKES THINGS GO UP AND WOULD MAKE THE CONDITION WORSE.

DATA FILE

Properties

Bitter, Acrid, Neutral

Channels

Lung

Functions and Uses

- Circulates the Lung qi, expels Phlegm and stops coughing: Jie Geng can be used to treat a wide variety of coughs, depending on the other herbs with which it is combined.
- Benefits the throat and opens the voice: used in many cases of sore throat and loss of voice, especially those caused by external Heat.
- Promotes the discharge of pus: use for expelling pus associated with Lung abscess or throat abscess.
- Makes herbs go to the upper body.

HOW TO USE

Like Xing Ren, Jie Geng can be used for a wide variety of coughs, especially for coughs caused by external pathogens, either Wind Cold or Wind Heat. It is useful for loss of voice, especially when this is caused by external Heat drying up the fluids in the throat. However, when combined carefully, it can be used for loss of voice due to Phlegm Heat or Yin Deficiency. It is often put into other prescriptions to direct herbs to the chest and head areas.

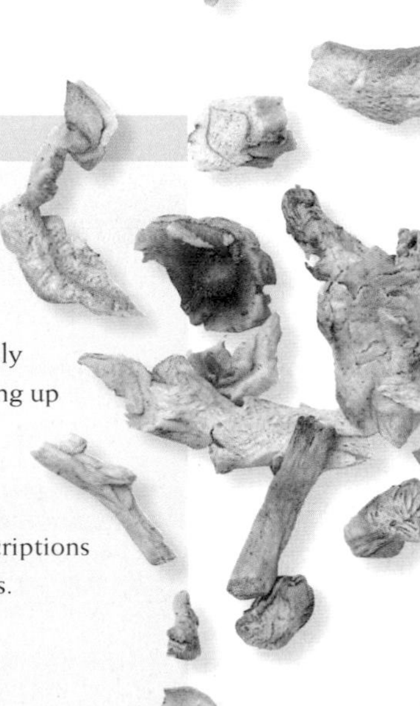

RIGHT *Jie Geng works on the Lung meridian, treating chest complaints.*

Polygala tenuifolia, Chinese senega root, polygala

YUAN ZHI

Yuan Zhi nourishes the Heart and calms the Spirit, or Shen, which is said to reside in the Heart. When the Shen is calm, personality is at its most potent.

HOW TO USE

❧ Yuan Zhi is used for insomnia, anxiety, palpitations, and forgetfulness. However, it differs from Suan Zao Ren in that it is most effective in cases when the patient thinks too much (excessive brooding), or for restlessness and disorientation. "Phlegm misting the Heart" implies quite serious psychological or psychiatric disturbances, when the Spirit is not clear and the patient loses touch with reality. It is also used for seizures and epilepsy. It is useful for coughs with copious sputum, especially when difficult to expectorate, and is applied topically for abscesses, sores, and swollen and painful breasts.

DATA FILE

Properties

Bitter, Acrid, slightly Warm

Channels

Heart, Lung, Kidney

Functions and Uses

❧ Calms the Spirit and quietens the Heart: use for pent-up emotions.

❧ Expels Phlegm and clears the orifices: when "mucus envelops the orifices of the Heart," with consequent emotional problems.

❧ Helps expel Phlegm from the Lungs.

❧ Reduces abscesses and dissipates swellings: use in powdered form, applied topically or mixed into a glass of wine.

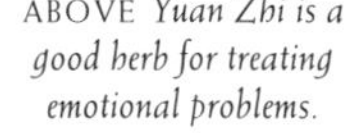

ABOVE *Yuan Zhi is a good herb for treating emotional problems.*

CAUTION

CONTRAINDICATED FOR YIN DEFICIENCY WITH HEAT SIGNS.

CAUTION SHOULD BE EXERCISED WITH ULCERS OR GASTRITIS.

Polygonum multiflorum, fleeceflower root

HE SHOU WU

This herb treats patterns of Blood Deficiency, and in TCM the two organs most affected by this disorder are the Heart and Liver, which direct and store the Blood, respectively.

HOW TO USE

❧ He Shou Wu is very commonly used, as it both tonifies and preserves the Kidney Jing-essence without being cloying. It is particularly used for premature graying or when the hair falls out (the name means "black hair"), as well as for dizziness, blurred vision, spots in front of the eyes, and a weak lower back and knees. It stops premature ejaculation, leaking of sperm, and vaginal discharge. Used raw, it is good for goiter and neck lumps, and as it moistens, is useful for constipation. It treats chronic malaria and prevents hardening of the arteries.

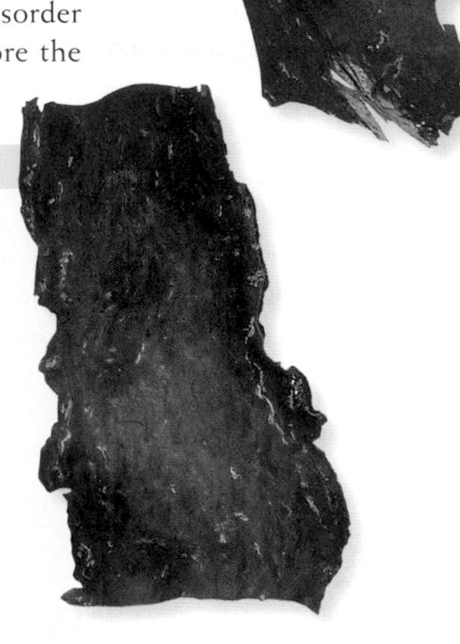

ABOVE *He Shou Wu strengthens the Jing and helps to prevent signs of aging.*

CAUTION

CONTRAINDICATED FOR SPLEEN DEFICIENCY, PHLEGM OR DIARRHEA.

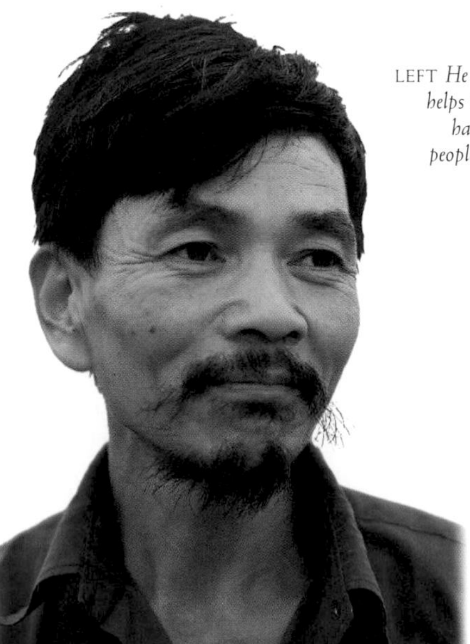

LEFT *He Shou Wu helps to preserve hair color as people get older.*

DATA FILE

Properties

Bitter, Sweet, Astringent, slightly Warm

Channels

Liver, Kidney

Functions and Uses

❧ Tonifies the Liver and Kidneys, nourishes the Blood and Jing-essence: used for treating Yin and Blood Deficiency.

❧ Firms the Jing and stops leakage: this refers to male sexual problems.

❧ Relieves Fire toxicity: use He Shou Wu raw for carbuncles and sores.

❧ Moistens the Intestines and unblocks the bowels.

❧ Expels Wind from the skin by nourishing the Blood: use for rashes that appear suddenly.

Polygonus multiflorum, fleeceflower vine

YE JIAO TENG

Ye Jiao Teng nourishes the Heart and calms the Spirit, which is said to reside in the Heart. It is therefore useful in tackling disturbed emotions.

HOW TO USE

Ye Jiao Teng is good for yin or Blood Deficiency patterns with insomnia, irritability, or emotional and nervous patients who cannot eat. It is especially useful for dream-disturbed sleep, and helps one feel comfortable in oneself. It also nourishes the Blood in the four limbs when the circulation is blocked or weak due to Blood Deficiency, and is used for such symptoms as generalized weakness, soreness, and aching or numb limbs. As it nourishes the Blood in the channels (meridians), it is also used externally as a wash for itching and skin rashes.

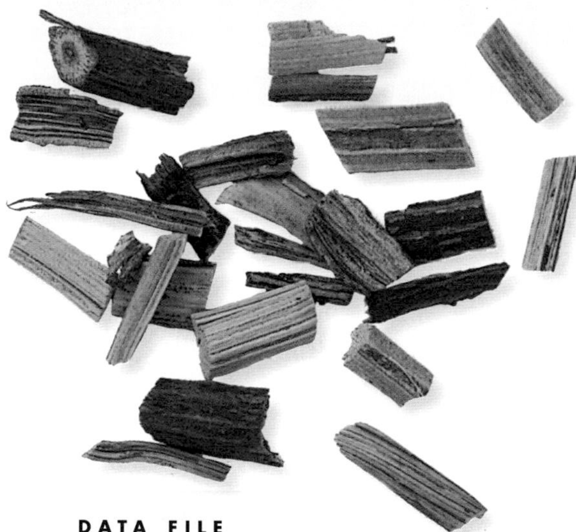

ABOVE *Ye Jiao Teng can be made into a decoction and applied to itchy skin rashes.*

DATA FILE

Properties

Sweet, slightly Bitter, Neutral

Channels

Heart, Liver

Functions and Uses

- Nourishes the Heart and Blood, and calms the Spirit.
- Activates Blood circulation and unblocks the channels.
- Alleviates itching: use as an external wash.

CAUTION

CONTRAINDICATED WITH DIARRHEA.

Poria cocos, tuckahoe, hoelen, bread root

FU LING

Fu Ling is a widely used herb that transforms Dampness, a "pathogenic influence" which creates stagnation in the Middle Burner, with various digestive or fluid-retaining effects.

ABOVE *Fu Ling is a neutral herb which is added to many prescription mixes.*

HOW TO USE

Fu Ling both strengthens the Spleen and gets rid of Dampness. It is good for difficulty with urination, diarrhea or edema (water retention), all symptoms of Dampness in the system. It helps with loss of appetite or bloating. Other symptoms of Phlegm include headaches or dizziness, and as it calms the Spirit it is good for palpitations, insomnia, or forgetfulness. It is a main ingredient in the qi-strengthening prescription Liu Jun Zi Wan ("Four Gentlemen") and is also essential in the main Yin-tonifying prescription, where it stops a person becoming too moist from the yin (fluid) tonifying herbs.

CAUTION

CONTRAINDICATED FOR COPIOUS URINE FROM DEFICIENT COLD.

DATA FILE

Properties

Sweet, Bland, Neutral

Channels

Heart, Spleen, Lung

Functions and Uses

- Promotes urination and leeches out Dampness by causing urination.
- Strengthens the Spleen and harmonizes the Middle area: helps prevent Dampness building up.
- Strengthens the Spleen and transforms Phlegm (congested fluids which can cause Heart palpitations and other symptoms).
- Quietens the Heart and calms the Spirit.

Prunus armenica, apricot kernel

XING REN

This herb is primarily used to treat coughing and wheezing. As it treats the manifestation (presenting symptoms) of the problem, it needs to be combined with other herbs that treat the root cause.

HOW TO USE

Xing Ren may be used for many kinds of coughing, whether from Heat or Cold, Exterior or Interior, depending on the combination with other herbs. Because the herb is moist in nature, it is useful for externally caught dry cough. It can be combined with Huo Ma Ren or Dang Gui for constipation due to Deficient Qi and dry Intestines.

CAUTION

USE WITH CAUTION FOR CHILDREN AND IN CASES OF DIARRHEA.

DATA FILE

Properties

Bitter, slightly Warm, slightly Toxic

Channels

Lung, Large Intestine

Functions and Uses

- Stops coughing and calms wheezing: Xing Ren is used widely for many kinds of cough.
- Moistens Intestines and unblocks the bowels: a secondary benefit due to the high oil content of Xing Ren.

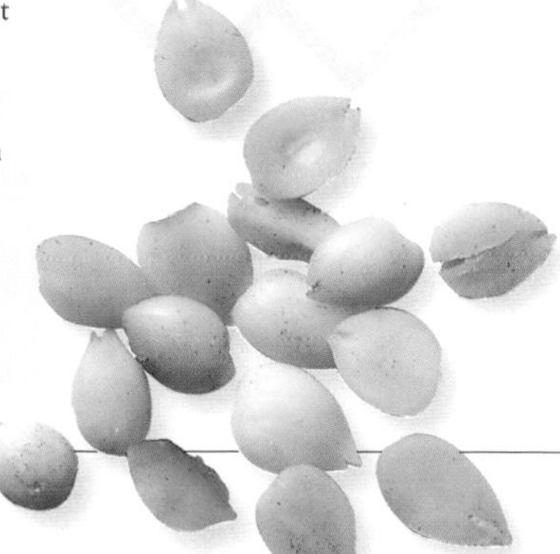

LEFT *Xing Ren is a valuable constituent of various herbal cough remedies.*

Prunus persica, peach kernel

TAO REN

This herb invigorates (or "regulates") the Blood, treating problems associated with Blood stasis. In TCM these disorders include pain and internal masses or growths.

HOW TO USE

❧ Tao Ren is a very strong herb. It breaks through Blood and is an important herb for hard abdominal masses and tumors, and for hypochondriac lumps such as enlarged Liver or Spleen, if there is Stagnant Blood present. It also treats congealed Blood amenorrhea and abdominal pain, or pain from injuries. It is good for psychosis caused by congealed Blood (according to TCM) or post-partum psychosis, and treats Lung and Intestinal abscesses. Like many seeds it is useful for constipation caused by dry Intestines.

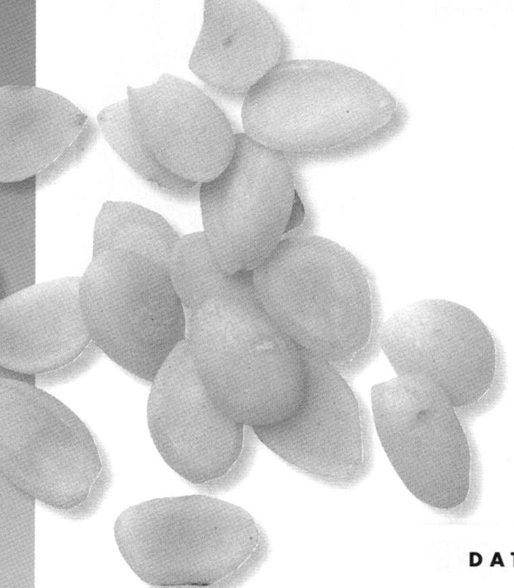

ABOVE *Tao Ren, the peach kernel, treats disorders of the Blood.*

DATA FILE

Properties

Bitter, Sweet, Neutral

Channels

Heart, Liver, Lung, Large Intestine

Functions and Uses

- Breaks up Blood stasis: it is a stronger herb than Hong Hua.
- Moistens the Intestines and moves stools.

CAUTION

CONTRAINDICATED DURING PREGNANCY.

CAUTION

CONTRAINDICATED IN CASES OF SPLEEN DEFICIENCY WITH DAMPNESS – SHENG DI HUANG IS TOO MOISTENING. ALSO CONTRAINDICATED IN THE PRESENCE OF PHLEGM.

Radix rehmannia glutinosa, Chinese foxglove root

SHENG DI HUANG

Sheng di Huang is one of a group of herbs that clear Heat: this includes febrile conditions and any illnesses with Heat signs. It can be used to treat diabetes, by addressing the Heat cause.

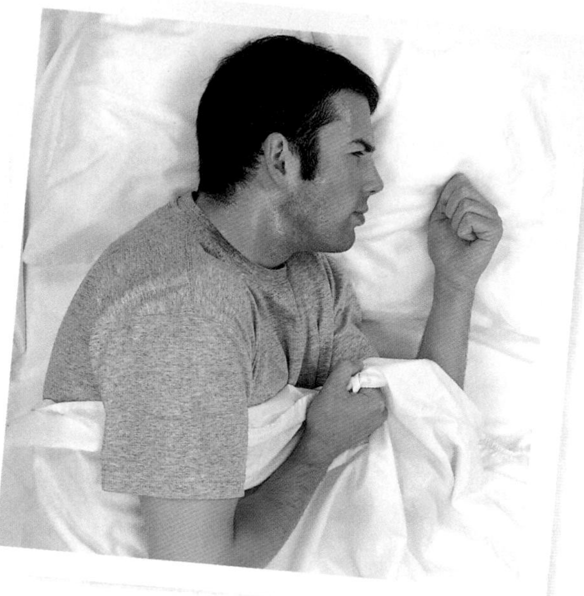

ABOVE *Feverish illnesses respond to treatment with Sheng di Huang, which is a cooling herb.*

DATA FILE

Properties

Sweet, Bitter, Cold

Channels

Heart, Liver, Kidney

Functions and Uses

- Clears Heat and cools the Blood: use in all febrile conditions where there is a very high fever, thirst, and a scarlet tongue. Also in hemorrhage when Heat enters the Blood level.
- Nourishes the yin and generates fluids: treats low-grade long-term fever with dry mouth, constipation, night sweats.
- Cools Heart Fire blazing: mouth and tongue ulcers, irritability, insomnia.
- Wasting–Thirsting syndrome, i.e. diabetes.

HOW TO USE

❧ Sheng di Huang is a very moistening as well as cooling herb. Therefore it is used in febrile illnesses where the Heat over a period has dried up the fluids in the body, causing thirst, irritability, and a scarlet tongue. It is also used, often with Bai Shao, when Heat in the Blood level causes hemorrhage from the vessels, leading to bloody urine, nosebleeds, and vomiting of blood. Untreated diabetes causes excessive thirst and urine – Sheng di Huang treats the Heat cause and helps the body replace the fluids.

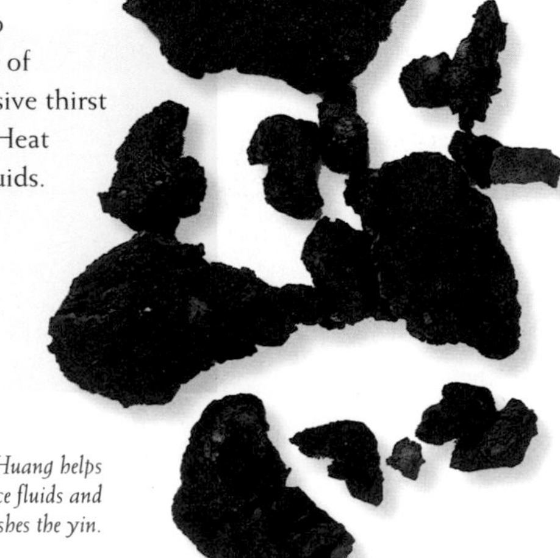

RIGHT *Sheng di Huang helps the body to replace fluids and nourishes the yin.*

Rehmannia glutinosa,
Chinese foxglove root cooked in wine

SHU DI HUANG

This herb treats patterns of Blood Deficiency, and in TCM the two organs most affected by this disorder are the Heart and Liver, which direct and store the Blood, respectively.

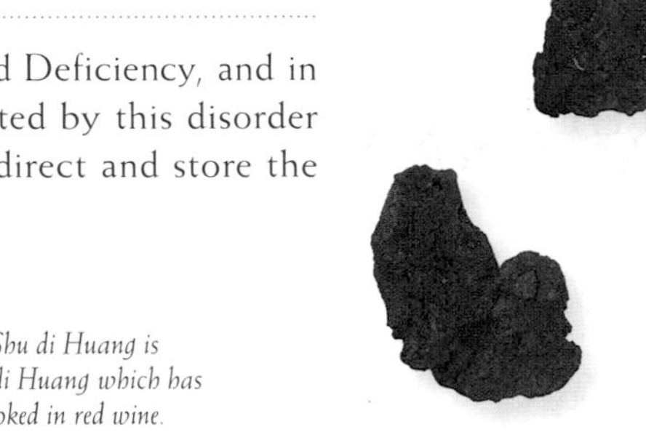

LEFT *Shu di Huang is Sheng di Huang which has been cooked in red wine.*

HOW TO USE

Shu di Huang is a very important herb – it is both a Blood and a yin tonic. Blood deficient symptoms include a pale complexion, dizziness, palpitations, and insomnia; also menstrual problems such as irregular bleeding, uterine bleeding, and amenorrhea (no menstruation). Kidney Yin Deficient patterns include night sweats, heat in the bones, nocturnal emissions (wet dreams), diabetes, and tinnitus (ringing in the ears). Jing Deficiency includes such Kidney symptoms as low back pain, weakness of the knees and legs, lightheadedness, deafness, and also premature graying of the hair.

DATA FILE

Properties
Sweet, slightly Warm

Channels
Heart, Kidney, Liver

Functions and Uses

- Tonifies the Blood: Blood deficient symptoms are similar to those of anemia.
- Nourishes the yin: use for treating Kidney Yin Deficient patterns.
- Nourishes the Blood and tonifies the Kidney essence (Jing) together: use it to treat Jing Deficient symptoms.

BELOW *Shu di Huang treats the symptoms caused by Blood Deficiency.*

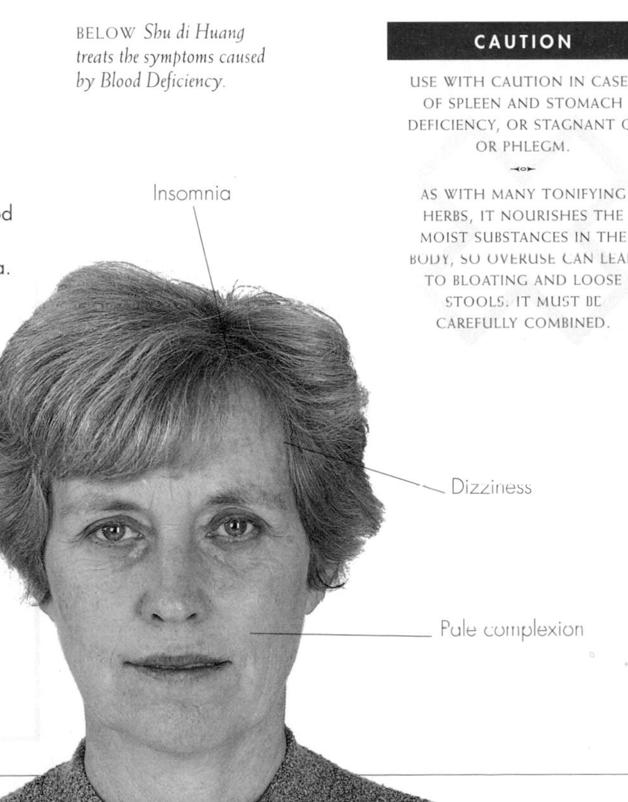

CAUTION

USE WITH CAUTION IN CASES OF SPLEEN AND STOMACH DEFICIENCY, OR STAGNANT QI OR PHLEGM.

AS WITH MANY TONIFYING HERBS, IT NOURISHES THE MOIST SUBSTANCES IN THE BODY, SO OVERUSE CAN LEAD TO BLOATING AND LOOSE STOOLS. IT MUST BE CAREFULLY COMBINED.

Rheum palmatum, rhubarb root and rhizome

DA HUANG

Da Huang comes into the category of Descending Downward: it facilitates the expulsion of stools in cases of constipation. This downward action clears Heat.

HOW TO USE

Da Huang (rhubarb) is a purgative. It has a strong downward action and clears Heat by acting as a powerful laxative. It treats Damp Heat jaundice, dysentery, and cystitis in the same way. It is good for Stagnant Blood complaints such as endometriosis, amenorrhea (lack of menstruation), and appendicitis.

THERAPY CONNECTIONS
RHUBARB
Herbalism p.127

DATA FILE

Properties
Bitter, Cold

Channels
Heart, Large Intestine, Liver, Stomach

Functions and Uses

- Drains Heat and purges accumulations: use for Full Heat conditions where there is fever, thirst, constipation, abdominal pain, a full pulse, and yellow fur on the patient's tongue.
- Drains Damp Heat via the stools.
- Clears Full Heat from the Blood: use for "reckless" bright red Blood that is flowing strongly, e.g. bleeding hemorrhoids (piles), nosebleeds.
- Invigorates the Blood: dispels Blood stagnation. Blood stasis can occur after traumatic injury, leading to a fixed pain.
- Clears Heat, resolves Fire Poison: use either topically or internally for boils, sores, burns, or Hot skin lesions (red lesions, giving off heat).

ABOVE *Da Huang is a Cold herb, used to treat Heat conditions by purging the body.*

CAUTION

CONTRAINDICATED IN THE FIRST STAGE OF INFECTIOUS DISEASES.

ALSO CONTRAINDICATED FOR QI OR BLOOD DEFICIENCY – IT DOESN'T TONIFY WEAKNESS BUT MAY BE ADDED TO A TONIFYING PRESCRIPTION TO CLEAR HEAT.

CONTRAINDICATED FOR COLD – IT IS A COLD HERB.

EXTREME CAUTION SHOULD BE EXERCISED DURING PREGNANCY, DURING MENSTRUATION, AND POST-PARTUM (AFTER BIRTH): IT HAS A STRONG DOWNWARD ACTION.

Schisandra chinensis, schisandra fruit

WU WEI ZI

Wu Wei Zi stabilizes and binds. It is a sour and astringent herb, and helps to keep leaking fluids and other substances within the body.

HOW TO USE

Wu Wei Zi is used for chronic coughs, wheezing, and asthma, especially with mucus, although it can also be used for dry coughs, as it nourishes the yin fluid. At the other end of the body, it is used for leaking of sperm, and urinary frequency or incontinence, vaginal discharges, especially watery and white (Cold), and daybreak diarrhea due to Spleen and Kidney Deficiency. It is indicated for excessive day or night sweating, with thirst and dry throat, but in common with other herbs in this category, it is not for sweat caused by outside infections. It also treats diabetes, the "wasting–thirsting" syndrome. Furthermore, it "holds the Heart yin in place," treating symptoms such as palpitations, irritability, dream-disturbed sleep, insomnia, forgetfulness, fear of ghosts, and of going outside. Basically, it helps keep a person feeling sane and calm.

ABOVE *Wu Wei Zi's uses include treatment of mental and physical disorders.*

BELOW *Wu Wei Zi helps to alleviate panic attacks of any kind.*

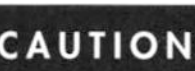

CAUTION

CONTRAINDICATED FOR EXTERNAL CONDITIONS, AND THE EARLY STAGES OF COUGHS AND RASHES – IT WILL KEEP THE "EXTERIOR PATHOGENIC FACTOR" INSIDE.

DATA FILE

Properties
Sour, Warm

Channels
Heart, Kidney, Lung

Functions and Uses

- Absorbs the leakage of Lung Qi and stops attacks of coughing.
- Firms the Kidneys, binds up Jing-essence and stops bouts of diarrhea.
- Absorbs sweating and generates fluids.
- Quietens the Spirit and calms the Heart.

THERAPY CONNECTIONS

SCHISANDRA
Herbalism p.130

SKULLCAP
Herbalism p.131

Scutellaria baicalensis, skullcap root

HUANG QIN

This herb is one that clears Heat: this includes febrile conditions and any illnesses with Heat signs. It is one of the "Three Yellows," which are often used together for severe infections.

HOW TO USE

Huang Qin mainly clears Heat in the chest and abdominal areas, so it is used for virulent diseases with high fever, irritability, thirst, cough, and expectoration (coughing up) of thick, yellow sputum. It can also be used topically on a dressing to clear red, hot swellings. It is used for dysentery and smelly diarrhea; also for febrile diseases which have a Damp element – symptoms such as a feeling of heaviness on the chest, and thirst with no desire to drink. It may be used for Damp Heat jaundice. It is one of the main herbs used in pregnancy to prevent miscarriage, and if toasted can stop Hot Bleeding from the nose, uterus, chest area, or in stools.

DATA FILE

Properties
Bitter, Cold

Channels
Heart, Lung, Gallbladder, Large Intestine

Functions and Uses

- Clears Heat, particularly in the Upper Burner (the upper third of the body, chest area).
- Clears Damp Heat: especially in the Stomach or Intestines. It is also used for Damp Heat in the Lower Burner, with symptoms such as cystitis.
- Clears Heat and calms the fetus.
- Stops bleeding due to Hot Blood: characterized as "the Blood becomes reckless with Heat and bursts out of its vessels."

CAUTION

CONTRAINDICATED FOR TUBERCULOSIS, WHICH IS A HEAT DEFICIENCY OF THE LUNGS, NOT A FULL HEAT, COLD DIARRHEA OR ANY COLD IN THE ABDOMEN, THREATENED MISCARRIAGE FROM A COLD CONDITION.

BELOW *Huang Qin comes from skullcap, a summer-flowering perennial.*

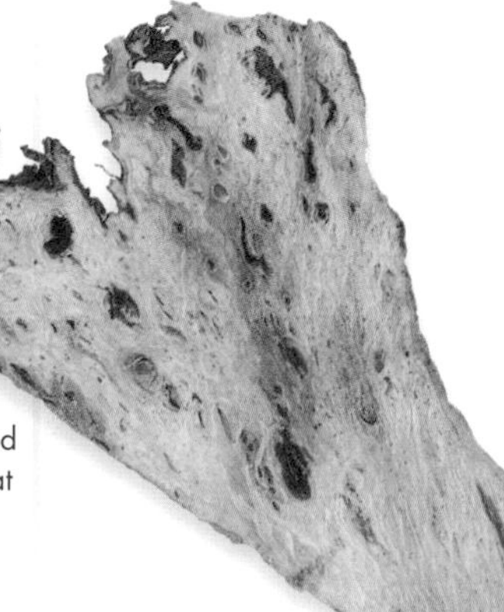

Stephania tetrandra, stephania root

HAN FANG JI

Like Wu Jia Pi, this herb dispels Wind Dampness from the muscles, joints, and bones. Whereas Wu Jia Pi is a Warm herb, however, Han Fang Ji is Cold. Wind Damp causes rheumatic and arthritic ailments.

CAUTION

USE WITH CAUTION IN CASES OF YIN DEFICIENCY, AS IT IS VERY DRYING.

DATA FILE

Properties

Bitter, Acrid, Cold

Channels

Bladder, Spleen, Kidney

Functions and Uses

- Expels Wind Dampness and alleviates pain: use for Wind–Damp–Heat in the channels, causing painful hot joints.
- Promotes urination; very effective at reducing edema – use Han Fang Ji whenever Damp collects.

BELOW *A colored X-ray of hands suffering from severe rheumatoid arthritis. Han Fang Ji relieves this condition.*

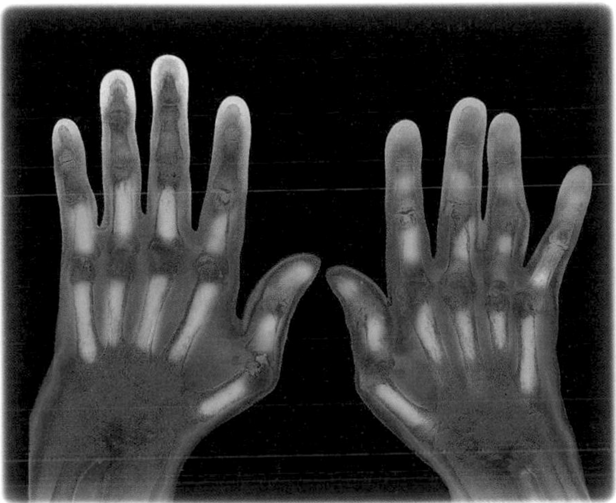

HOW TO USE

As a Cold herb, Han Fang Ji treats hot, painful swollen joints, such as in an acute attack of rheumatoid arthritis. It has an analgesic (pain relieving) and anti-inflammatory effect. It is very good in treating edema, especially of the lower body and legs, gurgling or ascites in the abdomen. It may also treat acute edema of the upper body (water on the lung).

Ziziphus spinosa, sour jujube seed

SUAN ZAO REN

This herb nourishes the Heart and calms the Spirit, which is said to reside in the Heart. Laboratory tests have proved that Suan Zao Ren has a sedative effect. It is used to treat emotional problems.

HOW TO USE

Suan Zao Ren is one of the main herbs used for calming the Heart by nourishing the Blood, treating symptoms such as irritability, insomnia, palpitations, and anxiety. It is also very good for both spontaneous and night sweating, and is used both in menopausal syndromes and withdrawal from addictive drugs, as well as many kinds of emotional problems.

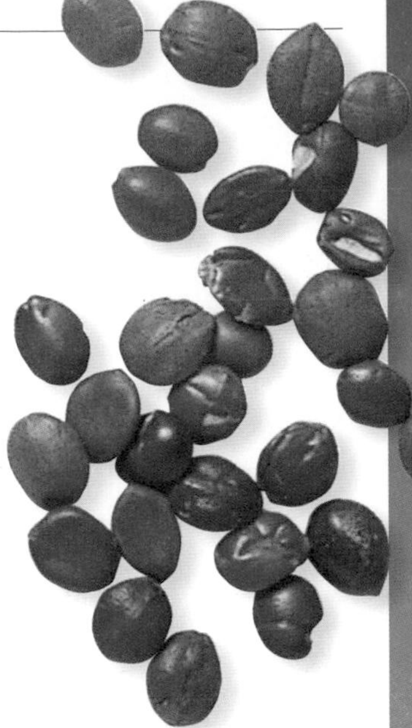

ABOVE *Suan Zao Ren acts via the Heart, Spleen, Gall-bladder, and Liver.*

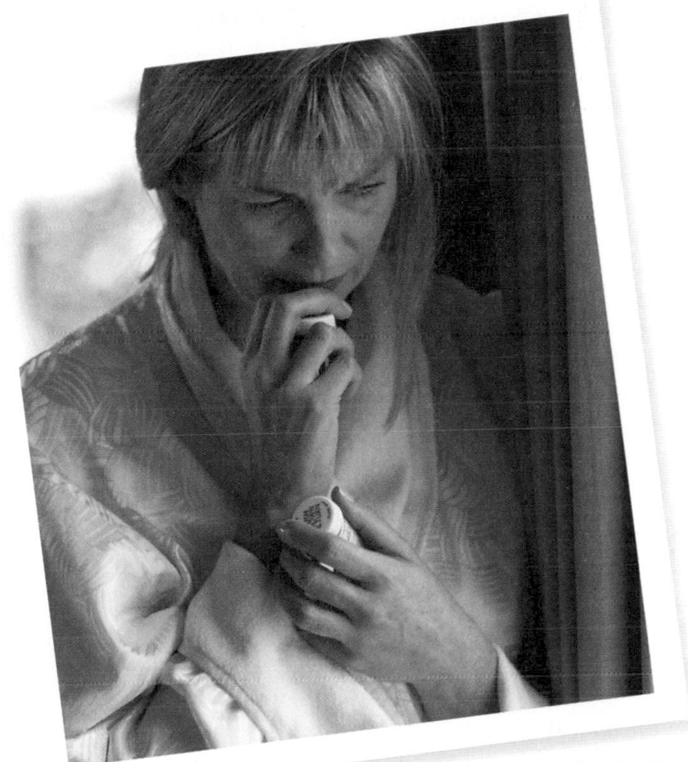

ABOVE *Suan Zao Ren is useful for fighting dependence or addictive drugs.*

DATA FILE

Properties

Sweet, Sour, Neutral

Channels

Liver, Gall Bladder, Heart, Spleen

Functions and Uses

- Nourishes the Heart yin and the Liver Blood, and calms the Spirit.
- Prevents occurrence of abnormal sweating.

CAUTION

CAUTION SHOULD BE EXERCISED IN CASES OF SEVERE DIARRHEA OR HEAT EXCESS.

TRADITIONAL HOME AND FOLK REMEDIES

Every culture, across the centuries, has had its own understanding and ways of healing. Local plants, customs, and beliefs determined the form it took, which varied across countries and between villages. Even today, away from the convenience of conventional physicians, villages around the world practise their own form of medicinal healing, using plants, age-old wisdom, and an instinctive and learned knowledge of their bodies as the tools.

TRADITIONAL REMEDIES

In times gone by, people more commonly tried to treat their ailments themselves, with remedies handed from generation to generation.

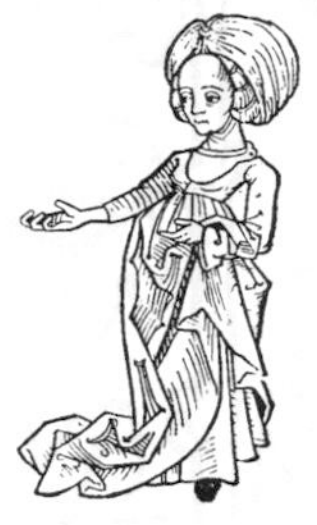

CONDITION *When illness struck, people treated themselves.*

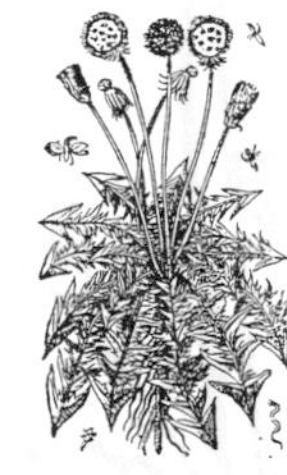

PLANT *Medicinal plants were gathered and prepared.*

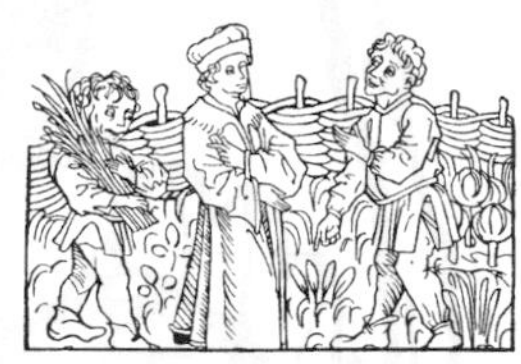

ADVICE *Most people had recipes for treating ailments.*

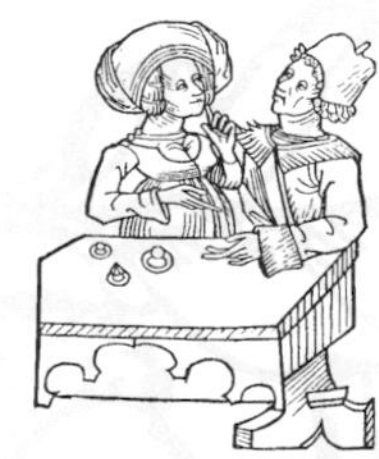

HEALING *People visited a healer if self-treatment failed.*

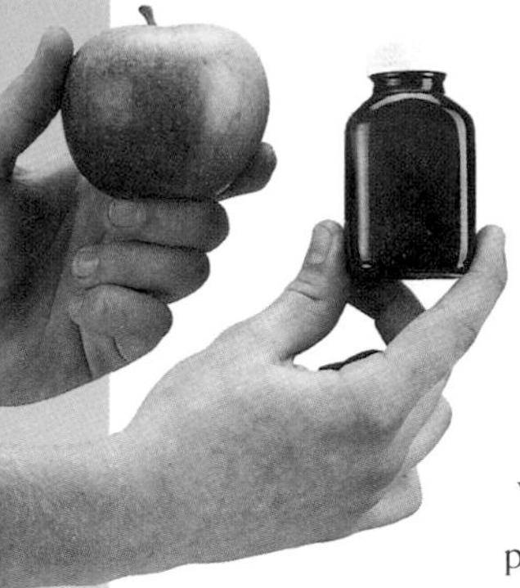

ABOVE *It's our choice: relying on conventional drugs, or reinvestigating alternative methods used for hundreds of years.*

A RETURN TO OLD WAYS

With the advent of technology and the growing dependence upon the miracles of modern medicine, most of us have lost the art of looking after ourselves. We have become dependent upon physicians, prescription drugs, store-bought preparations, and, through that, have lost an understanding of our bodies and how they work. Somewhere along the line we have put not only our faith but our independence in the hands of others. When we have a cold, a rash, even painful joints, we go straight to the medicine cabinet, or ring to arrange an appointment at the physician's surgery. The use of natural preparations, and the number of people addressing minor complaints in their own homes, hit an all-time low over the past decades, and only now are we experiencing a renaissance of natural healing and home remedies, as it becomes clear that conventional medicine, for all its wonders, is not the answer to everything.

Busy Western physicians have little time to spend diagnosing their patients, and our Western approach to pathology and anatomy is based on the theory that we are all the same. Individual personalities, lifestyles, emotions, spirituality, and indeed physical bodies are not taken into consideration for most conventional treatment, but we have now learnt that it is the complex combination of these very things that can make us sick or well. Treatment, therefore, needs to examine a wider picture.

In the past, many of us had the knowledge and the wherewithal to treat ourselves, using foodstuffs in our larders, and plants growing in our yards and fields. There would have been a village healer or physician who could be called upon in times of emergency, but for day-to-day and common ailments, treatment was undertaken at home.

While our understanding of biochemistry could not match that of a modern physician, our knowledge of how plants and various substances work in our bodies, and, indeed, how our bodies respond in various situations, and to different treatments, was much more profound. Women instinctively treated their children and their families – recognizing a bad temper as the onset of illness, perhaps, and being capable of addressing the cause of an illness according to a more general knowledge of our holistic being.

Today, most drugs on the market tend to deal with symptoms, rather than the root cause of an illness. Conditions and symptoms such as asthma, eczema, ME (CFS), headaches, and menstrual problems are controlled rather than cured. We take a tablet to ease the pain of a headache, but we do not stop and consider why we have a headache. We apply creams to stop the itching of eczema, but we do nothing to address the cause. In the past, we had a much greater general understanding of the causes and effects of illness, and a much more instinctive approach to treatment. Folk medicine and home remedies kept the majority of people healthy and it is that tradition to which many people are increasingly returning today.

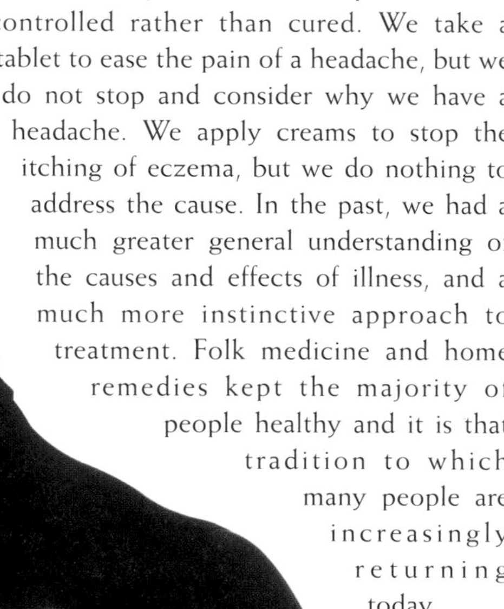

ABOVE *Exercise and diet are important when aspiring to adopt a more holistic lifestyle.*

CONVENTIONAL MEDICINE AND THE FOLK TRADITION

Physicians' offices are overwhelmed by the constant needs and demands of people suffering from minor illnesses. Conventional medicine has its place, and no one can deny that it has extended our lifespans and improved our chances of surviving serious illnesses. But it has its own drawbacks, one of the first and foremost being our dependence upon it. The majority of us are not able to listen to our bodies, and to take responsibility for our own health, in our own environment. Even conventional physicians welcome simple remedies to deal with the recurrent hazards of everyday life – coughs and colds, sore throats, cuts, bruises, skin infections, and many others – because it takes the pressure off medical systems and allows them to spend more time with more serious cases.

In the past, when conventional medicine did not have as much to offer and people could not afford to visit a physician, there was a commonsense approach to minor ailments. Indeed, many of the same remedies used have been adopted and adapted by conventional Western medicine. The popularity of these remedies is, quite simply, due to the fact that they are effective. They do, on many occasions, work better or at least as well as some of the pharmaceuticals of the modern age, and treatment is less likely to be complicated by side-effects. Their wider use means that we are less dependent upon conventional medical expertise and more self-confident. The power shifts from the physician back to the patient, which is both time- and cost-effective for everyone, and gives us a stake in our own health. Once learned, folk and home remedies can be used again and again.

PREVENTING ILLNESS

Natural medicine in the home is more than just first aid for common and minor ailments. It can be preventive, using some of the most common items in the larder – onions, garlic, thyme, mint, sage, chamomile – to protect against many illnesses. Modern research – particularly over the last three decades – is now justifying the use of plants and household items, things that have been used for centuries in both folk medicine and traditional cookery. For example, mint calms the digestive system, lemon is a great detoxifier, helping the liver and kidneys to function effectively, rosemary has profound antiseptic powers and is a natural stimulant, and caraway seeds will prevent flatulence. By incorporating some of these elements in your day-to-day meals, you not only add flavor and variety, but also provide the systems of your body with nourishment and support. These remedies have a beneficial effect on our general health and deal with specific problems, something that conventional drugs do not. Most available drugs work to address specific systems and do nothing for our overall health; many of them have side-effects that are more dangerous than the symptoms they are addressing. Traditional folk and home remedies tend to work with our bodies, allowing them to heal themselves by keeping them strong and healthy.

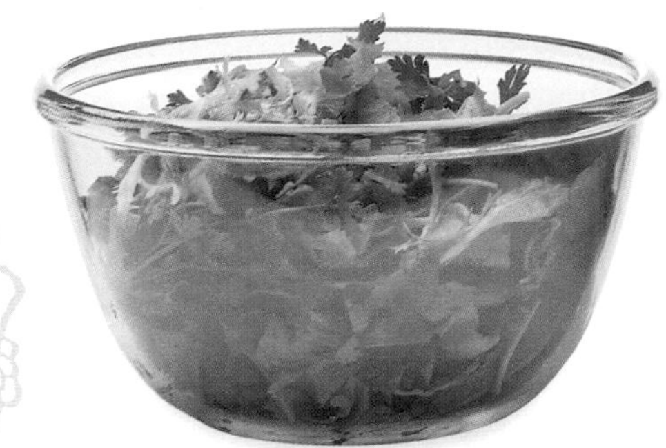

ABOVE *Adding beneficial herbs, such as mint, sage, and thyme to a salad, is an easy way to maintain health.*

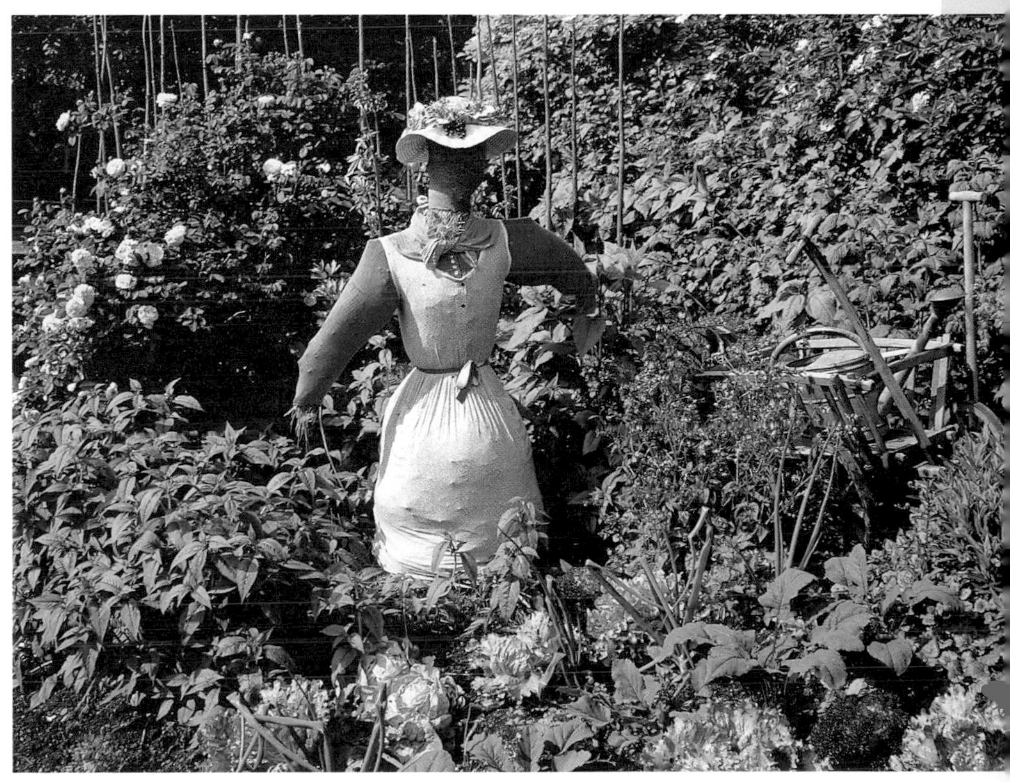

BELOW *The cottage garden was designed to provide a source of medicinal plants, as well as vegetables and beautiful flowers.*

WHAT IS FOLK MEDICINE?

The term "folk medicine" refers to the traditional beliefs, practices, and materials that people use to maintain health and cope with disease, outside of an organized relationship with academic, professionally recognized, and established medical systems and treatments.

The beliefs and practices that make up a system of folk medicine are very closely related to the history, traditions, and life of a recognizable social group. Many people practise folk medicine today, generally working in an environment where they share the belief system of their patients, and their approach to maintaining health and treating disease.

A HISTORICAL PERSPECTIVE

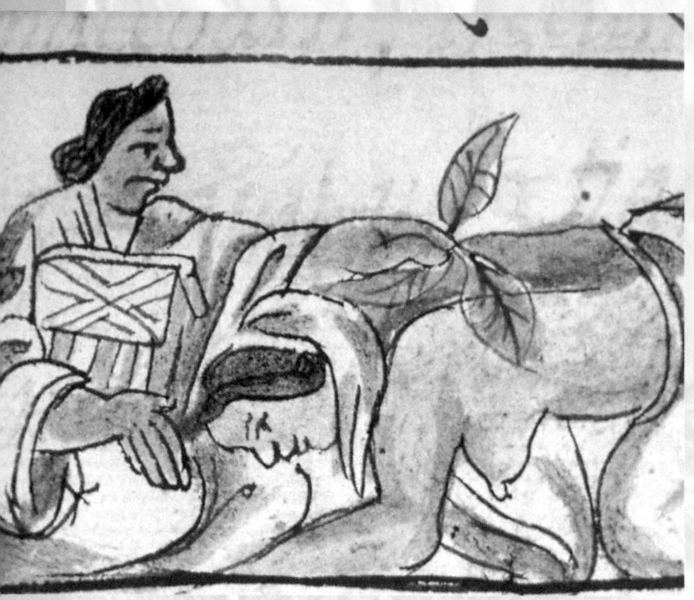

ABOVE *The Aztecs used certain plants to numb the pain of childbirth.*

Whenever possible, a system of folk medicine is best understood as a dynamic in a historical context. The Aztecs in Mexico provide a good example of how conventional medical systems can go hand in hand with folk medicine, feeding from one another and allowing both to grow according to the needs of the population.

Aztec establishment (as opposed to folk) medicine was highly organized, with a herbarium, a zoo, an intellectual elite, and a training and certification academy. It was based on a complex theoretical structure and experimental research. Some segments of the population, however, had only limited access to this medicine. They relied instead on traditional treatments and medicines.

Aztec establishment medicine was eliminated when the Spanish conquerors killed the medical personnel and introduced their own medicine. This intrusive system became the new medicine of the Aztec establishment. The system still offered limited access. Some elements of the European approach, however, were compatible with the folk medical practice of the Native Americans and were therefore incorporated into a new folk system. Mexican folk medicine thrived and continued to incorporate elements of the new establishment medicine.

Similarly, Native North American systems, while not highly organized and academic, were the establishment medicine in their own societies before conquest. Europeans brought diseases that decimated populations and challenged indigenous medical systems. The social and moral bases of the systems came under attack by missionaries and governments, even as immigrants began to adopt the ideas and materials from native systems. Again, this intrusive medicine became the establishment medicine, and Native American medicine, incorporating some Euro-American elements, became folk medicine.

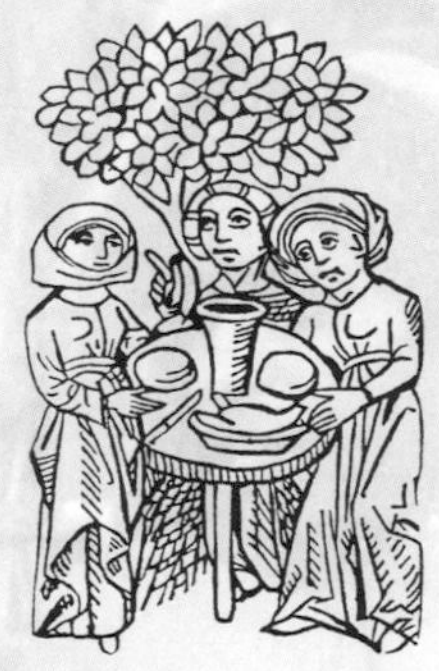

ABOVE *Medieval herbalists studying the properties of medicinal plants.*

DISCOVERING PLANT BENEFITS

But the history of using plants for medicine and healing goes back to the beginning of humankind. In their search for nourishment, primitive humans sampled many kinds of plants. Those that were palatable were used for food, while plants with toxic or unpleasant effects were avoided or used against enemies. Other plants that produced physiological effects such as perspiration, defecation, healing, or hallucinations were saved for medicinal purposes and divination. Over the course of thousands of years, people have learnt to use a wide variety of plants as medicines for different ailments.

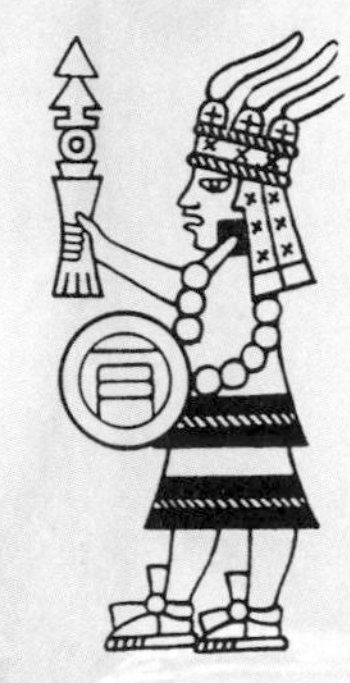

ABOVE *Aztec healers from the upper classes were highly trained.*

More than 4,000 years ago, the Chinese emperor Qien Nong (Chi'en Nung) put together a book of medicinal plants called *Ben Zao (Pen Tsao)*. It contained descriptions of more than 300 plants, several of which are still used in medicine. The Sumerians, at the same time and later, were recording prescriptions on clay tablets, and the Egyptians were writing their medical systems on rolls of papyrus. The oldest such document, known as the *Papyrus Kahun*, dates from the time of King Amenemhet III (1840–1792 B.C.E.) and contains information about women's diseases and medical conditions.

The most famous of these medical papyri, the so-called *Ebers Papyrus*, reports voluminously on the pharmaceutical prescriptions of the era. It includes specific information on how plants are to be used, for example, in the treatment of parasite worms or of stomach ailments. Some of these plants are still used today – in folk and conventional medicine.

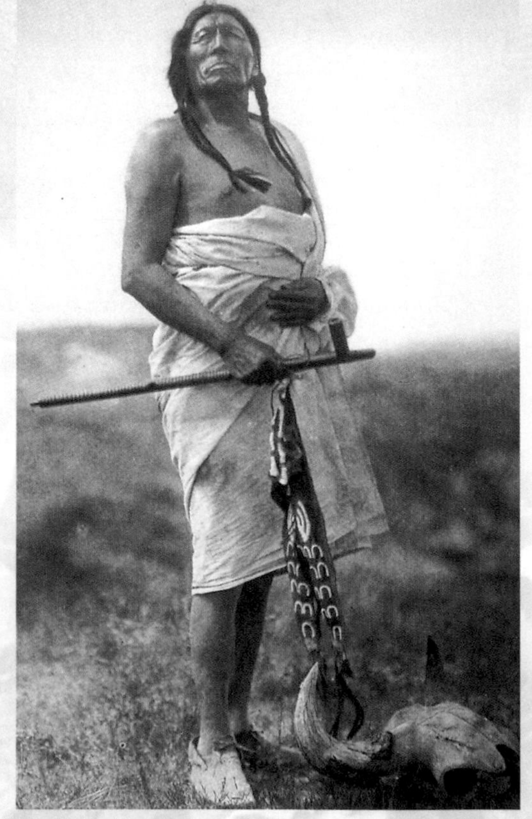

RIGHT *In Native North American tribes, healing was the domain of a shaman.*

TRADITIONAL FOLK MEDICINE TODAY

The growing concern about the side-effects of medicinal drugs, including the tragedies caused by compounds like thalidomide, has meant that herbalism has been called upon once more to provide natural medicines. In particular, pregnant women, children, people with chronic conditions (including chronic stress) that have refused to be shifted by orthodox medicine, and those with immunosuppressed conditions have had successful – and, most importantly, safe – treatment without the use of toxic drugs. Environmental pollution, food additives, contaminated water, and many other factors put massive stress on our bodies and on our immune systems, and it is now more important than ever to take a step back from chemical preparations and find ways to support our bodies against the demands of contemporary living.

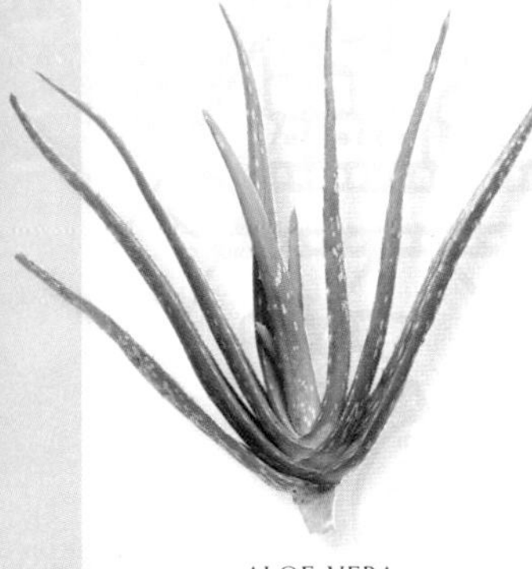

ALOE VERA

As research into the active constituents of herbs continues, increasing numbers of ancient treatments and tonics are being rediscovered and recognized, and brought back into widespread use. The global transport network means that we now have access to treatments used in countries around the world – bringing us a variety of amazing plants such as ginseng, guarana, tea tree oil, aloe vera, and ginkgo biloba.

Much of the pharmacopoeia of academic medicine – including aspirin (from the white willow) – has been derived from folk remedies, even as academic medicine has disparaged the folk reasons for their use. In the past this process has mostly been haphazard, but since the Second World War there has been an intensified, systematic investigation of tribal and folk medicines in the search for new preparations. More than 120 current prescription drugs are obtained from plants, and about 25 percent of all prescriptions contain one or more active ingredients from plants. There are plenty of herbal remedies already in use within orthodox medicine; for example, components of the yew tree have been used successfully to halt cancer, and the rosy periwinkle is used to control leukemia, especially leukemia in children.

Comparison and evaluation of folk and academic medical systems and practices is difficult. On the one hand, indiscriminate interpretation of folk medicine may result in inappropriate rejection of proven establishment methods – for example, some immunization, and drugs required to treat chronic and serious illness that may not have existed in the past. On the other hand, the dangerous aspects of folk medicine have often been emphasized, usually without recognizing the contributions of folk to conventional medicine and the similarities between them.

Today, there is a greater understanding of the power of natural remedies, and their use slowly accepted and indeed encouraged – particularly for ailments that people can safely and appropriately treat at home, such as headaches and upset stomachs, or sore throats. Disorders of the liver, heart, kidneys, etc., as well as severe illness – particularly in small children – are too serious for home treatment, and should be referred to a professional practitioner.

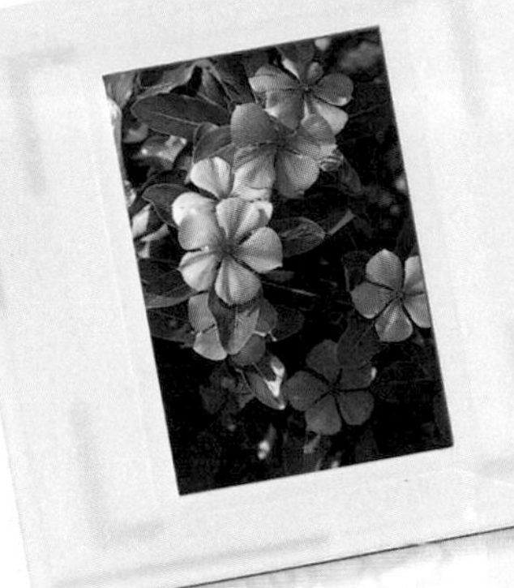

ROSY PERIWINKLE

The Greeks and the Romans derived some of their herbal knowledge from these early civilizations. Their contributions are recorded in Dioscorides' *De Materia Medica* and the 37-volume natural history written by Pliny the Elder. Some of these works are known to us through translations into Arabic by Rhazes and Avicenna. The knowledge of medicinal plants was further nurtured by monks in Europe who grew medicinal plants and translated the Arabic works.The first recognized apothecaries opened in Baghdad in the 9th century. By the 13th century, London became a major trading center in herbs and spices.

In the Dark Ages, the belief of the Christian Church that disease was punishment for sin caused a great setback in medical progress. Women in childbirth welcomed the pain as an opportunity to atone for their sins. Only in monasteries did herbals and other documented sources of natural medicine continue to be painstakingly translated.

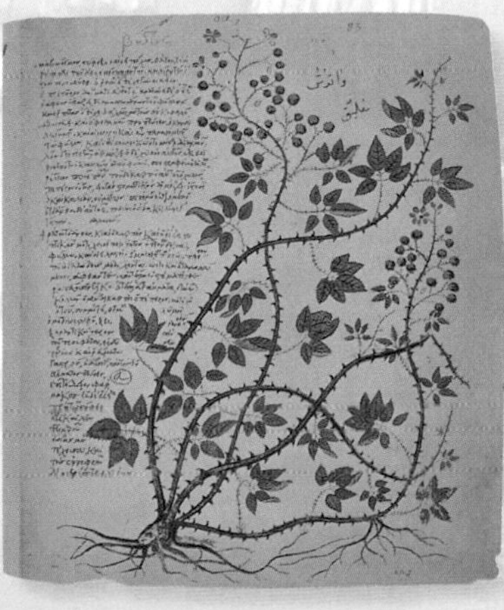

LEFT *A page from* De Materia Medica, *written by Dioscorides. Herbal knowledge was passed on from one civilization to another and expanded.*

The Renaissance provided a new forum for the development of the folk tradition. William Caxton printed dozens of medical manuals and Nicholas Culpeper translated the entire physicians' pharmacopoeia *The English Physician and Complete Herbals* in 1653. It is still in print.

The advent of alchemy, and the split between the "new philosophy" of reason and experiment, and the previous tradition of "science" (ancient medical doctrines, herbalism, astrology, and the occult) ended the golden age of herbals. Witch hunts disposed of village "healing women"; women were forbidden to study and all nonprofessional healers were declared heretics. The use of herbs became associated with magic and the occult, an uneasy alliance that has been difficult to shake. Herbalism was effectively dropped from mainstream medical training, though folk advice and treatment from the apothecary herbalist continued to be available, especially in less well-off areas.

CAUTION

THERE ARE SYMPTOMS WHICH COULD INDICATE A SERIOUS MEDICAL PROBLEM, AND FOR WHICH PROFESSIONAL ADVICE SHOULD BE SOUGHT IMMEDIATELY. THESE INCLUDE UNUSUAL OR PERSISTENT HEADACHES, CHRONIC PAIN, BLOOD IN THE URINE, FECES, OR MUCUS, PERSISTENT FATIGUE OR WEIGHT LOSS, AND BLEEDING BETWEEN MENSTRUAL PERIODS. THAT IS NOT TO SAY THAT HOME REMEDIES CANNOT BE USED TO TREAT THE PAIN AND DISCOMFORT OF SERIOUS PROBLEMS – FOLK AND HOME TREATMENT CAN GO HAND IN HAND WITH CONVENTIONAL MEDICINE, AND MANY REMEDIES ARE SAFE TO TAKE ALONGSIDE MEDICATION.

LEARNING ABOUT FOLK MEDICINE

Take time to learn about the various properties of the products available, and experiment until you find remedies that suit you and your family. Retrain yourself to consider the underlying causes of illness before seeking an instant relief from symptoms. Many of the home remedies work as fast as conventional drugs to bring relief, but the treatment of chronic disorders, such as bronchitis or rheumatism, will be slow, gentle, and cumulative, working to strengthen and stimulate various parts of the body over a long period of time. It is important to remember that the fresher or more recently picked the herb, the stronger its active properties. Dried herbs are more readily available and are about one-third as strong as the fresh product – and in some cases are better for the condition.

WHO CAN BENEFIT?

Folk medicine and home remedies do not provide a miracle cure, but almost anyone can benefit from the prudent use of herbs, plants, and household items as a form of restorative and preventive medicine. Most plants offer a rich source of vitamins and minerals, aside from having healing properties, and can be an important part of the daily diet, eaten fresh, or perhaps drunk as a tisane. A herbal tonic is useful, for example, in the winter months, when fresh fruit and green vegetables are not a regular part of our diets. Or plants like echinacea or garlic can be taken daily to improve the general efficiency of the immune system.

Some of the most common conditions that respond to home treatment include: hay fever, colds and respiratory disorders, digestive disorders (like constipation and ulcers), cardiovascular disease, headaches, anxiety, depression, chronic infections, rheumatism, arthritis, skin problems, anemia, and many hormonal, menstrual, menopausal, and pregnancy problems. On top of that are minor ailments such as scrapes, bruises, burns, swellings, sprains, and bites and stings.

Herbs do affect the way in which the body works, and although they are natural, they will have a profound effect on its functions. It is essential that you read the labels of any herbal products you have purchased, and follow carefully the advice of your herbalist. More is not better; although herbs don't have the side-effects of orthodox drugs, they have equally strong medicinal properties and can be toxic when taken in excess, causing liver failure, miscarriage, and heart attack, among other things.

TREATING YOURSELF AT HOME

Treatment is designed to help our bodies as a whole, and to stimulate their responses in order to cure disease. There are a variety of forms in which treatment can be offered, depending on the condition and your individual needs. Look at the "Preparing Remedies" box alongside. Many remedies are easily and quickly made. Some can be prepared in advance and stored for future use.

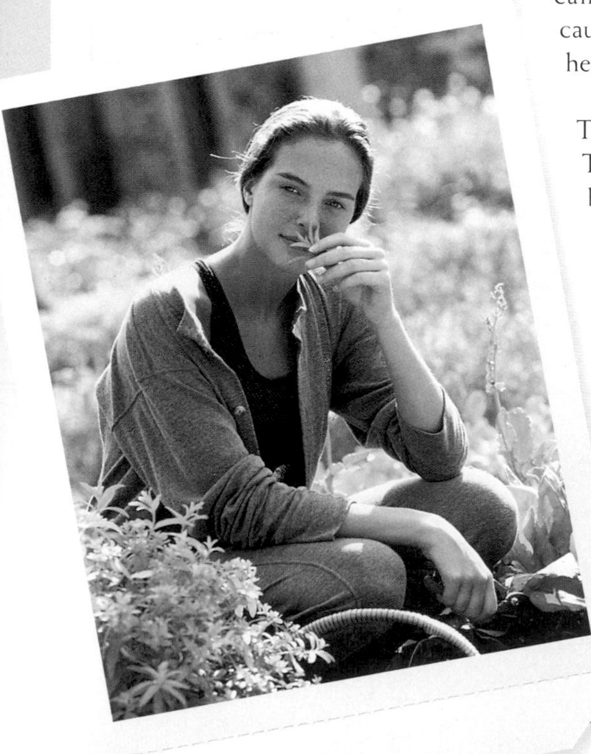

LEFT *Everybody can use traditional home remedies, along with conventional medicine if necessary.*

PREPARING REMEDIES

- **TISANES** Tisanes are mild infusions, usually prepackaged and sold in the form of a tea bag, which are boiled for a much shorter period than an infusion.
- **POWDERS** Plants in this form can be added to food or drinks, or put into capsules for easier consumption. Make your own powder by crushing dried plant parts.
- **PILLS** Plant remedies only rarely take this form since it is difficult to mix more than one herb and control the quantities. Some of the more common remedies will be available from professional herbalists or health food stores, or you can press your own with a domestic press.
- **COMPRESSES AND POULTICES** Compresses and poultices are for external use, and can be extremely effective, the active parts of the herb reach the affected area without being altered by the digestive process. A poultice is made up of a plant which has been crushed and then applied whole to the affected areas. You can also boil crushed plant parts for a few minutes to make a pulp, which will act as a poultice, or use a powdered herb and mix with boiling water. Because they are most often applied with heat and use fresh parts of the plant, they are more potent than compresses *(see below)*. Poultices are particularly useful for conditions like bruises, wounds, and abscesses, helping to soothe and to draw out impurities. A compress is usually made from an infusion or decoction, which is used to soak a linen or muslin cloth. The cloth is then placed on the affected area, where it can be held in place by a bandage or plastic wrap. Compresses can be hot or cold and are generally milder than poultices.
- **ESSENTIAL OILS** Often used in other therapies, like aromatherapy (*see page 140*), the essential oils of a plant are those which contain its "essence," or some of its most active principles. Useful for making tinctures and ointments.
- **BATHS** Plants and other items can be added to bath water for therapeutic effect – inhalation (through the steam) and by entering the bloodstream through the skin. An oatmeal bath, for instance, would work topically on eczema, and a chamomile bath would both soothe skin, and calm and relax.
- **INHALATIONS** Warm moist air can relieve many respiratory problems and allow the healing properties of plants and other products to enter the bloodstream through the lungs. To prepare an inhalation, half fill a big bowl with steaming water, and add a herbal infusion or decoction, or 2–3 drops of an essential oil.

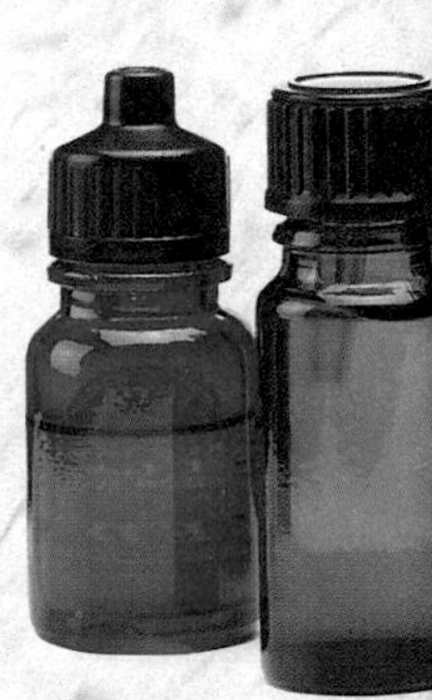

ESSENTIAL OILS

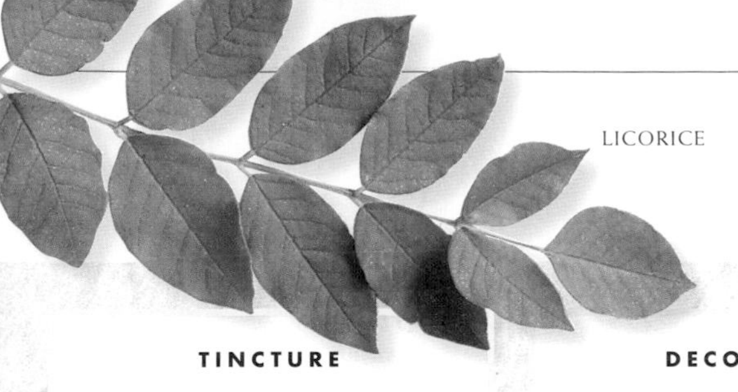

LICORICE

SUNFLOWER OIL

TINCTURE

Powdered, fresh, or dried herbs are placed in an airtight container with alcohol and left for a period of time. Alcohol extracts the valuable or essential parts of the plant and preserves them for the longest possible time.

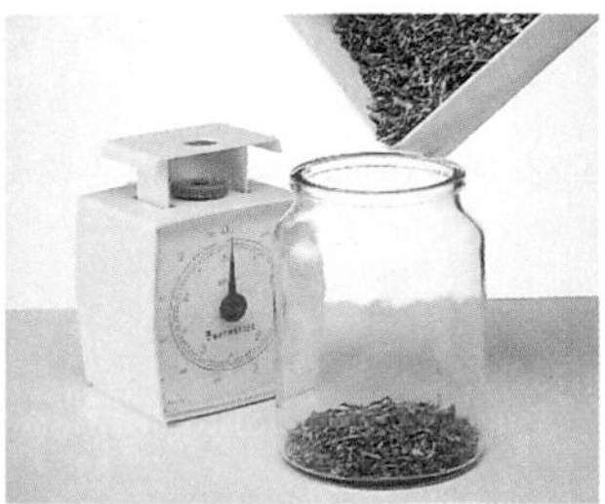

1 You can make your own tincture at home by crushing the parts of the plants you wish to use (about 1oz. [25g.] will do).

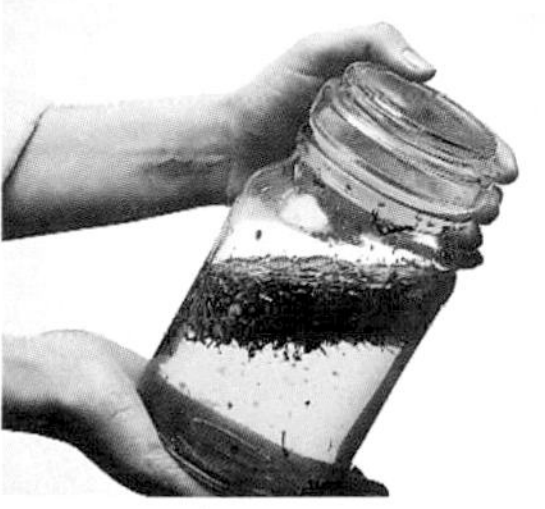

2 Suspend the plants in alcohol (about 1–1⅓pt. [600ml.] of vodka or any 40 percent spirit) for about two weeks, shaking occasionally. Dried or powdered herbs (about 4oz. [100g.]) may also be used, with the same amount of alcohol.

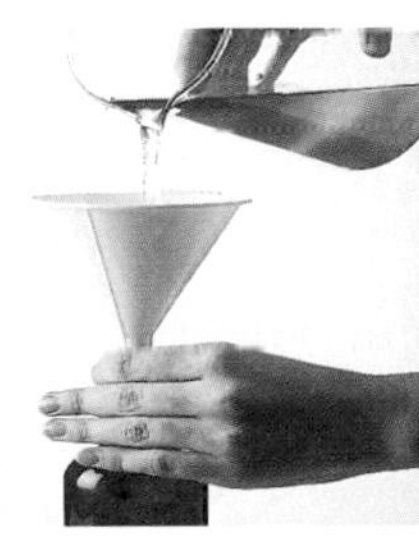

3 After straining, the tincture should be stored in a dark glass airtight jar. Doses are usually 5–20 drops, which can be taken directly or added to water.

DECOCTION

The roots, twigs, berries, seeds, and bark of a plant are used, and much like an infusion, they are boiled in water to extract the plants' ingredients. The liquid is strained and taken with honey or brown sugar as prescribed.

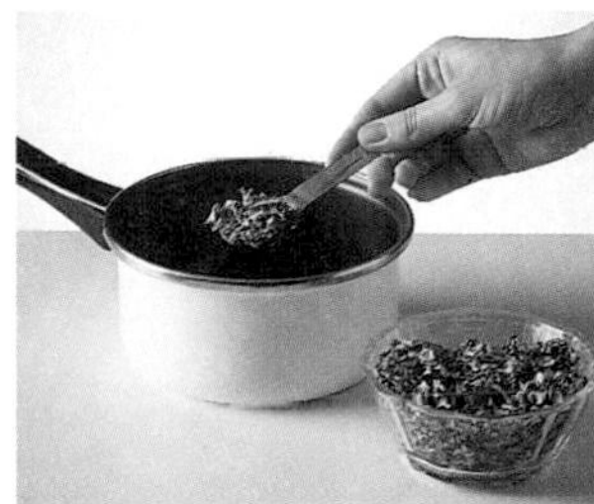

1 Put 1 teaspoonful of dried herb or 3 teaspoonfuls of fresh herb (for each cup) into a pan. Fresh herbs should be cut into small pieces.

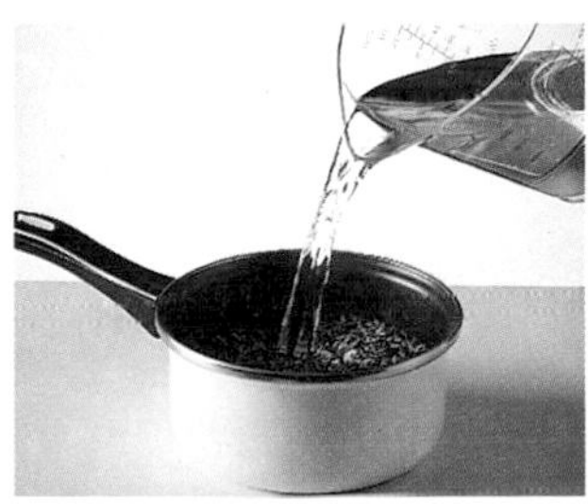

2 Add some water to the herbs. If making large quantities, use 1oz. (30g.) dried herb for each 1pt. (500ml.) of water. The container should be glass, ceramic, or earthenware. Metal pans should be enameled. Do not use aluminum.

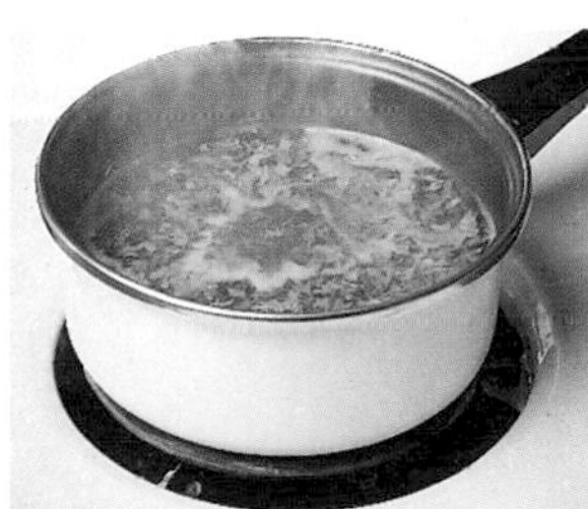

3 Bring to the boil and simmer for 10–15 minutes. If the herb contains volatile oils, cover the pan. Strain, cool, and refrigerate. The decoction will keep for about three days.

INFUSION

Effectively another word for tea, an infusion uses dried herbs, or in some instances fresh, which are steeped in boiled water for about 10 minutes. Infusions may be drunk hot, which is normally best for medicinal teas, or cold, with ice.

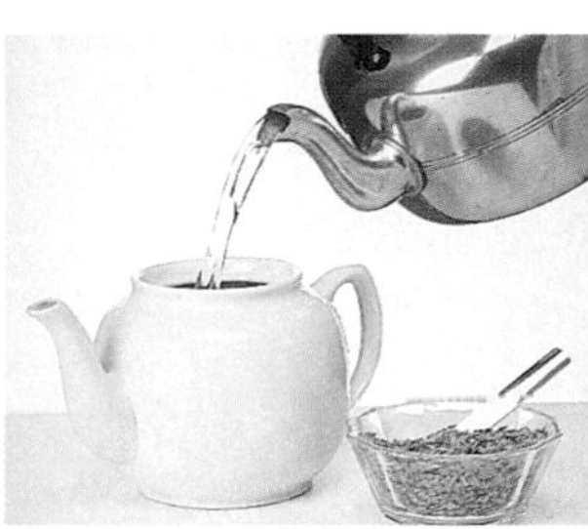

1 Put 1 teaspoonful of the herb or herb mixture into a china or glass teapot, for each cup of tea that is required. Add boiling water.

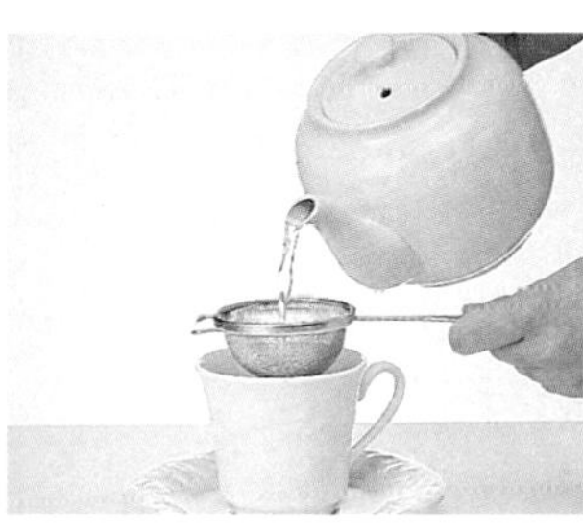

2 Add 1 cup of boiling water to the pot for each teaspoonful of herb that has been used. Keep the pot covered and always use the purest water available, which will ensure that the medicinal properties of the plant are effectively obtained. Strain the infusion and drink hot or cold either sweetened or unsweetened. Use licorice root, honey, or brown sugar to sweeten. Infusions should be made fresh each day, if possible. Infusions are most suitable for plants from which the leaves and flowers have been used, since their properties are more easily extracted by gentle boiling.

OINTMENT

For external use, ointments and creams are often prescribed. You can make your own by boiling the plant parts to extract the active properties, and adding a few ounces (grams) of pure oils (such as olive or sunflower).

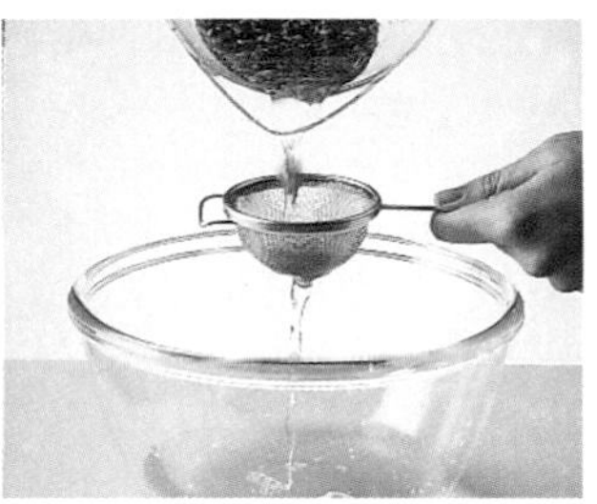

1 Make 1pt. (500ml.) of infusion or decoction (depending on what is appropriate for the herb), and strain. Reserve the liquid.

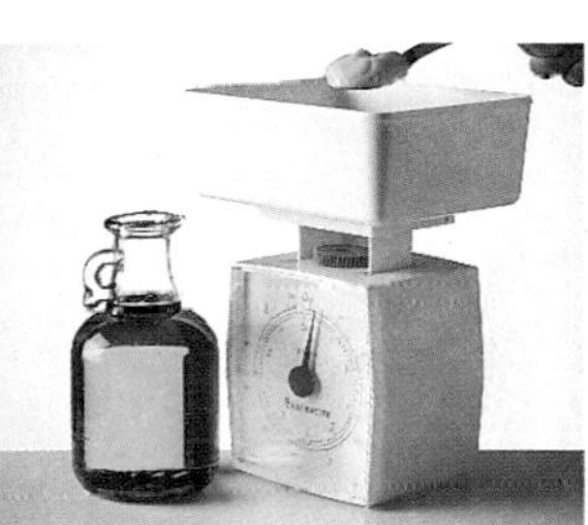

2 Pour 3fl.oz. oil (90ml.) into a pan. Mix 3oz. of fat into the oil. If a perishable base fat is used (such as lard), a drop of tincture of benzoin should be added for each 1oz. (30g.) of base. Add liquid.

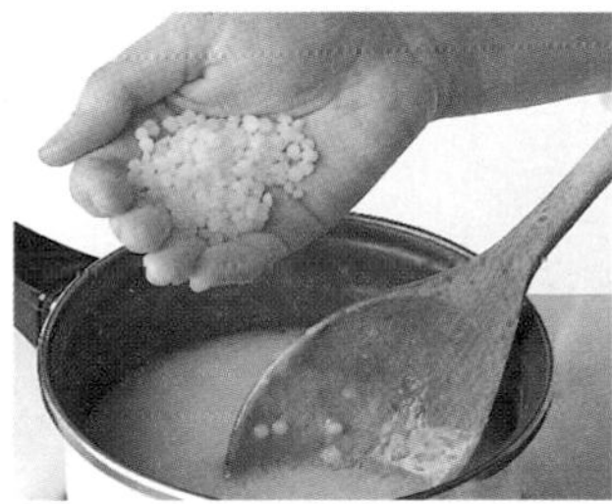

3 Simmer until the water has evaporated. Stiffen the mixture with a little beeswax or cocoa butter to make a cream. Melt in slowly.

OINTMENT

TRADITIONAL HOME AND FOLK REMEDY SOURCES

Allium cepa

ONIONS

The onion is by far the most important bulb vegetable in terms of its healing properties. It is used both in its green stage as a scallion, or green onion, and in its mature stage as a bulb – the tightly packed globe of food-storage leaves containing the volatile oil that is the source of the onion's pungent flavor. Thought to have originated in Asia, the onion has been cultivated since ancient times. The bulb of the onion is used in cooking and medicinally; like garlic, it warms the body and stimulates the circulation. Onions have long been considered the mainstay of every household remedy chest.

ABOVE *Grow your own: onions can be harvested 22 weeks after sowing.*

BELOW *Macerated raw onion can be used to heal a painful burn. It stimulates circulation and is antiseptic.*

DATA FILE

Properties

- Onions cause the body to "weep," which helps to release toxins
- Onion increases blood circulation and can relax the muscles
- Expectorant and diuretic
- Helps to reduce serum cholesterol after a fatty meal
- May provide some protection against cancer
- Antibiotic, draws out infection
- Warming
- Strengthens the lungs
- Cleanses the intestines and helps to maintain balance of bacteria

Uses

- Apply fresh onion to an abscessed tooth or a boil to draw out infection and help to encourage circulation to the area, which will facilitate quick healing.
- Mix onion juice with honey to relieve the symptoms of a cold.
- Taken daily, onions can help to prevent cancers of the digestive tract.
- The regular consumption of onions can reduce nervous debility.
- Onion poultices are used to treat bronchitis and can also help in the treatment of acne and boils.
- Onions are often recommended for gastric infections; onions will be effective cooked and raw.
- Use a poultice of roasted onion for earaches.
- Apply raw, macerated onions on sprains, bruises, and unbroken chilblains.
- Eat daily if you are at risk of heart disease or circulatory disorders.

Allium sativum

GARLIC

Garlic belongs to the onion family, and is one of the best-known and most-used medicinal plants. It has a strong odor, which many people find off-putting, but its health-giving and preventive properties make it well worth suffering the effects. Garlic has been shown to lower total serum cholesterol as well as LDL cholesterol in human clinical trials. Effective herbal preparations of garlic can be used at less cost and with fewer side-effects than most pharmaceutical drugs, and its use has recently been applauded by the conventional medical establishment.

DATA FILE

Properties

- Cleanses the blood and helps to create and maintain healthy bacteria population (flora) in the gut
- Helps to bring down fever
- Antiseptic
- Antibiotic
- Antifungal
- Tones the heart and circulatory system
- Boosts the immune system
- May help to reduce high blood pressure
- May prevent some cancers, in particular stomach cancer
- Treats infections of the stomach and respiratory system
- Helps prevent heart disease and reduces the risk of atherosclerosis
- Antioxidant
- Decongestant

Uses

- Fresh garlic, eaten daily, can reduce chronic acidity of the stomach.
- Eat crushed garlic for sexual debility.
- May help to reduce attacks of allergic asthma and hay fever.
- Garlic-infused oil can be used as a chest rub for respiratory or digestive ailments, or in the ear to reduce inflammation.
- Fresh garlic, eaten regularly, will reduce the need for antibiotics.
- Garlic syrup can be used to treat bronchitis, lung infections, and digestive disorders.
- Fresh garlic juice is antifungal, and can be applied neat to infections such as athlete's foot.
- Chew whole roasted garlic cloves to improve circulation.
- The intestinal tract can be cleansed by adding several mashed, raw garlic cloves to salads. Excellent in combination with red onion.

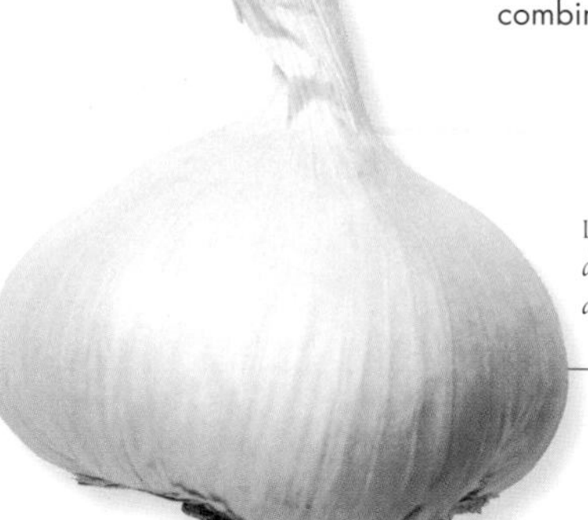

LEFT *Garlic bulbs are delicious roasted whole, as an unusual starter.*

TIP

THE SMELL OF GARLIC ON THE BREATH CAN BE REDUCED BY EATING AN APPLE, DRINKING A LITTLE FRESH LEMON JUICE, OR EATING FRESH PARSLEY.

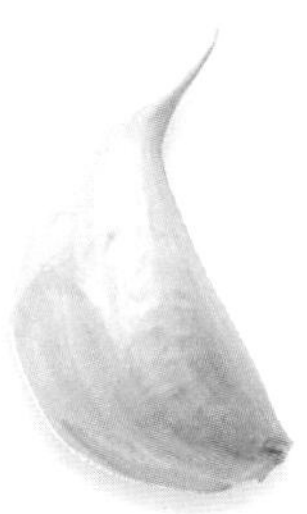

GARLIC SYRUP

Garlic syrup relieves bronchitis, and lung infections. You need some honey and a fresh garlic bulb.

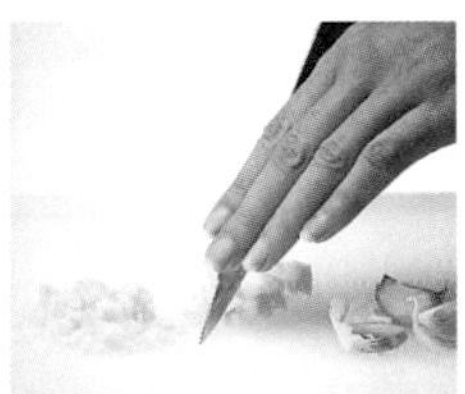

Peel and chop 6–8 cloves of fresh garlic.

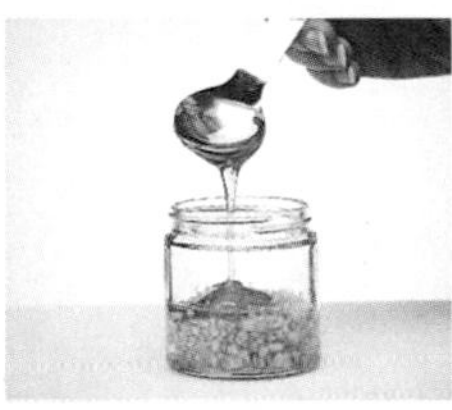

Place the chopped garlic in a jar, and cover with 8 tablespoons of honey. Let it stand for several days, and then strain. The garlic-infused honey can be given by the teaspoonful (1 for children, 4 for adults) to boost the immune system and treat infections.

Apium graveolens

CELERY

Hippocrates, the father of medicine, wrote that celery could be used to calm the nerves, and, indeed, its very high calcium level is likely to be the reason for this phenomenon. The seeds, leaves, and edible root of the plant are used. Celery is best eaten raw, and its juice is particularly useful. The seeds are rich in iron and many vitamins, including A, B, and C, and can be used in the treatment of liver problems and high blood pressure.

ABOVE *Celery is a popular vegetable; the leaves may also be used in cooking.*

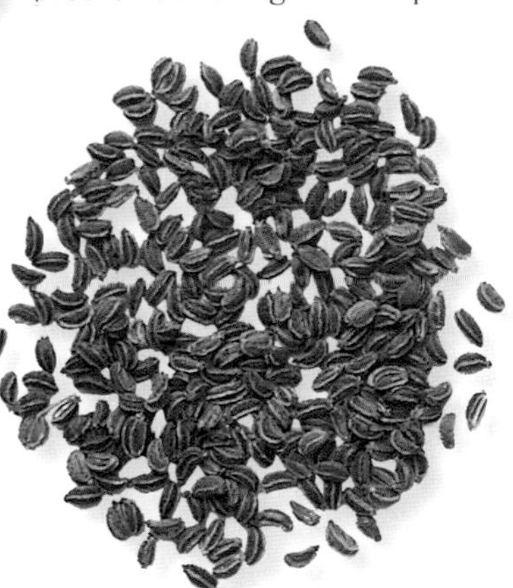

LEFT *Celery seeds are rich in vitamins and iron.*

CAUTION

BECAUSE CELERY MAY CAUSE THE UTERUS TO CONTRACT, IT SHOULD NOT BE EATEN DURING PREGNANCY.

DATA FILE

Properties

- Celery helps to reduce high blood pressure
- Digestive, reducing spasm in the muscle of the intestinal tract and acting as an anti-inflammatory agent
- Purifies the blood
- May help in the treatment of arthritis and rheumatic disorders; in Japan, rheumatic patients are sometimes put on a celery-only diet
- Celery seeds also have anti-inflammatory properties
- Stimulates the thyroid and pituitary glands
- Possibly antioxidant
- Celery clears uric acid from painful joints
- Acts on the kidneys and is a mild diuretic

Uses

- Eat the seeds to treat arthritis (for which they act as an anti-inflammatory) and to relieve muscle spasms (antispasmodic action).
- Grated, raw celery can be used as a poultice to apply to swollen glands.
- Raw, whole celery can be eaten regularly to reduce high blood pressure, and to act as a tonic for the liver.
- Celery juice or an infusion of celery seeds may be drunk to alleviate sciatica.
- Drink celery juice before meals to suppress the appetite. Chew celery seeds after a meal as a digestive.
- Celery root is said to be an aphrodisiac.

THERAPY CONNECTIONS

CELERY
Ayurveda p.29
Aromatherapy p.146

ONION
Ayurveda p.25
Homeopathy p.178

GARLIC
Ayurveda p.26
Herbalism p.113

CELERY TONIC

Celery seeds can be used to make a tonic that benefits the kidneys. You will need a bottle of brandy, and celery seeds.

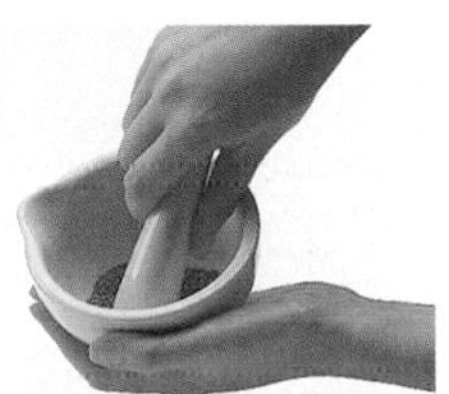

Steep 2 tablespoons of bruised celery seeds in 1pt. (500ml.) of brandy.

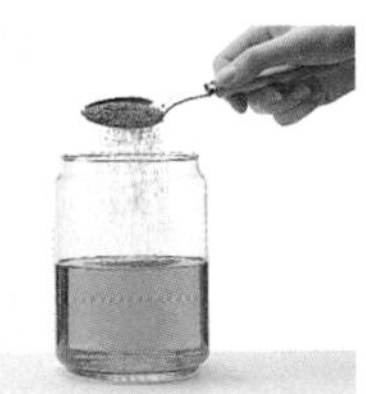

Take 1 tablespoon of the infused brandy, mixed with 2 tablespoons of water, three times daily.

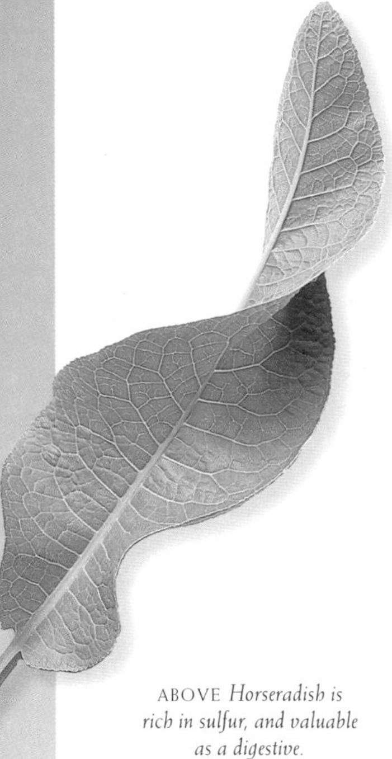
ABOVE *Horseradish is rich in sulfur, and valuable as a digestive.*

Armoracia rusticana

HORSERADISH

Horseradish is a member of the mustard family, and is native to southeastern Europe. It is widely cultivated for its pungent, fleshy root. Japanese horseradish, or wasabi (*Wasabid japonica*), is used both for cooking and for therapeutic purposes, and the grated rhizomes are often sold as a dry, green-colored powder. Horseradish root has been used for centuries in folk medicine, particularly to clear nasal passages. It also has a powerful diuretic effect.

CAUTION

TOO MUCH HORSERADISH TAKEN INTERNALLY CAN CAUSE NIGHT SWEATS, AND OCCASIONALLY DIARRHEA AND ABDOMINAL CRAMPING.

DATA FILE

Properties

- Diuretic
- Stimulant
- Clears nasal passages
- Warming
- Antiseptic
- Stimulates blood flow

Uses

- Apply tincture of horseradish root to skin eruptions, including those associated with acne, to draw out the infection and encourage healing.
- Add some horseradish root to your toothpaste to clean teeth effectively, kill bacteria, and control mouth ulcers.
- Eat fresh horseradish, mixed with a little lemon juice, for the relief of sinus infections and nasal blockages.
- Eat freshly grated horseradish root for the edema and swelling associated with PMS.
- A horseradish poultice can be applied to chilblains and hemorrhoids to encourage healing and improve the circulation of the blood.
- Chronic rheumatism may respond to an old remedy: eat tiny pieces of horseradish root without chewing, and continue for several weeks.

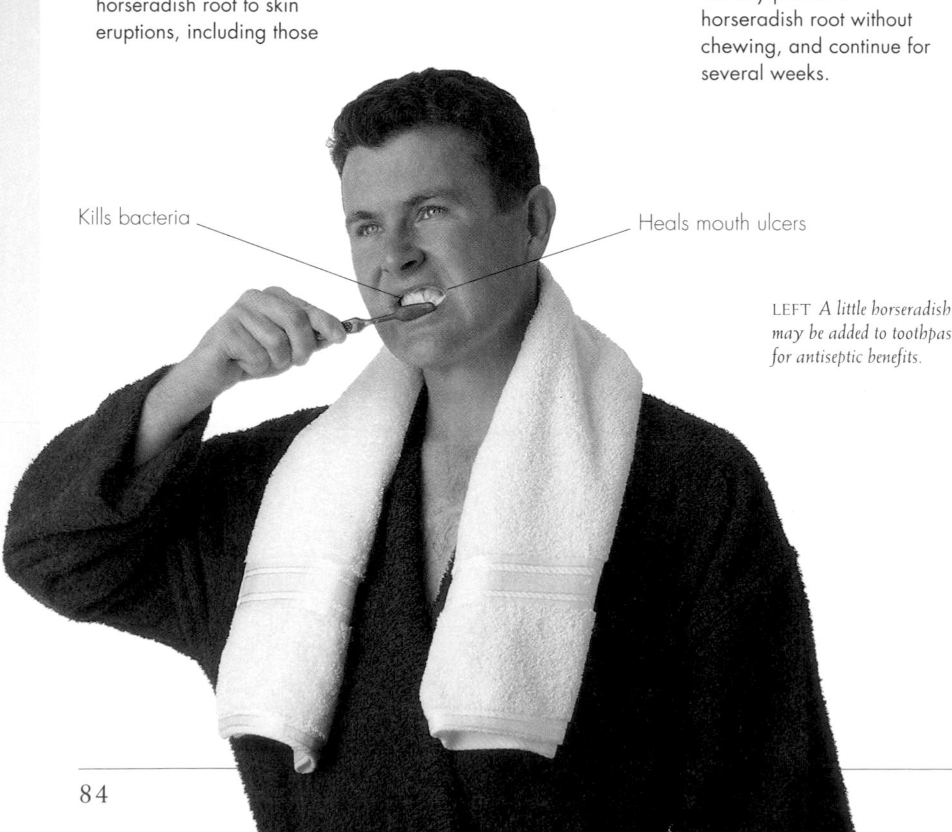

LEFT *A little horseradish may be added to toothpaste for antiseptic benefits.*

Avena sativum

OATS

Oats are a cereal plant, and are both extremely nutritious and useful therapeutically. Oats are one of the best sources of inositol, which is important for maintaining optimum blood cholesterol levels. Eaten daily, they provide a wealth of excellent effects.

DATA FILE

Properties

- A tonic for general debility, and used in the treatment of anorexia, also helpful for convalescence and fatigue
- Oats lower blood cholesterol levels
- Oats help to control hormonal activity
- Cleansing – internally and externally; may protect against bowel cancer when taken internally
- Used in the treatment of eczema
- Extremely rich in B vitamins and minerals
- Antidepressant, and can be used to treat depression, stress, and nervous disorders
- Often used in the treatment of addictions

Uses

- Eat raw oats as a source of fiber to ease constipation.
- Oatmeal (unrefined) can be eaten on a regular basis to reduce the effects of stress and nervous disorders.
- Cooked oats will relieve fatigue.
- A compress of oatmeal or an oatmeal bath soothes eczema and other problem skin conditions.
- Boil a tablespoon of oats in ½pt. (250ml.) of water for several minutes and drain; use as a nerve tonic and for its nourishing properties.
- Use the tincture for stress, addictions, eating disorders, and depression.
- Eat oats daily to lower blood cholesterol and to experience tonic effects.

CAUTION

OATS CONTAIN GLUTEN WHICH CAUSES AN ALLERGIC REACTION IN SOME INDIVIDUALS.

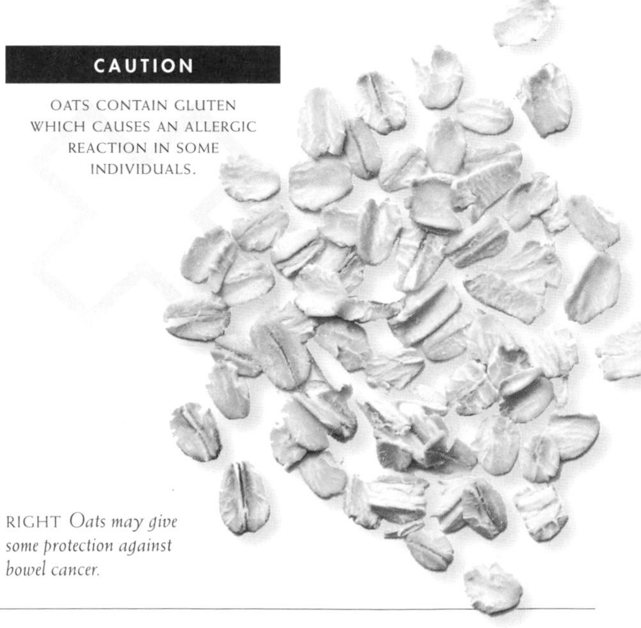
RIGHT *Oats may give some protection against bowel cancer.*

Asparagus officinalis

ASPARAGUS

A herbaceous perennial of the *Liliaceae* family, asparagus is cultivated for its tender shoots, which appear in early spring. In 1806 the French chemist Louis Nicolas Vauquelin, who discovered the elements chromium and beryllium, isolated asparagine, the first amino acid to be discovered, from the asparagus plant. Asparagus is a liver tonic, and promotes elimination (through the urine).

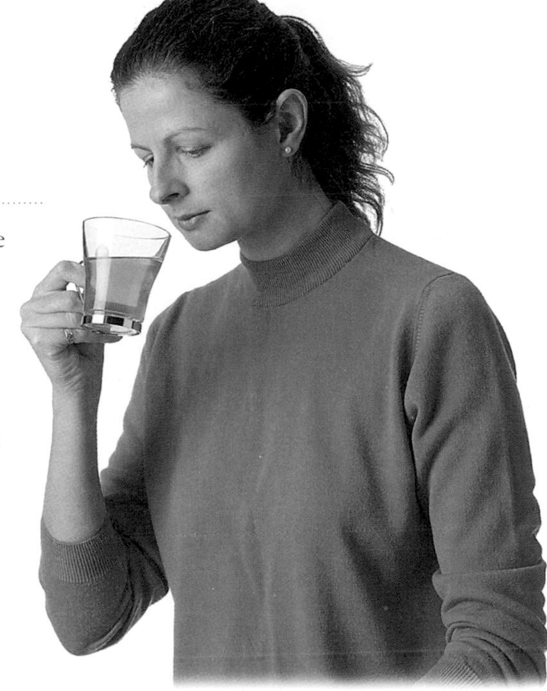

ABOVE *The water left after cooking asparagus treats urinary problems.*

CAUTION

ASPARAGUS IS HIGH IN PURINES, AND ANYONE SUFFERING FROM GOUT SHOULD AVOID IT.

DATA FILE

Properties

- Encourages the flow of urine, making asparagus a useful diuretic
- Acts as a tonic to the liver
- Aids digestion
- May help control the symptoms of PMS, including breast tenderness and abdominal bloating

Uses

- Drink asparagus water (the water remaining after steaming asparagus spears) for urinary complaints, arthritis, and rheumatism.
- Freshly cooked asparagus will tonify the liver, and may be used in cases of liver congestion and conditions such as hepatitis to encourage healing.
- Asparagus tincture can be added to food and drinks to encourage the elimination of urine.

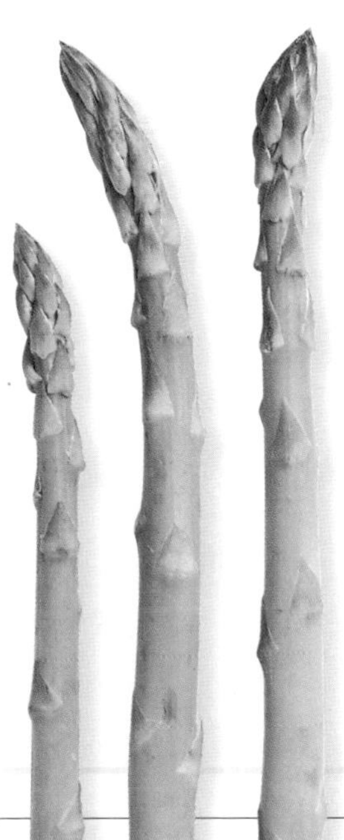

ASPARAGUS

Brassica oleracea

CABBAGE

Cabbage has traditionally been used for medicinal purposes as well as for cooking. It has anti-inflammatory properties, and contains chemicals which can prevent cancer. The ancient Greeks used fresh white cabbage juice to relieve sore or infected eyes, and juice from the cabbage stem is a good remedy for ulcers. Traditionally, the Romans and Egyptians would drink cabbage juice before big dinners to prevent intoxication; cabbage seeds are said to prevent hangovers.

DATA FILE

Properties

- An excellent anti-inflammatory
- Cabbage contains lactic acid, which acts to disinfect the colon
- Used to reduce the pain of headaches and rheumatic disorders
- Soothes eczema and other itching or weeping skin conditions
- Anticancer
- Draws out infection
- Red cabbage leaves are the basic ingredient of a good cough syrup

Uses

- Make cabbage a regular part of your diet to reduce the risk of cancer.
- A cabbage poultice can be applied to boils and infected cuts to draw out the infection and disperse pus.
- Applied to bruises and swelling, macerated cabbage leaves will encourage healing.
- Dab white cabbage juice on mouth ulcers, and gargle for sore throats.
- A warm cabbage compress, on the affected area, reduces the pain of headaches and some kinds of neuralgia.
- Drink fresh cabbage juice daily to reduce the discomfort of gastric ulcers and bronchial infections.
- A cabbage leaf, lightly pounded, can be placed directly on the breast to relieve mastitis.
- Raw cabbage juice is said to be useful for the treatment of ulcers, psoriasis, chronic headaches, asthma, cystitis, and bronchitis. Drink 1–2fl. oz. (25–50ml.) daily to get the best effects.

ABOVE *Cabbage leaves are excellent for bringing down swelling and drawing out infection.*

CAUTION

DO NOT EAT RED CABBAGE RAW, BECAUSE THE HIGH LEVELS OF IRON CAN INTERFERE WITH GUT ABSORPTION AND IRRITATE THE GUT, CAUSING CONSTIPATION.

AVOID CABBAGE IF YOU SUFFER FROM GOITER, OR TAKE MAOI ANTIDEPRESSANTS.

RED CABBAGE (COOKED) CAN CAUSE CONSTIPATION AND IRRITATION OF THE COLON, DUE TO THE LARGE QUANTITIES OF IRON.

Camellia sinensis

TEA

Tea is the beverage made when the processed leaves of the tea plant are infused with boiling water. Native to Southeast Asia, the tea plant is a small, shrub-like, evergreen tree that belongs to the family *Theaceae*; its seeds contain a volatile oil, and its leaves contain the chemicals caffeine and tannin. Green tea is made from the tips, or shoots, of the shrub *Camellia sinensis*; black tea is made from the fermented dried leaves. An essential oil, called tea absolute, is distilled from black tea. Both the leaves and the oil are used for medicinal purposes. Fruit teas do not actually contain tea but can also be beneficial to the health.

ABOVE *Tea also contains caffeine, which is a stimulant.*

DATA FILE

Properties

- Provides folic acid (vitamin B9), some potassium, and also magnesium
- Contains fluoride (a trace)
- Acts on the nervous system to control the respiratory and digestive systems
- Diuretic and astringent
- Antioxidants called polyphenols have beneficial effects on the circulatory system, while flavonoids act on the immune system
- Tannins may help to prevent heart disease and halt the course of, and prevent, some cancers

Uses

- The fluoride in tea may be beneficial in preventing dental caries.
- Tea may help in the treatment of diarrhea, dysentery, hepatitis, and gastroenteritis.
- The flavonoids contained in tea may destroy harmful bacteria and viruses.
- Cold, steeped tea bags placed over the eyes will soothe soreness and irritation. Tea's astringent properties also make tea bags useful for treating minor injuries and insect bites.
- The leaves of green and black tea may be beneficial in the prevention of heart disease and stroke.
- Raspberry leaf tea is a well-known tonic when taken during pregnancy. It also helps prepare the breasts for breast-feeding.
- Green tea may help to prevent cancer if it is drunk on a regular basis.

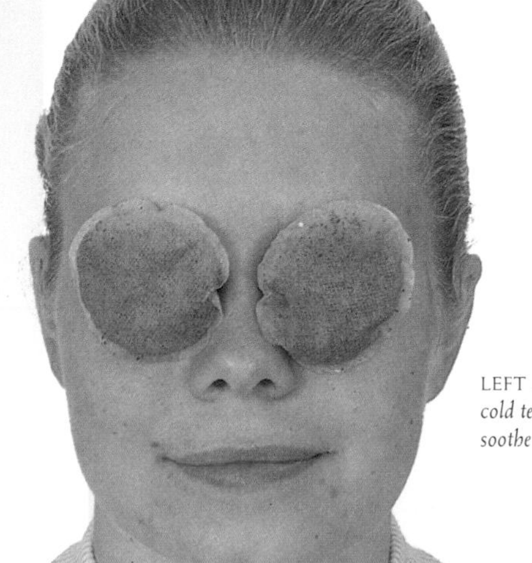

LEFT *A resourceful use of cold tea bags! They will soothe sore eyes.*

CAUTION

TEA CAN INTERFERE WITH THE EFFECTIVENESS OF DRUGS SUCH AS ALLOPURINOL (FOR THE TREATMENT OF GOUT), ANTIBIOTICS, ANTIULCER DRUGS, AND THE DRUG THEOPHYLKLINE, PRESCRIBED FOR ASTHMA.

IT CAN PREVENT THE ABSORPTION OF IRON AND INTERFERE WITH THE EFFECTIVENESS OF SEDATIVE DRUGS.

DRINKING TEA TO EXCESS CAN CAUSE CONSTIPATION, INDIGESTION, DIZZINESS, PALPITATIONS, IRRITABILITY, AND INSOMNIA.

Capsicum annuum var. annuum

RED PEPPER

The red pepper is also known variously as bell pepper, sweet pepper, and capsicum. It is one of five different types (grossum type) of Capsicum *annuum* var. *annuum*; the peppers from which the spices cayenne and chili are produced are longum peppers. Red peppers, which are the ripened fruit (some varieties ripen to yellow or purple), are used in the manufacture of paprika, cayenne, and chili powder. Green peppers are immature fruit. Other related peppers used for culinary and therapeutic purposes include *C. baccatum*, *C. chines* and *C. frutescens*, the Tabasco or hot pepper.

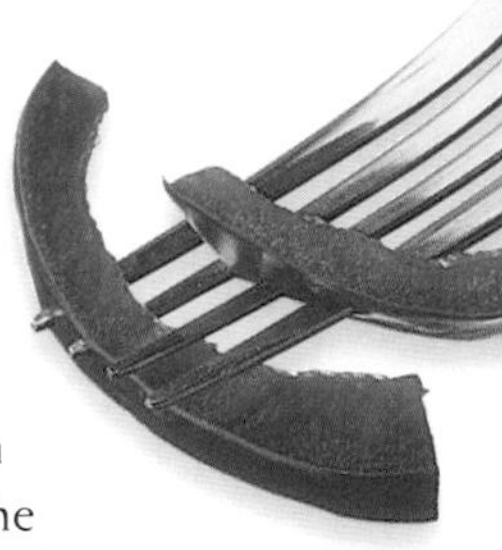

ABOVE *Peppers are rich in vitamins A and C. Add them to salads.*

CAUTION

PUNGENT PEPPERS SUCH AS CHILI PEPPERS MAY CAUSE SKIN IRRITATION AND PAINFUL INFLAMMATION WHEN USED IN EXCESS OR WHEN IN CONTACT WITH THE EYES AND BROKEN SKIN.

THE SEEDS ARE PARTICULARLY POWERFUL. STRONG PEPPERS MAY ALSO TEMPORARILY IRRITATE THE URINARY SYSTEM AS THE OILS ARE EXCRETED IN URINE.

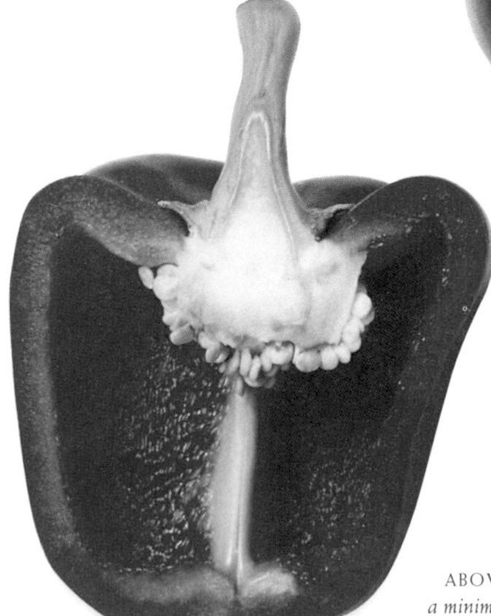

ABOVE *Peppers need a minimum temperature of 4°C (39°F) to grow.*

DATA FILE

Properties

- Peppers are an excellent source of vitamin C (a fresh green pepper contains 10 percent vitamin C)
- All peppers also contribute small amounts of iron and vitamin A: the largest amounts of vitamin A are found in fresh red peppers, while paprika and chili powder are also very rich in this vitamin
- Peppers are a good source of potassium, and have low levels of sodium and fiber
- They act as a tonic, have antiseptic effects, and are stimulating to the circulatory and digestive systems
- Peppers also have anesthetic properties

Uses

- Peppers increase perspiration and therefore have a cooling effect on the body.
- They may be effective in the treatment of varicose veins, asthma, and digestive complaints.
- Peppers reduce sensitivity to pain by irritating the tissues and increasing blood supply to the affected area, which then effectively numbs the pain.
- Cayenne acts as a tonic for those suffering from tiredness and cold. It can also induce a feeling of well-being. It is an expectorant and has been effective in treating catarrh and sinus problems.
- Peppers also help to eliminate various toxins from the body.

Citrus limon

LEMON

Lemons are the most widely grown acid species belonging to the citrus group of fruits. They rank third among all citrus fruits in tonnage produced, and have been used for generations for their therapeutic properties. Lemons are rich in vitamin C, and have a cleansing effect on the digestive system. They have a wide range of therapeutic properties, making them the mainstay of any good home remedy chest. The leaves and the whole fruit may be used, according to requirements.

THERAPY CONNECTIONS

LEMON

Aromatherapy *p.154*

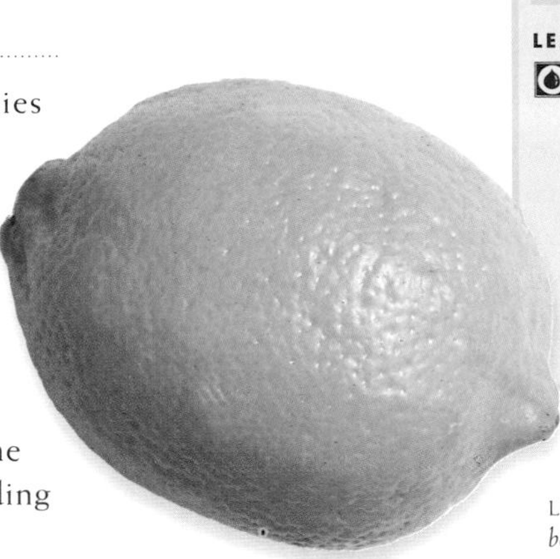

LEFT *Neat lemon juice can be dabbed on cold sores.*

DATA FILE

Properties

- Blood purifier, improves the body's ability to expel toxins; useful for skin problems like acne and boils
- Rich in vitamins B and C
- Antifungal
- Antacid
- Antiseptic
- Aids digestion
- One of the most powerful natural styptics; use on cuts and grazes to stop bleeding
- Antibacterial and antiviral properties. Lemons are excellent for halting the progression of infections
- Controls bladder and kidney infections

Uses

- The high potassium content of lemons will encourage the heart action, so lemons are a useful tonic for anyone with heart problems.
- Lemons are a natural insecticide and will discourage mosquitoes, black flies, and house flies.
- Drink fresh lemon juice (lemon in hot water will do) to cleanse the system.
- Drink lemon juice in hot or warm water first thing in the morning as a liver tonic.
- Lemon juice taken in hot water will ease stomach acidity; when drunk before going to bed it may help to relieve cramp and "restless legs" syndrome.
- Lemon strengthens the immune system and helps relieve the symptoms of colds and flu. It can also be beneficial in the treatment of other infections.
- Add slices of lemon to food on a daily basis to strengthen the circulatory system.
- Apply pure lemon juice to a wasp sting to relieve the pain.
- Regular intake of fresh lemons may be useful in the treatment of hemorrhoids, and kidney stones; also for varicose veins.
- Drinking lemon juice mixed with olive oil may help to dissolve gallstones.
- To help cure cold sores, put a few drops of undiluted lemon juice on the affected area. Repeat several times a day until the sore goes.
- A drop of lemon juice will also benefit ulcers on the tongue and in the mouth.

BELOW *For a lemon drink, boil 3 sliced lemons in 1pt. (600ml.) water, until the liquid is reduced by half. Add honey to taste.*

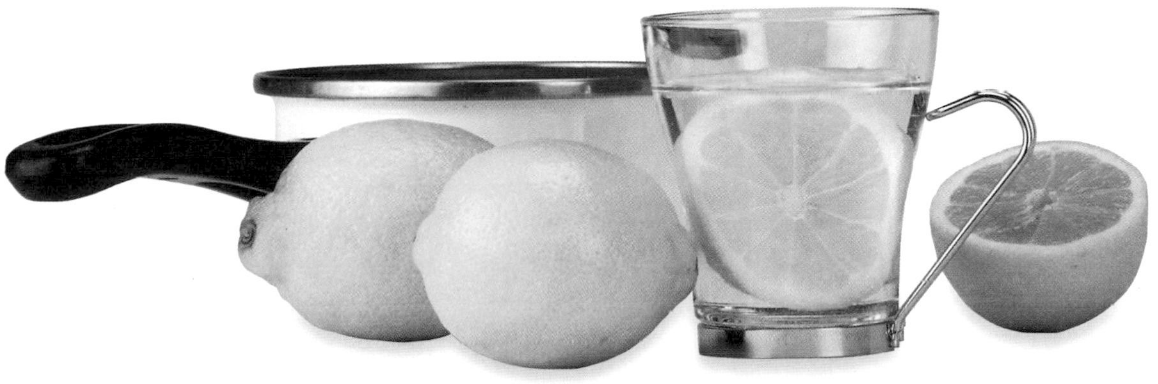

Citrus paradisi

GRAPEFRUIT

The grapefruit is an evergreen tree, *Citrus paradisi*, of the *Rutaceae* family, and its fruit is the largest of the commercially grown citrus fruits. Like all citrus fruit, grapefruit is rich in vitamin C and potassium. Pink grapefruit is rich in vitamin A, and acts as a natural antioxidant. Grapefruit is an excellent cleanser for the digestive and urinary systems, and the peel has many therapeutic properties.

THERAPY CONNECTIONS

GRAPEFRUIT

Aromatherapy *p.155*

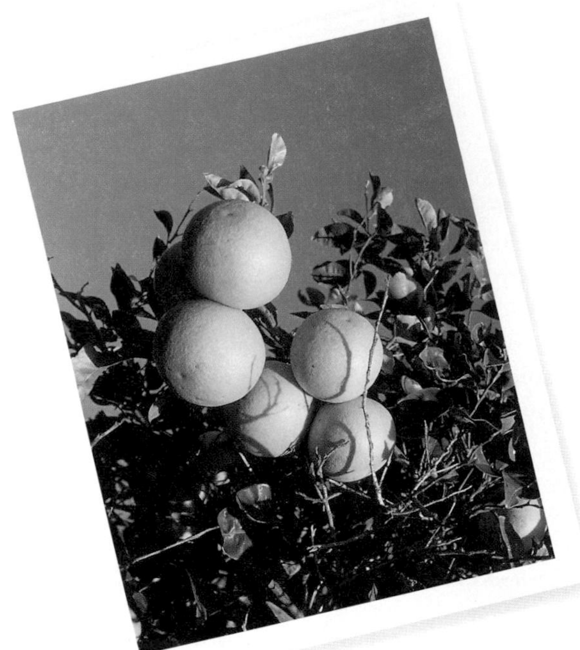

LEFT *Citrus requires a temperature of 15–30°C to grow well.*

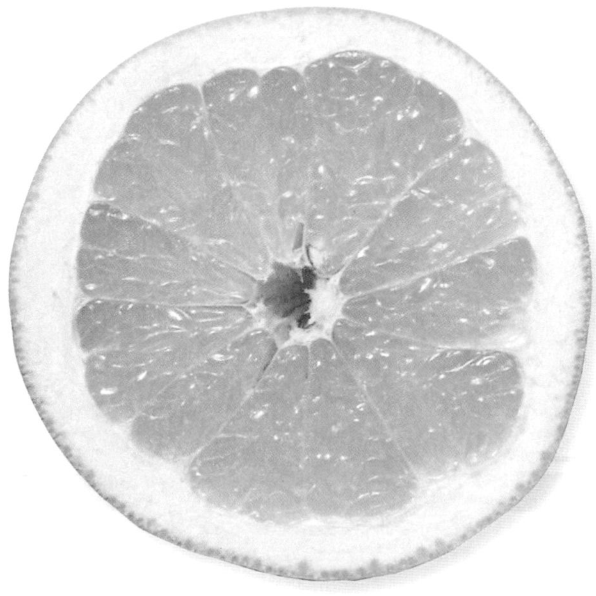

LEFT *Start the day the healthy way. Grapefruit is high in vitamin C and helps ward off colds.*

Properties

- Grapefruit cleanses the digestive and urinary systems, and is therefore often recommended by naturopaths
- Reduces appetite
- Aids in the breakdown of fats in the body
- Strengthens the respiratory system and aids respiration
- Invigorating tonic
- Relieves symptoms of colds and flu
- May help in the treatment of osteoarthritis
- Helps to balance the nervous system

Uses

- Eat grapefruit seeds to rid the body of worms.
- Grapefruit pith and membranes lower cholesterol in the blood.
- Drinking grapefruit juice can encourage healthy skin; used in the treatment of acne for its mild exfoliating properties.
- Grapefruit juice cleanses the kidneys and helps to eliminate toxins from the body.
- Aromatherapy massage with grapefruit oil is invigorating and uplifting, and may help to treat depression.
- Local massage, with a few drops of essential oil blended in a carrier oil, will relieve the severity of a headache.

DATA FILE

- Drinking grapefruit juice with iron supplements or foods rich in iron increases the absorption of iron in the body.
- Detoxifies the liver, and can ease chronic liver conditions. May help to reduce the severity of a hangover.
- Massage with grapefruit essential oil stimulates the immune system, which is particularly useful when suffering from infections.
- Used in steam inhalation or burnt in a room, grapefruit oil is beneficial in the treatment of colds, flu, and general respiratory problems.

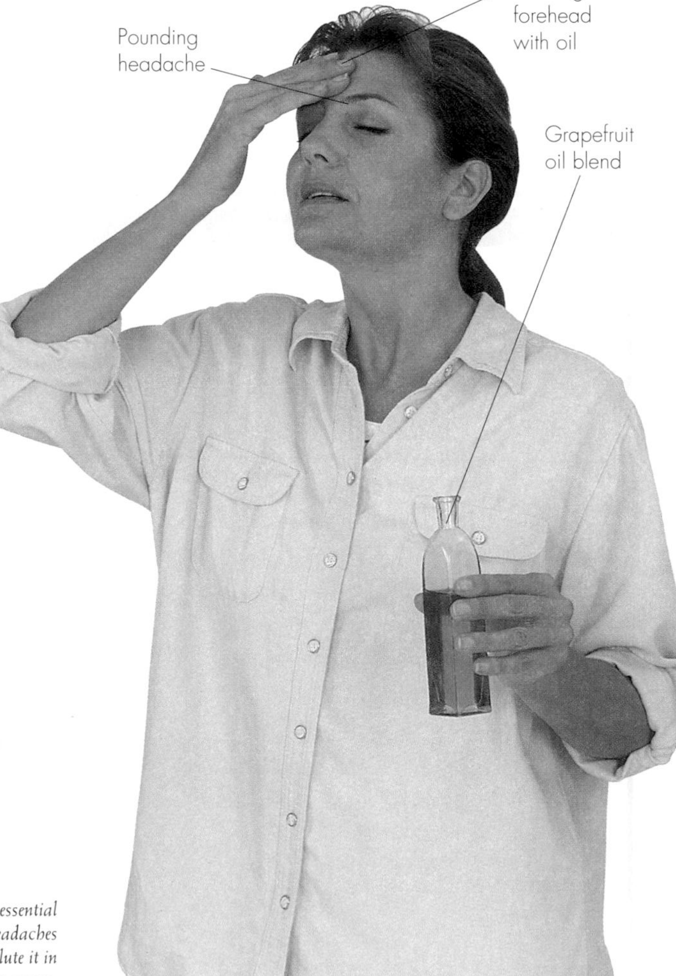

RIGHT *Grapefruit essential oil is excellent for headaches and hangovers. Dilute it in a carrier oil for massage.*

Cucumis sativis

CUCUMBER

The cucumber, *Cucumis sativis,* is a vine fruit that can be eaten fresh or pickled. A member of the *Cucurbitaceae* family, it is related to melons and squash. Cucumbers were native to northwestern India but have long been distributed throughout Asia, Europe, and Africa. Cucumber is a popular vegetable, which has been widely used in folk medicine to reduce heat and inflammation. It is a rich source of vitamin C, and can be used externally to cool and cleanse.

LEFT *To soothe the eyes, lie down for half an hour with a slice of cucumber on each eye.*

DATA FILE

Properties

- Diuretic
- Cooling
- Cleansing, particularly for skin disorders
- Used in the treatment of gout and arthritis
- Anti-inflammatory – soothes inflamed skin
- May help to treat lung and chest disorders
- Drink cucumber juice for inflammatory conditions such as arthritis

Uses

- Drink cucumber juice or eat fresh cucumber to soothe heartburn or to improve an acid stomach.
- Drink 3–5fl. oz. (100–150ml.) of cucumber juice every two hours for a gastric or duodenal ulcer.
- For strained or inflamed eyes, place a slice of cucumber on each eyelid to reduce swelling and soothe.
- Apply fresh cucumber or cucumber juice to sunburned skin to cool it down.
- Ground dried cucumber seeds are used to treat tapeworm.
- Cucumber juice, drunk daily, may help to control eczema, arthritis, and gout.
- Skin conditions respond to cucumber. Include fresh cucumber in your diet as much as possible.
- Cucumber juice acts as a kidney tonic.
- Use cucumber ointment externally on inflammatory skin conditions.
- Fresh cucumber juice, or the whole raw vegetable, is a mild diuretic and is cleansing. Use to treat lung and chest infections, and to bring down fever.

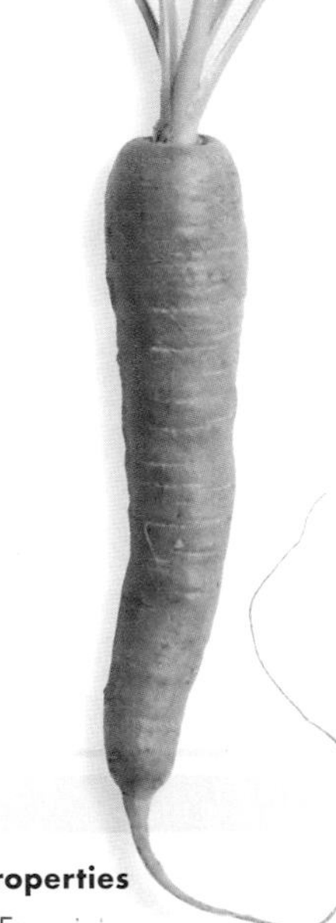

Daucus carota

CARROT

The carrot is a member of the *Umbelliferae* family, which also includes celery and parsnip. Carrots were first used as medicinal herbs rather than as vegetables, and they have the dual purpose of acting as therapeutic agents, and providing the best source of beta carotene (a form of vitamin A) in the human diet. They are rich in vitamins A, B, C, and E, and the minerals phosphorus, potassium, and calcium. Chinese medical practitioners suggest eating carrots for Liver energy.

DATA FILE

Properties

- Energizing
- Carrot cleanses the system of impurities
- Contains calcium, which will encourage health of skin, hair, and bones
- May help in the treatment of eye problems
- Useful in the treatment of respiratory conditions
- Carrot may help to relieve skin disorders
- May help to overcome many glandular disorders
- Taken daily, carrots may help to regulate the menstrual cycle
- Anti-inflammatory
- Antiseptic

CAUTION

EATING AN EXCESSIVE QUANTITY OF CARROTS MAY CAUSE THE SKIN TO YELLOW TEMPORARILY.

CARROT SEEDS ARE A NERVE TONIC AND WILL ALSO INDUCE ABORTION; AVOID DURING PREGNANCY.

Uses

- Drink fresh, raw carrot juice daily to energize and cleanse the body. It will help to relieve the effects of stress, and fatigue, and boost the body after illness.
- Carrot soup is a traditional home remedy for infant diarrhea – it soothes the bowel and slows down bacterial growth.
- Raw, grated carrots or cooked, mashed carrots can be applied to wounds, cuts, inflammations, and abscesses to discourage infection and encourage healing.
- Dried carrot powder will restore energy, and can help to treat infections, glandular problems, headaches, or joint problems
- The antioxidant *(see Glossary, page 472)* qualities of carrots will help to prevent some of the damage caused by smoking.

Relieves stress
Improves skin
Traditionally recommended for eyes
Treats glandular problems

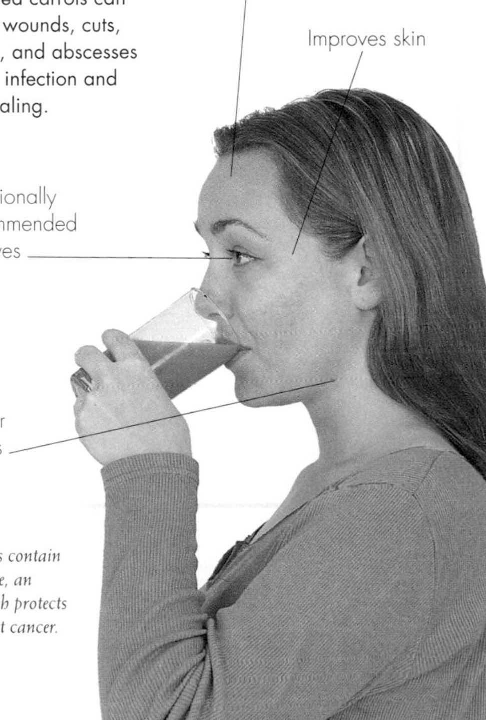

ABOVE *Carrots contain beta carotene, an antioxidant which protects the body against cancer.*

RIGHT *Make your own carrot juice daily for a cleansing, nutritious, energizing drink.*

Eugenica caryophyllata

CLOVES

Cloves are the dried buds of a tree of the myrtle family, *Syzygium aromaticum*. The tree, which may reach a height of 40ft. (12m.), produces abundant clusters of small red flower buds that are gathered before opening and dried to produce the dark brown, nail-shaped spice, clove. Whole and ground cloves used as food seasonings account for half the world production of cloves. Ground cloves are also used in a type of tobacco popular in Asia. Almost 20 percent of the clove's weight is essential oil, obtained by distilling, and used in perfumes, blends of spices, medications, and candies.

CAUTION

CLOVES CAN CAUSE UTERINE CONTRACTIONS, AND SHOULD NOT BE USED IN PREGNANCY.

DATA FILE

Properties

- Antiseptic and powerfully analgesic – particularly to the gums and teeth
- Cloves are warming, and useful for people who are prone to colds
- Anti-inflammatory, when used locally on swellings
- Cloves are calming to the digestive system
- Eliminate parasites from the body

Uses

- Oil of cloves can be placed directly on a sore tooth or mouth abscess to draw out the infection and ease the pain. Chew cloves for the same effect.
- Dab a tiny amount of neat oil on insect bites.
- Clove tea is warming, and can encourage the body to sweat, which is helpful for high fever or vomiting.
- Oil of cloves may be used during a long labor to hasten birth.
- Clove tea can be used to soothe wind and ease nausea – particularly the nausea of travel sickness.
- Inhale an infusion of cloves to clear the lungs and refresh the airways.
- A clove and orange pomander can be hung in cupboards as an effective insect repellent.
- Steep cloves in boiling water and then simmer. Strain and use the remaining liquid as a mild sedative and to soothe an acid stomach.
- Clove tea may be used in the treatment of depression – a cup a day can be uplifting for sufferers.

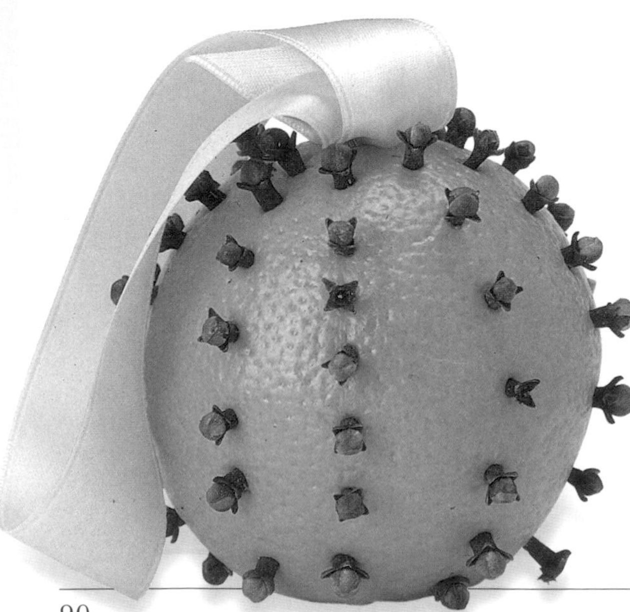

LEFT *Make a fragrant pomander by pushing cloves into an orange. Attach a piece of ribbon to hang it up.*

Ficus carica

FIG

Figs comprise a large family of deciduous and evergreen tropical and subtropical trees, shrubs, and vines belonging to the mulberry family, *Moraceae*. The most important fig is *Ficus carica*, the tree that produces the edible fig fruit. Figs are a nutritious and sustaining food, with a long history of medicinal use. For example, there are several references in the bible to figs being used to treat infections.

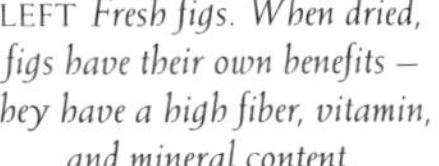

LEFT *Fresh figs. When dried, figs have their own benefits – they have a high fiber, vitamin, and mineral content.*

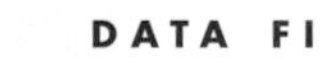

DATA FILE

Properties

- Highly alkaline
- Contains a powerful healing agent
- Soothes mucous membranes, particularly in the respiratory system
- The stem of the fresh fruit is antifungal, and can be used to treat warts
- Anticancer
- Contains ficin, which aids the digestion
- Contains a bactericide
- Reduces body heat, and helps to ease inflammation

Uses

- Eat dried figs to ease constipation.
- To bring a boil to a head, split a fig, heat it, and place it directly on the boil – this is a particularly good method for treating boils and ulcers in the mouth.
- Fig juice can be drunk daily as a cancer preventive.
- Digestive troubles can be eased by eating fresh figs after light meals or just prior to heavy meals.
- Roasted figs can be used as a poultice on boils and hemorrhoids in order to encourage healing and to draw out infection.
- Fresh figs can soothe respiratory ailments by acting as an anti-inflammatory agent.
- Boil four or five fresh figs in about 1pt. (500ml.) of water; bring to the boil, strain, cool, and drink the liquid for sore throats.

Glycyrrhiza glabra

LICORICE

Licorice is a pretty blue-flowered perennial, grown mainly in Europe. The roots are crushed, ground, and boiled to extract the juice, which is then thickened to produce hard black sticks of paste known as black sugar. The bittersweet flavoring is used in candy and tobacco, as a soothing ingredient in cough lozenges and syrups, as a laxative, and in the manufacture of shoe polish. Licorice is also an excellent source of iron.

LEFT *The leaves of the licorice plant, a perennial. The root of the plant is used for treatments.*

DATA FILE

Properties

- Expectorant and anti-inflammatory, making it excellent for stubborn coughs and lung infections
- Mild laxative
- Adrenal tonic
- Detoxifies the body. In the Far East, licorice is used to rid the body of poisons such as salmonella or as an antidote to overuse of drugs
- Raises blood pressure. Can be used in the treatment of low blood pressure
- Inhibits gastric secretions, making it useful in the treatment of gastric ulcers
- Stimulates the kidneys and the bowels

Uses

- Licorice syrup can be used to treat persistent coughs, and to reduce the incidence of asthma attacks.
- A strong infusion can protect against and heal ulcers. Drink it three times each day.
- Steep licorice root with a blend of other soothing herb teas to treat gastric disorders, and to stimulate kidneys and bowel.
- Used with other strengthening herbs such as ginseng for exhaustion.
- Licorice is used in creams or pastes for the relief of inflamed psoriasis and hot and weepy skin conditions.

CAUTION

LARGE DOSES OF LICORICE CAN CAUSE WATER RETENTION AND EXACERBATE HIGH BLOOD PRESSURE.

AVOID IN PREGNANCY.

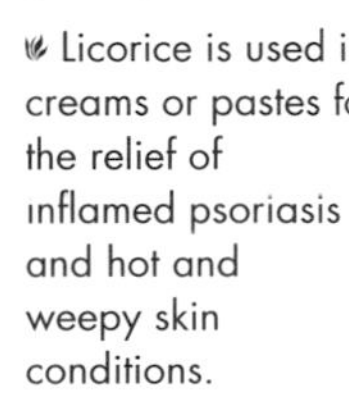

RIGHT *Children enjoy the taste of licorice. It is used to flavor candy and some medicines.*

THERAPY CONNECTIONS

CLOVES
Ayurveda p.38

LICORICE
Ayurveda p.39
Herbalism p.122
Chinese Herbal Medicine p.64

WITCH HAZEL
Herbalism p.123
Homeopathy p.197

Hamamelis virginiana

WITCH HAZEL

Witch hazel is a common tree grown in the U.S. Its leaves or roots are used for medicinal purposes. The common name arose as a result of the remarkable medicinal properties of the alcoholic extract from the leaves and bark of the plant, which is used on bruises and inflammations, and as a rubbing lotion.

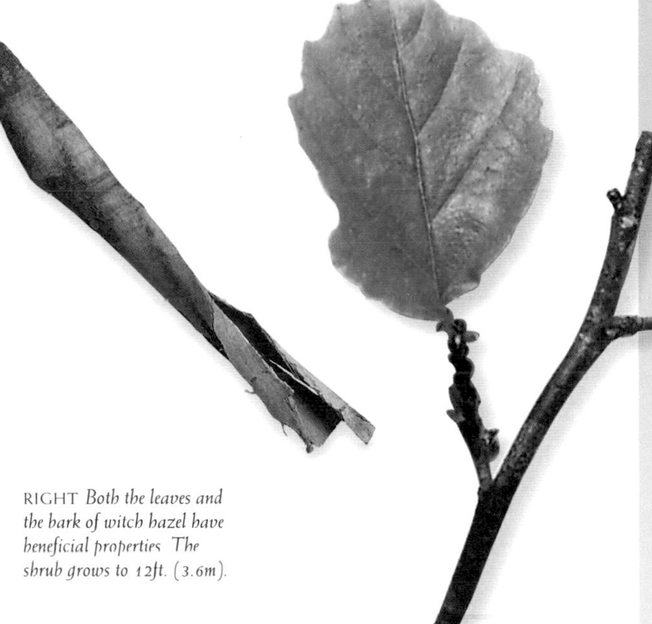

RIGHT *Both the leaves and the bark of witch hazel have beneficial properties. The shrub grows to 12ft. (3.6m).*

DATA FILE

Properties

- Analgesic
- Antiseptic – witch hazel can be used as a facial wash, and diluted to wash cuts and grazes
- Helps to control diarrhea when taken internally, and can encourage the health of the digestive tract
- Witch hazel soothes swellings, and reduces inflammation and bleeding, internally and externally
- Will encourage healing of bruises, sprains, and bleeding hemorrhoids

Uses

- Drink an infusion two or three times daily when there is inflammation (such as that of arthritis or rheumatism, sprains, or bruising) and for internal bleeding.
- Apply externally (as a decoction, tincture, or cream) for the treatment of bruising, hemorrhoids, or varicose veins.
- Use as a compress for sprains and strains.
- Dilute one part witch hazel to 20 parts boiled, cooled water, and use as an eyewash for sore and inflamed eyes.
- Add to the bath to reduce the aches and pains of rheumatic conditions.
- Witch hazel ointment can be used for painful joints, bruising (applied very gently), and local pain.

Hordeum sativum vulgare

BARLEY

Barley is rich in minerals (calcium and potassium) and B-complex vitamins, which makes it useful for convalescents or people suffering from stress. Barley has been used for its restorative qualities, in medicine and in cooking, for thousands of years. Malt is produced from barley.

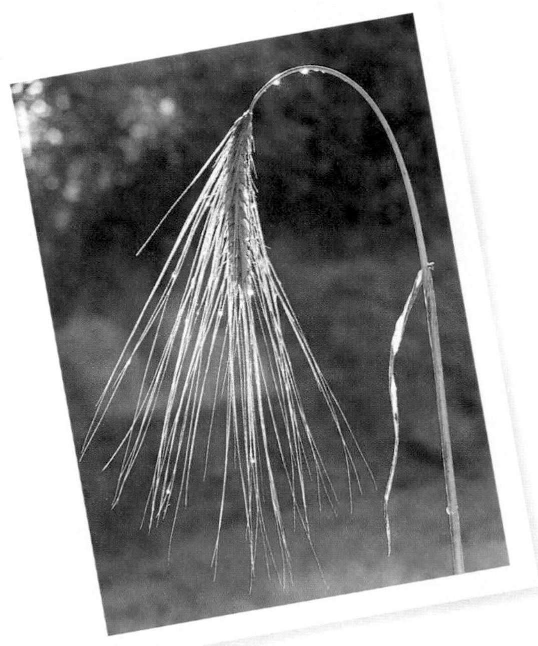

RECIPE

Barley Water

Add 2 tablespoons of pearl barley to 1pt. (500ml.) of water and boil for 10 minutes. Strain, and add barley to a fresh pint of water. Boil for another 10 minutes. Strain barley and serve water warm or cold, with lemon and honey.

ABOVE *Barley is a cereal crop cultivated for humans and animals.*

RIGHT *Barley water is delicious served with lemon. It helps relieve cystitis.*

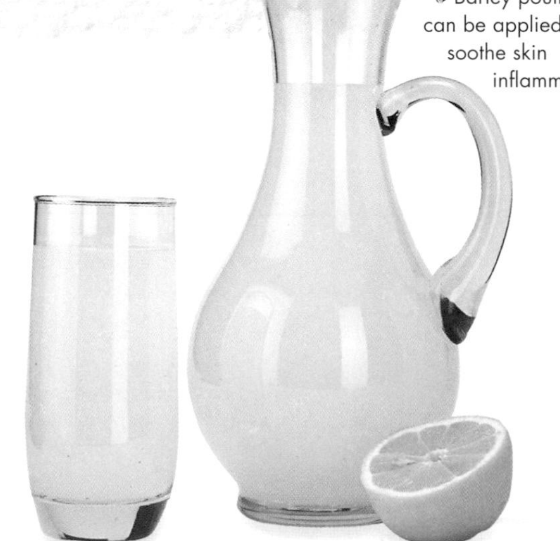

THERAPY CONNECTIONS

WALNUT

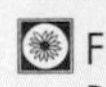 Flower Remedies p.232

DATA FILE

Properties

- Nutritious
- Anti-inflammatory, particularly to the urinary and digestive systems
- Used in the treatment of respiratory disorders
- Taken daily, it may lower cholesterol levels

Uses

- Barley water can be used in the treatment of respiratory disorders, and eases dry, tickling coughs.
- Barley water can be used for urinary tract infections and cystitis, and can ease flatulence and colic.
- Cooked barley is easily digested and nutritious, and is a traditional remedy for constipation and diarrhea.
- Barley water reduces acid in the spleen if drunk twice a day for a month.
- Make a poultice of barley flour to reduce inflammation of the skin.
- Barley may help to prevent heart disease, as it promotes the normal functioning of the heart and is able to stabilize blood pressure.
- Eat in soups and stews when convalescing.
- Barley poultices can be applied to soothe skin inflammation.

Juglans regia

WALNUT

Walnut is the common name for about 20 species of deciduous trees in the walnut family, *Juglandaceae*. The fruit has an outer leathery husk and an inner hard and furrowed stone, or nut. Walnuts are rich in protein, and high in potassium and other minerals such as zinc and iron. The bark of the walnut tree is used to treat gum disease, among other things.

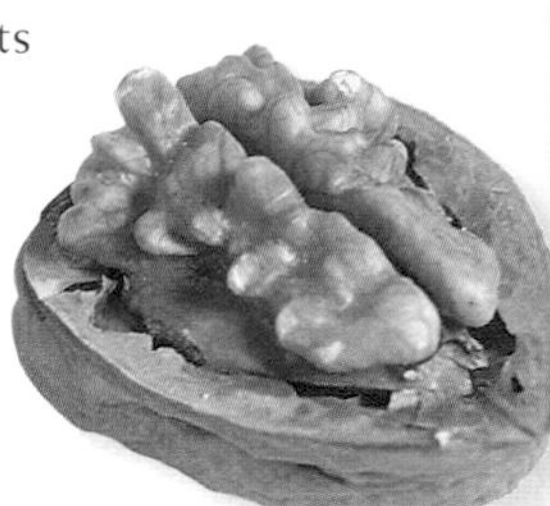

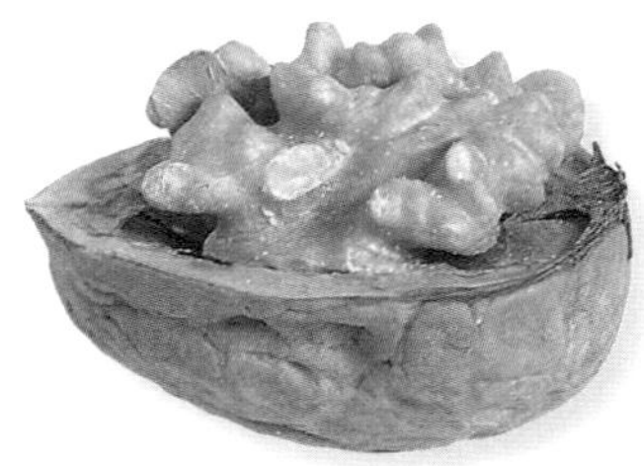

ABOVE *Walnuts are the fruit of a 50ft. (15m.) deciduous tree. Walnut leaves can be rubbed on a pet's coat to repel fleas.*

DATA FILE

Properties

- The bark of the walnut tree is astringent and cleansing
- Walnut bark strengthens the gums and acts as an anti-inflammatory
- The bark discourages milk flow in nursing mothers
- The nuts are aphrodisiac and mildly laxative
- The nuts prevent worms
- The nuts are soothing and a natural digestive

Uses

- Eat daily while convalescing to relieve fatigue and generally strengthen the body.
- Fresh walnuts and walnut oil can encourage circulation, and because they are rich in potassium, will keep the heart healthy.
- Add walnut bark to the bath for rheumatism, and sore and aching muscles and joints.
- Apply walnut bark tincture, in a little carrier oil, to swellings and skin problems, in order to encourage healing.
- Eat walnuts for heartburn and diarrhea.
- Fresh walnuts can help to soothe colic and dispel gas in the abdomen.
- Walnut oil, added to salads and vegetables, will help to ease the discomfort of irritable bowel syndrome and act as a mild laxative.

Lactobacillus

YOGURT

Yogurt is a fermented, slightly acidic food product made from milk. Its origins are unknown (although the name is Turkish), and it resembles the many other fermented milk foods made throughout the world, such as kefir and kumiss. Unlike many of these foods, however, yogurt is usually made from a concentrated milk and is soured by a specific bacillus, *Lactobacillus bulgaricus*. As a food, yogurt is a rich source of protein, and contains all of the vitamins and minerals found in milk. Live yogurt, which contains active bacteria, is most often used therapeutically, and should be eaten to increase the healthy bacteria in the body, to help it fight infection.

ABOVE *Make your own yogurt. Add 3 teaspoons of live yogurt to 1pt. (600ml.) milk. Leave to set.*

CAUTION

LIVE YOGURT IS NOT EFFECTIVE WHEN MIXED WITH SWEETENERS; FOR BEST EFFECT MAKE YOUR OWN YOGURT AND FLAVOR WITH A LITTLE UNPASTEURIZED HONEY AND A BANANA.

DATA FILE

Properties

- Live yogurt is antifungal, and can be used in the treatment of thrush
- Live yogurt may help to reduce cholesterol levels
- Encourages the growth of healthy bacteria in the bowels, which aids absorption of nutrients and helps to prevent infection
- Helps to produce vitamin B
- Yogurt stimulates bowel movements
- Helps to prevent and control the growth of cancerous cells
- Aids digestion

Uses

- Live yogurt should be eaten to increase beneficial bacteria following a course of antibiotics. Eat daily for two to three weeks.
- Apply live yogurt to areas affected by thrush; it can also be used internally as a douche.
- Daily intake of yogurt may prevent heart disease.
- Cleanse the skin with yogurt, which is a natural moisturizer.
- Eat live yogurt for chronic constipation and dyspepsia.
- Eat daily as a cancer preventive.

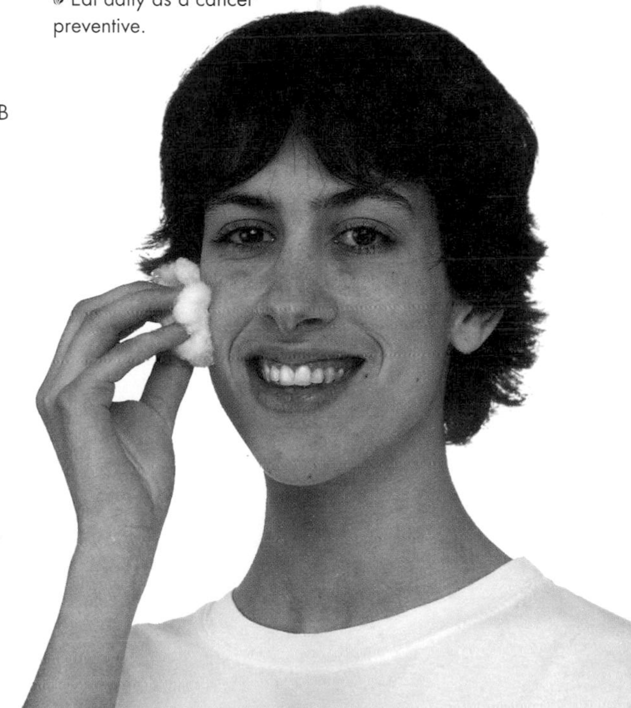

BELOW *Natural yogurt is a good facial cleanser and moisturizer. Apply to the skin with cotton wool*

Linum usitatissimum

FLAXSEED

Flax is a group of annual and perennial plants from the *Linaceae* family. Several varieties of one species, *L. usitatissimum*, are grown primarily for their fiber, used in making linen, or for their seeds, the source of linseed oil. The seeds contain a remarkable healing oil which can be used both internally and externally. Flaxseed is also known as linseed, but should not be confused with the "boiled" linseed oil available from building merchants. As far back as Hippocrates, flaxseed tea has been used to treat sore throats, hoarseness, and bronchial spasms.

CAUTION

COMMERCIALLY PRODUCED LINSEED OIL IS USED IN PROTECTIVE COATINGS SUCH AS PAINTS AND VARNISHES BECAUSE IT HAS A DRYING ACTION. IT IS NOT SUITABLE FOR HUMAN CONSUMPTION!

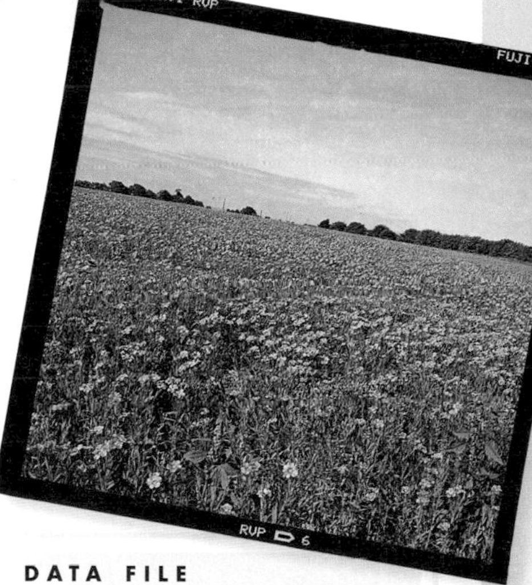

RIGHT *A field of flax grown for commercial purposes. Flax is used to make linen and linseed oil.*

DATA FILE

Properties

- Mildly laxative
- Tonic for the kidneys and encourages their action
- Encourages healing
- Analgesic
- Antispasmodic

Uses

- Apply the oil to sprains to reduce inflammation and ease the pain.
- Mix flaxseed with lime water to reduce the pain of burns.
- Flaxseed (linseed) tea can be used for mild constipation, and to encourage kidney function. The tea also works to ease kidney pains and cramping.
- The tea can be drunk during bouts of bronchitis to reduce inflammation of the lungs and prevent spasm.
- Add lemon and honey to flaxseed tea to encourage its action and improve taste.

Malus species, including Malus pumila

APPLE

The apple has many uses in traditional medicine, and the old adage "To eat an apple going to bed will make the physician beg his bread" has been justified by its many health-giving properties. Research shows that apples are excellent detoxifiers, and apple juice – even store bought – can destroy viruses in the body.

CAUTION

APPLE SEEDS CAN BE TOXIC WHEN TAKEN IN LARGE AMOUNTS.

DATA FILE

Properties

- Cleans teeth and strengthens gums
- Lowers cholesterol levels
- Antiviral action
- Detoxifies
- Protects from pollution, binding to toxins in the body and carrying them out
- Neutralizes indigestion
- Prevents constipation
- Soothing and antiseptic

Uses

- Eat raw apples regularly, as a detoxificant, for gout and rheumatism.
- To prevent viruses from settling in, and to reduce their duration, eat an apple (or drink a glass of apple juice) three times a day.
- Raw, peeled, and grated apples can be used as a poultice for sprains.
- For indigestion, heartburn, and other digestive disorders, eat an apple with meals.
- Use an apple poultice for treating rheumatic and weak eyes.
- Two apples a day can reduce cholesterol levels by up to 10 percent.
- As a treatment for intestinal infections, hoarseness, rheumatism, and fatigue, increase your daily intake to as much as 2lb. (1kg.).
- For curative purposes, as an alternative to eating the whole fruit, drink 1pt. (500ml.) of naturally sweet apple juice a day.
- Grated apple, mixed with live yogurt, may be helpful in cases of diarrhea.

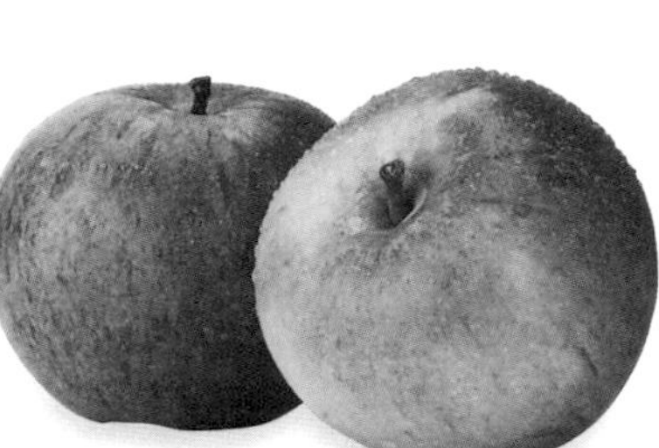

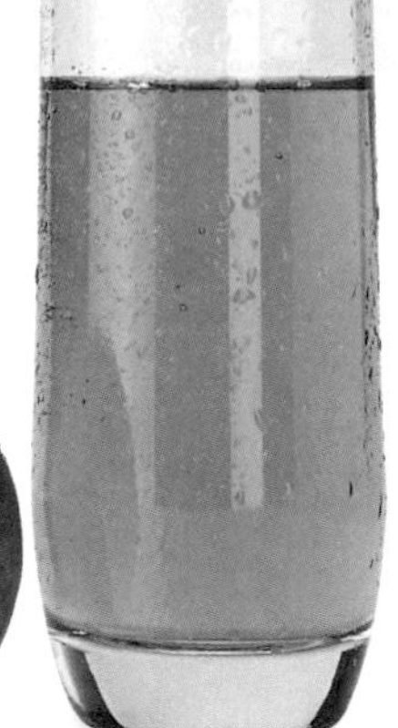

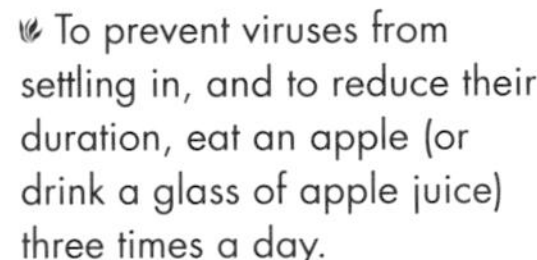

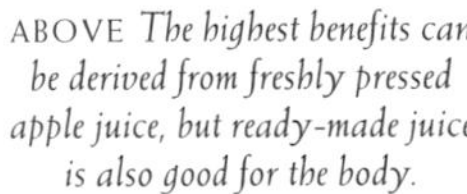

ABOVE *The highest benefits can be derived from freshly pressed apple juice, but ready-made juice is also good for the body.*

ABOVE *Apples have long been known to be beneficial to health and should be eaten regularly.*

THERAPY CONNECTIONS

APPLE
Flower Remedies p.234

OLIVE
Flower Remedies p.235

Nasturtium officinalis

WATERCRESS

Watercress is a floating or creeping water plant of the mustard family, *Cruciferae*. A perennial, it grows best in fresh water, particularly in cool streams and ponds, and in wet soil. Its round, edible leaves are pungent to the taste, and commonly used as salad greens or as a garnish. It is a rich source of vitamin C.

DATA FILE

Properties

- Contains benzyl mustard oil, which is powerfully antibiotic, but does not harm our healthy bacteria (flora)
- Beneficial to the health of the intestines
- Encourages immune activity in the body
- Provides good supplies of the vitamins C, A, and B (thiamine and riboflavin), iron, potassium, and calcium
- Stimulates digestion
- Anti-inflammatory, diuretic, expectorant, antiseptic

Uses

- Sometimes recommended for gall bladder complaints and anemia.
- The bruised leaves are said to remove pimples and to fade freckling. Eat to help skin eruptions.
- Eat fresh daily: may help to prevent migraine. Eat with a meal if you have a tendency towards heartburn or dyspepsia.
- High levels of potassium may help to prevent insomnia – eat some fresh leaves an hour before bedtime, and often throughout the day.
- Watercress may help in the treatment of edema.
- It is used to treat respiratory ailments such as coughs, catarrh, and bronchitis – eat fresh until symptoms improve. Can be useful as a preventive measure for chronic respiratory conditions.
- Watercress may strengthen the whole body system in cases of debility caused by chronic illness. It can also help to relieve stress.

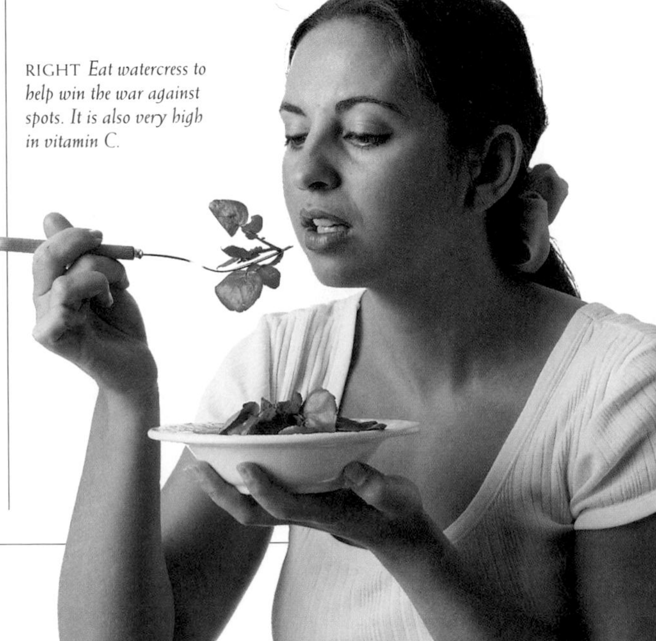

RIGHT *Eat watercress to help win the war against spots. It is also very high in vitamin C.*

Olea europea

OLIVE

The olive is a handsome, long-lived, evergreen, subtropical tree, and has been cultivated for at least 4,000 years for its edible fruit and its valuable oil. It is native to the eastern Mediterranean region, where its culture may have been begun by Semitic people as long ago as 3500 B.C.E. Its leaves and the oil of its fruit are used in cooking and medicinally, and studies show that it has powerful anticholesterol action in the body, making it a useful addition to any home medicine cabinet. Only cold-pressed olive oil is suitable for therapeutic use.

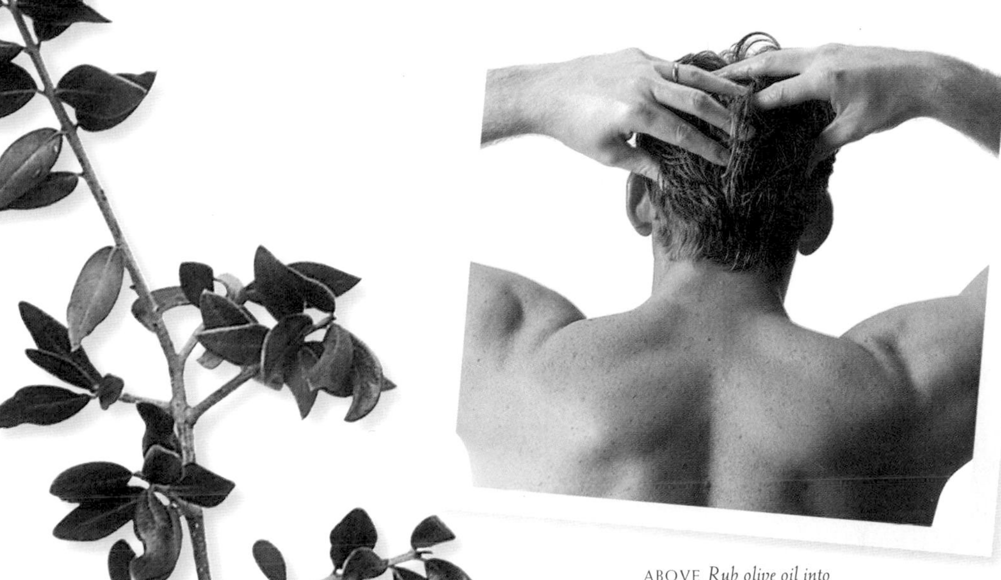

RIGHT *The olive branch is an ancient symbol of peace. Olive is reputed to calm nervous disorders.*

ABOVE *Rub olive oil into the scalp to improve problems such as itchy dandruff, eczema, and psoriasis.*

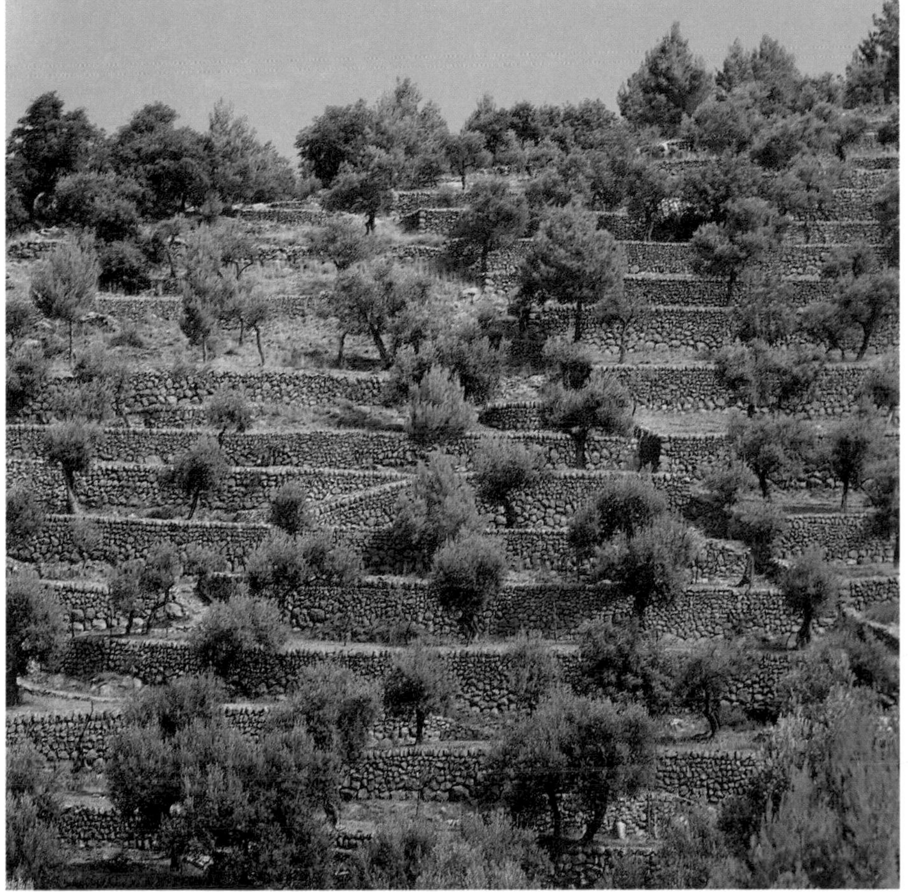

LEFT *A Mediterranean olive grove. The slow-growing trees thrive in a warm, sunny climate.*

DATA FILE

Properties

- Antioxidant
- Anticancer
- Emollient – particularly useful for skin conditions
- Olive oil can be used to treat constipation
- Soothes the itching of eczema, and moisturizes dry skin, hair, and scalp
- Olive oil is rich in vitamin E, and is now known to help lower cholesterol levels in the body
- It may reduce the risk of circulatory disease and nervous disorders
- Useful in the treatment of gastric disorders because it reduces the secretion of gastric juices

Uses

- Rub olive oil into patches of eczema, dandruff, and psoriasis to reduce itching and encourage healing.
- Olive oil, eaten daily, can reduce the risk of heart disease and help to slow down the degenerative effects of aging.
- Drink a little extra virgin olive oil to cure a hangover.
- Olives and olive oil, as part of a daily diet, will help to prevent and treat circulatory problems, and lower cholesterol levels.
- Eat olives for constipation.
- Olives are said to counteract poisoning from mushrooms or fish – drink a little extra virgin, cold-pressed oil when symptoms present themselves.

Oyrza sativa

RICE

Rice is the cereal that is a staple food to more than half of the world's peoples. It also has important medicinal uses, for which the rhizomes, seeds (the grains), and germinated seeds are used. White rice is the grain that is left after the bran and germ have been removed; brown rice retains the bran and germ. Rice is available as a breakfast cereal (the grains are "puffed" during manufacture), and is fermented to produce rice wine, called *saki* by the Japanese.

DATA FILE

Properties

- Rice contains high levels of carbohydrates (87 percent of white, uncooked rice)
- Rich in B vitamins (folic acid and pyridoxine), iron, and potassium. Brown rice also contains the B vitamin thiamine, which is present in the bran.
- White rice has 1 percent of fat; in brown rice the amount of fat is higher
- Rice contains low amounts of sodium and is also free from cholesterol
- A natural tonic
- Diuretic
- Digestive
- Controls sweating
- Lowers blood pressure
- Anti-inflammatory

Uses

- Eat rice daily if you suffer from chronic dyspepsia – excellent for heartburn, particularly that associated with pregnancy.
- Use rice bran for the treatment of hyperalcuria.
- Use rice flour to make a poultice for relieving inflammation of the skin, including acne, measles, burns, and hemorrhoids.
- A natural diuretic – increase your intake prior to menstruation if you suffer from bloating and symptoms of PMS. Eaten regularly, rice can prevent edema.
- The seeds are used to treat urinary ailments.
- Rice water helps to overcome stomach upsets.
- Rice and rice flour are used as substitutes for wheat and some other cereals by people who cannot tolerate gluten and gliadin, such as those with celiac disease.
- Germinated rice seeds may help in the treatment of abdominal bloating, lack of appetite, and indigestion.

LEFT *and* ABOVE *Brown rice and white rice. Brown, unpolished rice contains more vitamins and fiber.*

CAUTION

DO NOT EAT AVOCADOS OR TAKE ANY PRODUCT CONTAINING AVOCADO IF YOU HAVE BEEN PRESCRIBED MAOI ANTIDEPRESSANTS.

Persica americana gratissima

AVOCADO

Avocados are the fruit of a small, subtropical tree. They are rich in vitamins A, some B-complex, C, and E vitamins, and potassium, and because they contain some protein and starch, as well as being a good source of monounsaturated fats, they are considered to be a perfect – or complete – food. Traditionally avocados have been used for skin problems. The pulp has both antibacterial and antifungal properties.

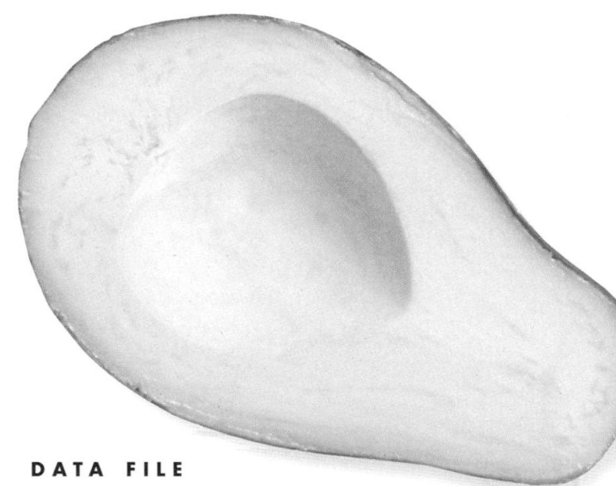

RIGHT *Avocados are full of vitamins and minerals, but they also have a high fat content.*

DATA FILE

Properties

- Excellent restorative food, particularly during convalescence
- Traditionally used for sexual problems
- Helps with skin disorders
- Antioxidant
- Used to treat circulatory problems
- Digestive
- Antibacterial
- Antifungal

Uses

- An avocado paste can be applied to rashes and rough skin to soothe and smooth.
- Avocado oil can be used as a base oil for massage.
- Eat an avocado each day when convalescing.
- The pulp, applied to grazes and shallow cuts, and covered with sterile gauze, can prevent infection entering the body and encourage healing.
- Eat regularly for digestive and circulatory problems.
- The flesh of a ripe avocado soothes sunburned skin. Cut an avocado in half and rub gently over the affected area.

BELOW *To make a face mask, mash a ripe avocado with a little olive oil and apply to the skin.*

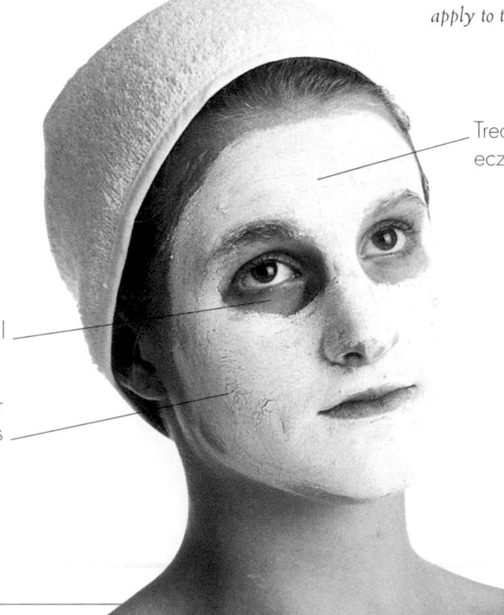

Piper negrum

BLACK PEPPER

Black pepper, a traditional seasoning for food, is a warm, aromatic, and comforting spice with therapeutic uses. The fruit, or corns, of the vine and the essential oil extracted from them are used. Black pepper is the whole, sun-dried, unripened fruit of the vine; white pepper is the ripe fruit, from which the skins have been removed.

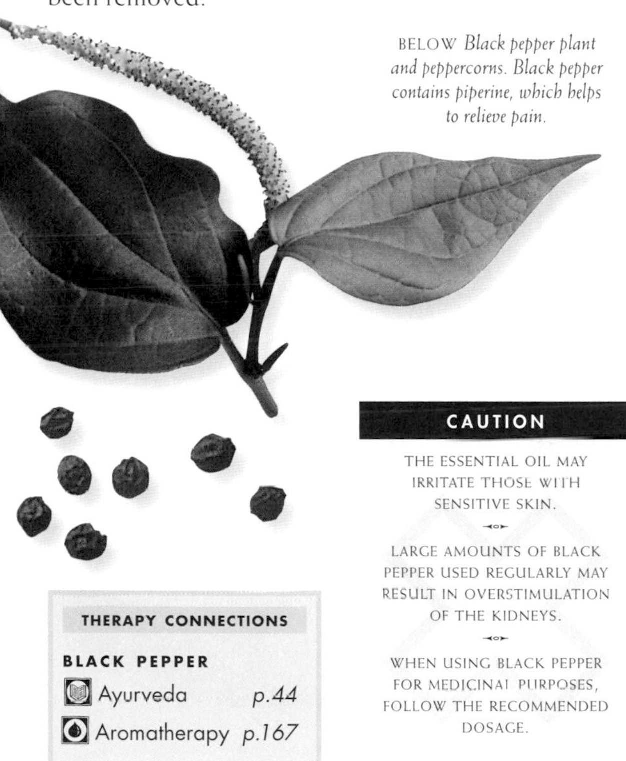

BELOW *Black pepper plant and peppercorns. Black pepper contains piperine, which helps to relieve pain.*

CAUTION

THE ESSENTIAL OIL MAY IRRITATE THOSE WITH SENSITIVE SKIN.

LARGE AMOUNTS OF BLACK PEPPER USED REGULARLY MAY RESULT IN OVERSTIMULATION OF THE KIDNEYS.

WHEN USING BLACK PEPPER FOR MEDICINAL PURPOSES, FOLLOW THE RECOMMENDED DOSAGE.

THERAPY CONNECTIONS

BLACK PEPPER

Ayurveda p.44

Aromatherapy p.167

DATA FILE

Properties

- Stimulating
- Expectorant
- Anesthetic
- Tranquilizing
- Analgesic

Uses

- Black pepper is useful for treating indigestion and flatulence – add to food daily for preventive action.
- Its essential oil eases muscular aches and pains, and is used to treat colds and flu.
- When used as a homeopathic remedy for fever, pepper can help to lower the body temperature.
- Pepper is an effective emetic and expectorant, and can be taken internally, or rubbed onto the chest (a tiny amount of oil in a suitable carrier oil) to prevent catarrh and to encourage healing.
- In Ayurvedic medicine, black pepper mixed with ghee is used to treat nasal congestion, sinusitis, and inflammation of the skin.

Prunus amygdalmus dulcis and Prunus amygdalmus amara

ALMOND

The almond tree produces the oldest and most widely grown of all of the world's nut crops, and is indigenous to western Asia and North Africa. Of the two major types of almonds grown, the sweet almond (*P. dulcis*) is cultivated for its edible nut. The bitter almond (*P. amara*) is inedible but contains an oil – also present in the sweet almond, and in the ripe kernels of the apricot and peach – which, when combined with water, yields hydrocyanic (prussic) acid and benzaldehyde, the essential oil of bitter almonds. The oil is used in making flavoring extracts and in some sedative medicines.

Almonds have been used for centuries to heal the body internally, and may be used ground in water to prevent fevers.

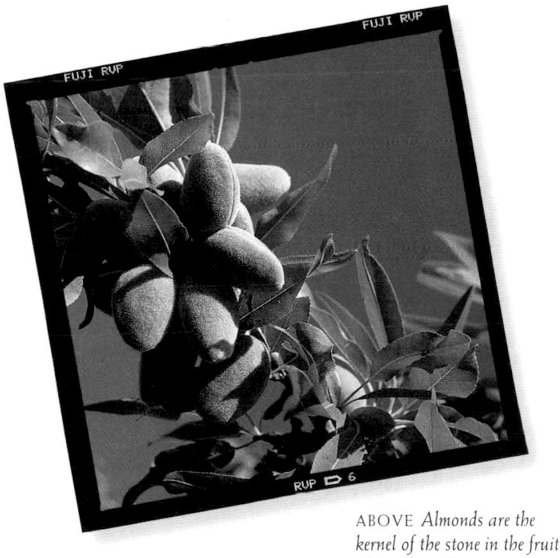

ABOVE *Almonds are the kernel of the stone in the fruit of the almond tree.*

DATA FILE

Properties

- Sweet almonds are high in protein
- Almonds reduce inflammation: used in the treatment of bronchitis
- Rich in protein, fat, zinc, potassium, iron, B vitamins, and magnesium
- Aids respiration
- Acts as a digestive

Uses

- Combine almond milk *(see right)* with barley water for urinary problems.
- Almond milk is an excellent tonic during convalescence.
- Drink almond milk daily to reduce frequency of digestive disorders, and to relieve respiratory problems.

SPECIAL NOTE

EAT ALMONDS WITH FOODS RICH IN VITAMIN C TO ENCOURAGE MAXIMUM ABSORPTION.

ALMOND MILK

Almond milk helps digestive, respiratory, and urinary problems. Drink it every day for the best results.

You will need almonds (6 tablespoonsful), water, and honey.

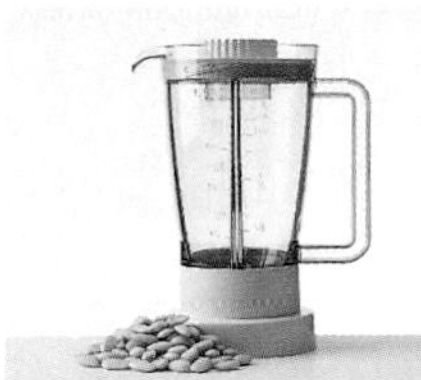

Blend the almonds in a food processor with 1pt. (500ml.) water. Grind until smooth.

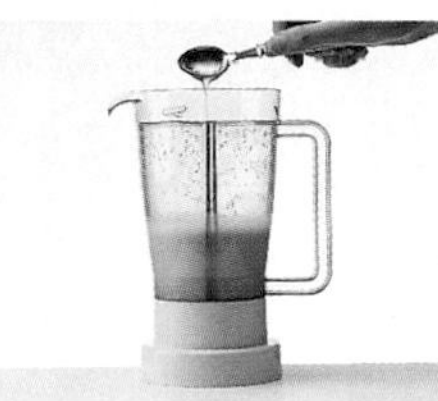

Add 1 teaspoonful of honey for flavor.

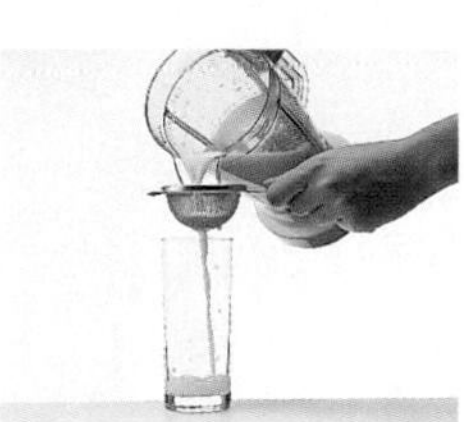

Strain the mixture through a sieve or fine cloth to drink. Store in a refrigerator.

Sinapis alba, Brassica nigra

MUSTARD

Black and white mustards are used for culinary and medicinal purposes. The leaves, flowers, seeds, and oils of the black mustard are used, while only the seeds of the white mustard are useful. Black mustard powder is an important herbal remedy because it draws blood to the surface of the skin quickly, which means that it is "rubefacient," and warming. Mustard oil is used as an ingredient in liniments, stomach stimulants, and emetics.

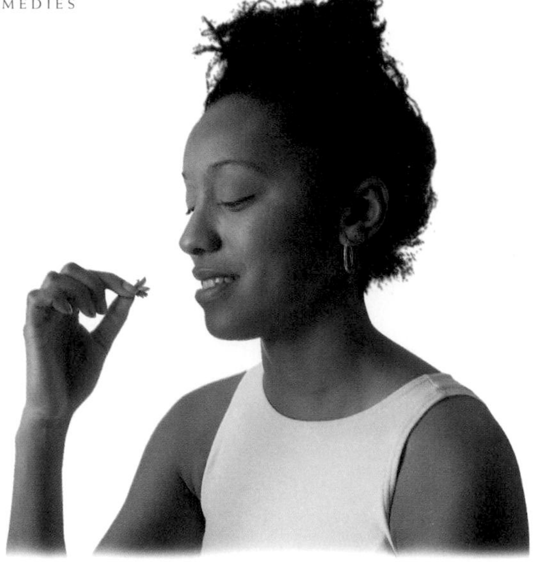

ABOVE *Mustard leaves are very nutritious, containing vitamin A, iron, and zinc.*

CAUTION

MUSTARD SEEDS CAN BURN THE SKIN; USE CAREFULLY.

AVOID CONTACT WITH THE MUCOUS MEMBRANES, AND WITH SENSITIVE SKIN.

DATA FILE

Properties

- Rich in calcium and iron
- Mustard helps to restore bacterial balance in the intestines
- Mustard greens are rich in vitamin A, iron, and zinc
- White mustard relieves pain, and is a diuretic and an antibiotic
- Mustard flour is an antiseptic and a deodorizer
- Mustard oil can be used for pain relief of arthritic conditions and chilblains
- An excellent expectorant
- A powerful emetic
- Black mustard and white mustard are warming and can be used to draw infection or congestion away from its source for nasal congestion, or for relief of an abscess
- Rubefacient qualities help respiratory and circulatory disorders, including heart problems

Uses

- Taken internally, mustard encourages the circulation, eases stomach and liver problems, and is able to stimulate the heart.
- Eat fresh mustard leaves when convalescing – they are nutritious and will help to encourage healing.
- A mustard foot bath (1 teaspoon of mustard powder added to a bowl of hot water) is a traditional remedy for colds, circulatory problems, and headaches.
- A mustard poultice on the chest relieves infection and congestion.
- Mustard essential oil can be used externally for neuralgia; massage a little oil gently into the affected area a few times a day.
- A poultice of mustard seeds or mustard essential oil is helpful when applied to areas of the body troubled by pain from rheumatism, sciatica, and lumbago.

THERAPY CONNECTIONS

MUSTARD

Ayurveda p.30

Flower Remedies p.239

BELOW *Powdered mustard seeds have no smell until water is added, and a pungent odor is released.*

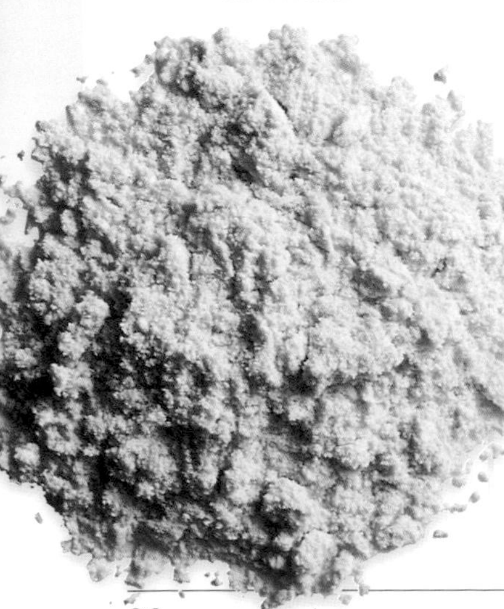

Solanum tuberosum

POTATO

The potato plant is native to the Peruvian Andes. It was supposedly endowed with powers such as the ability to cure impotence, and so long as the plant remained rare in Europe, its price often reached astronomical heights. Potatoes have been used for medicinal purposes for hundreds of years, and are extremely nutritious, supplying fiber, B vitamins, minerals, and vitamin C. The peels are high in potassium, and potato-peel tea has been traditionally used around the world for high blood pressure. The juice of raw potatoes is most useful, and can be added to soups, juices, or stews to disguise the taste.

ABOVE *At one time, a raw potato was carried in a garment pocket to protect against rheumatism.*

CAUTION

POISONOUS ALKALOIDS ARE PRESENT IN MOST NIGHTSHADE PLANTS, INCLUDING THE COMMON POTATO, BUT IT IS PERFECTLY SAFE TO EAT IF COOKED, AND IN SMALL AMOUNTS WHEN RAW.

SPROUTING POTATOES ARE POISONOUS AND SHOULD NOT BE EATEN.

Potato pulp

RIGHT *The pulp of a hot baked potato helps to relieve tennis elbow and other joint pain.*

DATA FILE

Properties

- Alkaline, which helps to detoxify the body
- Antiulcer
- Helps relieve inflammation and pain.
- The skin contains chlorogenic acid, which can help to prevent cell mutation causing cancer
- Encourages healthy blood circulation

Uses

- The juice of the raw potato can be used for stomach ulcers and to relieve the inflammation of arthritis.
- Make a potato poultice for healing a bruise or sprain of any kind.
- Raw, grated potatoes can relieve the pain of a burn.
- Apply hot baked potato pulp for tennis elbow and other joint pain.
- Boiled potato peel is said to be useful for inflammation of the prostate. Apply as a poultice to the affected area.
- Eaten daily, potatoes can help to prevent premature aging and heart disease.
- Regular consumption can prevent constipation and help to ease inflammation associated with irritable bowel syndrome.

Vaccinium oxycoccus var. palustris

CRANBERRY

Cranberries are small acidic berries which are rich in vitamins C and A, and contain an excellent infection-fighting ingredient. The commercial cranberry, *Vaccinium macrocarpon*, is a creeping evergreen plant of the heath family, whose red, acidic fruit is used in sauces and jellies served with savory and sweet foods and in a variety of fruit juice beverages.

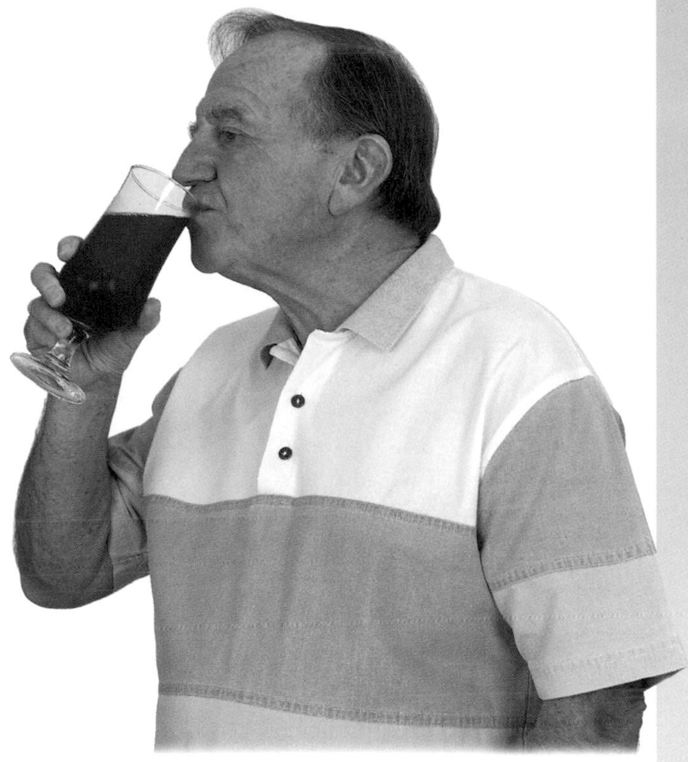

ABOVE *The prostate gland may cause urinary problems in later life. Fresh cranberry juice will help.*

DATA FILE

Properties

- An antiseptic action on the urinary system
- Used to control asthma
- Improves the health of the circulatory system
- Aids in the treatment of kidney stones

Uses

- Cranberries contain a substance which affects the acidity of the urine and acts as a bactericide. A daily glass of cranberry juice will prevent and treat cystitis, and discourage kidney stones. Fresh cranberries and cranberry juice are used in the treatment of prostate problems, and urinary tract infections.
- Crushed cranberries, boiled in distilled water and skinned, can be added to a cup of warm water to overcome an asthma attack. The berries contain an active ingredient similar to that in the drugs used to control asthma.

CAUTION

CRANBERRIES CONTAIN LARGE AMOUNTS OF OXALIC ACID, AND SHOULD NOT BE EATEN RAW.

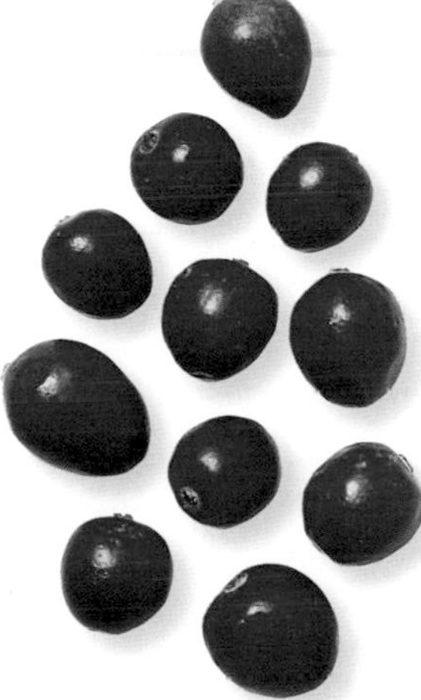

ABOVE *Cranberries are the fruits of an ericaceous shrub. They prevent harmful bacteria attaching to the bladder walls.*

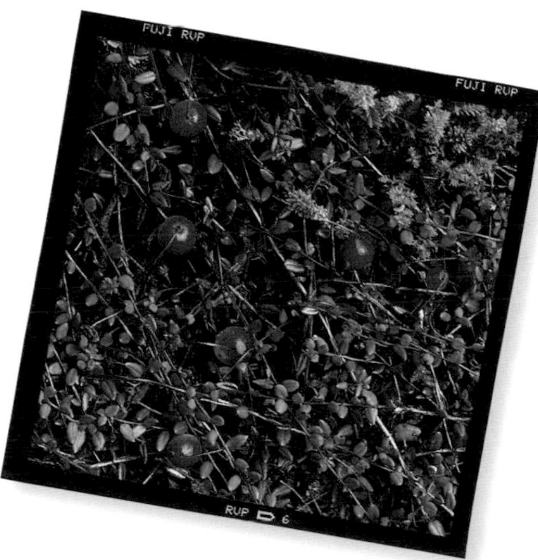

ABOVE *The juice extracted from cranberries contains oxalic acid, which discourages the formation of kidney stones.*

Zea mays

CORN

Archeological evidence indicates that a type of primitive corn was used as a food in Mexico at least 7,000 years ago. The kernels of corn have a translucent, horny appearance when immature and are wrinkled when dry. The ears are eaten fresh or frozen, or are canned. Corn, or maize, is known primarily as a staple food, but it also has therapeutic properties. The corn silk (stigmas and styles of female flowers), fruit, seeds, and oil are used. Corn is particularly useful as a remedy for urinary problems.

CAUTION

PEOPLE SUFFERING FROM PELLAGRA (A NIACIN-DEFICIENCY DISEASE) MAY BE ADVISED TO ELIMINATE CORN AND CORN PRODUCTS FROM THEIR DIET.

SOME PEOPLE ARE ALLERGIC TO CORN – IF YOU SUFFER A RASH, HEADACHES, OR ANY OTHER SYMPTOMS, AVOID CORN AND CORN PRODUCTS.

ABOVE *Corn silk refers to the hairs covering the corn: save these for making into herbal tea.*

DATA FILE

Properties

- Corn provides carbohydrates, B vitamins (thiamine and riboflavin), vitamin C, vitamin A, potassium, and zinc
- Stimulating and cooling
- Used in Chinese medicine for treating urinary and kidney problems
- Corn silk cleanses the kidneys and the urinary tract

Uses

- A tea made by infusing corn silk in hot water may help in the treatment of kidney stones. Drink three times a day.
- Corn silk is also a good cleanser of the urinary tract. A little of it eaten raw, with or without the corn kernels, will benefit the whole urinary system and may help to prevent cystitis.
- Corn and its products may be beneficial in the treatment of bedwetting in children, disorders of the prostate and cystitis, and inflammation of the urethra.
- Cornstarch, manufactured from the inner part of the corn kernel, makes a fine powder suitable for use as a face or bath powder.

Bicarbonate of soda

BAKING SODA

Baking soda is a white powder that is traditionally used as a raising agent for baking. It is used in many natural remedies, and on its own for its soothing and neutralizing properties.

DATA FILE

Properties

- Anti-inflammatory, particularly useful for skin conditions
- Natural bleach for teeth
- Alkaline (neutralizes acids)

Uses

- Salt and baking soda in the bath may reduce the effect of minor exposure to X-rays.
- A paste of baking soda and water can be applied to diaper rash to reduce skin inflammation and irritation.
- Drink a solution of baking soda and hot water (1 teaspoon to ½pt. [250ml.]) to reduce flatulence and ease indigestion.
- For bee stings, extract the sting and apply a paste of baking soda and water to neutralize it.
- The juice of half a lemon mixed with 1 teaspoon of baking soda and warm water will help ease a headache. Drink every 15 minutes until the pain begins to recede.
- Brush your teeth with baking soda, a natural whitener which reduces agents causing bad breath.

ABOVE *Take a teaspoonful of bicarbonate of soda in water to treat cystitis.*

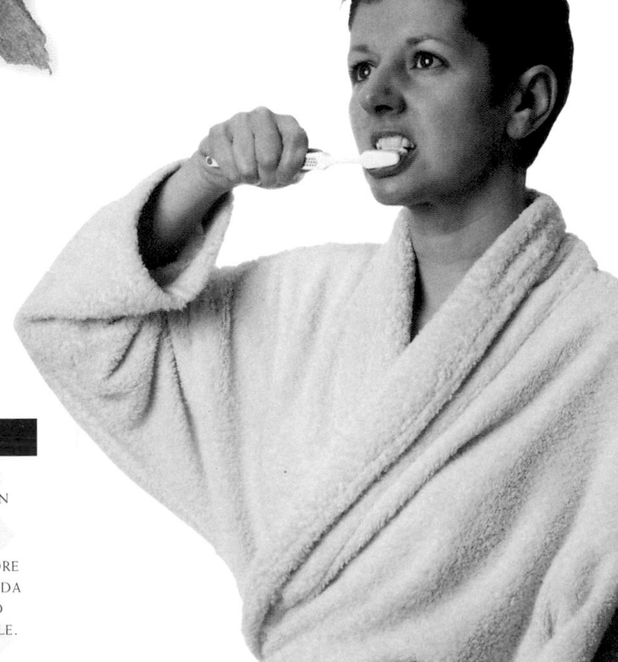

RIGHT *Baking soda toothpaste helps to whiten the teeth.*

CAUTION

BAKING SODA SHOULD BE USED ONLY EXTERNALLY ON CHILDREN AND BABIES.

CONSULT A PHYSICIAN BEFORE TAKING BICARBONATE OF SODA IF YOU HAVE HIGH BLOOD PRESSURE OR HEART TROUBLE.

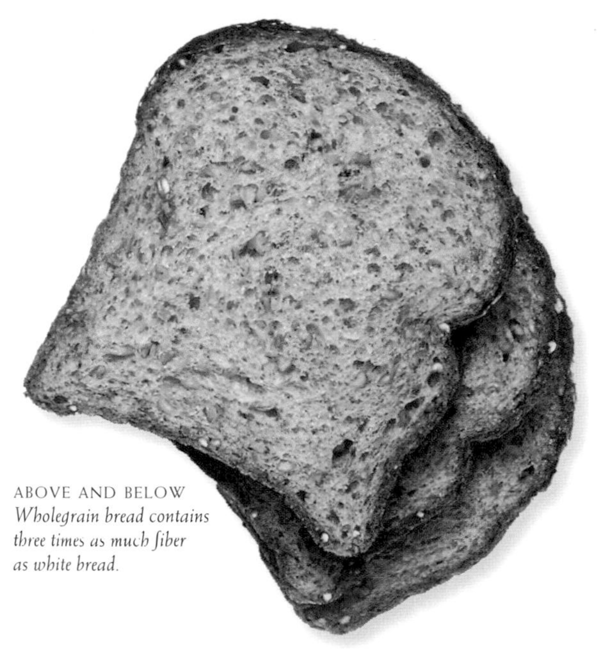

ABOVE AND BELOW *Wholegrain bread contains three times as much fiber as white bread.*

BREAD

Bread – particularly wholegrain bread – is an excellent source of carbohydrates and B-complex vitamins, which maintain the health of the nervous system and ensure the healthy functioning of body systems. Traditionally, bread was used as a poultice, and applied as a styptic to stop the bleeding of wounds.

DATA FILE

Properties

- Nutritious
- Anti-inflammatory
- Styptic (stops bleeding)

Uses

- Apply cold bread to closed eyes to reduce the inflammation of conjunctivitis and soothe itching.
- Apply a warm bread poultice to infected cuts to reduce itching and pain.
- Apply fresh bread to shallow wounds to help stop the bleeding.
- Ease the pain, and help to bring out a boil by applying a hot bread poultice.
- Eat wholegrain bread while convalescing and when under stress – it is rich in B vitamins that feed the nervous system.

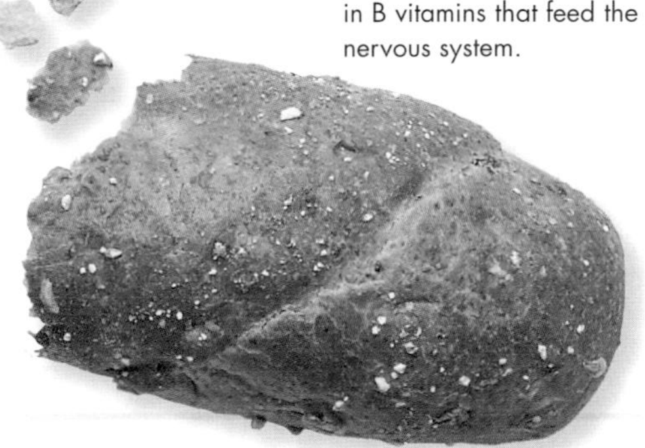

HONEY

Honey is the sweet liquid produced by bees from the nectar of flowers. The source of the nectar the honey is made from determines its color and flavor. For centuries honey has been used as an antiseptic, for external and internal conditions, and as a tonic for overall good health. Each country has a distinctive type of honey, dependent on the local flowers upon which the bees feed. All honeys are complex mixtures of the sugars fructose and glucose with water, organic acids, and mineral and vitamin traces, as well as some plant pigments.

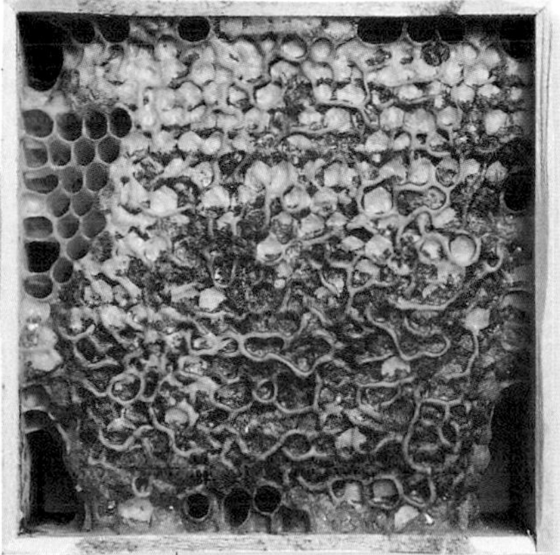

CAUTION

UNPASTEURIZED HONEY SHOULD NOT BE EATEN BY PREGNANT WOMEN, AND ONLY SPARINGLY BY CHILDREN. HOWEVER, ENSURE THAT YOU BUY COLD-PRESSED HONEY, BECAUSE HEATED HONEY CONTAINS ADDITIVES AND LOSES ITS HEALING PROPERTIES.

ABOVE *Honey ointment helps to heal sore places in the mouth.*

LEFT *Bees make honeycomb – where honey is stored, and eggs are laid.*

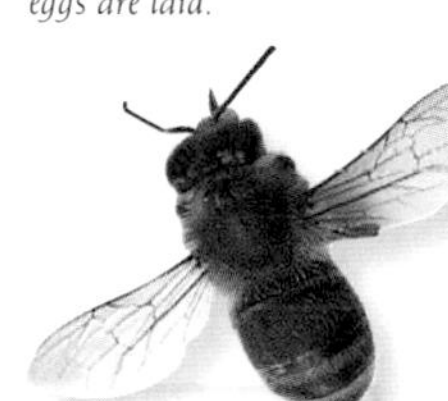

DATA FILE

Properties

- Soothes raw tissues
- Helps to retain calcium in the body
- Honey helps to balance acid accumulations in the body (because of the significant amount of potassium it contains)
- Sedative
- Antifungal
- Possibly aphrodisiac
- Nourishing – some minerals and vitamins, along with amino acids
- Antibacterial, for external and internal infections; unpasteurized honey has antibiotic properties

Uses

- Honey water can be used as an eye lotion (particularly good for conjunctivitis and other infectious conditions).
- Gargle with honey water to soothe a sore throat and ease respiratory problems.
- Honey and lemon mixed together are a traditional remedy for coughs.
- Mix with apple cider vinegar as a tonic or "rebalancer." This may also help to relieve the symptoms of arthritis and reduce arthritic deposits.
- Honey ointment can soothe and encourage healing of sores in the mouth or vagina.
- Honey is an excellent moisturizer, and can be rubbed into the skin as a revitalizing mask.
- Honey warmed with a little milk can be used as a gentle sedative.
- Eating a little local honey will sensitize you to pollens in the area – acting as a natural remedy for hay fever and all its symptoms.
- Apply a honey compress to cuts and bruises to soothe, encourage healing, and prevent infection.
- Smear set honey on ringworm or athlete's foot several times a day. Leave the foot uncovered.

Acetic acid

VINEGAR

Vinegar (from the French *vinaigre*, "sour wine") is an acidic liquid obtained from the fermentation of alcohol, and used either as a condiment or a preservative. Vinegar usually has an acid content of 4–8 percent; in flavor it may be sharp, rich, or mellow. Vinegar is often used to preserve herbs, and used on its own for medicinal purposes. Apple cider vinegar is the most useful medicinally.

DATA FILE

Properties

- Helps to make more efficient use of calcium in the body, and can help to encourage strong bones, hair, and nails
- Vinegar is antiseptic, astringent, and excellent for urinary tract infections
- Antispasmodic
- Antibacterial
- Improves functioning and adjustment of the body so that there is efficient use of the food you eat (i.e. it balances metabolic activity)
- Antifungal, used in the treatment of thrush
- Apple cider is a good tonic, and can help to relieve a sore throat

Uses

- Sip first thing in the morning, and just prior to meals to reduce appetite and encourage efficient digestion.
- Simmer cider vinegar in a pan, cover with a towel, and inhale to reduce the spasms of bronchitis and to help reduce any excess catarrh.
- Drink a glass of warm apple cider vinegar with honey a half-hour before bed to encourage restful sleep.
- Vinegar can be drunk (warm with a little honey) to treat digestive disorders and urinary infections.
- Apply vinegar to wasp stings to reduce swelling and ease discomfort.
- Coughs, colds, and infections will respond to a cup of warm water with 2 tablespoons of vinegar and some honey. Arthritis and asthma may also be treated with the same drink, adding slightly more vinegar.
- Apply cider vinegar to the skin to treat athlete's foot, ringworm, and eczema.
- Drink vinegar daily to treat thrush, and apply to the exterior of the vagina (mixed with a little warm water) to ease itching.
- Add vinegar to bath water to soothe skin problems, help to draw out toxins from the skin, and ease thrush.

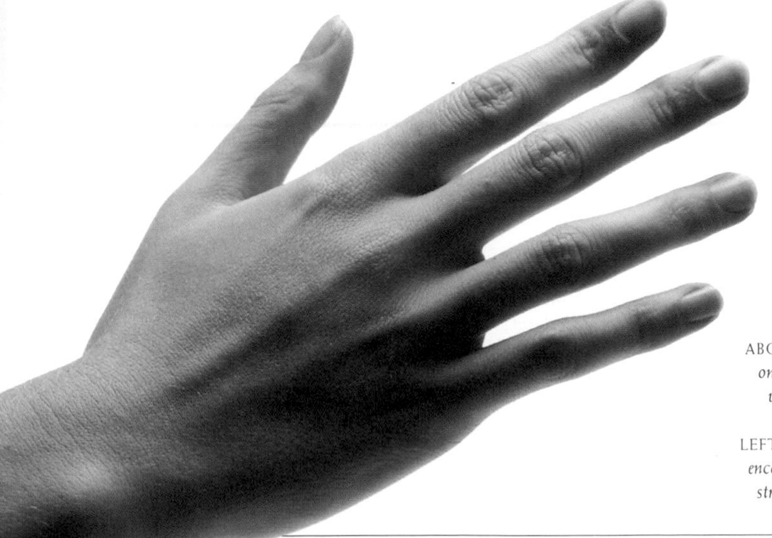

ABOVE *Malt vinegar is one of many types of vinegar available.*

LEFT *Vinegar can help to encourage the growth of strong, healthy nails.*

INHALATION

Vinegar is antispasmodic, and is useful for treating the bronchospasms common to bronchitis sufferers. Bronchitis is the inflammation of the bronchi, which link the windpipe to the lungs. It causes production of thick phlegm, and gives rise to bouts of coughing.

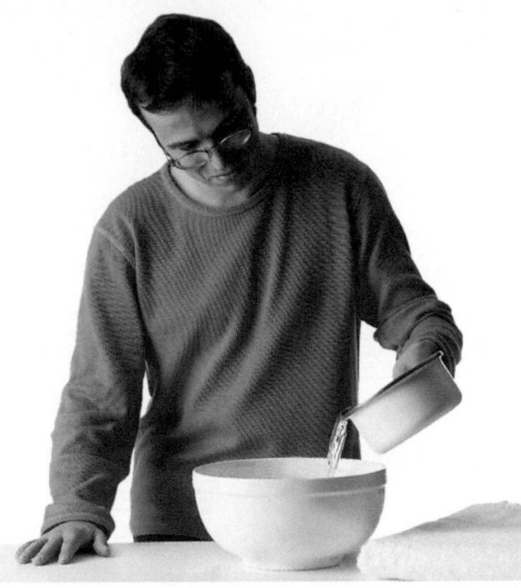

Inhaling the steam given off by hot cider vinegar will soothe spasms. Pour some apple cider vinegar into a pan and put it on the cooker to heat. Bring to the boil and simmer for a few minutes. Remove from the heat and pour into a medium-sized bowl.

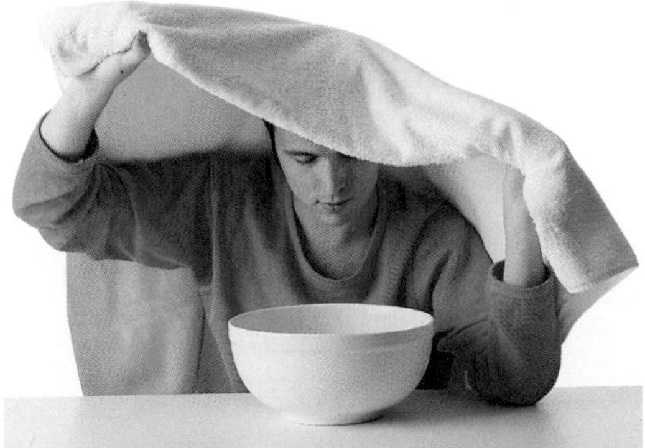

Take the bowl to your kitchen table and sit down with it in front of you. Drape a large towel over your head and the bowl, making a tent. Inhale deeply while the steam continues to be produced. This will also help catarrh.

Hydrogen dioxide

WATER

Pure water is a clear, colorless liquid made up of oxygen and hydrogen. It is the most common substance on the Earth's surface, covering more than 70 percent of the planet. It is also present in the atmosphere as a gas (water vapor or steam). Water is essential to life on Earth and constitutes a large part of most living things. Human beings are comprised of about 75 percent water. Water is necessary for maintaining the correct osmotic pressure in cells, and is needed for many other body processes, such as transporting nutrients and waste products around the body in the blood (blood is about 80 percent water). Water that has been cooled or heated to form ice, hot water, or steam can be used to treat minor complaints.

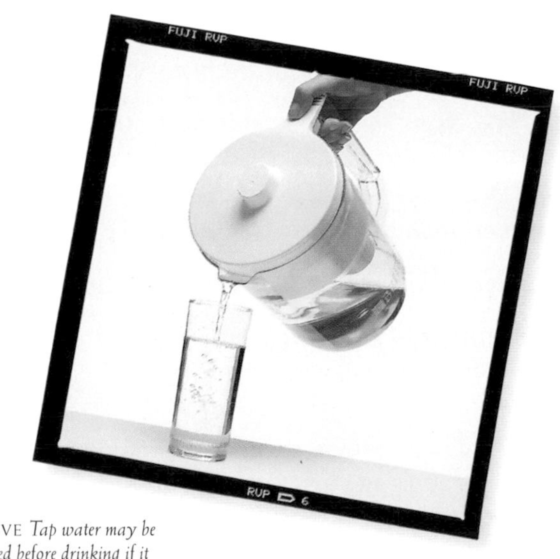

ABOVE *Tap water may be filtered before drinking if it is thought to contain a lot of impurities.*

DATA FILE

Properties

- Essential for life
- Dilutes toxins in the body, and expels them
- A natural diuretic
- Salt water is antiseptic
- Aids kidney action
- Prevents constipation
- May contain some naturally occurring fluoride
- Prevents dehydration

Uses

- Drink plenty of fresh water if you suffer from edema.
- Drink water to counter the effects of a hangover, and during illness to encourage the expulsion of toxins. People who drink excessive amounts of alcohol or coffee, or who smoke, should drink at least eight glasses of water daily.
- It can help to prevent tooth decay when sufficient fluoride is present.
- Water acts as a diuretic and a mild laxative – it adds water to stools and may stimulate muscle contraction in the digestive tract.
- Hard water may play a role in preventing hypertension and heart disease.
- Ice reduces swellings and is particularly beneficial for sprains. Ice packs help to relieve backache.
- Cold compresses placed around the throat may ease an attack of croup.
- Children suffering from croup will get relief when placed in a steamy bathroom. This is best achieved by running the hot water faucet or the shower.
- Swallowing cracked ice may be beneficial in relieving morning sickness and motion sickness.
- A hot compress can help to reduce skin inflammations caused by infection. Dip a face cloth or other thick cloth in hot water and wring out before applying.
- Bathing in warm water can encourage relaxation. Hot baths may help to soothe muscular aches and pains. A cool bath can be soothing for sufferers of prickly heat

LEFT *Gather some ice cubes from the freezer and wrap in a cloth. Hold against the back to relieve backache.*

CAUTION

WATER SHOULD BE FILTERED BEFORE IT IS DRUNK IF IT CONTAINS IMPURITIES.

BOTTLED MINERAL WATERS MAY BE HIGH IN SODIUM.

HERBALISM

SACRED HERBS

The Saxons had nine sacred herbs which they used for rituals and the treatment of disease. The herbs included hawthorn, yarrow, and marigold.

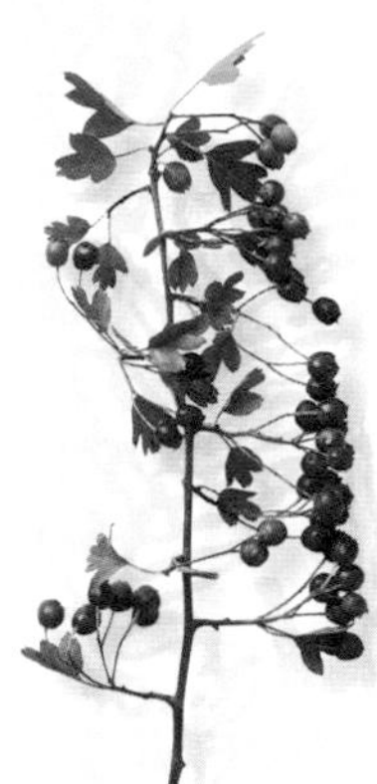

HAWTHORN
Hawthorn berries work to improve the functioning of the heart.

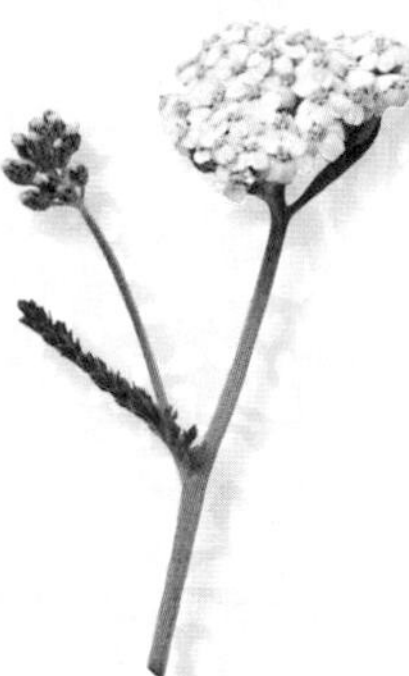

YARROW
Yarrow reduces fever, heals wounds, and lowers blood pressure.

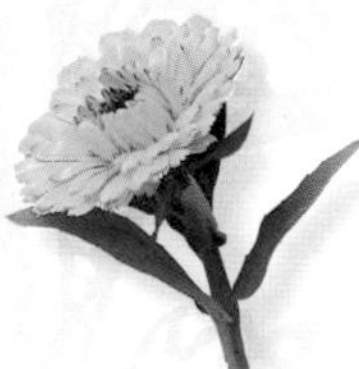

MARIGOLD
Calendula is antifungal, and treats wounds, burns, and indigestion.

Since before recorded history humans have used plants for food, medicines, shelter, clothing, dyes, weapons, musical instruments, and transportation. The cultural development of different countries and the rise and fall of empires have often been linked to the understanding and exploitation of plants. Herbalism, the use of plants for medicinal purposes, has been common to all peoples of the world. Our understanding of herbalism has been passed down by word of mouth from generation to generation.

It is the most natural thing in the world to use local flora for food and medicine, and list this knowledge for posterity. All native cultures have a well-developed understanding of local plants, and most of the world, even today, relies on herbal expertise for its primary healthcare. Shamans, wise women, bush doctors, traditional healers, and native medicine workers carry on a tradition thousands of years old.

Herbalism is the oldest, most tested, and proven form of medicine in the world. The *Ebers Papyrus* of the ancient Egyptians lists 85 herbs, some of which, like mint, are used in a similar way today. The Chinese herbal, *Pen Tsao*, contains over a thousand herbal remedies. The Assyrian and Babylonian scribes wrote herbal recipes on cuneiform tablets. The Greek Hippocrates (477–360 B.C.E) mentions herbs, remedies, and treatment stratagems which are still valid. Indeed, there is much practical and theoretical knowledge to be rediscovered. Globally, herbal lore is a treasure chest beyond price.

In the West, the Saxons wrote the *Leech Book of Bald*, a mixture of remedies and ritual. Their nine sacred herbs included yarrow, marigold, and hawthorn. A modern practitioner of herbal medicine would rate them equally highly. The golden age of herbals was precipitated by the development of the printing press. Culpeper printed the *London Dispensary* (1653) in English (it had previously been printed in Latin), and later published his *Complete Herbal*, a book, he boasted, from which any man (or woman) could find out how to cure themselves for less than three pennies! Culpeper's herbal was immensely popular and is still available, having gone through over 40 reprints.

Botanical medicine was regarded as fringe medicine for many years. It was valued as a starting place for modern research, but thought to have nothing to offer Western society as a therapy in itself. Pharmaceutical companies identified the active therapeutic principles of many plants, synthesized commercial analogues, and patented new drugs. But in doing so they often missed the major principles of using natural sources for therapeutic purposes. Herbalism, when practised properly, is marked by a completely different attitude from orthodox medicine. It is a holistic system that uses plants, or plant parts, in a nonintrusive way. Herbalists believe that the constituents of a plant work synergistically to stimulate the natural healing process.

THE TENETS OF HERBALISM

- The whole plant is better than an isolated extract.
- Treat the whole person not just the symptoms.
- Practise minimum effective treatment and minimum intervention.
- Strengthen the body and encourage it to heal itself.

Today there is a worldwide renaissance in therapeutic systems which use herbs as their major source of medicines. Modern science is validating traditional practices, precipitating a general reappraisal. Tibetan, Chinese, Native American, Indian, and Western systems are all examining their philosophical roots in a cross-cultural examination which is enriching to all. Many people now use herbs because they are felt to be safer, cheaper, more natural, and to have fewer side-effects. This is not always the case. Any substance can trigger an idiosyncratic response. Herbs must be given with knowledge and responsibility. But by following a few rules and using common sense, we add to our health, our sense of belonging, and our pleasure at being on the planet.

RIGHT *Really getting to know plants and the therapeutic actions of the remedies they provide is crucial to a sound practice of herbalism.*

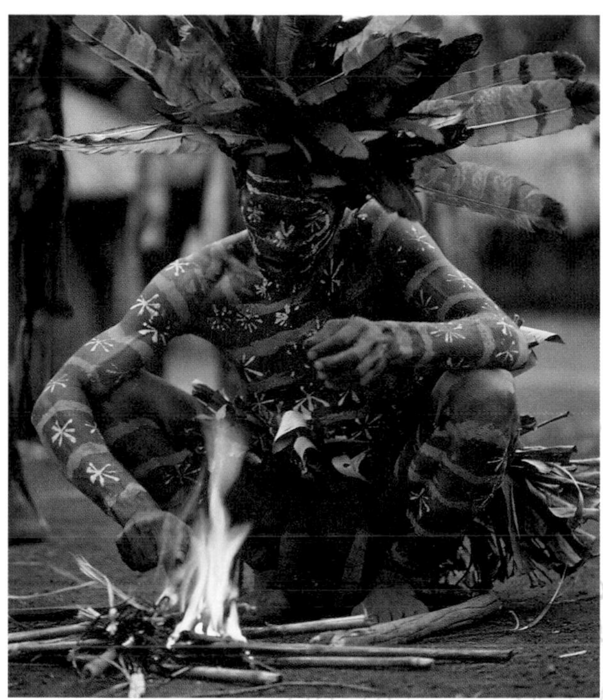

ABOVE *Native cultures have preserved the knowledge and practice of herbal treatments.*

THE TWO LEVELS IN MODERN HERBALISM

Modern herbalism is practised on two levels. These differ in the range of herbs which can be used, the results that can be achieved, and the amount of responsibility taken for treatment:

AS A PROFESSION

Western consultant medical herbalists act in just the same way as orthodox practitioners. They are trained in orthodox medical diagnosis and can provide a complete alternative. They also work with physicians to offer a complementary service. A medical herbalist will sometimes use some powerful herbs which are restricted by law, or only available after a personal consultation, in the same way as an orthodox practitioner will use prescription-only medicines. A good medical herbalist will have undergone extensive training and he or she will certainly belong to an established body of practitioners. (*For a list of organizations which keep a register of qualified herbal practitioners, see Useful Addresses, page 486.*)

AS A SELF-HELP SYSTEM

Herbs are ideal as a simple system of home care for first aid, everyday ailments, the management of chronic conditions, strengthening of the body, and preventive treatment. Herbs can be safely taken as long as a few simple rules are followed (*see The Rules of Safe Home Treatment, page 106*).

HERBALISM AND CONSERVATION

One hundred years ago, a person could have walked into the garden or local woods and returned with a remedy for the baby's gripe, a stomachache, sprained ankle, stiffening gout, or any number of ailments. Today we can walk into the local store and find the shelves full of natural ingredients from all corners of the world – from carrots and cabbage to precious spices like cinnamon. This array would have been the envy of a medieval apothecary; but while the stock is available, the knowledge is scarce. The culture of responsibility, self-care, and interaction with nature has largely been lost. It must be rediscovered if herbs and their proper uses are to be properly understood.

A herb has a taste, color, smell, texture, and history. The antiseptic calendula lotion applied to a spot was once an orange marigold growing clear and open-faced in a sunny meadow. The lavender used to reduce the tension of a pounding headache and bring sleep once shimmered in a soporific violet-purple haze on a French mountainside. Such pictures are part of the heritage of healing, and help us to remember and understand the actions of herbs and the way they work within the body.

Part of the beauty of herbalism lies in the many different possible methods of taking herbs. The skill in choosing the best method for a specific individual and condition is part of the art of caring. Hand baths, foot baths, skin washes, rubs, massage oils, eye baths, compresses, and fomentations are undervalued. Local treatments allow the herb to act exactly where it is needed, avoid affecting the whole system, and are comforting and effective. Remember that in all herbal preparations it is best to use organic herbs.

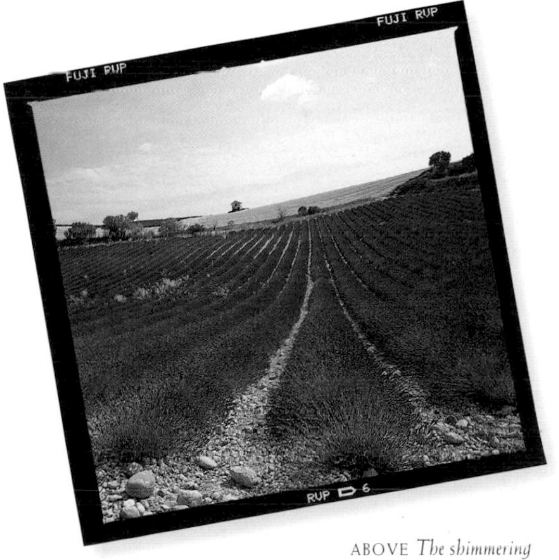

ABOVE *The shimmering violet-purple haze of a lavender field.*

A LONG HISTORY

Herbal remedies have been around for a long time. A walk in the garden or woods could provide a remedy for a baby's gripe, stomachache, or gout.

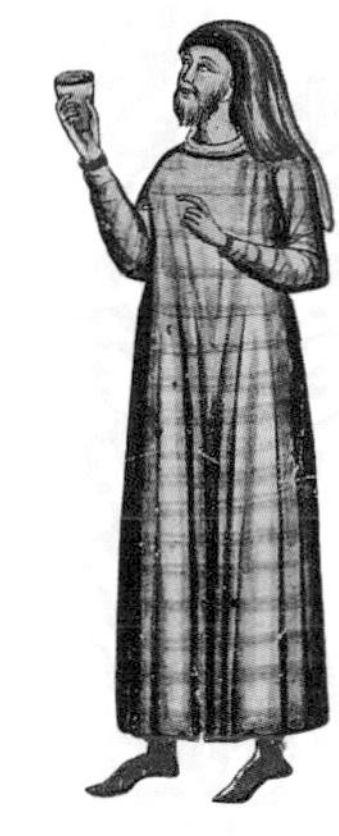

HIPPOCRATES
Hippocrates (477–360 B.C.E.) is known as the "father of medicine." He used herbal treatments.

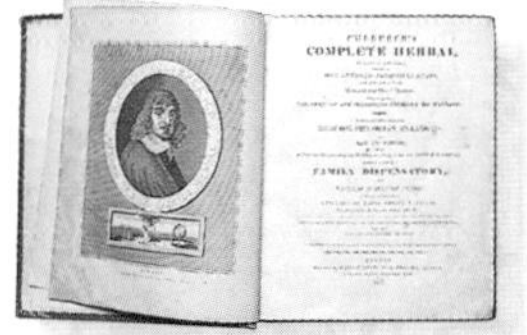

CULPEPER
Culpeper wrote a comprehensive guide to herbalism in the 17th century.

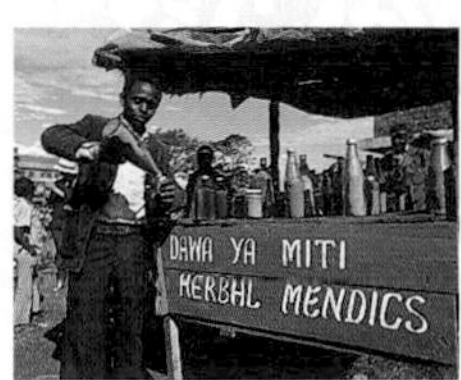

TRADITION
Many herbal remedies have been in use for hundreds of years and are still popular.

USING HERBS AT HOME

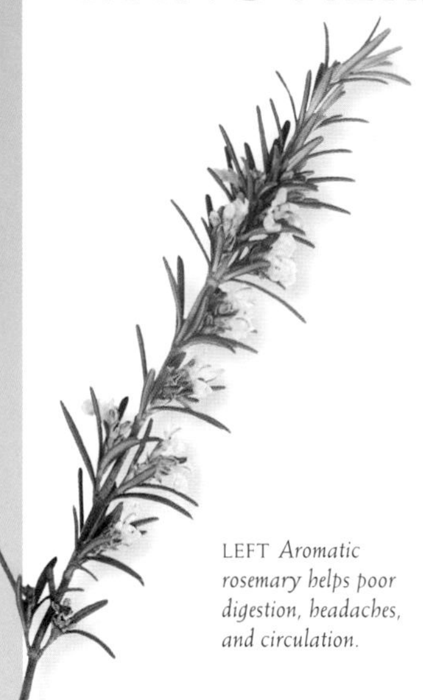

LEFT *Aromatic rosemary helps poor digestion, headaches, and circulation.*

To be able to care for yourself and your family by making natural remedies is a pleasure, and the benefits are legion. The organic chemistry of remedy-making is an extension of cooking, and the same principles and skills apply. For success, use the best-quality ingredients, practise absolute cleanliness, and follow the instructions carefully.

It is important to remember that several herbs may be recommended for a particular ailment; all are slightly different. For example, would rose, lavender, rosemary, or chamomile be best for your headache? Would a cool compress be best, or a long soak in a rosemary bath? Knowledge of the herb, the individual, and the different methods must be combined to prescribe remedies that will be really effective.

THE RULES OF SAFE HOME TREATMENT

- Consider the whole body and person first. Is medication needed? Consider a change of rest, diet, or exercise before prescribing the patient any remedy.
- Use simple remedies internally and externally. This will encourage the body to heal itself.
- Make a list. Know what you are taking and what to expect. Keep a note of all remedies taken. This will be useful if you need help later.
- Take as recommended. Remember the herbal tenet of minimum effective dosage and intervention. Stick to the standard dosages. Doubling does not double effectiveness, it may put an extra burden on a body that is already sick.
- TLC. Use lots of Tender Loving Care. A positive and loving attitude helps to make the illness more bearable, and may even speed up the healing process.
- Monitor progress after a few days.
- Stop treatment if there is any adverse reaction. Remember, people are all individuals; children, especially, respond quickly, so be alert for changes or new symptoms.
- Seek professional help if in any doubt. Assessing your own symptoms is different from making a diagnosis, which needs an objective eye.

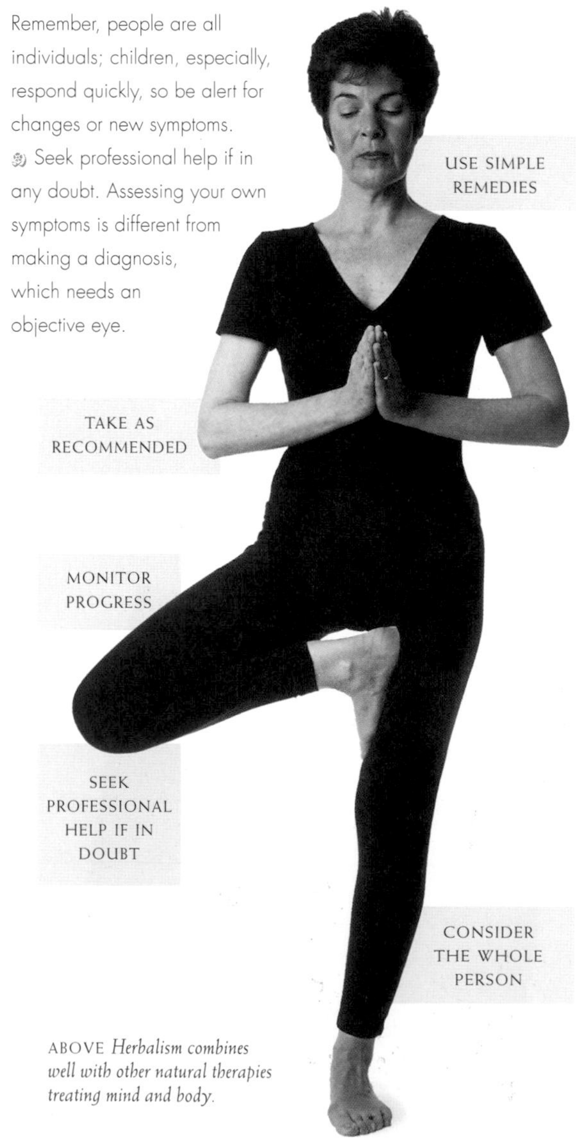

ABOVE *Herbalism combines well with other natural therapies treating mind and body.*

WHAT IS A HERB?

Herbage, like foliage, refers to plants with green leaves, but in herbal remedies more than leaves are used. Indeed, any part of a plant can be used:

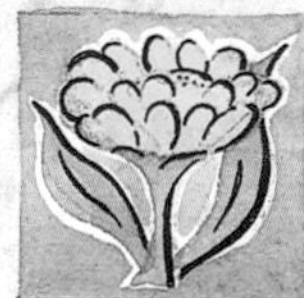

FLOWERS
Chamomile, marigold, linden, St. John's wort

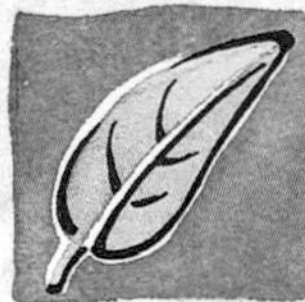

LEAVES
Peppermint, sage, thyme, comfrey

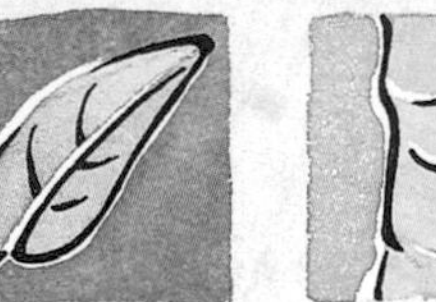

BARK
Willow, oak, cinnamon

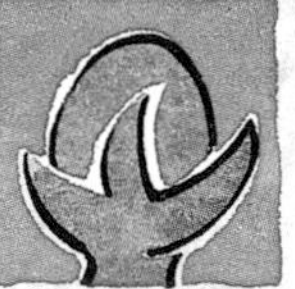

BUDS
Cloves

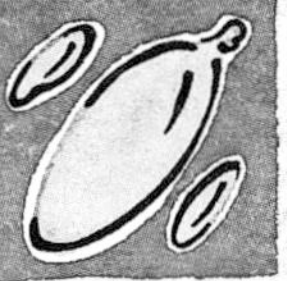

SEEDS
Fennel, cardamom

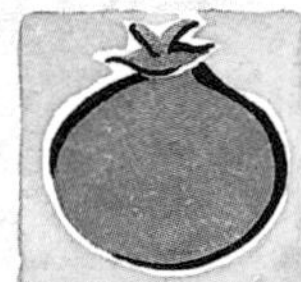

FRUITS
Cayenne, rose hips

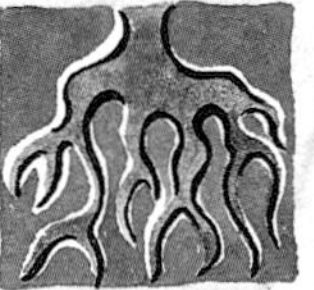

ROOT
Dandelion, marshmallow

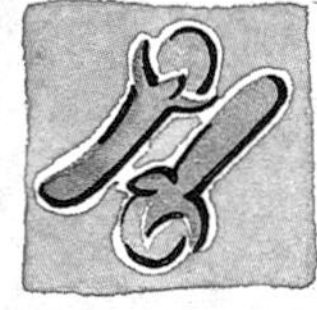
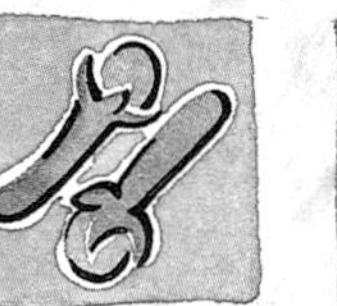

INNER SAP/GEL
Clove, Aloe Vera

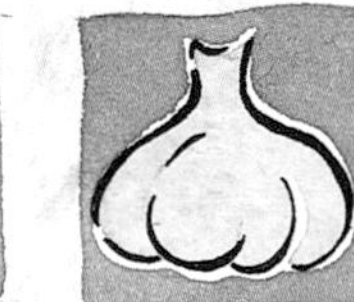

BULB
Garlic

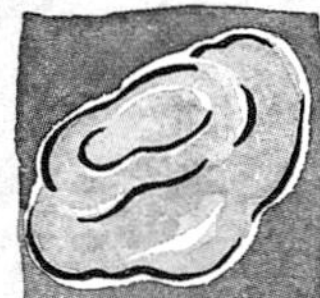

WOOD
Pau D'arco

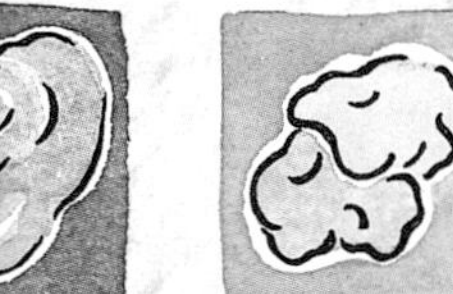

RESIN
Myrrh, frankincense

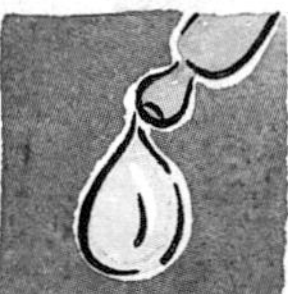

ESSENTIAL OIL
Rose, rosemary, lavender

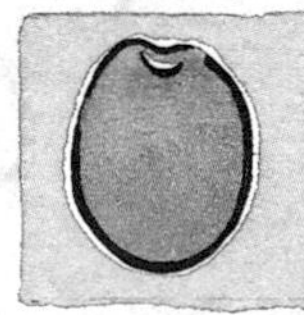

FIXED OIL
Olive oil, St. John's wort

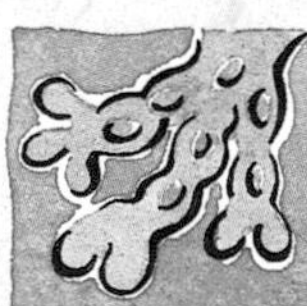

SEAWEED
Kelp, bladderwrack

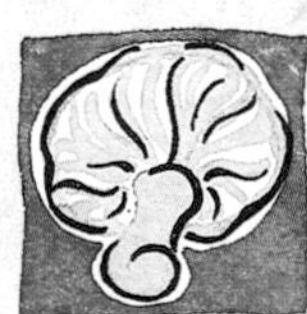

MUSHROOMS
Ganoderma (reishi), oyster

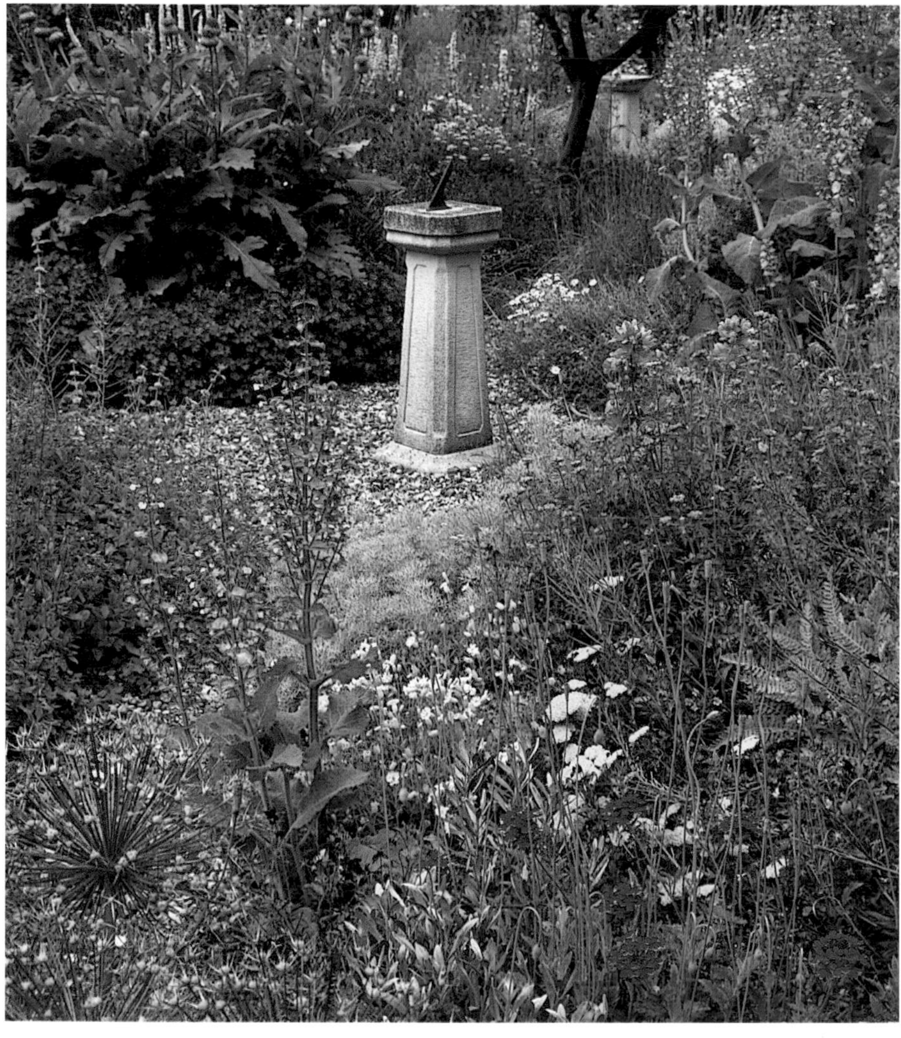

ABOVE *A dedicated herb garden close to the house is the best way to grow herbs.*

WHERE TO GET HERBS

Many herbs and herbal products are freely available. Plants or seeds can be bought from garden centers (always check the Latin name) and grown in the garden or in a window box.

Dried herbs are available from herb stores and some wholefood outlets. Always specify the herb (the Latin name if possible) and the part of the plant to be used – root, bark, leaf, or flower.

Herbal products, remedies, tinctures, tablets, etc. are available from wholefood stores, and some pharmacies and general food stores. Read the label and instructions carefully.

Regarding plants picked from the wild, countries have different rules and some plants are protected by law. Check the legal situation and get permission from the landowner. Check identification carefully and pick the minimum required, with proper regard for conservation. Never gather roots from the side of the road, by recently sprayed crops or foliage, or from sick-looking plants.

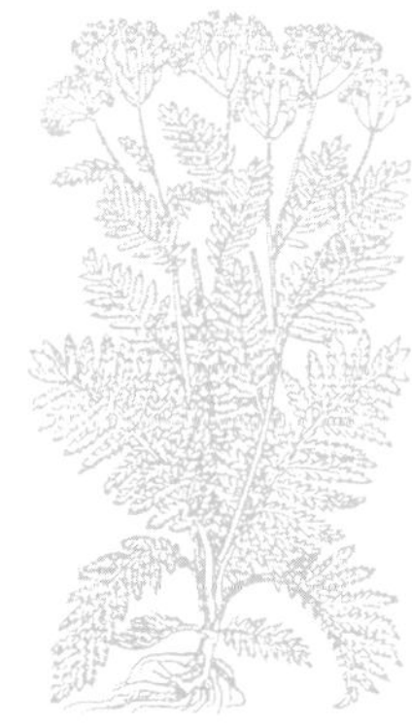

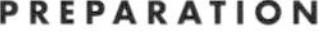

PREPARATION

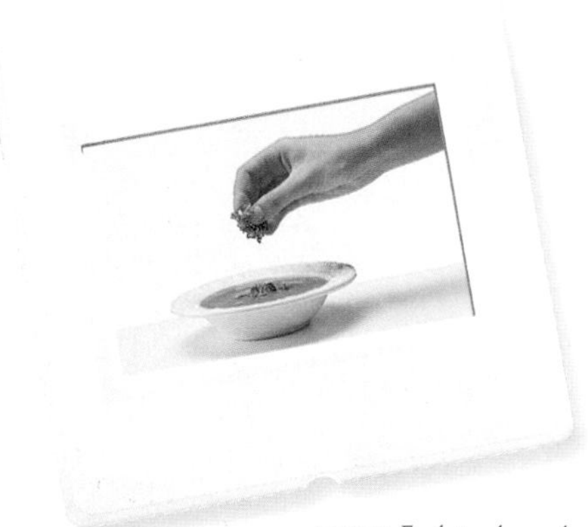

ABOVE *Fresh parsley makes a tasty addition to soup, and is high in vitamin C.*

THE FRESH PLANT

The easiest way to take a herb is to pick it directly from the plant.

Leaves can be used in salads, sandwiches, or soups. Chickweed, chicory, dandelion, and marigold make excellent salad additions. Nettle is traditional for green soup. Elderflower fritters are fun.

Chewing a few fresh leaves of marjoram will help clear the head. Horseradish leaves will clear sinuses. Sage eases mouth sores and sore throats.

Fresh leaves can also be used to make water infusions (teas), decoctions, tinctures, infused oils, and creams. Follow standard recipes and dosages. Most recipes give the amounts for dried herbs. When using fresh material add one-third more, as fresh plants contain a considerable amount of water.

IMMEDIATE RESPONSE

For cuts, grazes, and stings, pick four or five leaves (dock is traditional when stung on countryside walks as it is so readily available) and rub the leaves together between the hands to bruise them and release the juices. When damp, apply to the affected area and hold in place. Poultices can be made in the same way.

RIGHT *Dock leaves can be used to treat a sting. Bruise and apply.*

PREPARATIONS

Most herbs are sold in dried form. In this form they can simply be powdered and sprinkled on to food (half a flat teaspoon twice daily), but most are prepared further. Herbs are prepared for:

- AVAILABILITY AND PRESERVATION – so that seasonal plants are available year round.
- CONVENIENCE, EASE OF USE – compressed tablets are often more convenient to take than a cup of tea.
- SPECIFIC USE, TO AID THE ACTION OF THE HERB – for example infused oils for rubs, honey for adding a soothing and demulcent quality to thyme.

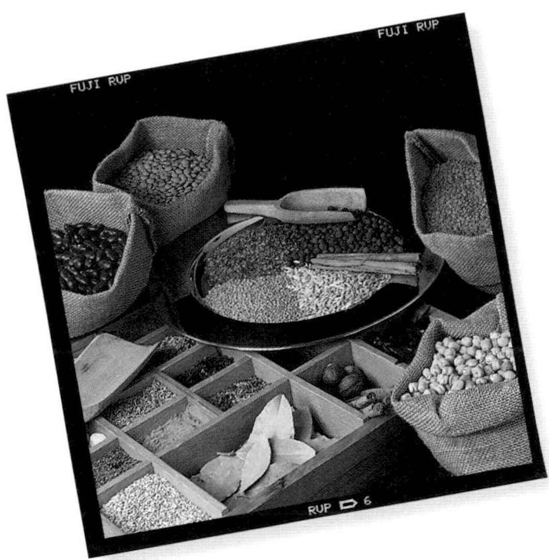

ABOVE *Dried herbs are most convenient for medicinal use, as they are readily available all year round.*

There are three main carriers for herbs, each of which adds a different quality:

- WATER – Infusions (teas). For flowers, leaves, some seeds, and fruit. Quickly assimilated and utilized by the body. Gentle for children, convalescents, and those with a delicate digestion. Ideal for diuretic, diaphoretic, cooling, and cleaning regimes. Decoctions are used for harder parts, like roots, and for stronger preparations.
- ALCOHOL – Tinctures and spiced wines. For all plant parts, especially hard parts. Alcohol adds some temporary heat and stimulation. It is convenient, although not for those intolerant of alcohol or for babies. Keeps indefinitely.
- OIL – Herbs infused in oil. For all parts of the plant. For rubs, massage oils, and liniments. Infused oils can be thickened with beeswax to make soothing and nourishing ointments and salves.

METHODS AND DOSAGES

WATER~INFUSIONS (TEAS)

STANDARD STRENGTH

1oz. (25g.) herb to 1pt. (500ml.) water; or 1 teaspoon herb to 1 cup water

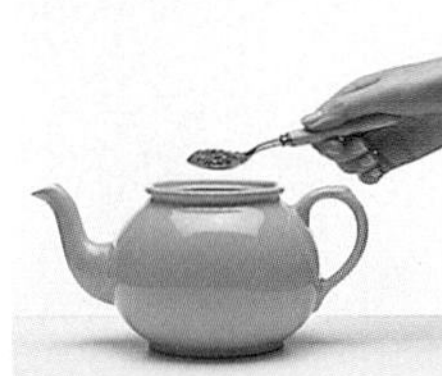

Use 1 teaspoon dried herb or (1½ teaspoon fresh) per cup required. Put the herb into a teapot.

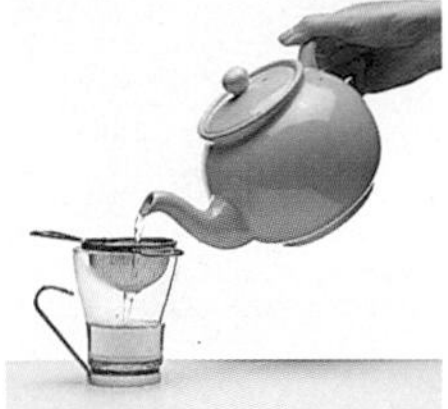

Pour on boiling water. Put on a tight lid. Brew for the required time (see below). *Strain and use.*

DOSE

Some herbs have specific indications and dosages; other herbs are not recommended at certain times, for example early pregnancy or when breast-feeding. Read the indications and contraindications of each herb carefully.

STANDARD ADULT DOSE

- 1 cup three times a day for normal conditions
- 1 cup up to six times a day, or every two hours, for acute conditions
- Drink 1 cup twice a day as a long-term strengthening tonic

CHILDREN'S DOSE

Reduce proportionally. Give a child of seven half the standard adult dose. At six months use 1 teaspoon of the standard strength tea. For breast-feeding infants give the remedy to the mother.

BREWING TIMES

To some extent this depends on personal taste, but the following is a good guide:

- up to 3 minutes for flowers and soft leaves
- up to 5 minutes for seeds and leaves
- up to 10 minutes for hard seeds, roots, and various barks

Water infusions at the standard strength are used as teas, gargles, as lotions for the skin, as compresses, and for fomentations. Dilute with an equal amount of water for hand or foot baths, douches, and enemas.

WATER~DECOCTIONS

STANDARD STRENGTH

- 1½oz. (40g.) herb to 1½pt. (750ml.) water

METHOD

- Put herb in saucepan
- Add 1½pt. (750ml.) water
- Put on a tight lid
- Bring to the boil, then turn down as low as possible and simmer for 10–15 minutes
- Strain thoroughly
- Discard herb
- Pour decoction into a clean bottle
- Will keep in a refrigerator for about two or three days

DOSE

- ½ cup twice a day for normal conditions, and as a tonic
- ½ cup three to six times a day for acute conditions

Decoctions can be diluted with an equal amount of water and used in the same ways as water infusions for hand baths, gargles, etc.

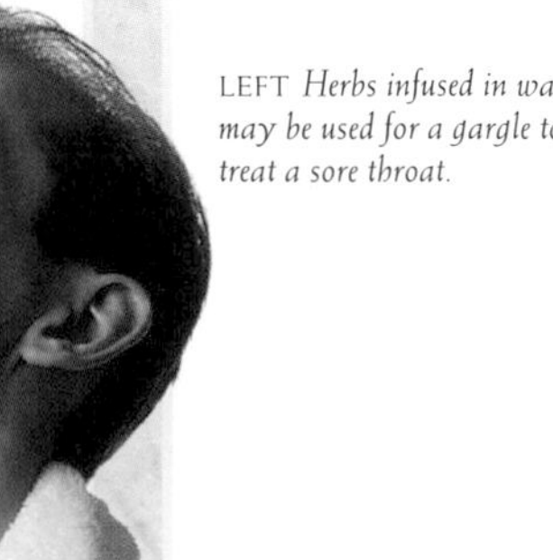

LEFT *Herbs infused in water may be used for a gargle to treat a sore throat.*

BEARBERRY

WATER~SIMPLE SYRUPS AND HONEYS

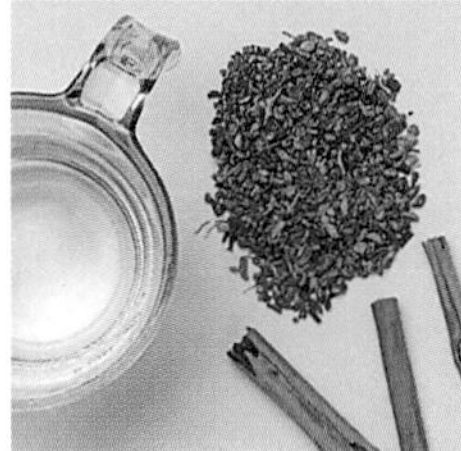

ABOVE *Ingredients for a laxative syrup: yellow dock root, cinnamon, and water.*

METHOD

- Make standard decoction with 1½oz. (40g.) herb and 1½pt. (750ml.) water
- Return to heat, remove lid, and simmer gently till liquid is reduced to ½pt. (250ml.), which may take a few hours
- Add 1¼lb. (600g.) honey or 1lb. (500g.) sugar, stirring until completely dissolved
- Pour into clean bottle, label, and date

STANDARD ADULT DOSE

- 1 dessertspoon 3 to 6 times a day

CHILDREN UNDER FIVE

- 1 teaspoon three times a day

Syrups and honeys can be used to sweeten other herbal preparations, or added to food or drink. They are ideal for children because they are sweet.

ALCOHOL~TINCTURES

A tincture is an alcohol-based herbal preparation. Tinctures can be made with fresh or dried herbs. The absolute strength of the alcohol needed varies slightly depending on the herb, but the method given below is sufficient for standard home use.

METHOD

To make 9fl.oz. (300ml.) of tincture:

- Chop ½oz. (12g.) dried or 1oz. (25g.) fresh herb
- Put in large glass jar
- Cover with 6fl.oz. (200ml.) alcohol, such as vodka or brandy, and 3fl.oz. (100ml.) water
- Put on a lid and leave for two weeks
- Shake occasionally
- After 2 weeks, strain well through a muslin bag
- Squeeze out the liquid
- Pour into clean, amber glass bottle
- Label and date
- Keep in a cool place away from children
- Will keep indefinitely

STANDARD ADULT DOSE

- 1 teaspoon 3 times a day, standard
- 5 drops to 1 teaspoon a day as a tonic
- 1 teaspoon 6 times a day for acute conditions

A tincture can be diluted with water: 1 dessertspoon to 1 cup water can be used as skin lotion, a wash, footbath, gargle, compress, or douche.

OIL~LINIMENT

A liniment is a soothing rub to relieve fatigued and stiff muscles and joints.

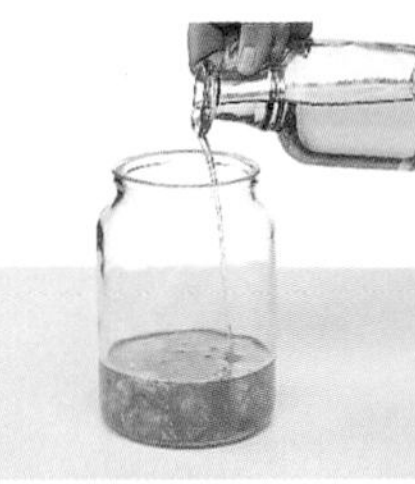

Put the fresh herb in a jar and cover with olive oil. Leave for up to 6 weeks.

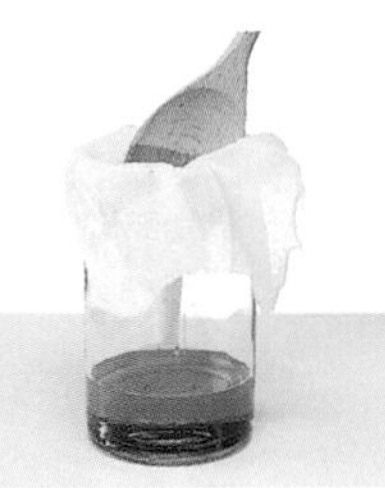

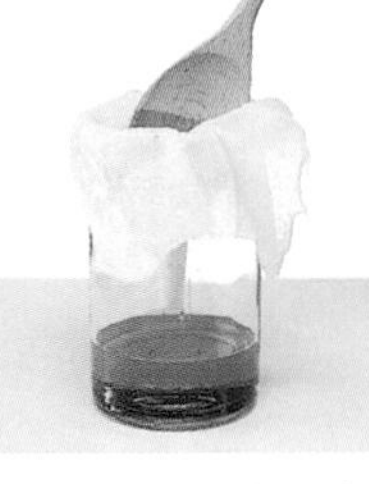

Strain the mixture through a cloth. Stand until the oil separates off: use this.

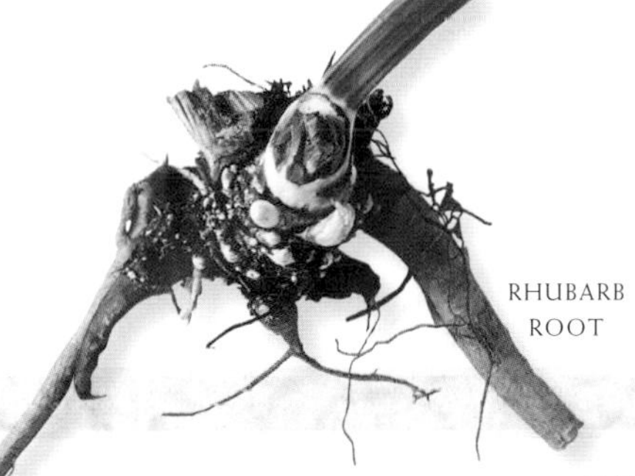

RHUBARB ROOT

OIL

Oil is soothing and nourishing for the skin, and acts as a lubricant to carry the active principles of the herbs in rubs, massage oils, and salves. There are two methods of infusion, hot and cold. Hot is used for thyme, rosemary, comfrey root, and spices such as Cayenne, Mustard, and Ginger. Cold is used for flowers (see St. John's wort, step-by-step, page 124).

INFUSED OIL

METHOD

To make ½pt. (250ml.):

- Chop 2–3oz. (50–75g.) dried herbs or spices, or 3–4oz. (75–100g.) fresh herbs
- Put half into a clean pan with a lid
- Cover with ½pt. (250ml.) pure vegetable oil (a pure and light vegetable oil is best).
- Put in a water bath and simmer gently for 2 hours (it is important that direct heat is not used, as this might burn the oil)
- Strain
- Throw away used herbs
- Put remaining half of unused herbs in pan
- Cover these with the oil (it will have changed color, having picked up some of the quality of the herbs)
- Replace lid and return pan to water bath for another couple of hours
- Strain
- Pour oil into clean bottles, label, and date

This double method makes a strong infused oil which can be used as it is, mixed with tincture for a liniment, or thickened with beeswax (for a thin cream, use 1 part beeswax to 10 parts infused oil; for a thick salve, use 1 part beeswax to 5 parts infused oil).

ALCOHOL~SPICED OR TONIC WINE

A good way to make a strengthening remedy for everyday use is to make a tonic wine. Spiced wines make good aperitifs, to stimulate and improve digestion.

METHOD

- 1oz. (25g.) herb(s)
- 1–2oz. (25–50g.) spices, depending on taste
- 4½pt. (2l.) of wine
- Stand for two weeks
- Strain and bottle

DOSE

¼ cup twice a day before meals (warm water can be added)

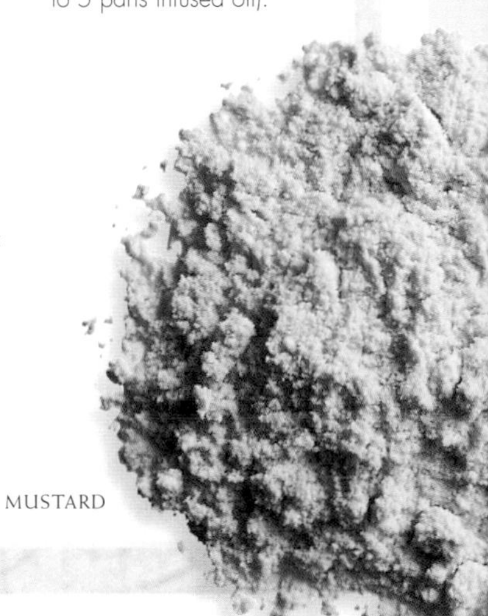

MUSTARD

THE REMEDIES

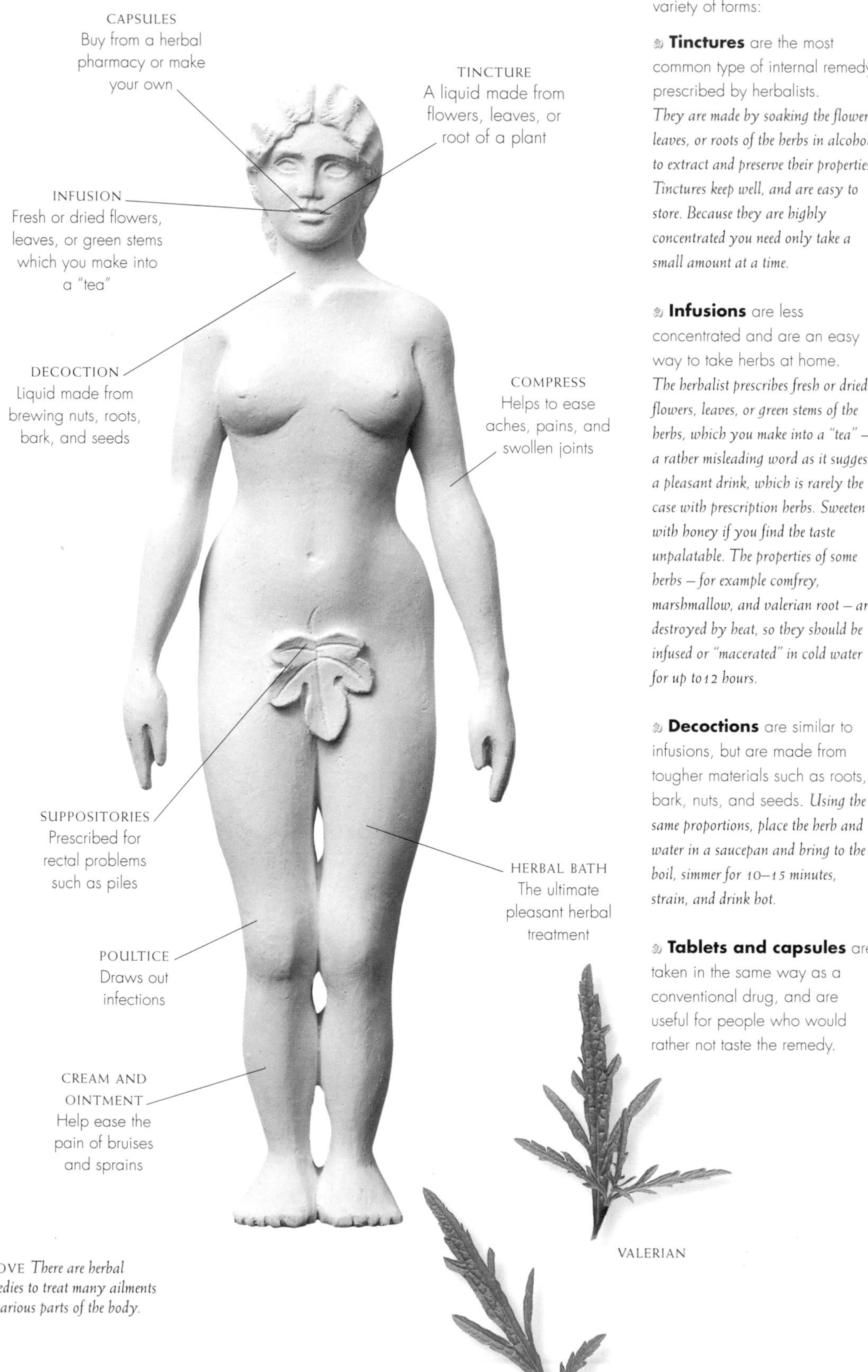

ABOVE *There are herbal remedies to treat many ailments in various parts of the body.*

VALERIAN

HERBAL REMEDY CARRIERS

Herbal remedies come in a variety of forms:

Tinctures are the most common type of internal remedy prescribed by herbalists. *They are made by soaking the flowers, leaves, or roots of the herbs in alcohol to extract and preserve their properties. Tinctures keep well, and are easy to store. Because they are highly concentrated you need only take a small amount at a time.*

Infusions are less concentrated and are an easy way to take herbs at home. *The herbalist prescribes fresh or dried flowers, leaves, or green stems of the herbs, which you make into a "tea" – a rather misleading word as it suggests a pleasant drink, which is rarely the case with prescription herbs. Sweeten with honey if you find the taste unpalatable. The properties of some herbs – for example comfrey, marshmallow, and valerian root – are destroyed by heat, so they should be infused or "macerated" in cold water for up to 12 hours.*

Decoctions are similar to infusions, but are made from tougher materials such as roots, bark, nuts, and seeds. *Using the same proportions, place the herb and water in a saucepan and bring to the boil, simmer for 10–15 minutes, strain, and drink hot.*

Tablets and capsules are taken in the same way as a conventional drug, and are useful for people who would rather not taste the remedy.

Creams and ointments are applied externally to soothe irritated or inflamed skin conditions, or ease the pain of sprains or bruises. *Cream moistens dry or cracked skin, and massaging the ointment into bruises and sprains helps to ease the pain. In both cases the active ingredients of the herb pass through the pores of the skin into the blood stream to encourage healing.*

Compresses, either hot or cold, help with aches, pains, and swollen joints. *Fold a clean piece of cotton into an infusion of the prescribed herb and apply to the point of pain. Repeat as the compress cools or, in the case of cold compresses, until the pain eases.*

Poultices, made from bruised fresh herbs or dried herbs moistened into a paste with hot water, are also good for painful joints or drawing out infection from boils, spots, or wounds. *Place the herb on a clean piece of cotton and bandage on to the affected area. Leave in place for around two hours or until symptoms ease.*

Suppositories and douches are sometimes prescribed for rectal problems such as piles, or vaginal infections, respectively. *The suppositories will come ready made for you to insert. Douches are made from an infusion or decoction that has been allowed to cool.*

Herbal baths are perhaps the most pleasant of the herbal remedies, and are a useful supplement to other forms of treatment. *The heat of the water activates the properties of the volatile oils so that they are absorbed through the pores of the skin and inhaled through the nose. In both cases they pass into the blood stream, and when inhaled they also pass through the nervous system to the brain, exerting a healing effect on both mind and body.*

SEEING A PROFESSIONAL

Professional consultant medical herbalists are usually trained in orthodox diagnosis and can treat all of the ailments treated by a family physician, or general practitioner. Accredited members of organizations such as the National Institute of Medical Herbalists have undergone four years of university or university-standard study and two years of supervision. They will understand all the indications and contraindications of herbs, and any problems which may arise from taking orthodox drugs. They will refer to other specialists if necessary. *(For a list of organizations which keep a register of qualified herbal practitioners, see Useful Addresses, page 486.)*

It is becoming more common for a patient to register with a herbalist in the same way as one would register with a physician – for a check-up and then to be on the books should the need arise. Such patients have yearly checks to maintain optimum health. Whole families register, as herbalism is especially suited to children and the elderly.

A consultation will take about an hour and consider all aspects of health, diet, exercise, and lifestyle. Your herbalist will take a "holistic" view, which means taking into consideration everything that affects your health on a physical, mental, and spiritual level.

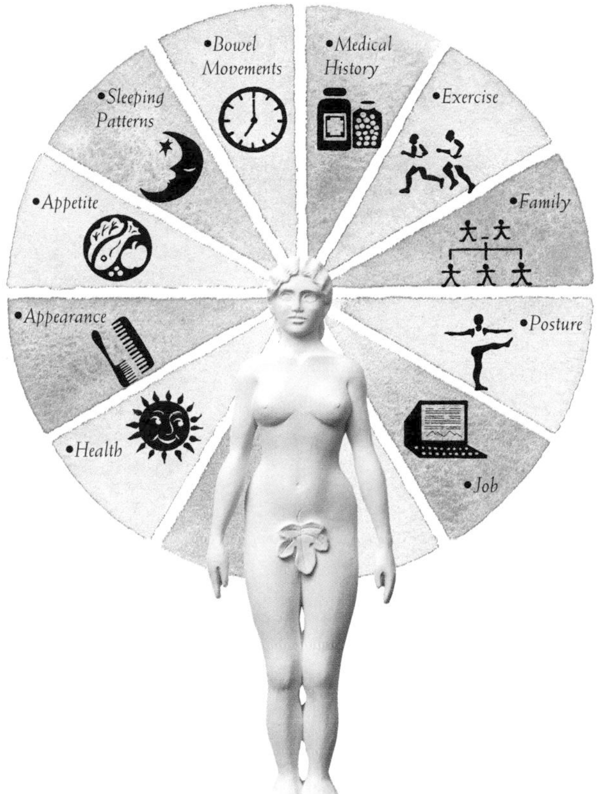

ABOVE *A consultation with a herbalist will cover a range of areas.*

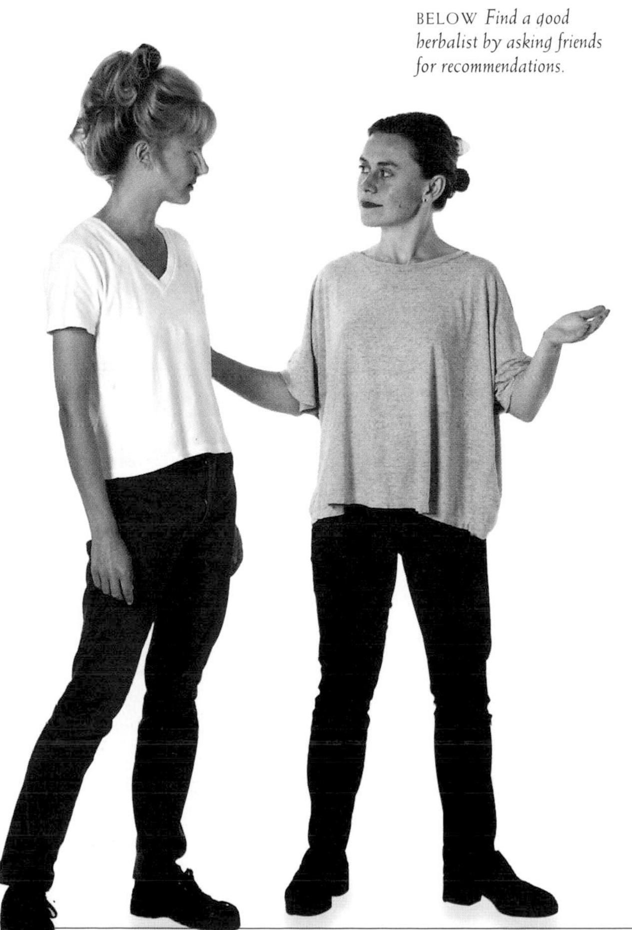

BELOW *Find a good herbalist by asking friends for recommendations.*

You will be asked questions about:
❀ age ❀ job ❀ personality and what is important to you ❀ concerns ❀ appetite ❀ sleeping patterns ❀ previous medicines and illnesses ❀ bowel movements ❀ family ❀ symptoms ❀ any other aspect that is relevant.

As well as what you say, your therapist will want to know how you feel and will note your appearance. The condition of your hair, skin, and facial expression, your posture, and how you move all provide important clues that will help with the diagnosis. There may also be a physical examination. Treatment will then be prescribed by the therapist.

Before a first visit it is worth spending some time considering your health and your expectations. It is useful to make a list of relevant points in your medical history and questions you want to ask, as these can easily be missed or forgotten in the stress of a first meeting. If for any reason you do not get on with the practitioner, try another one. It is important that there is a relationship of mutual trust and respect.

Many of the herbs prescribed will be familiar, but some will be unknown to you. After a consultation, a herbalist is able to prescribe herbs which are limited by law and not freely available over the counter to the general public.

WHO CAN IT HELP?

Every member of the family can benefit from herbal treatments.

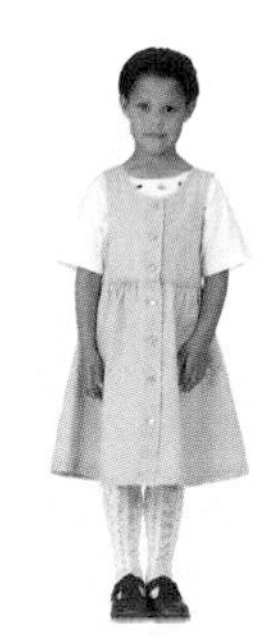

CHILDREN
Children respond especially well to herbal remedies.

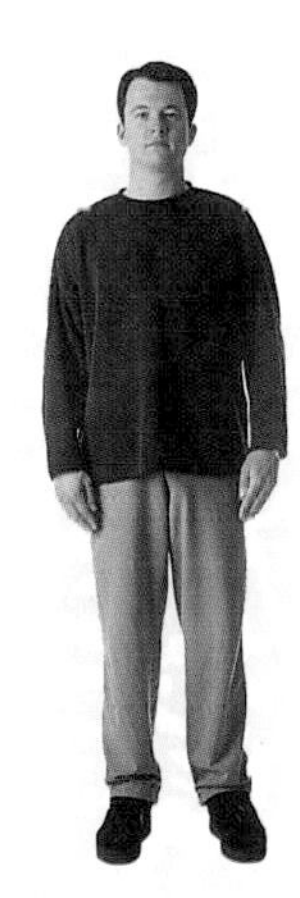

ADULTS
More and more people favor a return to natural treatments.

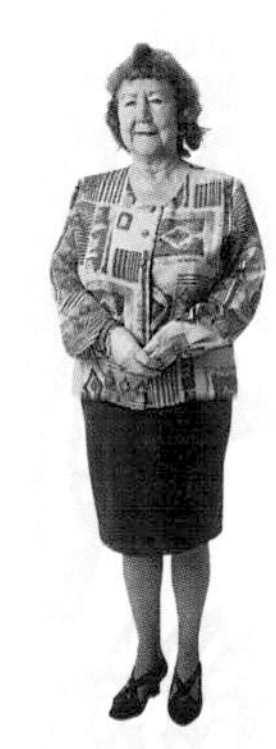

THE ELDERLY
Older people welcome the opportunity to cut down on prescribed drugs.

HERBAL REMEDY SOURCES

Achillea millefolium

YARROW

A common wild plant with feathery leaves and white or pink flowers. Often found on lawns. In Greek myth, *achillea* is said to have been used by Achilles to treat his army's wounds.

DATA FILE

Properties

- Diaphoretic
- Anti-inflammatory
- Antiseptic
- Antispasmodic
- Styptic
- Gentle bitter tonic

Uses

- Early stages of fevers, especially with hot, dry skin.
- Catarrh, sinusitis, hay fever, and dust allergies.
- For high blood pressure, with hawthorn and linden.
- With a little ginger for cold feet.
- Internal and external use for varicose veins and spontaneous bruising.
- Useful for thrombosis, to prevent blood clots.
- Supportive for people undergoing radiotherapy and intestinal infections.
- Diarrhea, liverishness, colic, and weak digestion.
- Irregular menstrual bleeding, cramps, and vaginal discharges.
- Helps pelvic circulation.
- With sage and marigold for pelvic infections and pelvic congestion with menstrual cramps, and pain before menstruation.
- Tea or tincture to disinfect wounds and stop bleeding.
- As a cream or compress for bleeding piles.
- Apply the infused oil to inflammations associated with varicose veins.
- In the bath to relieve aches and pains.

NOTES AND DOSAGES

Standard doses (*see pages 108–9*). **Take freely for fevers and acute complaints.**

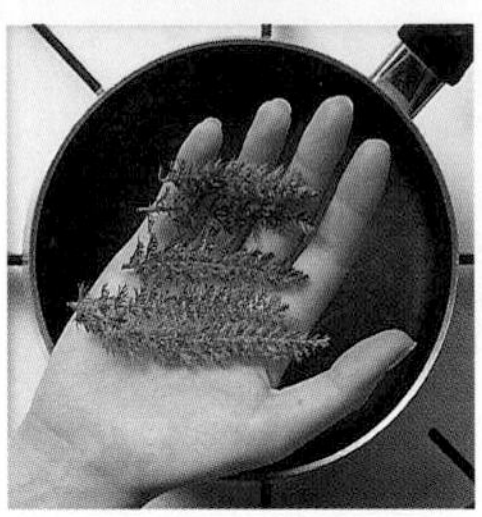

For a bath, simmer a handful of fresh leaves in 1pt. (500ml.) water for 15 minutes. Strain and add to your bath water. Chew a fresh leaf and apply to cuts to stop bleeding. Wash fresh root and chew for toothache.

It is said that one famous herbalist, when asked for suggestions for various ailments, said, "Go to bed with Yarrow tea and a hot brick." Yarrow is very versatile. The tea is excellent, on its own, for all feverish conditions, and can be mixed with other herbs, such as elderflower and peppermint, to treat colds and flu.

CAUTION

AVOID LARGE DOSES IN PREGNANCY. SMALL AMOUNTS ARE SAFE, BUT IF IN DOUBT CONSULT A PROFESSIONAL HERBALIST.

SOME PEOPLE DEVELOP AN ALLERGIC RASH IF THEY HANDLE THE FRESH HERB IN SUNLIGHT.

THERAPY CONNECTIONS

YARROW
Ayurveda p.24

AGRIMONY
Flower Remedies p.225

GARLIC
Ayurveda p.26
Traditional Home and Folk Remedies p.82

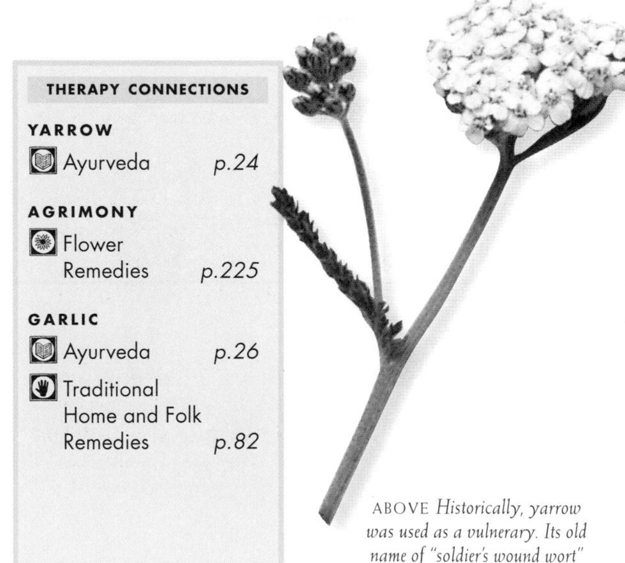

ABOVE *Historically, yarrow was used as a vulnerary. Its old name of "soldier's wound wort" gives a clue to this.*

Agrimonia eupatoria

AGRIMONY

A common wild plant with slender spikes of bright yellow flowers. The whole herb is used. Culpeper recommended it for gout "used outwardly in an oil or ointment, or inwardly, in a syrup or juice."

RECIPE

Agrimony Digestive Tonic

Combine equal parts of agrimony, raspberry leaf, and lemon balm (*Melissa officinalis*). Store away from the light. Make a tea from 1 teaspoon of the mixture to 1 cup of boiling water, and drink freely for colicky pains with looseness and nervous diarrhea.

DATA FILE

Properties

- Astringent and tonic
- Tones and strengthens the digestive system and liver
- A wound herb

Uses

- As a tea or tincture for indigestion, heartburn, diarrhea, and liverish feelings. Especially helpful for people suffering from food allergies – on a long-term basis.
- With St. John's wort and horsetail for bedwetting and chronic cystitis.
- As a lotion for the cleansing of wounds.
- As an eyewash for sore and inflamed eyes.

NOTES AND DOSAGES

Standard doses (*see pages 108–9*).

Agrimony makes a tasty substitute for ordinary tea.

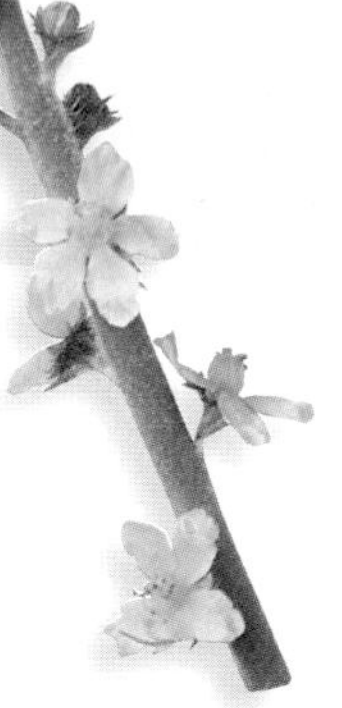

ABOVE *The word "agrimony" comes from a Greek word describing plants which healed the eyes.*

CAUTION

MAY AGGRAVATE CONSTIPATION, BUT OTHERWISE A SAFE AND GENTLE HERB TO USE.

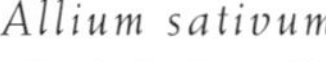

Alchemilla vulgaris

LADY'S MANTLE

A wild plant of wayside and meadows. Grows well in shady gardens, and bears sprays of greenish-yellow flowers.

CAUTION

DO NOT USE IN PREGNANCY EXCEPT UNDER PROFESSIONAL GUIDANCE, BUT OTHERWISE A SAFE HERB.

ALWAYS SEEK MEDICAL ADVICE FOR BLEEDING IN MID-MENSTRUAL CYCLE.

DATA FILE

Properties

- Astringent
- Tones and strengthens the womb

Uses

- Heavy menstrual bleeding, either alone or with an equal part of shepherd's purse or yarrow. Also for bleeding in the middle of the menstrual cycle and for irregular menstruation.
- To prevent menstrual cramps and for PMS, taken during the second half of the menstrual cycle.
- Thrush and other vaginal discharges, taken as a tea or douche.
- Traditional treatment for infertility in women with no obvious cause.
- Children's diarrhea.

ABOVE *The whole herb is gathered when the plant is in flower.*

NOTES AND DOSAGES

Standard doses. It is a pleasant drinking tea.

RECIPE

Lady's Mantle and Chamomile Wash

Make a strong tea with 1 cup of boiling water to 1 teaspoon of lady's mantle and 2 teaspoons of chamomile flowers. Infuse in a covered vessel for 15 minutes. Use this as a soothing wash for itchy genitals, in men and women.

Allium sativum

GARLIC

The familiar cooking herb. Garlic can be harvested about six to eight months after planting, in the summer. Bulbs not needed immediately can be dried in the sun and stored.

DATA FILE

Properties

- Antiseptic
- Antibiotic
- Expectorant
- Fungicide
- Antihistamine
- Lowers blood pressure and cholesterol

Uses

- Beneficial in cases of thrombosis, hardening of the arteries, high blood pressure, and high cholesterol.
- For chest infections, asthma, flu, colds, and ear infections. Combines well with echinacea.
- For intestinal worms and fungal infections.

ABOVE RIGHT *The active properties of garlic are due to its volatile oil.*

CAUTION

SAFE TO USE BUT MAY BE TOO HOT FOR SOME CONSTITUTIONS, IN WHICH CASE USE WITH MILK.

ENTERIC COATED TABLETS ARE AVAILABLE. THESE ARE EASIER ON THE DIGESTION.

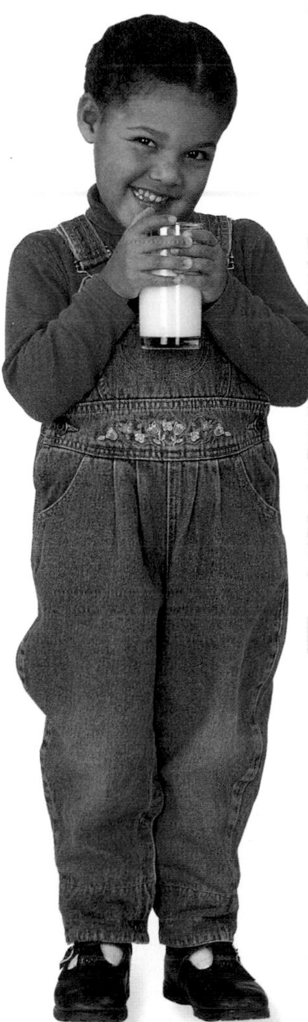

ABOVE *Garlic milk will help to relieve children's fevers and croup.*

RECIPE

Garlic or Onion Milk

Put 1 onion or 3 cloves of garlic, thinly sliced, into a pan with 2 cups of milk (cow's, goat's, sheep's, soy milk, or nut milk). Simmer over a very low heat for 20 minutes. Strain. Can be stored in a refrigerator for 2 or 3 days. *Dose:* Infants 1 or 2 dessertspoons every four hours. Young children can drink freely if feverish and croupy.

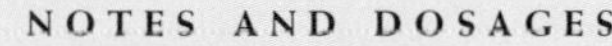

NOTES AND DOSAGES

Tablets are easy to take. Follow the instructions on the box. **Mix chopped garlic with an equal amount of honey and take 1 teaspoon 3 to 6 times daily. Half dose for children.** The infused oil can be applied to the skin, ear, and chest, to fight infections. **Regular dietary use benefits the circulation.**

Garlic is an exceptional respiratory disinfectant, but it is often too strong for young children. **Onions and leek are in the same family and have similar but milder actions.** Onion or garlic milk is an ideal remedy for infants and small children.

Aloe vera

ALOE VERA

A succulent, tropical plant that has been used for centuries to heal both externally and internally. Aloes are resistant to drought, taking in water very easily and losing moisture very slowly.

DATA FILE

Properties

- Soothing
- Cooling
- Antiseptic
- Antifungal

Uses

- Applied to burns and sunburn, ringworm, infected cuts, acne, shingles, eczema, wrinkles, and areas of dry, itchy skin.
- Use as a mouthwash for sore gums.
- As an internal medicine for candidiasis (thrush).

NOTES AND DOSAGES

Aloes are easily grown as a house plant. Cut the leaf and apply the gel directly to the skin, or take 1 tablespoon, twice daily, as an internal medicine. The cut leaves will keep and can be used again. There are many excellent preparations of aloe in the stores – follow the instructions on the packet.

The fresh aloe is unsurpassed for burns, irritable rashes, and sunburn. Keep some in the freezer for immediate use.

CAUTION

THE GEL IS SAFE, BUT PREPARATIONS OF THE WHOLE LEAF ARE STRONGLY LAXATIVE AND SHOULD NOT BE USED FOR LONG PERIODS OR IN PREGNANCY.

LEFT *Grow aloe inside, in a sunny position with a minimum temperature of 10°C (50°F).*

RECIPE

Aloe Gel

Wash the leaves. Cut into 2in. (5cm.) lengths. Slice each piece in half, to expose the largest amount of gel. Wrap each piece in plastic wrap and date. To use: remove plastic and apply the gel side of the leaf to the skin. Smear over the affected area, or hold in place with a bandage.

Althea officinalis

MARSHMALLOW

A wild plant easily grown in gardens. Use the root and leaves. It grows up to 4ft. (1.5m.) tall, with pale pink flowers. Its name comes from the Greek word *altho*, meaning "to cure."

DATA FILE

Properties

- Soothing
- Mucilaginous

Uses

- For acid stomach, heartburn, ulcers, hiatus hernia, and irritable bowel.
- Helps nonproductive and dry coughs.
- Irritable bladder.
- Dry skin, taken as a tea.
- Powdered root mixed into a cream or added to water to make a paste for insect bites and weeping eczema.

LEFT AND BELOW *Marshmallow leaves and root are used. Both have a high mucilage (a glutinous substance) content.*

NOTES AND DOSAGES

Can be taken freely. For best results soak 1oz. (25g.) cut root or leaf in 1pt. (500ml.) cold water overnight. Strain and drink 3 cups daily.

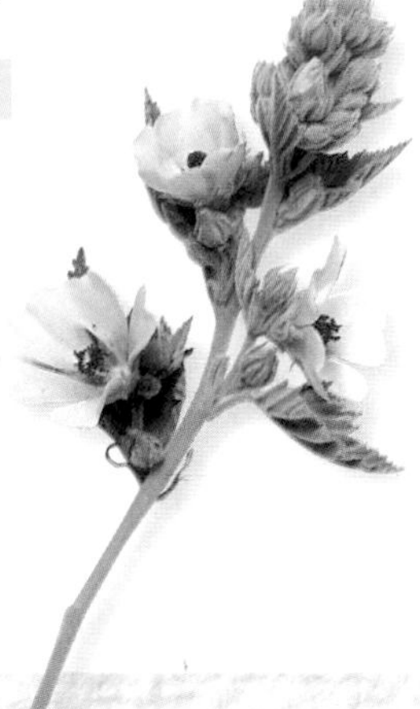

RECIPE

Marshmallow Paste

THIS IS AN ESPECIALLY EFFECTIVE PREPARATION FOR INSECT BITES AND STINGS.

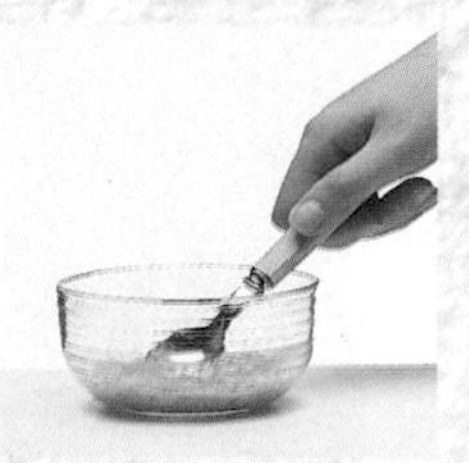

Take enough marshmallow root powder to cover the affected area, and add cold water to make a stiff paste.

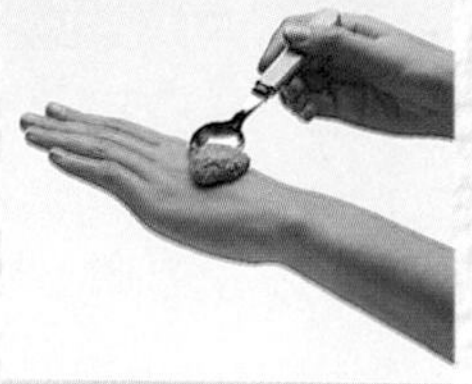

Apply thickly and allow to dry. Wash off and replace the paste every 2 or 3 hours.

Angelica archangelica and *Angelica sinensis*

ANGELICA ROOT

A tall, stately plant, popular in large gardens. The root should be dug up in the fall of the plant's first year, dried quickly, and stored in an airtight container. It will retain its medicinal properties for several years.

RECIPE

Candied Angelica

Cut the stems into 1in. (2.5cm.) lengths and simmer in sugar water until they are soft. Strain. Simmer in a sugar syrup (1lb. [500g.] sugar in ½pt. [250ml.] water) for an hour. Strain and allow to dry. Sprinkle with confectioner's sugar and store in an airtight tin. Dose: 2in. (5cm.) strip every few hours.

DATA FILE

Properties

- Warming and restorative
- Antiseptic
- Diuretic
- Diaphoretic
- Expectorant
- Relaxes spasm and strengthens digestion
- An excellent general tonic for those run down by chronic disease

Uses

- Tincture or decoction for convalescence, persistent fevers, indigestion, and weak digestion in general, colic and cramping pains, coughs, poor circulation, and general weakness with feelings of cold.
- Chinese angelica (Dang gui or *Angelica sinensis*) is an especially good tonic for women. In China it is called the women's ginseng. It is used for menstrual cramps and pains, anemia, and general debility in women.

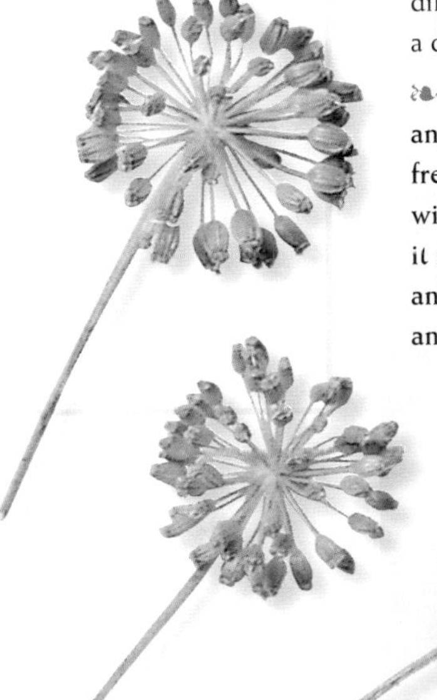

ABOVE Angelica archangelica *bears large umbels of yellow flowers from late spring to summer.*

THERAPY CONNECTIONS

ALOE VERA
Ayurveda p.27

ANGELICA
Ayurveda p.28
Chinese Herbal Medicine p.55
Aromatherapy p.146

CAUTION

ANGELICA ROOT IS CONTRAINDICATED IN DIABETES, AS IT INCREASES THE SUGAR LEVEL IN THE BLOOD.

AVOID LARGE DOSES IN PREGNANCY, EXCEPT AS ADVISED BY A QUALIFIED HERBALIST.

THE AMOUNTS TAKEN IN FOOD ARE HARMLESS.

SOME PEOPLE ARE SENSITIVE TO HANDLING THE FRESH PLANT.

NOTES AND DOSAGES

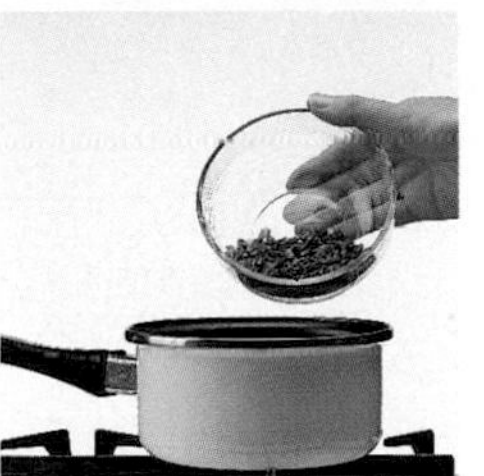

- Decoct 1oz. (30g.) of the root to 1pt. (500ml.) of water and take 2 or 3 times daily, or take up to ½ teaspoon (1–2ml.) diluted in water 3 times a day.
- **Crystallizing angelica preserves its fresh qualities for winter. When chewed it soothes the throat, and warms the chest and digestion.**

Arctium lappa or *Arctium minus*

BURDOCK

A common wayside plant with large leaves and purple flowers. The root is commonly used. Combined with yellow dock and sarsaparilla, it treats eczema.

NOTES AND DOSAGES

- Take 2 teaspoons of dried root, decocted, daily, or 1 teaspoon of the tincture twice daily for some months. For lack of appetite take the tincture 3 times daily, before meals, in a little water or fruit juice, 5–10 drops for children and 20 drops for adults.

Pickled burdock root makes a good daily tonic, digestive, and blood strengthener. It is a useful way to use the roots after weeding.

ABOVE *Burdock has large wavy leaves and round heads of purple flowers.*

CAUTION

LARGE DOSES MAY CAUSE A CLEANSING RASH. IT IS BEST TO START WITH SMALL DOSES AND THEN SLOWLY INCREASE THEM.

AVOID IN EARLY PREGNANCY EXCEPT WITH EXPERT ADVICE.

DATA FILE

Properties

- Blood cleanser
- Alterative
- Diuretic
- Lymphatic cleanser

Uses

- For "eruptive" and stubborn skin conditions, especially when hot and inflamed-looking – for example acne, spots, boils, rashes, psoriasis, rheumatism, and gout.
- With dandelion root for skin and liver problems.
- Chronic cystitis and loss of appetite

RECIPE

Pickled Burdock Root

Wash the root and cut into small rounds. Simmer in water until soft. Strain and put into a clean jar. Pour hot cider vinegar over the root. Label and date. Dose: As a tonic chew a piece first thing every morning. As a digestive, chew a piece 20 minutes before your meals.

Arctostaphylos uva-ursi

UVA URSI LEAVES

A small evergreen shrub of moors and mountains, also known as bearberry. The leaves are astringent and have a high tannin content.

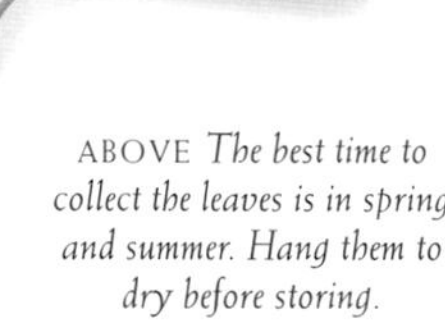

ABOVE *The best time to collect the leaves is in spring and summer. Hang them to dry before storing.*

DATA FILE

Properties

- Diuretic
- Urinary antiseptic
- Astringent

Uses

- For cystitis, together with soothing herbal remedies such as marshmallow.
- With horsetail or nettle for irritable bladder with persistent frequency.
- With lady's mantle or shepherd's purse for thick, white vaginal discharges.
- Take along with agrimony for diarrhea.

CAUTION

DO NOT USE DURING PREGNANCY OR BREAST-FEEDING, OR DURING KIDNEY DISEASE.

DO NOT USE FOR MORE THAN TWO WEEKS WITHOUT CONSULTING A PROFESSIONAL HERBALIST.

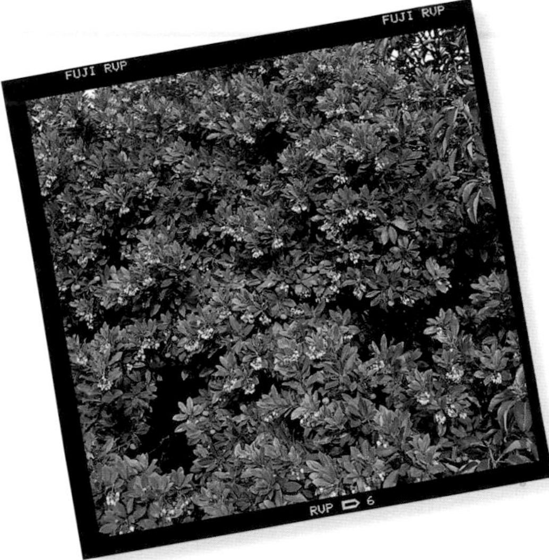

ABOVE *Bearberry leaves can be collected all year round, but are best in spring and summer.*

NOTES AND DOSAGES

For tea, use 1 teaspoon dried leaves to 1 cup water and infuse for 10 minutes. **For acute cystitis, take 1 cup of tea, or 1 teaspoon of tincture, 2 or 3 times daily for up to a week.** Take in combination with the suggested herbs for long-term use.

RECIPE

Tincture of Bearberries

Fill a jam jar with fresh or dried bearberries. Pour vodka over the berries until they are well covered. Store in a cool place for three weeks. Shake well every few days. Strain and store in a dark bottle. Dose: 30 drops. Use for bladder and intestinal infections. Blueberries or cranberries can also be used.

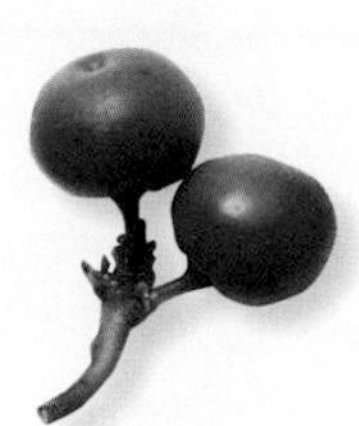

BEARBERRIES

Astragalus membranaceus

ASTRAGALUS

A herbaceous perennial plant of the pea family. The root is used for therapeutic purposes.

ABOVE *Dried astragalus root, sold in Chinese herb stores as Huang Qi. Use for decoctions.*

NOTES AND DOSAGES

Standard doses (*see pages 108–9*). Called Huang Qi. **The root can be bought in Chinese herb stores.** It is often used as a soup stock with other nourishing herbs for people with severe immune deficiencies.

Immune-enhancing soups can be made using astragalus root, which has a mild, sweet taste.

CAUTION

A SAFE HERB FOR HOME USE, BUT SEVERELY DEBILITATED PATIENTS SHOULD ALWAYS BE SEEN BY A PROFESSIONAL HERBALIST, WHO WILL PRESCRIBE ACCORDING TO THE INDIVIDUAL'S CONDITION AND CIRCUMSTANCES.

ALWAYS TELL THE HOSPITAL IF YOU ARE TAKING HERBAL MEDICINE IN CONJUNCTION WITH THEIR TREATMENT.

DATA FILE

Properties

- Helps to strengthen the immune system.
- A famous Chinese tonic.

Uses

- Decoction or tincture for chronic fatigue, persistent infections, night sweats, multiple allergies, and glandular fever.
- Modern research shows that the herb helps to counteract tiredness and lack of appetite in patients undergoing chemotherapy and radiotherapy for cancer.
- Soothing and healing for stomach ulcers.

RECIPE

Immune-enhancing Soup

Put 1oz. (25g.) of the chopped root in a pan. Simmer for one hour in 1pt. (500ml.) of water. Use as a stock for vegetable soups or for cooking brown rice. Take this every day. The soup has a mild, sweet taste that goes well with a range of vegetables.

Calendula officinalis

MARIGOLD FLOWERS

A popular garden plant with orange or yellow flowers. Do not confuse it with French and African marigolds (*Tagetes* species), which must not be taken internally.

NOTES AND DOSAGES

❧ Add 2 or 3 flowers to 1 cup of boiling water. Infuse for 10 minutes. Drink 3 cups a day, or 1 cup every 3 hours for acute complaints. Half dose for children over five years old. Give infants 3 or 4 teaspoons of a weak tea in fruit juice.

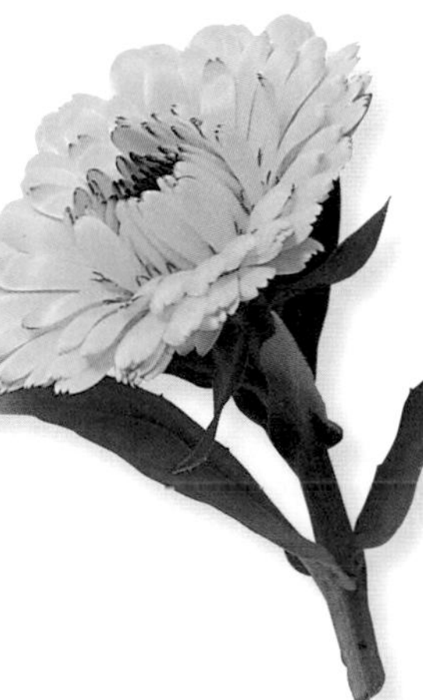

ABOVE *Calendula-infused oil helps cradle cap. Add a few teaspoonsful to the bath, for dry skin.*

DATA FILE

Properties

- Lifts the spirits
- Antispasmodic
- Antiseptic
- Antifungal
- Healing and anti-inflammatory

Uses

- Digestive colic, stomach, and duodenal ulcers.
- Speeds post-operative healing, reduces adhesions.
- Children's infections and fevers, as a gargle for sore throats, and tonsillitis.
- Wash, cream, or compress for boils, spots, inflamed wounds, painful varicose veins, leg ulcers, sore nipples in nursing mothers, and sore eyes.
- Douche or bath for thrush and vaginal infections.
- Lotion or cream for itchy skin rashes, grazes, cuts, broken chilblains, eczema, and fungal infections.
- Ideal first-aid remedy.

RECIPE

Marigold Tincture

Also sold as calendula lotion. Compresses and fomentations: 1 dessertspoon tincture to 1 cup water. Dip cloth into water, wring out. Use cold water to soothe and draw heat, for sprains, congestive pain, and hot joints. Use hot water (compress is called a fomentation) to relax and encourage circulation. For spasm, stiffness, and cold joints. Wrap around affected part. Cover.

Avena futua

WILD OATS

A wild grass. The origin of cultivated oats (*Avena sativa*). The whole plant (called oat straw) is used, picked while still green. Cultivated oats may be substituted. Groats, or oat grains, may be substituted, although they are not quite as good.

DATA FILE

Properties

- Nourishing and restorative to nerves and reproductive organs
- Antidepressant
- Strengthening

Uses

- Weakness and nervous exhaustion. A good remedy for helping to "keep on the go."
- Restless sleep from overexcitement.
- With valerian to ease the symptoms of withdrawal from tranquilizers.
- With vervain for weakness following illness.
- PMS with scanty menstruation and cramps.
- For exhaustion after childbirth and during breast-feeding.
- Addresses loss of libido in both sexes.
- With horsetail to strengthen the bones of children and the elderly.
- Baths and lotions are very soothing for eczema.

NOTES AND DOSAGES

❧ For oat straw, make a tea with 2 teaspoons to 1 cup of water. Infuse for 15 minutes. ❧ **For oats in general, buy the tincture. Use 20 drops every 2 hours when you need to keep going or 1 teaspoon 3 times daily for weakened states.** ❧ Eating porridge is beneficial to the nervous system and helps lower cholesterol levels. ❧ **For a bath, fill a muslin bag with porridge oats and hang it under the hot faucet, so that the water flows through it.** ❧ Preparations of oats for making baths can also be bought at general and herbal pharmacies.

BELOW *The wild oat grass benefits the nervous system.*

RECIPE

Oat Water

Take 1 dessertspoon of porridge oats and rub well between your fingers. Add to 1 cup of cold water. Stir well and leave for 20 minutes. Stir again and pass through a tea strainer. Makes a soothing drink for diarrhea, cystitis, and stomach upsets caused by antibiotics.

THERAPY CONNECTIONS

MARIGOLD

Aromatherapy p.148
Homeopathy p.187

WILD OATS

Flower Remedies p.226

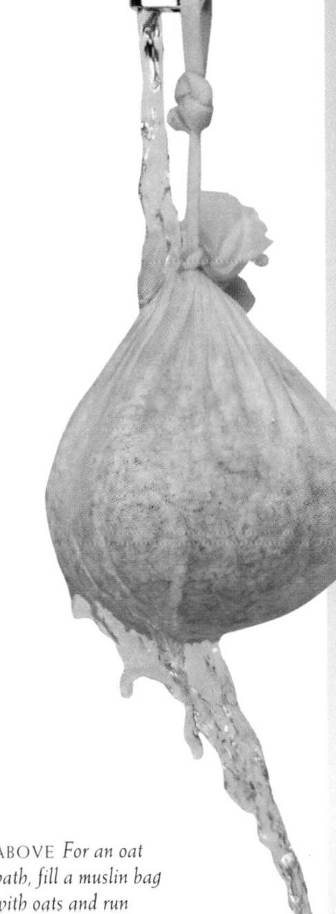

ABOVE *For an oat bath, fill a muslin bag with oats and run water through it.*

Capsicum minimum

CAYENNE

The kitchen spice, also called chili pepper. There are many different types of pepper spices made from red peppers, varying in strength from the mild paprika to the hottest cayenne.

NOTES AND DOSAGES

❧ People with poor circulation can add capsicum to any herbal medicines, with benefit. ❧ **Capsicum-based creams, liniments, and infused oils should only be used on small areas and rubbed in well.** ❧ Post-shingles neuralgia and chronic back pain may take a week or two to improve. ❧ **Useful for unbroken chilblains.** ❧ Hot oil is so called because it is hot to the taste and not because it is applied hot. It is a warming antispasmodic rub, improving circulation, and relaxing tension and spasm.

DATA FILE

Properties

- Circulatory stimulant
- Antispasmodic
- Carminative

Uses

- Poor circulation, chills, and inefficient digestion in the elderly.
- Externally for cramps and muscle spasm, aches and pains, cold and stiff joints, post-shingles neuralgia, and for unbroken chilblains.

CAUTION

USE ONLY IN VERY SMALL QUANTITIES. A SMALL PINCH OF THE POWDER OR 5–10 DROPS OF THE TINCTURE IS SUFFICIENT FOR A SINGLE DOSE.

AVOID APPLYING TO INFLAMED AREAS. AVOID GETTING IT INTO YOUR EYES.

CAN AGGRAVATE ACIDITY AND HEARTBURN.

RECIPE

Hot Oil

Make an infused oil using: 1 dessertspoon cayenne pepper, 2 dessertspoons powdered mustard seed, 2 teaspoons powdered ginger root, 1 cup unblended vegetable oil, sunflower or grapeseed oil. Use as a rub for cold joints and muscle spasm.

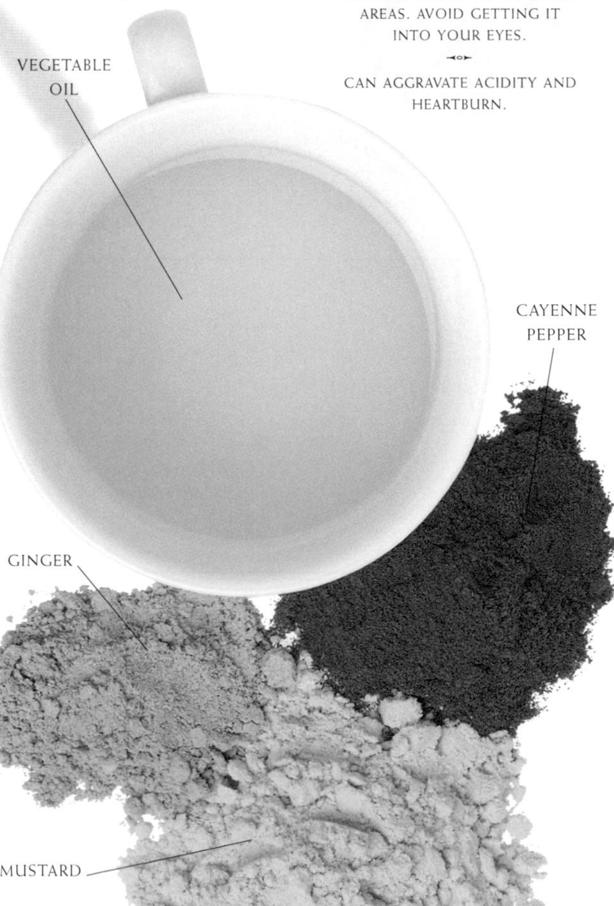

BELOW *Blend together these ingredients for a warming muscle rub.*

THERAPY CONNECTIONS

CAYENNE PEPPER
Ayurveda *p.31*

CHAMOMILE
Aromatherapy *p.150*
Homeopathy *p.204*

HAWTHORN
Chinese Herbal Medicine *p.61*

Codonopsis pilosula

CODONOPSIS

A sprawling herb with yellow, bell-shaped flowers, grown in China. The roots of this plant are used for medicinal purposes. Codonopsis can be purchased in Chinese herbal pharmacies as Dang Shen.

DATA FILE

Properties

- Soothing and strengthening
- An immune system tonic

Uses

- For general debility, exhaustion, weakness, lack of appetite, chronic diarrhea, excessive perspiration, acidity, chronic coughs, asthma, and shortness of breath.
- Used as a decoction, a tincture, or as a powder sprinkled on food.

ABOVE *Codonopsis root. In Chinese medicine it is used for digestive problems and as a tonic.*

CAUTION

SAFE BUT BEST USED FOR LONG-TERM DEBILITY. USE OTHER HERBS IN ACUTE CONDITIONS.

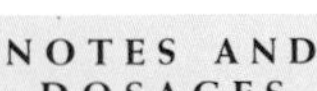

NOTES AND DOSAGES

❧ Take 1oz. (25g.) of the powder daily, sprinkled onto soups or made into a decoction. ❧ **Also called Dang Shen in Chinese herb stores.** ❧ Codonopsis is also known as the poor man's ginseng.

RECIPE

Soup of the Four Gentlemen

This is a famous traditional Chinese digestive and energy tonic. It is made from codonopsis, white atractylodes (Bai Zhu), Chinese angelica (Dang Gui), poria (Fu Ling), and licorice. Add 1oz. (25g.) of the herb mixture to 1pt. (500ml.) of water. Simmer for 15 minutes, strain, and drink daily.

Chamomilla recutita

CHAMOMILE

A wild plant with small, daisy-like flowers. It is the flowers that are most often used for therapeutic purposes. Chamomile is an aromatic plant, and it was used as a strewing herb in the Middle Ages.

NOTES AND DOSAGES

❧ May be taken freely. ❧ **As a sedative make a double-strength tea, using 2 teaspoons of flowers or 2 tea bags. Use a covered vessel, so the steam does not escape.** ❧ Linden flowers, chamomile, and four cloves makes an effective drink before bed, relaxing the body and the mind, and bringing satisfying sleep. ❧ **For infants, make an ordinary strength tea and give them 2 or 3 teaspoons to drink, either directly or in some pure fruit juice.** ❧ For times of severe stress make a mixture of three parts chamomile to two parts sage and one part basil (a pinch of ginger powder is optional). ❧ **Take twice a day to reduce tension and husband resources.**

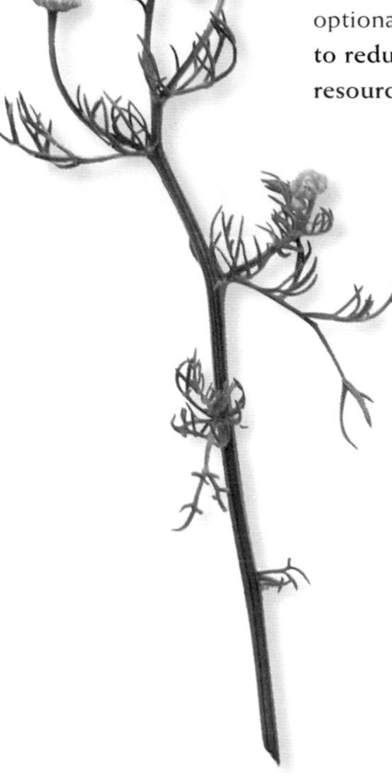

LEFT *Chamomile has a long history. The Egyptians used it to cure fever.*

DATA FILE

Properties

- Calming and soothing
- Anti-inflammatory
- Antiseptic
- Antispasmodic
- Digestive

Uses

- Anxiety, tension, headaches, and insomnia.
- For any kind of digestive upset – acidity, heartburn, wind, and colic.
- Lotion, cream, or bath for itchy skin conditions.
- For restless and overexcitable children, and for most children's complaints, including fevers and teething troubles. Especially helpful for infants.
- Although chamomile is sold in tea bags as a herbal drink for everyday use, it should not be overlooked as a medicinal herb, for it is gentle but very powerful.

RECIPE

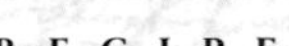

Chamomile Compress for Sore and Inflamed Eyes or Skin

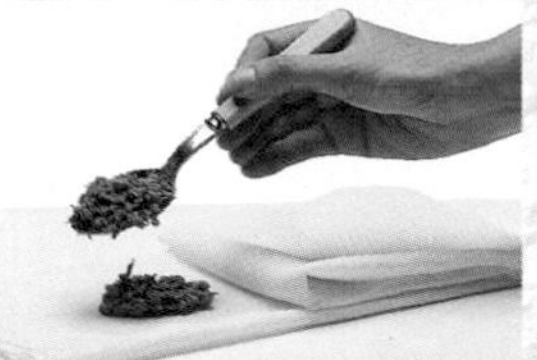

Put a handful of dried chamomile flowers into a bowl. Slowly pour on boiled water, stirring all the time until they make a mush. Allow to cool. Wrap in a length of cotton and apply. Leave on for at least 15 minutes.

CAUTION

CAN CAUSE AN ALLERGIC RASH, BUT THIS DISAPPEARS ON STOPPING USE OF THE HERB.

Crataegus oxycantha or *Crataegus monogyna*

HAWTHORN BERRIES AND FLOWERING TOPS

The berries and flowering tops of the common may tree. Hawthorn's Latin name comes from Greek words meaning hard (wood), sharp, and thorn.

DATA FILE

Properties

- Strengthens the heart
- Lowers blood pressure
- Relaxes arteries

Uses

- Heart failure. If you are taking drugs for heart problems, seek professional advice before taking any herbal medicine.
- Irregular heartbeat.
- Helpful for angina and high blood pressure, as part of an overall strategy.
- With nervine herbs such as valerian and linden, for anxiety with palpitations.

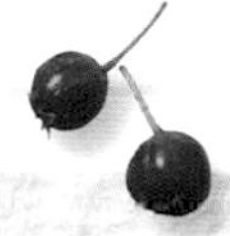

RECIPE

Hawthorn Brandy

This is the nicest way of taking hawthorn as a heart-strengthening tonic. Pick the flowering shoots (with flowers and leaves), wash, dry, and pack into a large jar. Cover with brandy and leave in a cool place for two weeks. Strain off the liquid, bottle, and label. Dose: 2 dessertspoons daily.

NOTES AND DOSAGES

❧ Standard dose (*see pages 108–9*). Make a tea of the flowering tops or a decoction of the berries. Tincture: take 1 teaspoon in a little water twice daily. For heart disease, take this dosage for at least 6 months.

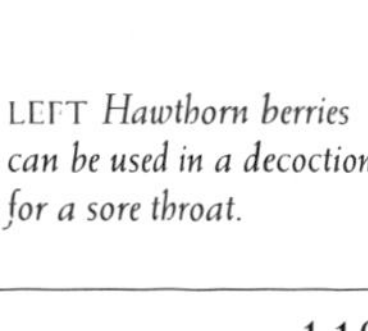

LEFT *Hawthorn berries can be used in a decoction for a sore throat.*

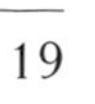

Dioscorea villosa

WILD YAMS

The rhizome of a Mexican wild yam. The dried root retains its medicinal value for up to a year.

WILD YAM ROOTS

DATA FILE

Properties

- Anti-inflammatory
- Antispasmodic

Uses

- Stomach cramps, nausea, vomiting, hiccups, recurrent colicky pains, pain of diverticulitis, and gall-bladder pains. With a little ginger for a quicker action.
- Menstrual cramps, and pain on ovulation.
- Menopausal symptoms, vaginal dryness.
- Useful for the treatment of rheumatoid arthritis.

ABOVE *Dried wild yam root, leaves, and fruit. The plant is dug up in the fall to harvest the root.*

NOTES AND DOSAGES

Standard doses (*see pages 108–9*). **Works especially well on persistent and recurrent problems.** Wild yam is the starting point for synthesization of hormones for the contraceptive pill and for "natural progesterone," used in a prescription cream for the menopause.

RECIPE

Decoction for Arthritic Pains

Take 1oz. (25g.) each of wild yam root and willow bark. Add to 3pt. (1.5l.) water. Simmer together for 20 minutes. Strain. The decoction will keep in the refrigerator for two or three days. Dose: ½ cup 3 times daily, adding honey to taste.

Echinacea angustifolia and *Echinacea purpurea*

ECHINACEA ROOT

Purple cone flower, a native plant of the U.S. Echinacea is the best way of ridding the body of microbial infections. It is effective against both bacteria and viruses.

DATA FILE

Properties

- Antiseptic
- Stimulates the immune system

Uses

- For a weak immune system where patient suffers chronic tiredness and is susceptible to minor infections.
- For boils, acne, duodenal ulcers, flu, herpes, and persistent infections.
- As a gargle and mouthwash for sore throats, tonsillitis, mouth ulcers, and gum infections.

NOTES AND DOSAGES

For acute conditions take large doses, 1 cup of the decoction or 1 teaspoon of the tincture every two hours for ten days. **For chronic conditions use in combinations and take ½ cup of the combined decoction or 1 teaspoon of the combined tincture, 3 times daily.**

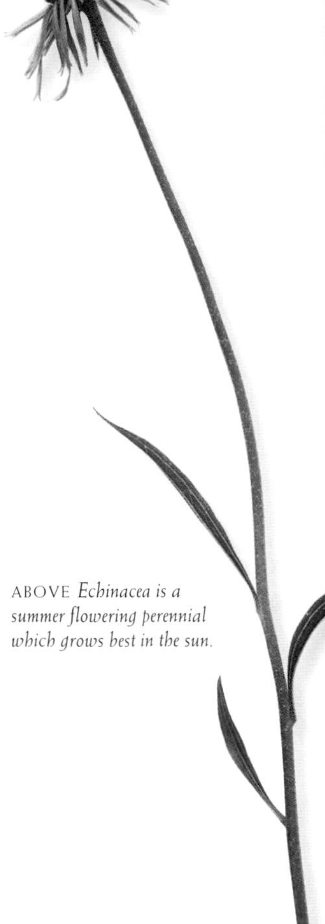

ABOVE *Echinacea is a summer flowering perennial which grows best in the sun.*

Equisetium arvense

HORSETAIL

A weed which is common on damp ground. Horsetail reproduces by spores, like ferns. Galen, a physician of Ancient Greece, used horsetail to heal sinews.

BELOW *Collect horsetail in early summer. Hang in large bunches and leave it to dry.*

CAUTION

AVOID LARGE DOSES IN EARLY PREGNANCY.

NOTES AND DOSAGES

The healing properties of horsetail are due to its high content of silica and zinc. **For a decoction, simmer 1 teaspoon in 2 cups of water for half an hour.** Drink twice daily for one month. **Make up a pitcher and keep it in the refrigerator.**

DATA FILE

Properties

- Styptic
- Diuretic
- Strengthens the bladder
- Antifungal

Uses

- For irritable bladder with urgency and frequency.
- For blood in the urine.
- For bedwetting problems, with cramp bark or St. John's wort.
- For arthritis.
- Strengthens nails and hair.
- Speeds healing after surgery.
- Compress for infected, weepy skin conditions.

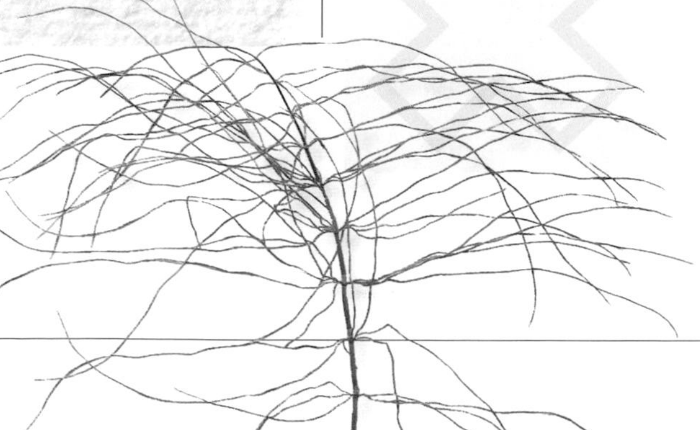

Filipendula ulmaria

MEADOWSWEET

The leaves, stalks, and flowers of a wild plant common in damp meadows. The flowers are very fragrant, and the plant was a medieval strewing herb. Culpeper described it as a help to acquiring a "merry heart."

DATA FILE

Properties

- Antacid
- Astringent
- Anti-inflammatory
- Diuretic
- Calming for overactive digestive systems

Uses

- Acid stomach, heartburn, ulcers, and hiatus hernia. Combines well with comfrey, marshmallow, and chamomile.
- With peppermint or chamomile for indigestion, diverticulitis, and wind.
- Helpful for rheumatism and arthritis. Clears sandy deposits in the urine.
- Excellent for summer diarrhea and fevers with an upset stomach in children.

RECIPE

Tea for Acid Stomachs

Take equal parts of meadowsweet, chamomile flowers, and comfrey leaves, dried. Mix together and store in a clean jar. Use 1 teaspoon of the mixture to 1 cup boiling water. Allow the tea to draw for 10 minutes. Drink 3–6 cups daily.

CAUTION

LARGE DOSES AND STRONG TEAS MAY CAUSE NAUSEA IN SOME PEOPLE.

NOTES AND DOSAGES

- Standard doses. Half dosages for children and elderly people. Will give quick relief for stomach pains, but best results come from long-term use.

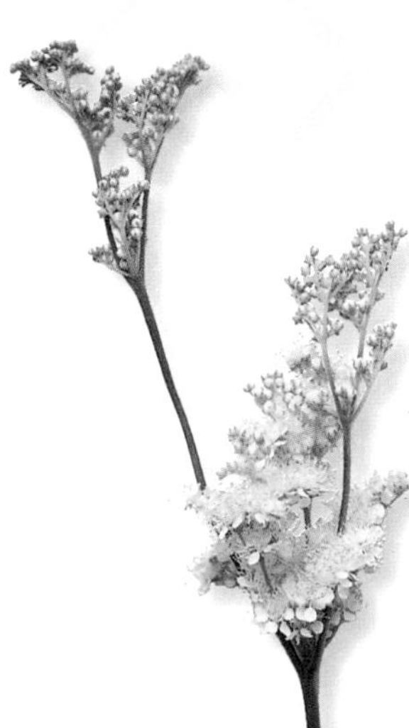
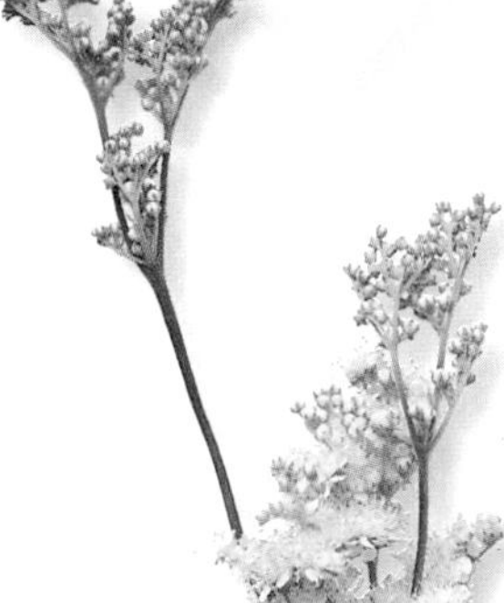

RIGHT *Filipendula bears cream flowers in summer and should be picked at this time.*

Foeniculum vulgare

FENNEL

A familiar cooking herb – the leaves and seeds are used. Fennel has feathery leaves and grows to about 6ft. (2m.). It was traditionally reputed to instil strength and courage.

ABOVE *Fennel seeds have an anise-like flavor, and help digestion.*

DATA FILE

Properties

- Warming
- Carminative
- Antispasmodic
- Antidepressant
- Promotes milk flow in nursing mothers

Uses

- For colic, wind, and irritable bowel.
- For breast-feeding; helps milk flow and reduces colic.
- For anxiety, depression, and disturbed spirits.
- For arthritis and water retention or edema.
- For griping in infants, give the tea in teaspoon doses, as much as they will take, or add 2 teaspoons to milk formulas.

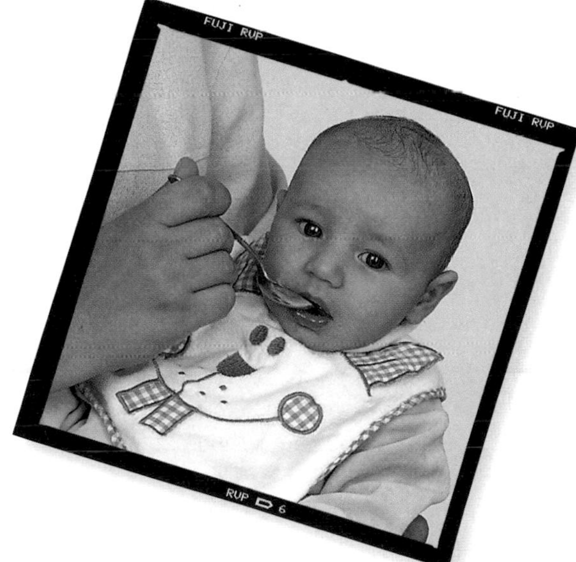

RIGHT *Fennel tea will soothe a baby's colic. Give by the teaspoonful.*

NOTES AND DOSAGES

- Standard doses.
- **Fennel seed tea bags are easily available – remember to cover the cup to avoid losing any goodness.**
- Traditionally taken during fasts to reduce hunger.

RECIPE

Fennel Eye Bath

Fennel tea, diluted 1:1 with water and with the addition of a pinch of salt helps ease tired, dry eyes and maintain clear vision. As with any liquid used for the eyes, absolute cleanliness must be observed. Strain the tea through a very fine strainer before use, and make fresh every day.

THERAPY CONNECTIONS

FENNEL

Aromatherapy *p.159*

CAUTION

REMEMBER THAT ANY BLOOD IN THE URINE SHOULD ALWAYS BE INVESTIGATED BY YOUR PHYSICIAN.

Fucus vesiculosis

BLADDERWRACK

A common dark brown seaweed found in the U.S and Europe. Also called kelp.

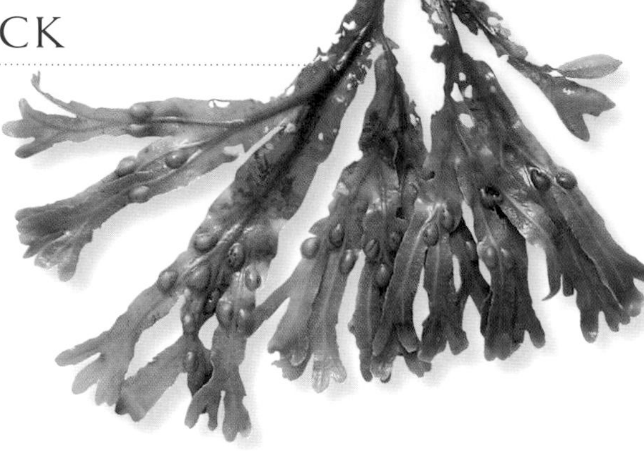

ABOVE *Gather bladderwrack from clean beaches, keeping away from sewage outlets.*

NOTES AND DOSAGES

- Take 1 tablet 3 times a day, or follow the instructions on the packet.
- **When using powder, 1 or 2 teaspoons may be sprinkled on to cooked meals or soups.**
- Half doses for children.

CAUTION

AVOID IN OVERACTIVE THYROID CONDITIONS, EXCEPT WITH PROFESSIONAL GUIDANCE.

NOT RECOMMENDED FOR CHILDREN UNDER FIVE.

IT IS BEST TO SEEK ADVICE BEFORE USING HERBS FOR WEIGHT LOSS.

DATA FILE

Properties

- Nourishing and soothing.
- Stimulates the thyroid gland.

Uses

- A nourishing tonic.
- Obesity with tiredness and dry skin.
- Cellulite, chronic dry skin, and stubborn constipation. Regular use will delay the progress of arthritis and hardening of the arteries. A good tonic for old age.
- For children with slow mental and physical development.

RECIPE

Bladderwrack Liniment

To make an excellent liniment for rheumatism and arthritis add 1oz. (25g.) of dried bladderwrack to 1pt. (500ml.) of water. Simmer for a half-hour. Strain and add to an equal amount of comfrey infused oil (*see page 132*). Shake before use and rub in well twice daily.

Ginkgo biloba

GINKGO LEAVES

The maidenhair tree, originally from China and often grown in parks. The tea, tincture, and tablets treat poor circulation, thrombosis, and varicose veins.

DATA FILE

Properties

- Improves blood flow
- Strengthens blood vessels
- Anti-inflammatory
- Relaxes the lungs

Uses

- For poor circulation, thrombosis, varicose veins, cramp which comes on walking, white finger, and spontaneous bruising.
- Especially helpful for failing circulation to the brain in elderly people.
- Strengthens memory.
- Often improves deafness, tinnitus, vertigo, and early senile dementia.
- Helpful in asthma.

NOTES AND DOSAGES

- The tea is best taken in large doses – at least 3 cups a day for some months. It is a pleasant drinking tea. Tablets are available – follow the dose on the packet.

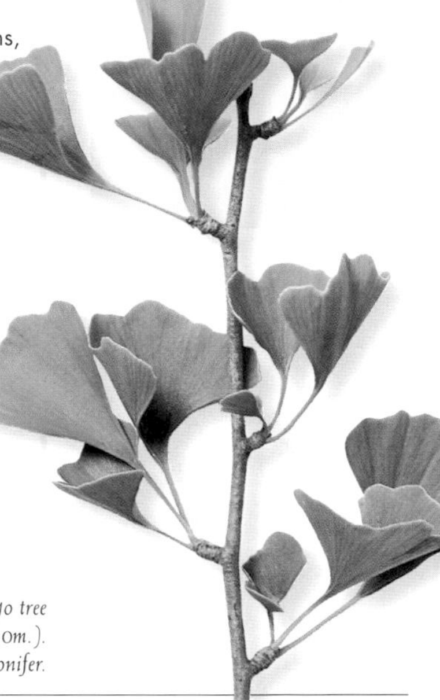

RIGHT *The ginkgo tree grows to almost 100ft. (30m.). It is a deciduous conifer.*

Glycyrrhiza glabra

LICORICE ROOT

A sweet root used in confectionery and medicine (often mixed with other herbs for long-term use).

CAUTION

CAN CAUSE WATER RETENTION AND RAISED BLOOD PRESSURE.

LARGE DOSES CAN BE LAXATIVE.

PROLONGED USE SHOULD BE AVOIDED IF YOU SUFFER FROM HIGH BLOOD PRESSURE.

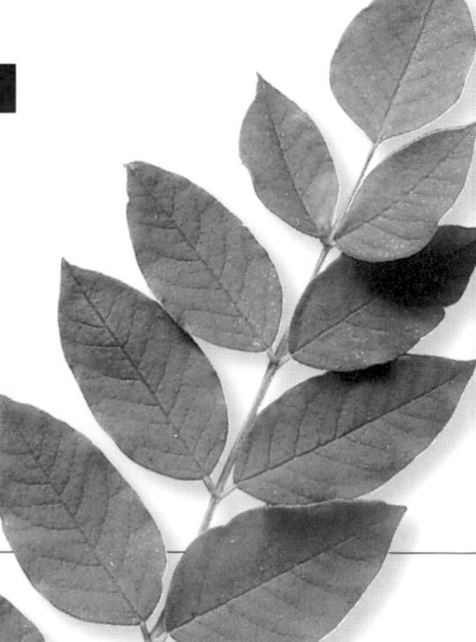

NOTES AND DOSAGES

- For bronchitis take ¼oz. (5g.) of the powdered root 3 times daily with honey or in capsules, for up to 2 weeks. For a decoction use ½ teaspoon to 1 cup of water – take 3 cups daily. Half this for long-term use. Boiling the decoction for an hour and then drying it out in a low oven produces an extract that is easy to take.

DATA FILE

Properties

- Soothing and anti-inflammatory
- Strengthening and up-building
- Expectorant

Uses

- Irritable, dry coughs and bronchitis.
- Stomach, acidity, heartburn, ulcers, colitis, and intestinal infections.
- With other strengthening herbs for exhaustion.
- In creams for inflamed psoriasis and hot and weepy skin conditions.

LEFT *The Greeks were using licorice in 3 B.C.E. for asthma and a dry cough.*

Harpagophytum procumbens

DEVIL'S CLAW

The tuber from a South African plant, which survives in very arid conditions. Devil's claw contains a glycoside called harpagoside that helps to reduce inflammation in the joints.

DATA FILE

Properties

- Bitter tonic and anti-inflammatory

Uses

- Decoction or tincture for all types of arthritis, especially for inflamed joints and arthritis affecting a number of joints.
- For gout, lumbago, sciatica, and rheumatism.
- For gall bladder inflammation, piles, and phlebitis (internally).
- For itchy skin with no obvious cause.

NOTES AND DOSAGES

Decoction: ½ teaspoon to 1 cup of water, 2 cups a day. Tincture: 1 teaspoon twice daily. Tablets are available in most health food stores – follow the dosage on the box. For acute flare-ups double the dosage for a week or two.

CAUTION

AVOID IN PREGNANCY.

MAY AGGRAVATE STOMACH ACIDITY.

DO NOT USE IN GASTRITIS AND WITH ULCERS.

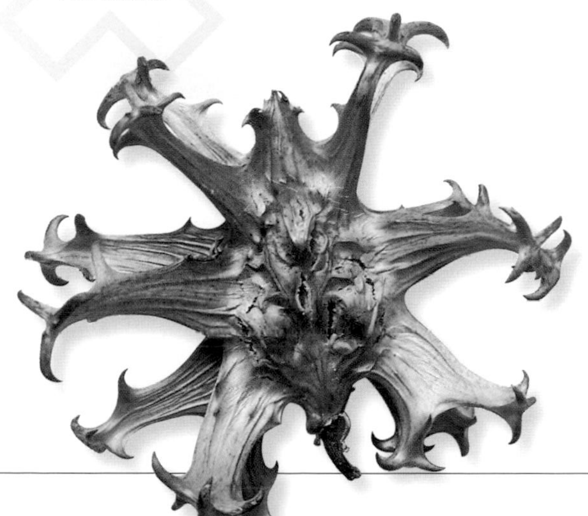
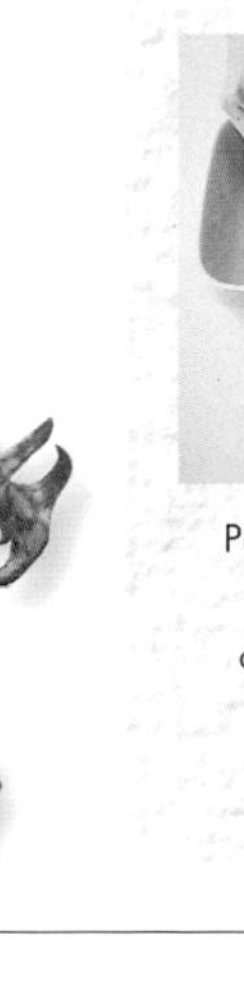

BELOW *Devil's claw tubers are dug up at the end of the rainy season and dried.*

RECIPE

Devil's Claw Capsules

Capsules are a good way of producing a customized remedy, and useful if you do not want to take a lot of liquid decoctions.

Dose: two capsules three times daily.

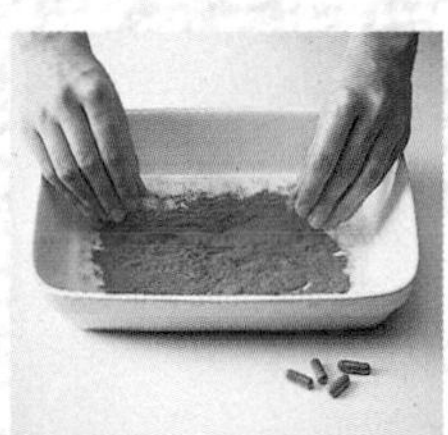

Buy 120 empty gelatin capsules from a herb store. Get out a flat dish and a coffee grinder.

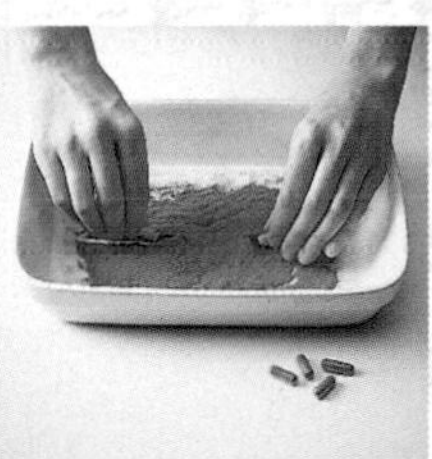

Powder 1oz. (25g.) chopped devil's claw in the coffee grinder (some stores sell it pre-ground).

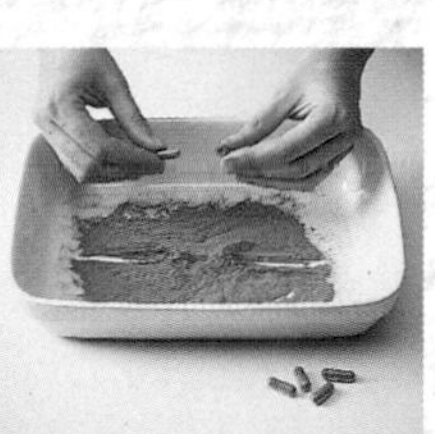

Put the powder in the dish. Fill each capsule by pushing the halves through the powder.

Hamamelis virginiana

WITCH HAZEL BARK AND LEAVES

A small U.S. tree often grown in gardens for its fragrant yellow spring flowers. The bark and leaves are used.

DATA FILE

Properties

- Astringent
- Anti-inflammatory
- Antiseptic
- Styptic

Uses

- External use only for bruises, cuts, oily skin, spots, broken capillaries, piles, and painful varicose veins.
- As a compress for sprains, phlebitis, sunburn, and hot swollen joints.
- As a compress and wash for hot and tired eyes.

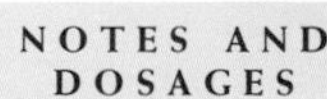

ABOVE *and* LEFT *Witch hazel's oval leaves turn yellow in the fall.*

NOTES AND DOSAGES

Distilled witch hazel and other preparations are easily available. The decoction and tincture are stronger but tend to stain clothes. Dilute the tincture with 3 parts of water to use as a compress or lotion.

THERAPY CONNECTIONS

WITCH HAZEL

Traditional Home and Folk Remedies *p.91*

Homeopathy *p.197*

LICORICE

Ayurveda *p.39*

Chinese Herbal Medicine *p.64*

Traditional Home and Folk Remedies *p.91*

RECIPE

Witch Hazel Compress

Take 1oz. (25g.) cut bark and 1pt. (500ml.) water. Simmer together for 10 minutes. Strain and allow to cool. Dip a cloth into the decoction, wring, and apply for a half-hour, wetting it again as needed. Suitable for sunburn, swollen and inflamed joints, and aching varicose veins.

Hypericum perforatum

ST. JOHN'S WORT

A common European wild plant, now a weed in many parts of the world. The tops of the plant are picked in full flower. It is easy to grow, but make sure you get the right species – *perforatum* has oil glands in the leaves which show up as transparent dots against the light.

DATA FILE

Properties

- Strengthens the nervous system and speeds healing
- Analgesic
- Antiviral
- Anti-inflammatory

Uses

- Neuralgia, sciatica, and back pain.
- Pain from deep wounds.
- Mild depression. (Not for severe depression.)
- Tincture for shingles, cold sores, and herpes.
- Cream for sore skin, inflamed rashes, and cuts.
- Infused oil as base oil for aromatherapy back massage, and with lavender essential oil for neuralgia.

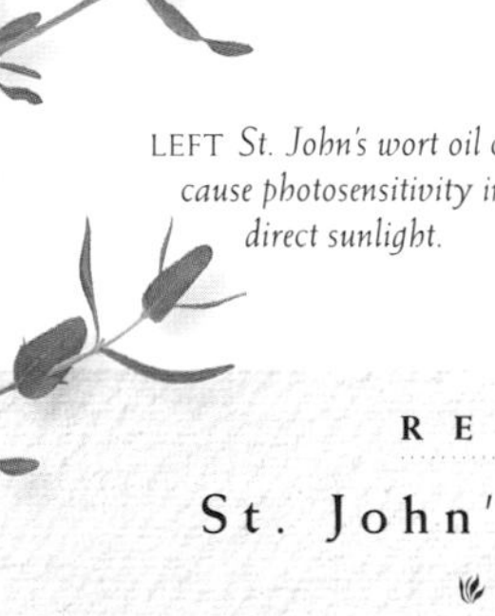

LEFT *St. John's wort oil can cause photosensitivity in direct sunlight.*

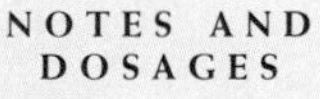

NOTES AND DOSAGES

Standard doses. It may be a week before depression begins to lift. The best preparations for external use are the infused oil and creams based on the infused oil *(see box)*. For nerve damage you may need to continue use for some months.

RECIPE

St. John's Wort Oil

Pick the flowering tops. Put into a pestle, add a small amount of a pure, light vegetable oil such as sunflower oil. Pour just enough to cover, then pound together to crush, bruise, and start releasing the oil. Put into a large clear glass jar. Cover with more oil so that all of the herb is well covered. Shake well. Then add another inch of oil. Leave outside in direct sunlight for 20 days. The oil will turn red when it is ready. Use for skin, healing nerve damage, as a base for massage oils, or as a salve.

ABOVE *Motherwort is especially good for female disorders – hence its name.*

Leonurus cardiaca

MOTHERWORT

A European wild plant with a tall spike of small pink flowers. Self-seeds readily in the garden. Culpeper wrote, "...there is no better herb to drive melancholy vapours from the heart ... and make the mind cheerful, blithe and merry."

DATA FILE

Properties

- Calms the heart and relaxes the womb
- Antispasmodic
- Emmenagogue

Uses

- Anxiety with palpitations and irregular heartbeat.
- Tachycardia from an overactive thyroid.
- With skullcap or valerian, for tranquilizer withdrawal.
- With vervain for anxiety from stress and overwork.
- With sage for menopausal hot flushes.
- For menstrual cramps, taken on a regular basis.
- Take daily during the last two weeks of pregnancy to help with the birth.

NOTES AND DOSAGES

Standard doses of decoction or tincture. May take a few weeks to work.

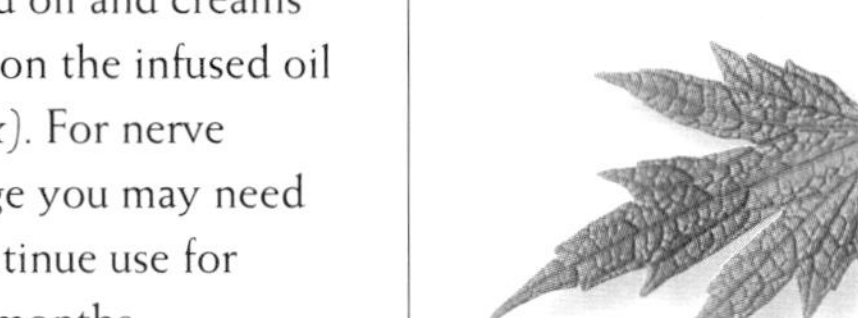

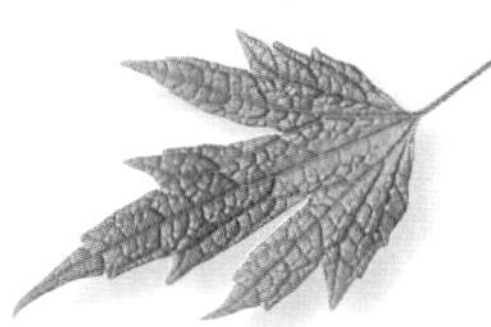

CAUTION

AVOID IN PREGNANCY, EXCEPT DURING THE LAST TWO WEEKS.

RECIPE

Motherwort and Lemon Balm Tea

Make an infusion, or tea, by pouring a cup of boiling water on to 1–2 teaspoonsful of the dried herb. Leave to infuse for 10–15 minutes. The tea should be drunk 3 times a day. Motherwort and lemon balm tea combines motherwort's sedative effect and lemon balm's antidepressant qualities.

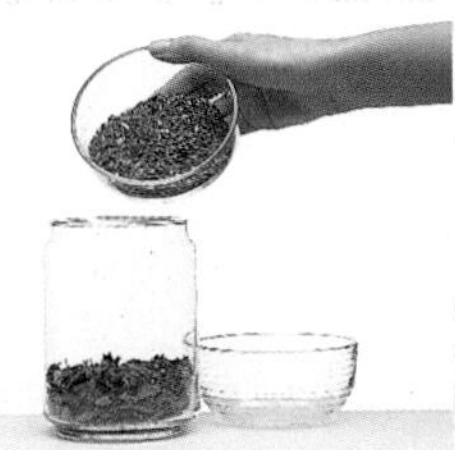

Mix together equal amounts of dried motherwort and lemon balm *(Melissa officinalis)* herbs. Store in a clean jar and label. Take as a regular tea for depression.

Lycium barbarum or *Lycium chinense*

LYCIUM FRUIT

The bright red fruit of a Chinese shrub, grown in Europe as a hedging plant. It is a deciduous shrub, growing to 8ft. (2.5m.) tall and spreading to about 15ft. (5m.). Lycium bears pinkish flowers and grows well even in poor soil.

DATA FILE

Properties

- Tonic for old age and associated weakness

Uses

- General weakness with vertigo, tinnitus, and recurrent headaches.
- For impotence and premature ejaculation.
- Convalescence, with equal parts of schisandra; improves skin color and restores strength.
- Failing eyesight.
- Aches and pains, especially backache, particularly in old age.

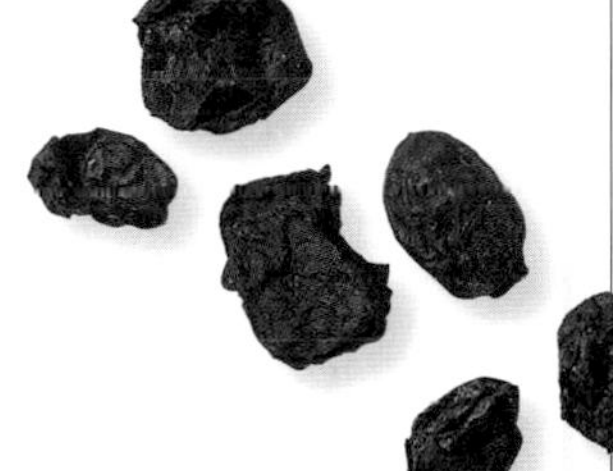

RIGHT *and* ABOVE *Lycium leaves and dried berries. The berries are favored for problems of old age.*

RECIPE

Eye-strengthening Soup

Take 1oz. (25g.) lycium fruit, 3 chopped carrots, and a sliced onion. Add to 1pt. (500ml.) soup stock made with chicken or vegetable stock cubes Simmer until the vegetables are cooked. Strain and blend. Take regularly to "nourish the vital essence and benefit vision."

NOTES AND DOSAGES

Also called wolfberry and the Duke of Argyle's tea plant. **Chinese herbalists call the berries Gou-qi-zi. Tincture: ½fl.oz. (15ml.) with a little water daily.** Dried fruit, ½oz. (10g.) daily chewed or in decoction. **Traditionally the berries are added to soup to help strengthen eyesight.**

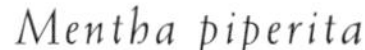

Mentha piperita

PEPPERMINT LEAVES

One of the most popular herb teas in the world. Easily grown in gardens, but is a rather invasive plant. Try growing it in a bucket buried in the ground, with the bottom knocked out.

LEFT *The leaves of peppermint are collected just before the flowers open.*

CAUTION

AVOID LARGE DOSES IN PREGNANCY.

THE AMOUNTS TAKEN IN FOOD ARE HARMLESS.

NOT SUITED TO INFANTS; USE CATMINT, WHICH HAS THE SAME PROPERTIES AND IS MORE SUITABLE.

DATA FILE

Properties

- Digestive
- Carminative
- Antispasmodic
- Mild stimulant
- Emmenagogue
- Cooling on the skin

Uses

- Indigestion, colic, wind, nausea, vomiting, depressed appetite, menstrual cramps, and gall bladder pain. Adding a couple of drops of the essential oil to hot water, and drinking it, or sucking a strong peppermint sweet, is also effective.
- With elderflower and yarrow for colds, sinus problems, and blocked nose. Inhale the steam as you drink.
- For hot, itchy skin problems, a strong tea used as a lotion.

NOTES AND DOSAGES

Take freely. A small amount of peppermint may be added to most herb teas for flavor.

RECIPE

Cooling Peppermint Drink for Hot Weather

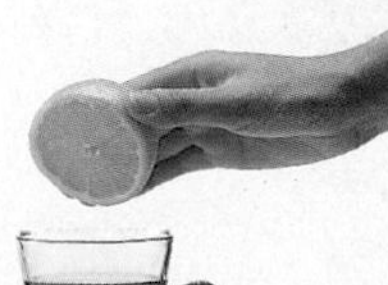

Make a weak peppermint tea using ½oz. (12g.) peppermint and 1pt. (500ml.) water. Add the juice of one lemon. Cool in the refrigerator, add ice and a sprig of fresh mint. Drink freely to avoid the debilitating effects of heat.

THERAPY CONNECTIONS

ST. JOHN'S WORT

Ayurveda p.40

Homeopathy p.199

PEPPERMINT

Aromatherapy p.164

Panax ginseng and *Eleutherococcus senticosus*

GINSENG AND SIBERIAN GINSENG ROOT

A famous tonic of the Far East, where it is very widely used. The word "ginseng" is said to mean "the wonder of the world."

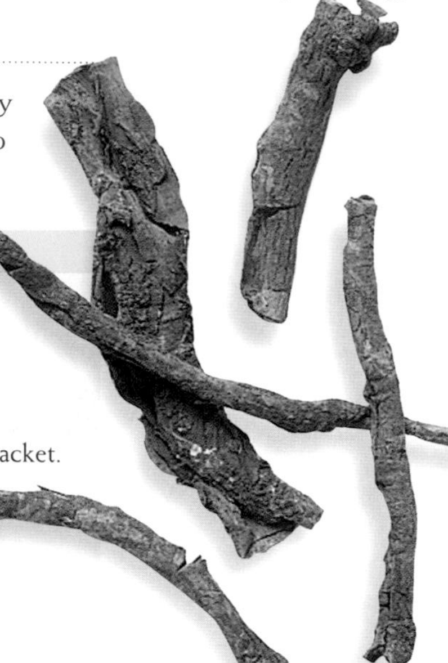

BELOW *Siberian ginseng root. Ginseng helps the body cope with stress and replenishes energy.*

NOTES AND DOSAGES

❧ Dose: 100mg. of powdered root, 300mg. of cut root in decoction, or 20–30 drops of the tincture twice daily. ❧ **Best suited to old and weakened people.** ❧ Many preparations are available in the stores – follow the dose on the packet.

CAUTION

NOT TO BE TAKEN IN PREGNANCY.

MAY AGGRAVATE ANXIETY AND IRRITABILITY.

AVOID WITH HIGH BLOOD PRESSURE.

DO NOT TAKE LARGE DOSES IN CONJUNCTION WITH STIMULANTS.

DO NOT TAKE CONSISTENTLY WITHOUT PROFESSIONAL ADVICE.

NOT FOR CHILDREN, EXCEPT UNDER PROFESSIONAL GUIDANCE.

DATA FILE

Properties

- Replenishes vital energy
- Strengthens the immune system
- Adaptogenic
- Increases concentration

Uses

- Convalescence, exhaustion, lack of concentration, weakness in old age.
- With other strengthening herbs for getting rid of persistent infections.
- Loss of sex drive in men.
- Helps the body to cope with the side-effects of chemotherapy for cancer.
- Jet lag.

THERAPY CONNECTIONS

GINSENG
Chinese Herbal Medicine p.67

RHUBARB
Chinese Herbal Medicine p.73

ROSEMARY
Aromatherapy p.168

RECIPE

Ginseng Tonic Wine

You can make a reviving tonic wine using this simple recipe.

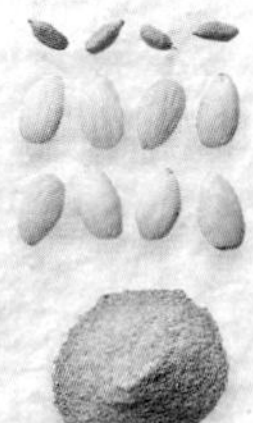

1oz. (25g.) powdered ginseng, 4 dried apricots, 8 blanched almonds, 4 cardamom pods (optional), 2pt. (1l.) red or white wine to taste. Put ingredients together, stand for 2 weeks, and strain. Drink a small glass (¼ cup) daily.

Plantago major or *Plantago lanceolata*

PLANTAIN LEAF

The broad-leaved plantain or the ribwort plantain are common weeds of pathways and lawns. It was said to spring up wherever the English established a colony, giving rise to its common name of "white man's foot."

DATA FILE

Properties

- Soothing
- Healing
- Astringent

Uses

- Running nose from allergies, irritation, and colds.
- Irritable bowel and irritable bladder.
- Compress or lotion for insect bites, allergic rashes, and infected eczema, cleaning wounds, drawing stings, and splinters.
- Soothes neuralgic pains and shingles rash.
- Cream or ointment for bleeding piles.
- The tea is a cooling drink for persistent fevers and is a useful addition to any medicine given to "hot" people.
- Mouthwash for sore and bleeding gums.

RECIPE

Plantain Lotion

Finely chop sufficient fresh plantain leaves to fill a small jar. Add sufficient glycerin to cover the leaves. Stand for 2 weeks, stirring from time to time. Strain and store in a dark bottle. Makes a soothing and healing lotion for weeping and itchy rashes, and insect bites.

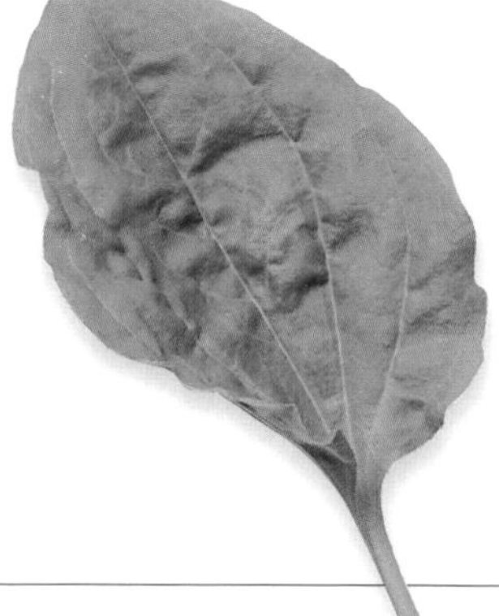

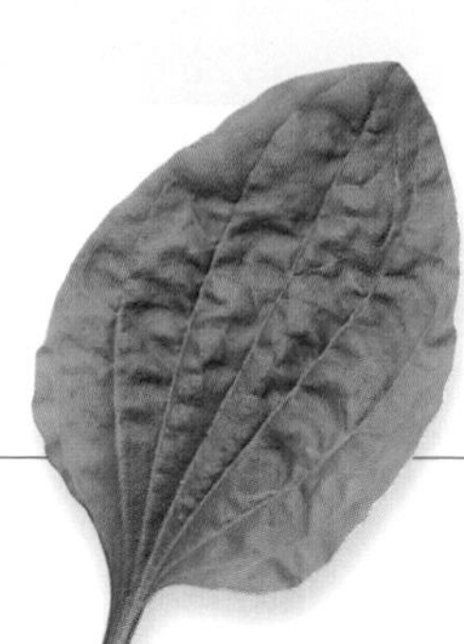

BELOW *In times past, plantain was reputed to cure mad dogs and snakebites.*

NOTES AND DOSAGES

❧ Double-strength tea (2 teaspoons per cup) for most purposes. Take it freely.

Rheum palmatum and *Rheum officinale*

RHUBARB ROOT

Chinese rhubarb, also called turkey rhubarb. Edible garden rhubarb is a hybrid of this. *Rheum palmatum* is a perennial growing to a height of 6ft. (2m.), with 2ft. (60cm.) leaves.

DATA FILE

Properties

- Laxative
- Astringent
- Bitter tonic
- Cooling

Uses

- Constipation, acute liver and gall bladder diseases.
- Feelings of congestion and fullness in the stomach.
- Stomach acidity.
- Gastroenteritis and diarrhea from food poisoning.
- Gout.
- Traditionally used in cancer.
- As a poultice for abscesses.

NOTES AND DOSAGES

Half the standard dose: ½ teaspoon to 1 cup of water for decoction, or 30–40 drops of the tincture, 3 times daily.

ABOVE *Rhubarb root may cause the urine to take on a reddish tinge.*

RECIPE

Laxative Wine

Warm a glass of white wine (don't boil). Pour on to 1 teaspoon of chopped rhubarb root. Add a good pinch of cinnamon powder and stand overnight. Strain and drink.

CAUTION

AVOID IN PREGNANCY, EXCEPT AS ADVISED BY A QUALIFIED HERBALIST.

NOT USED IN BOWEL SPASM OR WHEN COLICKY PAINS ARE PRESENT.

AVOID TAKING LAXATIVES FOR LONG PERIODS.

DO NOT EAT RHUBARB LEAVES.

Rosmarinus officinalis

ROSEMARY LEAVES

Late-flowering woody shrub. The whole plant smells, and it is almost impossible to pass by a rosemary bush without pinching a few leaves and rubbing them between the fingers to release the smell. Rosemary has many traditional uses and stories. It is planted in cemeteries for remembrance, and it does enhance the memory by improving the circulation. Rosemary vinegar is a powerful disinfectant.

NOTES AND DOSAGES

Standard doses used freely. Add 15 drops of essential oil to a bath to ease muscular tension, improve circulation, and boost spirits. **Rosemary tea can be used as a conditioning hair rinse.** For dandruff but also for gloriously glossy hair (especially for dark hair), use rosemary vinegar.

CAUTION

AVOID LARGE DOSES IN PREGNANCY, EXCEPT AS ADVISED BY A QUALIFIED HERBALIST.

DO NOT USE FOR TREATING HEADACHES AND MIGRAINES THAT FEEL "HOT."

THE AMOUNTS TAKEN IN FOOD ARE HARMLESS.

BELOW *In times of plague, rosemary was carried to ward off infection.*

DATA FILE

Properties

- Lifts the spirits
- Improves circulation
- Carminative
- Gentle bitter tonic

Uses

- Depression.
- Headaches associated with gastric upsets. Take rosemary with chamomile for stress-related headaches.
- Poor circulation, taken regularly. A useful addition to any herbal medicine for conditions associated with cold and poor circulation.
- Poor digestion, gall bladder inflammation, gallstones, and general feeling of liverishness.
- As a gargle for sore throats. Useful substitute for sage during pregnancy.
- With horsetail for hair loss due to stress and worry.
- As an infused oil for massage of cold limbs and aches and pains.
- Rosemary will encourage the circulation.
- Good circulation to the head strengthens the brain and improves the quality and strength of hair. Two cups of rosemary tea a day will prevent hair loss through poor circulation and restimulate growth after chemotherapy.

RECIPE

Rosemary Vinegar

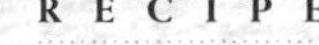

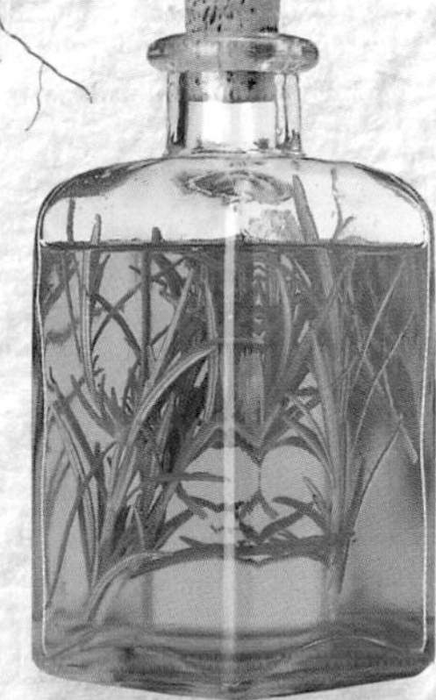

Take 1oz. (25g.) rosemary and 2pt. (1l.) cider vinegar. Leave the rosemary to steep in the vinegar for two weeks. Shake occasionally. After two weeks, strain, bottle, label, and date. Use 1–2 dessertspoons in the final rinsing water when washing hair. For dandruff, massage rosemary vinegar thoroughly into the scalp 20 minutes before washing.

Rubus idaeus

RASPBERRY LEAVES

The leaves from the raspberry bush. Raspberries grow best in rich, moist, well-drained soil, and prefer a sunny position.

DATA FILE

Properties

- Astringent
- Antispasmodic
- Especially applicable to the womb

Uses

- To promote an easy birth by tonifying the uterus.
- A mouthwash for sore mouths, sore throats, weak gums, and mouth ulcers.
- With marshmallow and peppermint for diverticulitis.
- Children's diarrhea and oral thrush. For infants put raspberry leaf tea in a sterilized spray bottle and spray into the mouth 3 or 4 times daily.

LEFT *When picking, make sure that the bush has not been sprayed with pesticide.*

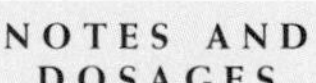

NOTES AND DOSAGES

Standard doses. For tablets, follow the dose on the packet. **To prepare for birth, the herb needs to be taken for at least 2 months.** Continue for 3 or 4 weeks afterward to re-tone the womb quickly.

CAUTION

AVOID IN EARLY PREGNANCY EXCEPT WITH PROFESSIONAL ADVICE – BEST TAKEN DURING THE LAST THREE MONTHS. OTHERWISE A SAFE HERB.

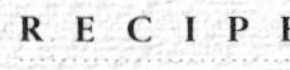

RECIPE

Raspberry Vinegar

This is made with the raspberry fruit. Fill a large jar with fresh raspberries. Cover with cider vinegar and stand in a cool place for two weeks. Strain and store in clean bottles. As a gargle for throats, dilute the vinegar with two parts of water to use.

Rumex crispus

YELLOW DOCK ROOT

A common wild plant, often used for blood and skin diseases. It contains anthraquinones which act on the bowel and relieve constipation.

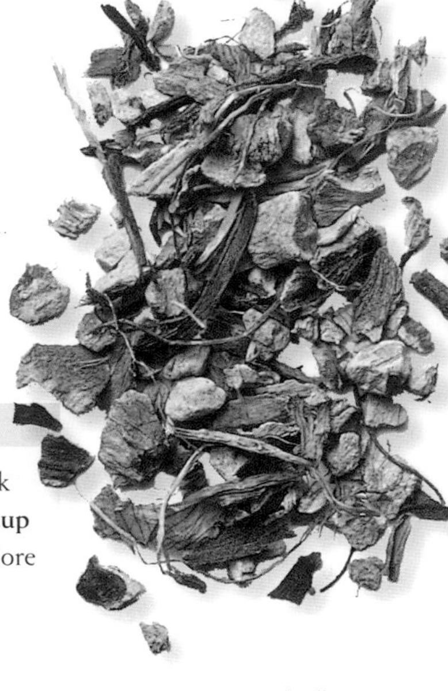

ABOVE *Dried yellow dock root. It is dug up in the fall.*

NOTES AND DOSAGES

Make the decoction using ½oz. (12g.) yellow dock root to 1pt. (500ml.) water. **For constipation, 1 cup of decoction or 2 teaspoons of tincture daily.** More might be needed for short periods. **Use half this dose for chronic conditions, for children, and for constipation in pregnancy.**

RECIPE

Laxative Syrup

Water
Sugar
Dried root
Cinnamon sticks

Take ½oz. (12g.) dried root, ½pt. (250ml.) of water and one stick of cinnamon. Simmer together for 20 minutes, then strain. Reduce over low heat to 2fl. oz. (50ml.). Add 4oz. (100g.) sugar. Stir over low heat until dissolved. Dose: 6 dessertspoons for adults, 3 for children and pregnant women.

CAUTION

ALWAYS CONSIDER DIETARY CHANGES FOR STUBBORN CONSTIPATION.

DATA FILE

Properties

- Astringent
- Laxative
- Bitter tonic
- Alterative

Uses

- Chronic constipation.
- Liver congestion with poor fat digestion, and for feelings of heaviness which come on after eating.
- Stomach acidity, and for irritable bowel syndrome with constipation.
- Food poisoning and intestinal infections, to clear the source of irritation out of the digestive system.
- With burdock for the relief of chronic, hot, and itchy skin diseases.

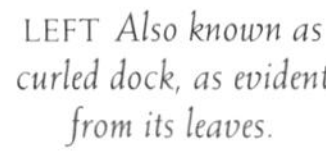

LEFT *Also known as curled dock, as evident from its leaves.*

Salix alba

WHITE WILLOW BARK

Bark from the willow tree. *Salix alba* is a 50ft. (15m.) silver-gray deciduous tree. A decoction or tincture of white willow treats arthritis, back pain, and lessens sexual desire.

DATA FILE

Properties

- Anti-inflammatory
- Mild painkiller
- Anaphrodisiac
- Tonic

Uses

- All types of arthritis, especially with inflamed joints, and for gout. With celery seed for multiple painful joints.
- With cramp bark for inflammatory back pain, and lumbago.
- Chronic diarrhea.
- Take together with rosemary for headaches.
- Sexual overstimulation, wet dreams, and for premature ejaculation.
- Convalescence and low-grade recurrent fevers; feeling of being overheated in the evenings.

NOTES AND DOSAGES

Take standard doses (*see pages 108–9*) and persist. **Willow bark contains aspirin-like compounds, but it does not upset the stomach.** It can be used to reduce dependency on aspirin and other anti-inflammatories.

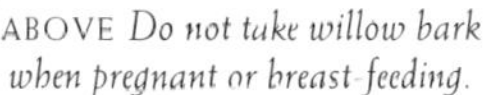

ABOVE *Do not take willow bark when pregnant or breast-feeding.*

RECIPE

Willow Bark and Ginger Decoction

Take 2 heaped teaspoons dried willow bark and 1 heaped teaspoon ginger powder. Add to 2 cups of water. Simmer together for 10 minutes. Strain. Add honey to taste and drink. Take freely, as needed, for chills, chronic diarrhea, and as a strengthening drink in convalescence.

Salvia officinalis

SAGE LEAVES

The common garden and cooking herb. The purple or red variety is stronger, but any variety will suffice. Sow seeds in late spring, in well-drained soil. Choose a sunny position. The plant grows to about 2ft. (60cm.).

NOTES AND DOSAGES

Standard doses (*see pages 108–9*). Traditionally, 1 cup a day maintains health in old age. **For an extra strength gargle add 5 drops of tincture of myrrh (from pharmacies or herb stores) to 1 cup of sage tea.** Sage tincture can be taken, instead of the cold tea, for stopping night sweats – 4 teaspoons daily, in a little water.

ABOVE RIGHT *Sage leaves may be added to meat, fish, egg, and vegetable dishes.*

DATA FILE

Properties

- Astringent
- Stimulant
- Antiseptic
- Carminative
- Antispasmodic
- Nervine
- Generally strengthening
- A woman's tonic

Uses

- Depression and nervous exhaustion, post-viral fatigue, general debility.
- Anxiety and confusion in elderly people, or accompanying exhaustion and weakened states.
- For indigestion, wind, loss of appetite, and mucus on the stomach.
- Excessive sweating and night sweats, tincture taken cold.
- Weak lungs with persistent and recurrent coughs and allergies.
- Menopausal hot flushes, menstrual cramps, and premenstrual painful breasts (as a tea and compress).
- Cold sage tea taken every few hours will usually dry up breast milk.
- As a gargle and mouthwash for sore throats, laryngitis, tonsillitis, mouth ulcers, and inflamed and tender gums.
- As an antiseptic wash for dirty wounds which are slow to heal.

THERAPY CONNECTIONS

WILLOW

Flower Remedies p.239

RECIPE

Sage and Vinegar Poultice

Bruise a handful of fresh sage leaves by flattening them with a rolling pin. Place in a pan and cover with cider vinegar. Simmer very gently until the leaves are soft. Wrap the leaves in a cloth and apply warm for bruises, swellings, and stings.

CAUTION

AVOID IF ALLERGIC TO SALICYLATES (ASPIRIN).

NOT SUITABLE FOR CHILDREN.

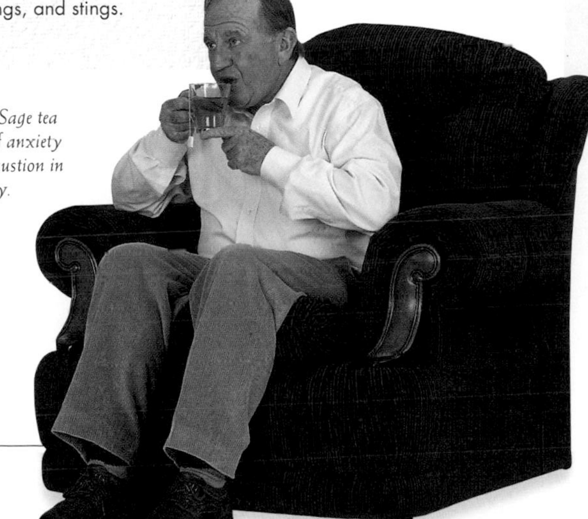

RIGHT *Sage tea wards off anxiety and exhaustion in the elderly.*

Sambucus nigra

ELDERFLOWERS

The creamy white flowers from a small tree common in hedgerows and on wasteland. The tree is in flower for only three weeks in summer. Elderflower ointment has long been a remedy for chilblains and chapped hands.

NOTES AND DOSAGES

❧ The hot tea is taken freely, up to 1 cup every 2 hours, for colds and fevers; 3 cups a day for chronic colds and sinusitis. ❧ **For children over five use half doses.** ❧ Eating fresh elderflowers will relieve the symptoms of hay fever, as will drinking a tea made with equal parts of elderflowers and eyebright (*Euphrasia officinalis*). ❧ **To prevent hay fever take 3 cups a day, starting two months before your regular season.** ❧ For colds and runny noses in infants add 3 or 4 cups of elderflower tea to their daily bath.

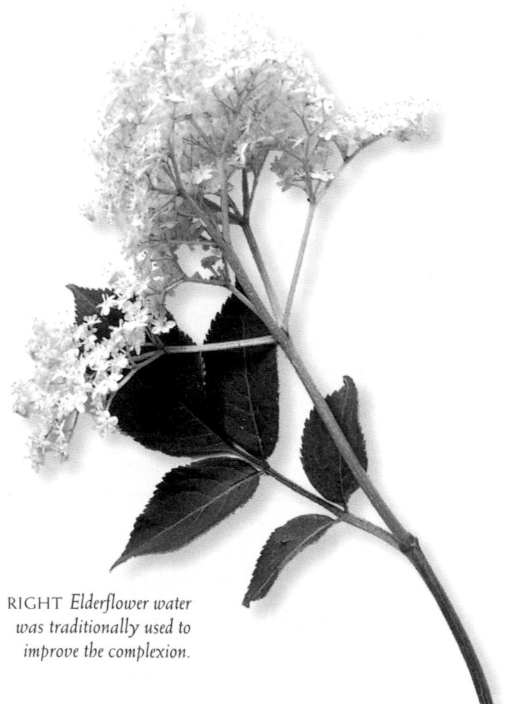

RIGHT *Elderflower water was traditionally used to improve the complexion.*

DATA FILE

Properties

- Restorative for mucous membrane and sinuses
- Diaphoretic
- Diuretic
- Anti-inflammatory

Uses

- Take the tea or tincture for sinusitis, colds, running nose, hay fever, and flu.
- To break a fever with hot, dry skin – it will induce sweating, bring down the temperature, and protect the kidneys.
- Suitable for use in children's fevers as a tea and as a lotion to soothe the rashes that often come with them.
- Lotion or compress for sore and runny eyes, eyestrain, and sunburn.
- Cream for chapped and discolored skin.

Schisandra chinensis

SCHISANDRA BERRIES

The red berries of an ornamental vine grown in China. The Chinese use schisandra berries to relieve spontaneous sweating.

NOTES AND DOSAGES

❧ Called Wu Wei Zi in Chinese herbalism. ❧ **Also available from specialist herb stores.** ❧ Dose: tincture – take 1 teaspoon three times daily; dried berries – take ½oz. (10g.) daily by decoction.

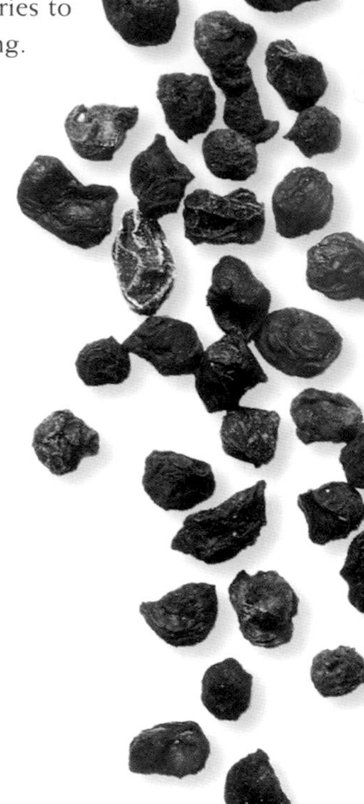

RIGHT *Dried schisandra berries are valued as a skin beautifier.*

DATA FILE

Properties

- Astringent
- Nourishing
- Soothing expectorant

Uses

- Weakness with nervous exhaustion and sleeplessness; exhaustion from prolonged hard work.
- Loss of sex drive in women and men; restores softness to the skin.
- Dry and chronic coughs, and asthma.
- Night sweats.

THERAPY CONNECTIONS

SCHISANDRA
Chinese Herbal Medicine p.74

SKULLCAP
Chinese Herbal Medicine p.74

RECIPE

Elderflower Nose Wash

Elderflower nose wash is useful for sinusitis and hay fever. Make a cupful of a strong infusion, allow it to cool to blood heat, and add a pinch of salt. Sniff the mixture up each nostril in turn, then allow it to run out or use a special nasal bath. Use daily during the hay fever season.

RECIPE

Schisandra Wine

Add 4oz. (100g.) dried schisandra berries to a bottle of rice wine. Store in a cool place for four weeks. Drink a small wine glass twice daily. For weak lungs with recurrent coughs, and to keep skin soft in old age.

Serenoa serrulata

SAW PALMETTO BERRIES

The fruit of a small palm-like plant grown in the West Indies and the U.S. The berries are gathered from early fall to the middle of winter, and dried for storage.

DATA FILE

Properties

- Strengthening tonic
- Urinary antiseptic
- Alterative
- Stimulates sex hormones

Uses

- Prostate enlargement and cystitis.
- With damiana for weakness and impotence in men.
- Helps restore weight after severe illness.
- Failure to thrive in children, with marshmallow; take 10–15 drops of the combined tincture three times daily in fruit juice.

NOTES AND DOSAGES

Decoction: ½ teaspoon of the crushed berries to 1 cup water. **Adult dose: 1 or 2 cups daily.** Tincture: 20–40 drops, in water, 3 times daily.

CAUTION

AVOID IN EARLY PREGNANCY, EXCEPT WITH PROFESSIONAL ADVICE.

ALWAYS HAVE SUSPECTED PROSTATE PROBLEMS MEDICALLY CHECKED.

RECIPE

Saw Palmetto and Nettle Root Tincture

Dig up, wash, and finely chop two or three handfuls of fresh nettle roots. Place in a jar and cover with saw palmetto tincture (available from specialist herb stores). Leave for two weeks, shaking from time to time. Strain and bottle. Dose: 30 drops, 3 times daily, for prostate problems.

BELOW *Saw palmetto berries are a diuretic and tissue builder*

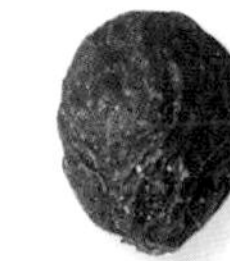

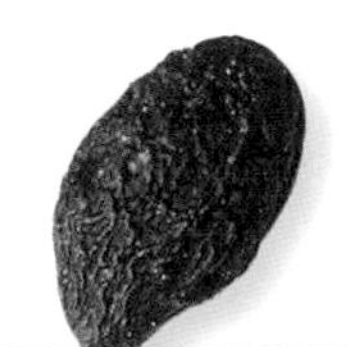

Silybum marianum

MILK THISTLE SEED

A tall, beautiful thistle that can easily be grown. The seeds resemble sunflower seeds. The seedheads are stored in a warm place to release the seeds.

NOTES AND DOSAGES

Standard decoction: ½ cup 3 times daily for at least six months. **Tablets are also available – follow the instructions on the box.** Recent research indicates it may be useful in hepatitis C.

BELOW *Milk thistle gets its name because it promotes milk production in nursing mothers.*

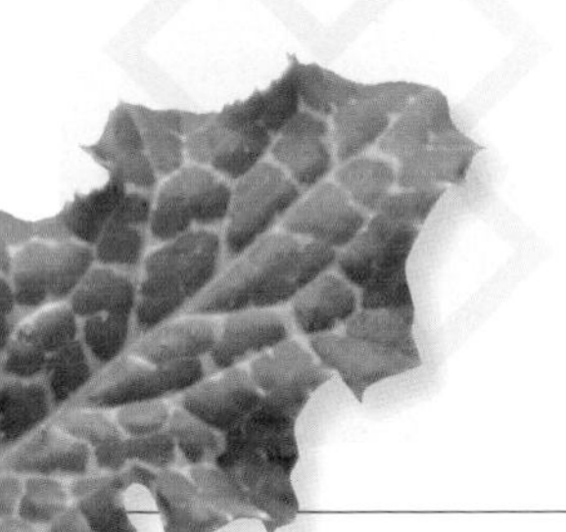

CAUTION

LIVER DISEASE SHOULD BE TREATED BY A PROFESSIONAL.

DATA FILE

Properties

- Strengthens and clears the liver and gall bladder.

Uses

- For "liverishness" and liver disease, poor fat tolerance, pale stools, and to protect the liver when taking strong drugs and medicines.
- Depression which comes on following hepatitis.
- For treating gallstones and for inflammation.
- Useful for Candida and food allergies.
- High blood pressure with liverish symptoms.

Scutellaria laterifolia or *Scutellaria galericulata*

SKULLCAP

U.S. skullcap, which is easily grown in gardens, or European skullcap, which grows wild on river banks.

DATA FILE

Properties

- Strengthens and calms the nervous system
- Antispasmodic

Uses

- Anxiety, tension headaches, PMS; for examination nerves, and to help fight off post-examination depression.
- With valerian or chamomile and linden flowers for insomnia and disturbed sleep, and for tranquilizer withdrawal.
- With vervain for workaholics, the mixture being relaxing without sedative effects.
- Supportive treatment in epilepsy and for people on major tranquilizers. Reduces anxiety without interfering with medication.

RIGHT *Skullcap prefers a sunny, open position in ordinary soil. The plant lives for about three years.*

CAUTION

SOME YEARS AGO COMMERCIAL PREPARATIONS WERE FOUND TO CONTAIN GERMANDER, WHICH IS SOMEWHAT POISONOUS. ALWAYS BUY YOUR HERBS AND HERBAL PREPARATIONS FROM A REPUTABLE FIRM.

NOTES AND DOSAGES

Standard doses (*see pages 108–9*). **There are many relaxing tablets available at various stores containing skullcap and other herbs** Follow the dosage on the box.

RECIPE

Examination Tea

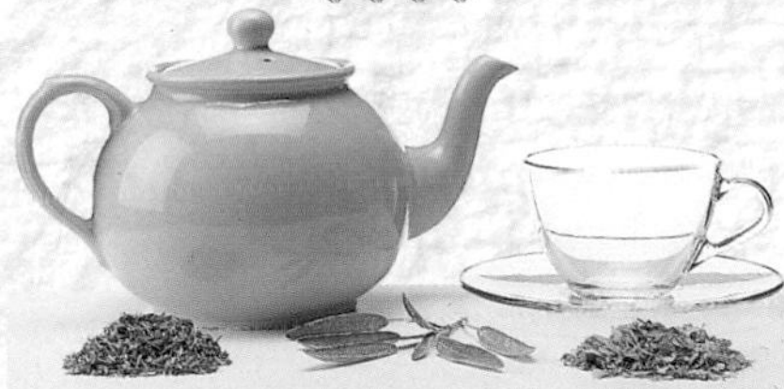

Mix together equal parts of dried skullcap, linden flowers, and sage leaf. Store in a jar in a dark place. Make a tea in the normal way, using 1 teaspoon of the mixture to 1 cup of boiling water. Drink 1 cup before examinations or 3 cups a day whilst studying.

Symphytum officinale

COMFREY

A common wild plant with large, bristly leaves and clusters of purple flowers. Comfrey root is used for treatment. One common name for comfrey is "knitbone," testifying to its healing powers.

DATA FILE

Properties

- Healing
- Mucilaginous

Uses

- Comfrey promotes rapid healing of cuts, wounds, sprains, and broken bones when taken as a tea or tincture, or used in poultices, creams, and liniments.
- Clean wounds well before applying comfrey.
- As a cream for cracked, dry skin.
- With chamomile and meadowsweet for hiatus hernia and stomach ulcers.

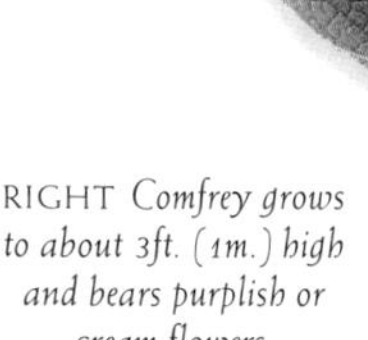

RIGHT *Comfrey grows to about 3ft. (1m.) high and bears purplish or cream flowers.*

NOTES AND DOSAGES

- Standard doses (*see pages 108–9*).
- **Add a few drops of a warming essential oil such as black pepper to the infused oil to make a good liniment for arthritis, bunions, and aches and pains arising from old injuries.**
- Comfrey ointment is a traditional soothing and healing preparation for sprains, and aches and pains.

CAUTION

THERE HAS BEEN SUSPICION OF LIVER DAMAGE FROM USING COMFREY ROOT AND FROM EATING LARGE AMOUNTS OF THE HERB.

THE HERB TEA AND TINCTURE ARE SAFE TO USE, BUT IT IS SENSIBLE TO AVOID THEM IN PREGNANCY, DURING BREAST-FEEDING, AND FOR INFANTS.

PREPARATIONS OF THE ROOT ARE NOT TAKEN INTERNALLY.

Tabebuia avellanedae

PAU D'ARCO

A tree from the South American rain forest. Also called lapacho and the Taheebo tree. It is particularly useful in the treatment of immunodeficiency diseases.

DATA FILE

Properties

- Immune tonic
- Antibiotic
- Antifungal

Uses

- Immune deficiency with susceptibility to infections.
- Good for diarrhea and intestinal infections.
- Traditionally used for cancer. Recent research has shown that the herb may be helpful for breast, liver, and prostate cancers. May be taken in conjunction with orthodox cancer treatment.
- For oral thrush, as a mouthwash; and to treat candidiasis, when taken as a decoction.

CAUTION

LARGE DOSES MAY CAUSE NAUSEA.

PEOPLE WITH BLOOD-CLOTTING DISORDERS SHOULD SEEK PROFESSIONAL ADVICE BEFORE TAKING THE HERB.

RECIPE

Tonic Soup

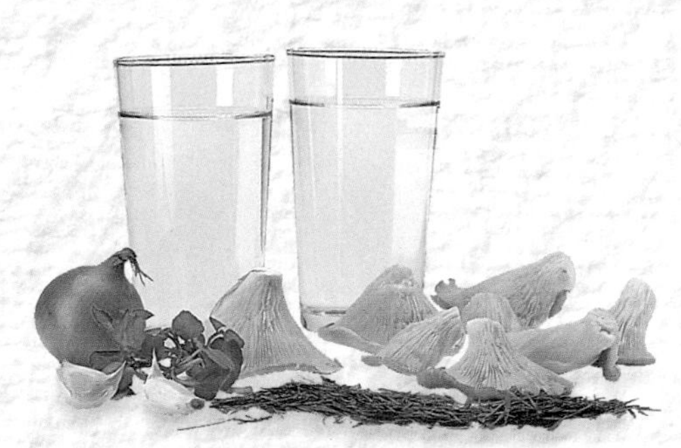

Make a decoction with ½oz. (12g.) Pau D'arco and 2pt. (1l.) water. Strain. Chop a small onion, two cloves of garlic, and a dozen oyster fungi. Simmer in the decoction until soft. Chop a small bunch of watercress and add to the soup just before serving. Eat daily for a weak immune system.

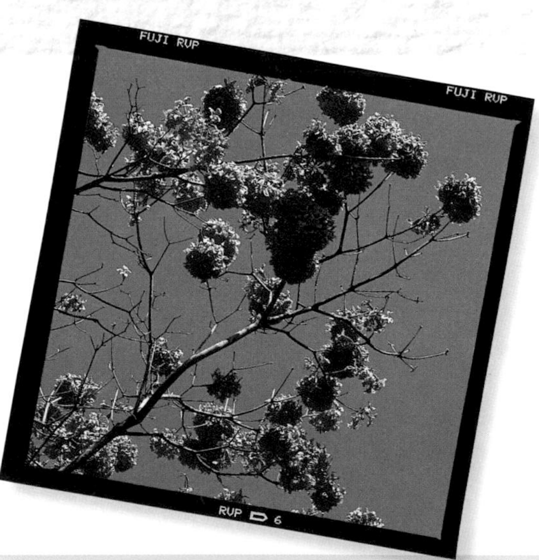

RIGHT *The inner bark of Pau D'arco is known to be an excellent antifungal agent.*

NOTES AND DOSAGES

- Make half-strength decoctions, ½oz. (12g.) Pau D'arco to 1pt. (500ml.) water.
- **Drink 3 cups daily.**
- Tablets and capsules are available – follow the doses on the packet.

Tanacetum parthenium

FEVERFEW

A small-flowered daisy, easily grown in gardens. Use the leaves, which should be picked just before the plant flowers. Feverfew is good for period pains, vertigo, and arthritis. The name is a corruption of the word "febrifuge."

DATA FILE

Properties

- Anti-inflammatory
- Antispasmodic
- Emmenagogue

Uses

- For migraine and arthritis.
- Combined with valerian for migraine linked with anxiety and tension.

ABOVE *Feverfew combined with skullcap relieves persistent headaches.*

NOTES AND DOSAGES

The best preparation is the tincture made from the fresh plant. **Dose: 1 teaspoon in a little water at the first signs of a migraine; repeat after 2 hours if necessary.** For repeated attacks and as a treatment for arthritis, take 1 teaspoon every morning. If you have a plant, 2 or 3 medium-sized leaves equal 1 teaspoon of tincture.

CAUTION

NOT TO BE TAKEN IN PREGNANCY OR DURING BREAST-FEEDING.

AVOID GIVING TO SMALL CHILDREN.

DO NOT TAKE IF USING BLOOD-THINNING DRUGS SUCH AS WARFARIN.

CHEWING THE LEAF CAN CAUSE MOUTH ULCERS IN SOME PEOPLE; IF THIS IS THE CASE, USE THE TINCTURE OR CAPSULES.

ABOVE *Make feverfew sandwiches, cut into cubes, and store in the freezer.*

RECIPE

Feverfew Preparations

There are many preparations of feverfew on the market, although many people still find that the fresh plant is the most effective. If it is not possible to keep a feverfew plant, make fresh feverfew sandwiches and keep them in the freezer.

Butter the bread. Cover one slice with a double layer of fresh feverfew leaves. Put on the top slice and press. Cut the sandwiches into small cubes. Each cube should have two or three medium-sized feverfew leaves. Wrap each cube in plastic wrap. Label, date, and freeze. Dose: one cube at the first sign of headache, then every two hours until the headache is over.

Taraxacum officinalis

DANDELION LEAF

The leaves from the familiar weed, which can be picked at any time. The leaves can be cooked and eaten like spinach, and are good for a springtime cleansing tonic. Dandelion leaf tea relieves edema and water retention.

DATA FILE

Properties

- A powerful diuretic
- Nourishing

Uses

- Tea for all types of water retention and edema, especially for swollen ankles which are associated with circulatory problems.
- Take with uva ursi or thyme for cystitis.

NOTES AND DOSAGES

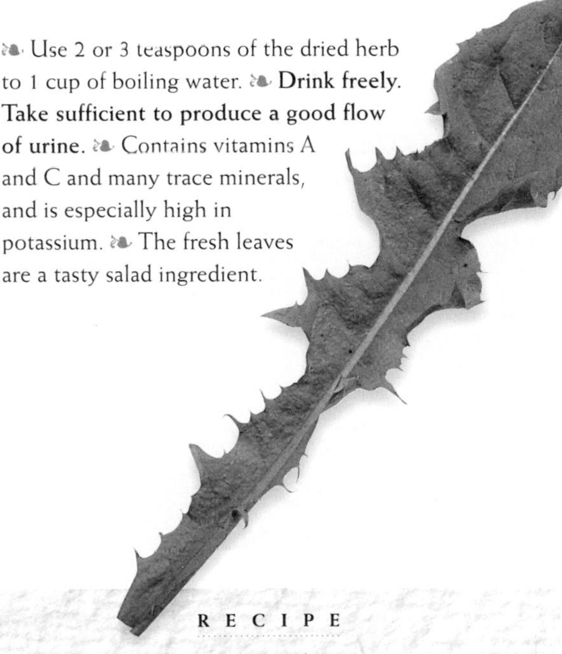

Use 2 or 3 teaspoons of the dried herb to 1 cup of boiling water. **Drink freely. Take sufficient to produce a good flow of urine.** Contains vitamins A and C and many trace minerals, and is especially high in potassium. The fresh leaves are a tasty salad ingredient.

RECIPE

Blanched Dandelion Leaf

This stimulates digestion and is excellent to include in daily salad for cases of poor appetite, weak digestion, and liver. General convalescence. Put a large pot upside down over a growing plant to keep out the light. Leave for two weeks or until the leaves are white. Dose: two leaves daily.

Taraxacum officinalis

DANDELION ROOT

The bitter dandelion root is a favorite in folk medicine, and particularly useful for stimulating a sluggish liver. The root of the dandelion is more effective than the leaves and stem in the treatment of liver problems. Coffee made from dandelion root is available, and it is thought to have a tonic effect on the pancreas, spleen, and female organs.

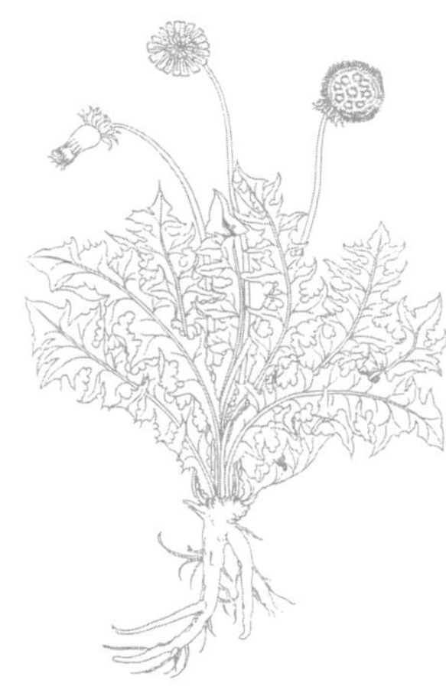

RIGHT *Dandelion root is a safe diuretic herb.*

DATA FILE

Properties

- Liver tonic
- Promotes good digestion
- Alterative

Uses

- For all types of liver and gall bladder problems.
- For indigestion, loss of appetite, and constipation in pregnancy.
- For arthritis and stubborn skin disease in combination with burdock.
- Research shows that regular use helps reduce blood cholesterol.
- The liver plays a crucial role in detoxification and nutrition, hence dandelion root is helpful in most chronic and wasting diseases, and helps the body to cope with strong chemical drugs.

RECIPE

Dandelion Coffee

Although dandelion is a wonderful plant it does not always grow where it is wanted. When weeding, keep the long taproots. Scrub all the dirt off the roots, chop into pieces, and roast in a medium oven until dry and slightly burnt. Make a decoction and take 1 or 2 cups a day as a liver strengthener and tonic.

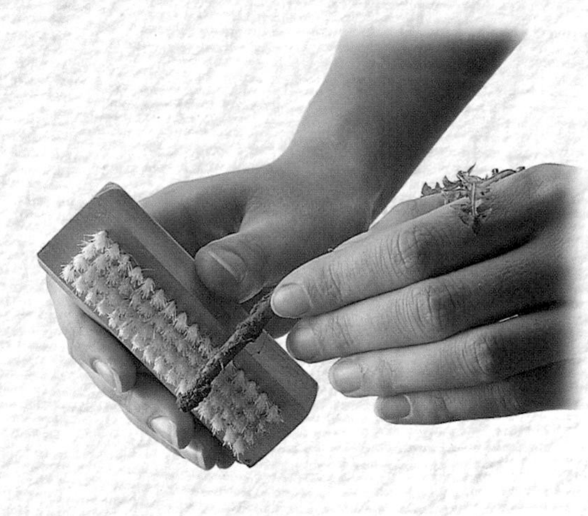

ABOVE *Do not slice the roots when you gather them, or the valuable sap will be lost.*

NOTES AND DOSAGES

At least 3 cups of decoction a day for 6 months. **Tincture: 4–6 teaspoons daily.** The decoction is best for liver problems.

Tilia europea

LINDEN

A tree often grown in parks and along streets. Its wood is good for carving, as it will take fine detail. Use the flowers, which are also called limeflowers. *Tilea europea* grows to 35m. (120 ft.). Its flowers are toxic to bees.

RIGHT *Limeflowers combined with elderflowers treat colds, and with hops treat nervous tension.*

DATA FILE

Properties

- Calming and soothing
- Strengthens nerves
- Antispasmodic
- Diaphoretic

Uses

- For anxiety, irritability, and insomnia. Long-term use strengthens the nervous system and improves tolerance of stress.
- Improves digestion, nervous indigestion.
- Induces sweating and reduces temperature in fevers. Suitable for children. Use at standard tea strength and take freely.
- Take linden with hawthorn tops as a tea for mild high blood pressure.

CAUTION

OLD OR IMPROPERLY DRIED FLOWERS ARE SAID TO BE SOMEWHAT NARCOTIC. REJECT STALE-SMELLING AND DISCOLORED FLOWERS. STORE CAREFULLY.

NOTES AND DOSAGES

- Standard doses (*see pages 108–9*). May be taken freely.
- **A popular every-day tea in France.**
- Linden mixes well with other herb teas.

RECIPE

Linden Flower Bath for Infants

Especially good for dry skin and eczema with irritability. Take ½oz. (12g.) dried linden flowers and 1pt. (500ml.) water. Put into pan and bring to the boil, cover, and allow to stand for 15 minutes. Add to the baby's bath.

Turnera diffusa

DAMIANA

A small, strongly aromatic shrub grown in South America. The leaves are used for therapeutic purposes. They treat depression, anxiety, poor digestion, cystitis, and are a tonic for the reproductive system.

DATA FILE

Properties

- Stimulant tonic for the nerves and reproductive system in both sexes
- Aphrodisiac

Uses

- For impotence and sterility associated with anxiety, especially in men.
- For physical weakness, depression, mental stupor, and nervous exhaustion in both sexes.
- For prostatitis and relief of chronic cystitis.
- For poor digestion with constipation and lack of appetite.

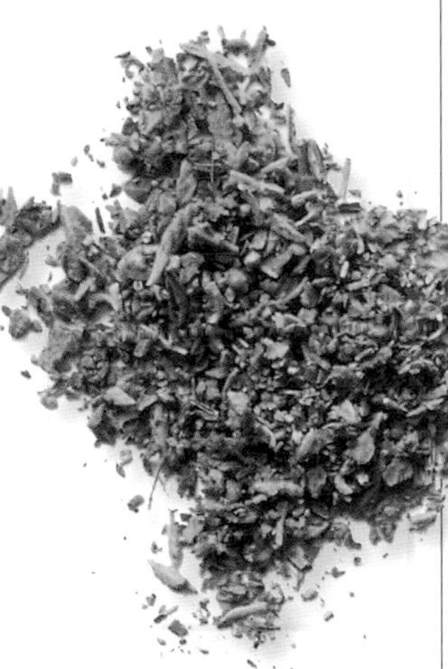

ABOVE *Dried damiana leaves and stems. These are gathered when the plant is in flower.*

NOTES AND DOSAGES

Take ½ cup of the tea or 1 teaspoon of the tincture twice daily. **Alternatively combine damiana with other herbs, such as wild oats or saw palmetto, and use 1 cup of the combination tea, or 1 teaspoon of tincture, twice daily.**

CAUTION

SAFE BUT QUITE STIMULATING.

DO NOT EXCEED THE RECOMMENDED DOSE.

RECIPE

Damiana Combination for Herpes

Combine equal parts of tinctures of damiana and echinacea. Dose: 1 teaspoon every four hours. This will often avert an attack, if taken at the first signs. Alternatively, make a decoction with equal parts of the herbs and take ½ cup every four hours.

Thymus vulgaris

THYME

The popular thyme used in cooking recipes. Thyme is an attractive small perennial herb. It is easy to grow and thrives in the rock garden or a sunny well-drained border. There are many different garden varieties.

NOTES AND DOSAGES

Take freely. Large doses might be needed for coughs. **For infants' coughs, 2 or 3 teaspoons of syrup up to 4 times daily. Make a chest rub from the infused oil. For children's worms, ¼–½ cup strong tea before breakfast, for 2 weeks.**

CAUTION

AVOID LARGE DOSES IN PREGNANCY, EXCEPT AS ADVISED BY A QUALIFIED HERBALIST.

THE AMOUNTS TAKEN IN FOOD ARE HARMLESS.

ASTHMA CAN BE SERIOUS AND SHOULD BE TREATED BY A PROFESSIONAL.

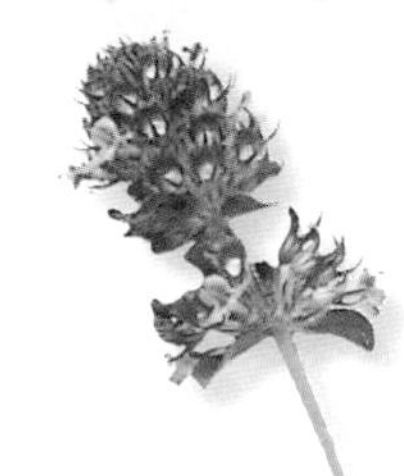

RECIPE

Thyme Syrup

Thyme makes an ideal antiseptic expectorant cough syrup. This recipe is for a tight chest and restless unproductive cough. Take ½oz. (12g.) thyme, 1oz. (25g.) chamomile, 1 teaspoon cinnamon, a pinch of cayenne or ginger (optional). Make a decoction, reduce, and add sugar or honey. Take as directed.

DATA FILE

Properties

- Antiseptic
- Antibacterial
- Antifungal
- Expectorant
- Digestive tonic

Uses

- For any cough with infected or tough phlegm.
- Helpful, if taken regularly, in asthma.
- Specific for the treatment of whooping cough.
- Indigestion, wind, and intestinal infections.
- Take along with marshmallow for cystitis.
- Fights distressing intestinal worms in children.
- Weak tea for nightmares.
- Thyme vinegar is antifungal for athlete's foot.
- Use thyme vinegar, diluted with an equal amount of water, for washes and douches for thrush.

THERAPY CONNECTIONS

THYME

Aromatherapy *p.170*

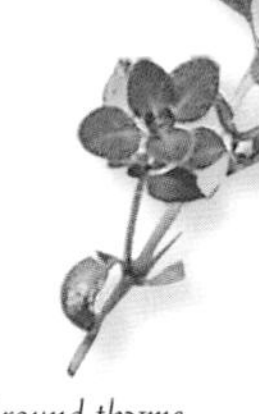

ABOVE *Ground thyme, with sage and chamomile, inhaled on a charcoal block, helps asthma.*

LEFT *Thyme cough syrup tastes pleasant and appeals to children.*

Ulmus fulva

SLIPPERY ELM BARK

The inner bark of a small U.S. tree, usually sold powdered. It smells rather like fenugreek, but tastes bland. It is very nutritious, as well as having healing properties.

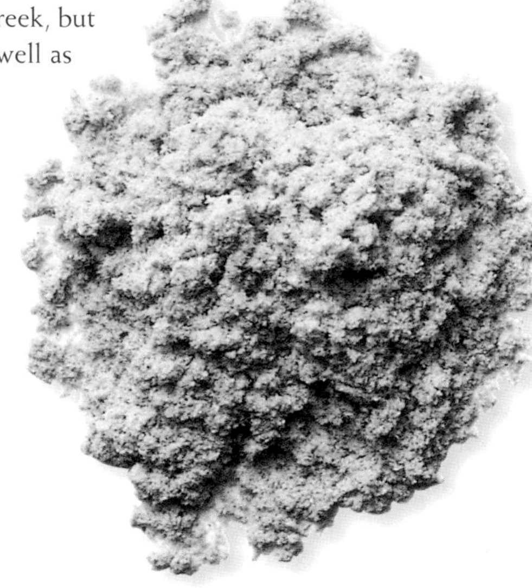

BELOW *Slippery elm is often used to back up other remedies. It is good for convalescents.*

DATA FILE

Properties

- Soothing
- Mucilaginous

Uses

- Any sort of inflammation or irritation in the digestive tract: nausea, indigestion, wind, food allergies, stomach ulcers, acidity, heartburn, hiatus hernia, colitis, diverticulitis, and diarrhea. One of the most useful herbs for treating digestive problems.
- Mix with sufficient water to make a paste for drawing splinters.

RECIPE

Slippery Elm and Chamomile Poultice

Mix together 2 dessertspoons each of slippery elm powder and dried chamomile flowers. Add hot water, slowly, stirring all the time to make a paste. Wrap the warm paste in light cotton and apply. Leave in place for a half-hour. Soothing and healing for any kind of painful swelling.

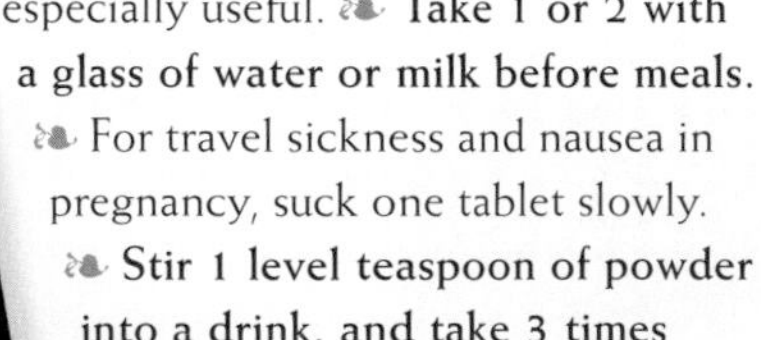

NOTES AND DOSAGES

Tablets flavored with carminative herbs are especially useful. **Take 1 or 2 with a glass of water or milk before meals.** For travel sickness and nausea in pregnancy, suck one tablet slowly. **Stir 1 level teaspoon of powder into a drink, and take 3 times daily before meals.**

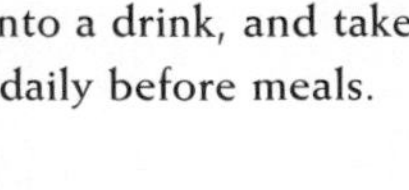

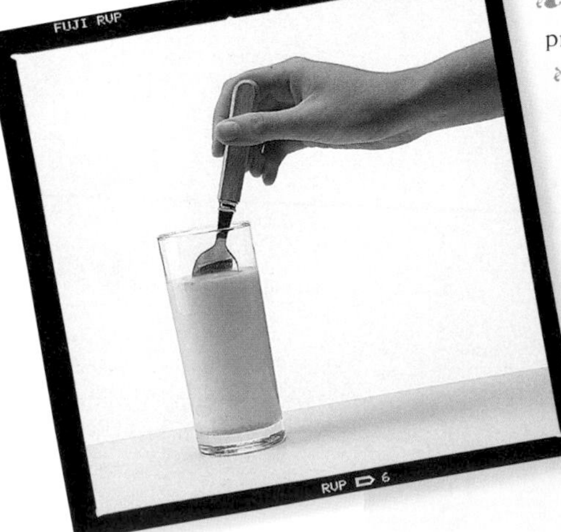

BELOW *Stir slippery elm powder into a glass of milk, and drink before meals to help digestion.*

Valeriana officinalis

VALERIAN ROOT

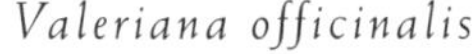

The root of a wild plant with pretty pink flowers. In the Middle Ages, it was used as a spice and a perfume, as well as a medicine.

NOTES AND DOSAGES

The cold decoction is best: soak 1 teaspoon in 1 cup of cold water overnight. **Dose: ½–1 cup.** Tincture: 20–60 drops 3 times daily. **More may be needed to help with tranquilizer withdrawal.** Relaxing tablets containing valerian are widely available.

ABOVE *Valerian leaves. The roots of the plant are used, and are dug up in the fall.*

CAUTION

A SAFE HERB IN GENERAL USE.

CAUSES HYPERACTIVITY IN SOME PEOPLE.

VERY LARGE DOSES CAN CAUSE TEMPORARY GIDDINESS.

DO NOT TAKE FOR LONG PERIODS WITHOUT EXAMINING WHY YOU ARE SO TENSE.

TRANQUILIZER WITHDRAWAL SHOULD ONLY BE UNDERTAKEN WITH PSYCHOLOGICAL SUPPORT.

DATA FILE

Properties

- Sedative
- Nerve restorative
- Calms the heart
- Antispasmodic
- Carminative

Uses

- Anxiety, confusion, migraines, insomnia, and depression with anxiety.
- Useful when flying.
- Palpitations.
- Helpful for withdrawal from tranquilizers.
- Good for high blood pressure from stress.
- With chamomile for colic and nervous indigestion.

BELOW *Valerian grows in damp ground, reaching 3ft. (1m.).*

RECIPE

Valerian Sleeping Mixture

Mix together equal amounts of tinctures of valerian root, dandelion root, and chamomile flowers (some specialist stores will make up the mixture for you). Store in a dark bottle and label. Adult dose: 1–3 teaspoons in a little water before bed for sleeplessness with tension or from indigestion.

Urtica dioica

NETTLE

The common stinging nettle, which grows all over the world. Plants have either male or female flowers, which is suggested by the name *dioica*, meaning "two houses." Nettles produce a good textile fiber.

DATA FILE

Properties

- Iron tonic
- Mild diuretic
- Antihistamine
- Strengthening
- Styptic

Uses

- Iron deficiency anemia. Nourishing and building, good to take in pregnancy.
- For lethargy, weakness, and feelings of heaviness in the body.
- Nettle rash, allergies to strawberries, and insect bites; as tea and lotion, and nervous eczema.
- Treats urinary gravel and water retention.
- Helpful for arthritis.
- Taken with cleavers as a spring tonic.

CAUTION

MAY BE TOO DRYING FOR SOME PEOPLE, IN WHICH CASE TAKE WITH MARSHMALLOW.

RIGHT *The juice of a nettle will relieve a nettle sting, strangely enough!*

NOTES AND DOSAGES

- Standard doses (*see pages 108–9*).
- **Leave to infuse for 15 minutes for best effect.**
- The tops can be cooked as spinach or made into soup.
- **Rubbing stiff joints with fresh nettles gives instant relief.**

RECIPE

Nettle Soup

Young nettle tops gathered in spring provide an unusual vegetable, which can be made into a nourishing soup. Pick 1pt. (500ml.) of the tops of young nettles, avoiding too much stem. Chop two medium potatoes, a carrot, and a small onion. Add the ingredients to twice as much water and boil until the potatoes are soft. Blend in a food processor. Serve seasoned to taste.

Verbascum thapsus

MULLEIN

A beautiful wild flower with a tall, thick spike of yellow flowers. Use the leaves and flowers. Mullein is demulcent, emollient, and astringent, good for lung complaints and diarrhea.

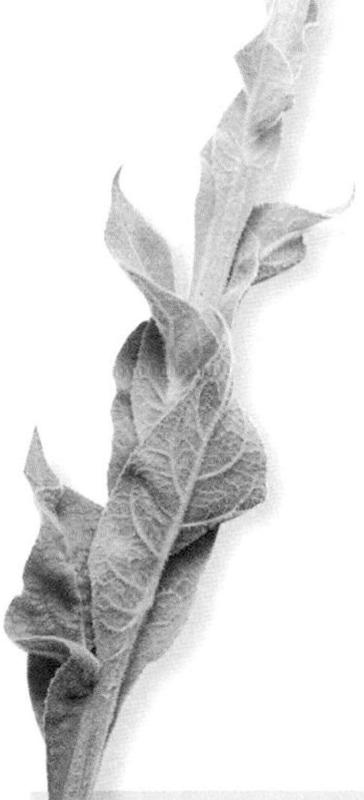

RIGHT *Mullein was also known as "bullock's lungwort" – it cured cattle's lung diseases.*

DATA FILE

Properties

- A soothing expectorant
- Clears mucus
- Heals wounds

Uses

- For deep and ticklish coughs and bronchitis. Helpful in asthma, by clearing sticky mucus.
- Mullein flower infused oil as ear drops for itchy ears and chronic earache, and as a salve for itchy eyelids.
- Mullein and garlic infused oil to soothe the pain of acute earache.
- Two drops of mullein flower infused oil, in a little juice, three times daily, is helpful for bedwetting.

CAUTION

DO NOT USE EAR DROPS IF THE EARDRUM HAS BURST.

NOTES AND DOSAGES

- The tea gives the best results for coughs.
- **Allow the mullein to infuse for a long time and drink freely.**

THERAPY CONNECTIONS

NETTLE

Homeopathy p.217

RECIPE

Mullein and Garlic Infused Oil

Pick the spike from a mullein in full flower. Make an infused oil (*see the instructions on page 109*). This is used for itchy ears. Fill a small jar with chopped garlic and cover it with the mullein oil. Leave overnight. Strain and use as drops for ear infections.

Verbena officinalis

VERVAIN

An unprepossessing wild plant with a spike of small, pale pink flowers. Often missed. Vervain is a nourishing tonic.

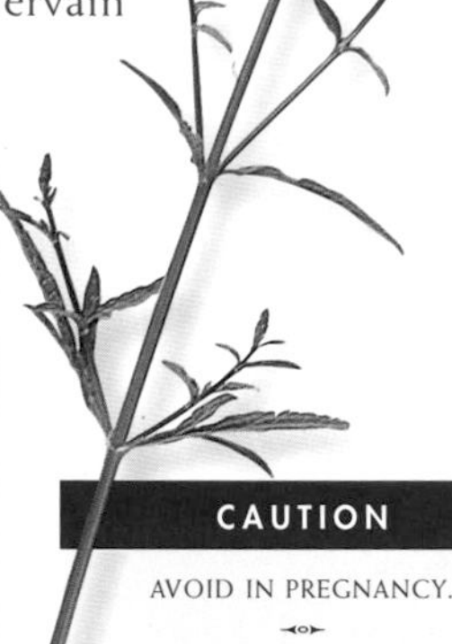

RECIPE

Combined Vervain Remedy

Prepare a vervain flower remedy (see page 241), or buy a bottle of the prepared flower remedy stock. Add 4 drops of this remedy to 1 cup of vervain tea, standard strength. Drink 2 or 3 cups daily to relieve tiredness and tension resulting from overwork.

CAUTION

AVOID IN PREGNANCY.

SAFE FOR CHILDREN AND WHEN BREAST-FEEDING.

LARGE DOSES OF THE TEA CAN CAUSE NAUSEA.

NOTES AND DOSAGES

Standard-strength teas taken every two hours in fevers, or 3 cups a day for chronic complaints. For worms and parasites, make double-strength tea and drink before breakfast for some weeks or until better. Vervain tea is an ideal restorative for people strained by overwork, especially mental work.

ABOVE LEFT *Both the leaves and the flowers of the vervain plant are used to make herbal remedies.*

BELOW *Vervain helps to treat depression and exhaustion.*

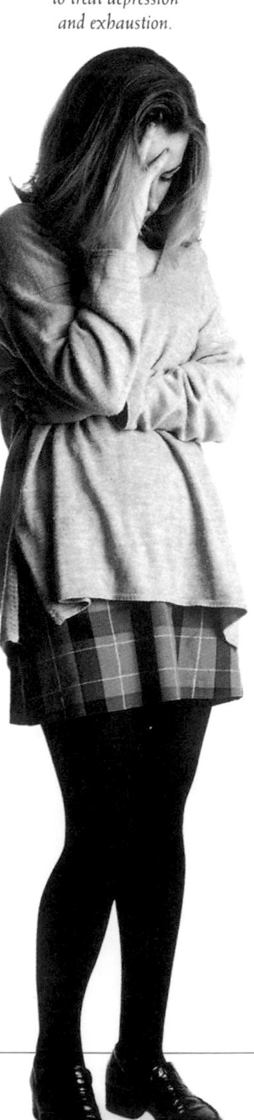

DATA FILE

Properties

- Tonic
- Fever herb
- Nerve restorative
- Antispasmodic
- Carminative
- Diuretic
- Promotes milk flow
- Emmenagogue

Uses

- Exhaustion and post-viral fatigue. Exhaustion from overwork. Vervain is a useful general tonic.
- Nervous depression.
- Fevers and flu, especially accompanied by headaches and nervous symptoms.
- Insomnia and excessive dreaming; also for feelings of paranoia.
- Good for "letting go."
- Indigestion, worms, and parasites; digestive discomfort following treatment for parasites.
- "Liverishness" with nausea, heavy headaches, and depression.
- Irritable bowel syndrome with mucus in the stools.
- Helpful in asthma – relieves chest tension.
- Sip the tea throughout labor to encourage regular contractions. Continue taking it after the birth to encourage milk flow.
- Post-natal depression.
- Menstrual cramps and to restore menstruation stopped by stress.
- Post-operative tiredness and depression.
- As a compress for inflamed eyes.

Viburnum opulus

CRAMP BARK

The bark from the wild form of the guelder rose. Treats nervous complaints, cramp, spasms, heart disease, and rheumatism.

ABOVE *The bark has a strong smell and is sold in thin strips. It is produced mainly in northern Europe.*

DATA FILE

Properties

- Relaxant
- Antispasmodic
- Mildly sedative

Uses

- For any sort of cramping pains, colic, menstrual cramps, muscle spasm, and shoulder and neck tension.
- Back pain usually involves some muscle spasm – often a dramatic improvement with cramp bark.
- For children when bedwetting is associated with tension and anxiety.

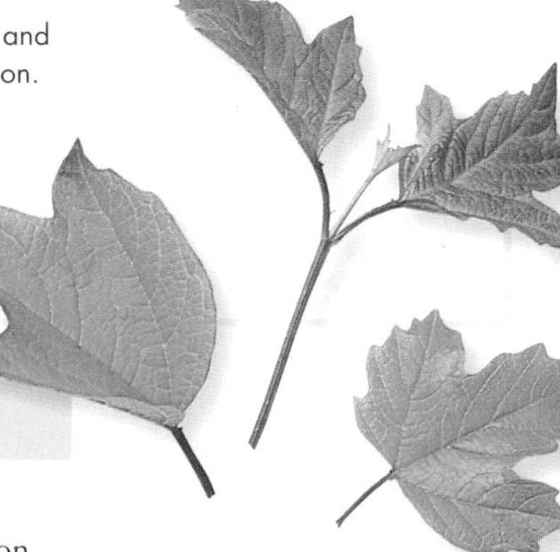

NOTES AND DOSAGES

Best taken freely, 1 cup of the decoction or 1–2 teaspoons of the tincture 4 or 5 times daily. May be improved by the addition of a little ginger. For children, give 30 drops of tincture, in fruit juice, three times daily.

CAUTION

SAFE IN GENERAL USE.

SOME PEOPLE FIND THAT LARGE DOSES WILL LOWER THEIR BLOOD PRESSURE, MAKING THEM FEEL A LITTLE FAINT.

RECIPE

Cramp Bark Capsules for Menstrual Cramps

Grind 1oz. (30g.) cramp bark and 1 teaspoon ginger powder together in a coffee grinder until you have a fine powder. Fill standard-sized gelatin capsules, available from herb suppliers. Take 2 or 3 capsules as required for quick relief from pain.

Vitex agnus-castus

AGNUS CASTUS BERRIES

The fruit of a pretty, half-hardy Mediterranean shrub. *Vitex agnus-castus* is also known as chaste tree, and is reputed both to increase sex drive, and also to damp it down, as indicated by its name!

DATA FILE

Properties

- Balances hormones

Uses

- PMS with irritability, breast pain, and water retention.
- Menopausal symptoms, especially with mood swings and depression. With sage for hot flushes.
- Helps restore a regular menstrual cycle when coming off the contraceptive pill or when the cycle has been disrupted.

CAUTION

MAY CAUSE CHANGES IN THE MENSTRUAL CYCLE. THIS IS A NATURAL PART OF THE WAY THE HERB WORKS.

AGNUS CASTUS MAY BE TAKEN IN CONJUNCTION WITH HORMONE DRUGS, BUT IT IS BEST TO SEEK THE ADVICE OF A PROFESSIONAL HERBALIST BEFORE DOING SO. NOT TO BE TAKEN WITH PROGESTERONE.

NOTES AND DOSAGES

The best time to take the berries is first thing in the morning, before breakfast. One cup of the decoction or 20–30 drops of the tincture in a little water, taken daily, will usually suffice.

RECIPE

Agnus Castus Pepper

The dried berries have a pleasant, peppery taste, and may be powdered in a coffee grinder and sprinkled on to meals. Dose: two good pinches or 1/4 flat teaspoon.

Agnus castus is still used in monasteries to help the monks keep to their vows of chastity, by balancing excess male hormones.

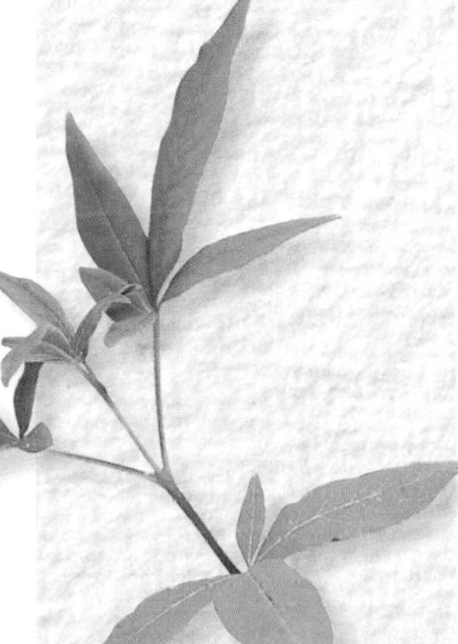

RIGHT *The leaves of the chaste tree. Berries should be picked in the fall and dried.*

Zingiber officinale

GINGER

Ginger is the spice made from the rhizome, or enlarged underground stem, of the herbaceous perennial plant *Zingiber officinale*, a member of the ginger family. Native to southern Asia, ginger is widely cultivated in Africa, Asia, Australia, and the West Indies, particularly Jamaica. Ginger is a warming, stimulating herb which is especially good for the circulation. The Chinese regularly use it in cooking.

RECIPE

Crystallized Ginger for Travel Sickness and Nausea

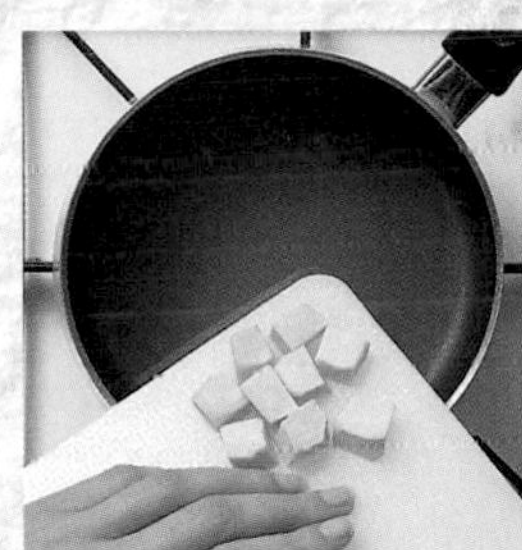

Peel a large piece of fresh ginger and chop it into small cubes. Make a syrup by dissolving 1 cup of sugar in 4 cups of water. Add the ginger and simmer gently until the root is soft. Leave in the syrup overnight, drain, and pack in sterilized jars.

DATA FILE

Properties

- Warming
- Carminative
- Antispasmodic
- Diaphoretic
- Anti-emetic

Uses

- For nausea and the nausea of pregnancy and travel sickness.
- For wind, colic, and irritable bowel.
- Good for chills, colds, and poor circulation.
- For fevers, added to elderflower or yarrow tea.
- For menstrual cramps, with cramp bark and as a compress of grated root.

CAUTION

AVOID TAKING GINGER IN ACUTE INFLAMMATORY CONDITIONS OR USING LOCALLY ON HOT AND INFLAMED AREAS. IT WILL BE TOO HEATING.

THERAPY CONNECTIONS

VERVAIN

Flower Remedies p.241

NOTES AND DOSAGES

More easily tolerated than cayenne. May be added to most remedies to improve absorption and activity. A mixture of ½ teaspoon of powder to 1 cup boiling water may be taken freely. Tincture: 5–20 drops in any herb tea. Crystallized ginger helps with the control of travel sickness.

ABOVE *Ginger root is dug up when the leaves have dried. It is then thoroughly washed.*

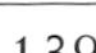

AROMATHERAPY

ESSENTIAL OILS

The practice of aromatherapy is based on the use of essential oils. The oils work on the whole body to treat specific ailments and restore the natural balance on both the physical and mental levels.

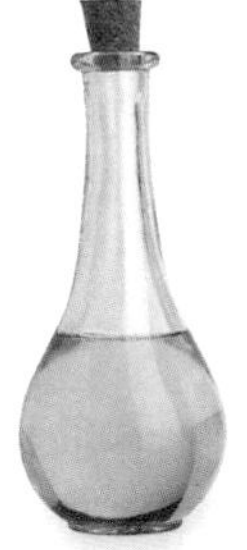

Each essential oil has its own individual scent and healing properties.

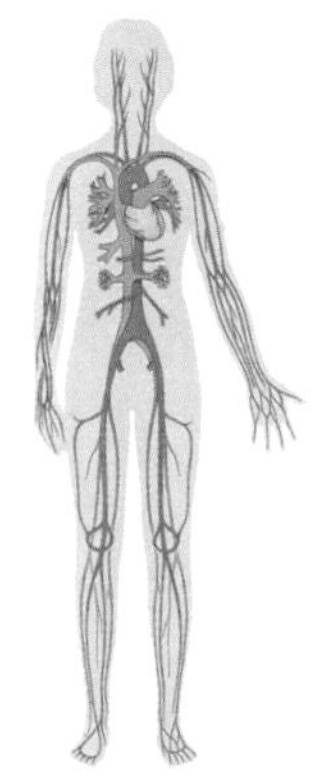

The oil molecules enter the bloodstream and are carried to every part of the body.

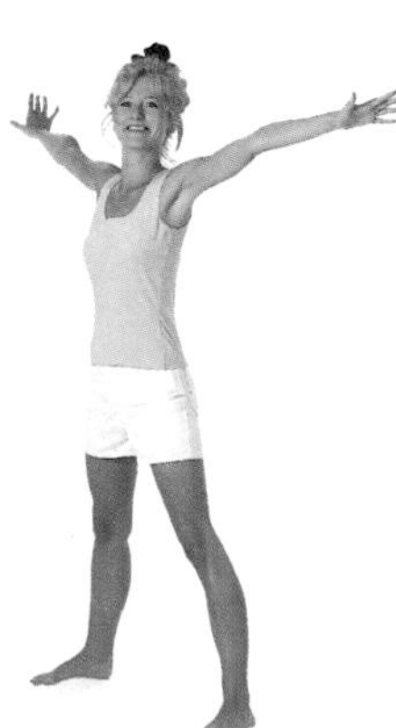

Oils affect both mind and spirit, restoring physical health and lifting the spirits.

The word aromatherapy means "treatment using scents." It refers to a particular branch of herbal medicine that uses concentrated plant oils called essential oils to improve physical and emotional health, and to restore balance to the whole person. Unlike the herbs used in herbal medicine, essential oils are not taken internally, but are inhaled or applied to the skin. Each oil has its own natural fragrance, and a gentle healing action that makes aromatherapy one of the most pleasant and popular of all the available complementary therapies.

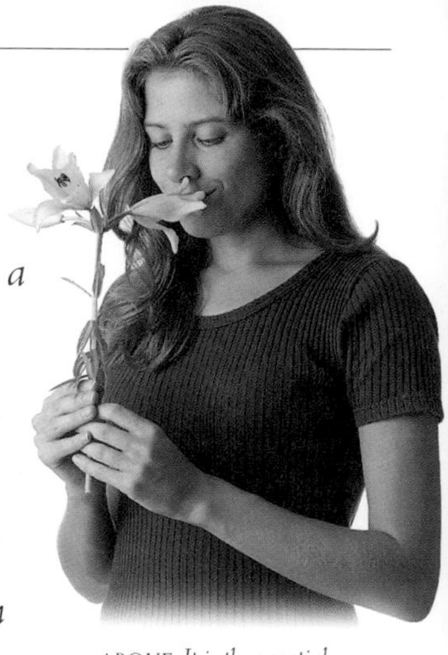

ABOVE *It is the essential, or volatile, oils of flowers, spices, and herbs that give them their unique fragrance.*

HOW AROMATHERAPY WORKS

Aromatherapy is subtle but effective when used correctly and given time to work. While one treatment may prove immediately relaxing or reviving, the effects tend to be short-lived. Regular treatments are needed to rebalance body systems and if you have been stressed or ill, it could take several weeks of treatment before you notice an improvement.The practice of aromatherapy involves using more than just the aroma of certain plant oils to treat mind and body. It is concerned with getting essential oils into the body in order to alter body chemistry, support body systems, and improve moods and emotions. This is done most effectively by massaging oils into the skin. Manipulating the soft tissues of the body has been shown to release emotional and physical tension, relieve pain, promote healthy circulation, and restore the whole person to a balanced state of health. Massage is the method of choice for professional aromatherapists. However, for home use oils can also be added to bathwater, or applied on hot or cold compresses to swollen, painful, or bruised areas.

When applied to the skin, essential oils start to work immediately on body tissues. The molecules in the oils are so small that they can be absorbed through the pores of the skin and into the bloodstream, by which means they are carried to every part of the body.

However, aroma is important. Inhalation can reinforce the effects of oils applied to the skin, and it is a safe way to benefit from the healing properties of oils that could cause irritation. No one knows exactly how aromas affect the mind, but it has been theorized that receptors in the nose convert smells into electrical impulses which are transmitted to the limbic system of the brain. Smells reaching the limbic system can directly affect our moods and emotions, and improve mental alertness and concentration.

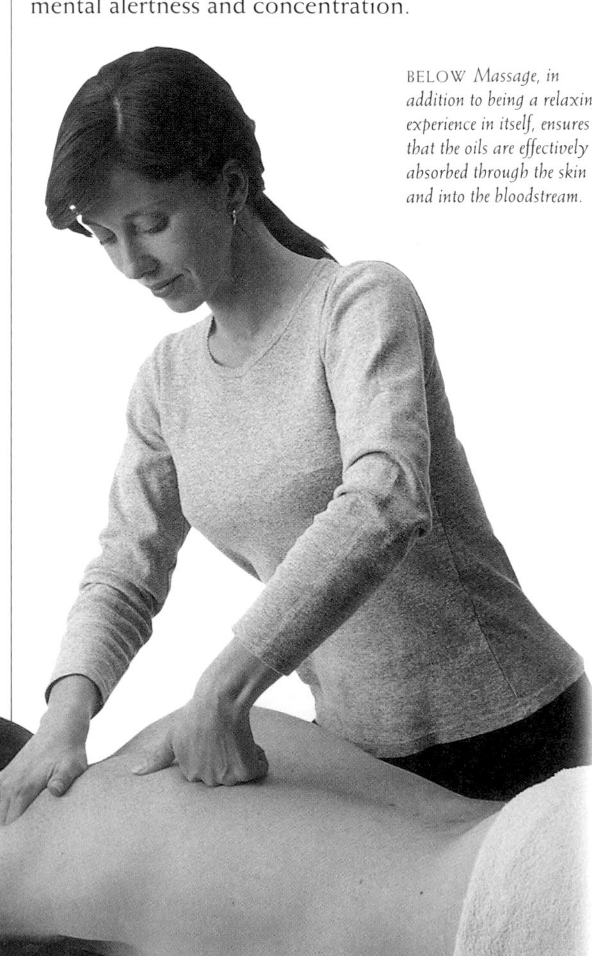

BELOW *Massage, in addition to being a relaxing experience in itself, ensures that the oils are effectively absorbed through the skin and into the bloodstream.*

LEFT *Essential oils are blended with a carrier oil for massage.*

THE BENEFITS OF AROMATHERAPY

Aromatherapy benefits people rather than illnesses. It is gentle enough to be used by people of all ages and states of health. It is nurturing for babies and children, and offers comfort and care to the elderly. Pregnant women and even seriously ill patients with cancer or AIDS can benefit from professional treatment. Aromatherapy is not recommended as a cure for any disease. Its most potent effect is that it relaxes mind and body, relieves pain, and restores body systems to a state of balance in which healing can best take place. It is also most effective when used as a preventive or to alleviate subclinical symptoms before they escalate into disease. The therapy has been shown to be particularly effective in preventing and treating stress and anxiety-related disorders, muscular and rheumatic pains, digestive problems, menstrual irregularities, menopausal complaints, insomnia, and depression.

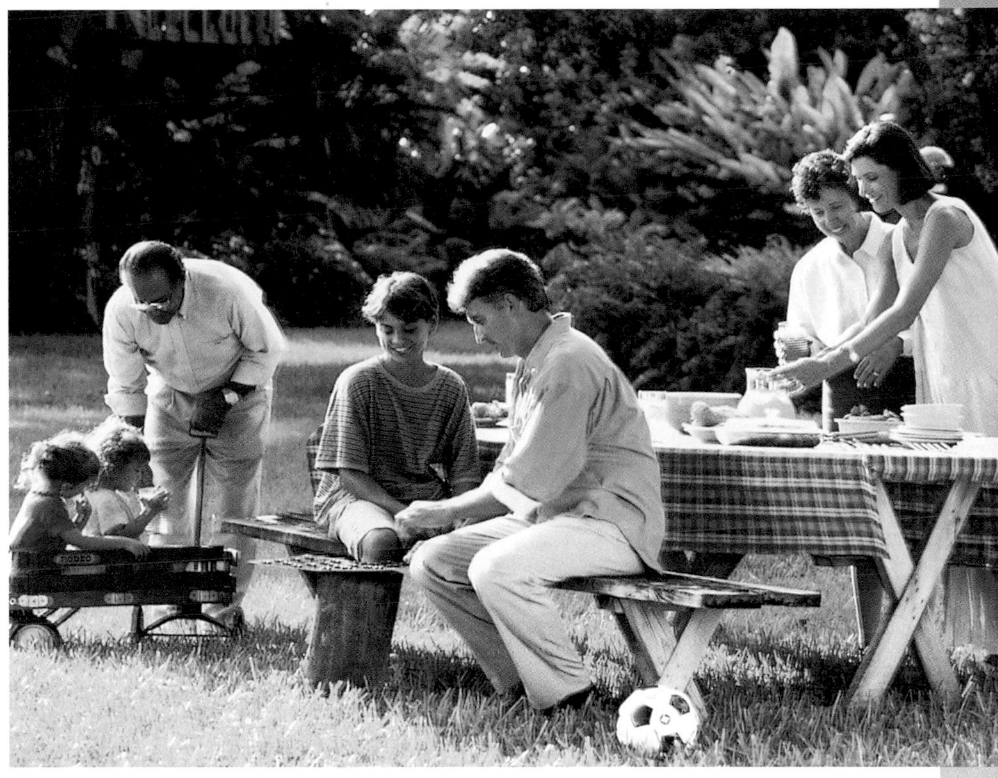

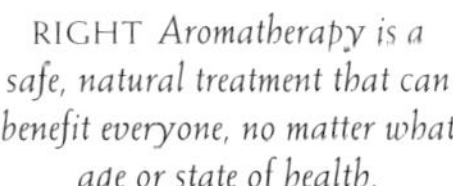

RIGHT *Aromatherapy is a safe, natural treatment that can benefit everyone, no matter what age or state of health.*

ANCIENT ORIGINS OF A MODERN THERAPY

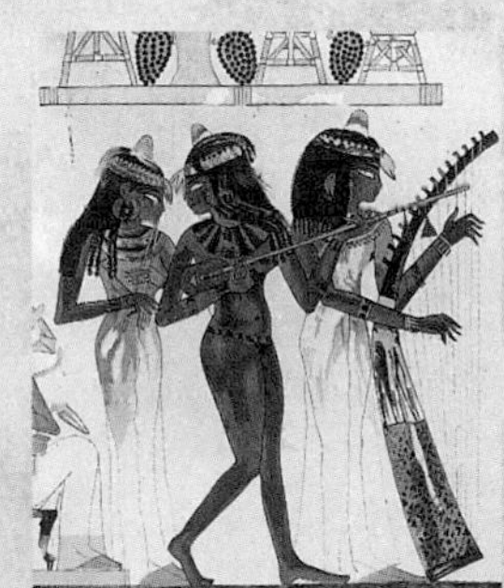

ABOVE *An ancient Egyptian wall painting showing women wearing perfume cones on their heads.*

Aromatic plant oils have been used therapeutically for thousands of years. The ancient Vedic literature of India, and historic Chinese and Arabic medical texts document the importance of aromatic oils for health and spirituality. In ancient Greece, Hippocrates, the "father of medicine," used fragrant fumigations to rid Athens of plague, and Roman soldiers kept up their strength by bathing in scented oil and having regular massages. However, the Egyptians were the most noted of the ancient aromatherapists. Physicians from all over the world are reputed to have traveled to Egypt to learn aromatic techniques.

Aromatherapy is believed to have come west at the time of the Crusades. Historical records show that essential oils were used during the plague in the 14th century. In the 16th and 17th centuries aromatherapy was popular among the great European herbalists. But it was not until the 18th and 19th centuries that scientists were able to identify many of the individual components of plant chemistry.

Research enabled scientists to extract the active components of medicinal plants. Ironically, this led to the development of pharmaceutical drugs and a rejection of plant medicine. However, in the 1920s the devotion of a French chemist, René Maurice Gattefossé, initiated a modest revival in plant oils. Gattefossé discovered that lavender oil quickly healed a burn on his hand, and went on to show that many essential oils were better antiseptics than their synthetic counterparts. He coined the term "aromathérapie" to encapsulate the healing effect of scented oils. Later, a French army surgeon, Dr. Jean Valnet, successfully used essential oils to treat soldiers wounded in battle and patients in a psychiatric hospital. In 1964 Valnet published *Aromathérapie*, still considered by many to be the bible of aromatherapy.

ABOVE *In the Middle Ages exotic essences, introduced into Europe by the Crusaders returning from the East, were used to treat many illnesses.*

In the 1950s Marguérite Maury, an Austrian beauty therapist and biochemist, introduced the concept of using essential oils in massage, and established the first aromatherapy clinics in Britain, France, and Switzerland. From this varied history, aromatherapy has evolved to become one of the most valued of modern complementary therapies.

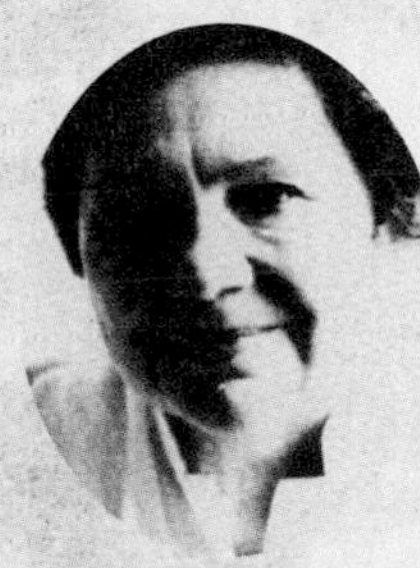

ABOVE *Marguérite Maury used aromatherapy in herbal beauty treatments to revitalize her clients.*

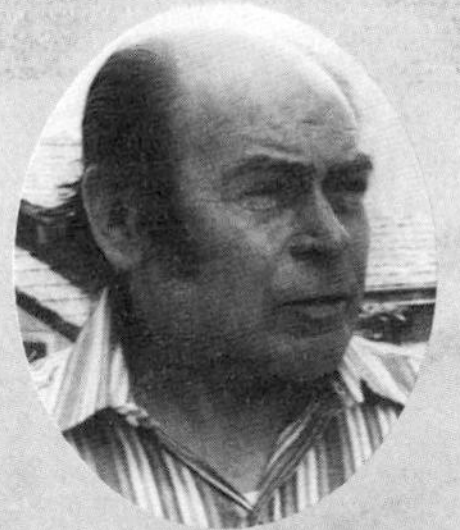

ABOVE *Jean Valnet used essential oils to treat specific medical and psychiatric disorders.*

ESSENTIAL OILS AND HOW THEY WORK

THE CHEMISTRY OF ESSENTIAL OILS

A single essential oil can be made up of many complex chemical components. The dominant characteristic and therapeutic potential of each oil is determined by its major ingredients.

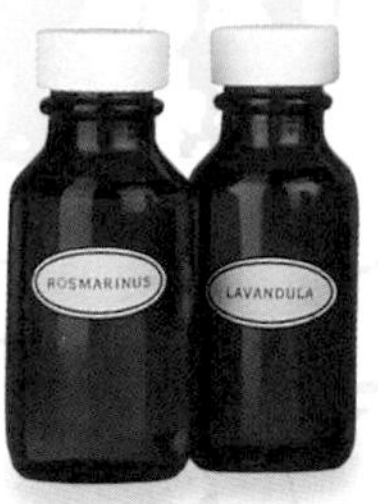

Essential oils should be stored in dark, well-stoppered, glass bottles, away from light and heat in order to maintain their potency.

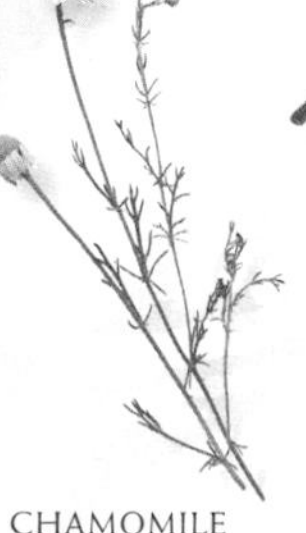

CHAMOMILE *Chamomile has long been appreciated for its calming and soothing properties.*

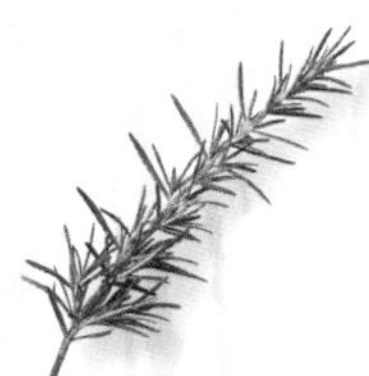

ROSEMARY *The dominant characteristic of rosemary oil is its stimulating effect.*

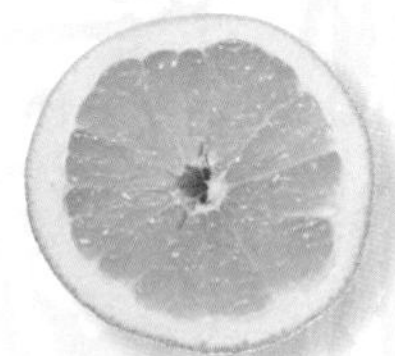

GRAPEFRUIT *Grapefruit oil, which is expressed from the peel of the fruit, refreshes the body and enlivens the mind.*

Essential oils are extracted from the aromatic essences of certain plants, trees, fruit, flowers, herbs, and spices. They are natural volatile oils with identifiable chemical and medicinal properties. Over 150 essential oils have been extracted, each one with its own scent and unique healing properties. Oils are sourced from plants as commonplace as parsley and as exquisite as jasmine. For optimum benefits, essential oils must be extracted from natural raw ingredients and remain as pure as possible.

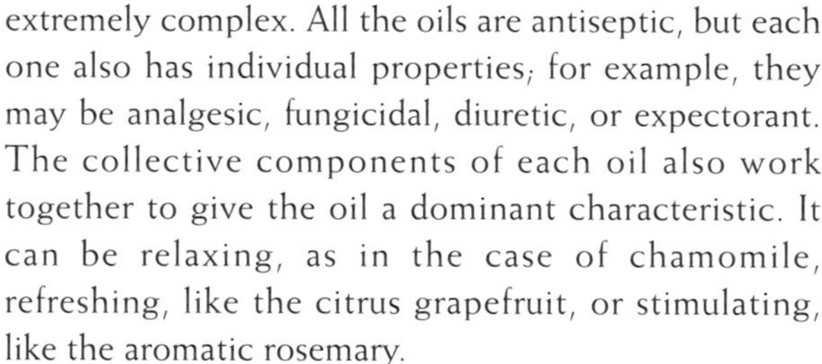

ABOVE *Jasmine, highly valued for its exquisite floral fragrance, is widely used in cosmetics and perfumes.*

ESSENTIAL OILS IN ACTION

Despite considerable research, the chemistry of essential oils is not fully understood. Each oil is composed of at least 100 different chemical constituents, which are classified as aldehydes, phenols, oxides, esters, ketones, alcohols, and terpenes. There may also be many chemical compounds that have yet to be identified. The oils and their actions are extremely complex. All the oils are antiseptic, but each one also has individual properties; for example, they may be analgesic, fungicidal, diuretic, or expectorant. The collective components of each oil also work together to give the oil a dominant characteristic. It can be relaxing, as in the case of chamomile, refreshing, like the citrus grapefruit, or stimulating, like the aromatic rosemary.

Within the body, essential oils are able to operate in three ways: pharmacologically, physiologically, and psychologically. From a pharmacological perspective, the chemical components of the oils react with body chemistry in a way that is similar to drugs, but slower, more sympathetic, and with fewer side-effects. Essential oils also have notable physiological effects. Certain oils have an affinity with particular areas of the body. For example, rose has an affinity with the female reproductive system, while spice oils tend to benefit the digestive system. The oil may also sedate an overactive system, or stimulate a different part of the body that is sluggish.

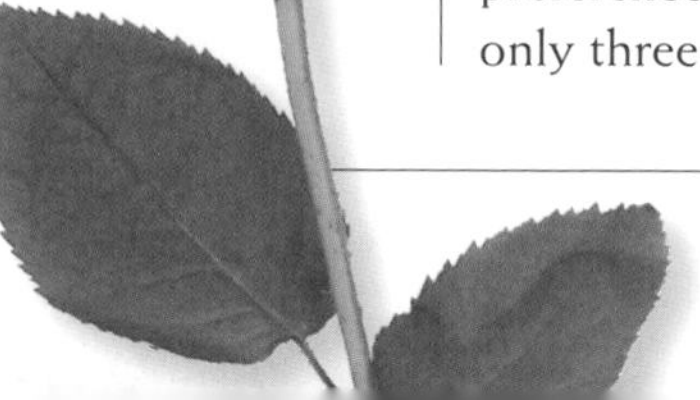

RIGHT *Rose, a perennial favorite as a perfume ingredient and cosmetic oil, also has an affinity with the female reproductive system.*

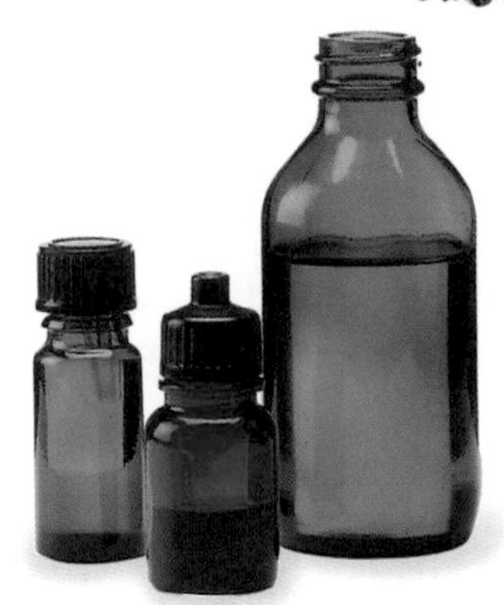

LEFT *Essential oils that share a high proportion of common constituents generally blend well together.*

Some oils, such as lavender, are known as adaptogens, meaning they do whatever the body requires of them at the time. The psychological response is triggered by the effect that the aromatic molecules have on the brain.

Essential oils are not all absorbed into the body at the same rate. They can take 20 minutes or several hours, depending on the oil and the individual body chemistry of the person being treated. On average, absorption takes about 90 minutes. After several hours, the oils leave the body. Most oils are exhaled, others are eliminated in urine, feces, and perspiration.

BLENDING AND USING ESSENTIAL OILS

Essential oils can be used alone or blended together. Oils are blended for two reasons: to create a more sophisticated fragrance, or to enhance or change the medicinal actions of the oils. Blending changes the molecular structure of essential oils, and when they are blended well, therapists can create a "synergistic" blend, where the oils work in harmony and to great effect. To create a blend, the therapist considers not only the symptoms and underlying causes of a patient's particular problem, but also the individual's biological and psychological make-up, and personal fragrance preferences. For therapeutic purposes it is usual to mix only three or four oils together.

ABOVE *Lavender is one of the most versatile essential oils because it responds to the body's particular needs at the time.*

METHODS OF EXTRACTION

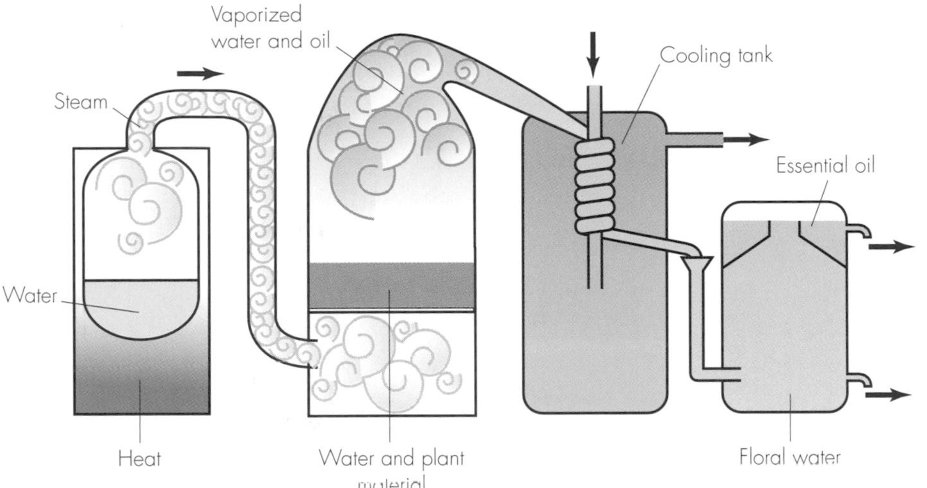

Essential oils are extracted from plants by a simple form of pressure known as expression, or by distillation. Most oils are extracted by steam distillation (*see above*). This involves steaming the parts of the plant to be used in order to break down the walls of the cells that store the essence. The released essence, combined with the steam, passes to cooling tanks, where the steam condenses to a watery liquid, and the essential oil floats on top. The oil is skimmed off and bottled, and the remaining liquid is sometimes used as flower or herbal water.

If you want to blend oils at home, choose two or three oils which you believe complement each other. In general, oils from the same groups (citrus, floral, spicy, etc.), and those which share similar constituents, blend well. Using the proportions detailed overleaf, mix a blend using small amounts of the strongest scented oils and more of the lighter fragrances. You can use the recipes for suggested blends in the remedies section, or create some of your own. Be guided by your own likes and dislikes – the best blend for you is often the one you find most appealing.

CREATING BLENDS

To use oils on the skin, choose a light cold-pressed vegetable oil such as grapeseed, sweet almond, or sunflower oil. For hair treatments choose a more penetrative oil, such as olive oil or jojoba. Where you need a slightly astringent oil, try hazelnut. Add your essential oils to the base oil a little at a time. Shake the bottle well and rub a little on the back of your hand to test the scent. Adjust the quantities until you achieve the blend you want. Add about 5 percent wheat germ oil to preserve the blend. Store blended oils in labeled dark bottles, out of children's reach, and use within three months.

BELOW *Essential oils can be used to treat skin disorders, but they are also appreciated purely for their unique scents.*

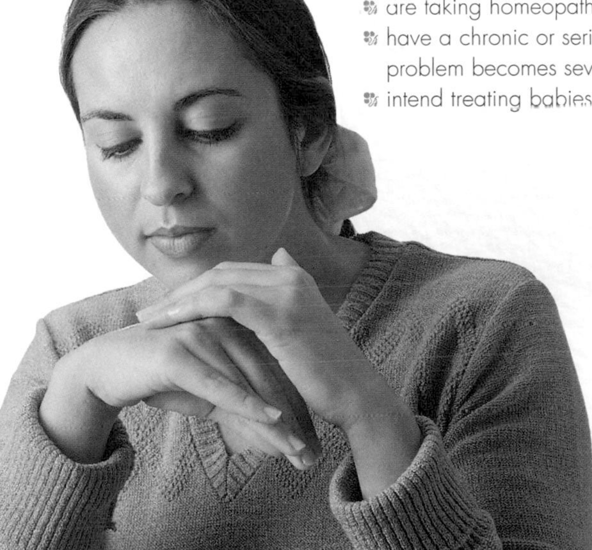

USING ESSENTIAL OILS SAFELY

Aromatherapy is compatible with conventional medicine and most other forms of holistic treatment. However, if you are taking medication consult your physician. Some oils are not compatible with homeopathic treatment. Aromatherapy is safe to use at home for minor or short-term problems, providing you follow certain guidelines.

- Do not take essential oils internally.
- Do not put essential oils in the eyes.
- Keep all oils away from children.
- Do not apply oils undiluted to the skin, unless it is stated that it is safe to do so.

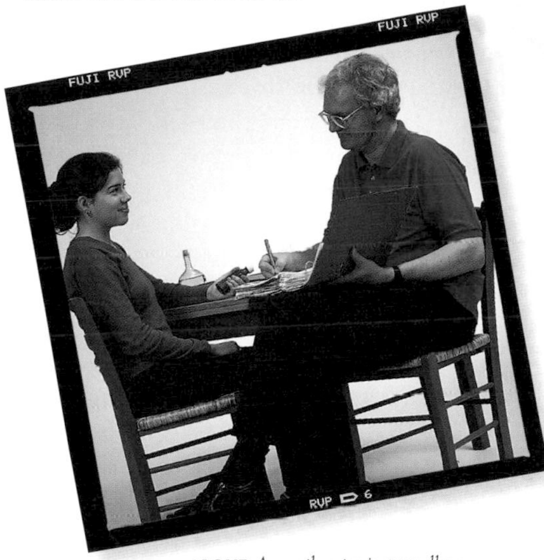

ABOVE *Aromatherapy is generally a safe form of home treatment, but there are certain situations when it is best to consult a qualified practitioner.*

Consult a qualified practitioner for advice and treatment if you:

- are pregnant;
- have an allergy;
- have a chronic medical condition such as high blood pressure or epilepsy;
- are receiving medical or psychiatric treatment;
- are taking homeopathic remedies;
- have a chronic or serious health problem or if a problem becomes severe or persistent;
- intend treating babies or very young children.

AROMATHERAPY TECHNIQUES

There are many ways to use essential oils to good effect. The most common form of treatment among professional aromatherapists is to apply diluted essential oils to the body in a full body massage. But therapists also encourage the use of essential oils at home. When massage is not possible or appropriate, there are many other ways for people to benefit from aromatherapy.

MASSAGE

Massage in itself is nurturing and therapeutic, and the rubbing action releases the fragrance of the oils and ensures that they are well absorbed into the skin. When combined with the medicinal properties of the oils, massage forms a potent healing treatment that can be relaxing or energizing; it can soothe the nervous system, or stimulate the blood and lymphatic systems to improve physical and psychological functioning. It eases pain and tension from tired, taut, or overworked muscles, and lifts the spirits. Whenever possible, try to include massage in your home aromatherapy treatments.

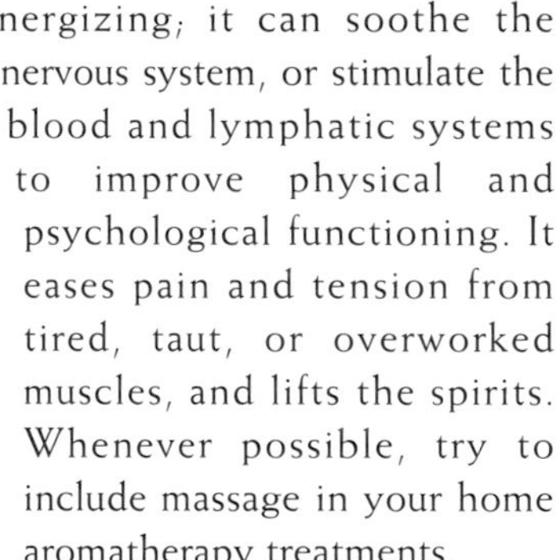
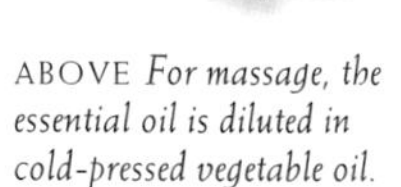

ABOVE *For massage, the essential oil is diluted in cold-pressed vegetable oil.*

❊ BASIC MEASUREMENTS *Dilute the essential oil in a cold-pressed vegetable carrier oil such as grapeseed, sweet almond, or sunflower oil. Use up to 5 drops of essential oil to 1 teaspoon of carrier oil for adults, half that strength for children under seven, and a quarter of the strength for children under three. The only essential oils suitable for babies are chamomile, rose, or lavender. Use only 1 drop to 1 teaspoon of carrier oil.*

BATHS

Aromatic baths are a simple, useful, and versatile way to use essential oils at home. They can be used to enhance moods, relax or stimulate body systems, treat skin disorders, and ease musculoskeletal pain. Essential oils do not dissolve in water, but form a thin film on the surface. The heat of the water releases their vapor and aids absorption into the skin.

❊ BASIC MEASUREMENTS *Fill the bath with warm water before you add the oils. For adults add 5–10 drops of essential oil to a full bath. Use less than 4 drops for children over two, and 1 drop for babies. Stir through the water with your hand.*

RIGHT *When used for skin care, the oils are best added to a cream or lotion.*

FORMS OF TREATMENT

Oils can be used in a variety of ways, depending on individual preferences and the type of ailment being treated.

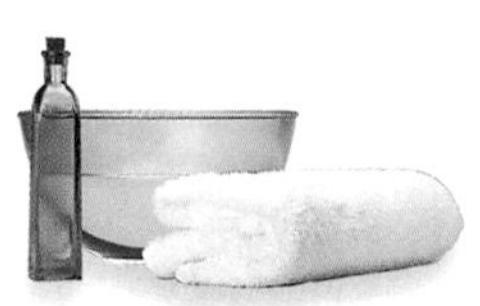

MASSAGE
Massage is one of the most popular and relaxing aromatherapy treatments.

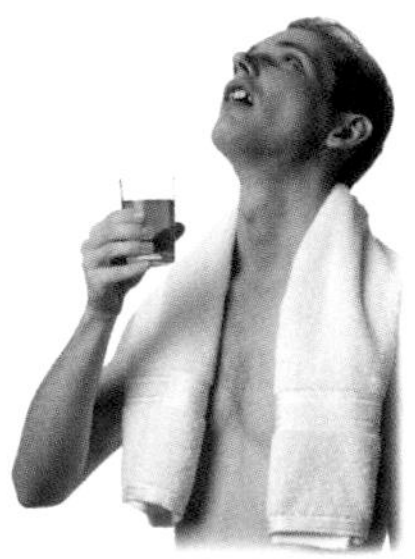

GARGLE
Antiseptic mouthwashes and gargles can be made with essential oils.

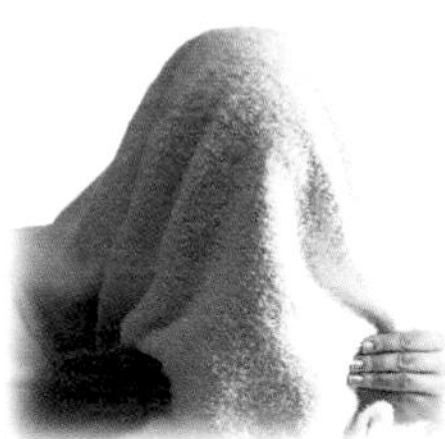

INHALATION
Steam inhalation of essential oils is suitable for sinus, throat, and chest problems.

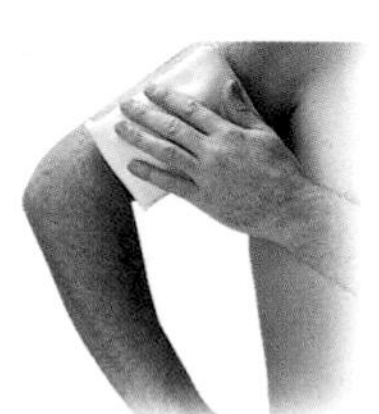

COMPRESS
Oils added to hot and cold compresses offer effective relief from pain and reduce inflammations.

ABOVE *A few drops of oil can be added directly to a bowl of boiling water for a steam inhalation.*

STEAM INHALATIONS

Inhalations are most beneficial for throat and respiratory infections, sinus and catarrhal congestion, and headaches. They are also effective for those oils that could cause irritation if applied to the skin. The steam releases the vapors of the oils. Steam inhalations are not always suitable for asthmatics or people with breathing difficulties, and they are not appropriate for treating children and infants.

❊ BASIC MEASUREMENTS *Add 3–4 drops of oil to a bowl of boiling water. Bend over the bowl, cover your head with a towel, and breathe deeply for a few minutes. You can also use this method as a facial sauna.*

VAPORIZERS

These can be electric, or a ceramic ring that is heated by a light bulb, but most are ceramic pots warmed by a small candle. They are a natural way to scent, deodorize, or disinfect a room, and are one of the best ways to use oils for enhancing mood and balancing the mind. Vaporizers are also useful for when young children have breathing difficulties.

❊ BASIC MEASUREMENTS *Add water and 6–8 drops of oil to the vaporizer. Alternatively, add the oil to a bowl of water and place by a radiator.*

CREAMS, LOTIONS, SHAMPOOS, AND GELS

One of the best ways to use oils for skin care and chronic skin complaints is to add them to a cream or lotion. This is more convenient and less greasy than massage, and it also means the oils can be applied when needed to wounds, bruises, or itchy skin. Adding oils to shampoos helps with everyday hair-care problems, and using essential oils with shower gels is excellent for fatigue and hangovers.

❊ BASIC MEASUREMENTS *Add 1 or 2 drops of essential oil to creams, lotions, and shampoos, and massage into the skin or scalp. Choose unscented products that are lanolin-free and made from good-quality natural ingredients.*

GARGLES AND MOUTHWASHES

Although essential oils should not be swallowed, mouthwashes and gargles are excellent ways to use antiseptic oils to treat mouth ulcers, gum disease, throat infections, and bad breath. These methods are not suitable for children.

❊ BASIC MEASUREMENTS *Dilute 4–5 drops of essential oil in a teaspoon of brandy. Mix into a glass of warm water and swish around the mouth or use as a gargle. Do not swallow.*

HOT AND COLD COMPRESSES

Compresses are an effective way of using essential oils to relieve pain and inflammation. They can be either hot or cold. Hot compresses are good for muscle pain, arthritis, rheumatism, toothache, earache, boils, and abscesses. Cold compresses benefit headaches, sprains, and swelling.

❁ BASIC MEASUREMENTS *Add 4–5 drops of essential oil to a bowl of hot or cold water. Soak a folded clean cotton cloth in the water, wring it out, and apply over the affected area. If using a hot compress, cover with a warm towel and repeat when it cools.*

❁ NEAT: *A few essential oils – such as lavender, tea tree oil, and sandalwood – can be applied undiluted to the skin. Most oils should not be used neat as they can cause irritation.*

❁ **NOTE: These are average safe dilutions for essential oils. In some of the following blends these measurements may vary slightly, but are still within safe guidelines.**

SEEING A PROFESSIONAL

A first appointment with an aromatherapist lasts between 60–90 minutes. It should take place in a warm, comfortable, subtly lit treatment room, containing a massage table, clean towels, and the therapist's stock of oils. The therapist may play soft music to create a relaxing atmosphere.

Every consultation begins with the therapist taking your case history. In order to provide safe, effective, holistic treatment he or she needs to know about your medical history and if you have come with a particular problem. As well as finding out which oils would be best to use, aromatherapists need to know which to avoid. If you are pregnant, have sensitive skin, high blood pressure, epilepsy, or have recently had an operation, some oils would be unsuitable to use. Pregnant women, for example, should avoid certain oils including thyme, basil, rosemary, clary sage, and juniper, because they may harm the fetus or induce miscarriage. The therapist will ask about your stress levels, and if you are using medication or taking homeopathic remedies. It is also important for the aromatherapist to know what sort of mood you are in and what kind of day you have had. This interview takes about 20 minutes and you may be asked to sign a consent form at the end of it.

Treatment usually involves massage. For this you will be asked to undress down to your underwear and lie on the massage table covered with a towel to keep you warm and prevent you from feeling exposed. The aromatherapist will move the towel as he or she works around your body, but will not remove it completely.

The therapist uses the information you have provided when deciding on a suitable blend of oils. Generally, the oils you like best are the ones that work best for you. Using the chosen blend the aromatherapist will begin your massage using gentle massage strokes and may also work on pressure points of the body. During the 30–45 minutes that it takes to give a full body massage the therapist will talk very little if at all, allowing you to relax completely.

At the end of your massage, you may be advised not to bathe or shower for several hours so that the oils can be fully absorbed. The therapist may conclude the visit by giving you oils to use at home.

AROMATHERAPY MASSAGE

The techniques of massage as we know it today in the West were developed in the nineteenth century by a Swedish professor, Pier Heidrich Ling, and his work is the basis for massage treatment today. Different strokes are appropriate to different areas of the body. Gentle strokes are used to commence a session to relax the superficial muscles, and more vigorous strokes then stimulate the deeper muscles.

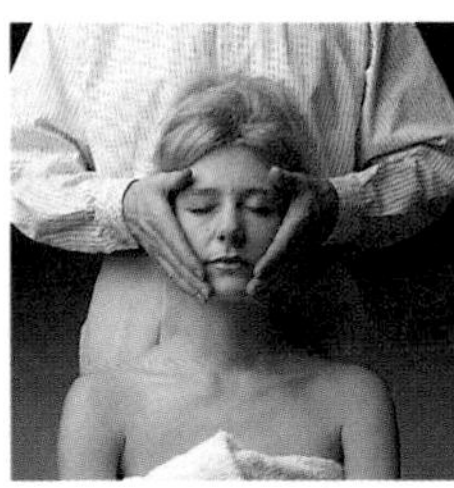

EFFLEURAGE

Effleurage is designed to sensitize your partner and prepare for the later strokes. It is particularly effective for the face. Place your hands on your partner's cheeks, fingers downward. Then stroke gently toward the ears, using the minimum pressure required to maintain contact. You can use this sliding stroke to massage the whole body if you vary the pressure and speed.

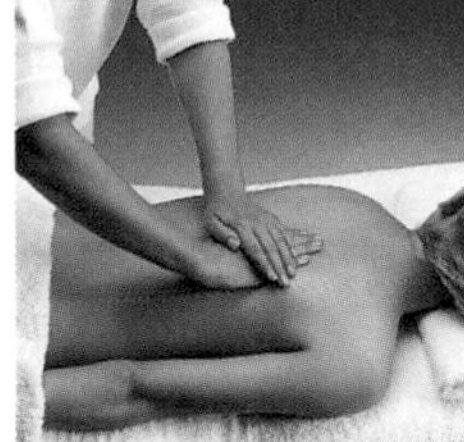

CIRCLING

Place both hands on your partner, a few inches apart, and stroke in a wide circular movement. Press into the upward stroke and glide back down. Your arms will cross as you make the circle, so just lift one hand over the other to continue. Circle lightly in a clockwise direction over the stomach to aid digestion.

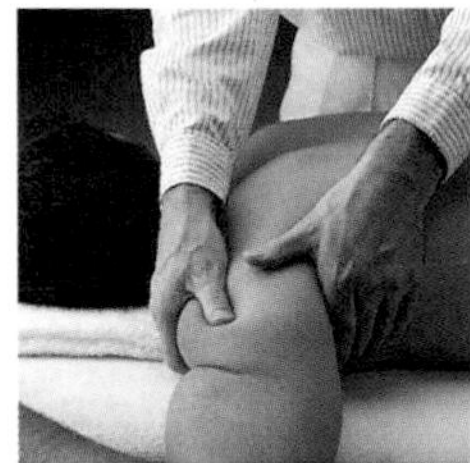

KNEADING

Place both hands on the area to be massaged with your fingers pointing away from you. Press into the body with the palm of one hand, pick up the flesh between your thumb and fingers, and press it toward the resting hand. Release and repeat with the other hand, as if you were kneading dough.

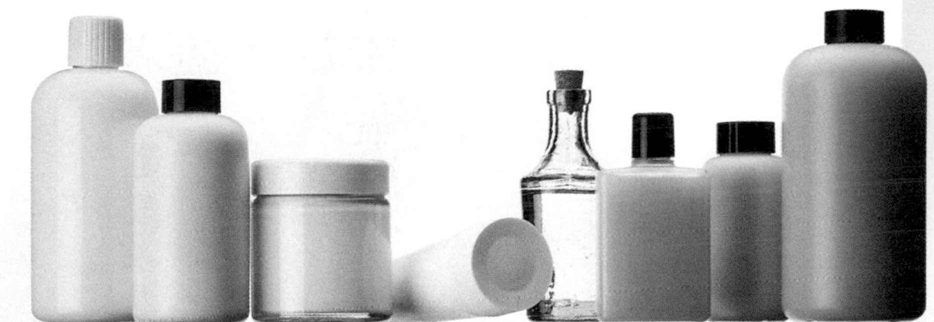

BELOW *The essential oils used for massage are always diluted in a carrier oil or lotion.*

ESSENTIAL OILS

Angelica archangelica

ANGELICA

The healing properties of angelica were so revered in antiquity that it was called the root of the Holy Spirit. There are over 30 varieties of angelica grown around the world; at least 10 are highly valued in Traditional Chinese Medicine. Angelica root and the seeds are used to produce the essential oil, which has a musky, sweet, woody scent.

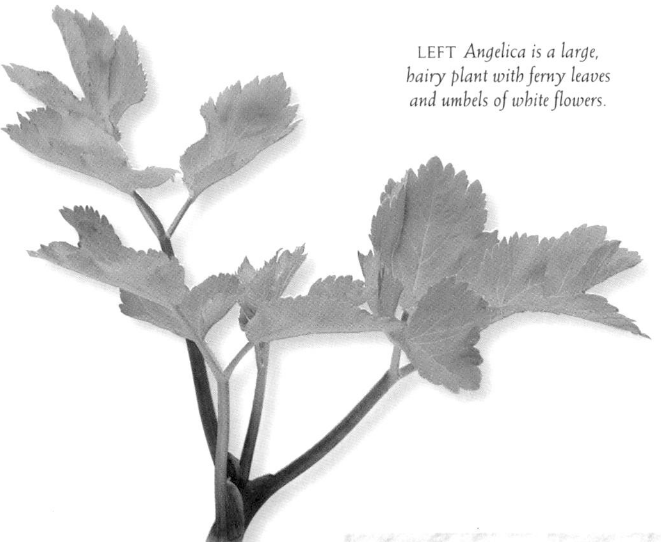

LEFT *Angelica is a large, hairy plant with ferny leaves and umbels of white flowers.*

DATA FILE

Properties and Uses

Angelica is a tonic and stimulant that seems to strengthen the immune system. Detoxifying and diuretic properties stimulate the circulation and lymphatic systems to eliminate toxins from the body, making it useful for cellulite, arthritis, and fluid retention. It relieves indigestion and flatulence, and alleviates digestive problems caused by stress. Angelica's expectorant properties are beneficial in treating colds, bronchitis, and respiratory infections. It is good for dull, congested, or irritated skin. Angelica is also believed to have an affinity with the female reproductive system.

CAUTION

DO NOT USE DURING PREGNANCY OR IF YOU ARE A DIABETIC.

DO NOT USE ON SKIN EXPOSED TO SUNLIGHT.

ANGELICA OIL ATTRACTS INSECTS.

RECIPE

Angelica Travel Oil

Add 5 drops angelica, 5 drops melissa, 5 drops peppermint, and 5 drops ginger to a small dropper bottle containing 1fl.oz. (30ml.) of sweet almond oil. Inhale or massage a few drops into the temples or around the back of the neck to relieve jet lag or headaches. A few drops massaged in a clockwise direction around the abdomen can ease stomachache.

INFORMATION

BLENDS WELL WITH CLARY SAGE, PATCHOULI, SANDALWOOD, VETIVER, BENZOIN, LEMON, AND OTHER CITRUS OILS.

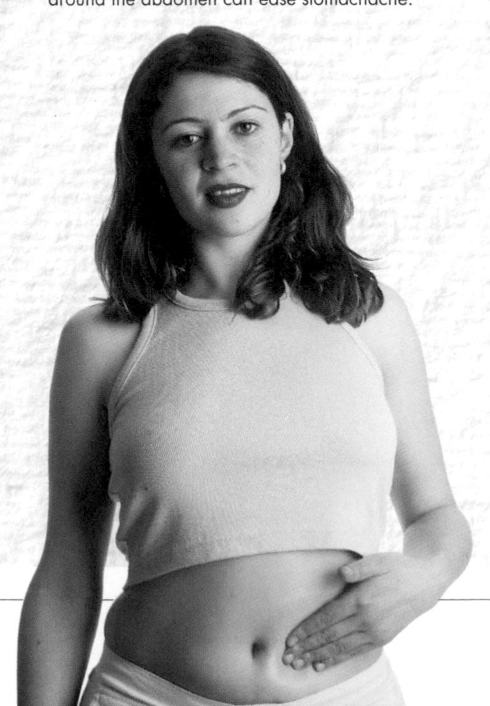

RIGHT *A few drops of blended angelica oil massaged around the abdomen soothes stomachache.*

Apium graveolens

CELERY SEED

Best known as a salad vegetable in Europe, celery is grown in India, China, the Netherlands, and Hungary for its essential oil. Celery seeds are crushed to produce the warm, spicy, scented essential oil. Celery has been valued throughout history for its use as a diuretic and a digestive aid.

RECIPE

Detoxifying Massage Blend

Add 4 drops celery, 3 drops juniper, 3 drops lemon to 4 teaspoons (20ml.) grapeseed oil, and use for a full body massage.

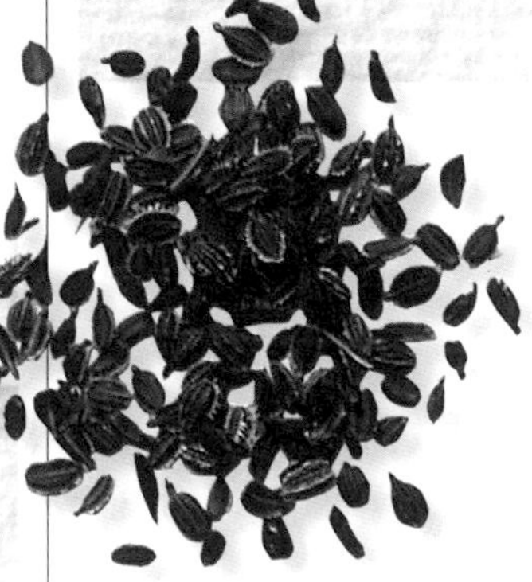

ABOVE *and* BELOW *Celery is a popular salad vegetable, and the seeds are widely used as a cooking spice.*

THERAPY CONNECTIONS

ANGELICA
Ayurveda p.28
Chinese Herbal Medicine p.55
Herbalism p.115

CELERY
Ayurveda p.29
Traditional Home and Folk Remedies p.83

INFORMATION

BLENDS WELL WITH LEMON, PEPPERMINT, JUNIPER, FENNEL, LAVENDER, BERGAMOT, PINE, TEA TREE, CINNAMON, AND OTHER SPICE OILS.

CAUTION

DO NOT USE DURING PREGNANCY.

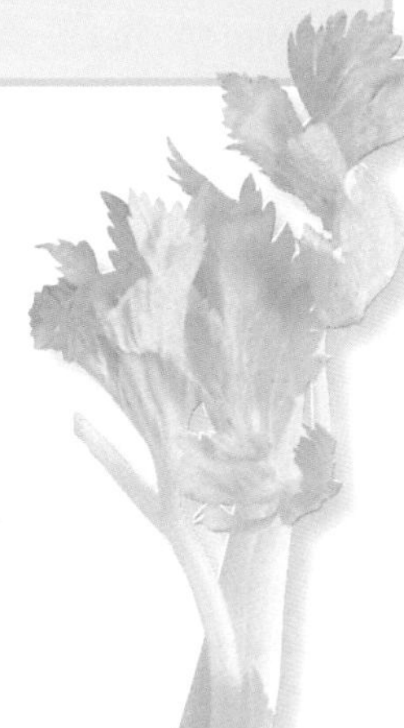

Aniba rosaeodora

ROSEWOOD

Most rosewood oil comes from Brazil, where it is distilled from the heartwood of the rosewood tree. Although distillation from wild trees contributes to the destruction of the rainforest, cultivated trees are also used in the production of rosewood essential oil. But for the sake of preserving the rainforests, it may be best to keep this oil, with its subtle woody floral fragrance, for special occasions, or for when no other oil is suitable.

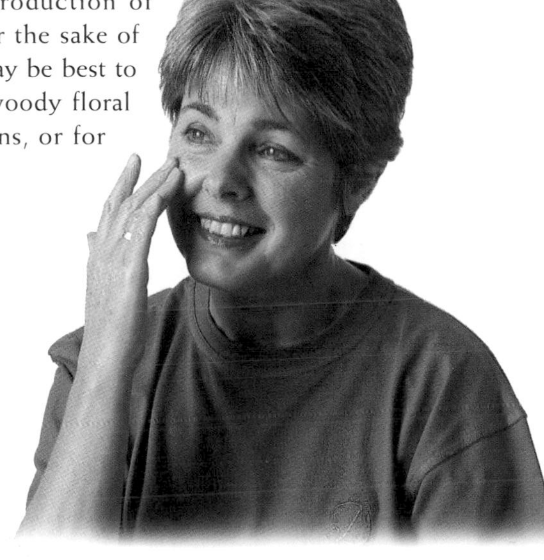

BELOW *Rosewood is especially beneficial for skin care.*

DATA FILE

Properties and Uses

Rosewood is a tonic and an immune stimulant, useful for infections or viruses such as colds or glandular fever. It can be used as a mild painkiller, an antidepressant, and an aphrodisiac. As a tissue regenerator it diminishes scars, wrinkles, and stretch marks. Because it is such a gentle oil rosewood benefits sensitive or irritated skin, and its antiseptic and bactericidal properties make it suitable for acne and wounds. The oil is also used to treat coughs and headaches, especially when accompanied by nausea. Rosewood is an emotionally uplifting and comforting oil that helps to rebalance the nervous system in times of stress. Rosewood is nonirritant nontoxic and nonsensitizing.

RECIPE

Replenishing Skin Care Oil

Pour 4 teaspoons sweet almond oil into a small, dark glass bottle. Add 4 drops rosewood, 3 drops sandalwood, 3 drops frankincense. Seal and shake well. Smooth over face, neck, and dry skin patches, using gentle circular movements.

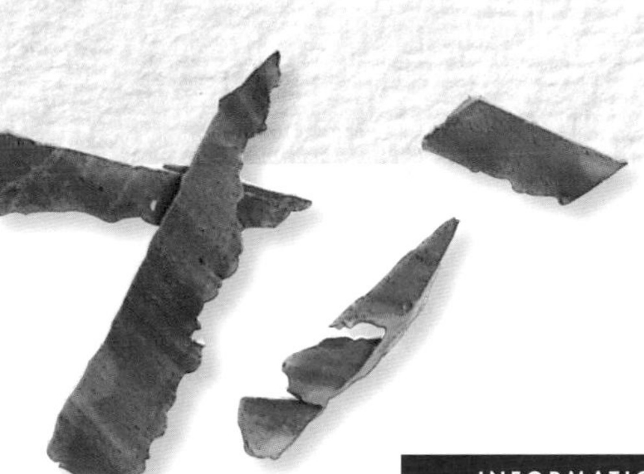

ABOVE *Rosewood oil is extracted by steam distillation from the wood chippings*

INFORMATION

BLENDS WELL WITH LAVENDER, SANDALWOOD, FRANKINCENSE, BASIL, PATCHOULI, CEDARWOOD, AND MOST WOODY, CITRUS, AND FLORAL OILS.

Boswellia carteri

FRANKINCENSE

Frankincense, also known as olibanum, is distilled from the resin produced by the bark of a small North African tree. Wonderfully calming and richly fragrant, the oil has a history of use as a fumigant, in embalming, and as incense. It is considered a spiritual oil, used by many to encourage meditation.

DATA FILE

Properties and Uses

Frankincense slows the breathing, and calms the nervous and digestive systems, relieving anxiety, depression, nervous tension, emotional upsets, and stress-related digestive problems. As an immune stimulant and an expectorant it can help respiratory and catarrhal conditions such as asthma, colds, chest infections, and chronic bronchitis. Frankincense has wound-healing, astringent, antiseptic, and anti-inflammatory properties, making it ideal for treating cuts, scars, blemishes, and inflammation, and it is recommended for firming aging skin. Frankincense is helpful for cystitis, as it has an affinity with the genitourinary system. Irregular or heavy menstrual bleeding and nosebleeds can also benefit from its gentle healing properties.

CAUTION

SAFE TO USE DURING PREGNANCY.

DO NOT TAKE IT INTERNALLY AND KEEP IT OUT OF CHILDREN'S REACH

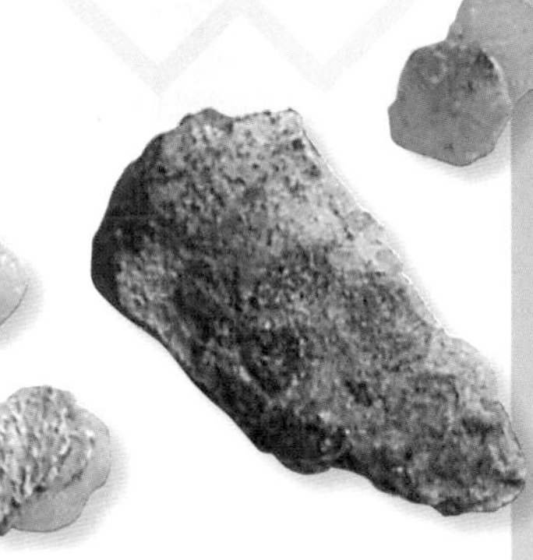

ABOVE *The gum resin used to make frankincense oozes out from the tree as a milky-white liquid and then solidifies into tear-shaped, amber to orange-brown lumps.*

INFORMATION

BLENDS WELL WITH ROSE, LAVENDER, GERANIUM, NEROLI, ORANGE, BERGAMOT, MANDARIN, SANDALWOOD, PINE, BLACK PEPPER, CINNAMON, AND OTHER SPICE OILS.

RECIPE

Inhalation for Dry Coughs

Add 2 drops frankincense, 2 drops lavender, 2 drops cypress to a bowl of steaming hot water. Lean over the bowl, cover your head with a towel, and inhale the aroma for 5–10 minutes.

Calendula officinalis

MARIGOLD

Calendula essential oil is not widely available, as the bright orange flowers of the common pot marigold yield only small amounts of oil. More common is infused oil of calendula, where the flowers are infused in warm oil, macerated, and strained. Marigold has had a variety of historical uses, treating anything from snake bites to toothache. The famous herbalists Nicholas Culpeper and John Gerard called the flower a "comforter of the heart and spirits."

CAUTION

DO NOT CONFUSE WITH AFRICAN MARIGOLD (TAGETES), WHICH IS TOXIC.

INFORMATION

BLENDS WELL WITH MOST FLORAL AND CITRUS OILS.

DATA FILE

Properties and Uses

As a soothing anti-inflammatory, antiseptic, and gentle astringent, calendula-infused oil is good for dry, cracked, or chapped skin, eczema, diaper rash, cracked nipples, and varicose veins. Because it helps to stop bleeding and has valuable wound-healing properties, it is a first-aid kit essential for cuts, grazes, wounds, and insect bites. Calendula has an affinity with the female reproductive system and has properties which help to regulate the menstrual cycle. The oil can also be used as a base for blending other essential oils.

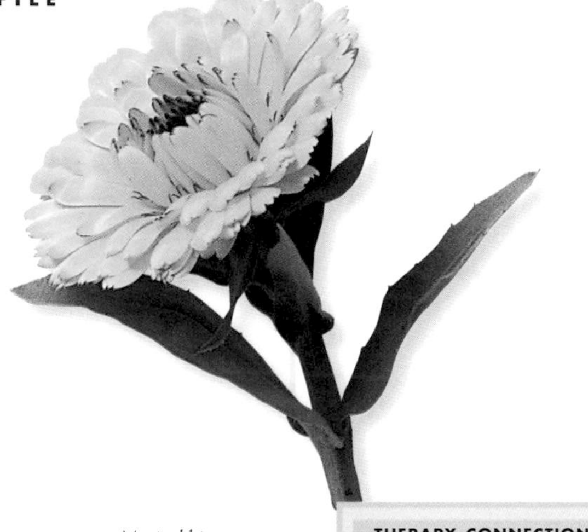

ABOVE *Marigold is an annual herb with bright orange, daisylike flowers; it has become naturalized throughout temperate regions of the world.*

THERAPY CONNECTIONS

MARIGOLD

Herbalism p.117

Homeopathy p.187

RECIPE

Calendula Cream

To make a soothing skin cream, add calendula oil drop by drop to any ready-made unperfumed pure plant cream, and blend thoroughly. Stop adding the oil when the cream reaches a soft usable consistency. Do not worry about adding too much calendula oil. Pure plant creams are often available from the suppliers of essential oils.

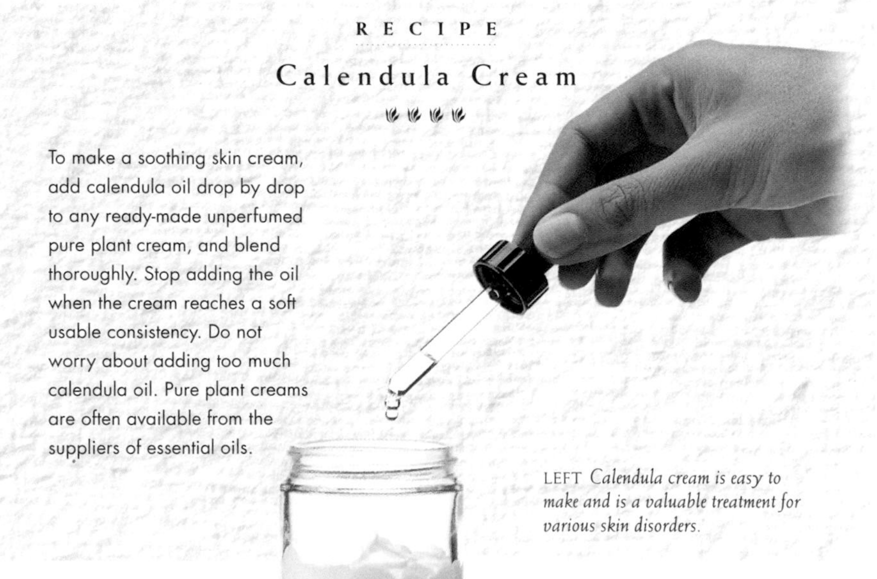

LEFT *Calendula cream is easy to make and is a valuable treatment for various skin disorders.*

Cananga odorata var. genuina

YLANG YLANG

This is extracted from a tropical tree that grows in the Philippines, Indonesia, the Comoros, and Madagascar. The name ylang ylang means "flower of flowers." The name suits the heady floral fragrance of this oil, which is distilled from the freshly picked flowers. Ylang ylang is a traditional tropical remedy for infections and skin diseases, but is also well known for its use in the Victorian hair preparation, Macassar oil.

DATA FILE

Properties and Uses

Ylang ylang is a sedative, an antidepressant, and a tonic for the nervous system. Depression, anxiety, tension, irritability, and stress-related insomnia can all benefit from its soothing properties. It helps to rebalance sebum production in oily skin, acne, and both dry and greasy scalps. It can also be used to calm irritated skin, as well as bites and stings. Ylang ylang is reputed to be an aphrodisiac. It can be used to treat sexual problems. It acts as a circulatory tonic and generally rebalances body functions. It can help to reduce blood pressure, and slow breathing and heart rate in cases of shock, panic, or rage.

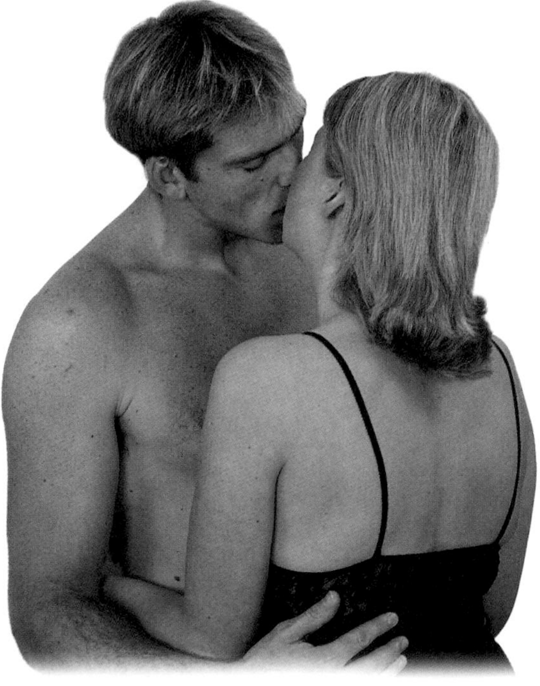

ABOVE *Ylang ylang is highly regarded as an aphrodisiac. In Indonesia, the ylang ylang flowers are spread out on the marriage bed of the bride and groom.*

RECIPE

Bath Blend for Nervous Tension

Add 3 drops ylang ylang, 2 drops rosewood, 3 drops lavender to 1½ teaspoons (8ml.) of a dispersible bath oil such as red turkey oil, and add to a warm bath, or drip the oils directly into the bath water and disperse with your hand. Relax in the bath for 10 minutes.

INFORMATION

BLENDS WELL WITH ROSEWOOD, ROSE, BERGAMOT, VETIVER, FRANKINCENSE, CHAMOMILE, LAVENDER, CEDARWOOD.

CAUTION

CAN CAUSE NAUSEA OR HEADACHES IN HIGH CONCENTRATIONS.

MAY IRRITATE SOME HYPERSENSITIVE PEOPLE.

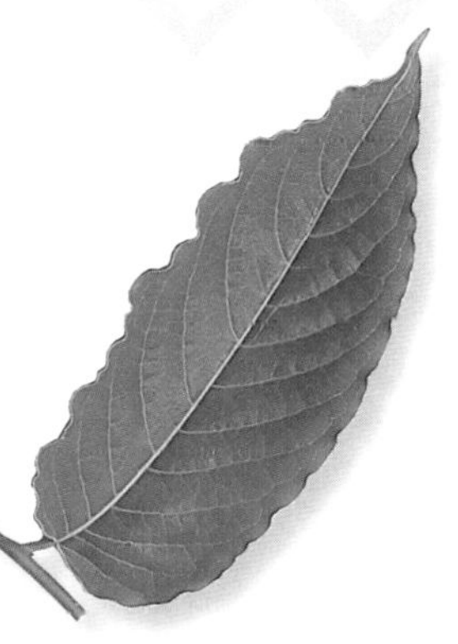

ABOVE *Leaves from the tropical ylang ylang tree.*

Cedrus atlantica

CEDARWOOD

The aromatic oil from the evergreen cedar tree was one of the first oils to be used in ancient medicine and ritual. Used by the ancient Egyptians for embalming, and by the people of the Middle East since biblical times, the wood still provides Tibetan monks with incense, burnt to aid meditation. Cedarwood oil is extracted by steam distillation from the wood chips. It has a rich, woody, masculine scent that is warming, physically cleansing, and emotionally grounding.

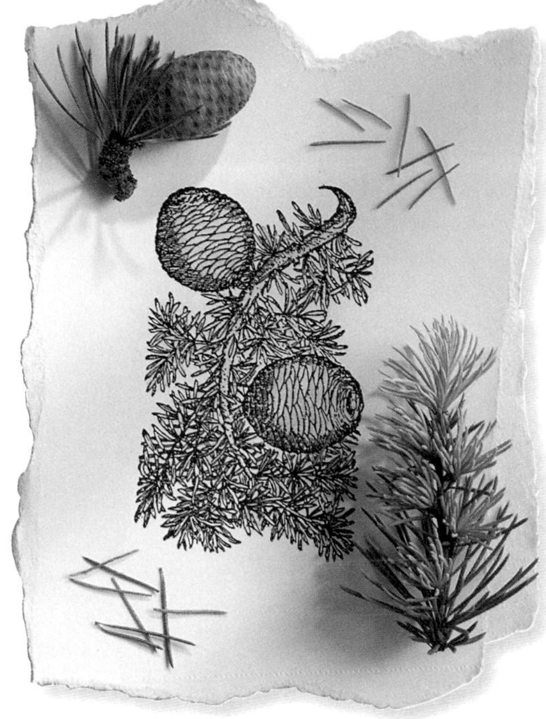

ABOVE *Cedar is a pyramid-shaped evergreen tree, up to 130 ft. (40m.) high. Its strongly aromatic wood contains a high percentage of essential oil.*

DATA FILE

Properties and Uses

The antiseptic, anti-seborrheic, and mild astringent properties of cedarwood make it a popular choice for treating acne, oily skin eruptions, and dandruff. It has diuretic properties which benefit the urinary system and help to relieve cystitis, and it is also used for vaginal infections and discharges. Cedarwood is an expectorant and mucolytic, which explains its traditional use in the treatment of catarrhal problems, especially bronchial congestion and infections. The oil is also valued for its ability both to stimulate the circulation and relax the nervous system, while having a tonic effect on the whole body.

On an emotional level, cedarwood can dispel gloomy or scattered thoughts, anxiety, obsessions, and fears.

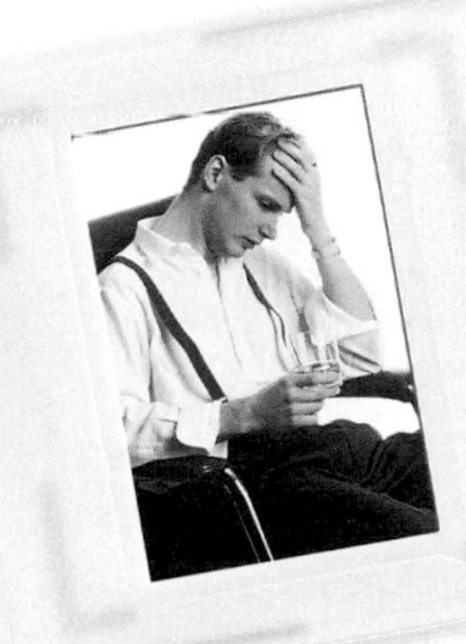

BELOW *Cedarwood oil helps to relieve nervous tension and stress-related conditions.*

CAUTION

DO NOT USE DURING PREGNANCY.

SEVERAL VARIETIES OF CEDAR TREES ARE USED TO PRODUCE OIL THAT IS SOLD AS CEDARWOOD. SOME OF THIS OIL IS VERY DIFFERENT FROM *CEDRUS ATLANTICA*. ALWAYS MAKE SURE YOU BUY ATLAS CEDARWOOD OIL.

INFORMATION

BLENDS WELL WITH NEROLI, JASMINE, JUNIPER, CHAMOMILE, GERANIUM, LAVENDER, FRANKINCENSE, ROSEMARY, YLANG YLANG, ROSEWOOD, VETIVER.

RECIPE

Antidandruff Treatment

Add 6 drops cedarwood, 6 drops rosemary, 4 drops cypress oil to 1½fl. oz. (50ml.) olive oil. Massage into the scalp with your fingertips, cover, and leave overnight, if possible. Shampoo thoroughly. Use half the recipe for children.

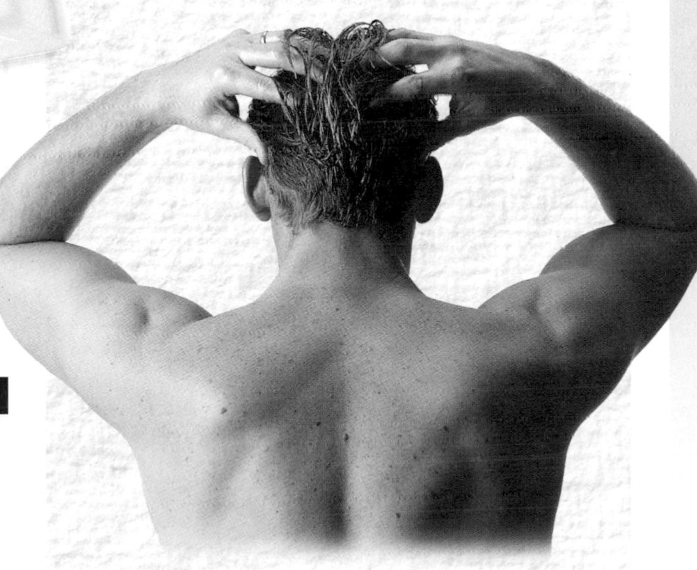

RIGHT *Cedarwood oil is used to treat dandruff.*

Chamaemelum nobile

ROMAN CHAMOMILE

Chamomile has a long history of use as a physical and emotional soother. It is one of the most gentle essential oils available, and particularly suitable for treating children. Massage can soothe fretful or colicky babies, and the diluted oil can be rubbed into the cheek to relieve teething pain. Of the many varieties of chamomile available, Roman chamomile is one of the most commonly used in aromatherapy.

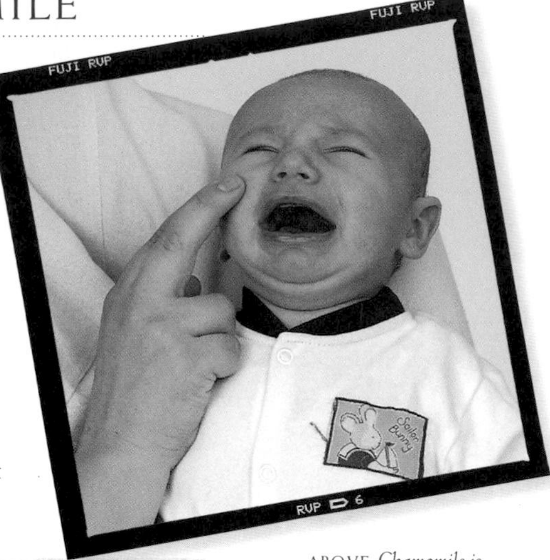

ABOVE *Chamomile is suitable for treating children and infants.*

RECIPE

Chamomile Compress

Fill a bowl with ice-cold or hot water and add 4–5 drops of chamomile oil. Soak a clean face cloth or folded piece of clean cotton in the bowl, and wring it out. Apply the compress to the affected area until it has cooled or warmed to body temperature. Repeat. Note: Use a cold compress for rashes, cuts, headaches, sprains, or swellings; a hot ompress for arthritic or rheumatic pain, boils, abscesses, earache, or toothache.

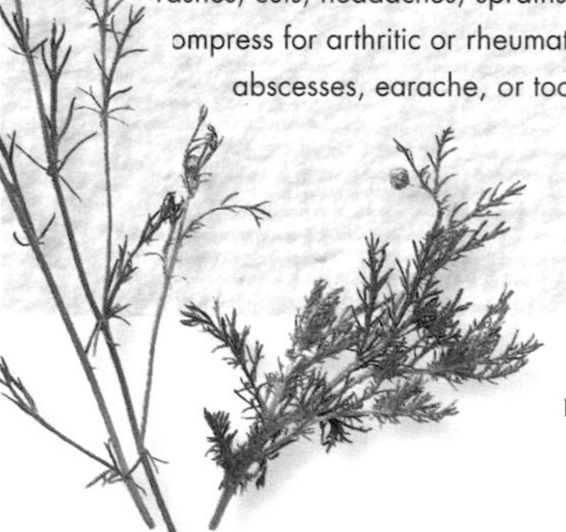

LEFT *Chamomile is a small perennial herb with daisy-like white flowers and feathery pennate leaves.*

CAUTION

DO NOT USE IN THE FIRST THREE MONTHS OF PREGNANCY.

DO NOT ALLOW CHAMOMILE ESSENTIAL OIL TO GET INTO THE EYES.

CAN CAUSE DERMATITIS IN SOME PEOPLE.

GERMAN CHAMOMILE MAY BE USED INSTEAD OF ROMAN CHAMOMILE, BUT NOT CHAMOMILE *MAROC ORMENIS MULTICAULIS*, WHICH IS NOT TRUE CHAMOMILE.

INFORMATION

BLENDS WELL WITH LAVENDER, GERANIUM, BERGAMOT, JASMINE, ROSE, NEROLI, CLARY SAGE, SANDALWOOD, MANDARIN.

DATA FILE

Properties and Uses

Chamomile calms the nervous system and induces sleep. It has valuable anti-inflammatory, antiseptic, and bactericidal properties. Chamomile prevents and eases spasms, relieves pain, settles digestion, and acts as a liver tonic. It can be used to relieve headaches, toothache, menstrual cramps, arthritis, and neuralgia. Indigestion, nausea, and flatulence can also benefit, and all manner of skin problems such as rashes, inflammation, cuts, boils, allergies, insect bites, and chilblains can be helped by a chamomile compress or bath. It also has a balancing effect on the menstrual cycle, reduces fluid retention, and acts as a gentle antidepressant and stress reliever. Chamomile also helps to reduce fever.

Cinnamomum zeylanicum

CINNAMON LEAF

Cinnamon is grown in India, Sri Lanka, Madagascar, the Comoros, and the Seychelles, but the best cinnamon oil is believed to come from Madagascar. Cinnamon was used by the Greeks, Romans, and ancient Egyptians, and its medicinal properties have long been valued by the people of India and China. The familiar warm, spicy fragrance is also reputed to enhance psychic ability.

RECIPE

Cinnamon Room Freshener

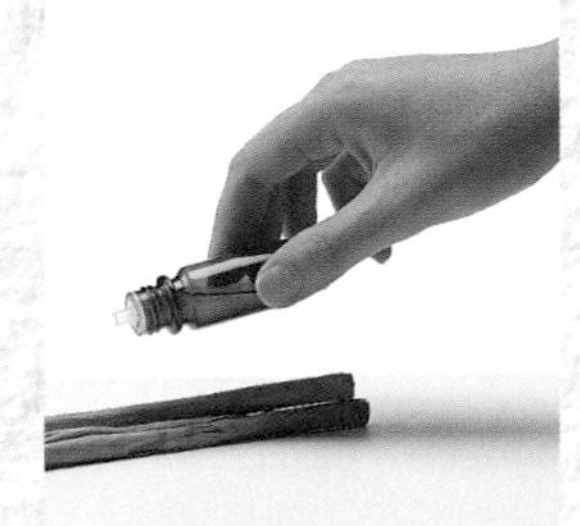

Sprinkle a few drops on rolled cinnamon sticks and add to potpourri made from dried orange peel, orange oil, and basil for a room freshener that stimulates and refreshes the mind, relieves tension, and soothes the nerves.

CAUTION

CINNAMON LEAF OIL MAY CAUSE SKIN IRRITATION.

USE ONLY IN A 1 PER CENT DILUTION, AND IN MODERATION.

DO NOT CONFUSE WITH CINNAMON BARK OIL, WHICH IS AN IRRITANT AND SHOULD NOT BE USED IN AROMATHERAPY.

INFORMATION

BLENDS WELL WITH YLANG YLANG, FRANKINCENSE, ORANGE, BENZOIN, MANDARIN, LEMON, BASIL, MYRRH, LAVENDER, GINGER.

BELOW *The inner bark of the new shoots of the cinnamon tree is gathered every two years and sold in the form of cinnamon sticks.*

DATA FILE

Properties and Uses

Cinnamon stimulates a sluggish digestion, relieves flatulence and spasms, and combats intestinal infection. It acts as a respiratory and circulatory stimulant, helping with rheumatic problems and chest infections. It helps to fortify the immune system against chills and infections, and has a cooling effect on fevers. Cinnamon also has antiseptic, antimicrobial, and parasiticidal properties, making it good for head lice, scabies, and other skin infections. Cinnamon can relieve mental fatigue, improve poor concentration and nervous exhaustion, and help to lift depression.

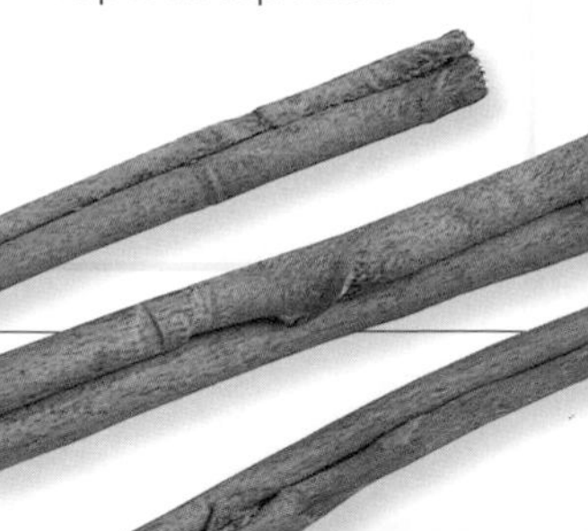

Citrus aurantifolia

LIME

Limes were traditionally used as a digestive remedy and to prevent scurvy among sailors. Lime has a fairly wide application in modern aromatherapy. It has properties similar to those of lemon, and the two oils are often used interchangeably. The essential oil is expressed from the peel of the fruit, or steam-distilled from the whole fruit.

DATA FILE

Properties and Uses

Lime acts as an appetite and digestive stimulant, and also helps to treat the symptoms of dyspepsia. Its antiseptic, anti-viral, bactericidal, and fever-reducing properties make it valuable in fighting colds, flu, fever, and chest and throat infections. It also helps to strengthen the immune system. Oily skin and conditions such as acne, boils, and warts can also benefit from these properties. Lime has a restorative, tonic effect on the whole person. It also has notable anti-rheumatic properties, and is known to increase mental alertness and assertiveness.

RECIPE

Stay-alert Diffuser Blend

Fill the dish of a pottery burner with water and add 4 drops lime, 2 drops black pepper, 2 drops peppermint. Light the night light and let the heat diffuse the oil into the air.

CAUTION

LIME INCREASES THE SKIN'S SENSITIVITY TO SUNLIGHT. DO NOT APPLY TO THE SKIN WITHIN TWO DAYS OF EXPOSURE TO SUNLIGHT

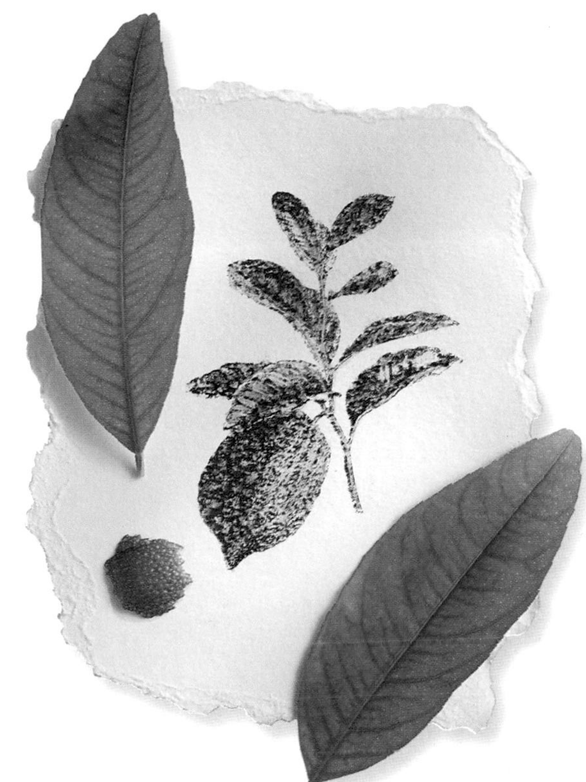

ABOVE *Lime is a small evergreen tree, up to 15 ft. (4.5 m.) tall, with stiff, sharp spines, smooth ovate leaves, and small white flowers. The pale green fruit is about the size of a lemon.*

INFORMATION

BLENDS WELL WITH LAVENDER, ROSEMARY, CLARY SAGE, BLACK PEPPER, BERGAMOT, AND OTHER CITRUS OILS.

Citrus aurantium var. amara, Citrus sinensis

ORANGE

Originally from China, oranges have a history of use in Traditional Chinese Medicine. Dried sweet orange is used to treat coughs and colds, while bitter orange is used to treat diarrhea. The outer peel of both bitter and sweet oranges is pressed to produce the sweet, fruity orange essential oil.

CAUTION

ORANGE OIL CAN INCREASE SKIN SENSITIVITY TO THE SUN.

MAY CAUSE CONTACT DERMATITIS IN SOME PEOPLE.

DO NOT USE MORE THAN FOUR DROPS IN THE BATH.

RECIPE

Massage Blend for Constipation

Mix 3 drops orange, 3 drops black pepper, 4 drops rosemary, 3 teaspoons (15ml.) sweet almond or grapeseed oil. Warm a little oil in the hands; massage into the abdomen clockwise.

BELOW *Both bitter and sweet orange trees are evergreen, but the sweet variety, shown here, is more hardy. Sweet oranges are larger and lighter in color than bitter oranges.*

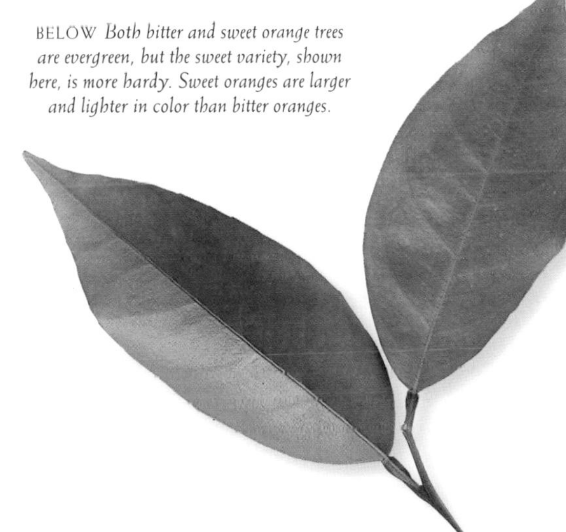

DATA FILE

Properties and Uses

As a sedative orange is good for nervous tension and related insomnia, either blended with lavender, or alternated with lavender or sandalwood. It is also a cheering oil, which enlivens the mind and dispels depression. Orange has a normalizing effect on intestinal peristalsis, making it beneficial for painful spasms, constipation, and diarrhea. It also helps to normalize blood pressure and circulation, and stimulates the lymphatic system to relieve water retention. Orange helps to fight chills, bronchitis, colds, and flu, especially when mixed with complementary winter spice oils such as cinnamon and clove.

THERAPY CONNECTIONS

CHAMOMILE
Herbalism p.119
Homeopathy p.204

CINNAMON
Ayurveda p.34
Chinese Herbal Medicine p.59

INFORMATION

BLENDS WELL WITH LAVENDER, YLANG YLANG, NEROLI, CINNAMON, BLACK PEPPER, CLARY SAGE, LEMON, MYRRH, CINNAMON, CLOVE.

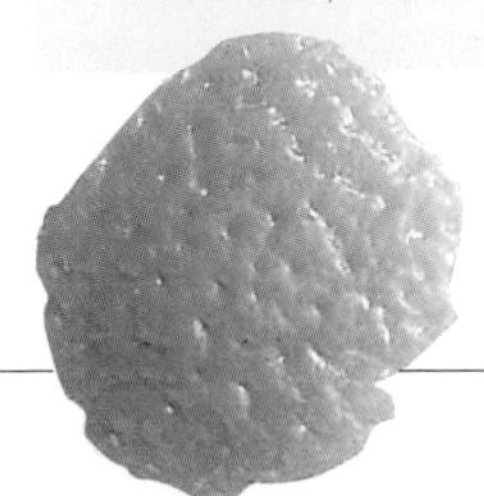

Citrus aurantium var. amara

NEROLI (ORANGE BLOSSOM)

The blossoms of the bitter orange tree yield this oil, which has an exquisite fresh floral fragrance. Neroli is named after an Italian princess, Anne-Marie of Nerola, who used it as a perfume. In folk traditions, orange flowers were included in bridal bouquets as a symbol of innocence and fertility, and to calm nervous couples on their wedding night.

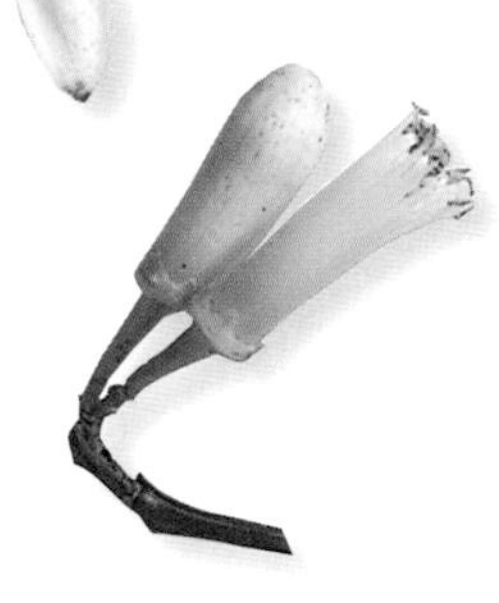

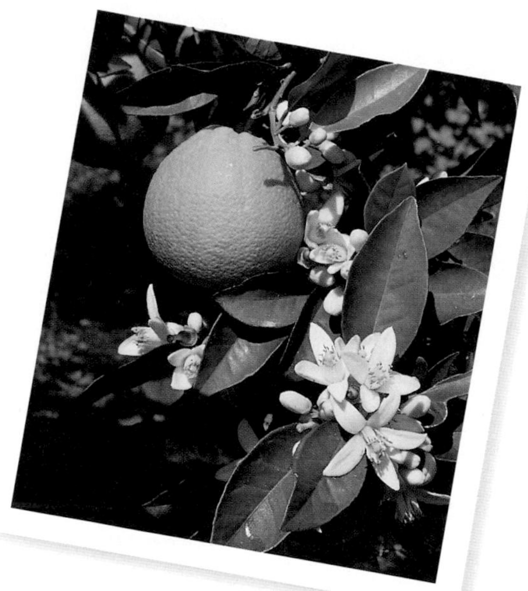

ABOVE *Orange blossoms and weddings have had a long association in folk tradition.*

RECIPE

Massage Blend for High Blood Pressure

Add 3 drops neroli, 3 drops celery, 4 drops rose to 1fl. oz. (25ml.) or 5 teaspoons grapeseed or other vegetable oil and use for gentle massage.

DATA FILE

Properties and Uses

Neroli tones the heart and circulatory system, and its carminative and antispasmodic properties can relieve digestive problems such as indigestion, diarrhea, flatulence, and stomach cramps. Neroli helps to tone the skin and improve elasticity. Added to cream or diluted in oil, it is used to prevent stretch marks, scarring, wrinkles, and to soothe sensitive skin. It is a gentle antidepressant and a nerve tonic, perhaps most helpful in treating anxiety, depression, nervous tension, and stress-related problems. As a sedative it can also help to combat associated insomnia.

CAUTION

KEEP ALL ESSENTIAL OILS OUT OF THE EYES AND NEVER TAKE THEM INTERNALLY.

INFORMATION

BLENDS WELL WITH LAVENDER, LEMON, BERGAMOT, ROSEMARY, ROSE, YLANG YLANG, CHAMOMILE, GERANIUM, BENZOIN, AND MOST OILS.

Citrus aurantium var. amara

PETITGRAIN

Fresh and flowery petitgrain is often regarded as a cheaper alternative to neroli. It is distilled from the leaves and twigs of the bitter orange tree, whereas neroli comes from the blossom. Both oils have similar properties and fragrances, but petitgrain is also a valuable oil in its own right, with a revitalizing and restorative character.

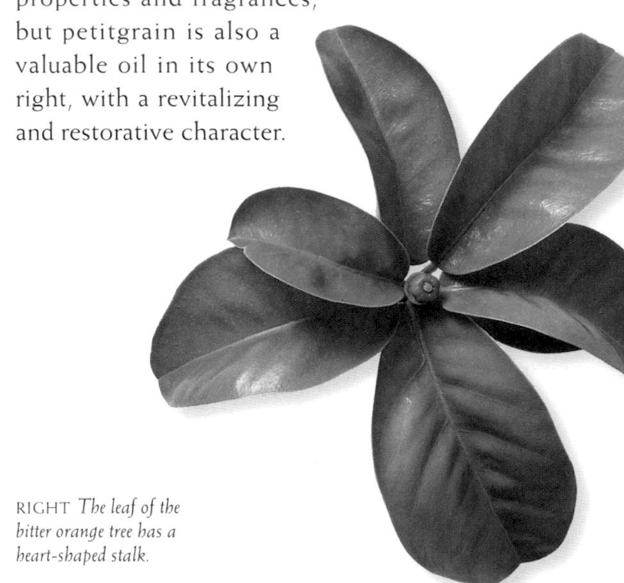

RIGHT *The leaf of the bitter orange tree has a heart-shaped stalk.*

RECIPE

Invigorating Room Fragrancer

Add 3 drops petitgrain, 3 drops lime, 2 drops cypress to a vaporizer dish filled with water. Light and burn for 10–15 minutes.

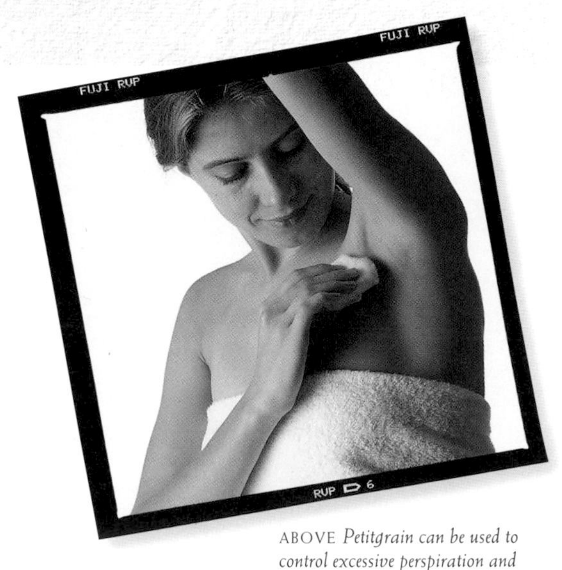

ABOVE *Petitgrain can be used to control excessive perspiration and is a gentle antiseptic.*

DATA FILE

Properties and Uses

Petitgrain can refresh or relax, depending on which oils it is blended with. It strengthens and tones the nervous system, and as such it can soothe many stress-related problems, such as nervous exhaustion and insomnia. Feelings of apathy, irritability, mild depression, anxiety, loneliness, and pessimism can all get a lift from petitgrain's antidepressant properties. This oil also has a tonic effect during convalescence, or when one is feeling "run down." It has a notable antispasmodic effect and helps to tone the digestive system, relieving flatulence and indigestion. Petitgrain is a deodorant, sometimes used to control excessive perspiration. It is also used to control the over-production of sebum in the skin and has gentle antiseptic properties, making it ideal for many greasy skin and scalp conditions, especially acne and greasy hair.

INFORMATION

BLENDS WELL WITH LAVENDER, GERANIUM, BERGAMOT, JASMINE, CLOVE, PALMAROSA, CLARY SAGE, AND OTHER ORANGE OILS.

CAUTION

KEEP OUT OF THE REACH OF CHILDREN.

Citrus bergamia

BERGAMOT

The bergamot tree was originally cultivated in Italy, where the fruit has a history of use in folk medicine. The refreshing essential oil is expressed from the peel of the fruit, which resembles a small yellow orange, when it is nearly ripe. Outside Italy, bergamot is perhaps best known as an ingredient in both Earl Grey tea and eau de Cologne.

INFORMATION

BLENDS WELL WITH CHAMOMILE, GERANIUM, LEMON, SANDALWOOD, MYRRH, JUNIPER, LAVENDER, NEROLI, CYPRESS, JASMINE, TEA TREE.

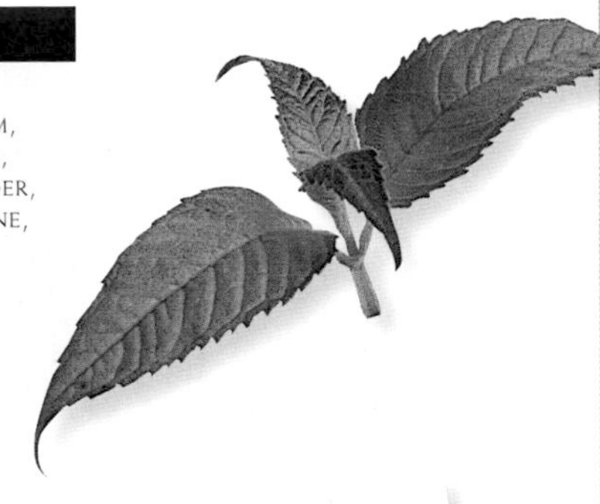

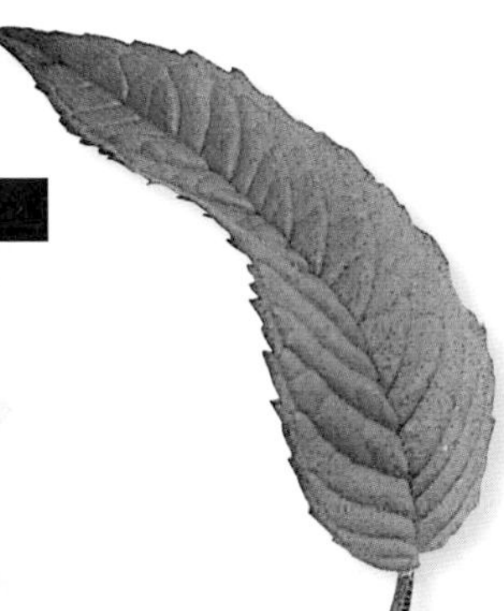

CAUTION

BERGAMOT INCREASES THE SKIN'S SENSITIVITY TO SUNLIGHT. NEVER USE UNDILUTED ON THE SKIN. AVOID IT IF YOU HAVE SENSITIVE SKIN.

MIX WITH A CARRIER OIL BEFORE ADDING TO BATH WATER TO ENSURE IT DISPERSES WELL IN THE WATER.

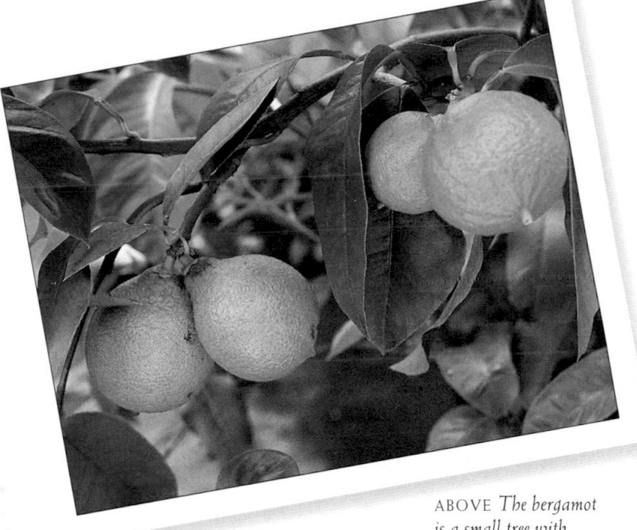

ABOVE *The bergamot is a small tree with fruits which are yellow when ripe.*

RECIPE

Bergamot Wash for Cystitis Relief

Cystitis is a bacterial infection causing inflammation of the bladder. This soothing wash will ease the characteristic burning sensation that occurs while urinating. You can also use absorbent cotton soaked in the solution to swab the opening of the urethra after passing water.

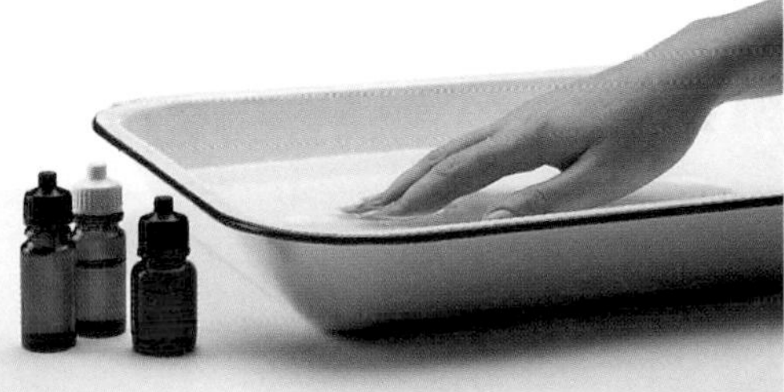

Add 3 drops bergamot, 3 drops lavender, 3 drops niaouli to a warm bath and soak for at least 10 minutes, or fill a bowl that is big enough to sit in with lukewarm water and add 1 drop of each oil. Agitate the water thoroughly with your hand to disperse the oil.

DATA FILE

Properties and Uses

Joyous and uplifting, bergamot is a powerful antidepressant which has a wonderfully balancing effect on moods. As an antiseptic it is good for acne and boils. Other skin complaints, such as oily skin, eczema, and psoriasis, cuts, and insect bites, can also respond well to bergamot. The oil inhibits viral activity; when diluted in alcohol it can be dabbed on cold sores, chicken pox, and shingles. The fragrance repels insects and the oil can be used to expel worms. Bergamot has an affinity with the genitourinary system. It is a diuretic and a powerful urinary disinfectant, particularly good for cystitis. It can also be used for thrush and other types of vaginal itching and discharge. As a digestive, bergamot is sometimes used to encourage appetite. It is also used to cool fevers.

Citrus limon

LEMON

The ancient Greeks and Romans included lemon in their medicine chest and it has a history of use in European folk medicine. The essential oil which is expressed from the fresh peel has many varied applications, making it invaluable in the home aromatherapy kit.

INFORMATION

BLENDS WELL WITH GERANIUM, FENNEL, JUNIPER, EUCALYPTUS, SANDALWOOD, FRANKINCENSE, CHAMOMILE, LAVENDER, YLANG YLANG, ROSE, NEROLI, AND OTHER CITRUS OILS.

CAUTION

CAN IRRITATE SENSITIVE SKIN.

DO NOT USE BEFORE SUNBATHING.

DILUTE WELL FOR MASSAGE AND BATH BLENDS, AND DO NOT USE FOR MORE THAN A FEW DAYS AT A TIME.

RECIPE

Hangover Bath Oil

Add 4 drops lemon, 2 drops fennel, 2 drops lavender to a warm bath and agitate the water with your hand. Relax for 10 minutes and inhale deeply.

DATA FILE

Properties and Uses

Lemon can stimulate the body's defenses to fight all kinds of infection. It is beneficial in treating inflamed or diseased gums, mouth ulcers, sore throats, and acne. It helps to clear colds, flu, and bronchitis, and can be used to remove warts and verrucae, and to clear herpes blisters. The oil has a tonic effect on the circulation and is often used to treat varicose veins, poor circulation, high blood pressure, and fluid retention. Lemon is both diuretic and laxative, and has the ability to stop bleeding in minor cuts and nosebleeds. As an astringent it benefits greasy skin and can also be used to reduce a fever. Because it also counteracts acidity in the body, lemon helps to relieve acid indigestion, arthritis, and rheumatism. On an emotional level, refreshing lemon dispels depression and indecision.

RIGHT *Lemon essential oil is expressed from the peel of the fresh fruit.*

Citrus reticulata

MANDARIN

As the name suggests, mandarin oil originated in China, where the small, sweet fruit was traditionally given as a gift to the Mandarin. The essential oil is expressed from the peel. It has delicate, fruity, floral aroma and a gentle healing action.

CAUTION

MANDARIN MAY INCREASE THE SKIN'S SENSITIVITY TO THE SUN.

INFORMATION

BLENDS WELL WITH FRANKINCENSE, CHAMOMILE, LAVENDER, ROSEWOOD, NEROLI, AND OTHER CITRUS OILS AND SPICE OILS, SUCH AS CLOVE AND CINNAMON.

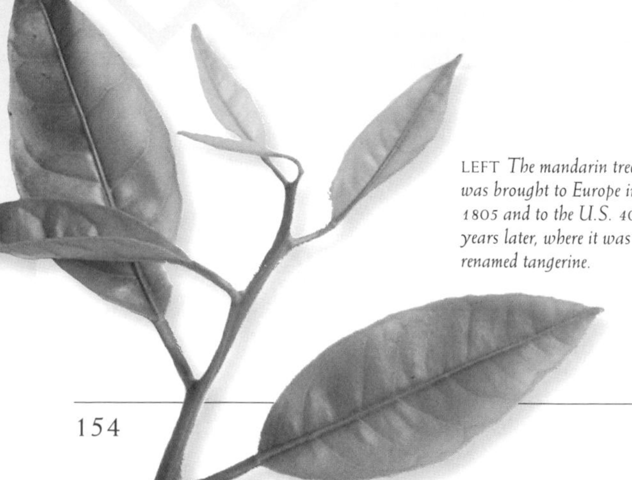

LEFT *The mandarin tree was brought to Europe in 1805 and to the U.S. 40 years later, where it was renamed tangerine.*

RECIPE

Oil to Prevent Stretch Marks

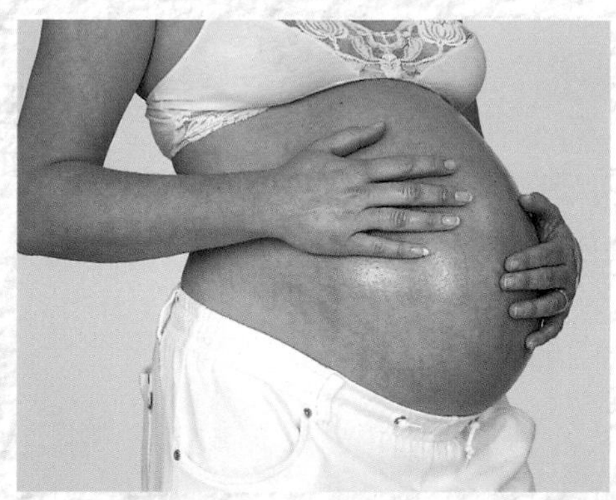

Add 4 drops mandarin, 3 drops neroli, 3 drops lavender to a bottle containing 1fl.oz. (25ml.) or 5 teaspoonsful sweet almond oil and 1 teaspoonful wheat germ oil. Massage into the abdomen twice a day from the fifth month of pregnancy.

DATA FILE

Properties and Uses

Mandarin is used mostly for treating digestive problems. It soothes indigestion and relieves intestinal spasms. It has a mild laxative effect and acts as a tonic for the stomach. It is gentle enough for children's digestive problems and hiccups. Mandarin also tones the liver, the body's main chemical processing and elimination organ. Because it is also a mild diuretic, mandarin can help to relieve fluid retention and stored toxins. The oil can be used as a skin toner for oily skin, acne, or congested pores. As a sedative it is also used to relieve nervous tension and insomnia during pregnancy, and can help to settle restless children.

Citrus x paradisi

GRAPEFRUIT

Refreshing grapefruit oil is expressed from the peel of the fruit, cultivated mainly in California, Brazil, Florida, and Israel. It has a fresh, tangy citrus scent that enlivens the mind and disperses feelings of gloom. Unlike many citrus oils, grapefruit does not increase the skin's sensitivity to sunlight.

RECIPE

Wake-up Shower Gel

Mix 2 drops grapefruit, 2 drops petitgrain, 1 drop rosemary with a dollop of unscented shower gel and work to a lather with a sponge.

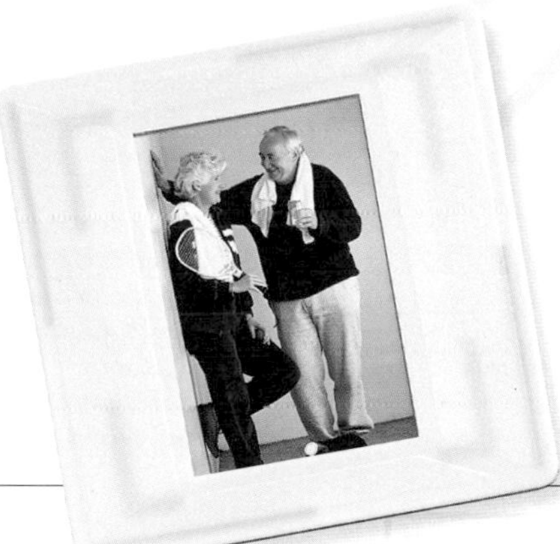

BELOW *A grapefruit oil massage helps to ease stiff muscles after exercise.*

INFORMATION

BLENDS WELL WITH ORANGE, LEMON, SANDALWOOD, BERGAMOT, NEROLI, LAVENDER, CYPRESS, ROSEMARY, GERANIUM, JUNIPER, CARDAMOM, CORIANDER, AND OTHER SPICE OILS.

CAUTION

DO NOT TAKE INTERNALLY.

KEEP OUT OF THE EYES.

DATA FILE

Properties and Uses

Grapefruit is diuretic, detoxifying, and cleansing to the kidneys. It also has a stimulating effect on the lymphatic system. Because of these properties it helps to relieve fluid retention and eliminate the toxins that cause cellulite. It is also beneficial in a massage blend to ease stiff muscles after exercise. Grapefruit tones an oily skin and scalp, is helpful in treating acne and congested pores, and can be applied neat to cold sores. It also stimulates digestion and improves immunity to infection. As an antidepressant, grapefruit oil enlivens the mind, relieves anxiety, and combats nervous exhaustion.

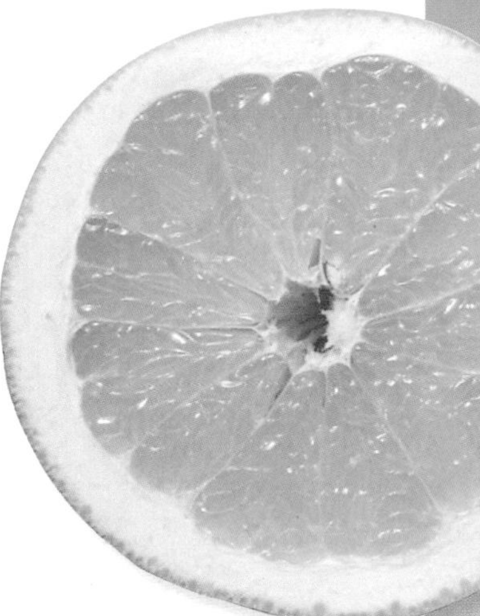

ABOVE *Grapefruit, like other citrus species, is high in vitamin C and is a good protection against infectious illnesses.*

Commiphora myrrha

MYRRH

Perhaps best known as one of the three gifts brought to the infant Jesus, myrrh was valued in ancient times as an ingredient in embalming preparations, incense, and as a medicine. According to legend, the soldiers of ancient Greece took myrrh ointment into battle to treat their wounds. Essential oil of myrrh has a musty, balsamic odor and is closely related to frankincense, with which it is often linked.

DATA FILE

Properties and Uses

Myrrh has an excellent soothing, antiseptic, and healing effect on sore or inflamed gums, mouth ulcers, wounds, and cracked or chapped skin. It can speed the healing of weepy eczema, and because of its antifungal properties it can be used as a vaginal wash for thrush or in a foot bath for athlete's foot. Myrrh is also an expectorant and a lung tonic, good for coughs, colds, bronchitis, and flu. It stimulates, tones, and soothes the digestive system, and is often used for diarrhea, hemorrhoids, and indigestion. The oil is a uterine tonic, which can be helpful for menstrual irregularities. Myrrh relieves agitation, calms fears and uncertainties, and has a positive, balancing effect on the emotions.

CAUTION

DO NOT USE IN HIGH DOSES.

DO NOT USE AT ALL DURING PREGNANCY.

INFORMATION

BLENDS WELL WITH FRANKINCENSE, SANDALWOOD, MANDARIN, LAVENDER, LEMON, ROSE, EUCALYPTUS, THYME, BENZOIN, GERANIUM, PEPPERMINT, CYPRESS, PINE, AND SPICE OILS.

RECIPE

Chapped Skin Cream

Add 5 drops myrrh, 5 drops benzoin, 4 drops geranium to 1oz. (30g.) of good unperfumed, lanolin-free cream. Mix well and apply to the skin.

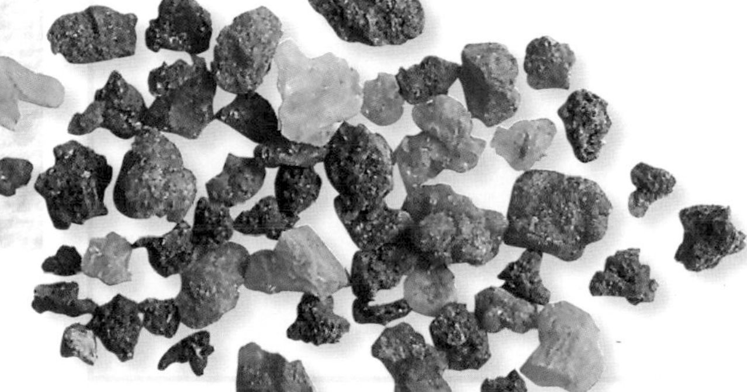

RIGHT *Myrrh is the hardened oleoresin from shrubs and small trees of the* Commiphora *species.*

THERAPY CONNECTIONS

LEMON
Traditional Home and Folk Remedies *p.87*

GRAPEFRUIT
Traditional Home and Folk Remedies *p.88*

MYRRH
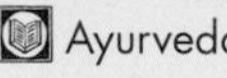
Ayurveda *p.34*

Coriandrum sativum

CORIANDER

Coriander is a highly aromatic annual herb. Coriander seeds were used by the ancient Greeks and have also been found in Egyptian tombs. The seeds and leaves are both used in cooking, and the Chinese use the whole herb for medicinal purposes. The essential oil, distilled from the crushed seeds, has a sweet and slightly musky, spicy, and woody aroma.

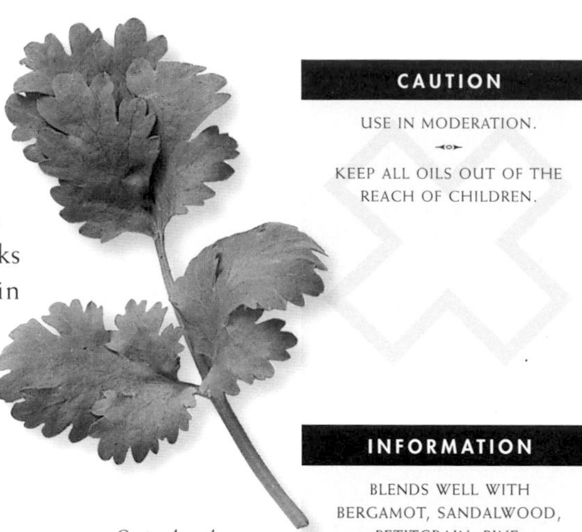

ABOVE *Coriander, also known as cilantro, is an annual herb with bright green, delicate leaves.*

CAUTION

USE IN MODERATION.

KEEP ALL OILS OUT OF THE REACH OF CHILDREN.

INFORMATION

BLENDS WELL WITH BERGAMOT, SANDALWOOD, PETITGRAIN, PINE, CITRONELLA, CLARY SAGE, GINGER, AND OTHER SPICE OILS.

DATA FILE

Properties and Uses

Coriander's pain-relieving properties make it suitable for headaches and neuralgia. It has a warming, antirheumatic effect, good for muscular pain and stiffness, arthritis, and rheumatism. Coriander is an effective digestive stimulant and tonic, used to relieve diarrhea, flatulence, nausea, painful spasms, and to stimulate appetite in cases of anorexia. It is also a nervous stimulant, beneficial for apathy, nervous exhaustion, and fatigue. The oil's stimulatory properties also work on the circulation. As such it is useful for hemorrhoids, poor circulation, and fluid retention. Coriander is an aphrodisiac which has a warming, stimulatory effect on the emotions.

RECIPE

Coriander Muscle Rub

Add 2 drops coriander, 4 drops juniper, 4 drops black pepper to 4 teaspoons (20ml.) grapeseed oil, and massage into tired and aching muscles.

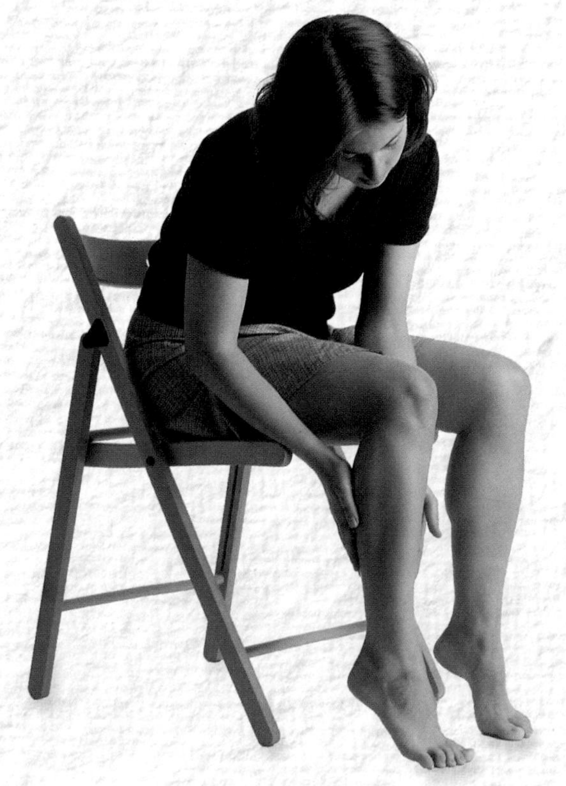

THERAPY CONNECTIONS

CORIANDER

Ayurveda *p.35*

Cupresses sempervirens

CYPRESS

Ancient civilizations used the tall evergreen cypress tree as a source of incense for religious ceremonies and for medicinal purposes. The oil, which is distilled from the twigs and needles of the cypress, has a pleasant, smoky, wood aroma, and a number of therapeutic uses.

DATA FILE

Properties and Uses

Cypress is an anti-spasmodic, useful in a vaporizer for respiratory problems such as bronchitis or asthma, or to prevent coughing attacks. Astringent properties make it suitable for use in a wash for hemorrhoids and for excessively oily skin. It can also be applied to cuts to stop bleeding and is used as a mouthwash for bleeding gums. Cypress is a circulatory tonic, which can improve poor circulation, relieve fluid retention, soothe muscular cramp, and can be applied gently to varicose veins. In a foot bath it counteracts excessively sweating and smelly feet. The oil is used to treat PMS, regulate the menstrual cycle, and counteract heavy bleeding. Menopausal symptoms such as hot flushes and irritability can also be alleviated by cypress.

CAUTION

DO NOT USE UNDILUTED ON THE SKIN.

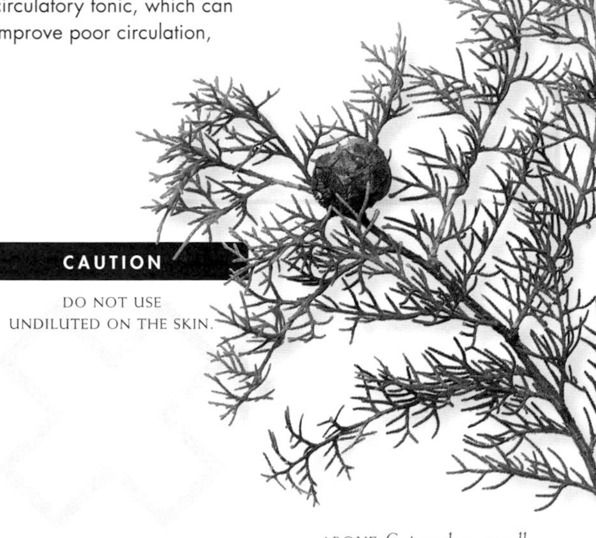

ABOVE *Cypress bears small flowers and round, brownish-gray cones or nuts.*

RECIPE

Varicose Vein Toner

Add 5 drops cypress and 10 drops geranium oil to 5 teaspoons (25ml.) vegetable oil. Starting at the ankle, gently stroke up the legs towards the heart.

INFORMATION

BLENDS WELL WITH JUNIPER, PINE, LAVENDER, SANDALWOOD, LEMON, MANDARIN, ORANGE, BERGAMOT, CLARY SAGE.

Cymbopogon citratus

LEMONGRASS

Lemongrass is a tall, aromatic grass. It is used as a flavoring in Thai cuisine and has been used in traditional Indian medicine for centuries. The essential oil is distilled from the grass leaves. It has a strong refreshing citrus smell that has many aromatherapy and domestic uses.

LEFT *The long, thin leaves of lemongrass are the source for its essential oil.*

DATA FILE

Properties and Uses

Lemongrass has a tonic effect on the nervous system and the body in general. It is also painkilling and antidepressant, good for headaches, lethargy, symptoms of stress, and beneficial for muscular pain and poor muscle tone. It has fever-reducing properties and helps the immune system to fight infections. As a deodorant, lemongrass can be used for excessive perspiration and sweaty feet, and its astringent properties make it an effective skin toner which helps to close open pores. Lemongrass is also an effective flea, lice, and tick repellent. Use it in a vaporizer to keep flies out of the kitchen in summer and to get rid of pet smells from the home.

INFORMATION

BLENDS WELL WITH LAVENDER, ORANGE, GERANIUM, JASMINE, ROSEMARY, NEROLI, BASIL, SANDALWOOD, EUCALYPTUS.

CAUTION

DILUTE WELL, AS LEMONGRASS MAY CAUSE SKIN IRRITATION IN SOME PEOPLE.

DO NOT USE ON BABIES OR CHILDREN.

DO NOT USE AROUND THE EYES.

RECIPE

Greasy Hair Shampoo

Add 2 drops of lemongrass to a normal dollop of mild, unscented shampoo, rub between your palms, and wash your hair as normal.

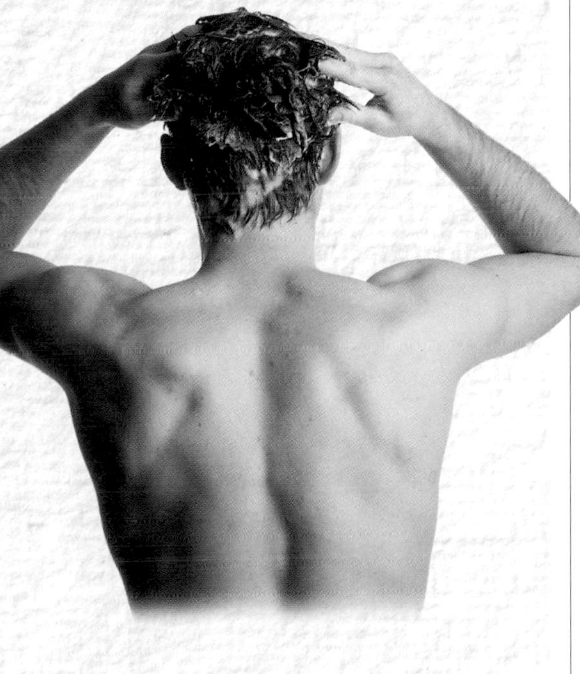

RIGHT *A few drops of lemongrass added to shampoo make an ideal greasy-hair formula.*

Cymbopogon martinii var. martinii

PALMAROSA

In Indian Ayurvedic medicine palmarosa has long been used to combat infectious diseases. Distilled from a fresh scented grass, similar to lemongrass, palmarosa has a gentle floral fragrance like a mix of rose and geranium. In the past it was also known as Indian or Turkish geranium.

RECIPE

Skin Rejuvenator

Add 6 drops palmarosa, 3 drops rose, 3 drops frankincense to a small bottle containing 5 drops evening primrose and 3 teaspoons (15ml.) apricot kernel oil. Shake well. Gently massage into the face at night.

DATA FILE

Properties and Uses

Palmarosa is a valuable oil in skin care. The diluted oil applied to the skin rebalances sebum production, thereby hydrating dry skin conditions. It also rejuvenates wrinkled or aging skin by promoting cellular regeneration, and it helps to heal wounds. Palmarosa is beneficial for acne, dermatitis, and skin infections because of its antiseptic properties. It has a stimulatory effect on the circulatory and digestive systems, helping to increase appetite and activate a sluggish digestion. As a bactericide, the oil prevents and treats intestinal infections. Palmarosa used in a massage blend is good for nervous exhaustion and stress-related problems.

RIGHT *Palmarosa is a perennial plant with long stems and terminal flowering tops.*

INFORMATION

BLENDS WELL WITH SANDALWOOD, LAVENDER, GERANIUM, ROSEWOOD, CEDARWOOD, FRANKINCENSE, LEMON, FLORAL, CITRUS OILS, AND WOODY OILS.

Cymbopogon nardus
CITRONELLA

The leaves of this tropical scented grass are valued in many countries for their medicinal properties. The essential oil, which is distilled from the dried leaves, has a strong, fresh, lemony scent. Although it is not widely used in aromatherapy, it is highly valued as a household disinfectant and insecticide.

RECIPE

Refreshing Foot Soak

Add 4 drops citronella, 2 drops tea tree, 3 drops cypress to a foot bath to refresh hot and sweaty feet.

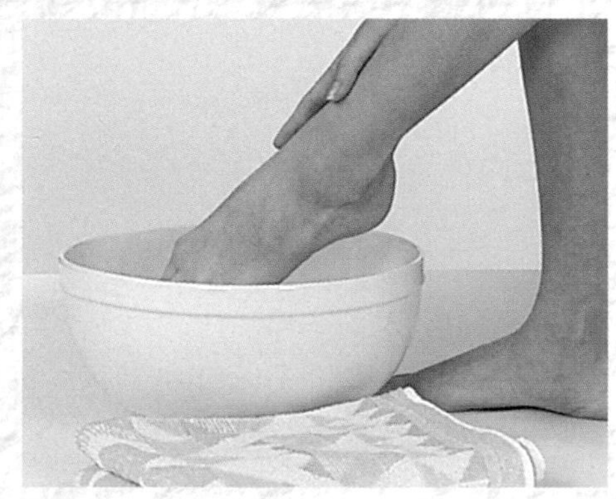

DATA FILE

Properties and Uses

Refreshing and uplifting, citronella helps to combat headaches, fatigue, and feelings of depression.
It has strong deodorant properties, which make it suitable for refreshing tired or sweaty feet, and for treating fungal infections such as athlete's foot. In Eastern cultures it is used to settle digestion and menstrual problems, and as a rub for rheumatic pain. It makes an excellent insect repellent, either used in a room spray, vaporizer, or dropped on to a square of cotton and added to a linen cupboard to keep clothes fresh and free from moths. Cats dislike the smell of citronella, so it can be used to keep them away from areas of the garden.

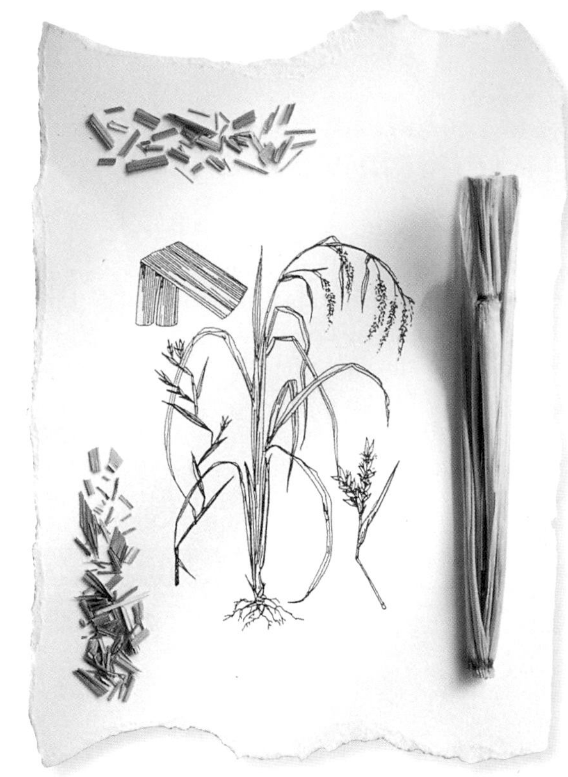

ABOVE *Citronella is a tall, aromatic, perennial grass derived from wild "managrass" found in Sri Lanka.*

CAUTION

DO NOT USE DURING PREGNANCY.

DILUTE WELL, AS IT MAY CAUSE IRRITATION TO SOME PEOPLE WITH SENSITIVE SKIN.

INFORMATION

BLENDS WELL WITH GERANIUM, LEMON, ORANGE, CEDARWOOD, CYPRESS, TEA TREE, BERGAMOT, EUCALYPTUS, PINE.

Elettaria cardamonum
CARDAMOM

This spice has been used since antiquity as a food flavoring, but it has also played a part in Indian Ayurvedic medicine for thousands of years. Hippocrates, a famous Greek physician known as the father of medicine, also acknowledged the therapeutic benefits of cardamom. The essential oil distilled from the seeds has a warm, sweet, spicy aroma and a warming quality similar to ginger.

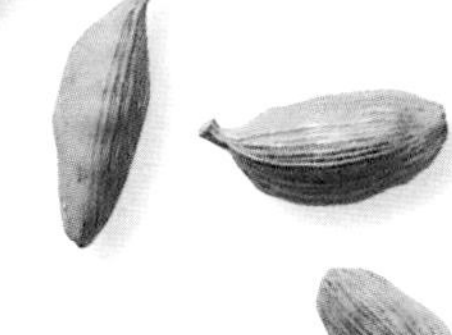

BELOW *and* ABOVE *Cardamom is a reedlike herb with long, blade-shaped leaves and yellowish flowers with purple tips, ripening into oblong seed pods.*

RECIPE

Massage Oil for Stomach Cramps

Add 1 drop cardamom, 1 drop basil, 2 drops marjoram to 2 teaspoons (10ml.) vegetable oil and massage in a clockwise direction over the stomach and abdominal area.

DATA FILE

Properties and Uses

Mainly used as a digestive remedy because of its soothing, antispasmodic, and digestive properties, cardamom is good for indigestion, flatulence, abdominal pain, heartburn, bloating, nausea, and bad breath. It has a diuretic effect which can help to relieve water retention. Cardamom also has a wonderful, stimulating, and tonic effect on mind and body; it makes a refreshing bath which can relieve fatigue and soothe strained nerves, and helps to clear the mind of confusion. In India cardamom is reputed to be an aphrodisiac.

INFORMATION

BLENDS WELL WITH BERGAMOT, ROSE, FRANKINCENSE, CLOVE, YLANG YLANG, NEROLI, BASIL, CEDARWOOD, FENNEL, LEMON, AND GINGER.

CAUTION

DO NOT TAKE INTERNALLY.

USE SPARINGLY, AS SPICY OILS MAY CAUSE IRRITATION IN SOME PEOPLE.

Eucalyptus globulus

BLUE GUM EUCALYPTUS

Several of the 700 species of eucalyptus are used to distill medicinal-quality essential oil, but the Australian "blue gum" is by far the most widely used. Eucalyptus is a traditional remedy in Australia and a familiar ingredient in numerous chest rubs and decongestants. The oil also eradicates lice and fleas.

BELOW *This evergreen tree bears long, narrow, yellowish leaves. Eucalyptus oil is extracted from the leaves and young twigs.*

INFORMATION

BLENDS WELL WITH PEPPERMINT, TEA TREE, ROSEMARY, THYME, LAVENDER, CEDARWOOD, LEMON, PINE.

DATA FILE

Properties and Uses

Eucalyptus is a powerful antiseptic and renowned decongestant, used mostly for coughs, colds, chest infections, and sinusitis. It alleviates inflammation generally, and is helpful in treating rheumatism, muscular aches and pains, and fibrositis. It is a diuretic and a deodorant, with strong antiviral and immune-stimulating properties, and is an effective local painkiller, especially for nerve pain. Urinary tract problems such as cystitis respond well to eucalyptus. The oil is also used to reduce fevers and treat skin infections, cuts, and blisters, genital and oral herpes, chickenpox, and shingles. Eucalyptus eases the pain of burns and helps new tissue to form. It is used to prevent and relieve insect bites and is an effective mosquito repellent.

RECIPE

Disinfectant Wash for Insect Bites

Add 3 drops eucalyptus, 3 drops thyme, 3 drops lavender to a bowl of clean water. Use cotton wool or a clean cotton cloth to dab repeatedly on the affected area.

CAUTION

DO NOT TAKE WHEN USING HOMEOPATHIC REMEDIES.

DO NOT USE FOR MORE THAN A FEW DAYS AT A TIME BECAUSE OF THE RISK OF TOXICITY.

DO NOT USE ON BABIES OR VERY YOUNG CHILDREN.

Foeniculum vulgare

FENNEL

In folklore fennel was believed to convey courage and strength and contribute to a long life. It also has a history of use as an antidote to poisons. The essential oil, distilled from the crushed seeds, is still valued for its detoxifying properties.

DATA FILE

Properties and Uses

Fennel appears to have a rebalancing effect on hormones, probably due to an estrogen-like plant hormone. As such it helps to stabilize hormone activity during the menopause and has traditionally been used to increase milk flow in breast-feeding mothers. It is a good diuretic, antimicrobial, and antiseptic which can help with premenstrual water retention and urinary tract infections. It helps to eliminate toxic wastes from the body, making it valuable in treating arthritis and cellulite. It reduces digestive spasms, calms and tones the stomach and digestive system, and has a slightly laxative effect, benefiting nausea, indigestion, constipation, and stomach cramps. Fennel also makes a good mouthwash for gum disease or infections.

THERAPY CONNECTIONS

CARDAMOM

Ayurveda p.38

Chinese Herbal Medicine p.55

FENNEL

Herbalism p.121

RECIPE

Anticellulite Massage Oil

Add 8 drops fennel, 8 drops juniper, 10 drops grapefruit oil to 5 teaspoons (25ml) sweet almond oil and 5 drops jojoba oil. Store in a dark glass bottle and massage into the affected area every day after your bath or shower.

LEFT *Fennel is a biennial or perennial herb with feathery leaves.*

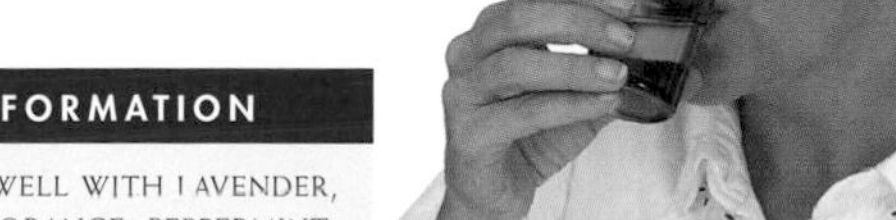

INFORMATION

BLENDS WELL WITH LAVENDER, LEMON, ORANGE, PEPPERMINT, ROSE, GERANIUM, JUNIPER, SANDALWOOD, ROSEMARY CYPRESS, CLARY SAGE.

CAUTION

USE ONLY SWEET FENNEL (ALSO KNOWN AS ROMAN OR FRENCH FENNEL), AS BITTER FENNEL SHOULD NOT BE USED ON THE SKIN.

DO NOT USE DURING PREGNANCY.

NOT SUITABLE FOR EPILEPTICS OR CHILDREN UNDER SIX YEARS OLD.

NARCOTIC IN LARGE DOSES.

LEFT *Fennel is used in mouthwashes to treat gum diseases and infections.*

Hyssopus officinalis

HYSSOP

Revered as a sacred cleansing herb by the Hebrews and the ancient Greeks, hyssop has also long been valued by herbalists for its medicinal properties. Both the leaves and the small blue or mauve flowers are distilled for their essential oil, which has a strong, spicy, herbaceous scent.

RECIPE

Inhalation for Chest Infections

Add 2 drops hyssop, 2 drops lavender, 2 drops benzoin to a bowl of steaming water. Cover your head with a towel, bend over the bowl, and inhale.

CAUTION

DILUTE WELL AND USE FOR NO MORE THAN A FEW DAYS AT A TIME BECAUSE THERE IS SOME RISK OF TOXICITY.

DO NOT USE DURING PREGNANCY.

DO NOT USE IF YOU ARE EPILEPTIC.

FOR PEOPLE WITH HIGH BLOOD PRESSURE HYSSOP SHOULD ONLY BE USED AS DIRECTED BY A QUALIFIED AROMATHERAPIST.

DATA FILE

Properties and Uses

Hyssop is an expectorant with antispasmodic, bactericidal, and antiseptic properties, which can be helpful for coughing, whooping cough, catarrh, sore throats, and chest infections. It can be used in skin care for cuts, bruises, and inflammation. Hyssop has hypertensive properties, making it useful in the treatment of low blood pressure, and has a general tonic effect on circulation. As an emmenagogue it can be used for scanty or no menstrual bleeding. The oil can also soothe indigestion and relieve colicky cramps. Hyssop's sedative and tonic properties can benefit stress- or anxiety-related problems. It helps to relieve fatigue, and increase alertness.

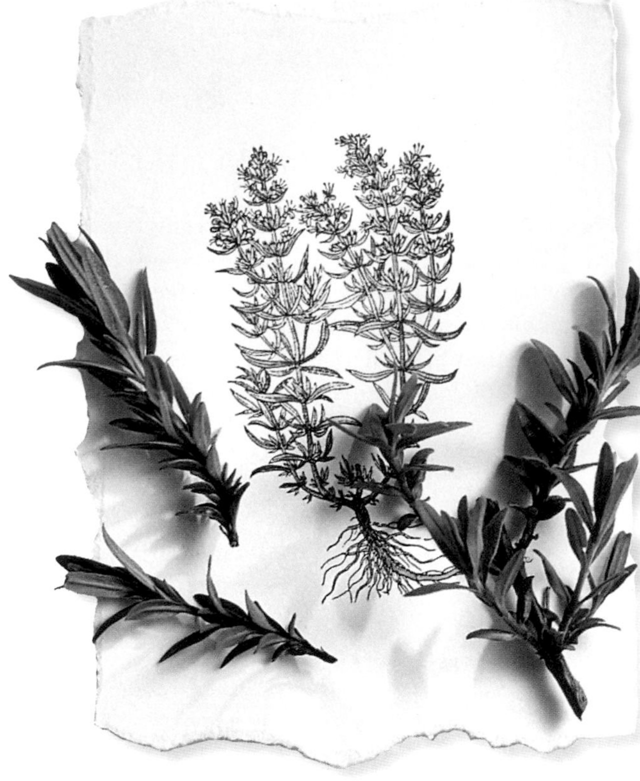

ABOVE *Hyssop is a perennial, almost evergreen shrub, with woody stems and small, lance-shaped leaves.*

INFORMATION

BLENDS WELL WITH SANDALWOOD, LAVENDER, YLANG YLANG, ROSEMARY, CLARY SAGE, CYPRESS, GERANIUM, LEMON, AND OTHER CITRUS OILS.

Juniperus communis

JUNIPER

Used in ancient Greece and Egypt to combat the spread of disease, juniper was still being used in French hospitals during the First World War. This warm woody-scented oil can be distilled from juniper berries and twigs, but the best oil is produced by distilling the ripe berries only.

CAUTION

DO NOT USE DURING PREGNANCY.

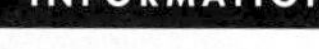

NOT SUITABLE FOR PEOPLE WITH KIDNEY DISEASE.

INFORMATION

BLENDS WELL WITH PINE, LAVENDER, CYPRESS, CLARY SAGE, SANDALWOOD, VETIVER, BENZOIN, ROSEMARY, FENNEL, GERANIUM, BERGAMOT, AND OTHER CITRUS OILS.

LEFT *Juniper is an evergreen shrub with bluish-green stiff needles.*

RIGHT *A hair and scalp tonic can be made with juniper oil.*

RECIPE

Hair and Scalp Tonic

Add 10 drops juniper, 8 drops rosemary, 7 drops cedarwood to 1½fl.oz. (50ml.) or 10 teaspoons olive oil and massage into your hair and scalp before you wash it. Wrap your hair in a warm towel and leave for about 2 hours. Wash out with a mild shampoo, massaging the shampoo into the hair before you wet it to remove all the oil.

DATA FILE

Properties and Uses

Juniper is physically and emotionally cleansing. It helps to detoxify the body of harmful waste products that contribute to problems such as rheumatoid arthritis and cellulite, and clears the mind of confusion and exhaustion. Juniper is also diuretic, has an affinity with the genitourinary system, and is excellent for treating cystitis. Skin problems, especially weepy eczema and acne, respond well to its toning, astringent, and antiseptic properties. Juniper is also good for hemorrhoids and hair loss, and assists with wound healing. In addition, it stimulates appetite, relieves nervous tension, and is an excellent disinfectant.

Jasminum officinale

JASMINE

It takes huge quantities of jasmine flowers to produce a small amount of this very expensive essential oil. However, very little is needed to produce an effect and the sensual floral perfume makes it a highly prized oil. In China the flowers and the root are used to treat conditions as diverse as liver cirrhosis and headaches.

CAUTION

JASMINE MAY CAUSE AN ALLERGIC REACTION IN RARE CASES.

RECIPE

Jasmine Massage for Menstrual Cramps

Add 4 drops jasmine, 4 drops clary sage, 2 drops lavender to 5 teaspoons (25ml.) sweet almond oil. Start the massage by sliding your hands from your hips across your abdomen. Gently stroke around the abdomen in a clockwise direction, sliding one hand after the other. Stroke your hands back up and around your hips, and around to the small of your back. Repeat.

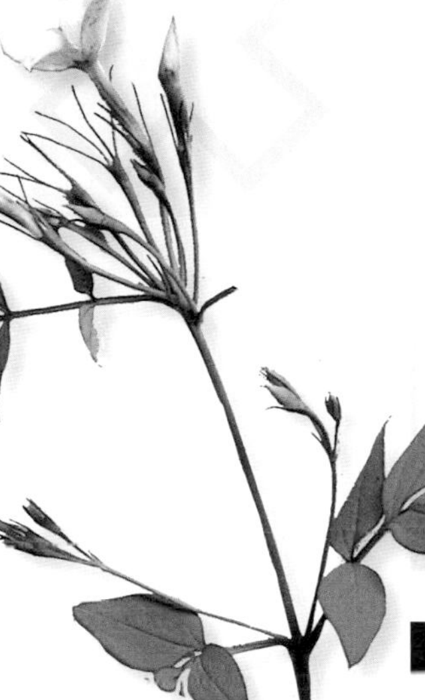

ABOVE *Jasmine is an evergreen shrub or vine, up to 33 ft. (10m.) high, with delicate leaves and highly fragrant flowers.*

DATA FILE

Properties and Uses

Jasmine has a reputation as an aphrodisiac, benefiting impotence in men and frigidity in women. It is also a uterine tonic which can help with menstrual cramp and disorders of the uterus. Its pain-relieving properties and ability to strengthen contractions make it one of the best oils to use during childbirth. It is also believed to strengthen male sex organs and has been used for prostate problems. Its relaxing and antidepressant effect helps to clear postnatal depression. It is excellent for stress relief and is uplifting during times of lethargy. Jasmine has a soothing, warming, and anti-inflammatory effect on joints and a rejuvenating effect on dry, wrinkled, or aging skin. Its antiseptic and expectorant properties also make it applicable for catarrh, and infections of the chest and throat.

INFORMATION

BLENDS WELL WITH LAVENDER, GERANIUM, CHAMOMILE, CLARY SAGE, SANDALWOOD, ROSE, NEROLI, AND OTHER CITRUS OILS.

THERAPY CONNECTIONS

HYSSOP
Chinese Herbal Medicine p.54

JASMINE
Homeopathy p.195

Lavendula augustifolia

LAVENDER

Of the several varieties of lavender used medicinally, *Lavendula augustifolia* is the most important. Lavender is the most versatile, best loved, and most widely therapeutic of all essential oils. Both the flowers and the leaves are highly aromatic, but only the flowers are used to make essential oil.

CAUTION

LAVENDER IS USUALLY SAFE FOR ALL AGE GROUPS, BUT SOME HAY FEVER OR ASTHMA SUFFERERS MAY BE ALLERGIC.

DILUTE WELL IF TAKING HOMEOPATHIC REMEDIES.

RECIPE

Bath or Massage Blend for Irritability

Add 3 drops lavender, 3 drops chamomile, 2 drops neroli directly to a warm bath and disperse with your hand. Alternatively, add to 3 teaspoons (15ml.) grapeseed or sweet almond oil for a soothing massage.

DATA FILE

Properties and Uses

Lavender is calming, soothing, antidepressant, and emotionally balancing. Its antiseptic, antibacterial, and painkilling properties make it valuable in treating cuts, wounds, burns, bruises, spots, allergies, insect bites, and throat infections. Because it is a decongestant it is also effective against colds, flu, and catarrhal conditions. Lavender lowers blood pressure, prevents and eases digestive spasms, nausea, and indigestion. It is antirheumatic and a tonic. Tension, depression, insomnia, headaches, stress, and hypertension respond particularly well to its soothing properties.

INFORMATION

BLENDS WELL WITH FLORALS SUCH AS ROSE, GERANIUM, YLANG YLANG, CHAMOMILE, JASMINE, CITRUS OILS SUCH AS ORANGE, LEMON, BERGAMOT, AND GRAPEFRUIT, ROSEMARY, MARJORAM, PATCHOULI, CLARY SAGE, CEDARWOOD, CLOVE, AND TEA TREE.

LEFT *Lavender is an evergreen woody shrub up to 3ft. (1m.) tall.*

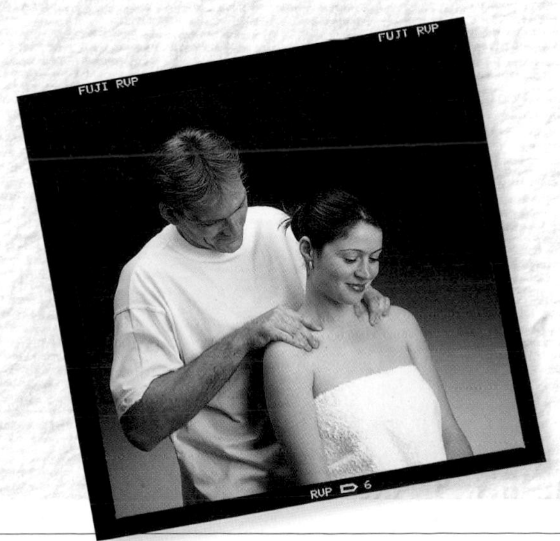

RIGHT *Lavender is a reviving yet soothing oil, an ideal ingredient for the bath or in a blend for massage.*

Melaleuca alternifolia

TEA TREE

This small tree or shrub is a traditional remedy among the Aboriginal people of Australia. Originally, the leaves were made into a tea, hence its name. More recently, scientific research has shown that tea tree oil can combat all types of infection.

DATA FILE

Properties and Uses

Primarily an anti-infection oil, tea tree has antifungal, antibacterial, and antiviral properties. It is frequently used for skin problems such as spots, acne, warts, verrucae, athlete's foot, rashes, insect bites, burns, and blisters. It is used to clean cuts and infected wounds, and it helps skin to heal by encouraging the formation of scar tissue. Tea tree is effective against dandruff, cold sores, and urinary or genital infections such as cystitis and thrush. It is an expectorant that also alleviates inflammation and is a valuable immune stimulant. It is an excellent choice when fighting colds, flu, respiratory infections, catarrhal problems, and infectious illnesses. Tea tree is also used to bring down a fever, to kill fleas and lice, and as a deodorant.

RECIPE

Treatment Oil for Acne

Add 4 drops tea tree, 3 drops bergamot, 3 drops lavender to 2 teaspoons (10ml.) jojoba oil, which is excellent for inflamed or acne-prone skin. Dab onto the affected areas.

INFORMATION

BLENDS WELL WITH LAVENDER, GERANIUM, CHAMOMILE, MYRRH, LEMON, ROSEMARY, MARJORAM CLARY SAGE, PINE, SPICE OILS SUCH AS CLOVE AND CINNAMON.

CAUTION

PEOPLE WITH SENSITIVE SKIN SHOULD INTRODUCE THE OIL WITH CAUTION.

DO NOT SWALLOW MOUTHWASHES OR GARGLES.

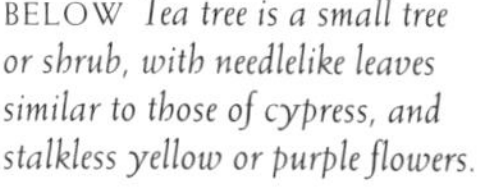

BELOW *Tea tree is a small tree or shrub, with needlelike leaves similar to those of cypress, and stalkless yellow or purple flowers.*

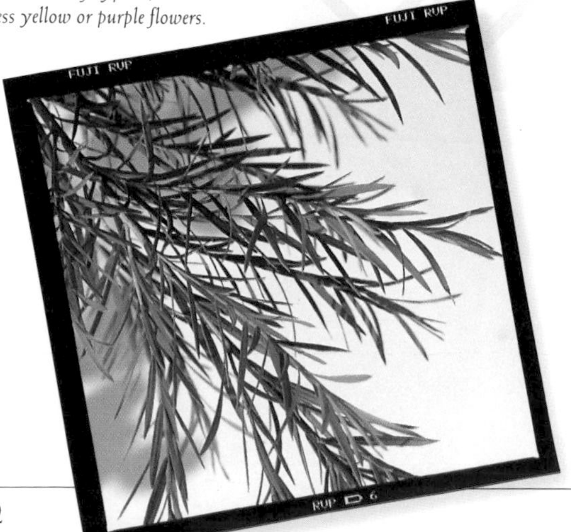

Melaleuca cajeputi

CAJEPUT

In Malaysia, the Philippines, Indonesia, and Australia, wild cajeput is used extensively for all manner of ills, from colds to toothache. Closely related to tea tree, this oil is distilled from the leaves and buds of cajeput, and has a distinctly medicinal camphorous odor.

RECIPE

Inhalation for Colds and Flu

Add 4 drops cajeput, 3 drops rosemary, 2 drops eucalyptus to a bowl of steaming water, cover your head with a towel, bend over the bowl, and inhale for 5–10 minutes.

BELOW *Cajeput is a tall, evergreen tree, up to 100ft. (30 m.) high, with thick pointed leaves and white flowers.*

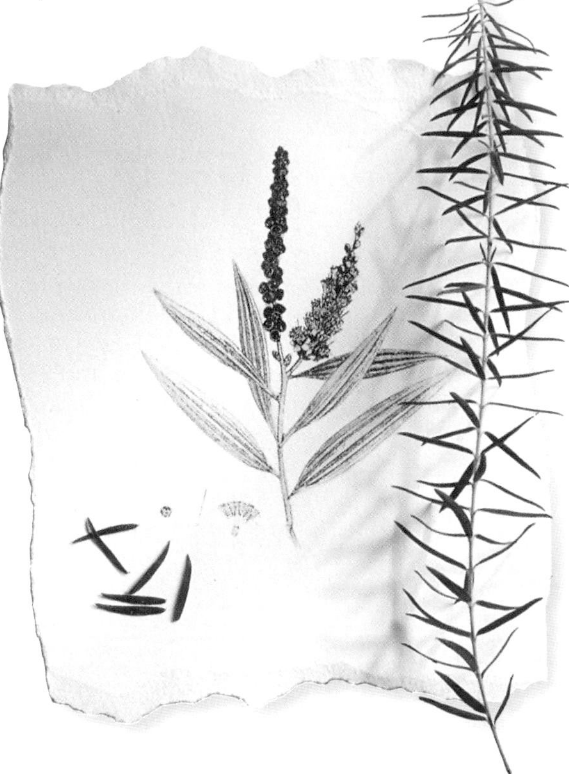

DATA FILE

Properties and Uses

Cajeput is antiseptic, antimicrobial, and it clears mucus. It is good to use in steam inhalations for colds, flu, sinusitis, asthma, bronchitis, and other respiratory infections. It has painkilling properties which can ease headaches and sore throats, and can be used to good effect on muscular and arthritic pain. The oil is also a urinary antiseptic. Used with care, it is effective against cystitis and other urinary infections. Cajeput can be used to soothe the stomach, counteract digestive spasms, and kill infections in the gastro-intestinal system. It is widely used for minor conditions such as insect bites and spots. Inhalation, which is one of the best ways to use this oil, helps to dispel mental fatigue and apathy.

CAUTION

DILUTE WELL, AS CAJEPUT IS A SKIN IRRITANT.

DO NOT USE AS A GARGLE OR AS A VAGINAL WASH AS THE OIL CAN IRRITATE THE MUCOUS MEMBRANES.

CAJEPUT IS A STIMULANT, AND SO IS BEST AVOIDED IN THE EVENING.

INFORMATION

BLENDS WELL WITH SANDALWOOD, JUNIPER, HYSSOP, LAVENDER, ROSEMARY, PINE, LEMON, EUCALYPTUS, MARJORAM.

Melaleuca viridiflora

NIAOULI

Closely related to cajeput and tea tree, niaouli is distilled from the leaves of a large tree grown in Australia and New Caledonia. It is a much more gentle oil than cajeput, and less likely to irritate the skin or mucous membranes. Niaouli, which has a strong medicinal odor, is sometimes labeled as "gomenol."

CAUTION

DILUTE WELL, AS IT MAY IRRITATE THE SKIN OF SOME PEOPLE.

DATA FILE

Properties and Uses

Antiseptic and bactericidal, niaouli is good for cystitis and other urinary infections. A few drops added to cooled boiled water also makes a healing antiseptic wash for cleaning minor wounds, cuts, or burns. Niaouli also stimulates the healing of burns and promotes the growth of new tissue. Oily skin, spots, acne, and insect bites can all be treated in this way. Inhalations of niaouli are helpful in all cases of colds, flu, respiratory, and catarrhal conditions. Added to a good chest rub, this oil helps to alleviate infections and stimulate the immune system. Because it is antispasmodic, niaouli can also benefit digestive problems. It has a general balancing and regulatory effect on body functions.

BELOW *The niaouli tree has pointed linear leaves and spikes of stalkless yellow flowers.*

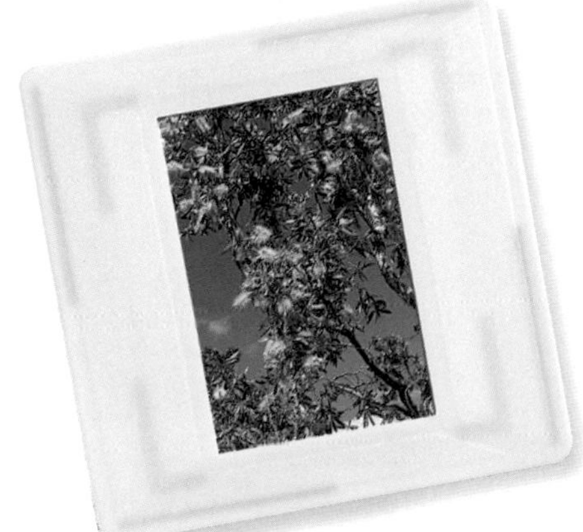

RECIPE

Chest Rub for Coughs

Add 3 drops niaouli, 2 drops hyssop, 1 drop myrrh to 3 teaspoons (15ml.) vegetable oil and rub into the chest.

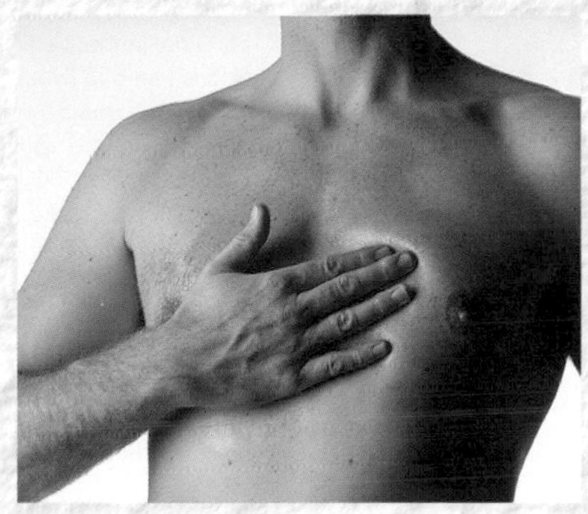

LEFT *A chest rub with niaouli oil will help to clear catarrh*

INFORMATION

BLENDS WELL WITH FRANKINCENSE, BASIL, CLARY SAGE, GERANIUM, LAVENDER, NEROLI, YLANG YLANG, AND OTHER FLORAL AND CITRUS OILS.

Melissa officinalis

LEMON BALM

Melissa, also known as "heart's delight," has been used medicinally since the 17th century. The fresh lemony essential oil is distilled from the leaves and flowering tops. Unfortunately, the plant yields very little essential oil, which is why true melissa is so expensive, and why most commercial melissa oil is adulterated with other lemon oils.

DATA FILE

Properties and Uses

Melissa helps to reduce high blood pressure, and because it also helps to calm palpitations and rapid breathing it is a good remedy for shock. The oil is often used for menstrual problems as it has a calming and regulating effect on the menstrual cycle, helps to ease menstrual cramps, and alleviates scanty menstruation and amenorrhea. Melissa can be used to reduce digestive spasms in colic, nausea, and indigestion. It can be used to relieve migraine and combat fever. Low dilutions can be beneficial for eczema and other skin problems. Allergies affecting the skin and the respiratory system can benefit from its antihistamine properties. Melissa calms the nervous system, relieves anxiety, and has an uplifting effect on the emotions, dispelling sadness and loss, and counteracting hysteria. It also has a general tonic effect on mind and body.

CAUTION

THIS OIL IS SOMETIMES ADULTERATED WITH OTHER LEMON OILS.

ABOVE *The lemon balm herb has bright green, serrated leaves and tiny white or pink flowers.*

INFORMATION

BLENDS WELL WITH LAVENDER, GERANIUM, PATCHOULI, TEA TREE, BERGAMOT, ROSEMARY, HYSSOP, PINE, PETITGRAIN.

RECIPE

Melissa Mind and Body Soother

For frazzled nerves, irritability, and exhaustion, dilute 3 drops melissa, 2 drops chamomile, 2 drops bergamot in 1 teaspoon (5ml.) of sweet almond oil and add to your bath water.

Mentha piperita

PEPPERMINT

Peppermint is best known as a remedy for digestive problems. It was used as such by the Romans and possibly the ancient Egyptians. Apart from its many therapeutic applications it is also used as a humane form of pest control. Peppermint grows throughout Europe, but most oil comes from the U.S.

RECIPE

Footbath for Chilblains

Add 3 drops peppermint, 3 drops lavender, and 5 drops rosemary to a bowl of lukewarm water and soak the feet for at least 10 minutes.

THERAPY CONNECTIONS

PEPPERMINT
Herbalism p.125

BASIL
Ayurveda p.42

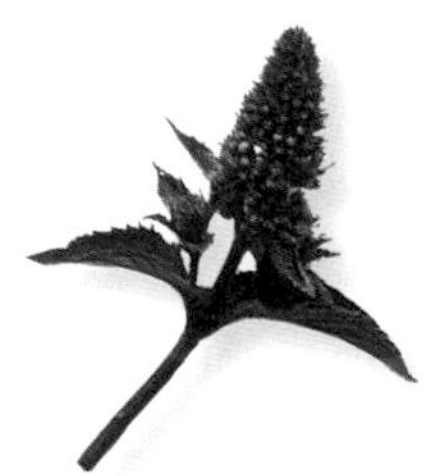

DATA FILE

Properties and Uses

Refreshing and stimulating, peppermint tones and settles the digestive system. It relieves indigestion, flatulence, spasms, diarrhea, nausea, stomach cramps, and travel sickness. It also helps to tone the liver, intestines, and the nervous system. It is a valuable expectorant in the treatment of bronchitis, colds, and flu, and it can reduce fevers by inducing sweating and cooling the body. Peppermint is a painkiller, beneficial for toothache, headaches, and some migraines. It relieves itching, is a useful antiseptic for acne and congested skin, and is an emergency remedy for shock. Muscle and mental fatigue are both relieved by peppermint.

INFORMATION

BLENDS WELL WITH LAVENDER, CHAMOMILE, ROSEMARY, LEMON, EUCALYPTUS, BENZOIN, SANDALWOOD, MARJORAM.

CAUTION

DO NOT USE DURING PREGNANCY.

MAY IRRITATE THE SKIN OF SENSITIVE PEOPLE.

DO NOT USE WHILE TAKING HOMEOPATHIC REMEDIES.

DO NOT USE FOR LONG PERIODS AT A TIME.

RIGHT *The peppermint plant has spikes of pink flowers.*

Ocimum basilicum

BASIL

The Greeks considered basil to be a regal plant. It is also valued and widely used in traditional Chinese and Indian Ayurvedic medicine. There are many varieties of basil, but French basil is the most commonly used in aromatherapy. This uplifting and refreshing oil has a strong spicy-sweet smell that is often most appealing in a blend with other oils.

INFORMATION

BLENDS WELL WITH LAVENDER, BERGAMOT, CEDARWOOD, LEMON, JUNIPER, ROSEMARY, TEA TREE, EUCALYPTUS, GERANIUM, CLARY SAGE, LIME, CITRONELLA.

CAUTION

DO NOT USE DURING PREGNANCY.

MAY IRRITATE PEOPLE WITH SENSITIVE SKIN.

DO NOT USE THE OIL FROM EXOTIC BASIL, WHICH IS SLIGHTLY TOXIC.

RIGHT *Basil is a tender annual herb with a powerful aromatic scent.*

RECIPE

Vaporizer Blend for Migraine

Add 3 drops basil, 4 drops lavender, 3 drops peppermint to vaporizer. Relax in a darkened room and inhale deeply.

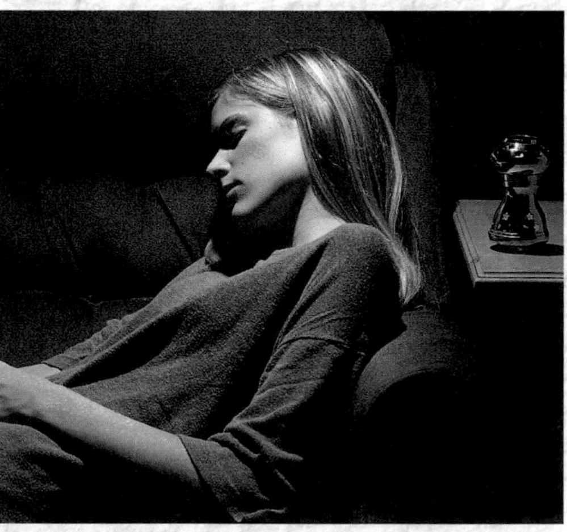

ABOVE *A dark room filled with the aroma of basil oil can bring relief from the misery of migraine.*

DATA FILE

Properties and Uses

Basil is a stimulating and antidepressant oil which relieves mental fatigue, clears the mind, and improves concentration. It is expectorant and antiseptic, used for all types of chest infections, also good for congested sinuses, chronic colds, head colds, and whooping cough. The antispasmodic and carminative properties of basil help to relieve abdominal pains, indigestion, and vomiting. It works well on tired muscles, especially in a massage oil used after hard physical work or strenuous exercise; it also eases arthritis and gout. It is reputed to be one of the best nerve tonics among all essential oils.

Origanum marjorana

SWEET MARJORAM

In ancient times marjoram was reputed to promote longevity, a belief that encouraged the ancient Greeks to include it in perfumes, cosmetics, and medicine. In folk tradition marjoram was believed to bring joy to newlyweds and peace to the dead. The essential oil, with its warm spicy scent, is still used to relieve agitation, dispel grief, and restore calm.

INFORMATION

BLENDS WELL WITH BERGAMOT, CHAMOMILE, FRANKINCENSE, ROSE, SANDALWOOD, LAVENDER, ROSEMARY, CEDARWOOD, JUNIPER, EUCALYPTUS, TEA TREE.

CAUTION

DO NOT USE DURING PREGNANCY.

DATA FILE

Properties and Uses

Marjoram is warming and pain-relieving. It also has antispasmodic properties, making it good for muscle spasms and strains. It is a sedative and nerve tonic which works to relieve nervous tension and promote restful sleep. Inhaling marjoram can help to relieve headaches and migraine. Antiviral and bactericidal properties help to fend off colds and infections, and its expectorant properties make it a useful oil to include in a steam inhalation for chest infections. Massaged into the chest or throat, marjoram can also relieve painful coughs. The oil is a vasodilator which is beneficial in treating high blood pressure and improving circulation. It also calms digestion, strengthens intestinal peristalsis, and eases menstrual cramps. Marjoram is a comforting oil that reduces sexual desire.

RECIPE

Marjoram Cold Cure

Add 4 drops marjoram and 2 drops eucalyptus to a hot bath to relieve cold symptoms, or add 2 drops to 1 teaspoon (5ml.) of vegetable oil and use as a chest rub.

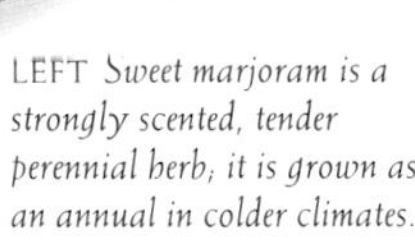

LEFT *Sweet marjoram is a strongly scented, tender perennial herb; it is grown as an annual in colder climates.*

Pelargonium graveolens

GERANIUM

Potted geraniums have a long history of medicinal use. Over 700 varieties exist, and their essential oils differ depending on where the plant is grown. Fresh and floral in fragrance, geranium was traditionally regarded as a feminine oil, a powerful healer, and a valuable insect repellent.

CAUTION

DO NOT USE DURING THE FIRST THREE MONTHS OF PREGNANCY AND NOT AT ALL IF THERE IS A HISTORY OF MISCARRIAGE.

INFORMATION

BLENDS WELL WITH LAVENDER, BERGAMOT, ROSE, ROSEWOOD, SANDALWOOD, PATCHOULI, FRANKINCENSE, LEMON, JASMINE, JUNIPER, TEA TREE, BENZOIN, BASIL, BLACK PEPPER.

ABOVE *Geranium oil is extracted from the leaves, stalk, and flowers of the plant.*

RECIPE

Massage Blend for PMS

Add 10 drops geranium, 10 drops clary sage, 10 drops bergamot to a bottle containing 1 fl. oz. (30ml.) or 6 teaspoons vegetable oil and shake well. Put 6–8 drops in your bath and use a little as a body oil to massage around your abdomen, hips, and lower back.

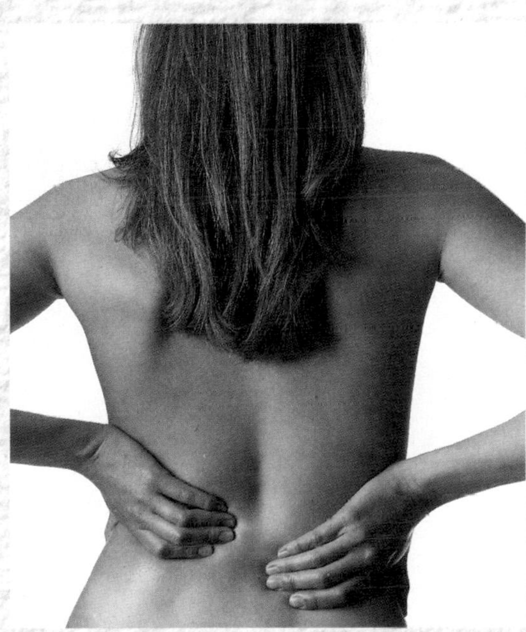

RIGHT *A massage with geranium oil helps to relieve premenstrual pain and tension.*

DATA FILE

Properties and Uses

Geranium is mentally uplifting and refreshing. It has a balancing effect on the nervous system, helping to alleviate apathy, anxiety, stress, hyperactivity, and depression. The anti-inflammatory, soothing, and astringent properties of geranium account for its success in treating arthritis, acne, diaper rash, burns, blisters, eczema, cuts, and congested pores. Antiseptic properties make it useful for cuts and infections, sore throats, and mouth ulcers. It is also a diuretic, used to relieve swollen breasts and fluid retention, and to stimulate sluggish lymph and blood circulation. Geranium helps to stop bleeding, and acts as a tonic for the liver and kidneys. It is used to treat PMS and menopausal problems, and has a balancing effect on mind and body.

Petroselimum sativum

PARSLEY

Common garden parsley is not only rich in vitamins, it also has significant therapeutic properties. The root is used in herbalism for digestive disorders, while the herb and seeds are used mainly for kidney and bladder problems. The essential oil, distilled mainly from the seeds, has a warm, spicy, herbaceous scent.

DATA FILE

Properties and Uses

Used mainly as a diuretic, parsley is good for fluid retention, PMS, and cellulite, and because of its antiseptic effect it also helps with cystitis. Parsley has a tonic effect on the reproductive system. It is sometimes used during labor and it helps to regulate the menstrual cycle. It has the ability to shrink small blood vessels and is helpful in treating piles, broken or thread veins, and bruising. Parsley is also used to stimulate appetite; it has a laxative effect on sluggish digestion, and it relieves flatulence, stomach cramps, and indigestion. Parsley has antirheumatic properties.

RECIPE

Parsley Bath for Water Retention

Add 2 drops parsley, 3 drops geranium, 3 drops fennel to a warm bath and swirl through the water with your hand.

CAUTION

USE IN MODERATION, AS PARSLEY CAN BE TOXIC AND IRRITANT.

DO NOT USE DURING PREGNANCY.

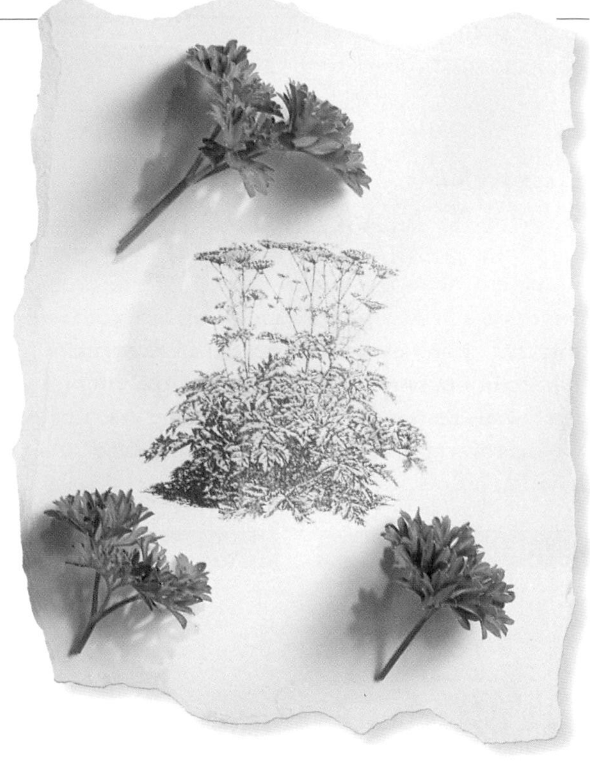

INFORMATION

BLENDS WELL WITH GERANIUM, ROSE, ROSEMARY, LAVENDER, BERGAMOT, LEMON, NEROLI, CLARY SAGE, TEA TREE, SPICE OILS.

ABOVE *Parsley has crinkly green foliage and small greenish-yellow flowers that produce small brown seeds.*

Pinus sylvestris

SCOTCH PINE

Perhaps one of the best-known natural fragrances is the fresh, invigorating aroma of pine. The Arabs, Greeks, and Romans all made use of its medicinal properties, while Native Americans are believed to have used pine to prevent scurvy and infestation with lice and fleas.

CAUTION

USE ONLY SMALL AMOUNTS IN THE BATH OR IN MASSAGE.

DO NOT USE IF YOU HAVE AN ALLERGIC SKIN CONDITION.

ALWAYS CHECK THE SOURCE OF YOUR OIL, AS OILS ARE DISTILLED FROM SEVERAL SPECIES OF PINE, SOME OF WHICH ARE UNSUITABLE FOR USE IN AROMATHERAPY.

INFORMATION

BLENDS WELL WITH LAVENDER, ROSEMARY, CEDARWOOD, EUCALYPTUS, TEA TREE, JUNIPER, SANDALWOOD.

RECIPE

Inhalation for Sinusitis and Stuffy Colds

Add 2 drops pine, 2 drops eucalyptus, 2 drops peppermint to a bowl of steaming hot water. Bend your head over the bowl and cover with a towel to keep in the steam. Inhale for 5–10 minutes. Do this five or six times a day.

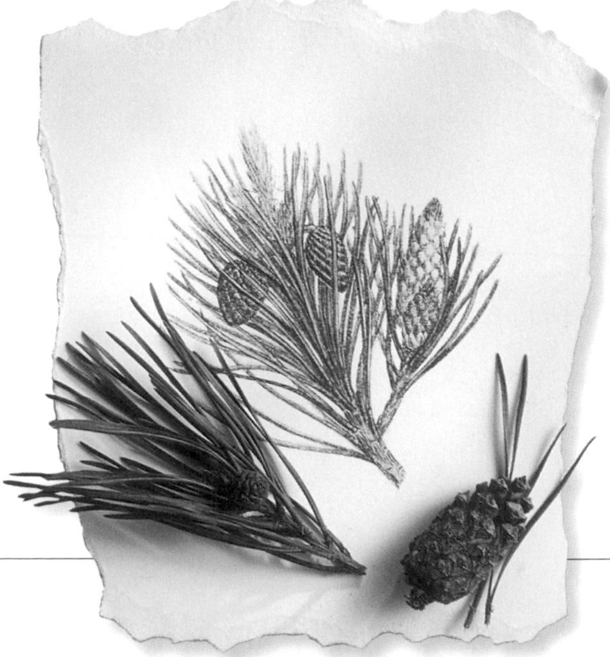

THERAPY CONNECTIONS

PINE
Flower Remedies p.236

BLACK PEPPER
Ayurveda p.44
Traditional Home and Folk Remedies p.97

LEFT *Scotch pine has long, stiff needles that grow in pairs and pointed, brown cones.*

DATA FILE

Properties and Uses

Inhalations of pine are wonderful for colds, catarrhal conditions, including hay fever, and sore throats. The oil, which is expectorant, antiseptic, and antiviral, helps to clear chest infections, sinuses, and ease breathing. Pine stimulates the circulation and helps to relieve rheumatic and muscular aches, pains, and stiffness. Pine is also deodorizing and insecticidal, good for excessive perspiration, and for clearing lice and scabies. The invigorating, refreshing aroma dispels apathy, relieves mental fatigue, nervous exhaustion, and stress-related problems.

Piper nigrum

BLACK PEPPER

Best known for its use in cooking, black pepper also has a 4,000-year-old medicinal history. Prized by the Chinese, the Romans, and the Greeks, pepper was one of the earliest spices ever used. The spicy-scented essential oil is extracted from dried, crushed black peppercorns.

RECIPE

Compress for Painful Joints

Add 3 drops black pepper, 2 drops chamomile, 2 drops marjoram to a bowl of hot or cold water and apply to the affected area as directed.

ABOVE *The berries of the pepper vine turn from red to black as they mature.*

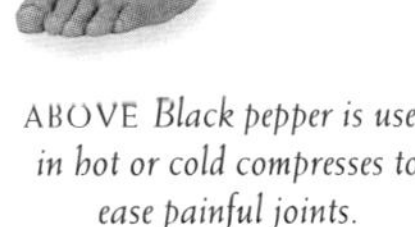

ABOVE *Black pepper is used in hot or cold compresses to ease painful joints.*

DATA FILE

Properties and Uses

Black pepper stimulates the nervous, digestive, and circulatory systems, which makes it good for poor circulation, constipation, sluggish digestion, and drowsiness. It also has a laxative effect, tones the muscles of the colon, soothes the stomach, helps to prevent food poisoning, and stimulates the appetite. As a rubefacient it helps with rheumatic and arthritic pain, poor muscle tone, and muscular aches and pains. It helps the immune system fight off infections and viruses, warms against chills, and as an expectorant it clear mucus from the chest. Black pepper helps prevent anemia and is credited with aphrodisiac properties.

CAUTION

DILUTE WELL WHEN USING ON THE SKIN.

DO NOT USE WHILE TAKING HOMEOPATHIC REMEDIES.

INFORMATION

BLENDS WELL WITH FRANKINCENSE, LAVENDER, ROSEMARY, MARJORAM, LAVENDER, LEMON, BENZOIN, CEDARWOOD, PARSLEY, FENNEL, SPICES, AND FLORALS.

Pogostemon cablin

PATCHOULI

The distinctive exotic and earthy aroma of patchouli is one that you either love or hate. Smell is important to the success of aromatherapy, so only use this oil if you like its scent. Patchouli has many uses, and is especially pleasant when used as part of a blend. It is an intense odor, which improves with age.

ABOVE *Patchouli is a perennial herb with large, fragrant, furry leaves.*

RIGHT *The oil extracted from dried patchouli leaves is good for aging skin.*

CAUTION

KEEP ALL ESSENTIAL OILS OUT OF THE REACH OF CHILDREN.

INFORMATION

BLENDS WELL WITH ROSE, GERANIUM, BERGAMOT, NEROLI, YLANG YLANG, LEMON, SANDALWOOD, CLARY SAGE, CLOVE, CEDARWOOD, LAVENDER.

RECIPE

Antiwrinkle Night Oil

Add 2 drops patchouli, 3 drops lemon, 5 drops rose to 2 drops evening primrose oil and 1 teaspoon (10ml.) sweet almond or hazelnut oil. Blend well and apply to the face and neck at night.

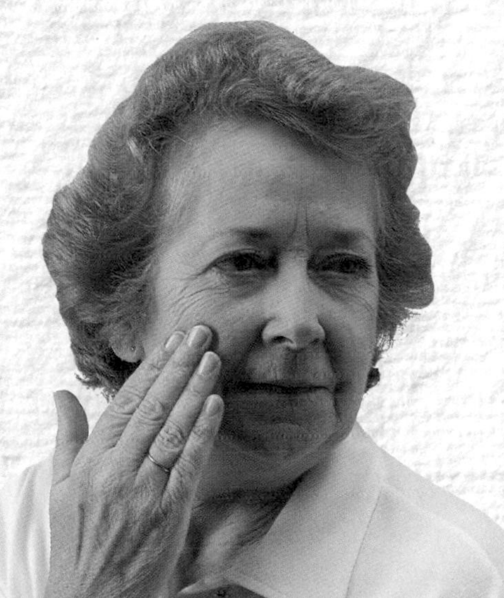

DATA FILE

Properties and Uses

An important anti-depressant, nervous tonic, and reputedly an aphrodisiac, patchouli is valued in treating depression, anxiety, nervous exhaustion, lack of interest in sex, and stress-related problems. It is astringent, anti-viral, antiseptic, and anti-inflammatory, good for chapped or cracked skin and open pores, and is also effective for acne, eczema, and dermatitis. It is one of the best choices for dandruff and fungal infections of the skin. It is a cell regenerator, good for aging skins, and it promotes wound-healing. Patchouli acts as a diuretic. It is often recommended for cellulite and as a general tonic.

Rosa centifolia, Rosa damascena

ROSE

Most of the rose oil used in aromatherapy is produced from two types of rose. They vary slightly in color and fragrance, but have similar properties and uses. Rose oil is expensive, but you need only use a little of this complex oil to reap the benefits.

DATA FILE

Properties and Uses

A renowned aphrodisiac, sedative, and a tonic with antidepressant properties, rose has an affinity with the female reproductive system, helping to regulate the menstrual cycle and alleviate PMS or post-natal depression. It benefits stress-related conditions such as insomnia and nervous tension, and is a powerful antiseptic against viruses and bacteria. Rose oil acts as a tonic for the heart, circulation, liver, stomach, and uterus, and helps to detoxify the blood and organs. It regulates the appetite, and prevents and relieves digestive spasms, constipation, and nausea. It soothes cracked, chapped, sensitive, dry, inflamed, or allergy-prone skin, stops bleeding, and encourages wound-healing. Broken veins, and aging or wrinkled skin also benefit. Rose is also useful in treating headaches, earache, conjunctivitis, coughs, and hay fever.

THERAPY CONNECTIONS

ROSE
Flower Remedies p.238

ROSEMARY
Herbalism p.127

SANDALWOOD
Ayurveda p.44

RECIPE

Comforting Massage Blend for Grief

Add 4 drops rose, 2 drops frankincense, 4 drops chamomile to 3 teaspoons (15ml.) sweet almond or grapeseed oil.

INFORMATION

BLENDS WELL WITH MOST OILS, ESPECIALLY CLARY SAGE, LAVENDER, SANDALWOOD, GERANIUM, BERGAMOT, PATCHOULI, YLANG YLANG.

BELOW *The healing virtues of the rose have been known since antiquity.*

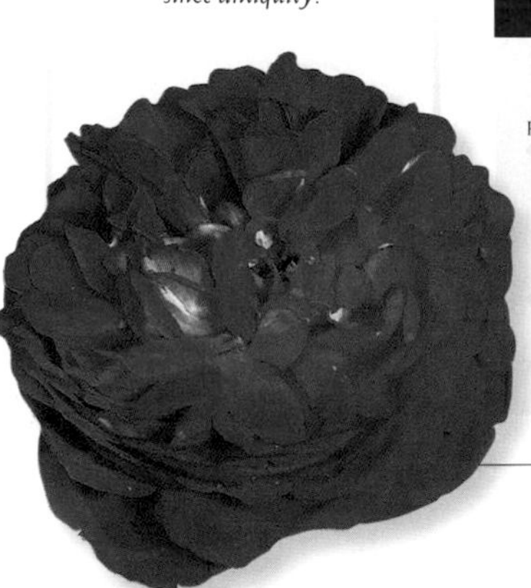

CAUTION

DO NOT USE DURING THE FIRST THREE MONTHS OF PREGNANCY AND NOT AT ALL IF THERE IS A HISTORY OF MISCARRIAGE.

CAUTION

DO NOT USE DURING PREGNANCY.

ROSEMARY IS NOT SUITABLE FOR PEOPLE WITH EPILEPSY OR HIGH BLOOD PRESSURE.

Rosmarinus officinalis

ROSEMARY

Rosemary was one of the first herbs to be used medicinally. Traditionally it was used to ward off evil, to offer protection from the plague, and to preserve and flavor meat. This strong distinctively scented oil is one of the most valuable of all essential oils.

RIGHT *Rosemary is an aromatic, evergreen bush, with silvery green leaves and pale blue flowers. The oil is usually extracted from fresh flowering tops.*

RECIPE

After-sport Shower Formula

Add 2 drops rosemary, 2 drops pine, 4 drops lemon to a large dollop of a gentle, unscented shower gel. Step into a hot shower and work into a lather using a sponge or flannel.

INFORMATION

BLENDS WELL WITH FRANKINCENSE, PETITGRAIN, BASIL, THYME, BERGAMOT, LAVENDER, PEPPERMINT, PINE, CEDARWOOD, CYPRESS, SPICE OILS SUCH AS CINNAMON, CLOVE, GINGER, AND BLACK PEPPER.

DATA FILE

Properties and Uses

Refreshing rosemary is a circulation stimulant, excellent for low blood pressure, muscle fatigue, poor circulation, aches, pains, and strains. It acts as a tonic for the nervous system and is anti-depressant. It relieves stress-related disorders, mental exhaustion, and promotes mental clarity. It also tones the skin, liver, and gall bladder. It is used for acne, eczema, dandruff, lice, and hair loss. Antiseptic and antibacterial, antifungal, and a diuretic, it is generally cleansing, and useful for fluid retention. It has properties that help to relieve painful menstruation and clear vaginal discharge, flatulence, indigestion, and constipation. Rosemary prevents and reduces digestive spasms, relieves wind, and regulates digestion. It helps to clear catarrh, coughs, colds, and headaches.

BELOW *Rosemary oil's stimulating effect on the circulatory system makes it an ideal remedy for muscle fatigue.*

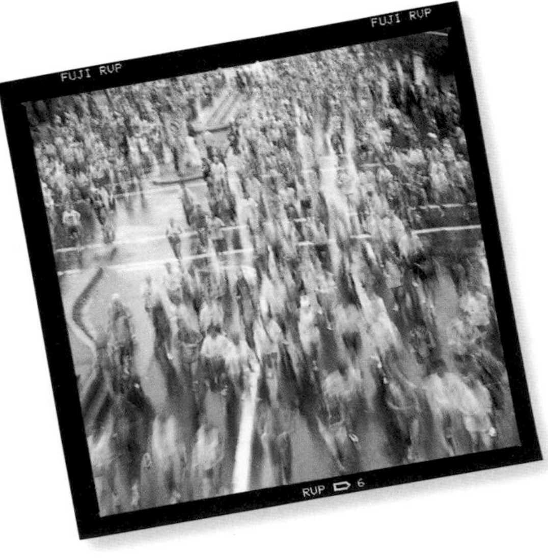

Salvia sclarea

CLARY SAGE

Affectionately known as "clear eye," clary sage was used in medieval times for clearing foreign bodies from the eyes. It remains popular in aromatherapy because of its gentle action and pleasant nutty fragrance. The oil is extracted from the flowering tops and leaves.

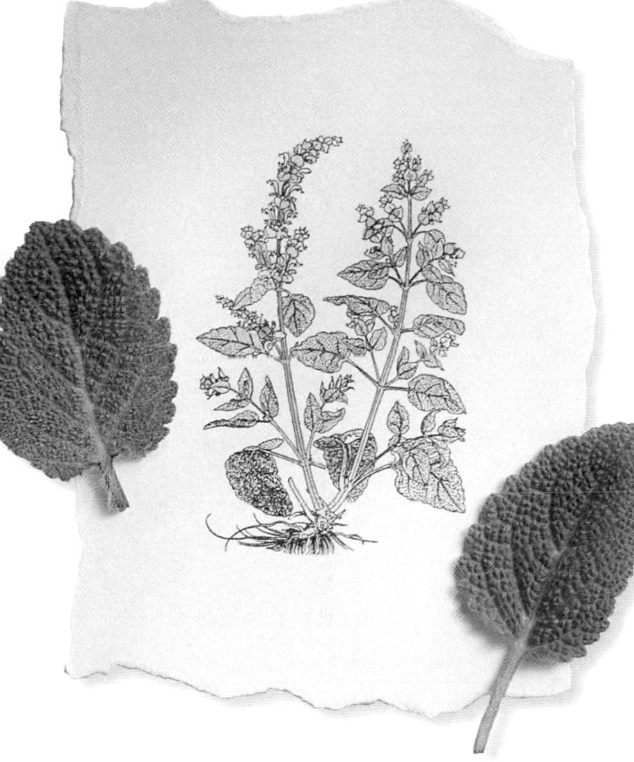

ABOVE *Clary sage is a biennial or perennial herb with large, hairy leaves, green with a hint of purple, and small blue flowers.*

DATA FILE

Properties and Uses

Clary is antidepressant, and sometimes described as euphoric. It helps to regulate the nervous system and is most beneficial in treating anxiety, depression, and stress-related problems. It acts as a powerful muscle relaxant, helping to ease muscular aches and pains, and benefits digestion, relieving indigestion and flatulence. Its astringent properties make it useful for oily skin and scalp conditions. Clary helps to prevent and arrest convulsions. It is antibacterial, and useful for throat and respiratory infections. Clary helps to lower blood pressure. It is recommended for absent or scanty menstruation and PMS, and is a renowned aphrodisiac that can benefit frigidity and impotence.

CAUTION

DO NOT USE DURING PREGNANCY.

DO NOT USE WHEN DRINKING ALCOHOL, AS IT CAN MAKE YOU DRUNK, DROWSY, AND CAN CAUSE NIGHTMARES.

INFORMATION

BLENDS WELL WITH LAVENDER, FRANKINCENSE, SANDALWOOD, CEDARWOOD, CITRUS OILS SUCH AS LEMON, ORANGE, AND BERGAMOT, GERANIUM, YLANG YLANG, JUNIPER, CORIANDER.

RECIPE

Premenstrual Bath Blend

Add 3 drops clary sage, 2 drops chamomile, 2 drops geranium to a warm bath, disperse with your hand, and relax for at least 10 minutes.

Santalum album

SANDALWOOD

The sweet, woody, oriental smell of sandalwood is one of the most appealing fragrances of all essential oils. The best sandalwood oil comes from India, where it has been used for at least 4,000 years for medicinal and religious purposes.

DATA FILE

Properties and Uses

Sandalwood is an antiseptic, especially effective for all urinary disorders, above all cystitis. It is bactericidal, astringent, and a trusted insect repellent. It clears catarrh and is effective for respiratory conditions such as bronchitis, dry coughs, and sore throats. The oil contains constituents that soothe the stomach, reduce digestive spasms, relieve fluid retention, and reduce inflammation. Sandalwood encourages wound-healing, and skin problems such as dry, chapped skin, acne, psoriasis, eczema, and shaving rash can all benefit from its soothing, rehydrating and antiseptic action. It is an anti-depressant oil that calms the nervous system. The fragrance can also help to lift depression and banish feelings of anxiety and lack of sexual desire.

BELOW *Sandalwood oil is extracted from the powdered and dried roots and heartwood of this small evergreen tree.*

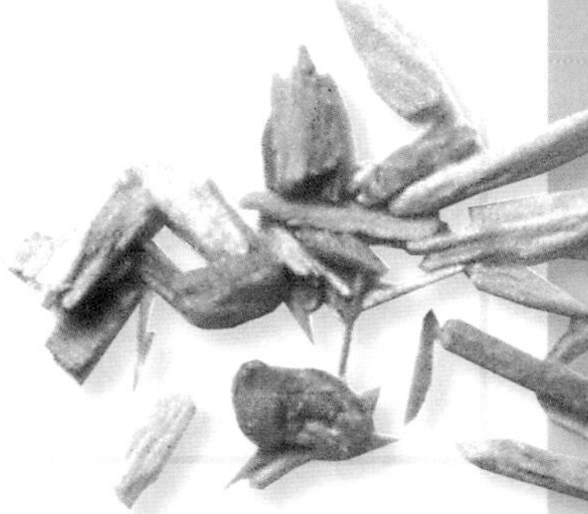

CAUTION

DO NOT USE UNDILUTED ON THE SKIN.

RECIPE

Aftershave Soother

Add 4 drops sandalwood, 6 drops benzoin, 4 drops chamomile to a bottle containing 4 teaspoons (20ml.) hazelnut oil. Warm a tiny amount in your hands and smooth into the face after shaving.

INFORMATION

BLENDS WELL WITH LAVENDER, ROSE, YLANG YLANG, GERANIUM, CHAMOMILE, PATCHOULI, BERGAMOT, FRANKINCENSE, BLACK PEPPER, BENZOIN, TEA TREE, JUNIPER, MYRRH, CYPRESS.

LEFT *Sandalwood is often used to fragrance cosmetics but its essential oil has the added benefit when used in aftershave of soothing the skin.*

Styrax benzoin

BENZOIN

Benzoin has been used in the East since antiquity as a medicine and as incense. It came into use in the West in the Middle Ages as a remedy for respiratory complaints. The oil, which has a sweet vanilla-like scent, is extracted from the resin of the tropical benzoin tree. It is not strictly an essential oil, but a resinoid dissolved in alcohol.

CAUTION

CAN CAUSE IRRITATION IN SOME SENSITIVE INDIVIDUALS.

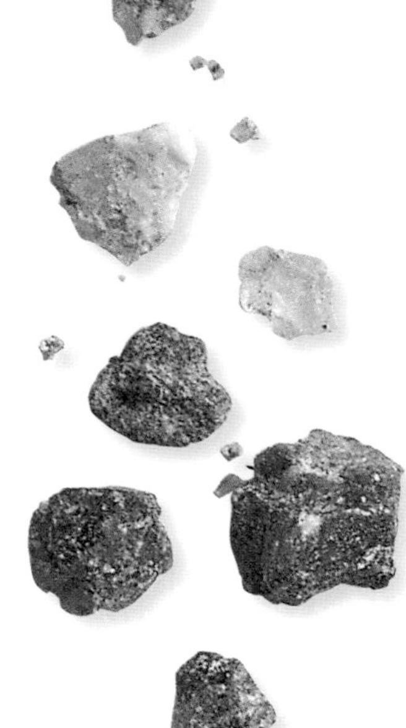

RIGHT *Crude benzoin is collected from the tree directly and made into benzoin resinoid using solvents, which are then removed.*

DATA FILE

Properties and Uses

Warming and decongestant, benzoin is helpful for colds and flu, and for clearing mucus from the system. Inhaled, it can soothe sore throats and help to restore a lost voice. Benzoin blended with cream or oil and rubbed into the skin soothes chapped or irritated skin on the hands, as well as cuts and skin inflammation. As a diuretic and antiseptic, benzoin is good for urinary tract infections. It also stimulates the circulation, and its anti-inflammatory action helps to alleviate arthritis and rheumatism. Benzoin is emotionally calming in a crisis, warming and comforting in times of loneliness, and helps to dispel depression, anxiety, and nervous tension.

RECIPE

Warming Winter Bath

Add 2 drops benzoin, 3 drops marjoram, 2 drops clary sage to a warm bath. Disperse with your hand, close the bathroom door to keep in the steam, and soak for at least 10 minutes.

INFORMATION

BLENDS WELL WITH SANDALWOOD, LEMON, ROSE, JUNIPER, MYRRH, FRANKINCENSE, JASMINE, CYPRESS, SPICE OILS.

RIGHT *Creams and oils containing benzoin help to soothe chapped skin and treat inflamed and irritated skin conditions.*

Thymus vulgaris

THYME

One of the most useful medicinal herbs in natural healthcare, thyme was also one of the first plants to be used for its healing properties. The oil, distilled from the leaves and tiny purple flowering tops of this sub-shrub, has a fresh green scent.

CAUTION

DILUTE WELL, AS THYME MAY CAUSE IRRITATION AND SENSITIZATION IN SOME PEOPLE.

DO NOT USE IF YOU HAVE HIGH BLOOD PRESSURE.

AVOID DURING PREGNANCY.

DO NOT USE IF YOU ARE TAKING HOMEOPATHIC REMEDIES.

DATA FILE

Properties and Uses

Thyme is antiseptic and antibiotic, disinfectant, and strongly germicidal. It is valuable for all infections, especially gastric and bladder infections, as it also has digestive and diuretic properties. The oil's antirheumatic and antitoxic properties are beneficial in treating arthritis, gout, and cellulite. Rubefacient and stimulant actions also help with muscle and joint pain, and poor circulation. Thyme stimulates the immune system to effectively fight off colds, flu, and catarrh, and ease coughing. The diluted oil is good for cleaning wounds, burns, bruises, and clearing lice. Used as a mouthwash it helps to soothe and heal abscesses and gum infections. Thyme has an uplifting fragrance, which can relieve depression, headaches, and stress.

RECIPE

Antiseptic Mouthwash

Add 10 drops thyme, 15 drops peppermint, 5 drops fennel, and 5 drops myrrh to a bottle containing 4fl.oz. (125ml.) of cheap brandy. Shake well and add 2 teaspoons (10ml.) of the mix to a glass of warm water. Rinse the mouth thoroughly, but do not swallow.

INFORMATION

BLENDS WELL WITH LEMON, BERGAMOT, ROSEMARY, LEMON BALM, LAVENDER, PINE, BLACK PEPPER, TEA TREE, LIME, CEDARWOOD, GRAPEFRUIT.

RIGHT *Thyme was used by the ancient Egyptians in the embalming process and by the ancient Greeks to fumigate against infectious diseases.*

Vetiveria zizanioides

VETIVER

In India and Sri Lanka, where vetiver grows, the essential oil is known as "the oil of tranquility." The tall grass is also cultivated in other countries, and the essential oil is distilled from the dried roots. The deep, smoky, earthy aroma of vetiver is wonderfully grounding and relaxing.

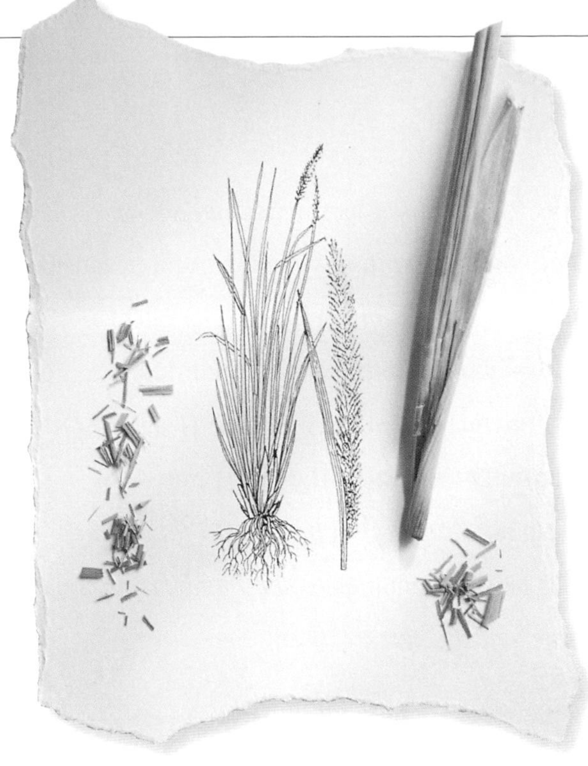

RIGHT *Vetiver is a tall, tufted, perennial, scented grass with straight stems and long, narrow leaves.*

DATA FILE

Properties and Uses

Valued most for its sedative properties, vetiver is used in massage and in baths to relieve stress, anxiety, nervous tension, and insomnia. It also helps to ground people who live too much in their head, or who need to feel stable after shock or a period of insecurity. Vetiver is a circulation stimulant and rubefacient, so it can provide relief from arthritis or rheumatism, and general muscular aches and pains. It is useful in skin care as an antiseptic, tonic, and detoxifier. It helps to clear acne, and because it promotes skin regeneration and strengthens the connective tissue, it assists with wound-healing and benefits aging skin.

THERAPY CONNECTIONS

THYME
Herbalism p.135

VETIVER
Ayurveda p.46

GINGER
Ayurveda p.47
Chinese Herbal Medicine p.57

INFORMATION

BLENDS WELL WITH JASMINE, CEDARWOOD, LAVENDER, SANDALWOOD, ROSE, YLANG YLANG, CLARY SAGE, PETITGRAIN, MANDARIN.

CAUTION

KEEP OUT OF THE EYES.

DO NOT TAKE INTERNALLY.

KEEP AWAY FROM CHILDREN.

RECIPE

Tranquility Bath Oil

Add 2 drops vetiver, 2 drops lavender, 4 drops rose to 2 teaspoons (10ml.) of sweet almond oil. Add to a running bath and disperse with your hand. Relax for at least 10 minutes.

Zingiber officinale

GINGER

Originally from India and China, warm, spicy ginger is now grown commercially throughout the tropics. It is a perennial herb with a thick, rhizomatus root. It has been used both to flavor food, and in medicine, for thousands of years, particularly by the Chinese. The essential oil distilled from the root smells similar to fresh root ginger.

CAUTION

USE SPARINGLY, AS HIGH CONCENTRATIONS OF GINGER CAN CAUSE IRRITATION IN SENSITIVE PEOPLE.

DO NOT USE IN EXCESSIVELY HOT OR INFLAMED CONDITIONS.

INFORMATION

BLENDS WELL WITH ROSE, CEDARWOOD, ROSEWOOD, FRANKINCENSE, VETIVER, PATCHOULI, PETITGRAIN, NEROLI, LIME, AND OTHER CITRUS OILS.

RECIPE

Ginger Throat Gargle

Add 2 drops of ginger oil to 1 teaspoon (5ml.) of vodka and dilute with hot water. When it has cooled sufficiently, use it as a gargle for a sore throat.

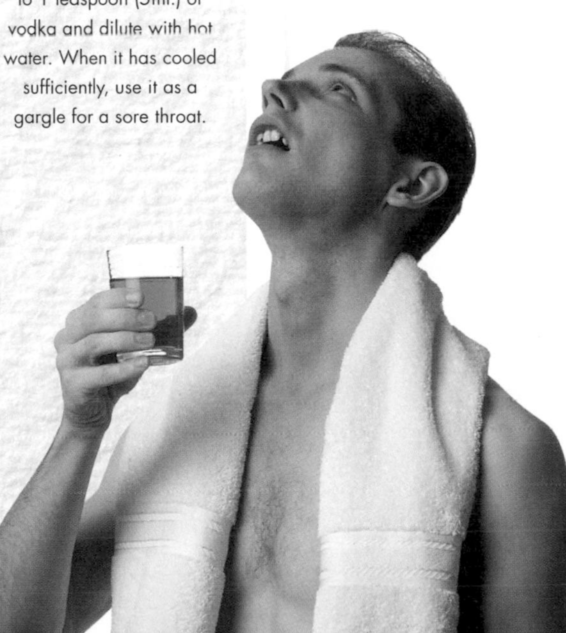

RIGHT *Ginger is used to prevent and treat colds and sore throats.*

DATA FILE

Properties and Uses

Ginger is a rubefacient which can effectively ease painful conditions such as arthritis, rheumatism, or muscle pain, and improve poor circulation. Massaged around the stomach and abdomen, diluted ginger calms the digestion, tones and soothes the stomach, and stimulates the appetite. It helps to alleviate nausea, travel sickness, indigestion, pain, and diarrhea. Ginger is pain-relieving, antiseptic, and antioxidant, valuable for preventing and treating colds, sore throats, and catarrhal congestion. It also eases coughing, and because it promotes sweating, it can be useful for flu. When inhaled, the warming ginger essence eases mental confusion, and helps to relieve fatigue and nervous exhaustion.

HOMEOPATHY

Homeopathy works by treating a person as a whole, or holistically, so although presenting symptoms will be looked at, the individual person – his or her mental, physical, emotional, and spiritual health – will be taken into account, too. Homeopathy is based on the principle that "like cures like" (from the Latin similia similibus curentur), meaning the treatment given is similar in substance to the illness it is helping. Although it has roots that go back many centuries, it began in its present form a mere two hundred years ago and today is popular as a safe and effective treatment.

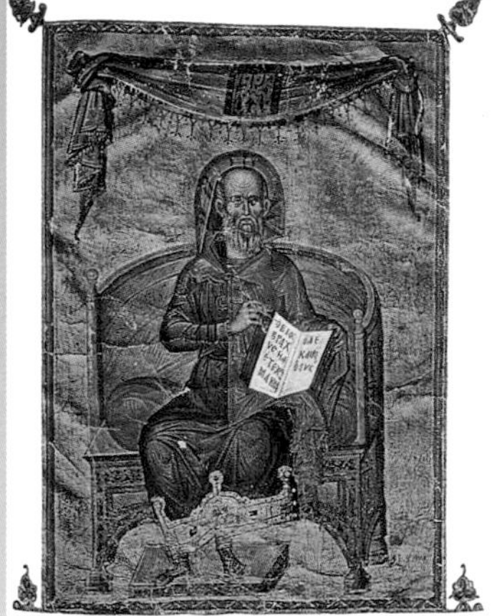

ABOVE *The Ancient Greek physician Hippocrates, whose theories had similarities with those of homeopathy.*

BELOW *Medical practices in the 18th century involved debilitating blood-letting as well as harsh drugs.*

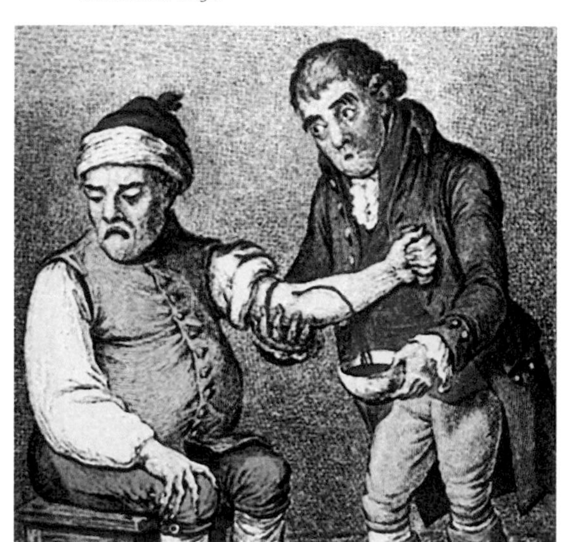

THE ORIGINS OF HOMEOPATHY

It was the Greek physician Hippocrates, known as the "father of medicine," who, in the 5th century B.C.E., was the first to understand the principle of treating the body with a remedy which will produce similar symptoms to the ailment suffered. He also believed that symptoms specific to an individual, that person's reactions to an ailment, and a person's own powers of healing were important in diagnosing and choosing a cure. On this basis, he built up his own medicine chest of homeopathic remedies. But it was the German physician Samuel Hahnemann (1755–1843) who first developed homeopathy as it is known and practised today. A prominent physician, chemist, and author, Hahnemann had become increasingly disillusioned with the methods of treatment of the day. These included harsh practices such as blood-letting and purging, and large doses of medicines that were often more debilitating than the illness itself. Yet it was obvious these practices were not working – disease was rampant. Hahnemann was one of the first physicians to advocate the improvement of poor hygiene, both in the home and in public places, and he stressed the importance of a good diet, fresh air, and higher standards of living for all. But disillusionment with the lack of response to his initiatives meant that he eventually decided to give up medical practice. In 1789, he moved to Leipzig where he became a translator of medical texts.

HOMEOPATHY V. ALLOPATHY

Homeopathy works on the principle of stimulating the body's defense mechanism by treating it with minute doses of a substance that produces symptoms similar to those of the illness. Allopathic, or conventional, treatment works by suppressing symptoms, so that diarrhea is treated by a substance that causes constipation and insomnia is treated with sedatives.

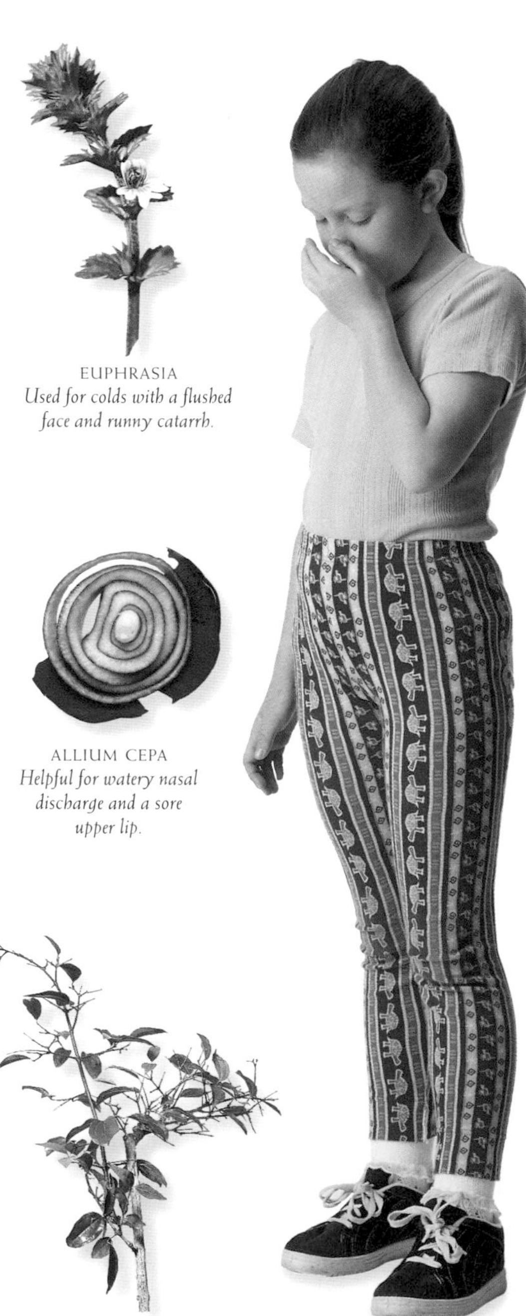

EUPHRASIA
Used for colds with a flushed face and runny catarrh.

ALLIUM CEPA
Helpful for watery nasal discharge and a sore upper lip.

NUX VOMICA
May be prescribed for patients who have a blocked nose at night and a runny nose during the day.

THE COMMON COLD
There are various possible homeopathic remedies for the common cold and the homeopath will select the most appropriate one in each case.

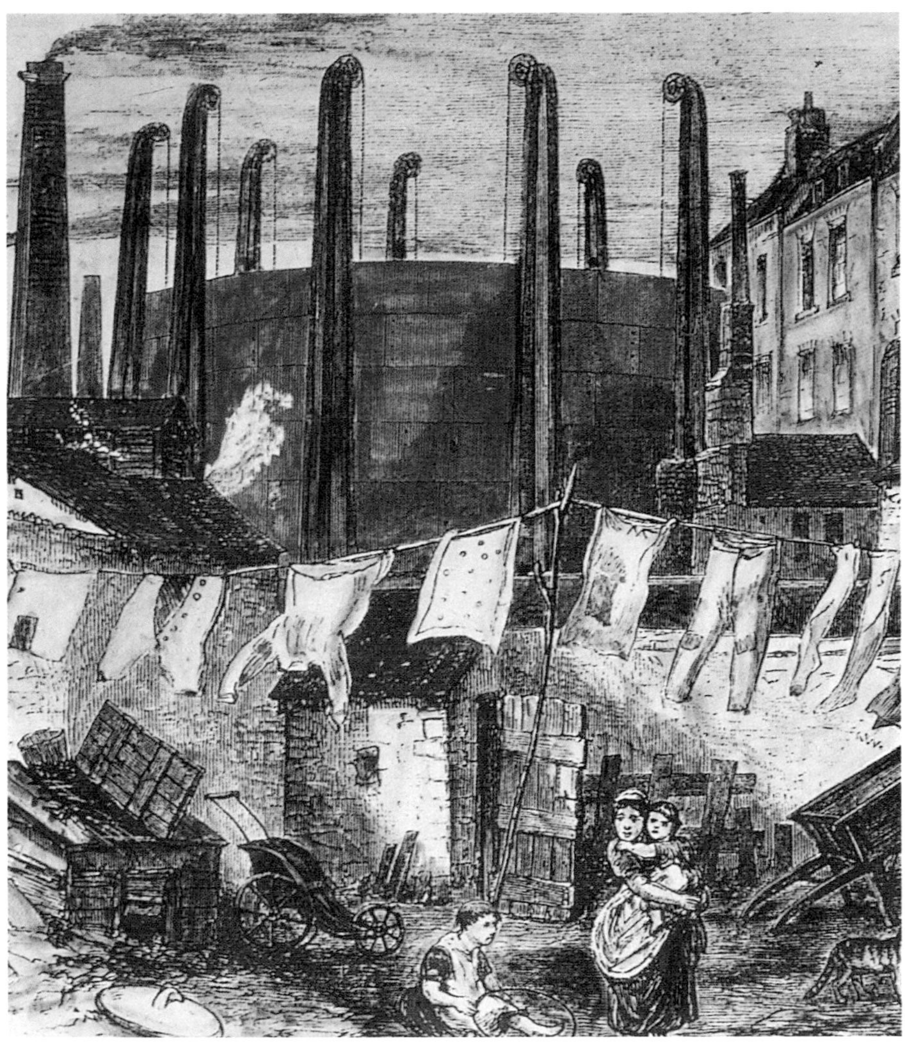

ABOVE *As Hippocrates had shown many centuries earlier, Hahnemann saw that the patient's circumstances can both cause and exacerbate disease.*

BELOW *Dr. William Cullen, a Scottish physician whose observations about the therapeutic effects of quinine stimulated Hahnemann's homeopathic experiments.*

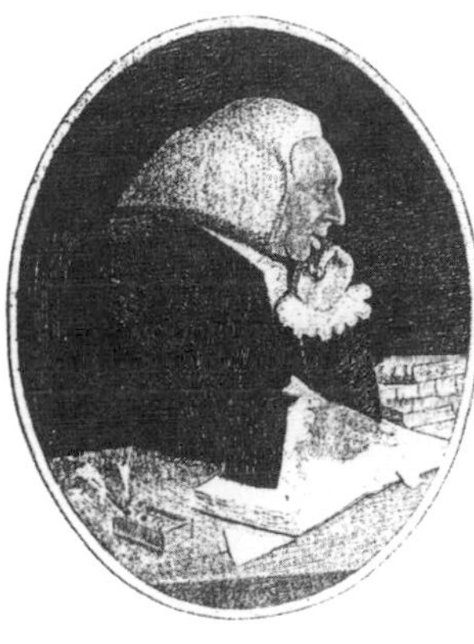

While translating one of these texts in 1790, *A Treatise on Materia Medica,* by Dr. William Cullen of London University, Hahnemann noticed an entry which was to set him on a path which would lead to the founding of homeopathic practice.

Cullen wrote that quinine (an extract of Peruvian bark) was an effective treatment for malaria because of its astringent qualities. As a chemist, Hahnemann knew quinine was effective against the disease, but doubted this was due to its astringency. He decided to explore this further and for days took doses of quinine himself and recorded his reactions. He found that he developed all the symptoms of malaria – palpitating heart, irregular pulse, drowsiness, and thirst – although he did not have the disease. Each time he took a new dose, the symptoms recurred. He speculated that it was the quinine's ability to induce the malarial symptoms that made it effective as a treatment. To back up his theory, he gave doses of quinine to volunteers, whom he called "provings," recorded their reactions, and found similar results.

A PICTURE OF SYMPTOMS

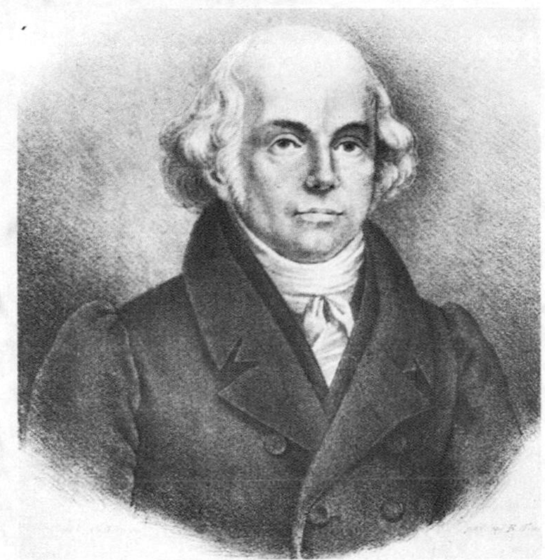

ABOVE *Samuel Hahnemann (1755–1843), who founded the system of homeopathy.*

Hahnemann experimented with other substances, as well as quinine, which were used as medicines at the time, such as arsenic, belladonna, and mercury. With each new substance given, he noted that individuals differed in their severity of symptoms and how they healed. Some showed few symptoms, while others suffered badly.

He found that some symptoms were commonly found after giving a substance. He called these first-line, or keynote, symptoms. The less common symptoms he called second-line and those that were more rare he called third-line symptoms. The combination of all these types of symptoms enabled him to build up a "drug picture" for each substance that he tested.

Following this, Hahnemann then went on to develop a "symptoms picture" of his patients. This included a physical examination, questions about their symptoms and general health, what made them feel better or worse, their likes and dislikes, and their lifestyle. He found that the more information he had about the patient, the more accurately he could match up the symptom picture to the remedy picture before prescribing, and therefore the more successful the eventual treatment. Hahnemann believed he had developed a new system of medicine, a system that worked on the principle that a substance and a disease that produce similar symptoms can negate each other, resulting in the full health of the patient. He called his new system "homeopathy," from the Greek words *homios*, meaning like, and *pathos*, meaning suffering.

WHAT IS HOMEOPATHY?

PREPARING THE REMEDIES

Homeopathic remedies are prepared in stages, involving repeated dilution and succussion over several days or even weeks.

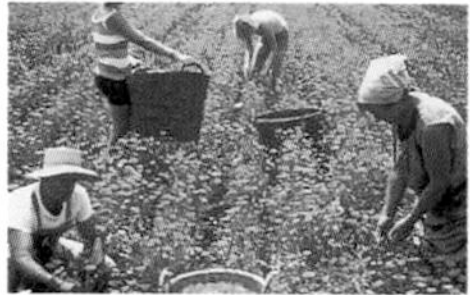

INGREDIENTS
Many remedies are prepared from plant material. After harvesting, the ingredients are steeped in alcohol to produce a tincture, which is then repeatedly diluted.

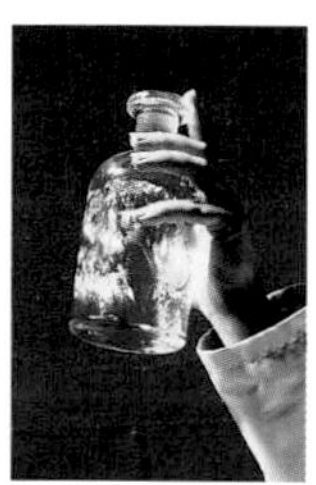

SUCCUSSION
Each time the tincture is further diluted it is subjected to succussion (vibration or shaking) to release its potency.

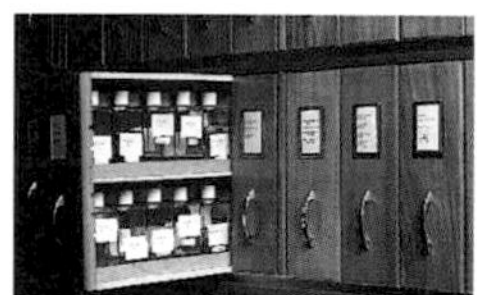

DISPENSARY
The dilution and succussion may be repeated up to 30 times to make a remedy of greater potency. The remedies are stored in sealed dark glass bottles in the dispensary.

The efficacy of homeopathy is proven by the popularity it has across the world, the number of practitioners and hospitals dedicated to homeopathic care, and the clinical trials that have been undertaken. Even so, it can be difficult to understand exactly how the principles of homeopathy actually work in practice, leading some modern doctors to remain skeptical about its effectiveness.

WHAT IS HOMEOPATHY?

From Hahnemann's first experiment with quinine, he went on to prove the efficacy of around 100 homeopathic remedies. There are now more than 2,000 available, with new ones continually being added. The remedies are made from animal, vegetable, and mineral sources, which are as varied as honey bees (including the sting), snake venom, and poison ivy leaves, onions, coffee beans, and daisies. But the amounts used are so minute that no substance can be tasted or side effects experienced, however poisonous or toxic the substance might be.

In his provings, Hahnemann had been worried by some patients who got worse before they got better after taking the substances given to them. To prevent this happening, he developed a new system of diluting the remedies. He diluted each remedy and then "successed" or shook it. He believed that doing this released the energy of the substance. He found not only that the new system of diluting prevented the worsening of symptoms, but also, to his astonishment, that the more diluted the substance, the better its effects. He called this method "potentization."

BELOW *Homeopathic remedies are usually offered as pills or powders, so they are very easy to take.*

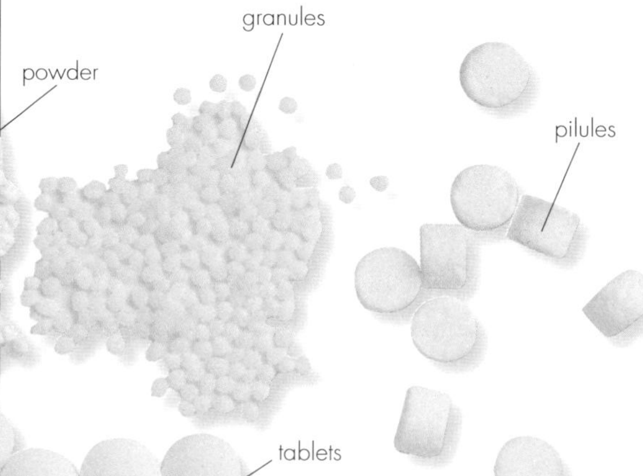

REMEDY SOURCES

Many of the ingredients used to make homeopathic remedies would be extremely harmful if ingested in their crude form. As well as plant material, substances of animal and mineral origin are used.

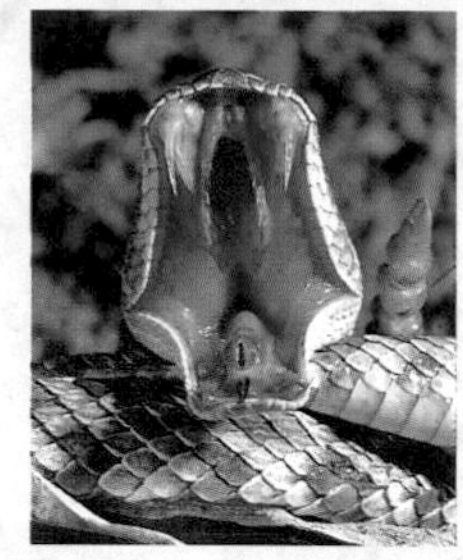

SNAKE VENOM
The venom of the North American rattlesnake is used to make a remedy known as Crotalis horridus, *used for shock and festering wounds.*

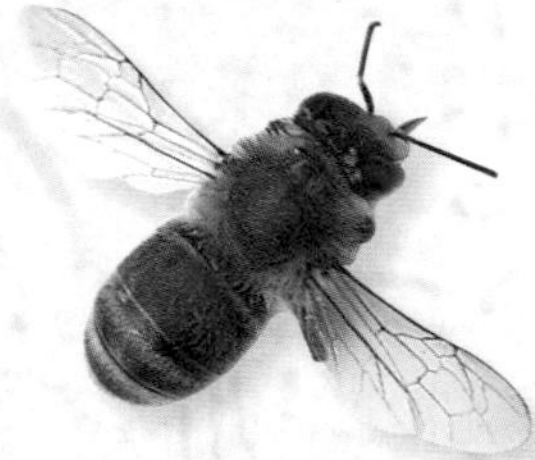

HONEY BEE
Whole bees and their stings are used to produce a remedy known as Apis mellifica. *This can be helpful in treating patients with rashes, especially where there is burning or stinging.*

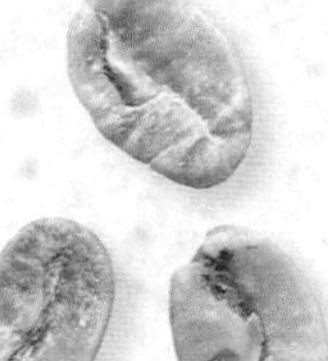

COFFEE
Coffee beans are used in the preparation of Coffea. This treats people who are mentally and physically overactive for any reason.

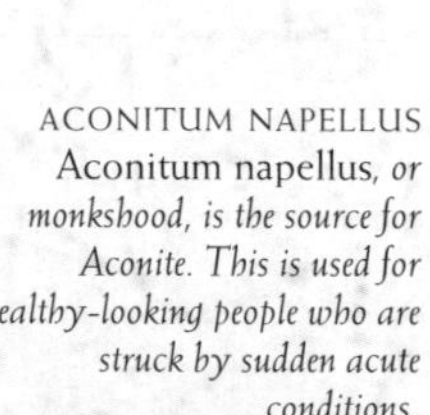

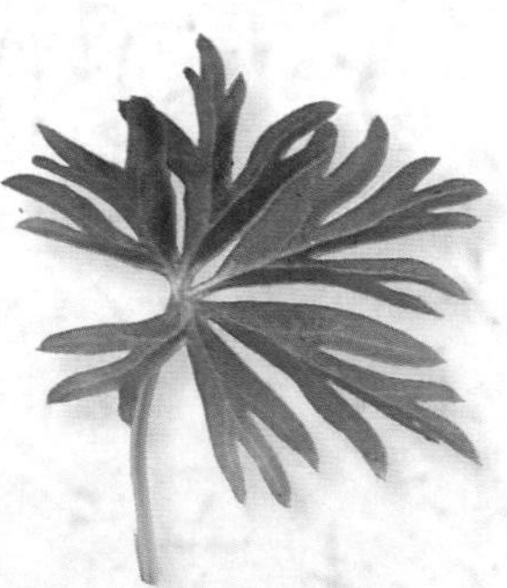

ACONITUM NAPELLUS
Aconitum napellus, *or monkshood, is the source for Aconite. This is used for healthy-looking people who are struck by sudden acute conditions.*

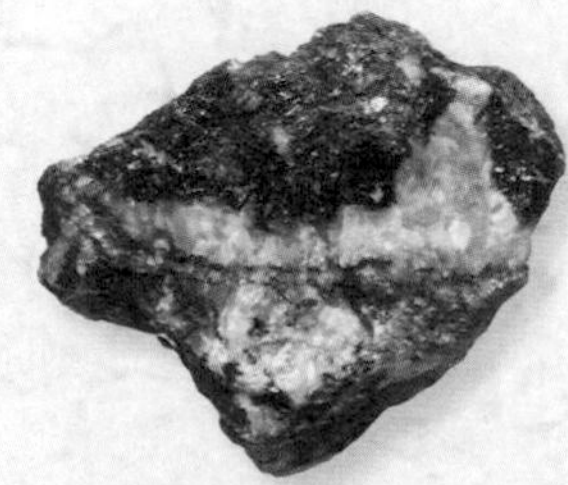

COPPER
Mineral sources include copper, which can be used to treat spasms, cramps, and convulsions.

DILUTION

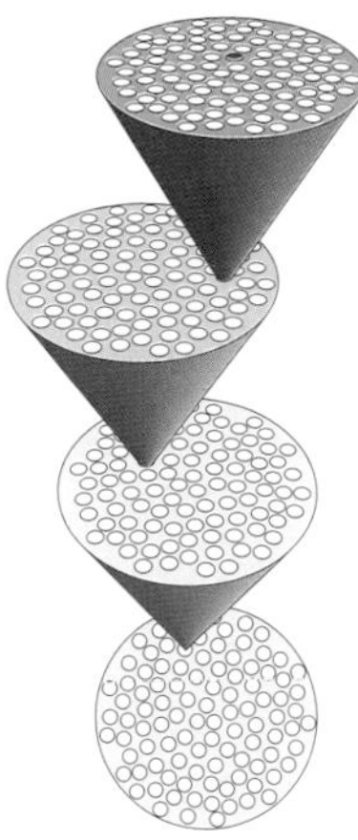

ABOVE *The more the remedy has been diluted, the higher the potency.*

The process of making the remedies is very precise. Soluble substances such as plant and animal extracts are dissolved in a solution of about 90 percent alcohol and 10 percent distilled water, depending on the substance. The mixture is kept in an airtight container and left to stand for two to four weeks, occasionally being shaken. Insoluble substances, such as gold, are first ground down into a fine powder until they become soluble, and then undergo the same process. The mixture is then strained, and the resulting solution is known as the mother tincture.

The mother tincture is then diluted again to produce the different potencies which make up the homeopathic remedies. The dilution is measured as either decimal (x) or centesimal (c). Decimal remedies are diluted to the ratio 1:10, while the centesimal ratio is 1:100. So to produce a 1c potency, one drop of the mother tincture is added to 99 drops of an alcohol and water solution, and then successed. To produce a 2c potency, one drop of the 1c solution is mixed with an alcohol and water solution, and then successed. By the time the remedy reaches a 12c potency it is unlikely that any of the original substance remains in the solution, and yet it remains effective. This is why some skeptics find it difficult to accept the efficacy of homeopathy. But the therapy's supporters believe that physics is not yet developed enough to explain the phenomenon. However, one theory is that the dilution process triggers an electromagnetic imprint which affects our own electromagnetic field; another is that the method of succussion creates and stores an electrochemical pattern in the solution which then spreads through the patient when taken. Once the solution has been successed and diluted to a certain level, the potentized remedy is then added to lactose, or milk sugar, in the form of tablets, pilules, granules, or powder and stored in a dark glass bottle, away from direct sunlight. For treatment purposes, different potencies are prescribed. For an acute illness, a low-potency remedy is recommended; for a chronic disease, a higher potency is more useful.

THE 12 TISSUE SALTS

In the 19th century Wilhelm Schussler identified twelve minerals that he believed to be vital to human health. When these are lacking they can be taken in the form of homeopathically prepared tissue salts.

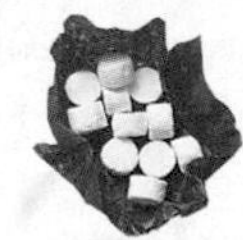

CALC. PHOS. *Produced from calcium phosphate*

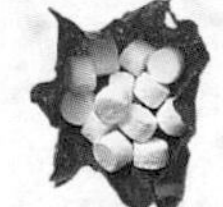

CALC. SULF. *Produced from calcium sulfate*

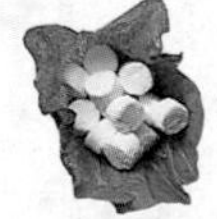

FERR. PHOS. *Produced from iron phosphate*

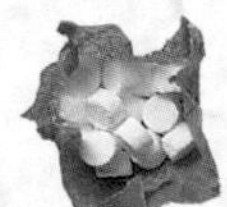

SIL. *Produced from silicon dioxide*

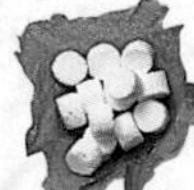

KALI MUR. *Produced from potassium chloride*

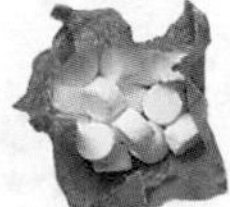

KALI PHOS. *Produced from potassium phosphate*

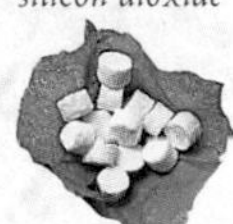

KALI SULF. *Produced from potassium sulfate*

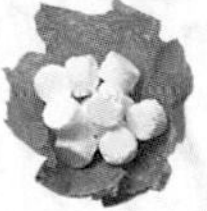

MAG. PHOS. *Produced from magnesium phosphate*

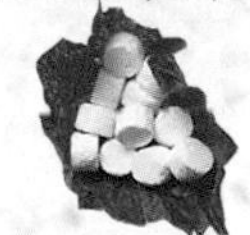

CALC. FLUOR. *Produced from calcium fluoride*

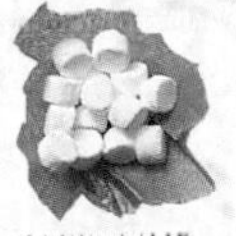

NAT. MUR. *From sodium chloride (common salt)*

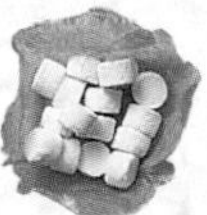

NAT. PHOS. *Produced from sodium phosphate*

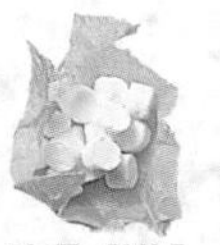

NAT. SULF. *Produced from sodium sulfate*

THE 12 TISSUE SALTS

Biochemic tissue salts are homeopathically prepared ingredients which were introduced at the end of the 19th century by a German physician, Wilhelm Schussler. He believed that many diseases were caused by a deficiency of one or more of 12 vital minerals. A deficiency in each salt would manifest as particular symptoms. Lack of calcarea phosphorica (Calc. phos.), for example, would show up as teething problems or an inability to absorb nutrients properly, while lack of magnesium phosphate (Mag. phos.) would affect nerve endings and muscles. Replacing the missing mineral with a minute dose of the tissue salt can correct the problem. Tissue salts are prepared only from mineral sources such as calcium, iron, and salt, but homeopathic remedies are made from animal, vegetable, and mineral sources. These can be as exotic and deadly as snake's venom or as common as the stinging nettle, but in all cases they are diluted to such an extent that there can be no possible side effects from even the most toxic substances.

THE VITAL FORCE

Hahnemann believed that we all have our own energy, or vital force. The force, which stimulates the body mentally, physically, and emotionally, can be disrupted by poor diet, stress, lack of exercise, pollution, and hereditary problems, weakening it so that illness results. The remedies stimulate the force, enabling the body to heal itself.

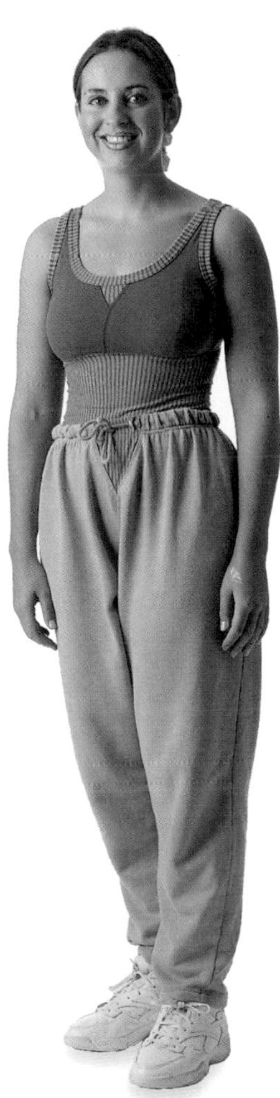

ABOVE *A healthy person has strong powers of self-healing. Illness is a sign that this vital force has been weakened.*

HOMEOPATHIC TECHNIQUES

Homeopathy can be safely used by anyone, from pregnant women, to babies and the elderly. Its popularity has grown in the U.K. since the first homeopathic hospital opened in 1849. It is widely used in Europe, particularly France and Germany, and in South America. It has spread, too, across continents, to Asia and India, where it is now officially recognized as a branch of medicine. In the U.S. homeopathy is becoming a recognized alternative to conventional healthcare, and homeopathic remedies are widely available in health stores.

HOW HOMEOPATHY WORKS

Homeopathy sees symptoms of disease as a positive outward sign that the body is trying to heal itself. Therefore, it holds that the symptoms should not be suppressed (as they are in allopathic medicine), and remedies are used which will help stimulate and support the healing process. In some cases, the symptoms will worsen before they improve.

A homeopath prescribes remedies for the "whole" person, basing his or her decision on Hahnemann's principles – the law of similars, the principle of minimum dose, and prescribing for the individual.

- THE LAW OF SIMILARS Formulated in 1796, it states that a substance that, in large doses, can produce symptoms of illness in a healthy person can cure similar symptoms in a sick person if used in minute doses. Hahnemann believed this was because nature allows for the existence of two similar diseases in the body at the same time. Homeopathic remedies work by introducing a similar artificial disease that negates the original disease, and yet its own effects are so minimal it causes no suffering.
- THE MINIMUM DOSE This states that successive dilutions enhance the curative properties of a substance, while eradicating any side effects. This means only the most minute dose of the substance is needed to help heal.
- WHOLE-PERSON PRESCRIBING Homeopaths believe that symptoms, pain, or diseases do not occur in isolation, but are an overall reflection of a person. They therefore do not just look at the problem presented to them, but at the person as a "whole." Each person is treated as an individual, and the homeopath will consider the patient's personality, temperament, emotional and physical state, likes and dislikes before prescribing a treatment. In this way, a homeopath might see two people with similar symptoms, but would treat them totally differently.

Homeopaths also believe treatment works according to a set of three rules known as the Laws of Cure. These are:

- *A remedy starts healing from the top of the body and works downward.*
- *It starts from within the body, working outward, and from major to minor organs.*
- *Symptoms clear up in reverse order to their manner of appearance.*

Homeopaths also believe that treatment should be prescribed according to a person's constitution, which is made up of inherited and acquired mental, physical, and emotional characteristics. These are matched to a remedy which will improve all-round health, no matter what illness the individual is suffering. This constitutional profile corresponds to a particular remedy, and a person might therefore be known as a Sepia type, or a Lachesis type.

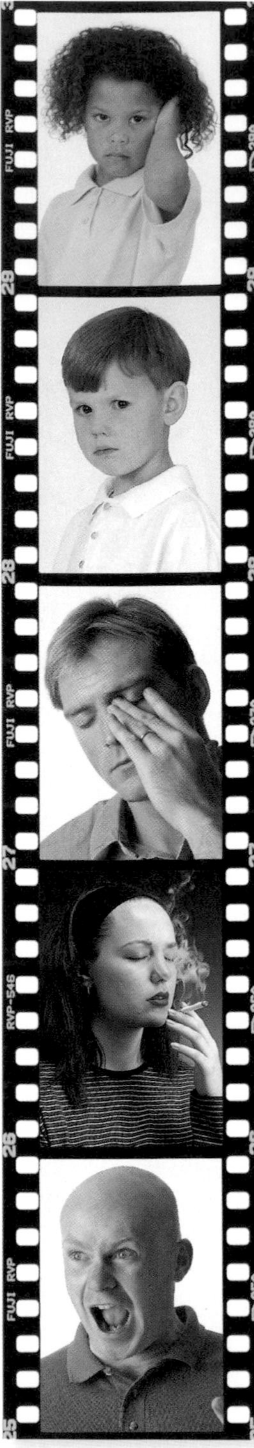

ABOVE *An illness and its remedies are affected by the constitution, character, diet, and lifestyle of the individual concerned.*

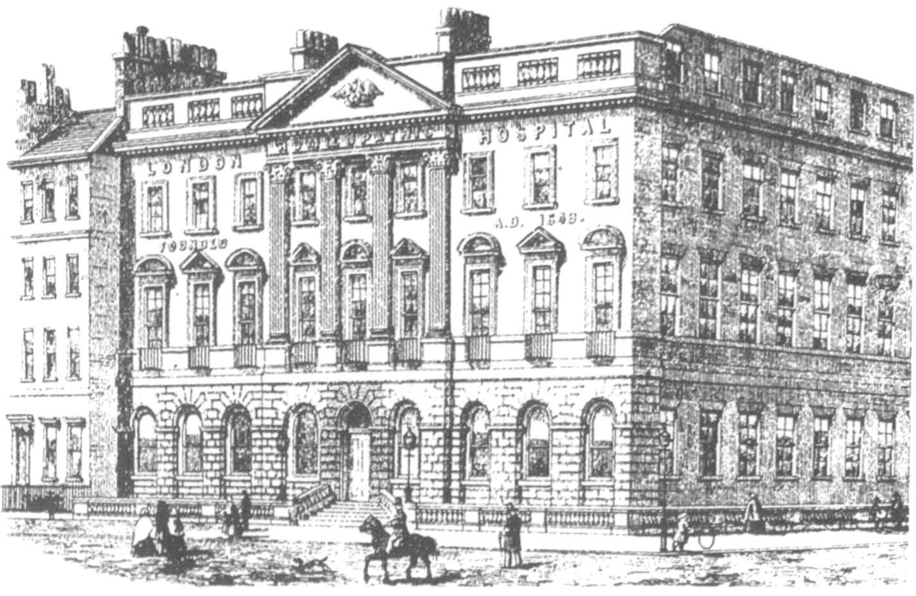

LEFT *The first homeopathic hospital in the U.K. opened in London in 1849, and the therapy has become steadily more popular across Europe and the U.S.*

HAHNEMANN'S CASE

Hahnemann used this wooden case to store hundreds of remedies in small glass vials. He continued to treat patients for many years, and died in 1843 at the age of 88.

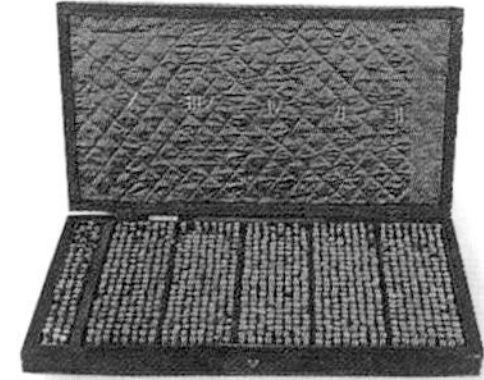

VISITING A HOMEOPATH

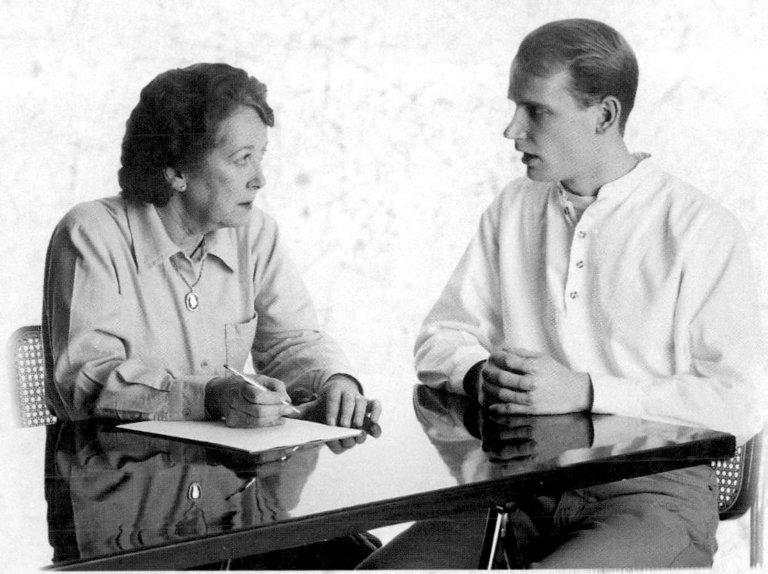

ABOVE *The first consultation with a homeopath involves many questions that will be seemingly unrelated to the health problem concerned. These enable the consultant to form a complete picture of the patient.*

A first visit may last around an hour, as the homeopath asks detailed questions to build up an overall picture of your mental, physical, emotional, spiritual, and general health. As well as questions about any inherited problems, past illnesses, and diet, you may also be asked which side you sleep on, what type of weather you prefer, and whether you have food preferences. Only then will the homeopath prescribe a remedy specifically to suit you. One remedy at a time is usually given, although the prescription may change as your symptoms change. You may not be told which remedy has been prescribed. This is because some people are not happy with the constitutional character type attributed to them. Diet and lifestyle changes may also be recommended.

The remedies should be handled as little as possible, so are usually taken on a spoon and slipped under the tongue to dissolve. Food and drink should be avoided for a half-hour before and afterward. You may also be advised to avoid coffee and peppermints as they may counteract the remedies.

A follow-up appointment will be made for about a month later to assess progress. You may only need two appointments, but chronic conditions tend to take longer. If there is no improvement after around four visits, think about trying alternative treatment. Once symptoms improve, the remedy should be stopped. The remedies are perfectly safe, and although "overdosing" will do no harm, as with any medicine it is best avoided. Treatment can be given alongside conventional medicine, although some drugs may affect the efficacy of homeopathic remedies.

HOME USE

The remedies can be used at home for simple ailments and first aid, but should not be taken as a substitute for professional care. As a general rule, low potencies (e.g. 6c) are used for chronic conditions, and higher potencies (e.g. 30c) for acute conditions such as a cold. Remedies for acute conditions are usually taken on a half-hourly basis at first, and then the intervals spread out to about 8–12 hours. More chronic conditions may combine both low and high potencies.

HOW TO TAKE AND STORE REMEDIES

- Take only one remedy at a time.
- Do not touch the remedies; empty them onto a teaspoon and put under the tongue, or tip them into the cap of the bottle to transfer them to the mouth.
- Take in a "clean mouth" at least 30 minutes after meals. If you need to take them sooner rinse your mouth out first with water. Avoid alcoholic drinks and cigarettes, spicy or minty foods while taking the remedies.
- Store in a cool dark place in tightly closed bottle away from strong smells such as perfumes, air fresheners, or essential oils. Stored correctly, remedies will keep for around five years.

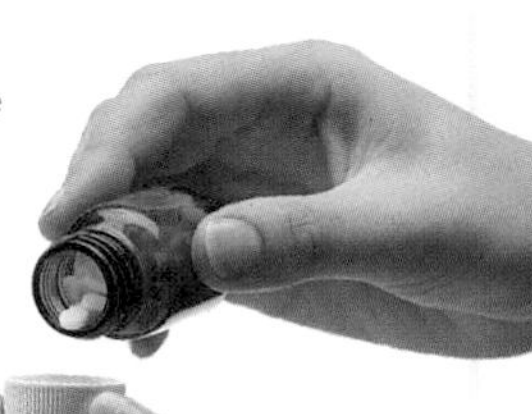

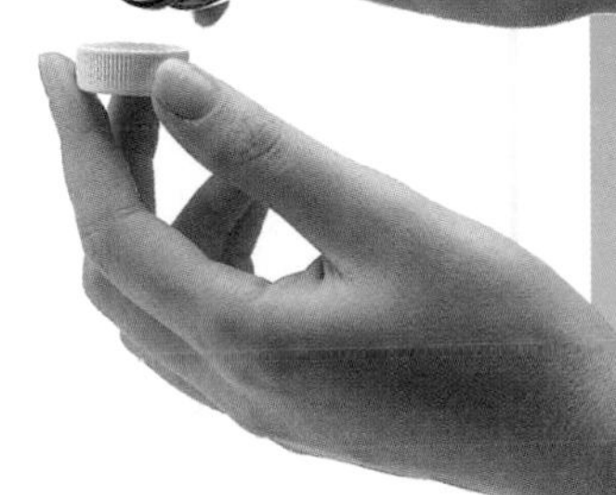

ABOVE *Remedies should not be touched by hand. Tap them out into the container lid or transfer them to a clean teaspoon.*

WHICH PROBLEMS CAN BE TREATED?

Homeopathy can successfully treat most complaints – physical, mental, and emotional – although some people respond better than others. Minor problems such as colds, diarrhea, and allergies, and more serious conditions such as rheumatoid arthritis, psoriasis, and depression can all improve with homeopathic treatment.

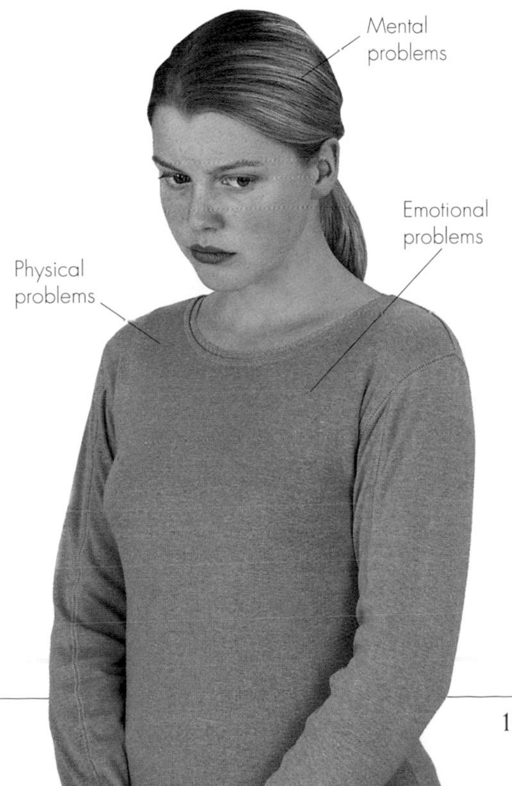

HOMEOPATHIC REMEDIES

Aconitum napellus, wolfsbane, blue monkshood, blue aconite

ACONITE

This deadly plant has been used for its poison for centuries. Saxon hunters dipped the tips of their arrows into its juice before hunting wolves, giving it one of its common names, wolfsbane, although its original title comes from the Latin word *acon*, meaning dart. It is grown in the European mountains, and the flowers, root, and leaves are used.

DATA FILE

Relieves

- acute conditions which begin suddenly and after shock or exposure to abrupt changes of climate
- skin irritations
- fears

Uses

Works well when given in the early stages of infections and inflammation, such as sore throats, coughs, and ear and eye problems and when the skin becomes hot, dry, and burning. Used for complaints which come on suddenly, for instance after shock or exposure to weather extremes. Also, when restlessness and fear accompany an illness or complaint, resulting in palpitations, panic attacks, or agoraphobia.

Which type of person?

- strong, full-blooded, healthy-looking
- when well, happiest in company, but may be malicious and insensitive to cover a lack of self-esteem
- when ill, avoid company
- do not handle shock well and fear dying, even to the extent of predicting their own time of death

SYMPTOMS

MENTAL

- mainly fears – general anxiety, of crowds, of dying

PHYSICAL

- infections or inflammation due to injury
- sudden fevers, accompanied by hot, dry skin
- tingling in hands and feet
- thirst

Symptoms improve in warmth and fresh air but worsen when listening to music, lying on the affected side, at night, and in airless rooms.

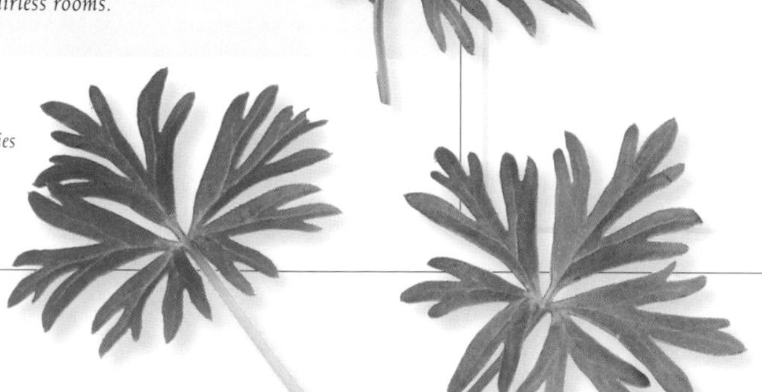

RIGHT *Aconite is one of Hahnemann's original remedies and is derived from the poisonous plant* Aconitum napellus *or monkshood.*

Allium cepa, red onion

ALLIUM

The onion, grown worldwide, has been used across many continents and by many religions for its healing properties. The whole red onion bulb is used, and its potent oil stimulates the tear glands and nasal mucous membranes, causing the eyes and nose to water. In homeopathy it is used to treat any condition which includes these symptoms, such as colds, allergies, and hay fever.

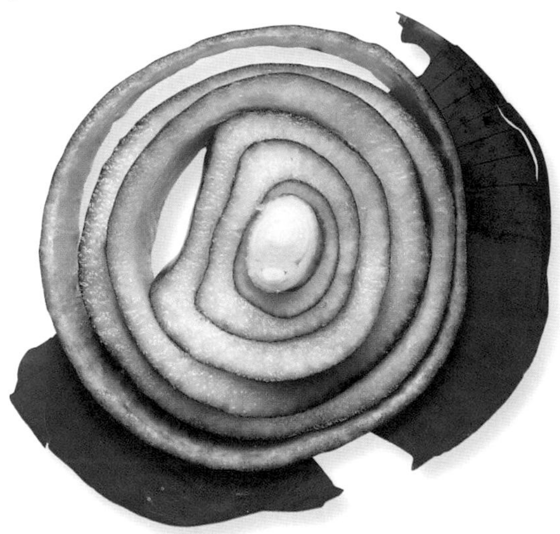

ABOVE *The red onion used in cooking is the source of the Allium remedy, used to treat coughs, colds, and hay fever.*

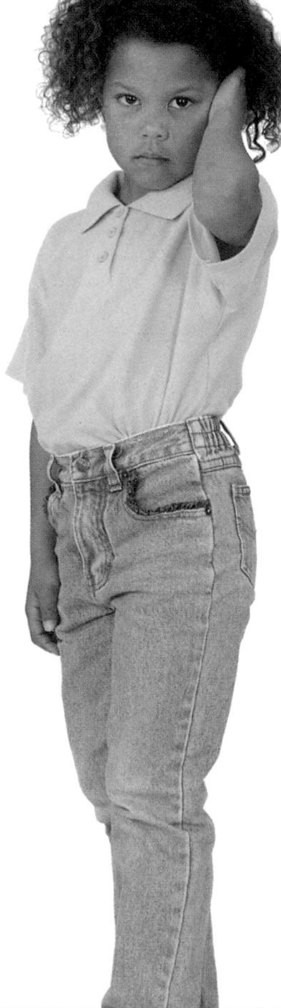

RIGHT *Allium is often used to treat earache and toothache in children, as well as the acute symptoms of a cold and related headaches.*

SYMPTOMS

MENTAL

- fear of pain

PHYSICAL

- profuse discharge from eyes and nose
- headache, toothache, earache in children, stuffiness, cough, neuralgia, colic in babies.

Symptoms improve in fresh, cool air, and worsen in warm, stuffy rooms, and in the cold and damp.

THERAPY CONNECTIONS

ONION

Ayurveda p.25

Traditional Home and Folk Remedies p.82

DATA FILE

Relieves

- streaming eyes and nose
- headaches, burning pain, and neuralgia
- pains that move from side to side, commonly from left to right

Uses

Particularly good for cold and hay fever symptoms – profuse discharge, smarting and swollen eyes, sneezing, sore nose and upper lip from irritation due to streaming. Also for burning or neuralgic pain that moves from side to side. Also, in children, neuralgic pain which accompanies earache, molar toothache which moves around, and headaches behind the forehead. Coughing and the early stages of laryngitis can also be helped.

Which type of person?

- no particular type

Anacardium orientale, Semecarpus anacardium, marking nut tree

ANACARD. OR.

Grown in the East Indies; the Hindus use the acrid black juice of this nut to burn away moles, warts, and other skin complaints. They also use it, mixed with ink, to make markings on linen. The Arabians used the juice for a number of conditions, such as mental illness, memory loss, and paralysis. Homeopathically, cardol, the juice extracted from the pith between the shell and kernel, is used to make the remedy which is given for "tight" feelings of pain.

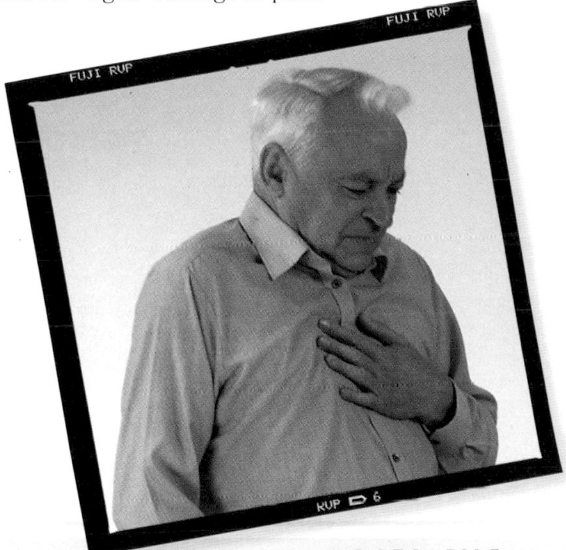

LEFT *Anacard. or. is used to treat "tight" feelings of pain or constriction.*

SYMPTOMS

MENTAL

- loss of memory, leading to instances of harsh behavior
- obsessive behavior
- fixations
- irritability
- nervous exhaustion

PHYSICAL

- tight feeling of constriction
- duodenal ulcers
- blocked gut or anus

Symptoms improve immediately after eating, when lying on the affected part, after rubbing, and worsen around midnight, after washing in hot water and using a compress.

DATA FILE

Relieves

- constricted pain
- plugged ear, nose, or back passage
- inferiority complex

Uses

This remedy is useful when there is a feeling of tightness or constricted pain. Other conditions that may be relieved are itchy skin; piles; constipation; indigestion; duodenal ulcers which feel better immediately after eating, but cause discomfort two hours later; and rheumatism. It is particularly beneficial for those who suffer an inferiority complex and who want to prove themselves, for those who feel possessed, or those who just don't quite feel themselves.

Which type of person?

- pale face
- blue rings around the eyes
- strong moral sense, so feel guilt acutely
- easily offended
- lack self-confidence
- like dairy products

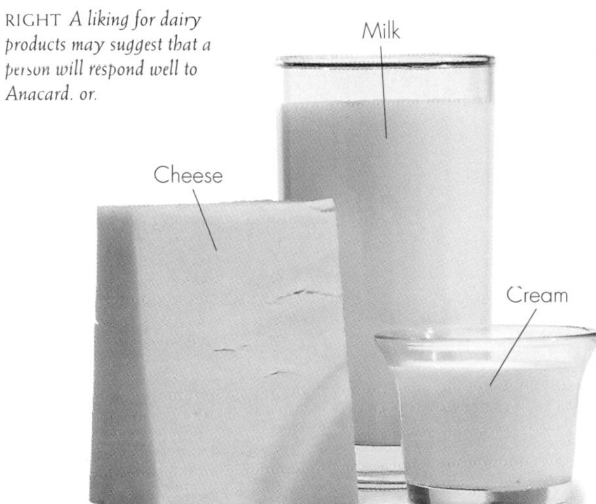

RIGHT *A liking for dairy products may suggest that a person will respond well to Anacard. or.*

Antimonium tartaricum, antimony potassium tartrate, tartar emetic

ANT. TART.

Antimony potassium tartrate is a poisonous crystalline salt which has no color or odor and is used as a fix for leather and textiles, and in insecticides. In the past it was used in conventional medicine as an emetic, and as an expectorant. Homeopathically, it is used to treat gastric disorders and chest complaints.

DATA FILE

Relieves

- chest conditions
- gastric or bowel complaints

Uses

This remedy is particularly good in the very young or very old who are too feeble or weak to help themselves, for instance by coughing up phlegm. Wet, cold conditions bring on excess thick mucus in the air passages, leading to rattling breathing. Sour food or drink can lead to gastric problems, intense nausea, and lack of thirst. Other symptoms treated include headaches with the feeling that there is a tight band around the head; a face cold to the touch; a thickly coated tongue; fluid retention leading to bloated legs; nausea.

Which type of person?

- pale, sickly looking
- dark rings around the eyes
- cold sweat on face
- look run down
- do not like being fussed over or interfered with when ill
- do not like being disturbed
- babies who whine, moan, want to be carried

BELOW *Tartar emetic is the source for Antimonium tartaricum, used for people who feel anxious and weak, especially old people and the very young.*

SYMPTOMS

MENTAL

- irritable and anxious
- despairing

PHYSICAL

- stomach upsets
- sweats
- build-up of mucus and phlegm
- off food and do not want to drink
- drowsy

Symptoms improve when sitting up, after vomiting, and in cold air, and worsen in stuffy rooms, if wearing too much, with movement, or when lying down.

Apis mellifica, Apis mellifera, honey bee

APIS

The bee is known for its unique ability to produce honey and for its painful sting. Bee products – honey, beeswax, propolis (resin used in the building of hives), and royal jelly (fed to queen bees) – are used in complementary medicine. In homeopathy, Apis is used to treat stinging pain and inflamed, burning skin which has swollen and is painful to touch. The honey bee is commonly found in Europe, Canada, and America. Homeopathically, the whole live bee is used, including the sting, and dissolved in alcohol. The remedy was first "proved" in the U.S., at the Central New York State Homeopathic Society.

BELOW *The Apis type will often spend hours trying irritably to achieve something without success.*

DATA FILE

Relieves

- hot, stinging pain
- smarting, watery swellings, which are sensitive to the touch
- fever with dry skin
- violent headache
- lack of thirst

Uses

Used for complaints such as bites, stings, and urticaria, when the skin becomes swollen, dry, and itchy, or burns and is sensitive to the touch. Also used for urinary tract infections, such as cystitis, and for urine and fluid retention. Allergic reactions which affect the nose, eyes, and throat, such as anaphylactic shock, when watery swelling occurs, and complaints where joints become swollen, such as arthritis, can also be treated. Also good for fever, accompanied by dry skin, sore throat, severe headache, and lack of thirst.

Which type of person?

- protective of own territory, resentful of outsiders
- irritable, agitated, and difficult to please
- love trying to organize other people's lives but have a "sting in the tail" for those who cross them, perhaps leading to the nickname "queen bee"
- spend hours trying to achieve things without making much headway

SYMPTOMS

MENTAL

- restlessness
- jealousy
- irritability
- sensitivity
- depression
- unpredictability

PHYSICAL

- watery swellings, from stings to edema
- fevers with dry, sensitive skin
- intense headaches
- lack of urination

Symptoms improve under cool conditions, but worsen when touched, in heat, or during sleep.

BELOW *This remedy is derived from the bodies of honey bees, including their stings.*

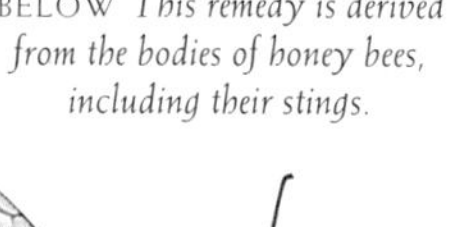

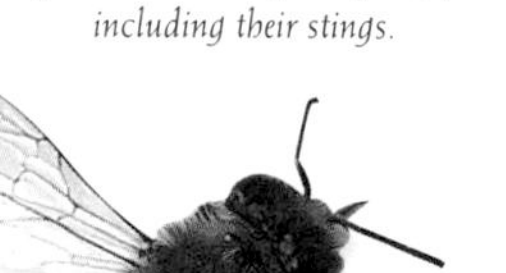

CAUTION

DURING PREGNANCY, AVOID APIS BELOW 30C POTENCY.

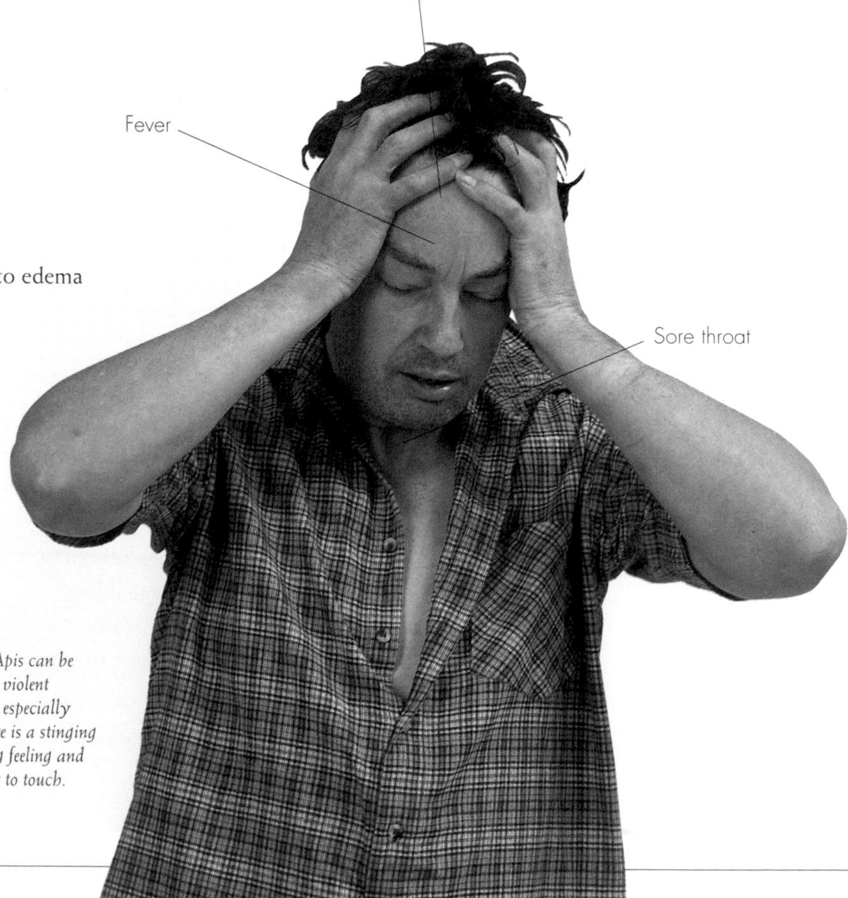

RIGHT *Apis can be tried for a violent headache, especially where there is a stinging or burning feeling and sensitivity to touch.*

Argentum nitricum, hell stone, devil's stone, lunar caustic

ARG. NIT.

Silver nitrate, the source of this remedy, was given the names "hell stone" or "devil's stone" because of its corrosive effect. Silver nitrate is extracted from the mineral acanthite, the main ore of silver, and is found in the U.S., South America, and Norway. In the past, due to its caustic and antibacterial qualities, it was used in medicine to cauterize wounds after surgery and treat conditions such as warts and eye infections. Although it is safe in small doses, large amounts are poisonous, causing breathing problems and damaging the kidneys, liver, spleen, and aorta, and overdosing affects the skin, turning it permanently blue. It has also long had a less lethal use – for making the backs of mirrors. In homeopathy, the remedy is most often used for nervous and digestive complaints.

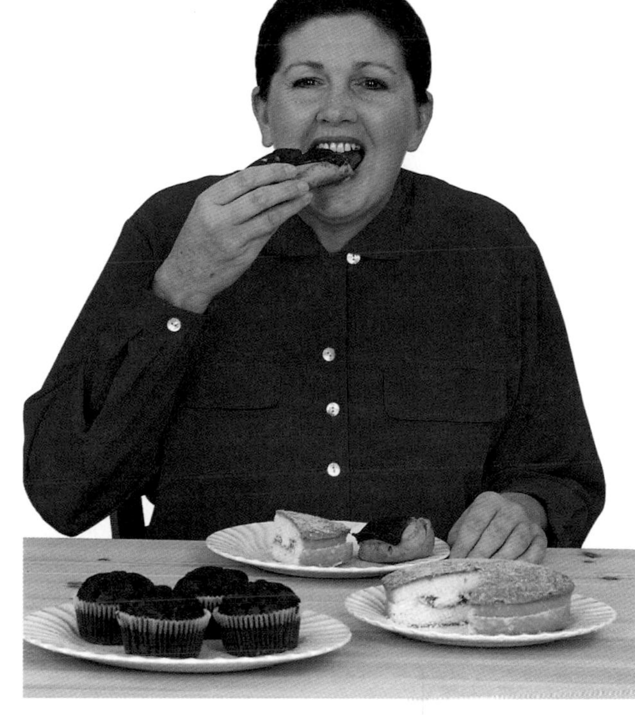

RIGHT *This treatment may suit impulsive people who can be irrational when under stress and binge on sweet foods.*

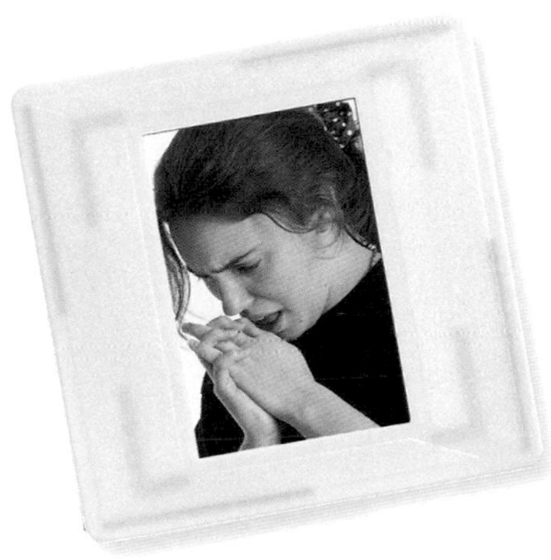

BELOW LEFT *Fears and anxiety, headache and neck tension, especially when under pressure, may be treated by Arg. nit.*

SYMPTOMS

MENTAL

- under stress, find it hard to control emotions, leading to irrational thoughts and impulses
- under pressure, and push themselves, because of a fear of failing

PHYSICAL

- headaches, brought on by overwork, excitement, and sweet foods, will be slow in onset then disappear
- tension in the neck
- weak areas: nerves, lining of the stomach, the left side of the body.

Symptoms improve in fresh air and in coolness, and if pressure is applied, but worsen in heat, at night, under stress, and if lying on the left side.

DATA FILE

Relieves

- fears, anxiety, phobias
- palpitations, sweating
- mental exhaustion
- digestive complaints brought on by nerves and other tension
- problems due to overconsumption of sweet, sugary foods
- vertigo

Uses

Arg. nit. is mainly used for fear and anxiety, usually brought on by stress, and can help with problems such as claustrophobia, dangerous impulses, such as throwing oneself off a bridge, and stage fright. It can also control superstition – the feeling that something awful is about to happen. It is also very useful for digestive problems, such as diarrhea and vomiting, particularly if brought on by nerves; and headaches which begin slowly and are caused by overeating sweet foods. It also helps other conditions such as asthma, colic in babies, epilepsy, warts, and sore throats. During labor, it can help bring relief when bearing down.

Which type of person?

- look fraught and prematurely old, with hollowed features, and an accumulation of wrinkles
- do work where quick thinking, rapid responses, and a good memory are necessary, such as acting, lecturing, or executive positions in business
- outwardly exuberant and happy, inwardly suffer from wild emotions, leading them to laugh, cry, or lose their tempers easily
- when worried and agitated, fret about what may go wrong in the future, even becoming irrational
- may break out in sudden nervous sweats
- prefer salty foods, dislike cold food, and crave sweetness, though causes stomach upset
- children look older than their years; may be sick through apprehension at the thought of school, and dislike airless rooms; overindulge in sweet or salty food, leading to diarrhea
- breast-fed babies will suffer diarrhea and colic if the mother eats sweet food

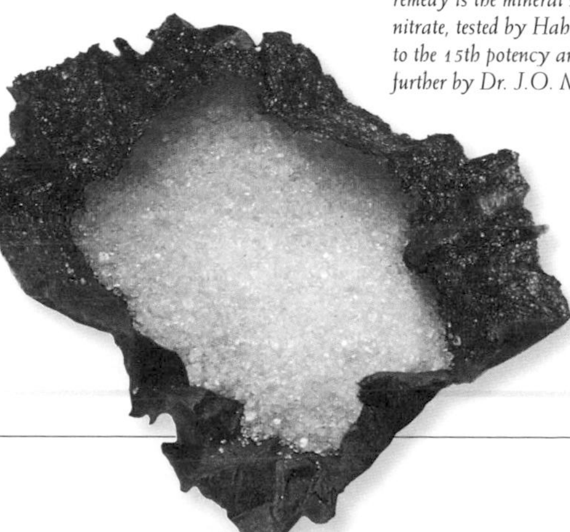

BELOW *The source of this remedy is the mineral silver nitrate, tested by Hahnemann to the 15th potency and proved further by Dr. J.O. Müller.*

Arnica montana, leopard's bane, mountain tobacco, sneezewort

ARNICA

Arnica has been used for its healing properties for centuries. It grows in the mountain regions of Europe and Siberia. In folk remedies it was used for aches and bruises, and in conventional medicine for rheumatism, gout, and dysentery. The South American Indians used it to treat injuries. Homeopathically, the remedy was first "proved" by Hahnemann. The whole fresh plant is used when in flower, externally as a cream for sprains and bruises, and internally for shock, often after the patient has suffered an injury.

CAUTION

DO NOT USE ARNICA CREAM ON BROKEN SKIN.

ABOVE *The flowers and rootstock of mountain arnica or leopard's bane, Arnica montana, have long been used in folk medicine.*

DATA FILE

Relieves

- bruises, sprains, pain
- shock from injury
- emotional shock, for instance after bereavement

Uses

Arnica is an effective first-aid treatment for sprains, strains, and bruising. Internally, it can help control bleeding and stimulates the healing of damaged tissue. It is also useful for shock, after either an injury or emotional trauma. It can be used for long-term joint and muscle complaints such as osteoarthritis. Internal treatment can aid external conditions such as eczema and boils.

Which type of person?

- morose, morbidly imaginative
- when ill deny there is a problem, refusing to see a doctor, and preferring to be left alone

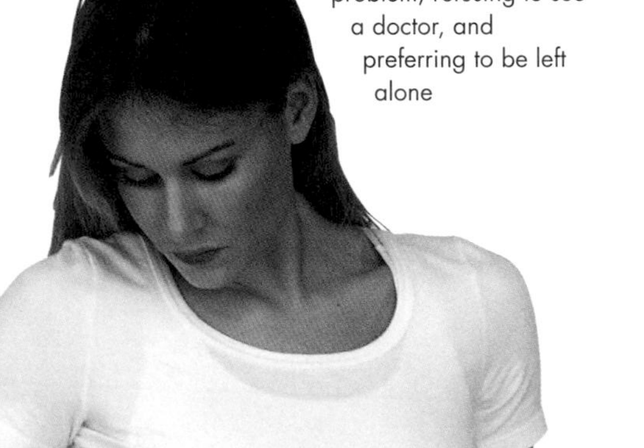

LEFT *Arnica cream is a well-tried first-aid remedy for sprains and bruises.*

SYMPTOMS

MENTAL

- hypochondria
- fear of being touched due to pain
- nightmares
- find it hard to concentrate because easily distracted
- impatient, indifferent, and restless, even in bed
- obstinate

PHYSICAL

- the head feels hot, the body cold
- severe fever
- broken capillaries
- sprained joints
- eczema

Symptoms improve during movement and lying down with the head lower than the feet, and worsen after prolonged movement or rest, under light pressure, in heat.

Arsenicum album, arsenic trioxide

ARS. ALB.

Arsenic has long been known as a useful poison for those intent on murder! These days, arsenic poisoning is more likely to be the result of accidental ingestion, for instance of agricultural pesticides. In large doses, swallowing arsenic leads to severe stomach upset, vomiting, convulsions, diarrhea, and, if not treated, death. In the past, small doses were given to treat syphilis, anthrax, and to improve stamina. Arsenic is contained in the mineral arsenopyrite, found in countries such as England, Canada, Germany, Norway, and Sweden. It is made up of metallic crystals which cannot be destroyed. In homeopathy, a minute compound of arsenic is used, which works beneficially on the sensitive lining of the digestive tract and respiratory system. Arsenic was first "proved" by Hahnemann.

SYMPTOMS

MENTAL

- fear being alone, burgled, dying
- anxiety leads to restlessness and irritability and a need to do everything meticulously
- possessive, hoard
- sensitive to touch, smell, cold

PHYSICAL

- digestive disorders
- headaches
- dizziness
- vomiting
- asthma which is triggered by anxiety
- fluid retention, diarrhea
- cracked lips, mouth ulcers

Symptoms improve with movement, in warmth, when lying down with the head propped up, and are worse on the right side, in the cold, after cold food and drink.

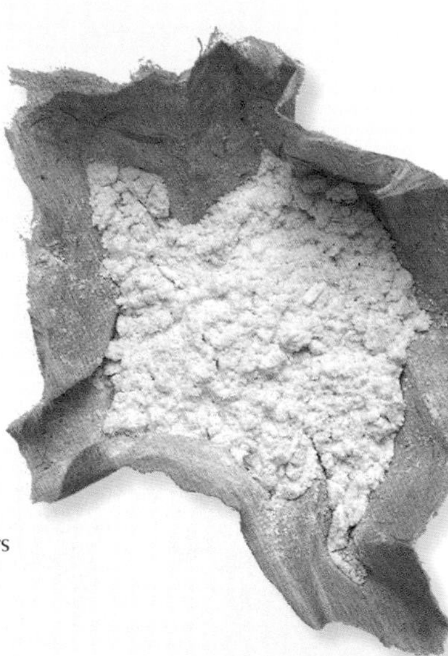

ABOVE *An oxide of arsenic, the powder known as white arsenic, is the source of this remedy.*

DATA FILE

Relieves

- digestive disorders
- fears and anxiety
- regular, painful headaches
- problems associated with burning pain

Uses

Ars. alb. is given to those suffering from fear – fear of going out alone, fear of the dark, fear of failure, and so on – which is caused by underlying feelings of insecurity. It is also useful for problems of the digestive system, such as indigestion, diarrhea, food poisoning, and excessive eating, such as overconsumption of fruit or ice cream, and drinking too much alcohol. Also, for a range of conditions which particularly sting or burn, such as mouth ulcers, sore lips, eye inflammation, vomiting, burning pains in the rectum. Asthma, fatigue, and fluid retention, especially around the ankles, can also be helped.

Which type of person?

- elegant, even dapper, everything in place
- attentive to detail, plan for every contingency as a way of covering up insecurity and lack of confidence
- strong ideas, making them intolerant of others, want everything to be done perfectly their way
- constant planning does nothing to relieve restlessness and worries, so fret about own health and the health of their family
- children are tidy, restless, and have a wild imagination
- prefer warm foods which are fatty, sweet, or sour; warm drinks, alcohol

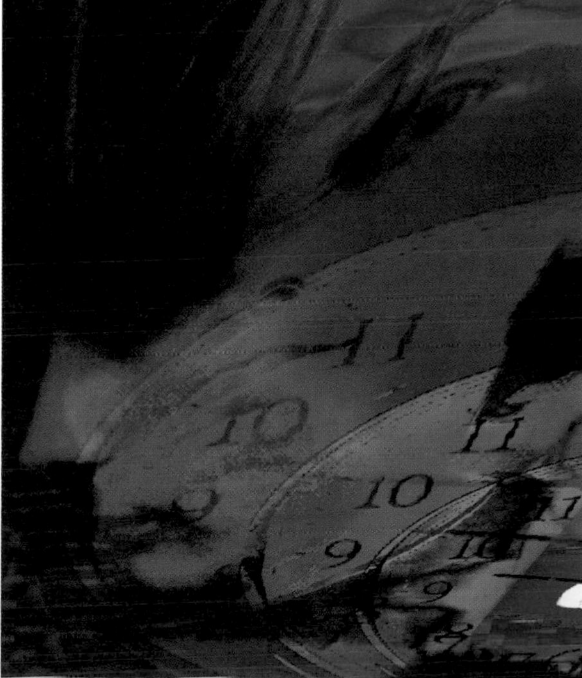

ABOVE *Fear of going out alone, fear of the dark, fear of failure, and so on – caused by underlying feelings of insecurity – are specific problems that can respond to Ars. alb.*

Atropa belladonna, deadly nightshade

BELLADONNA

It was thought that deadly nightshade was used in witchcraft during the Middle Ages. In Italian "bella donna" means beautiful woman, and Italian women used it in eye drops to enlarge their pupils to make themselves more attractive. In conventional medicine, the plant's alkaloid properties of atropine, hyoscamine, and scopolamine are used to treat spasms and nausea. It is grown throughout Europe, and in homeopathy the fresh leaves and flowers are used. Hahnemann first "proved" the remedy in the year 1799.

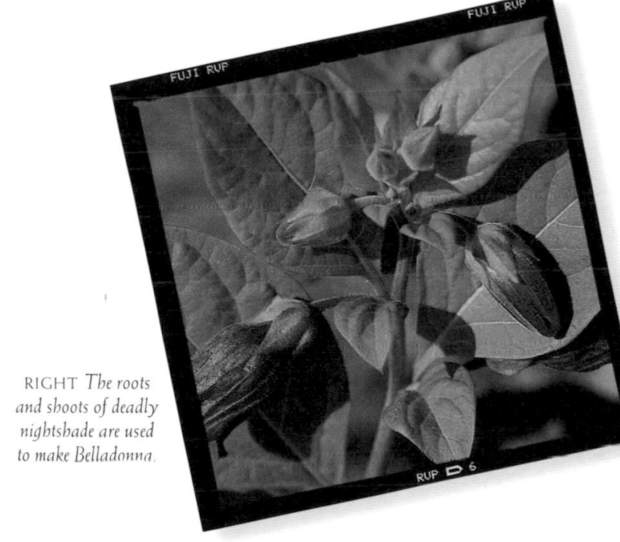

RIGHT *The roots and shoots of deadly nightshade are used to make Belladonna.*

SYMPTOMS

MENTAL

- restless
- excitable behavior
- wild imagination, even hallucinations, nightmares
- fear when approached

PHYSICAL

- very sensitive to light, touch, and movement
- throbbing headaches
- earache, especially on the right side of the head
- hot, dry face, bright red tongue

Symptoms improve in warmth, when standing up, with warm compresses, and worsen when cool, on the right side, at night, with movement, noise, light, pressure.

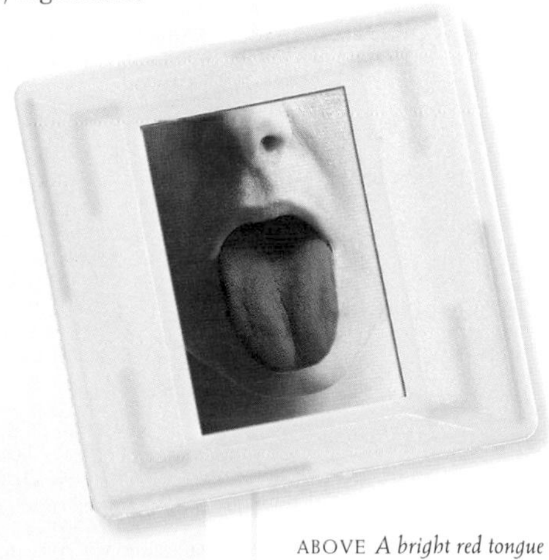

ABOVE *A bright red tongue can indicate the need for the Belladonna remedy, especially if the face is hot and dry.*

DATA FILE

Relieves

- sudden, violent complaints, with flushing and throbbing, due to increased circulation
- ailments which include sensitivity to light, noise, pressure, touch
- fever, with staring eyes, dilated pupils

Uses

Commonly used for complaints with sudden onset, inflamed infections, such as fever, tonsillitis, flu, earache – particularly on the right side. Helps severe, pounding headaches jarred by eye movement; boils; labor pain; sore breasts from breast-feeding; fits; cystitis; teething babies.

Which type of person?

- fit, healthy, normally strong in mind and body
- lively and entertaining when well
- agitated, restless, stubborn, and maybe violent when ill
- extremely sensitive to light, touch, movement, and noise

Aurum metallicum, gold

AURUM MET.

In the 12th century, gold was used by Arabian physicians to treat heart conditions. In the early 20th century, it was used in diagnosing syphilis and treating tuberculosis, and today is used for treating cancer and rheumatoid arthritis. It is found in Canada, America, South Africa, and Australia. Homeopathically, it is given to treat a range of clinical complaints, such as heart disease and depression.

DATA FILE

Relieves

- depression
- ailments accompanied by sensitivity to touch, taste, smell, noise
- vascular complaints

Uses

Useful for mental conditions such as depression and suicidal tendencies. Also for ailments where an increase in blood circulation leads to congestion in the head, as in pulsating headaches, or other organs. Symptoms of heart disease, such as chest pain and breathlessness, can also be helped. Liver problems and sinusitis can be relieved.

Which type of person?

- workaholics who set themselves high goals
- deep sense of duty
- sensitive to the opinions of others as never feel they have achieved as much as they should
- feelings of failure can lead to depression, and even suicidal thoughts

SYMPTOMS

MENTAL

- depression, even suicidal leanings
- explosive behavior if contradicted

PHYSICAL

- red flushes when angry
- blood congestion in organs, such as liver and heart
- inflammation of testes in young boys

Symptoms improve in fresh air and when walking, after washing in cold water and resting, and worsen after mental exertion, when emotionally upset, and at night.

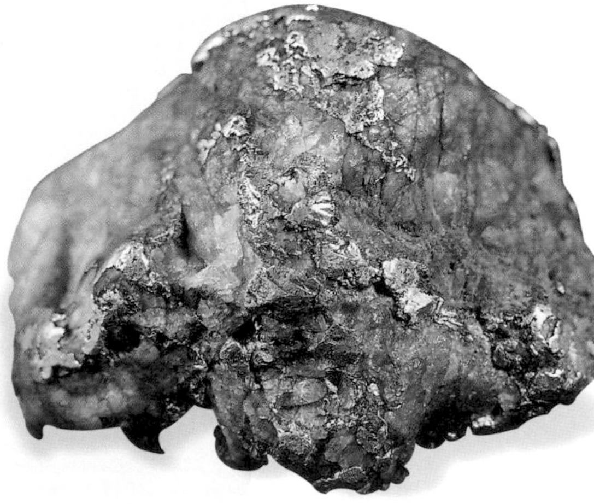

BELOW *Aurum. met. is derived from the precious metal, gold, and is used by homeopaths for a variety of complaints.*

Baptisia tinctoria, wild indigo, horsefly weed, rattlebush

BAPTISIA

Wild indigo is a perennial plant which is native to the U.S. and Canada. Poisonous if ingested in high doses, causing gastrointestinal problems, its medicinal properties were first discovered by Native Americans, who also used it as the basis for indigo dye. It is also used in herbal medicine as a cooling agent, and as an antiseptic and an antibacterial treatment. Homeopathically, the fresh root is used. The remedy was originally "proved" using only seven volunteers, the results being published in the *North American Journal of Homeopathy* in 1857 and 1859.

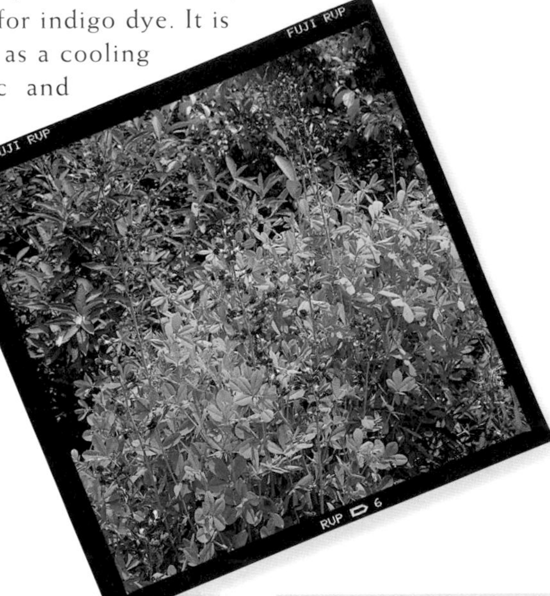

BELOW *The native American plant wild indigo, used to make blue dye, is the source of Baptisia. The plant root is the source of the remedy.*

CAUTION

A PATIENT NEEDING BAPTISIA IS USUALLY SEVERELY ILL AND WILL NEED PROFESSIONAL MEDICAL CARE.

DATA FILE

Relieves

- toxic and septic conditions
- acute feverish illness

Uses

This remedy is mainly used for complaints which have quickly deteriorated into a serious condition, such as acute flu and typhoid fever. Symptoms treated include a rambling mind; restlessness; severe aches and tenderness; prostration and falling asleep mid-sentence; inability to sleep because of delirious mind; foul-smelling breath and stools; dry, coated tongue; mouth ulcers; and persistent ear infections.

Which type of person?

- no particular type, but will be very ill, with puffy face and a drugged look

SYMPTOMS

MENTAL

- restlessness
- confused, wandering mind and talk
- fear of poisoning from food

PHYSICAL

- unable to move around to make themselves more comfortable
- ulcers of the mouth and throat
- foul breath
- coated tongue
- gum sores
- breathing difficulties

Symptoms improve with walking in fresh air and worsen in humidity.

Baryta carbonica, barium carbonate, witherite

BARYTA CARB.

The source of barium carbonate, a poisonous alkaline soluble salt, is barite and witherite, found in the earth's crust in the U.S. and parts of Europe. When heated, it glows and is a useful tool in radiology. Witherite obtains its name from the man who first discovered it in 1783, William Withering. It was given medicinally to treat glandular swellings and tuberculosis. Homeopathically, it was first "proved" by Hahnemann, and the remedy is used mainly for children and the elderly.

ABOVE *Barium carbonate, used in some rat poisons, is the source for Baryta carbonica, one of the remedies proved by Hahnemann.*

DATA FILE

Relieves

- enlarged glands
- headaches
- slow development

Uses

This is a particularly useful remedy for children, adults who have immature tendencies as if going through a second childhood, and the elderly. Children who are shy, are late in walking and talking, are slow to develop physically. Those who are slow intellectually, physically, and emotionally respond well. As they are susceptible to infection, they suffer recurrent problems such as sore throats. The elderly, suffering from senile dementia or a stroke, also respond well.

Which type of person?

- tend to be overweight
- dry, lined skin
- mentally dull, may be mentally challenged
- forgetful, with a short attention span
- children are timid and slow developers
- like cold food

RIGHT *Children, especially those who are shy or slow to develop, are often responsive to Baryta carb.*

SYMPTOMS

MENTAL

- fear of strangers, minor things, things that may happen
- memory loss
- tendency to dwell on past problems
- confusion
- lack of self-confidence
- odd sensations such as cobwebs on face or as if inhaling smoke

PHYSICAL

- recurrent sore throats, accompanied by enlarged glands
- palpitations when lying on the left side
- frequent urination
- constipation

Symptoms improve in the open air, when warmly wrapped, and worsen when thinking about problems, after washing, when lying on the affected side, with exposure to cold or damp.

Bryonia alba, common bryony, white bryony, wild hops

BRYONIA

The Greek physician Hippocrates was one of the first physicians to use bryony, in the 5th century B.C.E. The Romans also used it to treat paralysis, gout, hysteria, and epilepsy. The plant has a deadly, bitter root which, if eaten, can kill within hours. The homeopathic remedy, in which the fresh root is first pounded to a pulp, was one of the first treatments to be "proved" by Hahnemann, in 1834.

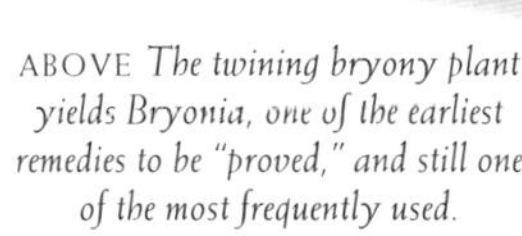

ABOVE *The twining bryony plant yields Bryonia, one of the earliest remedies to be "proved," and still one of the most frequently used.*

DATA FILE

Relieves

- acute complaints with slow onset, painful with movement, thirst
- ailments accompanied by dryness of the mouth, lips, eyes, chest

Uses

Often used for coughs, colds, headaches, and flu which develop slowly and are accompanied by dryness, for instance in the throat, and great thirst. The condition worsens with movement. Also useful for joint inflammation such as rheumatism and osteoarthritis; chest and abdominal inflammation; pleurisy; pneumonia; constipation; mastitis.

Which type of person?

- fear poverty, so materialistic
- worry about financial security, even if well-off; anxious, irritable if security is threatened
- plod, but straightforward, reliable
- meticulous, critical
- usually have dark hair and complexion

SYMPTOMS

MENTAL

- reluctant to speak or to move
- irritable, heavy-headed
- want things, but do not know what, then refuse it when offered
- fears of not getting better, even of dying
- worry about finances and job

PHYSICAL

- excessive sweating
- dryness, constricted throat, thirst
- stabbing headaches
- heavy eyelids
- cravings

Symptoms improve after rest, when pressure is applied, and worsen with movement.

Calcarea carbonica, calcium carbonate

CALC. CARB.

The source of this remedy is the mother-of-pearl in oyster shells. Mother-of-pearl was commonly used for its beauty to adorn combs and the backs of hairbrushes. In homeopathy it also has wide-ranging uses, but is most often used for problems relating to the teeth and bones. It is particularly good for broken bones which are slow to heal, backache, and joint pain.

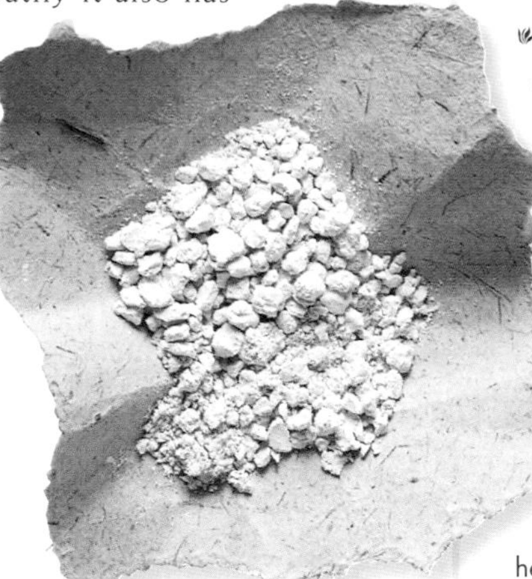

RIGHT *Calc. carb. is the homeopathically potentized version of common chalk or calcium carbonate.*

SYMPTOMS

MENTAL

- fear of poverty, illness, and death
- swing from being productive at work to lazy
- fear of the dark, ghosts
- dislike small spaces, thunderstorms, mice
- discuss every detail of each illness to the irritation of others

PHYSICAL

- sensitive to cold
- often tired and anxious
- excessive, sour-smelling sweat, even after light exertion
- constipated, but feel better for it

Symptoms improve when lying on the affected side, late morning, and in dry weather, and worsen with sweating, after exertion, in the damp and cold, on waking, and before menstruation.

LEFT *Oyster shells are the usual source of Calc. carb., which has an affinity for bone and joint problems, and people who like oysters.*

DATA FILE

Relieves

- aches and pains in the bones and joints
- slow development of teeth and bones
- excessive sweating
- fears, anxieties

Uses

Used to treat bones and joints which are slow to develop, or slow to heal after injury. Also relieves complaints which may be due to this, such as backache. Also helps slow-growing teeth and pain during teething. Eye infections characterized by redness, particularly in the right eye, and ear infections accompanied by unpleasant-smelling discharge are also treated. Right-sided headaches, premenstrual tension, heavy menstruation, the menopause, thrush, eczema, and digestive problems can also be helped by Calc. carb.

Which type of person?

- shy, quiet, sensitive
- seem withdrawn, but are more afraid of making a fool of themselves
- when well, happy and work hard; when ill, slightly depressed and need constant reassurance
- although generally healthy, tend to be overweight, leading to sloth
- prefer sweet, sour, and starchy foods, cold drinks, oysters, and dislike coffee and milk; suffer unusual cravings, chalk, for instance

Calcarea phosphorica, calcium phosphate

CALC. PHOS.

Calcium phosphate is a mineral salt which is the main constituent, along with collagen, of bones and teeth. A natural version is the mineral apatite. For homeopathic use, it is prepared chemically from dilute phosphoric acid and calcium hydroxide, which form fine particles of calcium phosphate. These are then filtered and dried. Calcium phosphate is also used in making porcelain and glass, and as plant food. The remedy is also used as a tissue salt, to treat complaints affecting the bones and teeth.

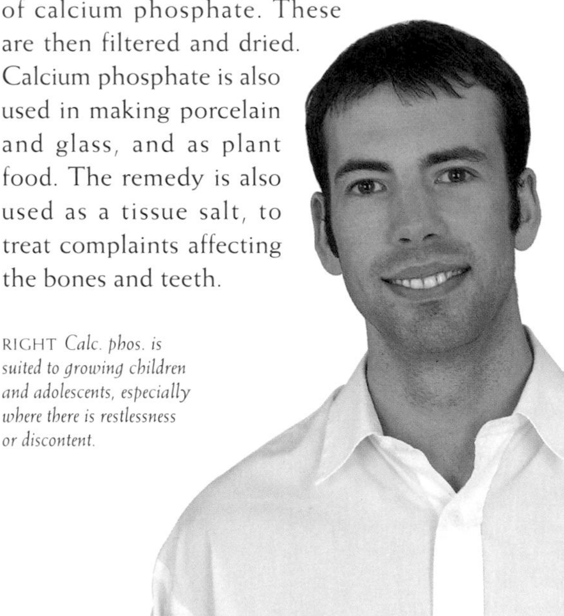

RIGHT *Calc. phos. is suited to growing children and adolescents, especially where there is restlessness or discontent.*

SYMPTOMS

MENTAL

- restless, dislike routine
- need constant stimulation
- hate getting up in the morning

PHYSICAL

- growing pains
- slow-healing fractures
- cravings
- weak digestion

Symptoms improve in dry, warm weather, and worsen in cold, damp weather, when worrying, after excessive sexual activity or other overexertion.

DATA FILE

Relieves

- painful teeth and bones
- digestive complaints
- growing pains

Uses

Used to treat slow growth and growing pains in children. For instance, a fontanel that is slow to close in a toddler, painful teething, numbness and tingling attributed to growing. Also used to treat bones and joints that are healing slowly; slow recovery after illness due to weakness and fatigue; for digestive problems such as diarrhea and indigestion; recurrent throat infections.

Which type of person?

- thin, with dark hair, long legs
- discontented, unhappy
- friendly, but always complaining
- dislike routine
- babies are irritable, needing constant attention; when older easily bored

BELOW *This remedy is prepared from phosphate of lime. Calcium phosphate occurs in animal and human bones as well as rocks.*

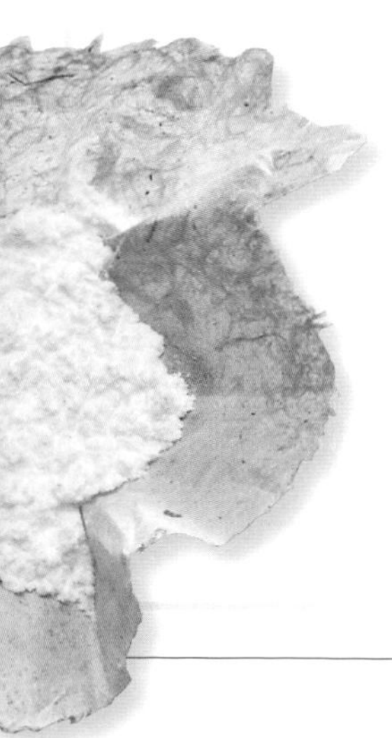

Calendula officinalis, marigold

CALENDULA

The common, or pot, marigold is a hardy annual bush which grows in southern Europe. It should not be confused with the African marigold, *tagetes*, which is toxic. *Calendula* has bright orange or yellow daisy-like flowers and narrow pale green leaves, and it grows to a height of about 2ft. (70cm.). The plant has been used for centuries for its healing properties. It is a popular herbal medicine, and is used for its anti-inflammatory and antimicrobial qualities in conditions ranging from skin complaints to cancer. It is a common first-aid treatment for cuts, grazes, and scalds in both herbal and homeopathic medicine. Homeopathically, the fresh leaves and flowers of the plant are used to make the remedy and a cream for external use.

SYMPTOMS

MENTAL

- none in particular, although patient may be irritable and frightened

PHYSICAL

- cuts, grazes, scalds
- perineal tears
- bleeding after tooth extraction

Symptoms improve when lying still or walking, and worsen in damp, cloudy weather; in draughts, and after eating.

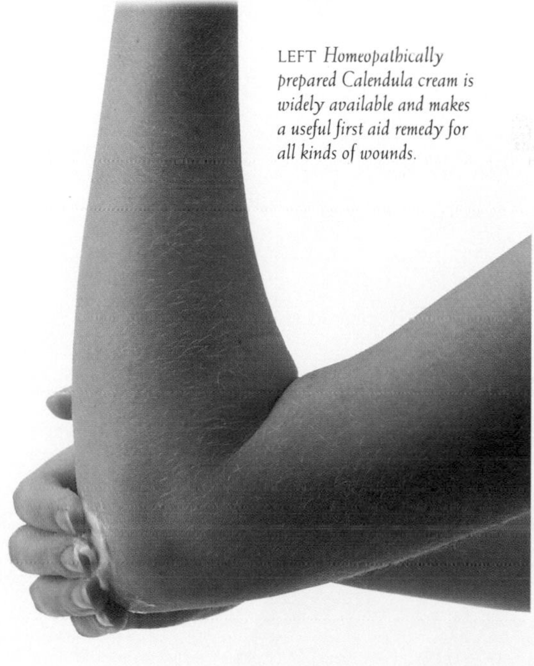

LEFT *Homeopathically prepared Calendula cream is widely available and makes a useful first aid remedy for all kinds of wounds.*

DATA FILE

Relieves

- cuts, grazes, minor wounds
- perineal tears, after childbirth
- mouth ulcers

Uses

An excellent first-aid treatment for small cuts, grazes, and scalds to help control bleeding, for its cleansing antiseptic qualities, and to promote healing by aiding clotting. Also, after childbirth it is used by midwives in baths or lotions to aid perineal tears. After tooth extraction profuse bleeding can be controlled by gargling with calendula in cooled boiled water. Other conditions which can be helped by calendula include fever accompanied by agitation; jaundice.

Which type of person?

- no particular type

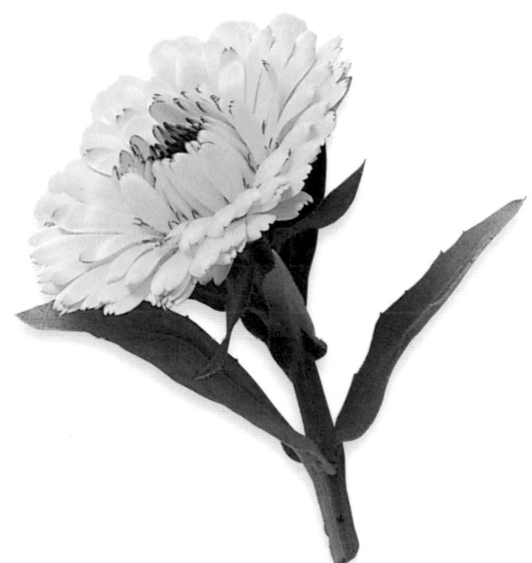

ABOVE *The leaves and flowers of calendula or pot marigold have been used for centuries by herbalists and also provide the basis for homeopathic preparations.*

CAUTION

ENSURE CUTS ARE CLEAN BEFORE USE SO THAT RAPID HEALING DOES NOT CLOSE IN DIRT OR GERMS. DO NOT USE FOR PUNCTURE WOUNDS OR DEEP CUTS AS RAPID HEALING MAY SEAL THE INFECTION INSIDE THE WOUND.

THERAPY CONNECTIONS

MARIGOLD

Herbalism p.117

Aromatherapy p.148

Cantharis vesicatoria, Lytta vesicatoria, Spanish fly, blister beetle

CANTHARIS

Spanish fly is in fact a bright green beetle which is native to southern Europe and western Asia. It emits a fast-acting irritant, cantharidin, causing blistering, hence its other common name. In the past, it was used as an aphrodisiac, causing sexual frenzy in some cases, and medicinally was used to treat a variety of ailments from warts to rheumatism. It was first "proved" by Hahnemann, and the remedy is made up from the whole beetle, dried, and then powdered. Homeopathically, it is used to treat complaints characterized by a burning sensation.

ABOVE *The Spanish fly or blister beetle is the source for Cantharis.*

SYMPTOMS

MENTAL

- irritability
- feels excessive sexual desire
- violent tendencies

PHYSICAL

- thirst, but no wish to drink
- loss of appetite
- burning sensation in the stomach
- sweating, and palpitations
- rapidly worsening infections

Symptoms improve in the warmth, with massage, after flatulence or burping, and at night, and worsen with movement, after drinking coffee or cold water, and in the afternoon.

BELOW *Conditions involving stinging or burning, especially in irritable people who tend to behave violently, can be helped by Cantharis.*

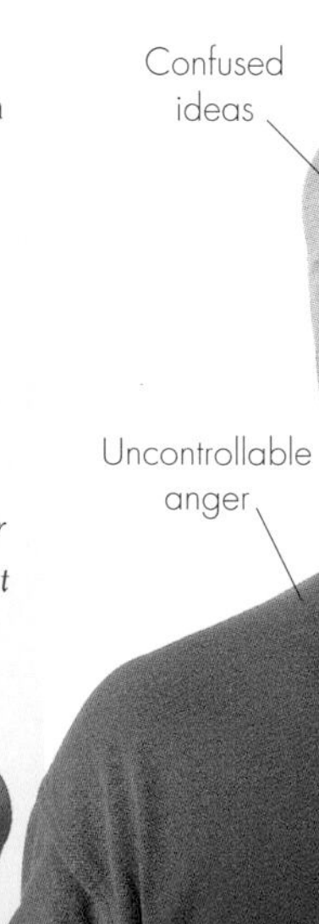

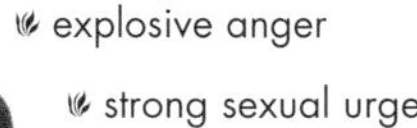

DATA FILE

Relieves

- conditions accompanied by stinging or a burning sensation
- rapidly spreading infection
- stings, burns

Uses

Ailments characterized by burning or stinging, particularly urinary tract infections such as cystitis, frequent but painful urination, insect bites, burns and scalds, infections, burning abdominal pains, and stinging diarrhea. Also for infections which spread rapidly, or conditions which quickly deteriorate. Other conditions which respond well include great thirst without a desire to drink because of breathlessness; pus-filled eruptions on hands; burning throat; burning soles of the feet; loss of appetite. Mental problems such as rage, agitation leading to violence, excessive sexual desire, and severe anxiety can be relieved by Cantharis.

Which type of person?

- have a head full of ideas, but are confused
- maniacal tendencies
- explosive anger
- strong sexual urges

Carbo vegitabilis, charcoal

CARB. VEG.

Charcoal is wood that has been burnt without air, forming a hard carbon. It has been used as a fuel, in explosives, for smelting, and as an absorbent. In the past, it was used medicinally for its deodorizing and disinfecting qualities, for septic conditions, and flatulence. Today, it is still used to treat the latter in conventional medicine. In homeopathy, charcoal from beech, poplar, and silver birch trees grown in the northern hemisphere is used, and the remedy was first "proved" by Hahnemann.

ABOVE *Charcoal, itself a classic remedy for certain types of digestive problems, is the source of Carb. veg. Beech wood is normally used.*

SYMPTOMS

MENTAL

- never quite feel well following an ailment
- lack mental energy
- fear of the supernatural

PHYSICAL

- burping, regurgitating food
- flatulence
- headaches, especially prevalent in the morning and after eating too much
- clammy hands
- indigestion
- poor circulation

Symptoms improve in cold, fresh air, and are relieved after burping, and worsen in warm, wet air, after fatty, milky foods and wine, and when lying down.

DATA FILE

Relieves

- lack of vitality; fatigue
- cold, clamminess externally, heat internally, associated with shock
- excess mucus from digestive system
- poor venous circulation

Uses

Used to aid recovery after an illness, when there is exhaustion and weakness, and for shock that may follow an operation which leaves the patient with cold, pale skin, but feeling hot inside. Also treats poor venous circulation, when the face, hands, or feet are cold and turn bluish; and bleeding varicose veins. Useful for digestive problems, such as indigestion and flatulence; asthma; whooping cough.

Which type of person?

- complain of never quite recovering after an illness
- prefer day to darkness
- fixed ideas
- mentally and physically tired and sluggish
- erratic memory

Causticum hahnemanni, potassium hydrate

CAUSTICUM

This remedy was invented and "proved" by Samuel Hahnemann himself and is unique to homeopathy. It is made chemically from quicklime (calcium oxide) and potassium bisulfate. He found that it caused a burning taste in the back of the mouth and an acerbic sensation. It is used for a set of symptoms known as the Causticum cough (*see Data File below*) and for various neuromuscular conditions.

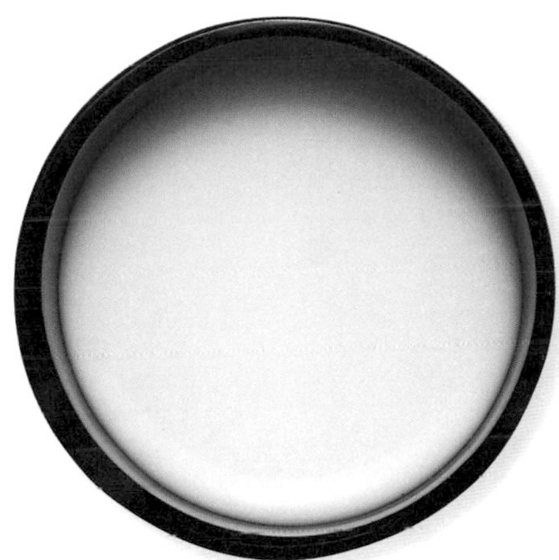

ABOVE *Quicklime (calcium oxide), which becomes slaked lime when combined with water, is used in the preparation of Causticum.*

SYMPTOMS

MENTAL

- fear animals, darkness, ghosts, strangers, death
- can be very critical of others
- empathize with the suffering of others
- despair of recovering from illness

PHYSICAL

- chilly
- prone to warts
- symptoms tend to come on slowly
- tearing, bursting pain in joints, muscles, and bones
- paralytic problems
- contractions of the muscles and tendons

Symptoms improve in warm, damp weather, after cold drinks and washing, and worsen in dry, cold winds, with movement.

DATA FILE

Relieves

- Causticum cough
- progressive weakness leading to paralysis
- burning, bursting pain

Uses

Symptoms of the Causticum cough include a raw, tickly throat with dry cough; burning in the throat; hard, racking cough; chest filled with mucus which is difficult to cough up; incontinence with each cough, and coughing which is worse on breathing out. Also helps neuromuscular problems such as weakness; stiffness; neuralgia; tearing pains in the joints, muscles, and bones; cramps, particularly affecting the vocal cords, bladder, larynx, or the right side of the face. Other conditions alleviated include dizziness when bending forward; heartburn in pregnancy; burning rheumatic pain; roaring sounds in the ears; nasal soreness; and tender scars and injury sites.

Which type of person?

- dark hair and eyes, with sallow skin
- often mentally and physically exhausted
- narrow-minded
- hypersensitive, weepy
- dislike the smell of food and feel worse after drinking coffee

Cephaelis ipecacuanha, ipecacuanha

IPECAC.

Ipecacuanha is a small, perennial shrub grown in the tropical rainforests of southern and central America. The first recorded medicinal use – for treating vomiting – was around 1600, by a Portuguese friar in Brazil. It was brought to Europe some 70 years later, where it was used as an anti-dysentery drug in France, as well as for a variety of ailments. It is still used in conventional medicine to induce vomiting in cases of drug overdoses or poisoning, and as an expectorant. Homeopathically, the root is used to treat nausea and vomiting. It is collected when the plant is in flower and then dried.

DATA FILE

Relieves

- persistent nausea
- breathing difficulties

Uses

Commonly used for nausea and vomiting, and accompanying sweats and clamminess. Also good for stomach complaints accompanied by salivating, lack of thirst, weak pulse, and fainting; conditions causing breathing difficulties, such as asthma and coughing; coughing and vomiting at the same time; persistent nausea.

Which type of person?

- no particular type

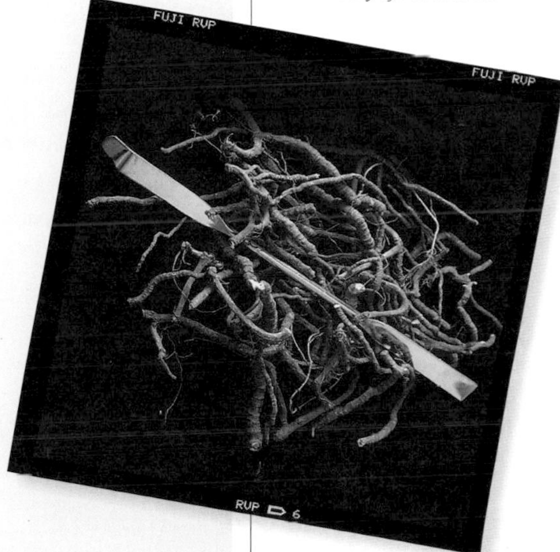

BELOW *Ipecac. is obtained from the dried root of the ipecacuanha plant that grows in Central America. The plant has a long history of medicinal use.*

SYMPTOMS

MENTAL

- contemptuous
- anxiety, including fear of death
- morose

PHYSICAL

- breathing difficulties
- constant nausea
- fainting, cold or hot sweats, clamminess
- bleeding
- weak pulse

Symptoms improve in fresh air, and worsen in warmth, in winter, when moving or lying down, and when under stress or embarrassed.

China officinalis, Cinchona succirubra, Peruvian bark, cinchona bark, Jesuits' bark

CHINA

The China remedy is made from Peruvian bark – grown in the tropical rainforests of South America, in India, and southeast Asia – which is stripped and dried. Quinine, an extract of the bark, was the first substance to be tested and "proven" by Hahnemann, in 1790. He used quinine on himself, noting that large doses caused similar symptoms to malaria, while small doses acted as an antidote. Quinine is still used in conventional medicine today as part of the treatment for malaria. Homeopathically, the dried bark of China is used for exhaustion.

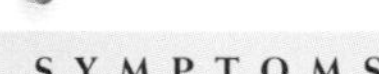

DATA FILE

Relieves

- nervous exhaustion after incapacitating illness
- weakness after vomiting, diarrhea, or sweating, as a result of loss of body fluids

Uses

Aids recovery from nervous exhaustion after debilitating illness and as a result of loss of fluids from vomiting, diarrhea, or sweating. Also for digestive conditions such as gastroenteritis, flatulence, and gallbladder problems; mental upsets such as lack of concentration, indifference, and outbursts that are out of character; also neuralgia, dizziness, tired and twitchy muscles, tinnitus, hemorrhages.

Which type of person?

- sensitive
- intense
- artistic
- idealistic
- their own intensity is tiring, making them lazy, depressed, sometimes violent
- find it difficult to express themselves to others so do so through their creativity
- prefer talking about meaningful issues, not trivia
- imaginative mind, fantasize about heroic deeds

ABOVE *People who are imaginative and artistic, especially if they are exhausted, weakened, or mentally tired out, may be helped by China.*

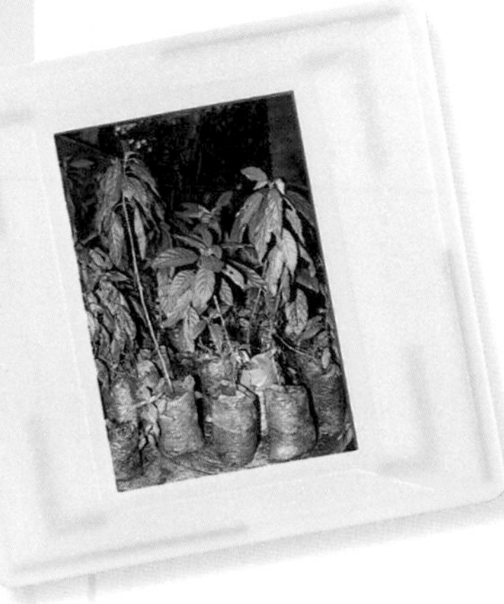

LEFT *The remedy is obtained from the bark of* China officinalis, *which also yields quinine.*

SYMPTOMS

MENTAL

- emotionally fragile
- difficulty in expressing feelings
- lacks concentration
- nervous exhaustion

PHYSICAL

- headaches, dizziness
- convulsions
- weak muscles
- sallow skin
- indigestion, flatulence, a feeling that food is stuck behind the breastbone

Symptoms improve in the warmth, when firm pressure is applied to the affected area, and after sleeping, and worsen in the cold or draughts, in the fall.

Cimicifuga racemosa, Actaea racemosa, Black cohosh, bugbane, black snakeroot, rattleroot

CIMIC.

Grown in the U.S. and Canada, the Native Americans used the rhizome or underground stem of this plant to cure rattlesnake bites, giving it one of its common names, rattleroot, and for rheumatism and gynecological problems. It has also been used for menstrual and labor pain as well as being chewed as a sedative to help with depression. Brewed in a tea which was then sprinkled around a room, it was said to prevent the presence of evil spirits. Homeopathically, it was "proved" in America. The fresh black root is commonly used for treating problems arising during pregnancy and childbirth.

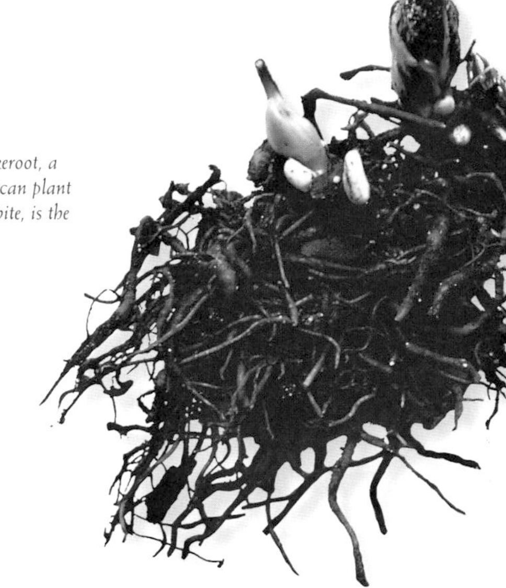

RIGHT *Black snakeroot, a native North American plant once used for snakebite, is the source for Cimic.*

SYMPTOMS

MENTAL

- emotional and highly strung
- sigh repeatedly when sad
- strong fears, such as insanity and death, particularly when menopausal

PHYSICAL

- cramps and backache when premenstrual
- nausea and vomiting in pregnancy
- depression after childbirth
- faints and flushes during menopause

Symptoms improve when warm, in fresh air, when pressure is applied, and with gentle movement, but worsen in cold, damp, draughty conditions, with alcohol or excitement.

DATA FILE

Relieves

- menstrual symptoms
- nausea, vomiting in pregnancy
- head, neck aches
- woefulness
- conditions accompanied by chills

Uses

Cimic. works well on the nerves and muscles of the uterus, making it useful for menstrual problems such as back cramps and headaches; early miscarriage; pregnancy complaints, such as pain in the uterus, difficulty in sleeping, nausea, and vomiting; and postnatal depression and menopausal problems, such as hot flushes. The upheaval in emotions associated with these problems, such as anxiety and irritability, can also be relieved.

Which type of person?

- mainly women
- often extrovert, talkative, and excitable
- when sad become depressed, often sigh
- experience strong, intense emotions
- fear death

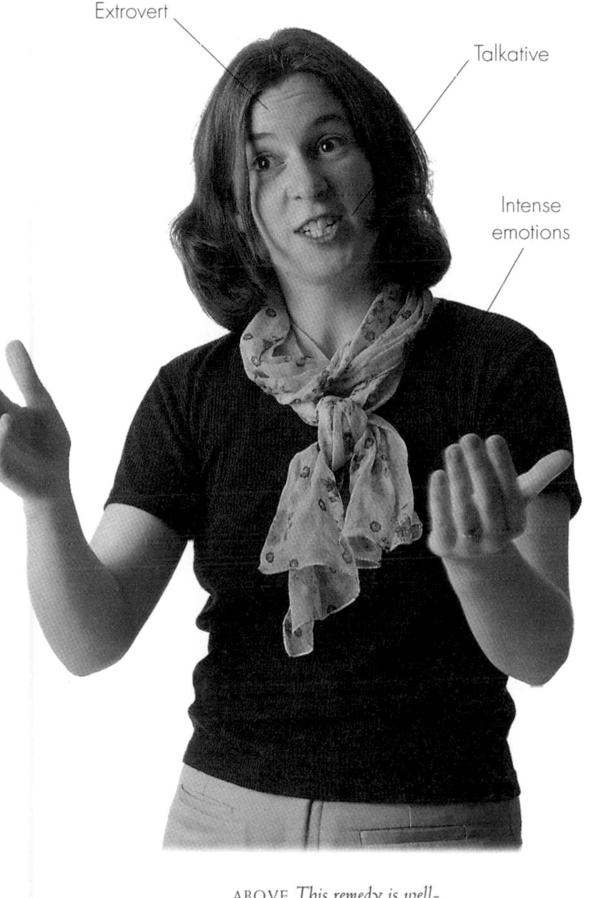

ABOVE *This remedy is well-suited to many female complaints, and can be helpful for women who appear restless and highly strung.*

Cucumis colocynthis, bitter apple, bitter cucumber

COLOCYNTHIS

Colocynthis, or Coloc., comes from a gourd, *Cucumis colocynthis*. In the past, the bitter apple, as it is also known, was used by Arab and ancient Greek physicians as a purgative (with radical results), in order to induce abortion, and to treat derangement, lethargy, and dropsy. The seeds alone are harmless, but when the whole fruit is eaten, it causes bowel inflammation and cramping pains, due to the release of a resin called colocynthin. Homeopathically, the fruit – which grows in hot, arid conditions – is dried and powdered, without the seeds. It was first used in 1834, and is given as treatment for digestive complaints and colic.

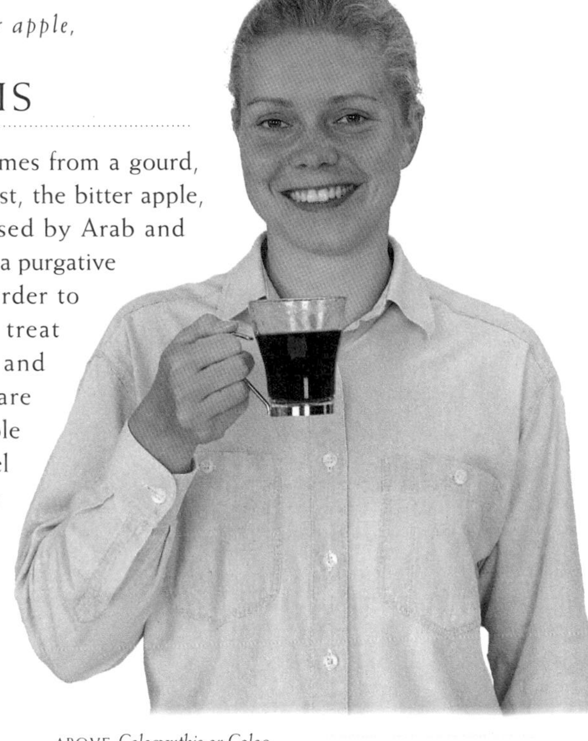

ABOVE *Colocynthis or Coloc. is often found suitable for people who are fair haired and fair-skinned, when their symptoms are related to anger.*

SYMPTOMS

MENTAL

- upset if contradicted, especially if feel humiliated
- keen for justice to be done

PHYSICAL

- digestive problems
- neuralgia and headaches
- abdominal pain

Symptoms improve in the warmth, after flatulence, or drinking coffee, but worsen after eating, when indignant or angry, and in damp, cold weather.

BELOW *The leaves of the bitter cucumber (also called bitter apple), whose fruit is the source of Coloc.*

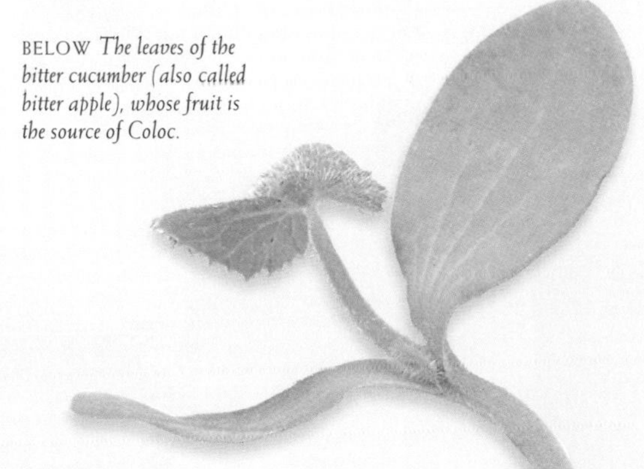

DATA FILE

Relieves

- digestive complaints
- neuralgia, headaches, and stomach pains brought on by anger

Uses

Mainly used to treat symptoms brought on by anger, particularly suppressed anger, such as neuralgia and abdominal pain; stomach pain, facial neuralgia, and headaches respond well, as does nerve pain in the ovaries or kidneys; gout, sciatica, and rheumatism symptoms can also be helped.

Which type of person?

- tend to be fair-haired and fair-skinned
- reserved
- have a strong sense of right and wrong
- dislike being contradicted
- suffer physical effects when angry or indignant

Coffea arabica, Coffea cruda, coffee

COFFEA

Coffee is native to Arabia and Ethiopia, and is thought to have been first drunk in Persia. Now grown in Central America and the West Indies, it has been used widely for medicinal purposes as a diuretic, painkiller, and to ease indigestion. It is also a well-known stimulant. Homeopathically, coffea is made from the raw berries of the coffee tree, and was first "proved" by Hahnemann himself and a handful of volunteers. It is mainly used to treat those who are excitable and mentally overstimulated.

SYMPTOMS

MENTAL

- irritable
- heightened senses
- mind buzzing with ideas
- anxiety leading to restlessness
- insomnia
- guilt

PHYSICAL

- trembling limbs
- toothache
- headaches
- palpitations
- hypersensitive skin

ABOVE *Raw coffee beans are the source of Coffea. Coffee has been used for a variety of medicinal purposes as well as in the production of caffeine.*

Symptoms improve in the warmth, after lying down, and when holding cold water in the mouth. They worsen with extreme emotions such as anger, with touch, smell, or noise, and during cold, windy weather.

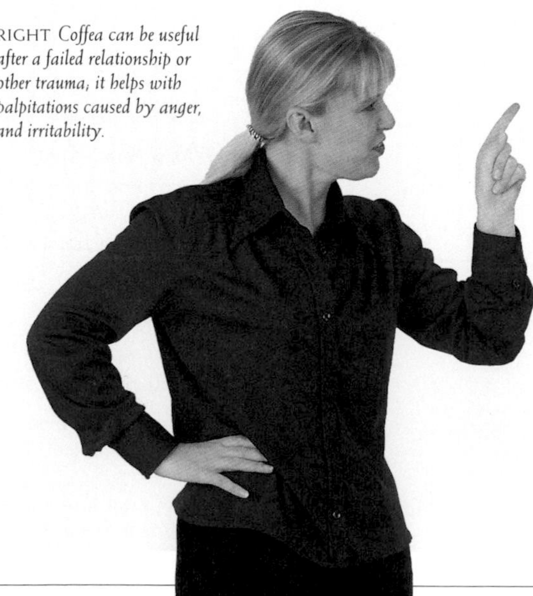

RIGHT *Coffea can be useful after a failed relationship or other trauma; it helps with palpitations caused by anger, and irritability.*

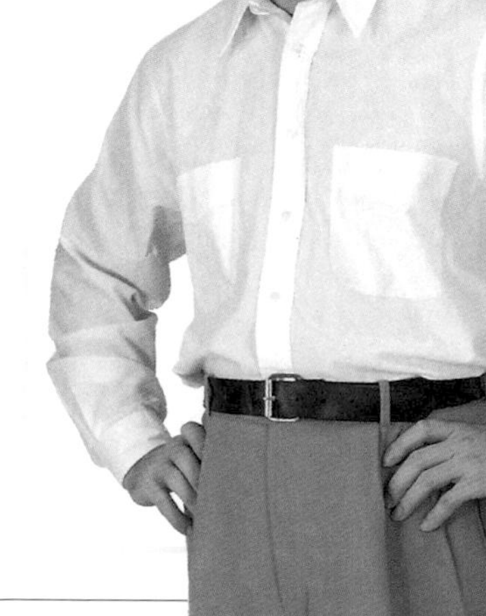

DATA FILE

Relieves

- excitability
- mental overstimulation
- sleeplessness

Uses

Commonly used to treat excessive mental activity when the mind seems to be buzzing; where the person is very excitable and hypersensitive, for instance with toothache or labor pain; when all the senses are acutely affected, making any noise, smell, or touch seem unbearable; headaches which are so severe it feels like a nail is being driven into the skull; palpitations when excited or angry; and for acute premenstrual symptoms.

Which type of person?

- tall, lean, with a tendency to stoop
- dark complexion
- symptoms may appear after a failed relationship, and with exhaustion or after a trauma
- on a high, but will then descend into despair
- tend to "burn out"

Cuprum mettalicum, copper

CUPRUM MET.

Copper, a red-gold metal, is often found in many tools and weapons. In the past, coppersmiths often suffered toxic poisoning due to working with the metal, falling ill with complaints such as coughs, malnutrition, colicky pain, and sometimes even paralysis and death. In the days when alcohol was often made secretly in home distilleries, poisoning occurred from the copper tubing. Small amounts were also used medicinally to help heal wounds. Homeopathically, it was first "proved" in 1834, and is used to treat respiratory problems and various complaints of the nervous system.

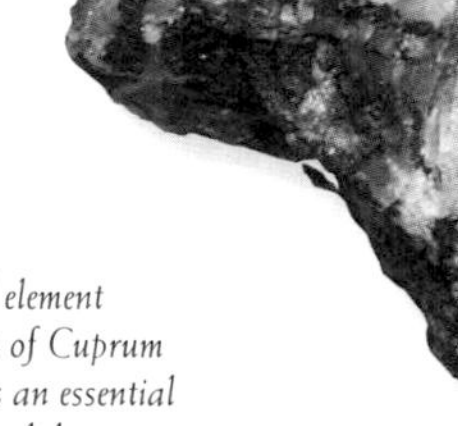

RIGHT *The metal element copper is the source of Cuprum met. Copper itself is an essential trace element although larger amounts are toxic.*

SYMPTOMS

MENTAL

- hide deep emotions
- suppression of feelings leads to physical problems
- cry, becoming morose

PHYSICAL

- twitches, jerks, convulsions
- erratic breathing
- pale color, sometimes turning blue

Symptoms improve after sweating and cold drinks, and worsen if emotions are being suppressed, in the heat, when touched, and after vomiting.

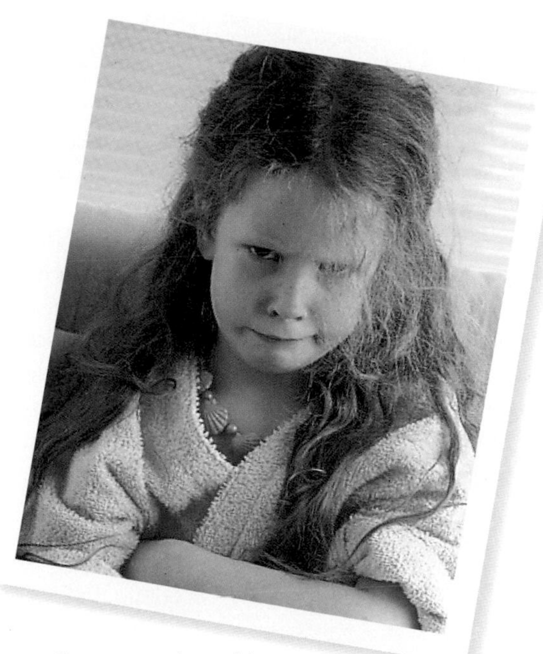

ABOVE *Cuprum met. can be a useful remedy for problems in children who have a destructive mentality, and when angry, hold their breath.*

DATA FILE

Relieves

- muscular spasm, cramp
- breathing problems
- tiredness associated with mental exhaustion

Uses

Problems of the nervous system are commonly treated. Tics, twitches – particularly those that start in a minor way and spread more deeply – and convulsions can be helped. Epilepsy responds well. Tiredness brought on after much mental activity can be treated, as can respiratory problems when breathing seems to be intermittent, such as with asthma.

Which type of person?

- intensely emotional, but suppress feelings, so may appear reserved
- serious, self-critical
- swing from being headstrong to submissive

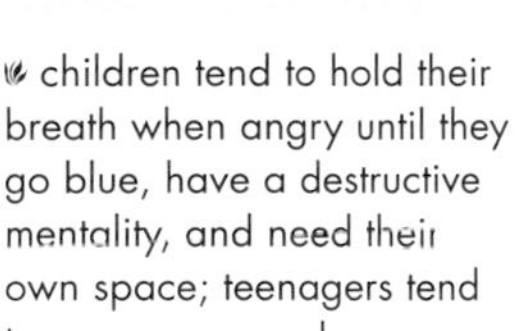

- children tend to hold their breath when angry until they go blue, have a destructive mentality, and need their own space; teenagers tend to suppress sexual urges

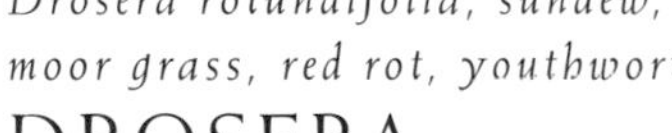

Drosera rotundifolia, sundew, moor grass, red rot, youthwort

DROSERA

The sundew is a carnivorous plant which grows widely in the heaths and boggy areas of Europe, South America, the U.S., China, and India. Insects are attracted by the long, red hairs on the leaves of the plant. Glands on the surface of the leaves then secrete a fluid which traps and breaks down the insect, digesting it. The juice of the plant is caustic, affecting the respiratory system, and when eaten by sheep, leads to a harsh, spasmodic cough. It was used in the Middle Ages to treat the plague, and 16th-century physicians used it for tuberculosis. Homeopathically, it was "proved" by Hahnemann, and the whole fresh plant is used, mainly to treat coughs.

SYMPTOMS

MENTAL

- feel persecuted
- difficulty in concentrating
- unable to settle, and become stubborn

PHYSICAL

- barking cough
- tingling in leg bones

Symptoms improve when walking, in fresh air, with pressure, when sitting up, and when quiet. They worsen after midnight, after cold food and drinking, when lying down, and if the bed is too warm.

DATA FILE

Relieves

- severe, spasmodic hollow-sounding cough
- breathing difficulties
- retching or the vomiting of mucus
- growing pains

Uses

Complaints such as whooping cough, characterized by a violent, spasmodic, hollow-sounding cough, triggered by a tickling sensation in the throat. The cough worsens after midnight, and at the acute stage is accompanied by retching and vomiting, cold sweats, and nose-bleeds, after which the patient becomes talkative. Also helps the uncomfortable tingling sensation associated with growing pains, stiffness, and a hoarse voice.

Which type of person?

- restless, obstinate when ill
- unable to concentrate
- dislike being left alone
- fear of ghosts
- worry about being given bad news

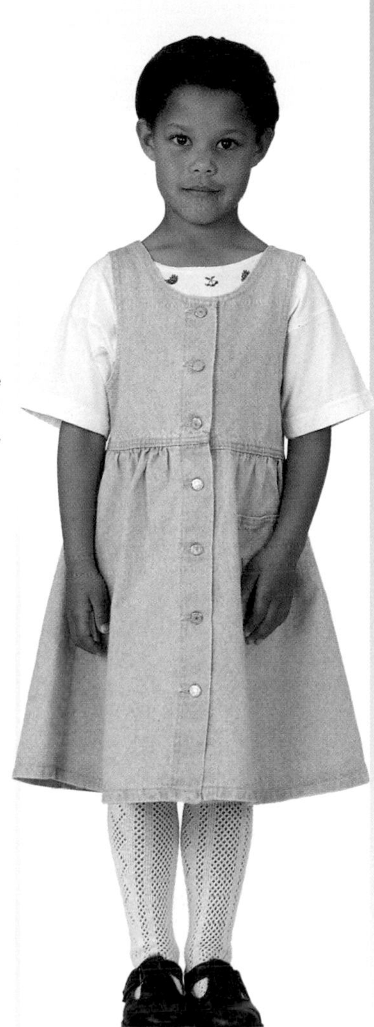

RIGHT *Children who find it hard to settle, especially when ill, may be cured of coughs by this remedy.*

LEFT Drosera rotundifolia, *the round-leaved sundew plant that is used to produce Drosera.*

Euphrasia officinalis, Euphrasia stricta, eyebright

EUPHRASIA

Grown in Europe and America, eyebright – as its name suggests – has been used for centuries to treat eye problems. It is believed the name comes from one of the Three Graces, Euphrosyne, who was known for her gladness and joy. First mentioned as an eye treatment in 1305, it was used in later centuries as an infusion for eyes, and in the 19th century was also used as a treatment for coughs, headaches, and earaches. It is commonly used in herbal medicine. Homeopathically, the whole fresh plant is used when in flower to make a remedy for sore, irritated eyes and eye injuries.

ABOVE *The flowering plant* Euphrasia officinalis *or eyebright is used by herbalists as well as in homeopathy.*

DATA FILE

Relieves

- stinging, watery discharge from the eyes
- inflammation or injury to the eyes
- running eyes associated with hay fever

Uses

Any eye irritation or inflammation, such as conjunctivitis, inflammation of the eyelid or iris, small blisters on the cornea. Also for dimmed vision; dislike of bright lights; watery, irritated eyes associated with hay fever sufferers, but accompanied by only bland nasal discharge; colds accompanied by flushed face and runny catarrh; eye injuries; dry eyes associated with the menopause. Also useful for constipation, exploding headaches, short painful menstruation, the early stages of measles, and, in men, inflammation of the prostate gland.

Which type of person?

- no particular type

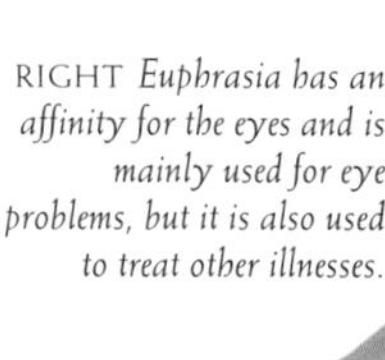

RIGHT *Euphrasia has an affinity for the eyes and is mainly used for eye problems, but it is also used to treat other illnesses.*

SYMPTOMS

MENTAL

- none in particular

PHYSICAL

- stinging discharge from the eyes
- watering eyes
- an intolerance of bright light
- hot cheeks
- bursting headaches

Symptoms improve after lying down in a darkened room and with drinking coffee, and worsen in bright light, in the evening, in enclosed spaces, and during warm, windy weather.

Ferrum phosphoricum, iron phosphate

FERR. PHOS.

The Ferr. phos. remedy is made from iron phosphate, which is a chemical combination of iron sulfate, sodium phosphate, and sodium acetate. It is one of the 12 biochemical tissue salts developed by the German physician Wilhelm Schussler between 1872 and 1898. Schussler believed many complaints were the result of a deficiency of minerals, and that by replacing these minerals, or tissue salts, health could be restored. Schussler found Ferr. phos. particularly useful in the early stages of inflammation, and the homeopathic remedy is used for similar purposes.

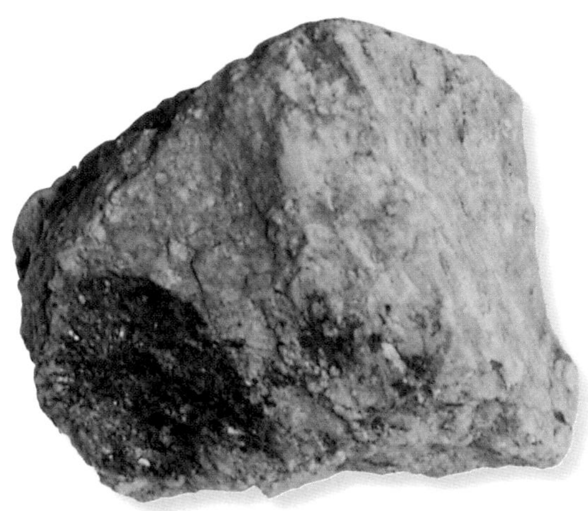

ABOVE *The mineral salt ferrous phosphate, from which Ferr. phos. is prepared, is a compound of iron, the white magnetic metal derived from iron ores.*

SYMPTOMS

MENTAL

- none in particular

PHYSICAL

- headaches and head colds
- dry, hacking cough, laryngitis, hoarseness
- shooting rheumatic pains
- facial flushing and rapid pulse
- chills starting in the early afternoon

Symptoms improve with gentle exercise and cold compresses, and worsen in the heat, with movement, when touched, lying on the right side, between 4 A.M. and 6 A.M., when suppressing sweating.

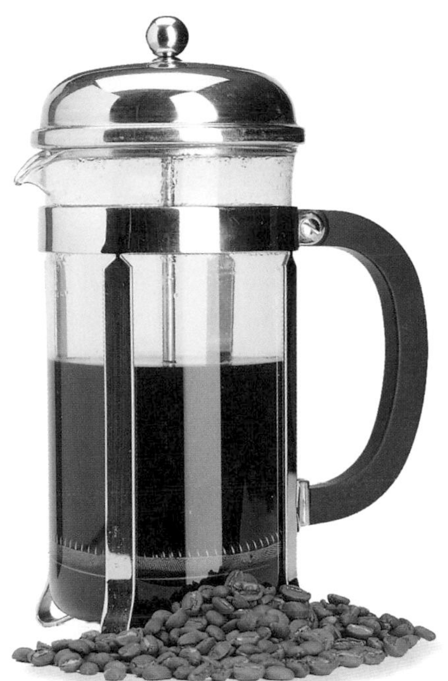

ABOVE *A craving for coffee may indicate Ferrum phosphoricum as an appropriate remedy.*

DATA FILE

Relieves

- early stages of inflammation or infection
- coughs and colds which come on slowly

Uses

First stages of inflammation or infection, when more blood is flowing to the affected areas, causing congestion, and before the onset of other symptoms. Also slow-starting colds accompanied by nosebleeds and fevers, with hacking coughs; headaches which are helped by cool water; rheumatic pain; gastritis including vomiting undigested food; indigestion with sour-tasting burps; hemorrhages; in women, intermittent, painful menstruation; stress incontinence; first stages of dysentery with bloody stools.

Which type of person?

- pale, anemic-looking
- full of ideas
- susceptible to sudden facial flushes
- complaining but good-natured
- dislike milk, meat, crave coffee
- tend to suffer respiratory and gastrointestinal complaints

Gelsemium sempervirens, yellow jasmine, Carolina jasmine, false jasmine

GELSEMIUM

ABOVE *Gelsemium is produced from the poisonous false jasmine* Gelsemium sempervirens, *also known as Carolina jasmine.*

This climbing plant, with its fragrant yellow flowers, is native to the southern states of the U.S. and, despite being attractive to look at, is poisonous if eaten. Ingesting large quantities will affect the respiratory system and movement, leading to shaking, inflammation, and paralysis. Historically, its medicinal uses were first noted when a farmer in Mississippi in the 1840s accidentally ate the plant's root and found his fever was cured. It was used as a treatment for fevers in herbalism before being "proven" in homeopathy.

SYMPTOMS

MENTAL

- fears and phobias, accompanied by trembling and need to urinate
- fears such as the dentist, falling or throwing oneself from a height
- dull and lethargic
- nervous and feel inadequate

PHYSICAL

- headaches causing tightness
- faintness
- facial flushing
- visual disturbances
- muscle pain
- trembling

Symptoms improve after urinating and perspiring, after alcohol or stimulants, and when bending forward. They worsen after physical exertion, in heat, humidity, damp, or fog, with excitement, worry, or stress about symptoms.

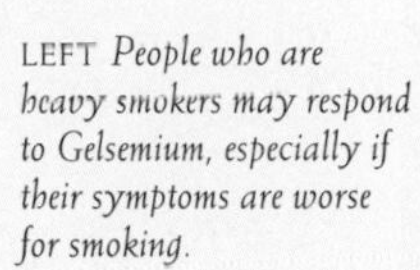

LEFT *People who are heavy smokers may respond to Gelsemium, especially if their symptoms are worse for smoking.*

DATA FILE

Relieves

- complaints of the nervous system
- fears and phobias
- colds, flu
- visual disturbances

Uses

Conditions which affect the nervous system respond well, such as problems of the nerves and muscles. Headaches which worsen with movement or light; muscle pain which accompanies fever; nervous disorders such as multiple sclerosis; nerve inflammation; right eye pain; heavy, drooping eyelids; inflamed tonsils and summer colds can all be helped. Also fevers, including flushing; an unpleasant taste in the mouth; twitchy muscles, and chills. It can help alleviate fears and shock accompanied by shaking or trembling. Visual disturbances and blurred vision can also be treated.

Which type of person?

- dull and heavy-looking, often with a blue tinge to the skin
- intelligence is often below average
- heavy smokers
- cowardly
- mentally weak

Glonoinum, nitroglycerine, glyceryl trinitrate

GLON.

Nitroglycerine, a thick, clear, toxic liquid, was discovered by the Italian chemist A. Sobrero in the mid-19th century. Two decades later, Swedish scientist Alfred Nobel used it as the explosive component in dynamite. In conventional medicine it is used to treat heart disease. Homeopathically, the remedy is made from glycerine, nitric and sulfuric acid. In Victorian times, typesetters and printers who worked under the powerful heat of incandescent gas lamps used it to treat the severe headaches they suffered. The remedy is mainly used for blood and circulation conditions.

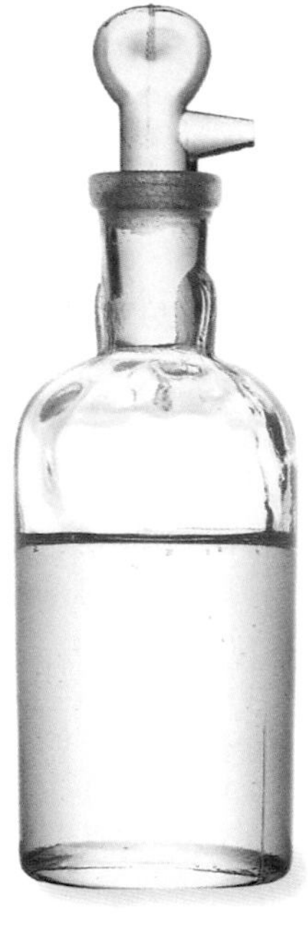

ABOVE *Glonoinum (also known as Glonoin) is based on nitroglycerine, which is produced from glycerine with nitric and sulfuric acid.*

DATA FILE

Relieves

- heatstroke
- headaches
- hot flushes

Uses

This is a useful remedy for heatstroke, when an increase in blood circulation flows to the head, causing flushes of heat and a painful bursting sensation in the head. It is also good for headaches and migraine when the head feels very hot and blood vessels seem to be expanding, the patient feels like vomiting, and pressure on the head is unbearable; dizziness; for headaches which are aggravated by heat or cold; and for the cessation of menstruation and the hot flushes often associated with the menopause.

Which type of person?

- no particular type

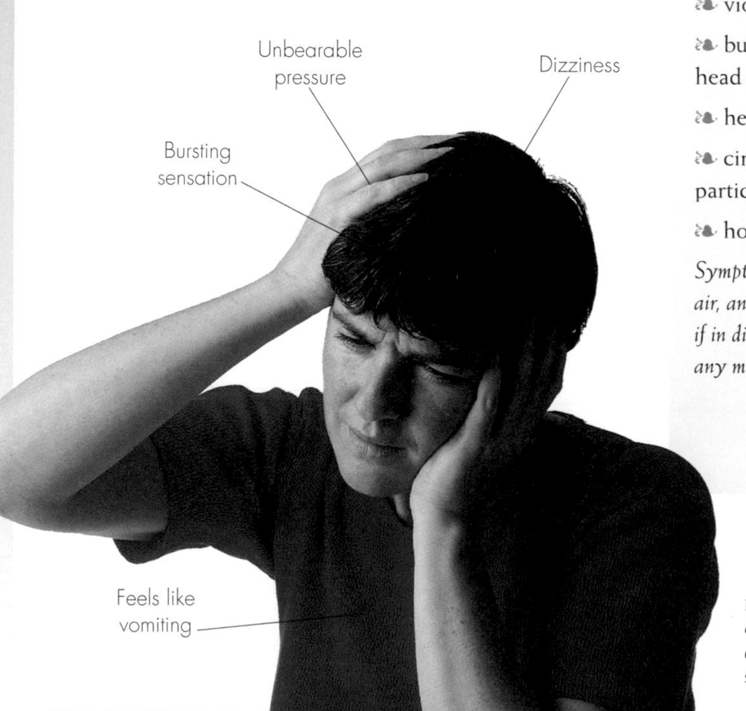

LEFT *Nitroglycerine is a characteristically unstable explosive and treats symptoms of the same sort.*

SYMPTOMS

MENTAL

- quick and violent
- expansive
- strong emotions
- confused
- lacks sense of direction in life

PHYSICAL

- violent symptoms
- bursting feeling in head and neck
- headaches, migraine
- circulation not particularly good
- hot flushes

Symptoms improve in fresh air, and worsen in the heat, if in direct sunlight, with any movement of the head.

Graphites, graphite, plumbago, black lead

GRAPH.

Graphite is a mineral found in marble, granite, and crystalline rocks, and is mined in Sri Lanka, Canada, the U.S., and Mexico. It is a mixture of carbon, iron, and silica, and is contained in products such as batteries, polishes, lubricants, and also pencils – its name comes from the Greek *graphein*, meaning to write. It was first "proved" by Hahnemann when he discovered that workmen were using black lead to heal cold sores. Homeopathically, graphite is ground to a powder to make the remedy, and is used to treat skin complaints and metabolic imbalances.

RIGHT *The remedy Graphite is obtained from the powdered natural mineral.*

DATA FILE

Relieves

- skin problems, nail malformation, and obesity, which have been triggered by metabolic imbalances
- menstrual problems
- stomach ulcers
- problems on the left side of the body

Uses

Commonly used for skin problems such as eczema, where the skin cracks in places such as the palms of the hands, behind the knees and ears, and a thick discharge oozes out. Skin complaints which have been triggered by a metabolic imbalance, such as psoriasis, where the skin becomes dry and cracked, and nail malformation; cuts and grazes that refuse to heal and become septic; inflamed, itchy scars, and obesity can be treated. Conditions that develop on the soft mucous membranes, for instance in the mouth or stomach, such as cold sores and ulcers can also be helped. Other conditions, such as hair loss, cramps in hands and feet, catarrh, swollen glands, and sweating after nosebleeds are responsive.

Which type of person?

- dark-haired, coarse-featured, with pale, dry skin
- overweight, even obese
- only able to concentrate for short periods
- moody, apprehensive, indecisive, slow reactions
- prefer sour and acidic cold drinks, dislike seafood, sweet and salty things
- grumpy on waking and become more irritable throughout the day
- prefer outdoor, manual employment
- children tend to be plump and pale-looking; pessimistic and anxious; prone to car sickness; and tend to have little stamina

SYMPTOMS

MENTAL

- fear of thunderstorms, insanity, death
- anxiety as do not feel mentally alert
- easily startled
- tend to be morose and occasionally depressed

PHYSICAL

- dry, rough skin
- flaky and crusted scalp
- easily flushed
- no stamina
- headaches if a meal is missed
- ulcers or cold sores
- problems tend to occur on left side

Symptoms improve in warm, fresh air, after eating or sleeping, and in the dark. They worsen in cold, damp air, in the morning and evening, during menstruation, after eating sweet food or seafood, and if the skin problems are suppressed, for instance with steroids.

BELOW *Fear of thunderstorms may be one of a number of symptoms that indicate Glycerine as an appropriate remedy.*

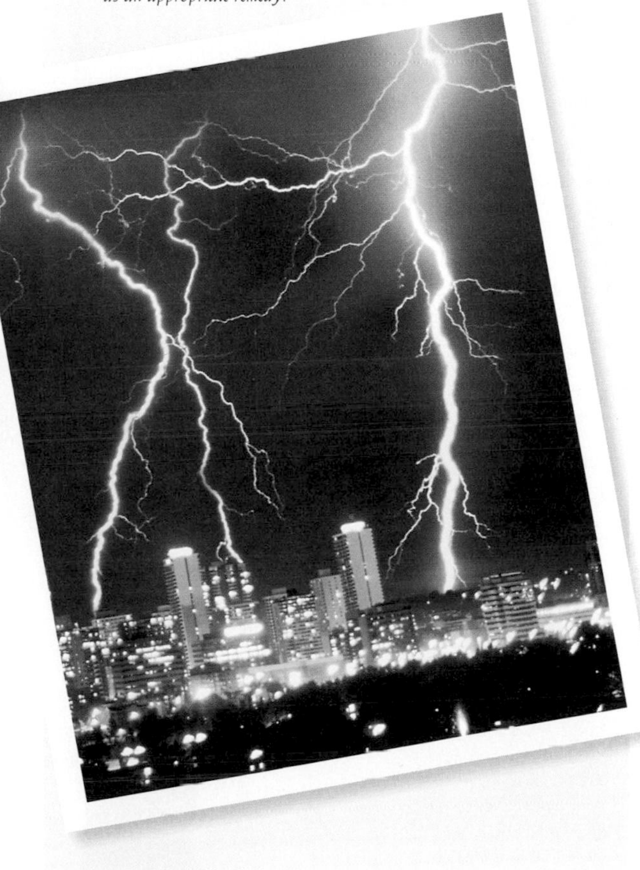

Hamamelis virginiana, witch hazel, snapping hazelnut, spotted alder

HAMAMELIS

Grown in parts of Canada, America, and Europe, witch hazel, which can come from a number of trees or shrubs in the *hamamelis* family, has historically been used for its astringent qualities. In conventional medicine, it has been used for treating minor cuts, burns, rashes, and insect bites. In the homeopathic remedy, the outer skin of the root and bark of the twigs are chopped and pounded to a pulp. The remedy was first "proved" in 1850 by Dr. Hering, an American follower of Hahnemann, and is commonly used to treat piles and varicose veins by improving venous circulation.

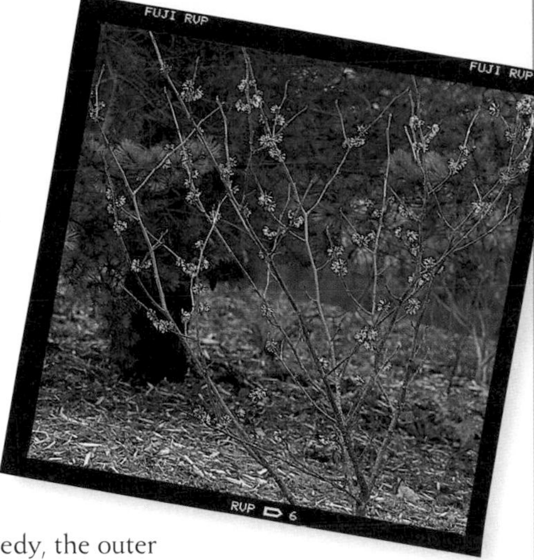

ABOVE Hamamelis *or witch hazel, the plant whose roots and bark are used for the Hamamelis remedy. The plant has long been used in herbal medicine.*

SYMPTOMS

MENTAL

- depression, wanting to be left alone
- restlessness and irritability
- demand respect
- big ideas

PHYSICAL

- piles, varicose veins
- painful bruising
- bloodshot eyes
- headaches, relieved by nosebleeds
- in women, inflammation of the ovaries or uterus
- heavy menstrual bleeding, pain at the time of ovulation

Symptoms improve in fresh air and after thinking about the problem, talking, or reading, and worsen in warm, damp air, and with pressure or movement.

DATA FILE

Relieves

- varicose veins, piles
- nosebleeds
- bruises
- depression

Uses

Primarily used to treat problems associated with bleeding, such as varicose veins and piles (hemorrhoids), which occur when the veins become weakened and swollen with blood; also when the fragile blood vessels in the nose rupture, causing nosebleeds; bruises and soreness due to injury; bloodshot eyes; phlegm dotted with blood after coughing. It is also used for heavy bleeding during menstruation and pain during ovulation, as well as being given to treat bouts of depression.

Which type of person?

- no particular type

THERAPY CONNECTIONS

WITCH HAZEL

Traditional Home and Folk Remedies p.91
Herbalism p.123

BELOW *Hamamelis is most often used to treat problems that involve bleeding, such as nosebleeds and bruising.*

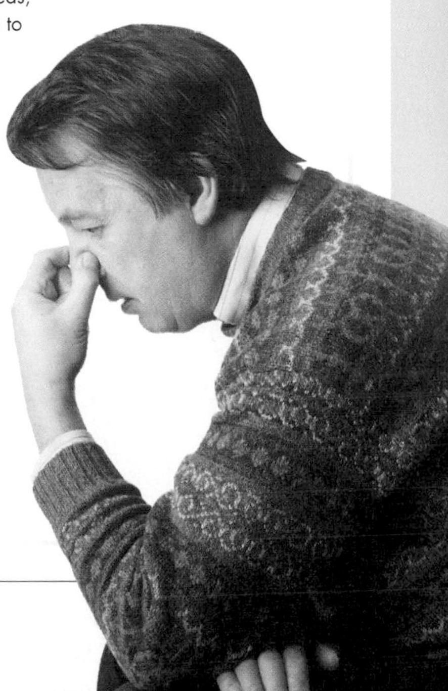

Hepar sulfuris calcareum, calcium sulfide

HEP. SULF.

Historically, calcium sulfide was used to treat a number of complaints such as rheumatism, gout, and itching. In conventional medicine it is used for skin conditions such as acne and boils. It was first "proved" by Hahnemann in 1794 and was used to counter the effects of mercury, which was often used to treat illnesses at that time. Homeopathically, the remedy, made from heating the calcareous inner layer of oyster shells with flowers of sulfur, is used to treat skin infections and ailments accompanied by a discharge.

ABOVE *Flowers of sulfur are used in the preparation of Hep. sulf., mixed in equal parts with powdered oyster shells.*

SYMPTOMS

MENTAL

- anxious and irritable
- tendency to be depressed
- sluggish
- sensitive to touch, pain, cold air, noise

PHYSICAL

- sour-smelling secretions – sweat, urine, stools
- skin moist and sensitive
- low pain threshold
- seeping ailments: ulcers, cold sores, acne, boils
- coughs, colds, sore throats, flu

Symptoms improve in warmth, after applying warm compresses, and after eating, and worsen in the morning, in the cold, when touching or lying on the affected parts.

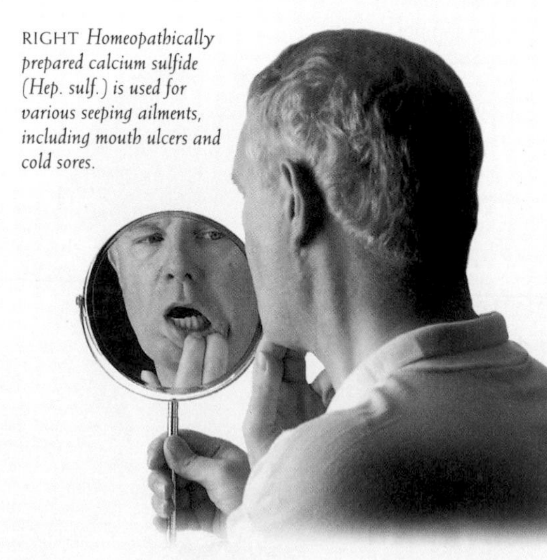

RIGHT *Homeopathically prepared calcium sulfide (Hep. sulf.) is used for various seeping ailments, including mouth ulcers and cold sores.*

DATA FILE

Relieves

- pus-producing infections
- skin infections
- conditions accompanied by sensitivity to touch

Uses

Commonly treats infections in which there is discharge, such as conjunctivitis, sinusitis, cold sores, and mouth ulcers, as well as general infections such as earache, tonsillitis, phlegm-filled chests, and flu. Also used for infections to aid in expelling pus, such as for acne where the spots are sensitive to touch. Other conditions which it can be used to help include colds accompanied by a tickly cough, and dry, hoarse coughs accompanied by a lot of phlegm.

Which type of person?

- tend to be flabby or are quite overweight
- pale-looking
- lethargic and listless
- have exaggerated likes and dislikes
- anxious and frequently bad-tempered
- fail to think things through properly
- easily offended

Hyoscyamus niger, henbane, black henbane, hog's bean, stinking Roger

HYOSCYAMUS

It is believed the Romans first brought this poisonous plant to Europe, although it is also grown in parts of the U.S., Canada, and Asia, thriving on rubbish heaps and cemeteries. In conventional medicine it was used as a painkiller, sedative, and anticonvulsant, and the drug hyoscine is currently given as an antispasmodic. Homeopathically, it was first "proved" by Hahnemann. The remedy is made by extracting juice from the whole fresh plant (which is of the same botanical family as Belladonna) when in flower. It is a useful remedy for the elderly due to its gentle approach.

DATA FILE

Relieves

- emotional problems
- twitches
- dry coughs

Uses

Used when emotions, such as jealousy or paranoia, seem to have taken over, and the sufferer feels that he or she is being watched or poisoned. The patient will be either silent or very talkative, with violent outbursts and foul language. Physical conditions are characterized by confusion and passive stupor, with the patient mumbling and weak; twitching and trembling may occur. Dry, spasmodic coughs, that are accompanied by twitching and jerking, and helped by sitting up, also respond.

Which type of person?

- lack of self-expression
- suspicious
- may hallucinate
- urge to count things

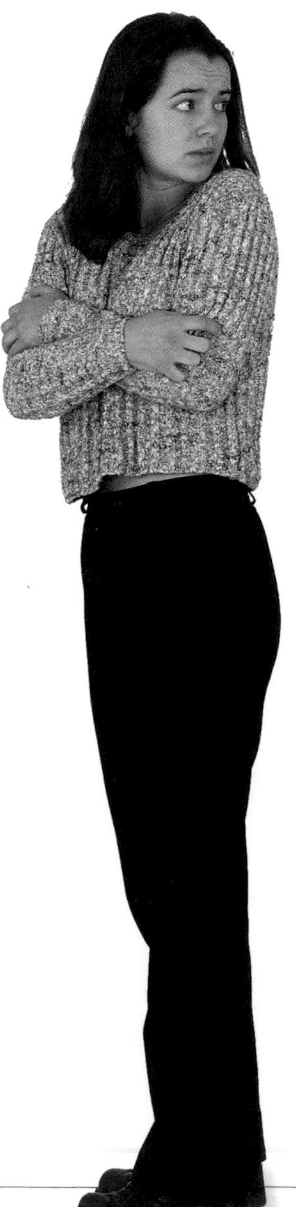

RIGHT *People with emotional problems verging on paranoia may be helped by this gentle remedy.*

SYMPTOMS

MENTAL

- talkative, even obscene
- want to expose body
- may laugh at anything
- fear of animals
- ritual behavior

PHYSICAL

- agitation
- muscle tremors, involuntary jerking
- cough
- sensitive skin
- urge to urinate, although little and infrequent flow

Symptoms improve when bending or sitting up, and worsen after emotional upset, when touched, after food, when lying down, and in the evening.

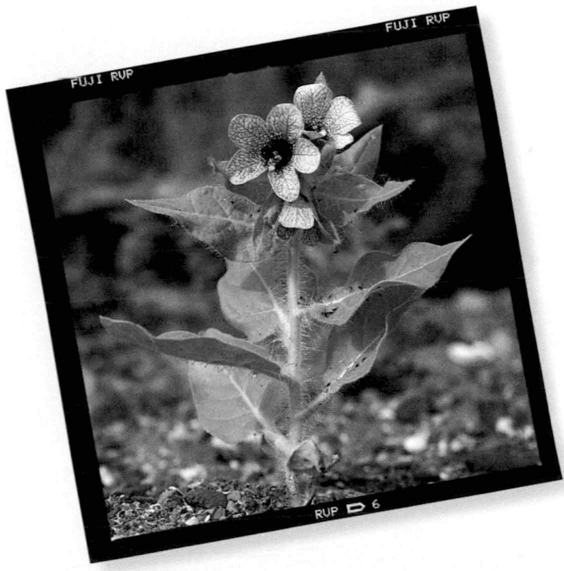

ABOVE *Black henbane, from the same family as Belladonna, is the source for the Hyoscyamus remedy.*

Hypericum perforatum, St. John's wort

HYPERICUM

The St. John's wort shrub is native to Asia and Europe, but is now grown worldwide. Its glandular leaves and yellow flowers secrete a blood-red juice, which led it to be used for cuts and wounds in the past. Its name comes from John the Baptist, and the black marks on the leaves were said to be a symbol of his beheading at the insistence of Herod's daughter, Salome. It is commonly used in herbal medicine, where, as in homeopathy, it is valued for its antidepressant action. In homeopathy, the whole fresh plant is used when in flower, and it is most often given to treat nerve pain following injury, due to its effective action on the central nervous system. Hypericum was "proved" by Dr. G. F. Mueller.

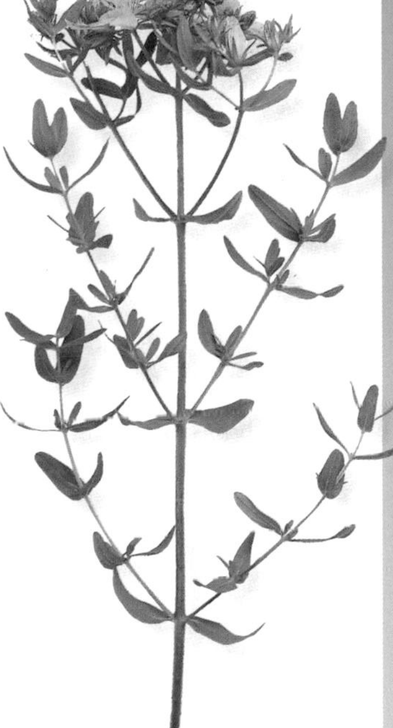

ABOVE *St. John's wort. All parts of the fresh, flowering plant are used to make the Hypericum remedy.*

SYMPTOMS

MENTAL

- depression
- sleepiness

PHYSICAL

- neuralgia
- concussion
- toothache
- severe shooting pains that travel upward
- cravings for hot drinks, wine

Symptoms improve when the head is tilted backward, but worsen in warm, stuffy rooms; in damp, cold, or foggy weather; when touched, or when the affected part is exposed.

BELOW *Hypericum can be used as a first aid remedy for all kinds of injury, including concussion.*

DATA FILE

Relieves

- nerve pain after injury
- head injuries
- shooting pains

Uses

Hypericum works well on any area affected by nerve pain and injury, but particularly on injuries to parts of the body where there are many nerve endings, such as the spine, head, fingers, toes, and lips. It can also help concussion, neuralgia, back pain, pain that shoots upward, pain after dentistry, small wounds such as bites or splinters, nausea, asthma which worsens in fog, painful piles, and rectal nerve pain. In women, late menstruation accompanied by headaches can also be alleviated.

Which type of person?

- no particular type

THERAPY CONNECTIONS

ST. JOHN'S WORT

Ayurveda p.40
Herbalism p.124

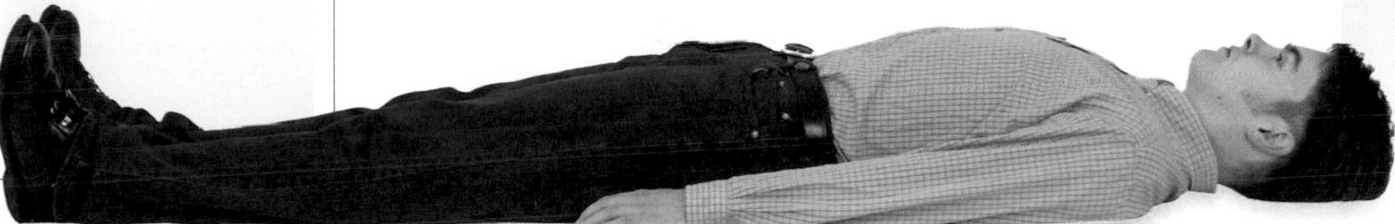

Ignatia amara, Strychnos ignatii, St. Ignatius' bean

IGNATIA

The Ignatia amara tree is found in the Philippines, the East Indies, and China. Its seeds have been used for centuries for healing, and native Filipinos wore them as amulets to ward off disease. The Spanish Jesuits brought the seeds to Europe in the 17th century, naming the tree after the Catholic priest Ignatius Loyola, who founded the Society of Jesus. In conventional medicine, they were used to treat cholera and epilepsy. Homeopathically, the seeds are separated from their pod and powdered. The remedy is used to treat emotional upsets, such as shock and grief, as the strychnine acts on the central nervous system.

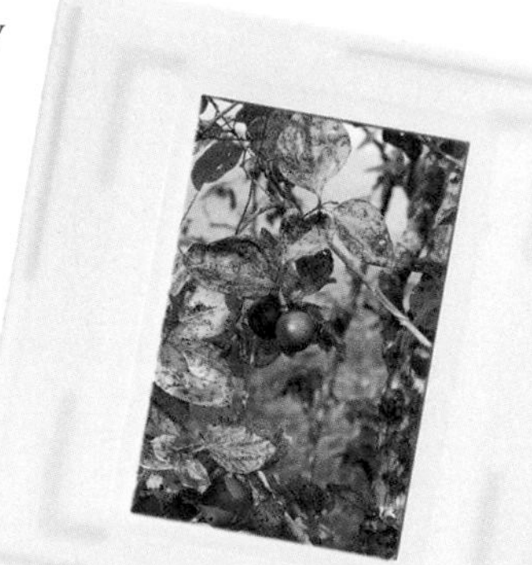

RIGHT *Ignatia amara is made from the fruits of* Strychnos ignatii; *also known as St. Ignatius' bean.*

DATA FILE

Relieves

- emotional traumas
- bereavement
- depression
- headaches
- changeable ailments

Uses

Ignatia is commonly used to treat shock, anger, and grief characterized by changes of mood, insomnia, and hysteria. All emotional upsets – mild depression, love traumas, self-pity, tearfulness, nervous headaches, fainting, sweating, choking, or a tickly cough – can be alleviated. Contradictory symptoms, for instance a sore throat which feels better after eating solids, are helped. In women, lack of menstruation, or uterine spasm during menstruation, constipation, piles, and shooting pain in a prolapsed rectum are relieved.

Which type of person?

- mainly thin, dark-haired women
- tired, look strained
- emotionally sensitive, artistic, nervous disposition
- unpredictable
- high expectations
- prefer sour food, dairy products, bread, coffee; dislike fruit, sweet food, and also alcohol
- children tend to be bright, excitable, highly strung; do not cope well with stress, becoming angry and scared. Suffer nervous headaches; are prone to nervous coughing

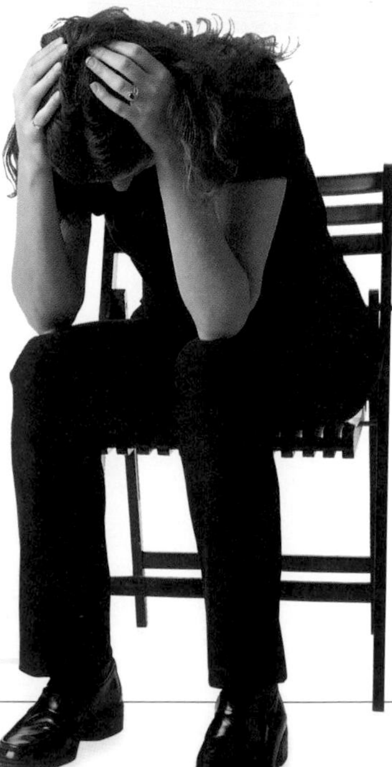

RIGHT *This remedy can help those in nervous or emotional states, perhaps caused by bereavement or the breakdown of a relationship.*

SYMPTOMS

MENTAL

- fears emotional hurt
- dislikes losing control, enclosed spaces, crowds
- difficulty in expressing emotions
- often contradictory
- sensitive to pain
- moody, laughs and cries at the same time

PHYSICAL

- yawns or sighs a lot
- intense headaches, spasmodic cough
- faints in small spaces
- food cravings, constipation

Symptoms improve after eating, urinating, with firm pressure, or lying on the affected side, with heat. They worsen in the cold, when touched, after emotional upset, when taking coffee or smoking, when exposed to strong odors.

Kali bichromicum, potassium dichromate, potassium bichromate

KALI BICH.

Potassium dichromate is an orange-red crystalline substance which has caustic and corrosive effects. It is used in a variety of manufacturing processes such as color dyeing, photography, calico printing, and as a bleaching agent. The homeopathic remedy was first "proved" in 1844, and is commonly given to treat ailments affecting the mucous membranes which lead to mucus and discharge, for example in the nose, throat, stomach, and vagina.

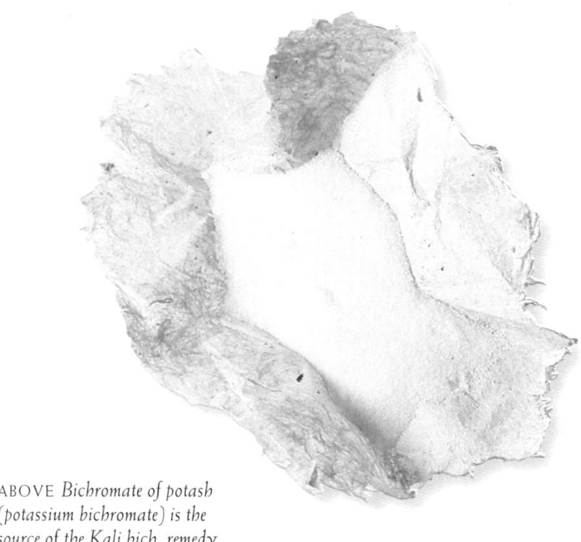

ABOVE *Bichromate of potash (potassium bichromate) is the source of the Kali bich. remedy.*

DATA FILE

Relieves

- all forms of mucus or discharge
- pain that moves about

Uses

This remedy is useful for any condition which affects the mucous membranes, leading to a stringy, yellow, or white discharge. It can help alleviate problems such as sinusitis; glue ear; coughs and colds accompanied by catarrh, where the affected areas feel congested and under pressure. Vomiting where the cause is a digestive disorder and yellow mucus is ejected can also be helped, as can rheumatic pain in joints when the pain tends to move about and becomes worse in hot weather. Migraines which begin at night, feel worse when bending, but better when pressure is applied to the base of the nose also respond well.

Which type of person?

- down-to-earth, straightforward
- high morals
- self-absorbed
- conservative
- like routine, pay attention to detail
- prefer orderliness

SYMPTOMS

MENTAL

- preoccupied with details
- dislike hot weather

PHYSICAL

- chilly and sensitive to cold when ill
- discharge from nose, throat, stomach, vagina
- catarrhal coughs
- heavy colds and blocked ears
- migraines

Symptoms improve in the warmth, after eating, vomiting, or moving. They worsen in cold, wet weather, after drinking, and on waking, between 3A.M. and 5A.M., in summer heat, and when feeling cold.

BELOW *A person needing this remedy tends to be chilly, feeling particularly cold in the neck area, and repeatedly suffering from catarrh and fits of coughing.*

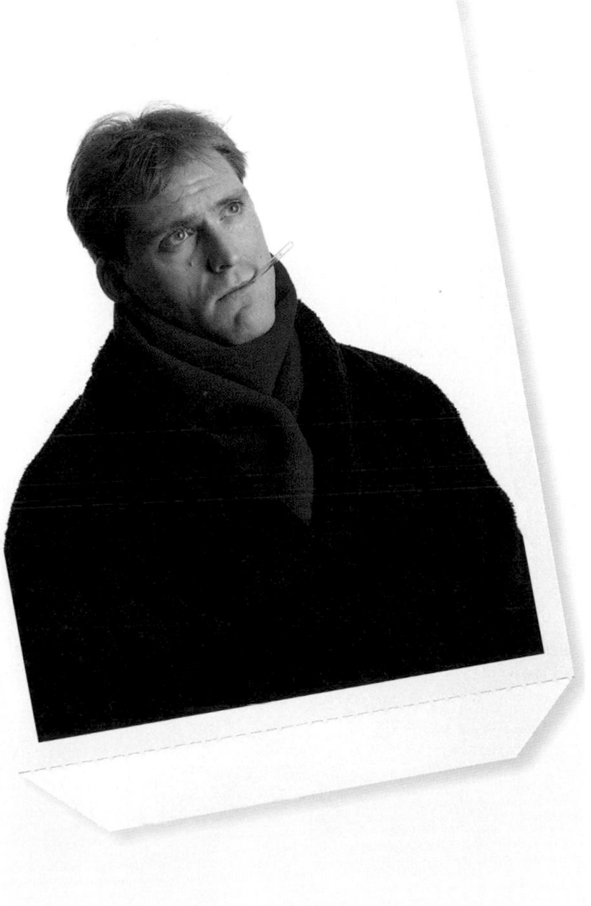

Kali phosphoricum, potassium phosphate, phosphate of potash

KALI PHOS.

BELOW *Kali phos. types are easily worn down by stress and overwork.*

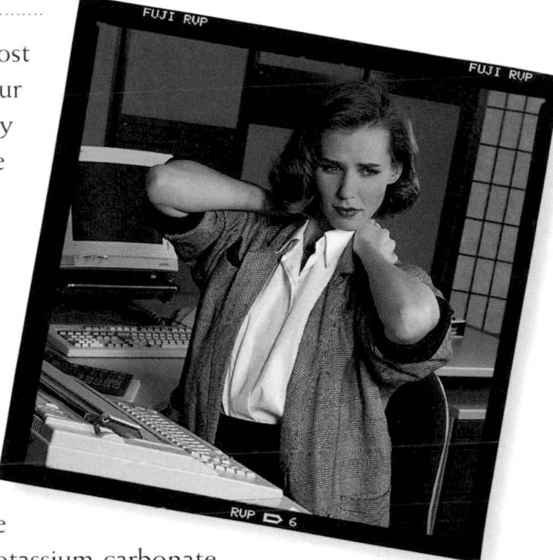

Potassium is found naturally in almost all foods and is an essential part of our diet. We need it to maintain healthy function of the brain and nerve cells. In conventional medicine it is given when levels of phosphorus are low, for instance after gastroenteritis or for those who need to be fed intravenously. Kali phos. is also one of the 12 tissue salts identified by the German physician Wilhelm Schussler. Homeopathically, it is prepared by adding dilute phosphoric acid to a solution of potassium carbonate (also known as potash), and is used to treat conditions affecting the nervous system, and for exhaustion.

SYMPTOMS

MENTAL

- worry
- stressed out
- easily upset on hearing sad news

PHYSICAL

- easily exhausted by hard work
- sensitive to disturbances and cold
- suffer a discharge from the bladder, vagina, or the lungs
- muscular weakness

Symptoms improve in the warmth, after eating or gentle movement, and in cloudy weather. They worsen in cold, dry conditions, in winter, after cold drinks, after physical exertion or talking, and when exposed to noise.

DATA FILE

Relieves

- physical and mental exhaustion
- disorders of the nervous system

Uses

Used to treat mental and physical exhaustion, particularly when the nerves become so frayed the patient is on edge, and sensitive to any disturbance or distraction. Sufferers wish to be left alone and become introverted. Conditions such as sensitivity to cold, pus or yellow vaginal discharge, discharge from the lungs or in the stools, muscle fatigue, unwelcome early morning awakening, and chronic fatigue syndrome can all be alleviated.

Which type of person?

- conservative but outgoing
- clear-sighted
- easily upset by bad or distressing news
- stress and overwork tire them out easily

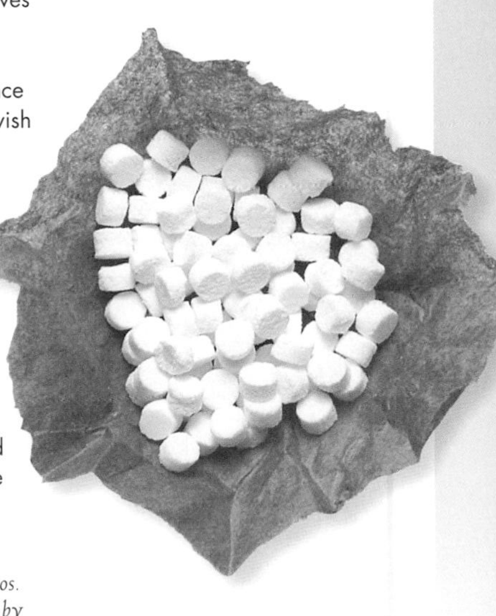

ABOVE RIGHT *The Kali phos. remedy is chemically prepared by adding phosphoric acid to potassium carbonate.*

Ledum palustre, wild rosemary, marsh tea

LEDUM

It is the fine, woolly hairs on the underside of the rosemary plant which give it its Greek name, *ledos*, meaning woolly robe. Wild rosemary has been used for its antiseptic qualities for centuries, and was used more than 700 years ago by the Finns to deter vermin. In the U.S. colonies it was first used in 1773 as a substitute for tea when the tea taxes were introduced. It grows in Ireland, Scandinavia, the U.S., and Canada. Homeopathically, Ledum is made from the whole fresh plant in flower, which is dried and powdered.

RIGHT Ledum palustre *is the plant known as wild rosemary, marsh tea or Labrador tea. The whole fresh plant or dried twigs may be used.*

DATA FILE

Relieves

- cuts, grazes, stings
- pain that moves about
- prevents wounds becoming infected

Uses

Ledum is a useful first-aid remedy and helps prevent infection in cuts and wounds. Complaints that need immediate treatment – such as stings, cuts, grazes, eye injuries, and puncture wounds – respond well, and Ledum is effective if there is accompanying bruising and the area becomes painful, swollen, and puffy. It can also help to alleviate rheumatic pain which starts in the feet and moves up; painful or injured joints which may look pale or bluish; and where the affected part feels cold to the touch, but the person feels hot inside.

Which type of person?

- no particular type

SYMPTOMS

MENTAL

- timid, but impatient
- morose and want to be left alone
- get extremely angry
- hate others

PHYSICAL

- stiff joints
- puffy, bluish skin
- night sweats
- black eyes

Symptoms improve when cold compresses are applied to the affected part, and if the area is left uncovered, and worsen if warm, touched, when in bed, and at night.

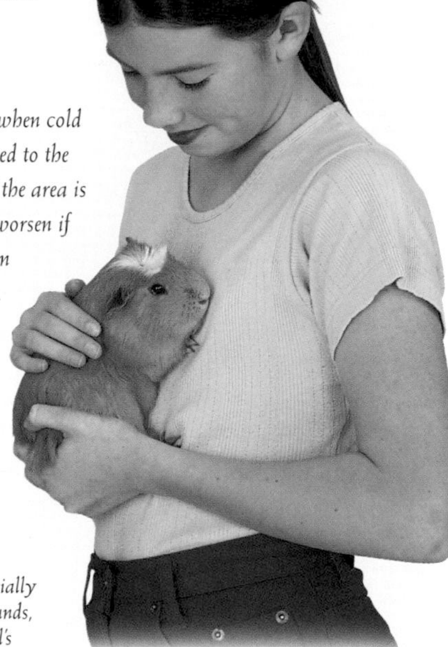

RIGHT *Ledum is especially useful for puncture wounds, such as from an animal's claws or teeth.*

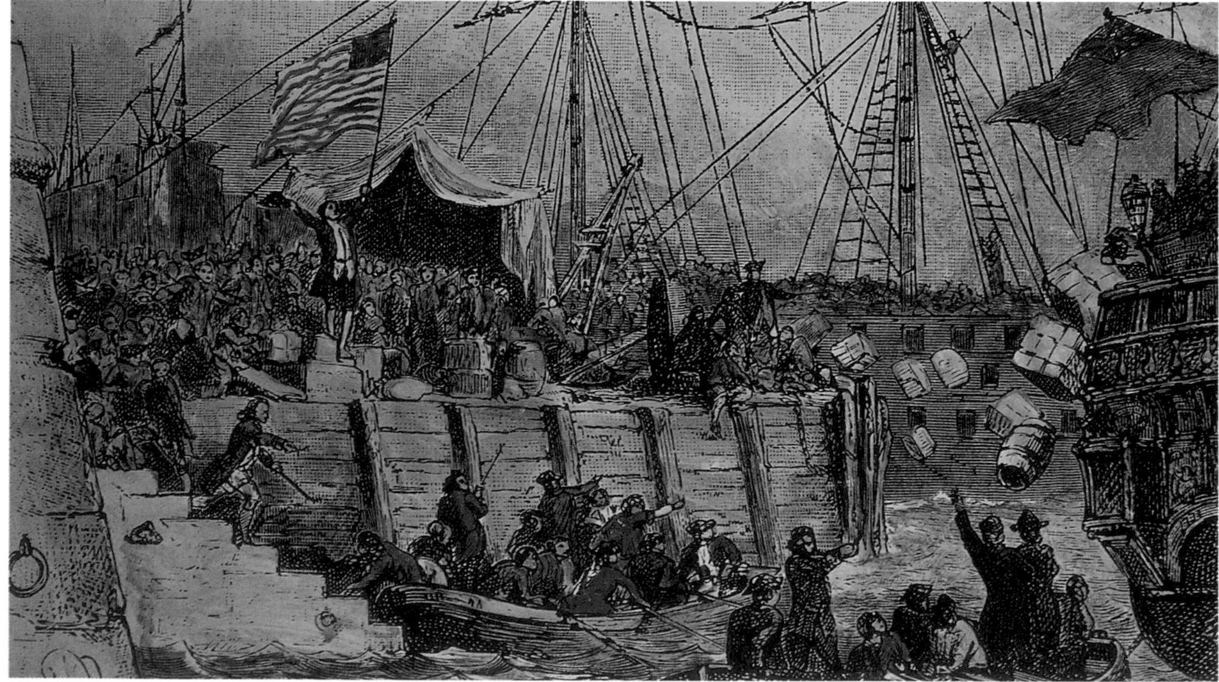

RIGHT *The Ledum plant was widely used in infusions, and in the 18th century it was imported to be sold as a substitute for tea in the U.S.*

THERAPY CONNECTIONS

ROSEMARY

Herbalism *p.127*

Aromatherapy *p.168*

Lycopodium clavatum, club moss, wolf's claw, stagshorn moss, running pine

LYCOPODIUM

This plant has long been used to treat stomach complaints and urinary disorders, and is grown in the mountains and forests of the northern hemisphere. Historically, Arabian physicians used it to disperse kidney stones, while 300 years ago its yellow pollen was used to treat urine retention and gout. It flares up when exposed to naked flame and in the past was used in fireworks. It is also water resistant and was used to coat pills to prevent them from gluing together. Lycopodium was first "proved" by Hahnemann, and for homeopathic use the pollen dust is shaken out of the spikes of the fresh plant.

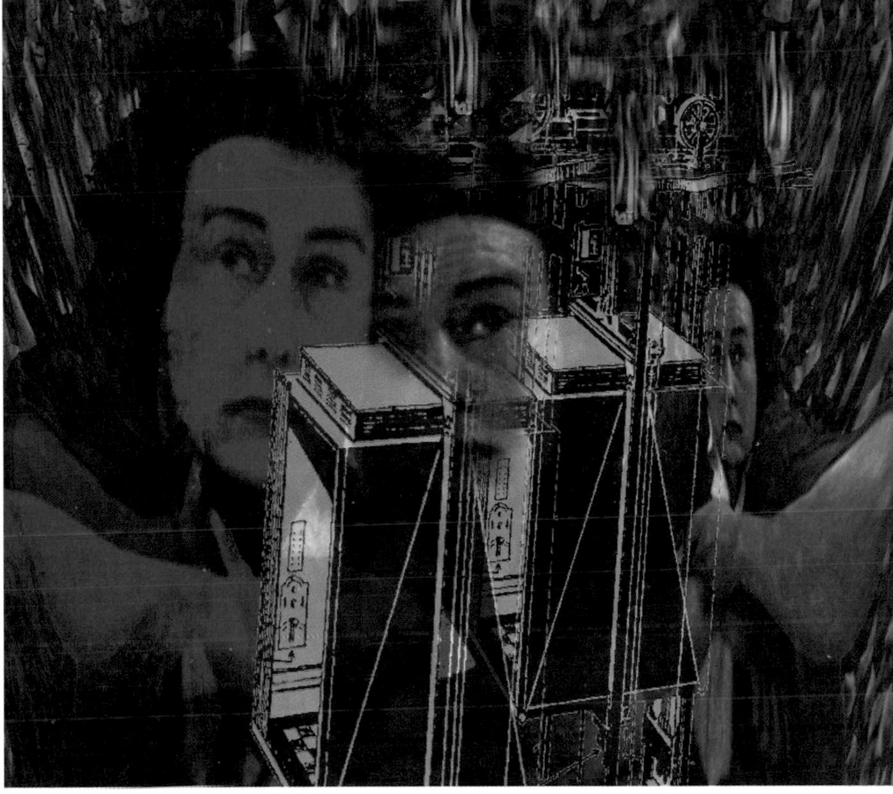

RIGHT *Lycopodium types fear being trapped in enclosed spaces, like elevators.*

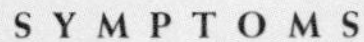

SYMPTOMS

MENTAL

- fear of being alone, enclosed spaces, crowds, death
- hatred of the thought of failure
- dislike of the dark
- intolerance of weakness in others and illness
- sexual promiscuity

PHYSICAL

- weakness on right side of body
- sensitive areas include the digestive organs, brain, lungs, skin, liver, kidneys, and bladder
- fatigue

Symptoms improve when in cool, fresh air, when wearing loose clothing, after hot food and drink, and at night. They are worse on the right side, in stuffy rooms, when wearing tight clothing, after overeating or not eating, between 4A.M. and 8A.M., and between 4P.M. and 8P.M.

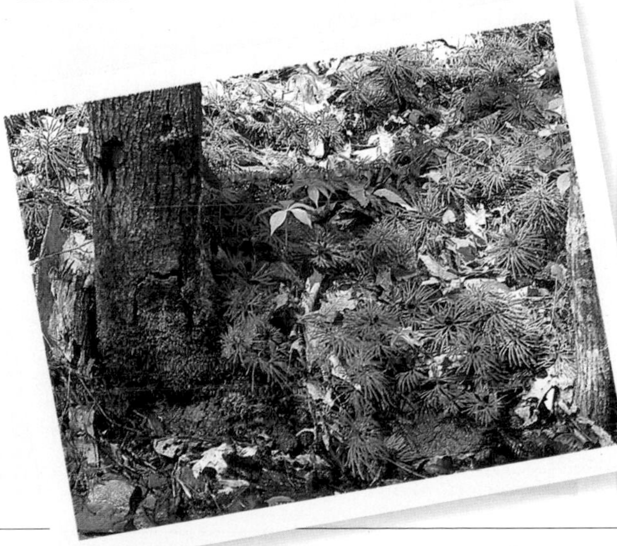

LEFT Lycopodium clavatum *is a moss which is found growing on mountain pastures and heaths.*

DATA FILE

Relieves

- stomach disorders
- digestive conditions
- complaints of the bladder and kidney
- problems on the right side
- in men, enlarged prostate, inability to have an erection
- emotional problems and anxiety caused by insecurity

Uses

This remedy is commonly used to treat digestive complaints, such as vomiting, indigestion, distended abdomen with flatulence, constipation, bleeding piles, and hunger which turns to discomfort after eating. Other problems that can be alleviated include swelling in the ankles, feet, or hands (edema); burst blood vessels in the eye; chronic catarrh; psoriasis on the hands; and pneumonia. Most problems tend to occur on the right side of the body, and are accompanied by cravings for sweet food. In men, the remedy is helpful for an enlarged prostate; urine which has a reddish tinge and contains a sandy sediment due to kidney stones; increased libido, but without the ability to achieve or sustain an erection.

Which type of person?

- distinguished appearance
- tall and lean in physique, but not physically strong
- deep facial frown lines, may also be prematurely bald or gray
- detached and poised
- hold important positions, e.g. diplomat or lawyer
- deep insecurity leads to gross exaggerations
- dislike change and having to face challenges
- enjoy company but avoid commitment
- prefer shellfish, sweet food, hot food and drink, cabbage, and onions
- children tend to be thin and sallow, are shy and lack confidence, prefer reading to outdoor activities, have a slightly distended abdomen, and although well behaved at school, are bossy at home

BELOW *People who benefit from Lycopodium may have a liking for shellfish, although they also like sweet food.*

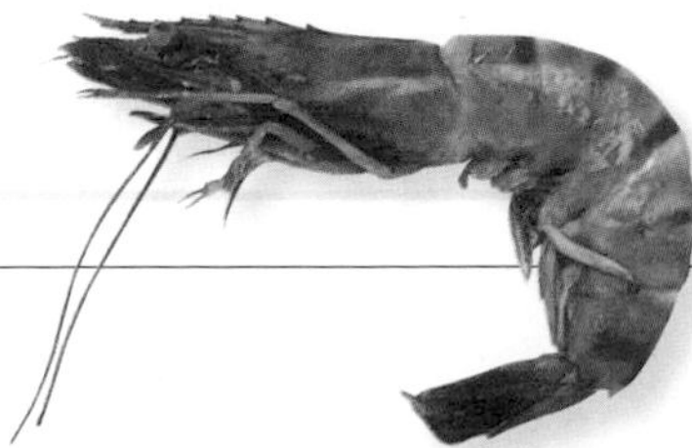

Magnesia phosphorica, magnesium phosphate, phosphate of magnesia

MAG. PHOS.

Magnesium phosphate is one of the homeopathically prepared tissue salts introduced by the German physician Wilhelm Schussler at the end of the 19th century. He believed a deficiency of a mineral salt such as Mag. phos., could lead to disease. In the case of Mag. phos., he found deficiency caused problems associated with muscular nerve endings and tissue. The homeopathic remedy is made chemically from magnesium sulfate and sodium phosphate, and has an antispasmodic effect. Magnesium phosphate is also found naturally in grain cereals like wheat and oats.

ABOVE *Magnesium phosphate occurs naturally in grain cereals.*

SYMPTOMS

MENTAL

- impulsive
- dislike mental effort
- may stammer
- forgetful

PHYSICAL

- complain of coldness in the spine
- headaches
- dizziness
- jerky movements
- pain on right side of body

Symptoms improve in the warmth, with pressure, hot compresses, and bending double, and are worse on the right side, when cool, when touched, and at night.

DATA FILE

Relieves

- cramps
- neuralgia
- pains on the right side

Uses

A useful remedy for any type of cramp from infant colic and abdominal cramp, to menstrual pains and writer's cramp, with the sufferer doubled up in pain.

Abdominal cramps are sharp and intense, with the pain jumping from one part to another, and may improve when bending, with heat, and hard pressure, and worsen in the cold, draughts, and at night. Certain types of headache and neuralgia can also be helped – when the head throbs, the face is flushed, and pain suddenly comes and goes – which improve in the warmth and if the head is bound, but worsen in the cold and draughts, and at night. Pains tend to be on the right side of the body.

Which type of person?

- thin, weak
- sensitive, artistic
- intellectual, intense
- restless and nervous

LEFT *Use of hands and fingers over a long period, whether in writing, playing a musical instrument, or using computer equipment, can cause the kind of cramps for which Mag. phos. is useful.*

Matricaria recutita, German chamomile, wild chamomile

CHAMOMILLA

Hippocrates was one of the first physicians to understand the medicinal benefits of chamomile. It is extensively used in herbal medicine to treat conditions such as asthma and eczema, and during childbirth to strengthen the uterus. Chamomile tea is a popular, soothing herbal drink. The plant is a member of the daisy family, and the aromatic flowers can be found all over Europe and America. Homeopathically, the juice is extracted from the whole fresh plant when it is in flower in the late spring, and the remedy is given for those who are sensitive and have a low pain threshold, and is particularly good for children.

DATA FILE

Relieves

- low pain tolerance
- nervous afflictions
- children's ailments

Uses

Chamomilla works well for those who are sensitive to pain and are unable to deal with their discomfort, being impatient, rude, and angry when ill. Often the reaction seems disproportionate to the amount of pain being felt. Even slight pain may cause sweats and fainting in women and children. Children particularly benefit from the remedy. Teething newborns, who are feverish and want to be held all the time, can be soothed; earache when the child is unable to sit still due to the pain and may scream, and toothache which makes one cheek red and hot can also be alleviated. Other conditions treated include heavy, painful menstruation, tinnitus, heartburn, and slimy green diarrhea.

Which type of person?

- low pain tolerance
- whining
- impatient
- never satisfied

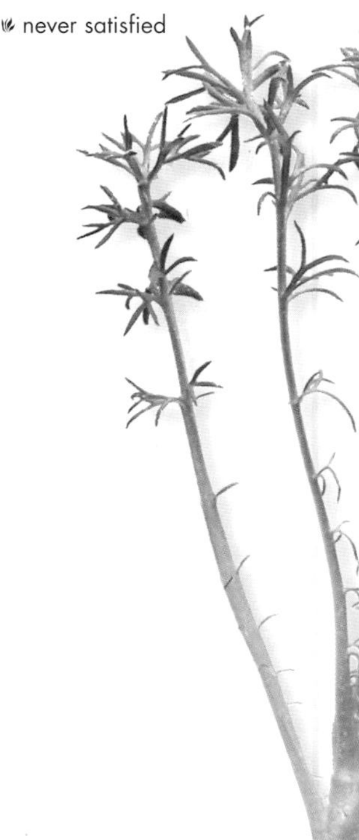

RIGHT *Wild chamomile is the source for Chamomilla. In herbalism and homeopathy alike it is widely used in treating children.*

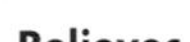

SYMPTOMS

MENTAL

- angry, irritable
- spiteful
- sensitive to people and surroundings
- cries in sleep

PHYSICAL

- restless
- teething
- earache
- toothache

Symptoms improve in the warmth, in wet weather, for not eating, and if carried (children). They worsen in heat, fresh air, cold winds, when angry, and after drinking coffee.

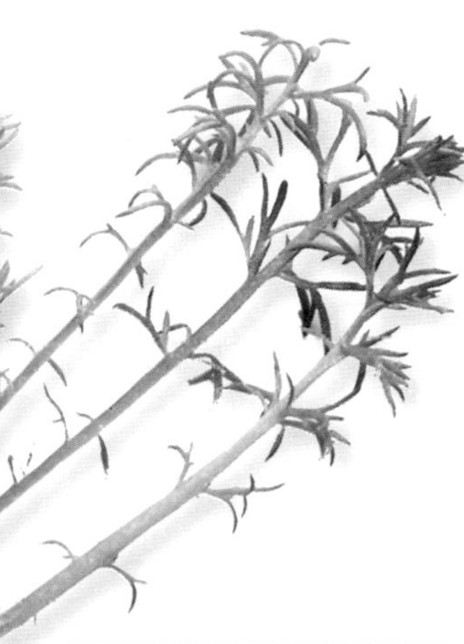

THERAPY CONNECTIONS

CHAMOMILE

Herbalism p.119
Aromatherapy p.150

Mercurius solubilis hahnemanni, mercury, quicksilver

MERC. SOL.

In Roman times Mercury was known as the messenger of the gods. In recent centuries the substance has been used for various medicinal purposes. Although it is toxic and if given in too large a dose causes salivation and vomiting, it was once used in small amounts to treat conditions such as syphilis and to encourage secretions. Mercury is usually found in cinnabar, a mineral which forms near hot springs and volcanoes. A silvery-white liquid metal, it is dissolved in dilute nitric acid, forming particles which are dried and powdered for homeopathic use. Although there are many *Mercurius* remedies, Merc. sol. is mainly used to treat conditions associated with foul-smelling secretions.

SYMPTOMS

MENTAL

- restlessness, anxiety
- worry about family becoming ill
- fear of insanity, death
- dislike of thunderstorms
- explosive anger, even murderous feelings if upset

PHYSICAL

- any complaint which is characterized by a strong-smelling discharge
- burning secretions
- eye complaints
- skin conditions
- aching joints
- weak areas include lining of the stomach and respiratory system, skin, bones and joints, blood, mouth and throat, liver

Symptoms improve in temperate weather and after rest, and worsen in changeable weather, when lying on the right side, if too hot in bed, when sweating, and at night.

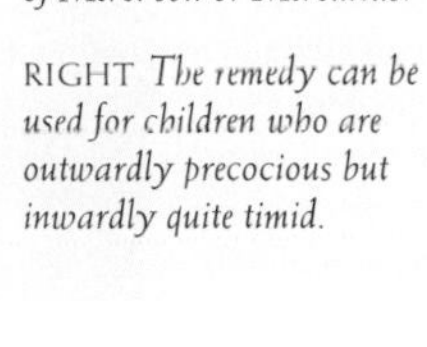

ABOVE *Metallic mercury or quicksilver is the source of Merc. sol. or Mercurius.*

RIGHT *The remedy can be used for children who are outwardly precocious but inwardly quite timid.*

DATA FILE

Relieves

- complaints accompanied by strong-smelling secretions
- conditions affecting the mouth and throat
- offensive sweating

Uses

Conditions characterized by a smelly discharge are helped by this remedy, including chronic conjunctivitis, pus secretions from the ears, watery catarrh, nasal cold sores, glutinous saliva which stains the pillow during sleep, throat ulcers which make swallowing painful, phlegmy cough which is worse in the warmth and at night, drenching sweats, pus-filled skin eruptions, sores, and, in women, excessive vaginal discharge and green-looking stools flecked with blood. In the mouth and throat, gingivitis, thrush, bad breath, loose teeth in infected gums, swollen tonsils, and ulcers can be helped. Other symptoms which can be alleviated are foul-smelling sweat which chills the skin as it dries, and oily sweats which make other symptoms worse; stinging, watery eyes and swollen lids due to conjunctivitis; burning nasal secretions; and blisters and scalp lesions.

Which type of person?

- fair-haired, with smooth, clear skin
- outwardly detached, yet sensitive to criticism
- inner sense of haste
- insecure, cautious, and suspicious of others
- dislike being contradicted and may react badly
- strong emotional undercurrents
- when ill, become slow, uncomprehending, forgetful, and lack will-power
- prefer cold drinks, lemons, bread and butter, dislike sweet food, alcohol (except beer), meat, salt
- children tend to appear very grown up, flirty, and precocious, but inwardly are cautious and easily upset; may also be shy and introverted with a tendency to stammer; prone to problems with ears, nose, and throat

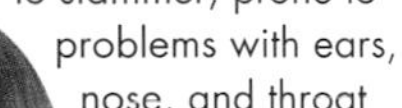

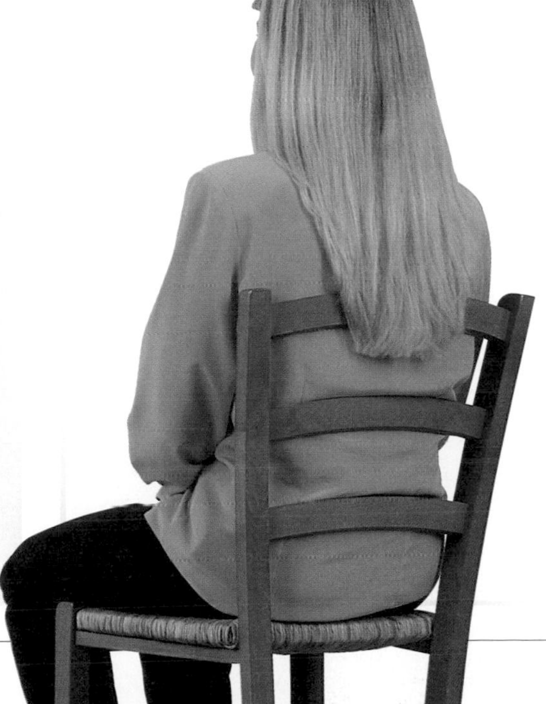

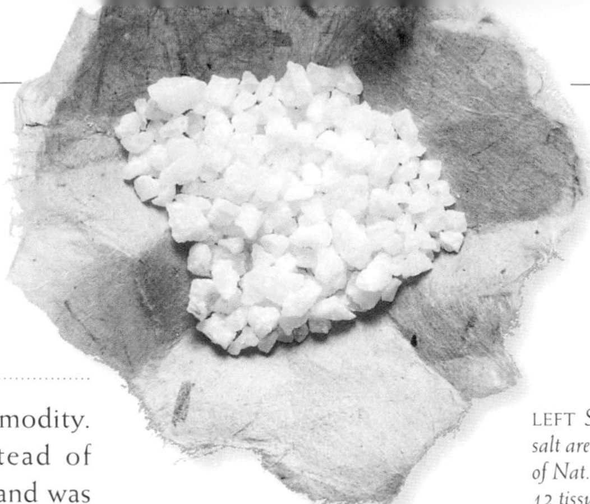

LEFT *Sea salt and rock salt are the usual sources of Nat. mur., one of the 12 tissue salts.*

Natrum muriaticum, rock salt, sodium chloride, halite

NAT. MUR.

Salt has long been a valuable commodity. In the past, it was used instead of money for trading purposes and was given as payment to soldiers for services, hence the word salary, which comes from the Latin *salarium*. Many people add salt to food for flavor, but in fact we get more than enough salt, or sodium chloride, naturally from what we eat. In conventional medicine salt is used in the form of saline solution, for instance, during surgery to replace fluids. Homeopathically, the Nat. mur. remedy is made from rock salt which is formed through the evaporation of salty water, leaving a crusty crystalline solid. The remedy is used to treat a number of conditions resulting from emotional problems and ailments characterized by a discharge. It is also one of the 12 tissue salts identified by Dr. Wilhelm Schussler.

ABOVE *People who may be helped by this remedy will either strongly like or strongly dislike table salt.*

SYMPTOMS

MENTAL

- impatient, easily upset when judged
- mildly depressed on waking
- fear enclosed spaces, crowds, business failure, insanity, death
- worry about losing self-control, and being hurt in the emotional sense
- dislike the dark, being late, thunderstorms

PHYSICAL

- lower lip often has a center crack
- headaches
- conditions accompanied by discharge
- constipation
- feel the cold but dislike heat

Symptoms improve with fresh air, after sweating, and avoiding food. They worsen in the cold, hot weather, sea air, between 9A.M. *and* 11A.M.*, after overexertion, if fussed over.*

DATA FILE

Relieves

- anxiety and depression from suppressed emotions
- conditions accompanied by secretions or discharge
- skin complaints
- in women, irregular or absent menstruation
- headaches

Uses

Nat. mur. works well for emotional problems, such as distress, restlessness, and depression, which tend to occur because of the suppression of other emotions, such as fear and grief. Conditions characterized by secretions or discharge, such as colds, catarrh, vaginismus, mouth ulcers, nasal boils, acne, cold sores, and other skin complaints such as hangnails, warts, and a cracked lower lip are alleviated. In women, it helps with erratic menstruation; menstruation which has stopped due to stress, shock, or grief; malaise or swollen ankles before and after menstruation; and a dry or sore vagina. Headaches respond well – those caused by trauma or exercise, explosive headaches, blinding migraines, headaches which feel like the head is being hammered, and are worse between 10A.M. and 11A.M., those that start on the left side.

Which type of person?

- mainly women
- usually have a square or pear-shaped figure
- sandy or dark hair
- greasy, pale, pasty skin
- watery, red-rimmed eyes
- civilized, sensitive
- when hurt, become quiet and introverted
- enjoy the company of others, but tend to be alone
- prefer sour food and beer, like but cannot tolerate starchy food and milk, dislike chicken and also coffee
- love or loathe salty food
- children tend to be slow walkers and talkers, small for their age, flush and sweat easily, are responsible and diligent, but timid and easily upset, although dislike fuss; prone to headaches and hangnails

RIGHT *A timid, oversensitive child will benefit from Nat. mur.*

SYMPTOMS

MENTAL

- sometimes have suicidal thoughts
- more depressed in the morning
- brood
- sensitive, sometimes cry on hearing music
- sad

PHYSICAL

- prone to asthma, brought on by damp
- tend to have profuse discharges of yellow-green mucus
- chest complaints
- triggered by damp

Symptoms improve in fresh air, dry atmosphere, and after changing position, and worsen in the morning, late evening, when lying on the back or left side, when listening to music, and in damp weather.

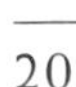

Natrum sulfuricum, sodium sulfate, Glauber's salt, sal mirabile

NAT. SULF.

Sodium sulfate, a white crystalline compound, is found naturally in spa waters, salt water lakes, and in mineral water. It is also known as Glauber's salt. Sodium sulfate is used in the manufacture of paper, detergents, and glass. It is naturally present in the body and helps to maintain water balance. Homeopathically, it was "proved" by Hahnemann's followers, Nenning and Shieler. It is one of the 12 tissue salts identified by Dr. Wilhelm Schussler.

DATA FILE

Relieves

- chest problems
- emotional changes after head injury
- headaches

Uses

Used to treat chest problems such as asthma, bronchitis, colds, and flu, where there is a build-up of thick yellowish catarrh, which comes from the nose; emotional trauma after an accident in which the head is injured, leading to depression and suicidal thoughts or other emotional changes; headaches which have a vice-like grip at the back of the head and behind the forehead. Other conditions treated include dry mouth, with the tongue having a dirty coating; biliousness; thirst and frequent urination, leading to an inability to deal with damp conditions and sharp liver pains.

Which type of person?

- flabby
- prefer cool weather, dislike damp and humidity
- materialistic
- sometimes sensitive and artistic
- restless
- serious, responsible
- discontented

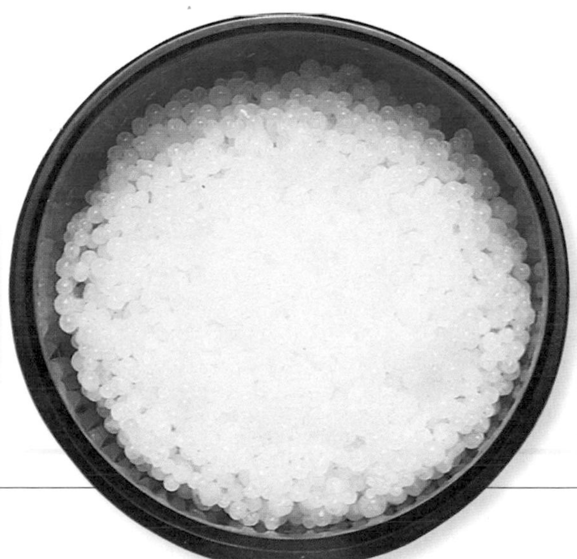

BELOW *Glauber's salt or sodium sulfate is the source of this remedy; it occurs naturally as the mineral, threnardite.*

Papaver somniferum, opium poppy

OPIUM

The opium poppy has grayish-green leaves and flowers which range from white to various shades of red. It is grown in Asia, India, Turkey, and Iran. Opium is a well-known painkiller and tranquilizer, and an addictive narcotic drug. The unripe seed capsules contain alkaloids such as codeine and morphine, derivatives of which are used in conventional medicine as analgesics and hypnotics. The homeopathic remedy is made from the dried milky juice excreted by the seed capsules.

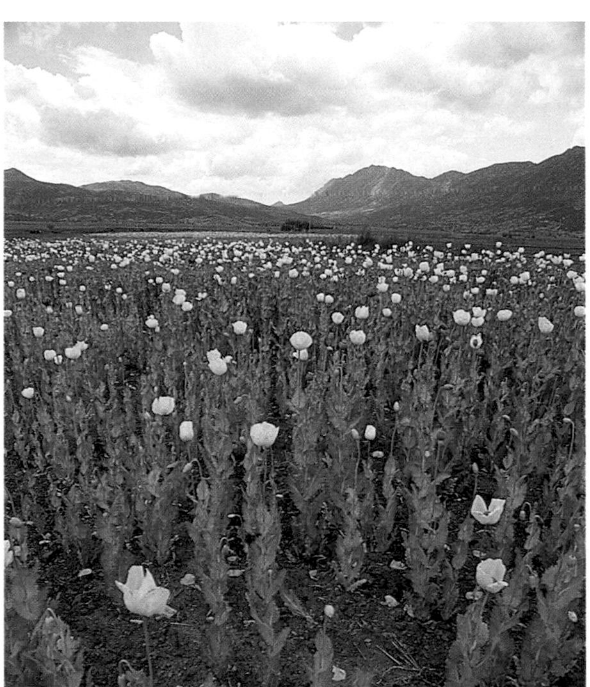

LEFT *A field of opium poppies, whose unripe seeds yield the addictive drug and are also the source of the Opium remedy.*

SYMPTOMS

MENTAL

- apathetic
- uncomprehending
- overexcited
- may be delirious
- panicky
- in shock
- frightened

PHYSICAL

- loss of appetite
- constipation
- infrequent urination
- stroke
- irregular breathing
- sweaty skin

Symptoms improve in cool surroundings and with movement, and worsen in the warmth, in heat, during and after sleep.

DATA FILE

Relieves

- apathy after shock
- excitability after shock

Uses

Commonly used as a treatment after a shock, such as bereavement, when the patient may be either listless and indifferent to what is going on, or overexcited, even appearing delirious, and unable to sleep; also the patient may not be aware of pain, is very sleepy, but has no recollection of dreams once awake, and perspires easily. It is also given for slow workings of the bowel and urinary system, which can lead to constipation and water retention. Stroke victims also respond well.

Which type of person?

- no particular type

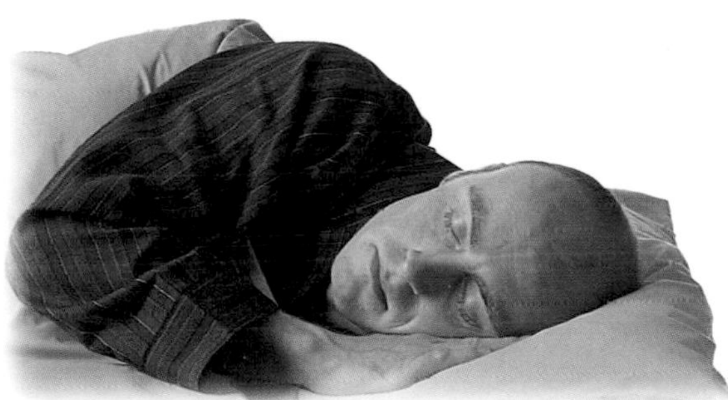

BELOW *The person needing Opium may feel desirous of sleep but unable to sleep, or may actually be sleepy.*

Phosphorus, phosphorus

PHOS.

The name phosphorus comes from the Greek, meaning "light-bringing." It is a yellowish-white nonmetallic element which occurs in phosphates and living matter. Because of its flammable properties, white phosphate, a toxic substance, was used to make matches and fireworks, but this was replaced by the nontoxic red phosphorus. Because of the ease with which it ignites, phosphorus is kept submerged in water. Our bodies need phosphorus for the healthy functioning of our teeth, bones, bodily fluids, and DNA. In conventional medicine it has been used to treat conditions as diverse as measles and malaria. As a homeopathic treatment, it is mainly given to those suffering from anxiety and digestive disorders.

LEFT *The source of the Phosphorus remedy is phosphorus obtained from bone ash.*

SYMPTOMS

MENTAL

- mentally alert
- nervous under pressure
- tend to bottle things up
- indifferent to family and friends when ill
- fear illness and death

PHYSICAL

- weak areas include digestive organs, circulation, nervous system, the left side of the body, liver
- bleeding, such as nosebleeds
- respiratory problems
- headaches

Symptoms improve in fresh air, after sleeping, when touched, and when lying on the right side. They worsen in the morning and evening, after mental or physical exertion, after hot food or drink, when lying on the left side, and in thunderstorms.

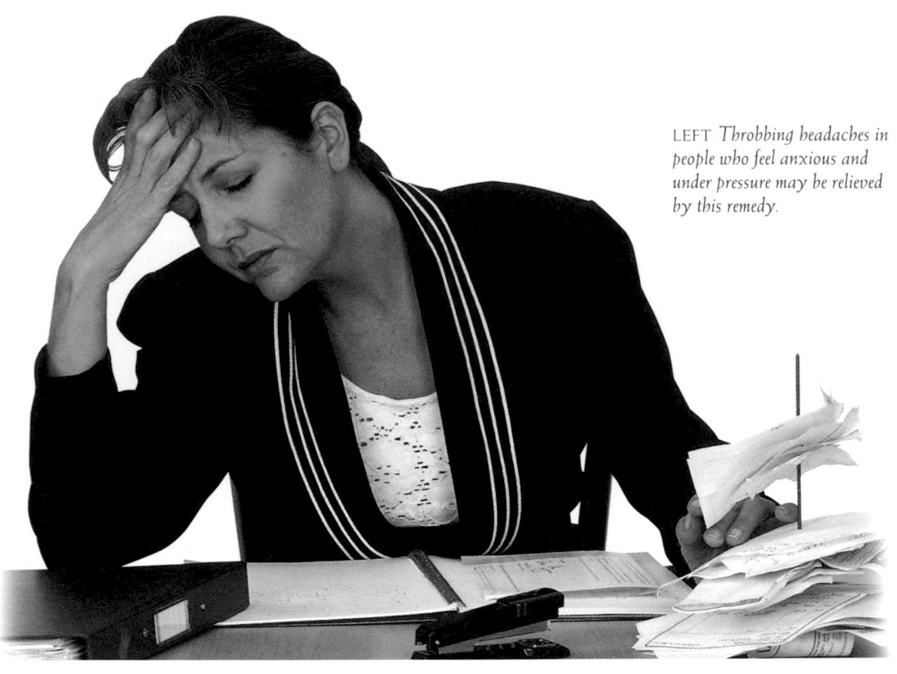

LEFT *Throbbing headaches in people who feel anxious and under pressure may be relieved by this remedy.*

DATA FILE

Relieves

- anxieties, fears
- digestive complaints
- circulatory conditions and those causing bleeding
- respiratory problems

Uses

Phosphorus is used to treat symptoms such as exhaustion, insomnia, nerves which are caused by underlying stress, anxiety, and fears, for instance due to exam pressure, overwork, fear of dying. Other problems that can be helped include digestive problems such as nausea and vomiting due to coughing, stress, or food poisoning, cravings for certain foods, and pressure in the stomach; poor circulation, such as cold or overheated fingers and toes; excessive bleeding, such as bleeding gums, nosebleeds, and heavy menstrual bleeding; respiratory problems such as acute bronchitis or asthma, difficulty in breathing, tight chest, pneumonia, dry tickly coughs, and red-tinged phlegm. Other conditions which can be alleviated include headaches which are worse in heat but improve after a cold compress or eating; dry skin; sensitive red eyes; perspiring under stress; fever with alternate sweating and shivering; cramps; unresolved sexual problems.

Which type of person?

- well proportioned, tall, and lean
- fine or dark hair, with reddish tinge
- pale skin, blush easily
- intelligent, outgoing, an eye for clothes, often artistic
- open and affectionate
- enthusiastic, but only in short spurts
- tend to offer more than can deliver
- imagination needs constant stimulation
- tend to crumble when subjected to pressure
- love attention, particularly when ill
- prefer spicy, salty, sweet foods, carbonated drinks, cheese, wine, and dislike fruit, fish, tomatoes
- children tend to be tall for their age, smooth-featured, but blush easily; prefer company but become restless and nervous; perceptive, artistic, and affectionate. They dislike doing homework, the dark, and thunderstorms

BELOW *The Phos. patient often has a preference for spicy foods such as curry.*

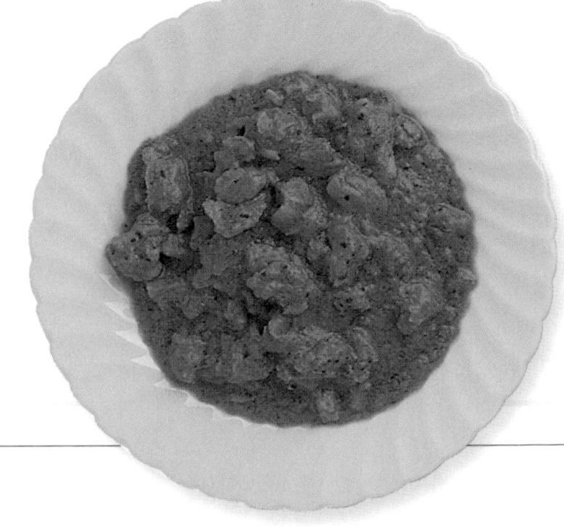

Pulsatilla nigricans, Anemone pratensis, pasque flower, paschal flower, meadow anemone, wind flower

PULSATILLA

The pasque flower is distinguishable from other members of the *Pulsatilla* family by its beautiful, deep-purple flowers. It is found growing in central and northern Europe, Russia, and western Asia. The name passe-fleur was given by the French in the 16th century, meaning "flower that excels." It took its later name, pasque or paschal flower, meaning Easter flower, because it usually blooms at that time. It has long been used medicinally for a number of ailments such as ulcers, tooth decay, and cataracts. In homeopathy, the whole fresh plant in flower is used to make the remedy, and it is given for a number of conditions, such as digestive disorders, depression, and gynecological problems.

SYMPTOMS

MENTAL

- avoid confronting people
- depressed
- self-conscious
- cry easily
- fear being alone, the dark, insanity, death
- lack of strength of character

PHYSICAL

- ailments characterized by discharge
- gynecological conditions
- digestive problems
- bad taste in mouth, dry mouth
- aching joints

Symptoms improve in fresh air, with gentle movement, and with sympathy, and worsen in the heat, on eating rich foods, after lengthy standing, when lying on the left side, and in the evening.

DATA FILE

Relieves

- digestive disorders
- gynecological conditions
- emotional traumas
- conditions accompanied by excessive discharge

Uses

Pulsatilla can help relieve a number of digestive problems, such as rich food causing lack of sleep, a stomach which is tight on waking in the morning and which reacts badly to rich or fatty food, particularly pork, heaviness under the breastbone after eating, cravings for sweet foods, and a rumbling stomach. In women it can be used to treat lack of or late menstruation, particularly if due to shock or illness, thick, stinging discharge, and menopausal problems, all of which tend to be accompanied by crying and depression. Moodiness, depression, and fear of being alone can also be treated. Ailments characterized by excessive discharge or secretions, such as conjunctivitis, catarrh with yellow phlegm, sinusitis, and a runny nose, can also be helped. Other troublesome conditions which respond well include headaches above the eyes, backache, rheumatism, varicose veins, corneal ulcers, loose coughs, palpitations, bedwetting.

Which type of person?

- usually women
- fair skin and fair hair, with blue eyes
- blush easily
- tend to be plump
- good-natured, kind, popular, easily influenced by, and depend on, others
- lack assertiveness, and avoid confrontation
- led by emotions rather than head
- relate to those in distress, including animals
- prefer sweet food, cold food and drink, dislike spicy food, pork, butter, fruit
- children tend to be either small and fair with delicate features, easygoing, affectionate yet shy, blushing easily; or darker-haired, small, listless, needing reassurance and attention, but slow in returning it. Both types are scared of the dark, dislike weather changes, particularly the cold, which can trigger ailments, and are prone to colds

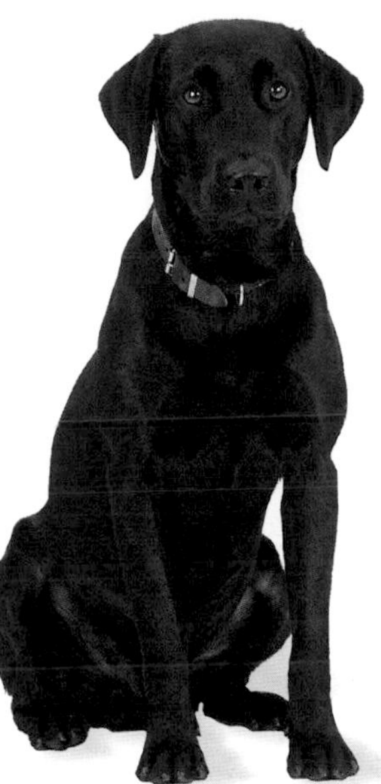

BELOW *The Pulsatilla type is likely to relate well to those in distress, including animals.*

ABOVE LEFT *The spring-flowering pasque flower, source of Pulsatilla, is also used by herbalists.*

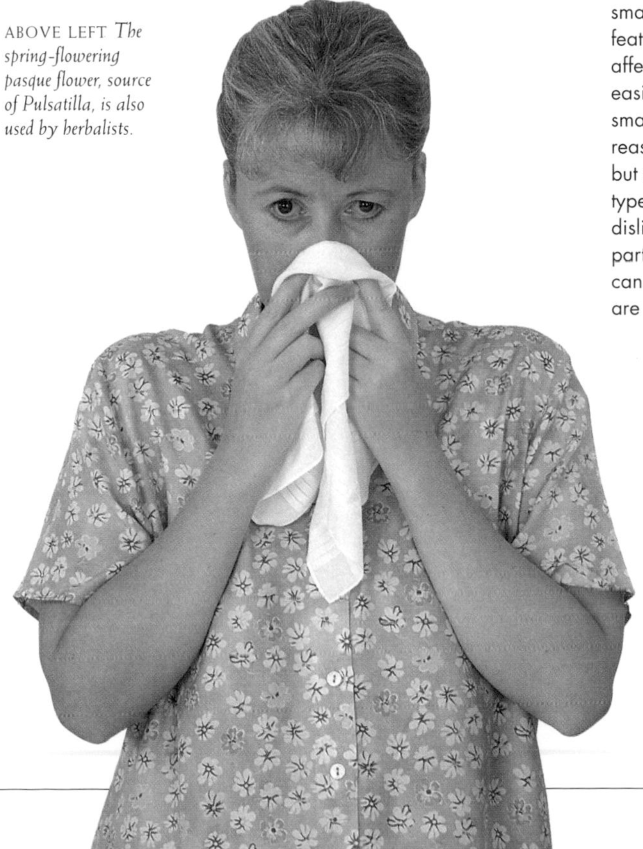

LEFT *Shifting symptoms, changeability and moodiness, with runny eyes and nose, may well indicate Pulsatilla.*

Ruta graveolens, rue, bitter herb, herb of grace

RUTA GRAV.

In the Middle Ages rue was used to ward off the plague. In the 16th and 17th centuries it was scattered over courtroom floors to prevent the spread of typhus, or jail fever, which was carried by the lice which thrived in the squalid jail conditions. It has also been used to treat croup, colic, headaches, and coughs, and was given as an antidote to mushroom poisoning. The homeopathic remedy is made from the juice of the whole plant, which is picked before it flowers. It is given mainly for bruising and restlessness.

DATA FILE

Relieves

- bruises, strained ligaments
- restlessness
- eye strain

Uses

The treatment of bruised bones and tendon injuries, aching bones, deep aching pain, rheumatism, sciatica which is worse when lying down, and the restlessness which goes with having to be still. Also good for eyestrain, when the eyes feel hot and sore from overuse or reading small print, and accompanying headaches. Other conditions treated include infection after tooth extraction; weak chest with breathing difficulties; prolapsed rectum; constipation with stools that are either large and difficult to pass or loose, containing blood and mucus.

Which type of person?

- no particular type

SYMPTOMS

MENTAL

- contradict, criticize others
- depressed when ill
- restless
- anxious, troubled
- dissatisfied with selves and with others

PHYSICAL

- painful, aching limbs
- bruises
- headaches due to eyestrain

Symptoms improve with movement and worsen in the cold and damp, when resting or lying down.

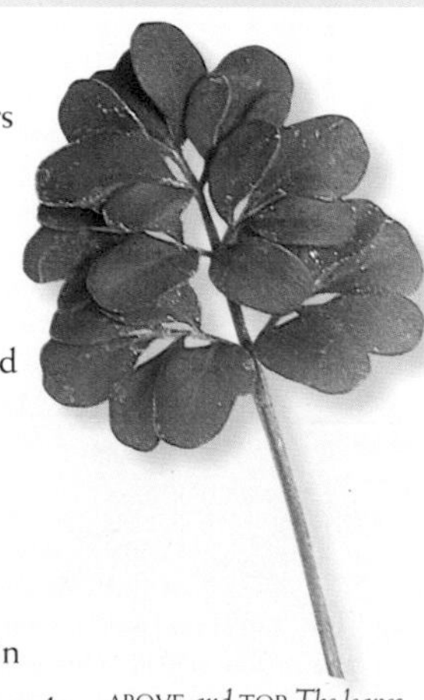

ABOVE *and* TOP *The leaves of rue (the herb* Ruta graveolens*), the plant used as the source of Ruta. grav.*

Rhus toxicodendron, Rhus radicans, poison ivy, poison oak

RHUS TOX.

Rhus tox. is made from both poison ivy, and a variety of it, poison oak, both of which are native to the U.S. and Canada. Brushing against the leaves can cause a severe skin reaction, as well as headache, swollen glands, and fever, as they contain a poisonous sap. In homeopathy, poison ivy was first "proved" by Hahnemann. The fresh leaves of the plant are collected before it flowers, when the poison is most potent, and pounded to a pulp. The remedy is used for skin conditions and rheumatic pain.

ABOVE *Twigs of poison ivy, whose leaves are used as the source of Rhus tox. Despite the plant being a native of North America, the remedy was "proved" by Hahnemann.*

DATA FILE

Relieves

- joint and muscle pain, and general stiffness
- red, itchy skin eruptions

Uses

It can be used to treat skin complaints characterized by red, itchy, puffy areas which feel like they are burning and which tend to form a scaly surface, such as eczema, herpes, diaper rash, and raised patches of skin where there is a clear demarcation line between the affected and unaffected part. Muscle and joint pain, such as that associated with rheumatism, osteoarthritis, cramps, restless legs, stiffness in the lower back, numbness in arms and legs, and strains can also be alleviated. Other complaints, such as headaches, dizziness, fever, stitch pains made worse by cold and damp, and abdominal pain, can also be relieved. In women, early, heavy, or prolonged menstrual bleeding and accompanying abdominal pain can be treated.

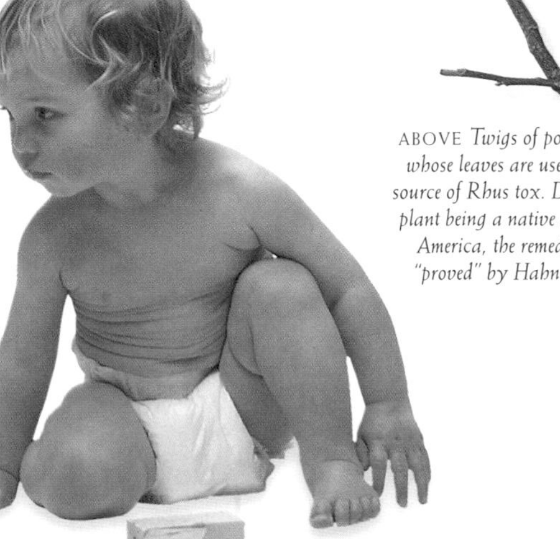

ABOVE *Infants with eczema or diaper rash can benefit from Rhus tox. treatment.*

Which type of person?

- lively, extrovert
- diligent workers
- restless
- cry for no reason
- anxious at night
- like milk, always thirsty

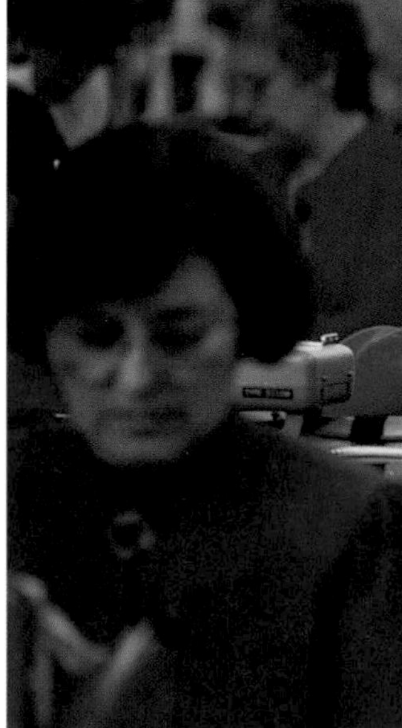

SYMPTOMS

MENTAL

- fear being poisoned
- anxious at night
- depressed and may contemplate suicide
- may act compulsively

PHYSICAL

- headaches after being cold or damp
- eyes are inflamed after being wet
- backache
- blistering skin

Symptoms improve in the warmth, with movement or after changing position, and after stretching. They worsen during cold, wet weather, with rest, when lying on the back or on the right side, and at night.

BELOW *The Rhus tox. remedy is suited to people who are diligent workers and has a wide range of applications.*

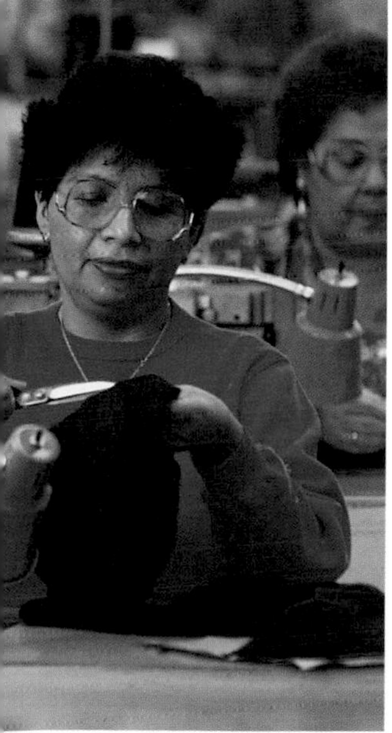

Silicea terra, quartz, silica, flint, rock crystal

SIL.

Silica, the main constituent of rock, is prepared from silicon dioxide, found in flint, quartz, and sandstone. Plants absorb it through their stems and in humans it is essential for the growth of bones, teeth, hair, and nails, and for the maintenance of connective tissue. In homeopathy, it is useful for problems of the digestive and nervous systems, bone and skin conditions, and for its ability to promote the expulsion of foreign bodies such as thorns and splinters. It is also one of the 12 tissue salts identified by Dr. Wilhelm Schussler.

SYMPTOMS

MENTAL

- fear of failure, exertion, sharp objects
- timidity, lack of self-confidence
- worry about future events
- fear of commitment because of being hurt

PHYSICAL

- feet often sweaty
- chills
- slow healing
- discharges
- cracked lips, brittle nails

Symptoms improve in heat and when wrapped up, and worsen in draughts, cold, and damp, when lying on the left side, after washing, by suppressing sweat, and in the morning.

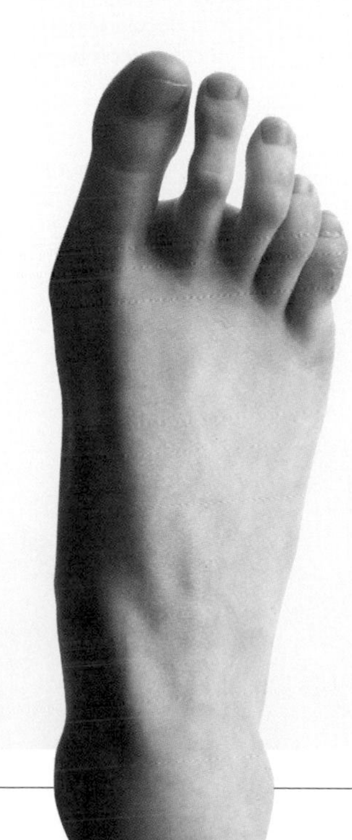

BELOW *Sweaty feet and problems that result from getting the feet wet can indicate the need for Sil.*

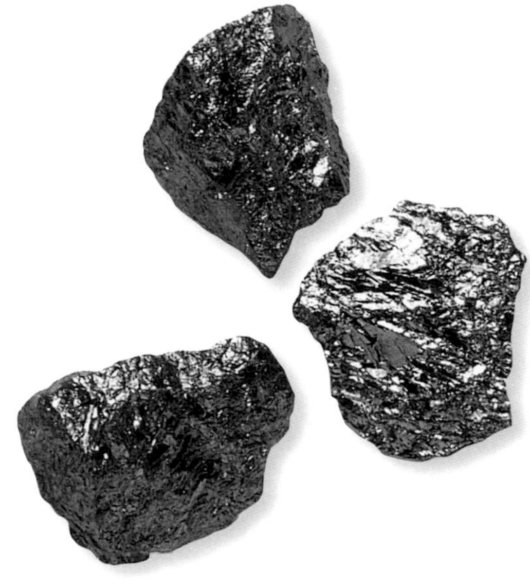

ABOVE *The crystalline form of the element silicon, the source of the homeopathic remedy and tissue salt, Silicea.*

DATA FILE

Relieves

- conditions caused by low immunity due to being malnourished
- bone and skin conditions
- assists in the expulsion of foreign bodies

Uses

Silica is good for complaints which have occurred as a result of low immunity due to lack of nourishment, such as colds, ear infections, catarrh. It can also be used to treat skin and bone conditions, such as acne, weak nails, slow growth, or fontanels which are slow to close in babies, slow-healing fractures; to assist in expelling splinters, glass shards, or thorns from body tissue; and to alleviate problems associated with the nervous system, such as colic and migraines. Other problems alleviated include catarrh with thick, yellow discharge, enlarged lymph nodes, offensive sweat, headaches which start at the back of the head and move over the forehead, glue ear, and restless sleep.

Which type of person?

- slim, small-boned, with lank hair
- neat appearance but prone to cracked lips, brittle, and uneven nails
- appear fragile and lack stamina, but are tenacious
- lack self-confidence, but are strong-willed
- often tired
- worry about new challenges, but take them on anyway
- prefer cold food and dislike milk, meat, cheese, warm food
- children tend to be neat, small, but with large sweaty heads, feel the cold easily, are shy but strong-willed, and conscientious but lacking in confidence

Sepia officinalis, cuttlefish

SEPIA

Historically, cuttlefish ink has been used medicinally to treat conditions such as kidney stones, hair loss, and gonorrhea. It is also used as a pigment in paint, which is where Hahnemann first came across it. He noticed that an artist he was treating for apathy and depression often sucked his brushes, which had been dipped in sepia paint. He published his findings in 1834 after "proving" the remedy. Today, sepia is most commonly taken by women, and is used to treat complaints such as menstrual problems and hormonal imbalances.

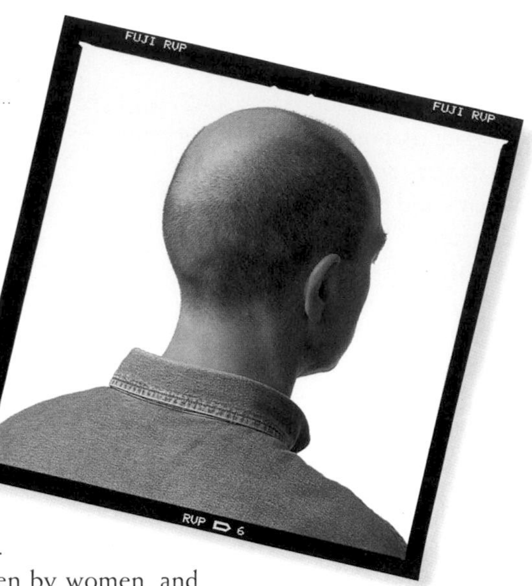

ABOVE *Although Sepia is mainly a women's remedy it is sometimes used for hair loss in either sex.*

SYMPTOMS

MENTAL

- fear poverty, being alone, insanity
- irritable with family, but good in company
- bottle up anger
- find it hard to conceal thoughts

PHYSICAL

- sudden weeping
- easily chilled
- dragging sensation in abdomen
- burning or throbbing pains

Symptoms improve after food, exertion, especially dancing, sleep, and in the warmth, and are worse on the left side, after physical and mental exertion, in the early morning and evening, in thundery weather, and if near tobacco.

DATA FILE

Relieves

- menstrual problems
- conditions associated with hormonal imbalance
- complaints accompanied by exhaustion

Uses

Useful for women who feel "dragged down," both physically and emotionally. Useful for complaints relating to the vagina, ovaries, and uterus, such as heavy or painful menstruation, PMS, menopausal hot flushes, thrush, conditions associated with pregnancy, and the feeling of a sagging abdomen, where the woman feels the need to cross her legs. Pain during sex, aversion to sex, or exhaustion afterward can also be treated. Also, any situation where the woman is feeling emotionally and physically tired, and lacking in energy. Also useful for headaches with nausea, hair loss, dizziness, offensive sweating, indigestion, skin discoloration, and circulatory problems.

Which type of person?

- mainly women
- tall, slim, dark hair and eyes, yellowish facial skin pigmentation
- dignified and attractive
- detached yet emotional
- martyr
- love dancing
- have strong opinions, hating to be contradicted
- resentful of responsibilities
- either career women who appear tough yet are vulnerable, or wives and mothers whose own needs are not met
- prefer sour and sweet foods, alcohol, and dislike milk and pork
- children tend to be sallow, sweaty-skinned, and tire easily; sensitive to weather; moody and negative, dislike parties and being left alone; tendency to constipation

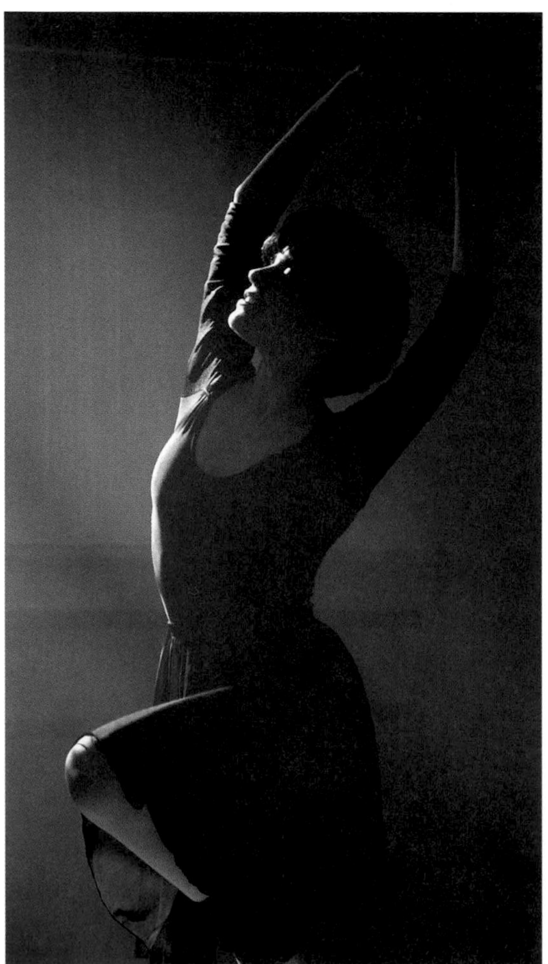

LEFT *A love of dancing may characterize the person who would benefit from treatment with Sepia.*

LEFT *The cuttlefish is the source of sepia used to color ink, and to make the Sepia remedy.*

Spongia tosta, sponge

SPONGIA

Sponge was first treasured for its medicinal properties more than 600 years ago, when it was used as a treatment for goiter, the swelling of the thyroid gland, which is brought on by a deficiency of iodine. Although it was not known then, sponge contains useful amounts of iodine and bromine. Homeopathically, the remedy was first "proved" by Hahnemann, and appears in the sixth volume of his *Materia Medica Pura*. The remedy is made by toasting and powdering the sponge, which is harvested from the waters of the Mediterranean.

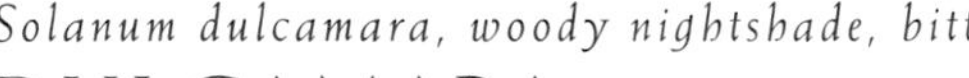

LEFT *Sea sponges, source of the remedy Spongia, were first used medicinally hundreds of years ago.*

RIGHT *Those who will benefit from Spongia usually find that their symptoms are soothed by warm drinks.*

DATA FILE

Relieves

- croup
- coughs
- laryngitis

Uses

This remedy works particularly well for children's croup, characterized by sneezing and a hoarse, dry barking cough, with the patient waking in alarm with the feeling of suffocation, later followed by thick mucus which is difficult to bring up. Associated symptoms of coughs, such as hoarseness, dryness of the larynx from a cold, headaches which are worse when lying down, but improve when sitting up, bronchitis, dry mucous membranes, and feelings of heaviness and exhaustion are also alleviated. Laryngitis, where the throat is raw and dry, and feels like it is burning, responds well. Sponge is also good if chest conditions or tuberculosis tend to run in the family.

Which type of person?

- light-haired, blue-eyed
- lean
- dried-up appearance

SYMPTOMS

MENTAL

- anxiety
- fear of suffocation, and death
- waking from sleep, feeling frightened

PHYSICAL

- congestion of the chest or heart region
- coughs
- palpitations
- laryngitis

Symptoms improve with warm food and drink, and when sitting up. They worsen when talking, swallowing, consuming sweet food or cold drinks, moving, touching the affected area, lying with the head lower than the feet, and around midnight.

Solanum dulcamara, woody nightshade, bittersweet

DULCAMARA

Woody nightshade has been used since Roman times as a remedy to help those suffering from conditions such as asthma, catarrh, rheumatism, and pneumonia resulting from the effects of cold and wet. It is also extensively used in herbal medicine, where it is known as bittersweet, for conditions such as eczema, psoriasis, and ulcers. The remedy, first "proved" by Hahnemann, is made from the green shoots and leaves of the flowering plant, and is given for complaints resulting from exposure to wet weather and temperature changes.

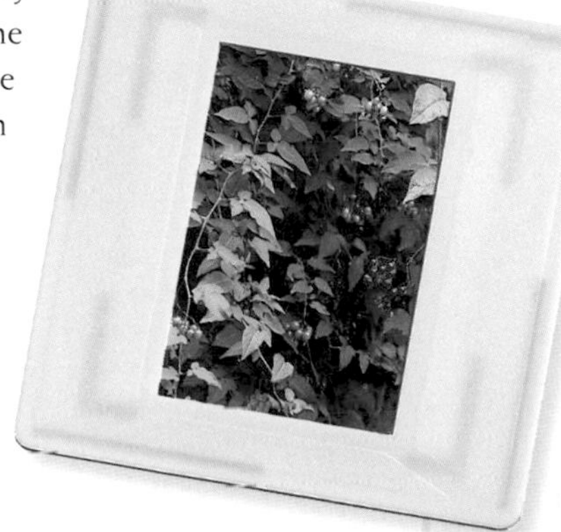

RIGHT *The green shoots and leaves of woody nightshade* (Solanum dulcamara), *a relative of Belladonna, are used to make Dulcamara.*

DATA FILE

Relieves

- conditions which are triggered by or worsen with temperature changes

Uses

Any condition which is brought on by exposure to cold, wet weather, weather changes, for instance from warm to cold or from cooling down too quickly after sweating, can be alleviated. Patients tend to be worse in the autumn and in damp, cold weather. Other problems brought on by weather conditions and helped by the remedy include diarrhea triggered by hot days and cold nights; back and neck pains from the damp; fevers due to exposure to the cold while the body is hot; congested eyes; ulcers; sore throat; frequent urination if chilled; and catarrhal, or dry, hoarse coughs. Skin conditions such as urticaria, crusty facial eruptions, fleshy or flat warts, and ringworm.

Which type of person?

- strong-minded, domineering personality
- possessive
- restless, confused
- keen to keep on the move
- eager for a thing, indifferent when get it

SYMPTOMS

MENTAL

- none in particular

PHYSICAL

- susceptible to cold and weather changes, leading to ailments such as conjunctivitis and diarrhea
- prone to colds
- hungry, but do not want food
- drowsy during the day, restless at night

Symptoms improve in the warmth and with movement, and worsen in the cold and damp, after sweating and then rapidly cooling down, in temperature extremes, and with lack of movement.

Strychnos nux vomica, poison nut, Quaker buttons

NUX VOMICA

The poison nut plant, native to the East Indies, contains strychnine, which is extracted from the seeds. In the past, it was a useful poison for murder. Medicinally, in small amounts, it can help relieve digestive problems, but large doses cause muscular spasm and death from respiratory failure. Strychnine was used during the Middle Ages to help treat sufferers of the plague. Homeopathically, it was first "proved" by Hahnemann. To make the remedy, which is mainly used for oversensitivity and digestive problems, the seeds are extracted from the soft, gelatinous pulp of the fruit and dried.

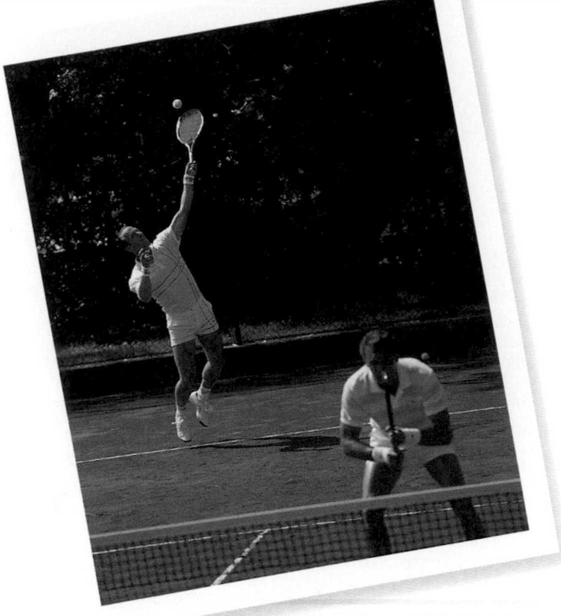

SYMPTOMS

MENTAL

- fear insects, failure, crowds, death
- quarrelsome
- critical of others
- fastidious
- prone to hypochondria

PHYSICAL

- chills
- sensitive to light, smell, noise
- upset by overindulgence in food, alcohol, coffee
- aching, bursting, burning pains

Symptoms improve when lying down and after sleep, in warmth and humidity, in the evening, after washing, and with pressure. They worsen in cold, windy weather, in the morning, in open air or under the sun, two hours after food, and after mental exhaustion.

ABOVE RIGHT *Men, particularly those who are competitive or aggressive, may be Nux vomica types.*

RIGHT *The remedy is derived from the poison nut plant,* Strychnos nux vomica, *from which strychnine is obtained.*

DATA FILE

Relieves

- digestive upsets
- oversensitivity
- chills

Uses

Commonly used to treat emotional problems such as irritability and oversensitivity, it works well for those who bottle up their anger, who are never satisfied, are prone to arguments, dislike having to depend on others, and prefer being left alone. Also used for digestive conditions, such as nausea, vomiting, diarrhea, indigestion, constipation, and piles, which may be brought on by overindulgence in certain foods, or due to suppressing the emotions, or from mental overwork. Other problems it can alleviate include flu, retching coughs, colds with a blocked nose at night and runny nose during the day, chills, headaches which are worse after mental exertion; in women, erratic, early, or heavy menstrual bleeding, morning sickness, constant urination, and labor pain.

Which type of person?

- mainly men
- hypersensitive
- strained-looking, lined face, sallow skin
- criticize, but cannot take criticism from others
- competitive, enjoy meeting challenges
- verbally and mentally alert, with quick wit
- intolerant of others, and easily angered
- may use stimulants to enhance performance
- disgruntled when ill
- prefer rich, fatty food, and like, but are upset by, alcohol and spicy foods
- children tend to be hyperactive and easily irritated, dislike being contradicted; prone to tantrums; diligent and competitive, but hate losing; moody on awakening; prone to stomach aches

SYMPTOMS

MENTAL

- selfishness, egotism
- argumentativeness, aggressiveness
- fear of ghosts, height, failure
- lethargic depression
- full of bright ideas which fade away

PHYSICAL

- burning, itching sensations
- inflammation of affected part
- offensive odors
- thirstiness
- weak areas include left side of the body, circulation, digestive organs, and skin

Symptoms improve when lying on the right side, in warm, dry, fresh air, after physical activity, and worsen in stuffy atmospheres, in the morning, particularly around 11 A.M.*, and at night, in the damp and cold, and after washing.*

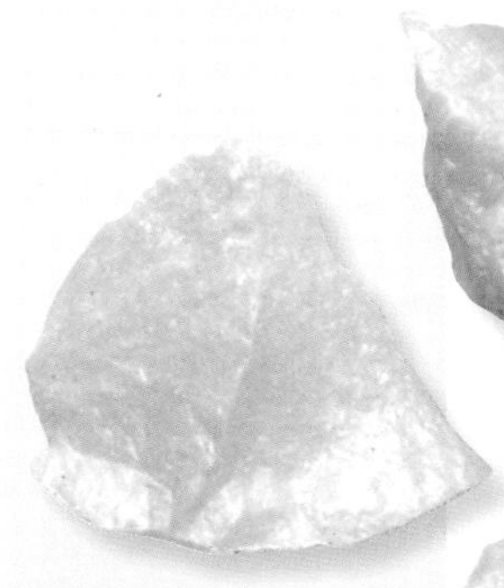

RIGHT *Sulfur, which has many medical and other uses, is the source of the Sulfur remedy.*

Sulfur, brimstone, flowers of sulfur

SULFUR

Sulfur is a mineral which is found in rock forms beside hot springs and in volcanic craters. It has been used medicinally for many centuries – in the 16th century flowers of sulfur was used to fumigate rooms where infection had been present. It was also used as a purgative and to treat rheumatism. Children used to be given brimstone and treacle to encourage bowel function. It has also been used in conventional medicine to treat skin problems such as acne. Homeopathically, it was first "proved" by Hahnemann. A fine, yellow powder is extracted from the mineral. The remedy treats digestive and skin disorders.

DATA FILE

Relieves

- inflamed, itchy skin conditions
- digestive complaints
- offensive odor
- women's conditions
- conditions other remedies do not seem to be helping

Uses

Sulfur can be used to soothe hot, red, itchy skin associated with problems such as eczema and diaper rash, digestive complaints such as vomiting and diarrhea which occur in the morning, indigestion which is made worse by drinking milk, and hunger pangs. It can also treat offensive odors, such as foul-smelling sweat or discharge; premenstrual symptoms such as irritability and headaches; and menopausal symptoms, such as flushing and dizzy spells. It is also useful when another remedy has not worked as hoped or if the picture remedy is not clear. Other problems, such as lack of energy, restless sleep, depression, fever, burning pains and eruptions, congestion, and back pain, can be helped.

Which type of person?

- either round and red-faced or lanky with bad posture
- dry, flaky skin, dull hair, unclean-looking
- selfish, self-centered, and egocentric, but can be giving and good-natured
- full of ideas, but unable to carry them out, because of a lack of will-power
- fuss over minor details
- quickly angered, but just as quickly calm down
- sensitive to smell
- prefer sweet, fatty, spicy, and sour foods, alcohol, stimulants, and dislike milk, hot drinks, and eggs
- children tend to be either well built, with thick hair and a rosy complexion, or thin and pale with dry skin; both types eat well, look disheveled, are happy when stimulated, take care of their possessions, and are difficult to get to go to bed

Tarentula hispanica, Lycosa tarentula, Spanish spider, wolf spider

TARENTULA

Tarentula gets its name from the Italian town of Taranto (Latin name *Tarentum*), where the wolf spider is commonly found. It was given the name wolf spider because of the way it chases after its prey rather than lying in wait on a web. The European wolf spider does not harm humans, unlike the bite of the poisonous South American tarantula, which was said to cause maniacal behavior, twitching, and the feeling of suffocating. The homeopathic remedy is made from the whole live spider and is used to treat restless, frantic behavior.

SYMPTOMS

MENTAL

- experience extreme mood swings
- edgy, restless
- manic laughter
- violent outbursts

PHYSICAL

- weak legs
- constricting pains
- restless legs
- rolling from side to side in order to alleviate symptoms

Symptoms improve in the open air, while listening to music, looking at bright colors, moving from side to side, and worsen with movement, noise, touch, on seeing others in trouble, and at a particular time each year.

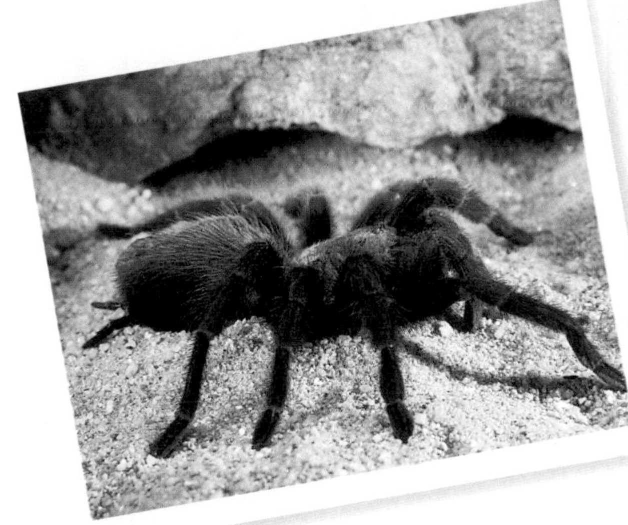

LEFT *The European wolf spider is the source of Tarentula. The whole spider is used in this preparation.*

DATA FILE

Relieves

- mental and physical restlessness
- mood swings
- heart complaints
- in women, ovarian disease, genital sensitivity

Uses

It can be used to treat nervous disorders, such as mental and physical agitation, twitchy, restless legs, numbness, extreme mood swings, and impatience. Angina and heart disease also respond well. In women, sensitivity of the genitalia, which become itchy, heavy menstrual bleeding, and ovarian disease which feels worse on the left side of the body can be alleviated.

Which type of person?

- hyperactive, behave destructively
- extremely impatient
- manipulative
- suffer vertigo
- workaholic

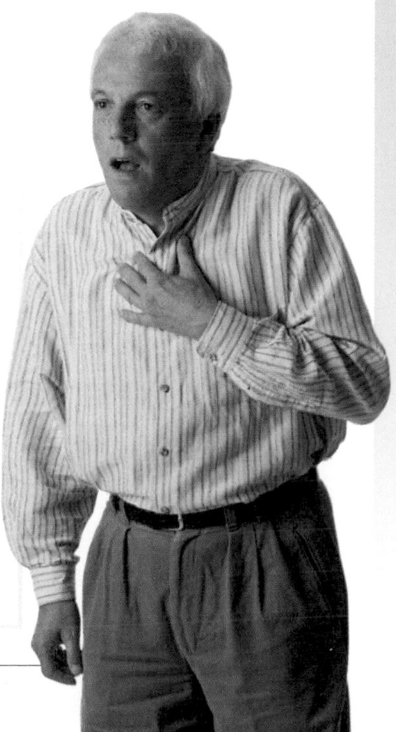

RIGHT *Choking and feelings of suffocation caused by heart problems can be helped by this remedy.*

Thuja occidentalis, arbor vitae, white cedar, tree of life

THUJA

The name thuja comes from the Greek word *thero*, meaning to sacrifice or fumigate. In pagan sacrifices, the tree was burnt when victims were executed. The evergreen tree is grown in Canada and the U.S., and native Americans used its twigs and leaves to treat rheumatism, gout, and malaria. In homeopathy, the scented leaves and twigs are pounded to a pulp to make both the remedy and a cream that is especially useful for rheumatic pain.

ABOVE *and* BELOW *Leaves of* Thuja occidentalis, *a member of the extensive Cupressus family, which is the source of Thuja.*

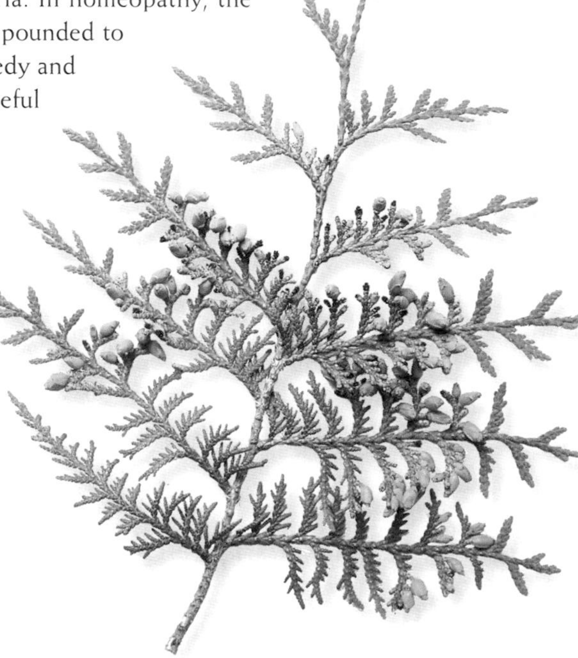

DATA FILE

Relieves

- inflamed, swollen joints
- skin complaints
- genitourinary infections

Uses

Thuja can be used for joints that have become swollen and inflamed, as in rheumatism; for skin complaints, particularly warts, and for pale, greasy skin which sweats when exposed; urinary infections; headaches brought on by stress or fatigue; yellow-green catarrh; foul-smelling perspiration; tooth decay; weak nails; in women, for uterine or vaginal infections, early or scant menstruation, and loss of appetite in the morning; gurgling bowels.

Which type of person?

- greasy, pale skin
- take little interest in physical appearance
- sensitive, weep easily
- prefer tea and dislike meat, potatoes, fat
- children are small, with a slim build, and are slow

SYMPTOMS

MENTAL

- paranoia that others are taking advantage
- anxiety
- fear of strangers
- odd fixations

PHYSICAL

- headaches
- warts
- weak nails
- urinary conditions
- catarrh

Symptoms improve when warm in bed and with movement, and worsen in the cold and damp, at night, and on the left side of the body.

Trigonocephalus lachesis, Lachesis muta, bushmaster snake, surukuku

LACHESIS

The South American bushmaster snake is extremely poisonous – one bite into a vein can cause immediate death – as the venom affects the heart and central nervous system. A lesser bite will cause bleeding and blood poisoning. The snake gets its other name, surukuku, from the humming sound it makes as it lies in wait for its prey. Homeopathically, it was first "proved" by Dr. Constantine Hering in 1837, who tested the venom on himself while in the Amazonian jungle. The remedy uses fresh venom, and treats wounds that are slow to heal or that bleed profusely.

SYMPTOMS

MENTAL

- fear of burglars, poisoning, water, suffocating, death
- disgruntled on waking
- strong ideas and philosophies
- suspicious of people
- jealous
- suffer nightmares
- prone to post-menopausal depression
- short-tempered

PHYSICAL

- blueness around skin problems
- bloating
- restlessness
- oversensitivity to touch and noise
- weak areas include the left side of the body, circulation, nervous system, and female reproductive organs

Symptoms improve after discharges, such as menstruation, nosebleeds, or bowel movements, in fresh air, and after a cold drink, and are worse on the left side, with sleep, when touched, with motion, in heat, and after hot drinks.

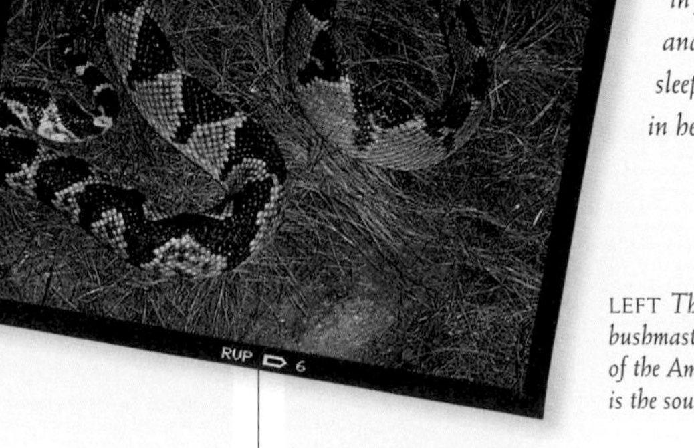

LEFT *The deadly bushmaster snake, native of the Amazonian jungle, is the source of Lachesis.*

DATA FILE

Relieves

- premenstrual and menopausal complaints
- circulatory and vascular problems
- left-sided complaints
- slow-healing wounds

Uses

Helpful for premenstrual problems such as erratic pain relieved by blood flow, and problems associated with the menopause, such as hot flushes and dizziness. It works well for any problems connected with blood flow and circulation, such as varicose veins, irregular pulse, angina, and palpitations. Problems which occur on the left side, for example earache, headaches, and sore throats, can be alleviated; wounds that are not healing well, such as bleeding piles, ulcers, and cuts are helped. Other conditions include nervous disorders such as fainting and petit mal epileptic attacks; blue wounds; purplish, bloated face; fever; sweats; any pulsations or throbbing; waking up with a sensation of choking; and glands which are swollen.

Which type of person?

- tend to be redheaded, freckled, pale-skinned
- puffy or bloated-looking
- egocentric, with no regard for others
- intuitive, creative, aspiring
- selfish, devious, jealous
- dislike commitment, blow hot and cold with partners
- dislike being restricted
- strong ideologists
- may be gloomy and quiet
- creativity is short-lived
- prefer sour and starchy foods and alcohol, and cannot tolerate hot drinks and wheat
- children tend to be hyperactive and difficult to control, prone to jealousy, possessive of friends, but may hurt them with their poisonous tongue

RIGHT *Urtica cream is available to alleviate rashes and stinging, smarting or burning skin conditions.*

Urtica urens, stinging nettle

URTICA

The stinging nettle, a common weed found in many countries, has been used for centuries for its medicinal properties. The Greek physician Dioscorides used it as a purgative and detoxification. It is commonly used in herbal medicine for conditions such as piles, nosebleeds, stomach conditions, and as a tea. The 16th-century herbalist John Gerard used it as an antidote to poison. The small plant is covered in soft, spiny hairs which secrete a sap that causes itching and inflammation if touched. In homeopathy, it was first "proved" by Hahnemann and is used to treat conditions which are accompanied by stinging or burning. Urtica can be used externally in the form of a cream, as well as taken internally.

ABOVE *Allergic reactions, to stings or to eating foods such as strawberries, can be helped by this remedy.*

THERAPY CONNECTIONS

NETTLE

Herbalism p.137

DATA FILE

Relieves

- stinging, burning conditions of the skin
- rheumatic pain
- neuralgia

Uses

Used both as an internal remedy and externally as a cream, Urtica is useful for skin conditions, particularly if the skin is stinging or has the sensation of burning. It is good for rashes where the skin is blotchy and blistered, such as urticaria (hives) and bee stings, or when there is an allergic reaction, for instance after eating strawberries. Other conditions which it can be used to alleviate include rheumatism, neuralgia, neuritis, gout, excess uric acid, and, in women, vulval itching and painful breasts when the milk flow is blocked.

Which type of person?

- no particular type

SYMPTOMS

MENTAL

- none in particular

PHYSICAL

- stinging, burning skin
- rheumatic pain
- cystitis
- gout

Symptoms improve after massaging the affected area and when lying down, and worsen in cold, damp air, if touched, and with water.

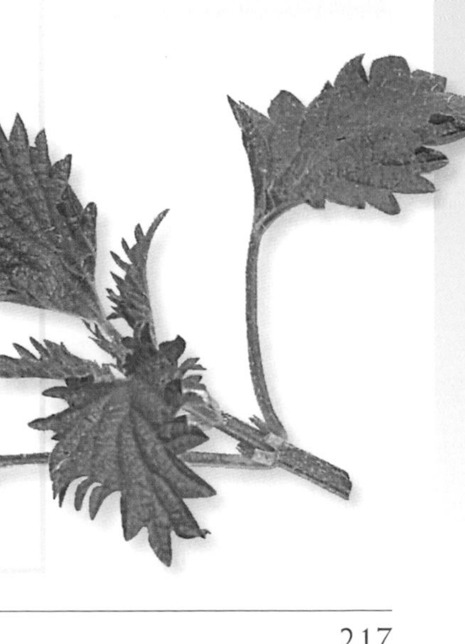

BELOW *The common stinging nettle is the source of Urtica, also known as Urtica urens and Urt. u.*

FLOWER REMEDIES

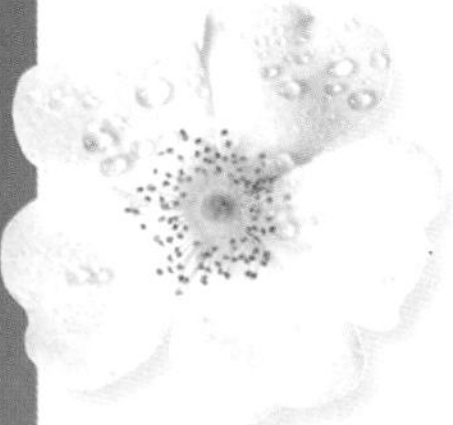

ABOVE *Flower remedies draw on the vibrational power of flowers like wild rose.*

Flower essences, or flower remedies, as they are more commonly known, are used therapeutically to harmonize the body, mind, and the spirit. The essences are said to contain the life force of the flowers used to make them. Thousands of essences are available in health food stores, and they work "vibrationally" on a mental and emotional level, to relieve negative feelings, encourage the healing process, and to balance the energy in the body.

Flower remedies are ideal for home use, being simple to make and use. They are prepared in water and preserved with alcohol. Historically, flower water and the morning dew collected from flower petals were thought to be imbued with magical properties. That flower remedies work is indisputable; no one knows how, so there is still an element of magic associated with their use – even today, when our understanding of vibrational medicine is growing.

Flower remedies are so simple that they are often dismissed as a placebo. They do not work in any biochemical way, and because no physical part of the plant remains in the remedy, its properties and actions cannot be detected or analyzed as if it were a drug or herbal preparation. Therapists believe the remedies contain the energy, or imprint, of the plant from which it was made and work in a way that is similar to homeopathic remedies. In this way a remedy is believed to provide the stimulus needed to kick-start your own healing mechanism.

DR. BACH

Until recently, the name Dr. Edward Bach was almost synonymous with flower remedies. His set of 38 remedies became the inspiration for the worldwide development of remedies. They are still the cornerstone of flower remedy therapy and easily available. While working in the London Homeopathic Hospital, just after the First World War, he noticed that people with similar attitudes often had similar complaints. He concluded that, independently of other factors, mood and a negative attitude predisposed people toward ill health, and that illness was a manifestation of a deeper disharmony or an indication that the personality was in conflict. Between 1928 and 1932 he identified seven main negative states and found the first twelve of the flower remedies he needed to address them. Over the subsequent few years, he dedicated himself to finding natural remedies from the countryside, and at his death had made 38 separate remedies. His successors at his house in Oxfordshire, Mount Vernon, continue to make his remedies today, and they are sold under the name Bach Flower Remedies.

OTHER REMEDIES

The Bach Flower Remedies are made from the trees and flowers Dr. Bach saw on his travels, which are native to England, with the exceptions of Olive and Vine. In the last twenty years, remedies from the U.S. and Australia have been made. Sometimes they are called flower essences (do not confuse them with essential oils), but they are said to work in the same way as the original flower remedies. They address the emotional self, unlocking repressions, liberating negativity, and encouraging positive well-being.

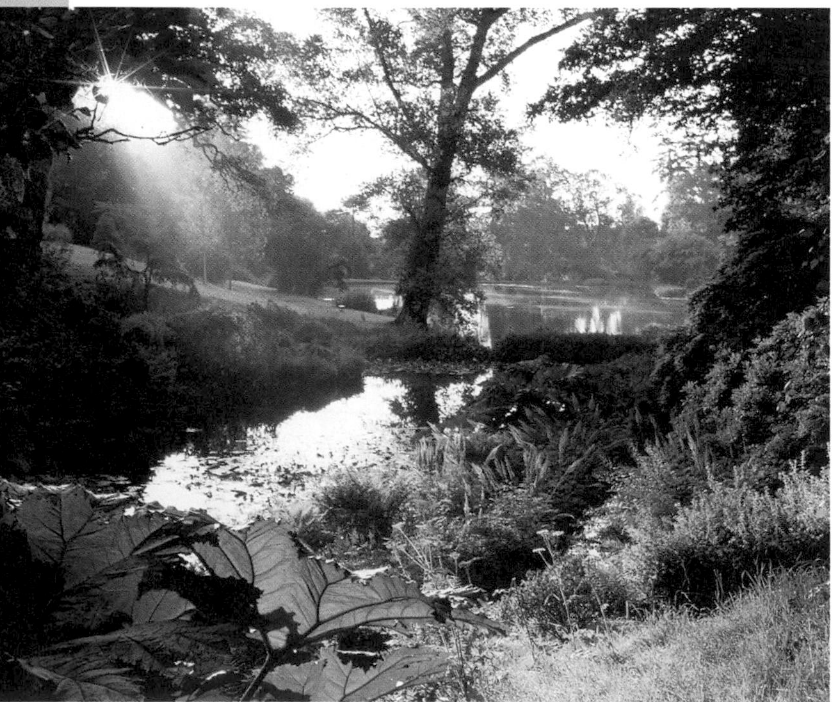

LEFT *Dr. Edward Bach, the originator of the Bach Flower Remedies, sought his ingredients in the English countryside and tested them all on himself.*

THE FUTURE

The world is more complex than it was in 1920, more is demanded, and people have to delve deeper to find the reserves to cope. Human nature has not changed, however, so the same 38 remedies Dr. Bach found still form a complete system that can address all human emotions. Nevertheless, many people have started to make new essences, and remedies are available now from all corners of the world.

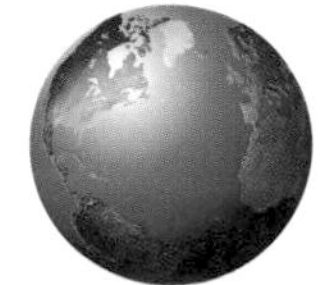

UNITED KINGDOM
It was in the U.K. that Dr. Edward Bach first identified and began to harness the healing power of flowers.

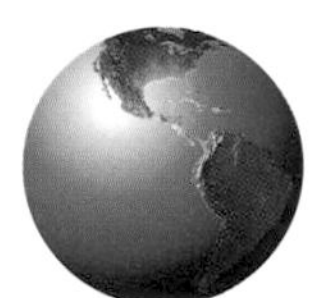

UNITED STATES
American flower essence makers have developed remedies according to the needs of late 20th-century society.

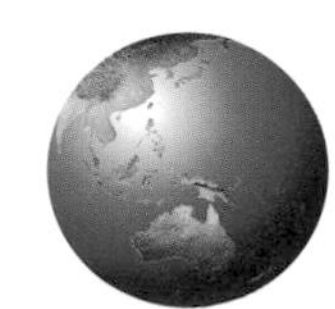

AUSTRALIA
Flower essence makers in Australia have used the natural fauna of their own country to create Australian Bush remedies.

NEGATIVITY CONTRIBUTES TO ILL HEALTH

Negative emotions depress the mind and immune system, repress activity, and contribute to ill health. All are rooted in one or more of the following, which are headings under which Dr. Bach grouped his 38 remedies:

- fear
- uncertainty
- insufficient interest in present circumstances
- loneliness
- oversensitivity to influences and ideas
- despondency or despair
- over-care for the welfare of others

By learning the healing capacity of peace, hope, joy, faith, certainty, wisdom, and love it is possible to develop a positive outlook and a sense of well-being.

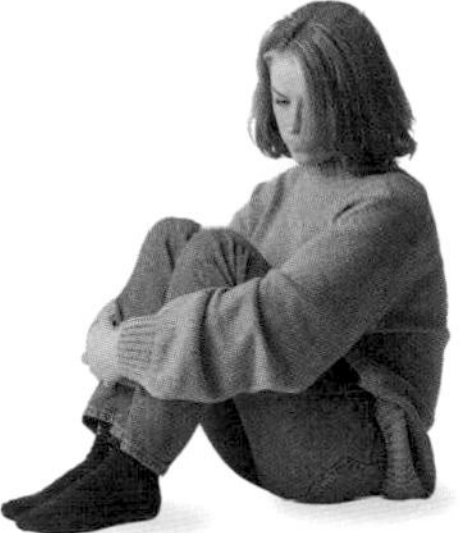

ABOVE *Negative emotions have a detrimental effect on the health.*

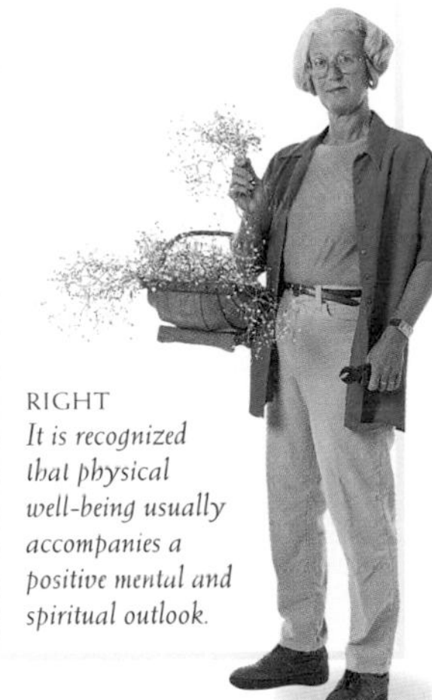

RIGHT *It is recognized that physical well-being usually accompanies a positive mental and spiritual outlook.*

THE BACH FLOWER REMEDIES: A QUICK GUIDE

- **AGRIMONY** For those who hide their feelings behind humor and put on a brave face.
- **ASPEN** For fear of the unknown; vague, unsettling fears which cannot be explained.
- **BEECH** For the perfectionist who tends to be intolerant of other people's methods and experience.
- **CENTAURY** For those who find it impossible to say no to the demands of others and thus exhaust themselves by doing too much.
- **CERATO** For those who lack confidence in themselves and are constantly seeking the advice of others, to make up their mind.
- **CHERRY PLUM** For the fear of loosing one's mind, and for irrational thoughts or behavior.
- **CHESTNUT BUD** For those who find it hard to learn from life and keep making the same mistakes.
- **CHICORY** For the self-obsessed, mothering type who is overprotective and possessive.
- **CLEMATIS** For the absent minded daydreamer who needs to be awake and focus the mind on the here and now.
- **CRAB APPLE** For those who feel unclean or polluted on any level, either physically, emotionally, or spiritually; Crab Apple is for those who feel they need purification.
- **ELM** For those who suffer temporary feelings of inadequacy brought on by all the responsibilities they have taken on.
- **GENTIAN** For despondency, and for those who are easily discouraged by a setback in life.
- **GORSE** For those who suffer feelings of hopelessness and despair, and who are stuck in a negative pattern; pessimism.
- **HEATHER** For those who like to be listened to when they talk constantly about themselves; for poor listeners and those who are self-obsessed.
- **HOLLY** For those who suffer dissipating bouts of hatred, jealousy, envy, and suspicion.
- **HONEYSUCKLE** For those who suffer from nostalgia or who dwell on the events of the past instead of living in the present.
- **HORNBEAM** For those who are stuck in a rut and feel tired, so that work which used to be fulfiling is now tiresome.
- **IMPATIENS** For impatience and irritability; Impatiens helps those for whom life is always a rush and who are too busy to slow down.
- **LARCH** For those who feel worthless and are suffering from lack of confidence or low self-esteem.
- **MIMULUS** For the fear of known things; for the strength to face everyday fears and all fears which can be named.
- **MUSTARD** For depression without cause, those who feel they are under a dark gloomy cloud for no apparent reason.
- **OAK** For the fighter who never gives in and is exhausting him or herself by being too persistent in the same old fight.
- **OLIVE** For those who are exhausted on all levels, fatigued, and drained of further optimism and spirit after a long struggle or effort.
- **PINE** For those who suffer self-reproach and guilt; for those who say sorry even when things are not their fault.
- **RED CHESTNUT** For those who are overanxious about the welfare of family or friends; for those who fear that something awful may happen to their loved ones.
- **ROCK ROSE** For those who feel helpless and experience extreme terror or panic, when there may or may not be a reason but the feeling is real.
- **ROCK WATER** For perfectionists who are hard on themselves and demand perfection in all things.
- **SCLERANTHUS** For those who suffer from indecision and who cannot make up their mind.
- **STAR OF BETHLEHEM** For shocks of all kinds, accidents, bad news, sudden startling noise, and trauma.
- **SWEET CHESTNUT** For utter despair and hopelessness; for when there seems no way out.
- **VERVAIN** For enthusiasts and those with a strong sense of justice; those who never rest in their pursuit of an aim.
- **VINE** For the over-strong and dominating leader who may tend toward tyranny; for bullying.
- **WALNUT** For change; for breaking links so that life may develop without hindrance.
- **WATER VIOLET** For people who are aloof, self-reliant, and self-contained; to relax the reserved and enable sharing.
- **WHITE CHESTNUT** For tiresome mental chatter and the overactive mind, full of persistent and unwanted patterns of thought.
- **WILD OAT** For those who need help in deciding on the path and purpose of their life.
- **WILD ROSE** For those who drift through life resigned to accept any eventuality; for fatalists and people too apathetic to try.
- **WILLOW** For those who feel they have been treated unfairly; for resentment and self-pity.

USING FLOWER REMEDIES

Flower remedies are simple and effective, and they can be used:

- *to support in times of crisis.*
- *to treat the emotional outlook produced by illness.*
- *to address a particular recurring emotional or behavioral pattern.*
- *to give strength during a temporary emotional setback.*
- *as a preventive remedy when things start to go out of balance.*

Remedies act swiftly for passing moods and there should be an improvement very quickly, although it may take months to start to change a long-standing pattern.

The flower remedies or essences bought in a store are sold in stock bottles. They can be used straight from the bottle, but it is better to make a personal remedy mix. Sometimes a single flower remedy is needed, but in most cases two or more are combined.

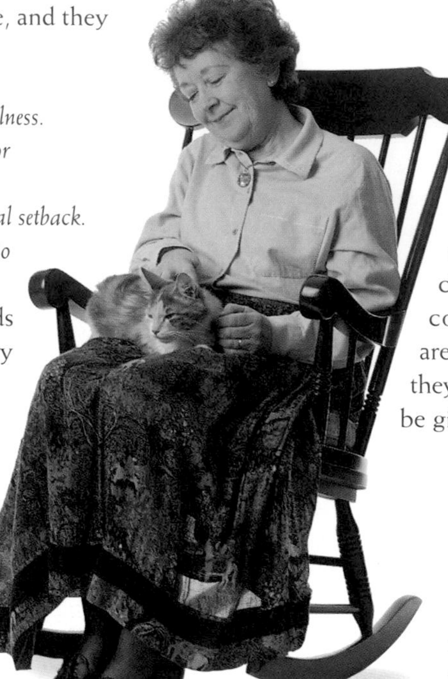

LEFT *Many claim that animals as well as people can be helped by flower remedies.*

ARE THEY SAFE?

The remedies are not addictive or dangerous, nor do they interfere with any other form of treatment. They are suitable for people of all ages. Pregnant women and children can take them with confidence. Flower remedies are safe for young babies, should they need them, and they can also be given to animals and plants.

WHICH PROBLEMS CAN THEY HELP?

All types of mental or emotional problems.

TO MAKE A PERSONAL REMEDY

You'll need:

- 1fl.oz. (30ml.) amber glass dropper bottle
- 1fl.oz. (30ml.) spring water; or 1 teaspoon (5ml.) brandy and 5 teaspoons (25ml.) spring water

- Decide on the remedies which are most applicable. Usually between one and six is enough. If you think you need several, simplify to a maximum of seven covering immediate issues, and check again in a few weeks.
- Put 2 drops of each remedy into a clean 1fl.oz. (30ml.) amber glass dropper bottle. This is the standard amount, but read the label, as occasionally some of the newer essences suggest you use 4 or 7 drops.
- If the remedies are to be used within a week, fill the bottle with clean spring water.
- If the remedies are to be taken for a prolonged period, add 1 teaspoonful (5ml.) of brandy to the bottle and then fill with spring water.
- Label the bottle with your name and the date.
- Give the remedy a title or a few words to remind you of the purpose. Would an affirmation be useful?
- Take as directed (*see below*).
- Keep remedies, like other medicines, out of the reach of children.

To use

- The standard dose is 4 drops, on or under the tongue, 4 times a day.
- At times of crisis, 2 drops from the stock bottle can be put into a glass of water (or, in an emergency, any drink) and sipped as needed.
- If for any reason it is impossible to take anything by mouth, put the drops on the skin or in washing water.

BELOW *Flower essences are usually added to water, up to six kinds are mixed.*

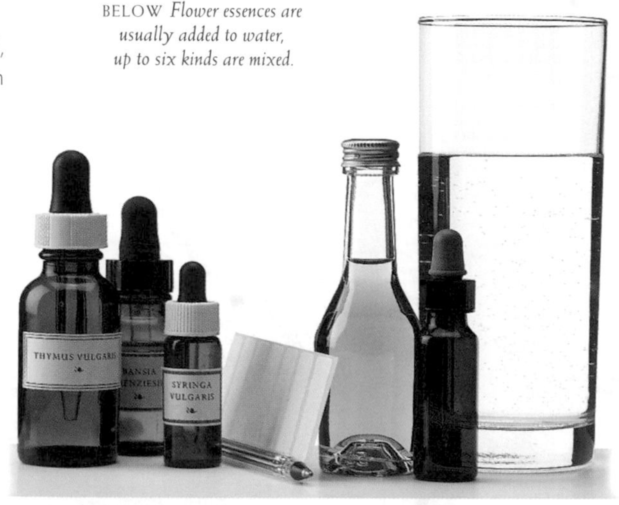

USING THE REMEDIES

Successful treatment depends on accurate diagnosis. Get to know the different essences available and then aim to match the remedies to the individual character.

FOR YOURSELF If you find it hard to decide on a remedy, make a note of the one you think you need and then ask yourself the same questions you would ask anyone for whom you were prescribing:

- How do you feel?
- Why are you feeling like that?
- How do the symptoms affect you?
- What could have caused the problem?

FOR CHILDREN Children show their nature in their behavior and play. Try to match the behavior of the child to the remedy:

- Is the child always active like Vervain?
- Timid and shy like Mimulus?
- Gentle and obedient like Centaury?
- Bossy like Vine?
- Or sulky like Willow?

FOR ANIMALS You need to know the animal's nature and note how differently it behaves when ill. For example, a dog which looks sorry for itself needs Willow; an aggressive one needs Holly or Vine; and cats often need Water Violet for their pride and independence. Add 4 drops to a small animal's drinking water, and 10 drops for large animals such as horses and cows. Add more drops whenever the water is replaced.

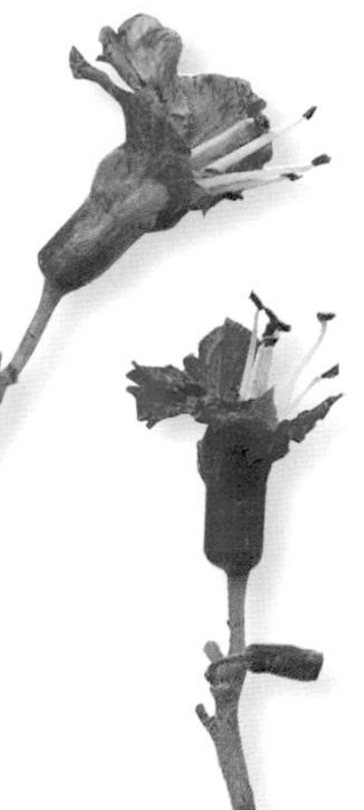

ABOVE *The flowers of Red Chestnut are a good remedy for parents who are over-anxious about their family's welfare.*

CHILDREN

- Flower remedies are ideal for children. Treat them as soon as you notice that something is "not quite right."
- Physical symptoms must be professionally treated. Consult a physician if in doubt.
- Listen and do not trivialize children's emotional lives. Be calm and methodical. Notice the mood or address a previously known pattern. Give the remedy for a day or two, then reassess. Moods in children may change rapidly.
- If worried about a child (or other family member) take Red Chestnut, Rescue Remedy, or any other remedy which seems relevant, to settle yourself before deciding on treatment.
- If the child is of breast feeding age, give the remedy to the mother. It may also be put in the bath, for example use Impatiens to treat the hot and restless frustration of a teething baby.
- Treat and support the parents. If home nursing, give Mimulus to minimize known fears. Give Rescue Remedy and Walnut if the child is hospitalized. Other remedies may be applicable.
- Treat the parents. Their emotional problems (even if suppressed) may be the root of a child's distress.

ATTITUDE AND AFFIRMATIONS

Flower remedies should not be taken without thought and due care.

Ask these questions:
- Why is it needed?
- What do I expect?

There should be a clear reason for taking a herb or remedy and a positive treatment aim or goal.

Some people recommend the use of affirmations, suggesting that an appropriate affirmation is written down several times a day for a week while taking the remedy. An example of a positive affirmation for the Clematis daydreamer would be: "I am awake (or becoming awake) and open to the experience of here and now."

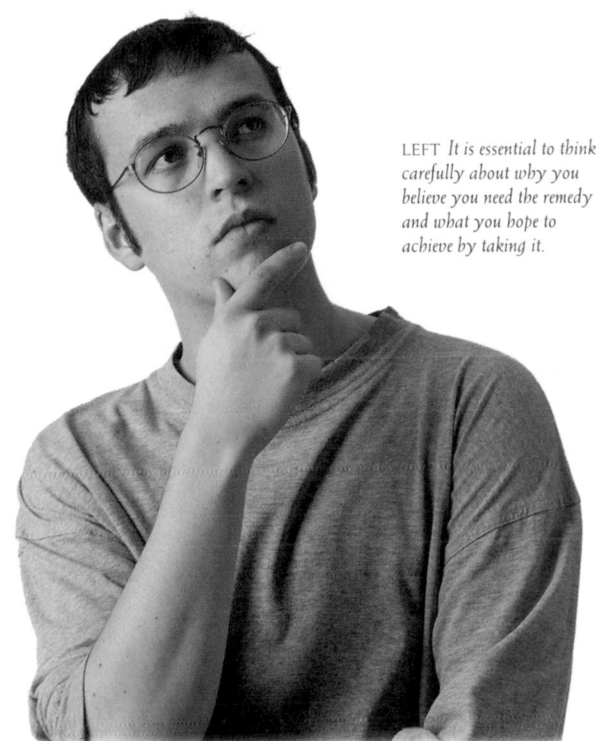

LEFT *It is essential to think carefully about why you believe you need the remedy and what you hope to achieve by taking it.*

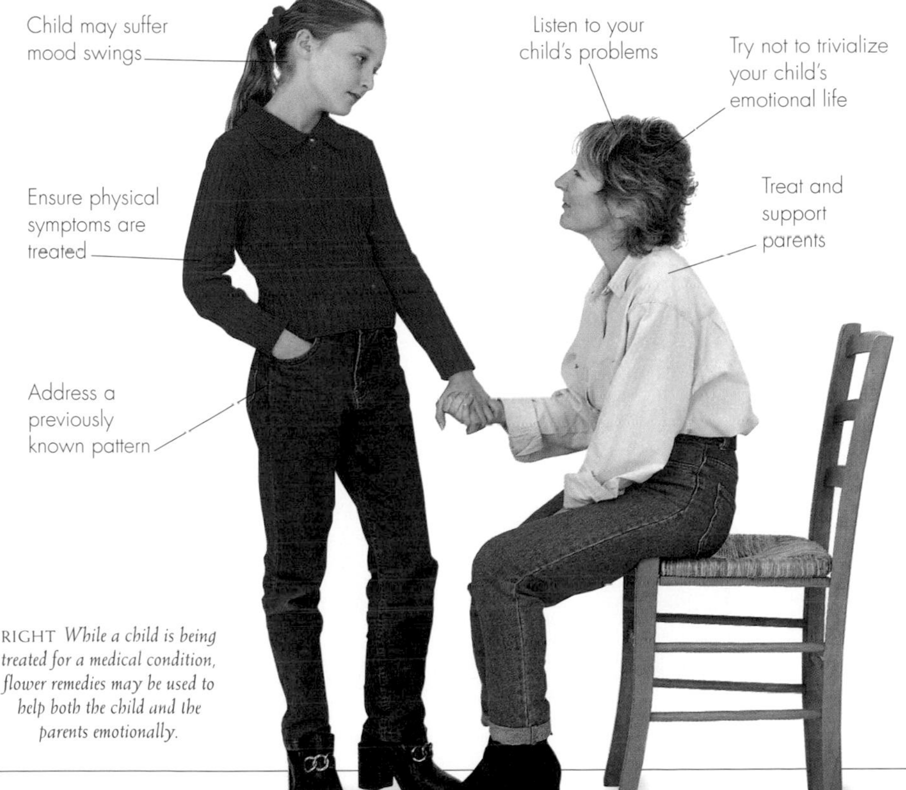

RIGHT *While a child is being treated for a medical condition, flower remedies may be used to help both the child and the parents emotionally.*

REMEDIES AND ALCOHOL

Flower remedies and essences are preserved in alcohol. The amount of alcohol in a personal remedy made solely with water is minute, but it is enough to upset those who are alcohol intolerant or recovering from alcoholism. Always check the status of those to whom you give a remedy. Thoughtlessness can do untold damage.

It is possible to remove the alcohol by putting the diluted drops of remedy in a boiling hot drink – the steam will evaporate the alcohol. Leave the remedy to cool before taking. Sip throughout the day.

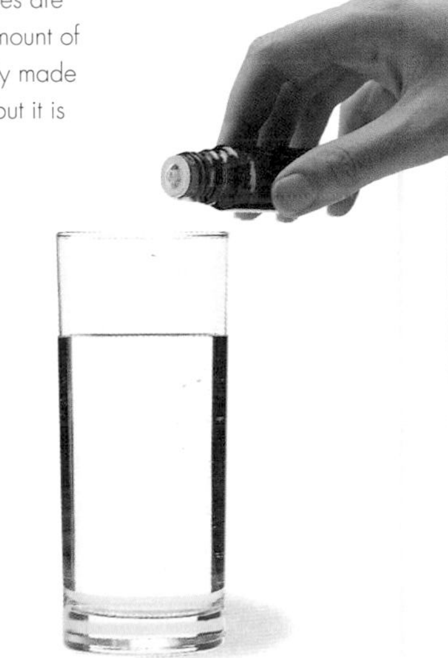

ABOVE *The remedies can be taken in hot or cold water as the patient prefers.*

MAKING THE REMEDIES

HOW TO MAKE FLOWER REMEDIES

Flower remedies are simple to make, and rewarding and effective to use. Remedies are made in two ways: the sun method and the boiling method.

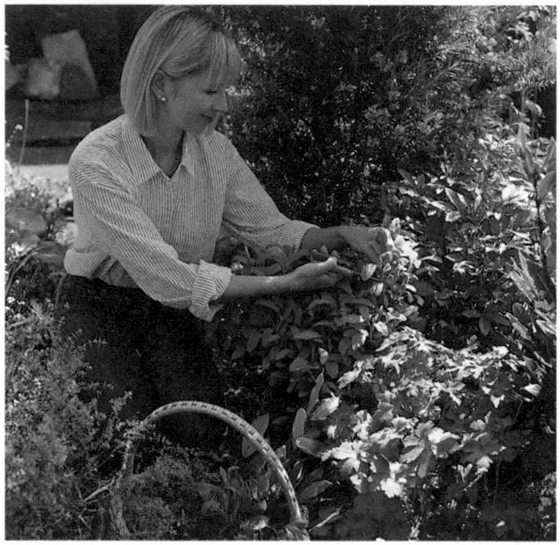

ABOVE *Whichever method you are using, collect your materials on a fine day, preferably before noon.*

Whatever the method there are a few basic rules:

CORRECT IDENTIFICATION Find the plant and site well before the day of picking. Make sure that it is legal to pick it or that you have the landowner's permission.

PREPARATION Collect essentials. Absolute cleanliness is essential. Wash your hands and rinse them several times. Utensils can be cleaned by boiling in spring or rain water for 20 minutes and then allowing them to drain dry. Wrap them in a clean cloth to keep them ready for a suitable day.

THE RIGHT DAY For sun method remedies, choose a warm, sunny day with no clouds. For boiling method remedies any bright, sunny day is good.

ON THE DAY Pick with respect. Remember that you are making a remedy and what the remedy is designed to treat. Pick flowers that you are drawn to. Pick from all sides of the plant, from the top and bottom branches of trees, or from a wide area with meadow plants. Work quickly so there is only a little time between picking the flowers and putting them into the water to make the remedy. If you need to carry the flowers, cover your palm with a large leaf (preferably from the plant being picked) to prevent the heat and oils from the hand contaminating the blossoms. Use a twig to stir and remove the flowers.

LABELING When you have finished, label and date your remedy clearly. Keep it in a cool, dark place, away from direct sunlight.

THE SUN METHOD

Pick when the flowers are coming into full bloom. This will depend on the climate and the type of season, but the following can serve as a general guide:

✣ EARLY SPRING: oak, gorse, olive, vine.

✣ LATE SPRING: white chestnut, water violet.

✣ SUMMER: rock water, mimulus, agrimony, rock rose, centaury.

✣ LATE SUMMER: scleranthus, wild oat, impatiens, chicory, vervain, clematis, heather.

✣ FALL: cerato, gentian.

A 3fl.oz. (100ml.) bottle of mother tincture will last the average family many years. The recipe can make more, up to six bottles. If you wish to make more for family or friends, prepare more bottles. Each 3fl.oz. (100ml.) should contain 1½fl.oz. (50ml.) of brandy and be made up as outlined below:

✣ You'll need:
- bottle of spring or mineral water
- plain glass bowl
- 3fl.oz. (100ml.) amber bottle(s)
- 1½fl.oz. (50ml.) brandy
- natural and unbleached filter paper
- pen and label

✣ Decide beforehand on the plants, where to pick from, and where to place the bowl, then wait for a suitable sunny day.

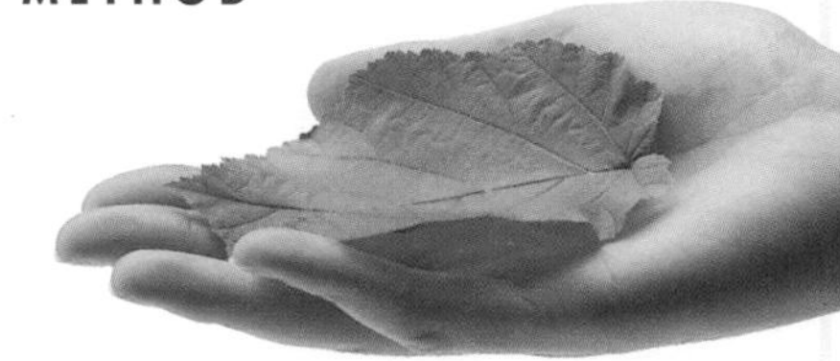

ABOVE *Use a leaf, ideally of the plant being picked, to protect the flowers from the heat of your hand.*

The bowl should be placed in a clear open place, as close to the plants as possible, but away from shadows and possible contamination.

✣ The best time of the day for harvesting the plants is between 9A.M. and midday. The flowers are dry from the dew, but not yet exhausted by the sun.

✣ Pick the flowers and put in the water as quickly as possible.

✣ Float the flowers on the water until the whole surface is covered. Use a twig or leaf to arrange them, not your fingers.

✣ Leave the bowl out in the open where it will receive direct sunshine for three hours.

✣ After 3 hours, remove the flowers with a twig and filter the liquid.

✣ Pour 1½fl.oz. (50ml.) of the water into the bottle with the brandy. Shake and label with the name, "flower essence mother tincture," and date.

This mother tincture will be used to prepare stock bottles and it will keep for many years. To prepare a stock bottle, put 2 drops of mother tincture into a 1fl.oz. (30ml.) dropper bottle, and top up with brandy. Then, from the stock bottle, use 2 drops to make up the treatment bottle as already described.

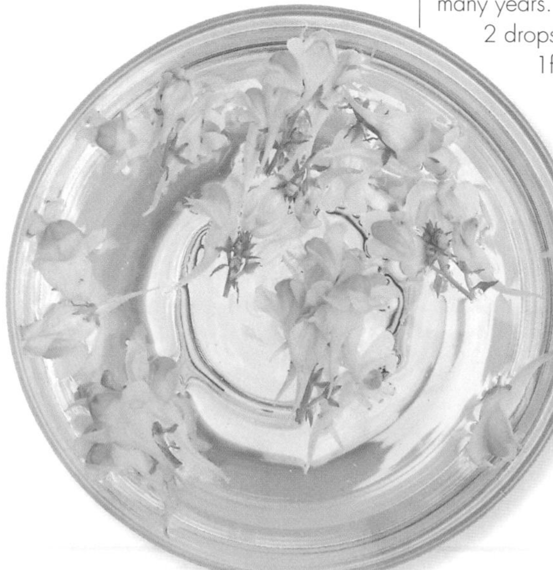

LEFT *Leave the flowers floating on the surface of the water in the sun.*

THE BOILING METHOD

The boiling method is mainly used for the flowers of trees. In any case, more than just the flower are picked – in addition, it is necessary to collect twigs that have a few leaves on them.

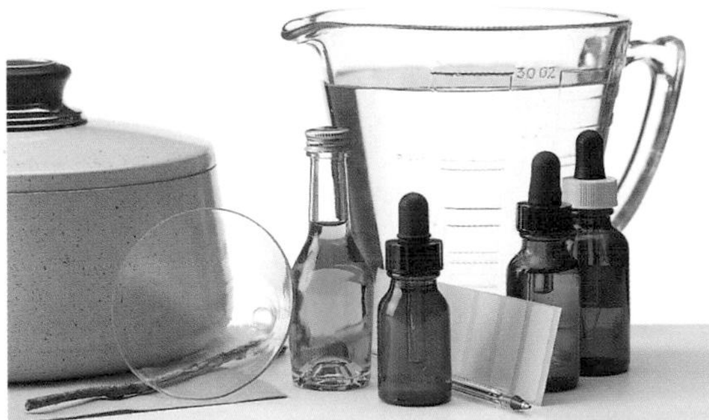

ABOVE *The equipment needed for the boiling method, which is used for the flowers of trees.*

Pick when the flowers are at their best:

- EARLY SPRING: cherry plum.
- SPRING: elm, aspen.
- LATE SPRING: beech, chestnut bud, hornbeam, larch, walnut, and Star of Bethlehem.
- LATE SPRING: holly, crab apple, willow.
- EARLY SUMMER: red chestnut, pine, mustard.
- SUMMER: honeysuckle, sweet chestnut, wild rose.

Again, cleanliness is vital to avoid contamination. Sterilize utensils.

- You'll need:
  - 6pt. (3l.) saucepan with lid (use an enamel, glass, or stainless steel pan; avoid copper, aluminum, and Teflon-coated pans)
  - a glass measuring jug
  - 2pt. (1l.) of cold water (rain water or mineral water)
  - 3fl.oz. (100ml.) amber glass bottle(s) (up to six)
  - 1½fl.oz. (50ml.) of brandy
  - natural and unbleached filter paper
  - pen and label

- Decide on the plants beforehand; prepare and clean the utensils. If you are going to boil the remedy outside, check your camping stove and equipment. Wait for the perfect day.
- Take everything into the field between 9A.M. and 11A.M. on a sunny day.
- Touch as little as possible. Pick twigs or flowers until the saucepan is three-quarters full; put on the lid and take to the heat source as quickly as possible.
- When the pan is on the heat source, cover the flowers and twigs with the cold water and bring to the boil.
- Once it has reached boiling point, simmer for a half-hour. Use a twig from the tree to push the twigs under the water.
- After a half-hour, remove the pan from the heat, put the lid on it, and stand it outside to cool.
- When cool, remove the twigs, then carefully filter the water into the jug.
- Put 1½fl.oz. (50ml.) of the flower water into the 3fl.oz. (100ml.) bottle(s) with the brandy. Label with the name, "flower essence mother tincture," and date.

This is the mother tincture from which a stock bottle is made. It will keep for many years, and is used to make up personal remedies as previously described.

SEEING A PROFESSIONAL

Flower remedies were created to be so simple to use that people could treat themselves. However, many practitioners of other disciplines – such as herbalism, homeopathy, and aromatherapy – use flower remedies to complement their own remedies, and a few flower essence therapists use the remedies exclusively.

Most therapists have their own ways of working. But every consultation should begin with an interview between you and the therapist. This can last from as little as 15 minutes to over an hour. During this time the therapist will explain the system to you if you do not already know how it works. He or she will ask why you have come to see a therapist and will listen while you talk about yourself and your worries. The therapist will observe your posture and appearance, and will listen to the tone of your voice and the way you say things, as these can be as revealing as what you say. While you chat, the therapist may take notes and ask questions to work out, by a process of elimination, which remedies would be best for you. He or she might ask questions about your fears, how you feel about your children or other family members, or how easily you give up when something you attempt does not work out. It is not enough for the therapist to know that you have a problem at home or at work.

At the end of the consultation the therapist will help you select the remedies. The number of remedies prescribed depends on the individual, but it is unlikely to be more than six, and will often be much fewer. Most people feel at least a little better at the end of the consultation because they have been able to talk through their problems.

The Dr. Edward Bach Foundation maintains an international register of qualified practitioners in the Bach Flower Remedies. A list of practitioners may be obtained from the Bach Center (*see page 478*).

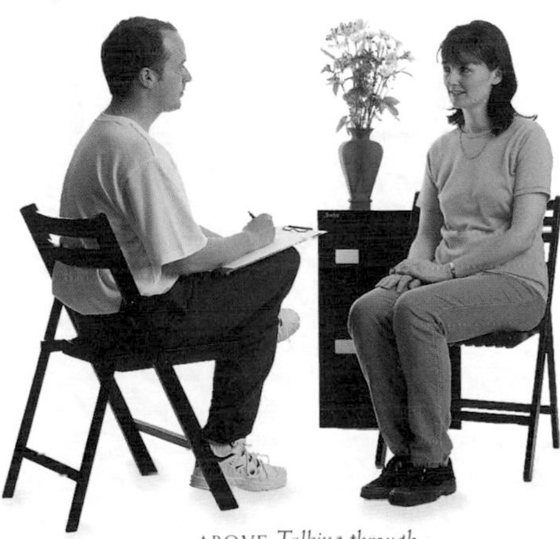

ABOVE *Talking through your problems is part of the consultation process.*

FLOWER ESSENCES

Aesculus carnea

RED CHESTNUT

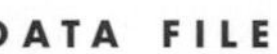

This essence is extracted from the pink-flowered chestnut tree, which is frequently grown for ornamental decoration in parks.

DATA FILE

Use

Red Chestnut is for those who suffer fear and anxiety for others. They may have forsaken worrying about themselves, but project their fear onto their loved ones. They often anticipate that some unfortunate accident or illness (the worst scenario) will befall friends and relations, and ceaselessly worry. This inappropriate fear limits the social interactions of both the sufferer and his or her loved ones. Red Chestnut helps us realize that the anxiety is a projection of personal fear. It brings the calm necessary to be sensitive to the real problems and concerns of our loved ones, and to give empathetic support.

Method

The boiling method *(see page 223)*

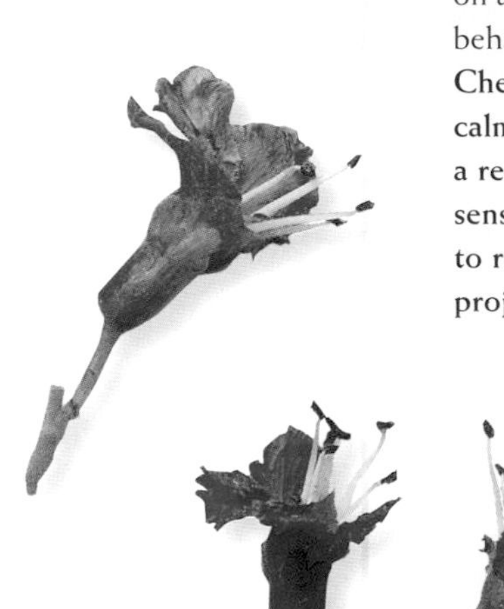

ABOVE *The red chestnut tree is often seen growing in parks.*

PROFILE

GOAL – Sensitivity to others **People who need Red Chestnut fear that something awful may happen to their loved ones.** They experience unnecessary fear, over-worry, even hypochondria on another person's behalf. **Red Chestnut encourages calm and rationality, a response based on sensitivity to others, to replace the projected fear.**

Aesculus hippocastanum

WHITE CHESTNUT

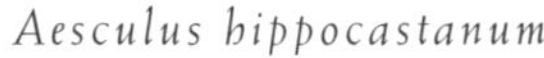

The common horse chestnut tree has distinctive, upright clusters of white flowers and divided spatulate leaves.

ABOVE *and* BELOW *The familiar leaves and fruit of the white chestnut (horse chestnut).*

DATA FILE

Use

When the mind is full of unwanted thoughts, ideas, or persistent and worrying mental arguments – overactive and exhausting mental chatter going round and round in a never-ending circle.

Method

The sun method *(see page 222)*

PROFILE

GOAL – Clear mind; clarity **For people who suffer from constant mental chatter, persistent thoughts, and worries.** For sleeplessness due to worry. **White Chestnut switches off unwanted thoughts so that it is possible to find peace and mental clarity.** Other remedies might be needed to address the root cause.

Aesculus hippocastanum

CHESTNUT BUD

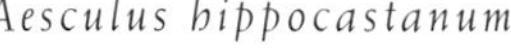

The white chestnut tree is used to make two remedies: White Chestnut and Chestnut Bud. The large leaf buds, called "sticky buds," are picked when they are just about to open to make this particular essence.

DATA FILE

Use

For those who make the same mistake over and over again, and who are slow to learn from experience. Chestnut Bud is for people who find themselves stuck in the same repeating pattern, who regretfully do not seem able to learn the lessons of past experience, events, and relationships.

Method

The boiling method *(see page 223)*

PROFILE

GOAL – Vision **The person who needs Chestnut Bud may suffer poor health, chronic conditions may continually "flare up," or they may suffer from preventable illness.** If the same pattern is continually repeated they are stuck in the energy of that moment. **Chestnut Bud helps focus the mind and enable us to see our path with greater objectivity.**

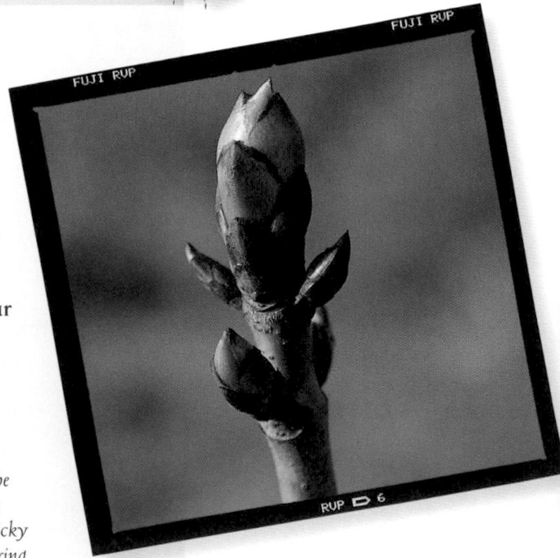

RIGHT *The leaves of the white chestnut or horse chestnut grow from the "sticky buds" produced in early spring.*

Agrimonia eupatoria

AGRIMONY

A wild plant with small yellow flowers on tapering spikes like church spires, sometimes known as "church steeples." The seed vessels are covered in hooked hairs and cling to animals coming into contact with them.

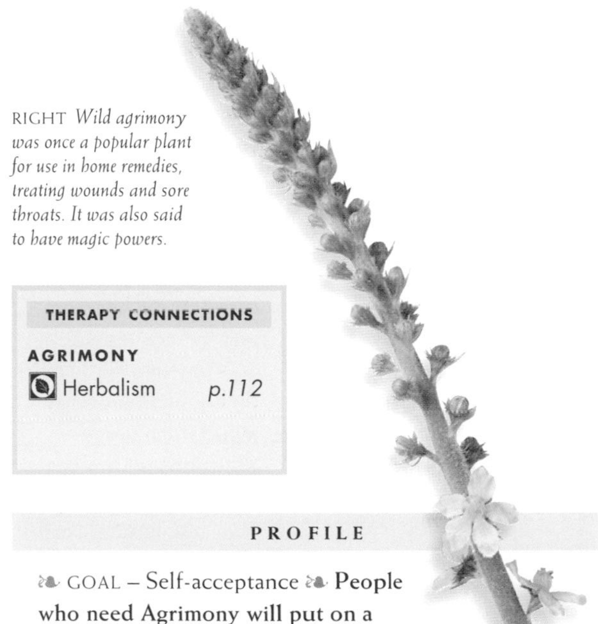

RIGHT *Wild agrimony was once a popular plant for use in home remedies, treating wounds and sore throats. It was also said to have magic powers.*

THERAPY CONNECTIONS

AGRIMONY

Herbalism p.112

PROFILE

❧ GOAL – Self-acceptance ❧ **People who need Agrimony will put on a brave face of cheerfulness. Laughter hides things as well as being distracting; other distractions may be drink, drugs, or dangerous or thrill-seeking hobbies or occupations.** ❧ They may be restless sleepers or unable to sleep without help. ❧ **Agrimony helps us to love ourselves as we are, and to put aside the mask. It helps us cope with the difficult sides of our nature and use humor appropriately.**

DATA FILE

Use

For those who hide their problems and inner selves behind a cheerful face, masking real feelings of unhappiness and unworthiness. They are the life and soul of a party, and will make jokes, perhaps even inappropriately. The person who needs Agrimony finds it hard to deal with the darker, less pleasant parts of life and extreme emotions. They are reluctant to burden others and dread arguments, pursuing peace at all costs. This can lead to an inner anguish that is often masked by alcohol or drugs.

Method

❧ The sun method *(see page 222)*

Anigozanthos manglesii

KANGAROO PAW

This large Australian perennial is one of the first plants to recolonize after bush fires. It is so named because the flowers at the end of the long stems resemble a kangaroo's front paw.

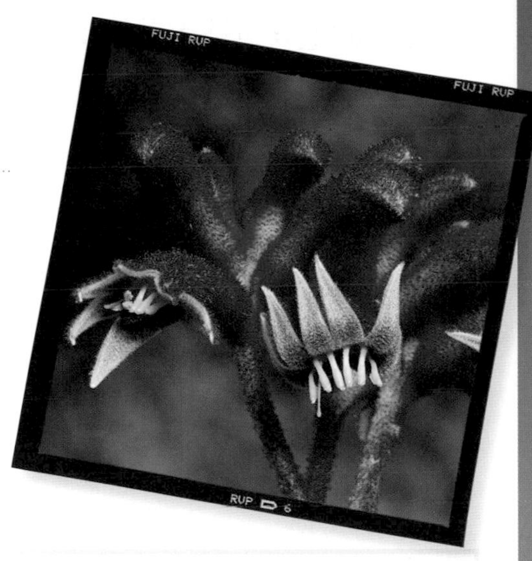

RIGHT *The flowers of kangaroo paw are a more recent addition to the list of available remedies.*

PROFILE

❧ GOAL – Kindness and sensitivity ❧ **For people who are inexperienced, socially inept, or embarrassed.** ❧ Associated symptoms include clumsiness, nervousness, stuttering, or stammering; blushing and embarrassment; shyness and timidity. ❧ **Kangaroo Paw encourages sensitivity and empathy, and gives us the courage to just be, to accept, and be kind to ourselves and others. It allows us to experience true two-way communication.**

DATA FILE

Use

For people who have poor social skills, and difficulties relating to and communicating with others, who are so self-conscious and self-aware that they feel "out of place" at work, at meetings, gatherings, or parties. This may be noticed by others and become a joke. Interactions feel like competitions, and they find it impossible to find the space to think before acting, or to be aware of other people's feelings. Kangaroo Paw makes it possible for them to relax and get in tune with themselves and others, and to become aware of their surroundings. It encourages sensitive and appropriate social interaction.

Method

❧ The sun method *(see page 222)*; pick the whole cluster (or paw) of flowers

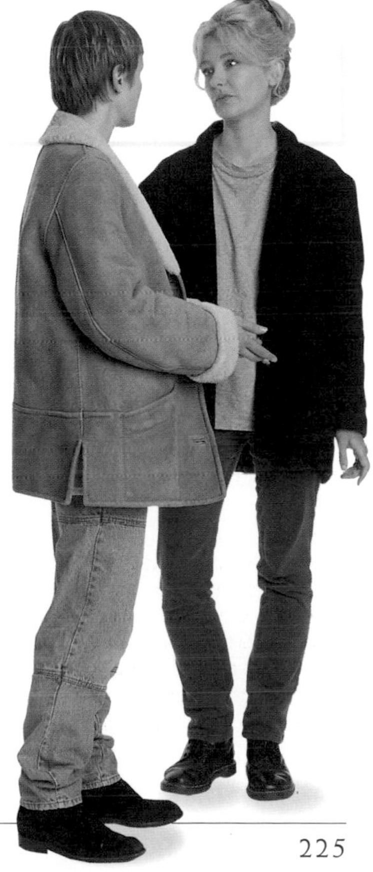

RIGHT *People who feel nervous and ill-at-ease with others can be helped to relax with Kangaroo Paw.*

Bromus ramosus

WILD OAT

An elegant woodland grass, wild oat stands between 2 and 5 feet (½–1½m.) high. The common name is hairy or wood brome grass, because of the soft, hairy leaves.

PROFILE

❧ GOAL – Meaningful purpose, a positive direction ❧ **Wild Oat is for uncertainty and frustration with current activities, when a person has the desire to find a purpose, yet is aimless, drifting from one job or relationship to another.** ❧ Wild Oat helps us listen to our calling, find our true vocation, and gives the strength of character to act on this.

DATA FILE

Use

Wild Oat is for capable people who have ambition to do something meaningful in their lives but have not yet found their true calling. They may have several choices or directions they could follow and may be working hard on a given path, but fundamentally they are dissatisfied and frustrated. Somewhere deep down they know that they have not found their true calling in life, and are emotionally or spiritually unsatisfied. Wild Oat helps to tune the heart to what will bring true meaning and purpose. It helps us to make choices, sometimes difficult, which unite all aspirations. It also helps us to balance the needs of spirituality and making a living.

Method

❧ The sun method *(see page 222)*

THERAPY CONNECTIONS

WILD OATS

Herbalism *p.117*

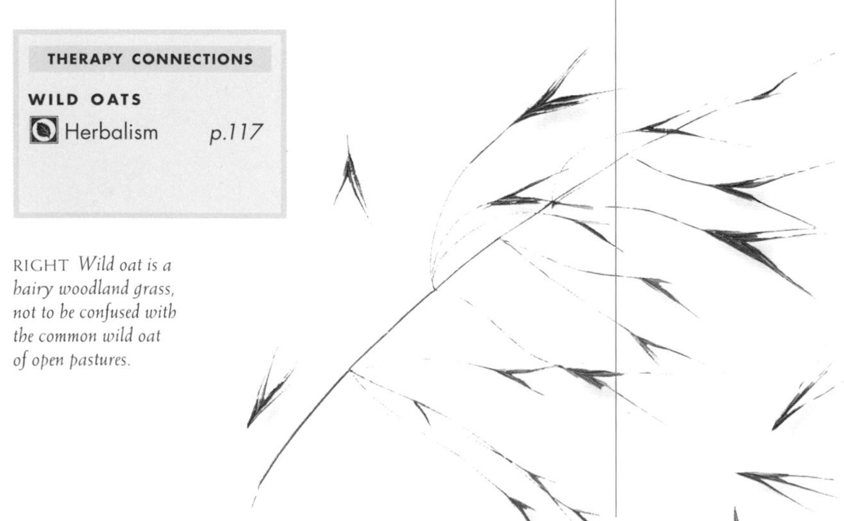

RIGHT *Wild oat is a hairy woodland grass, not to be confused with the common wild oat of open pastures.*

Calluna vulgaris

HEATHER

This common plant is often found in Alpine areas, on heaths, and waste ground. *Calluna* prefers acid soil. According to variety, flowers are produced from summer to fall.

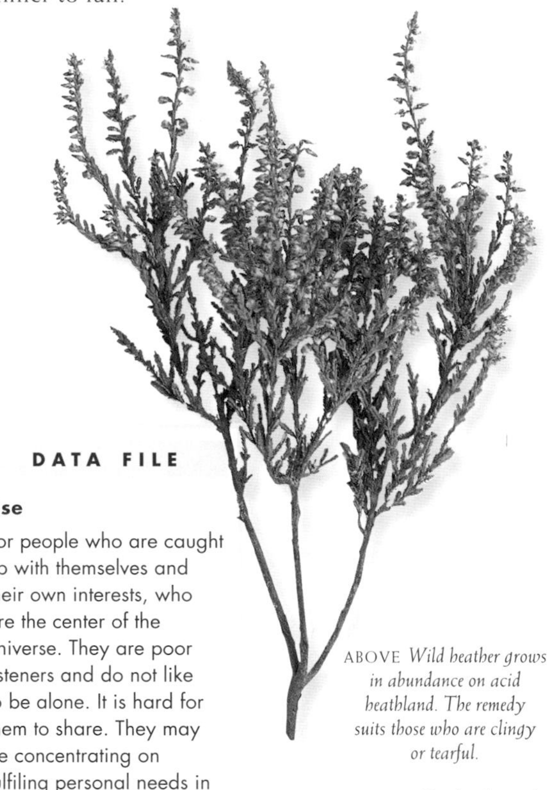

ABOVE *Wild heather grows in abundance on acid heathland. The remedy suits those who are clingy or tearful.*

DATA FILE

Use

For people who are caught up with themselves and their own interests, who are the center of the universe. They are poor listeners and do not like to be alone. It is hard for them to share. They may be concentrating on fulfiling personal needs in order to avoid loneliness.

Method

❧ The sun method *(see page 222)*

PROFILE

❧ GOAL – Love with space to share; to listen: A useful affirmation might be: "I am listening and letting the love of the world nourish my heart." ❧ **People who need Heather can be self-centered and self-obsessed. They may intrude into other people's personal space, cling, or be aggressively talkative.** ❧ They can be weepy and hypochondriac. ❧ **They may be lonely, as friends may avoid them because they demand too much.** ❧ We should love and nurture ourselves. Heather helps us to look after ourselves without being obsessed with our own personal needs. It gives us the space to listen to others, and experience genuine love and companionship.

BELOW *People who need Heather often become isolated from others because they are self-obsessed or demanding.*

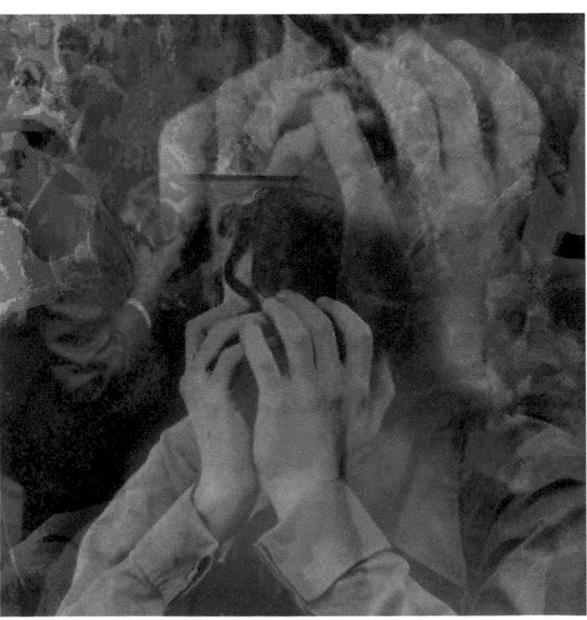

Carpinus betulus

HORNBEAM

A medium-sized, deciduous tree common in woods. It grows well in a sunny or lightly shaded position, and its leaves turn a rich yellow-orange in the fall.

DATA FILE

Use

Hornbeam is for those who feel that they do not possess enough strength to fulfill the responsibilities of daily life, for the "Monday morning blues." This feeling often comes from boredom or some basic dissatisfaction with the work they are doing. These people might feel that they are in the wrong job, or in some way not fully expressing their creative potential.

Hornbeam restores confidence and optimism, and helps us find the satisfaction in the mundane "nine-to-five" aspects of our lives.

Method

The boiling method *(see page 223)*

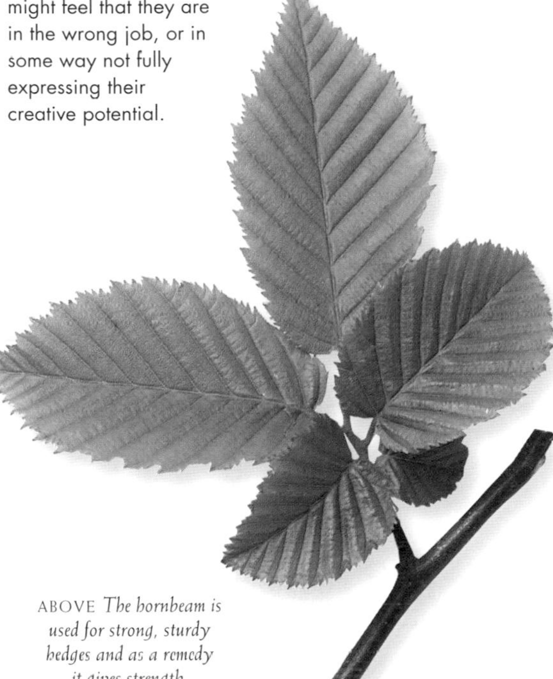

ABOVE *The hornbeam is used for strong, sturdy hedges and as a remedy it gives strength.*

PROFILE

- GOAL – Strength to carry out daily tasks
- **People who need Hornbeam feel exhausted at the thought of working. They may feel stuck in a rut.**
- Procrastination is a common avoidance stratagem.
- **Hornbeam is usually for a temporary feeling. If the weakness is a regular occurrence, the person may be exhausting him or herself in the wrong direction, and other remedies may be needed.**

Castanea sativa

SWEET CHESTNUT

This chestnut tree produces edible fruits after its creamy flowers. The tree grows to 100ft. (30m.) and is deciduous.

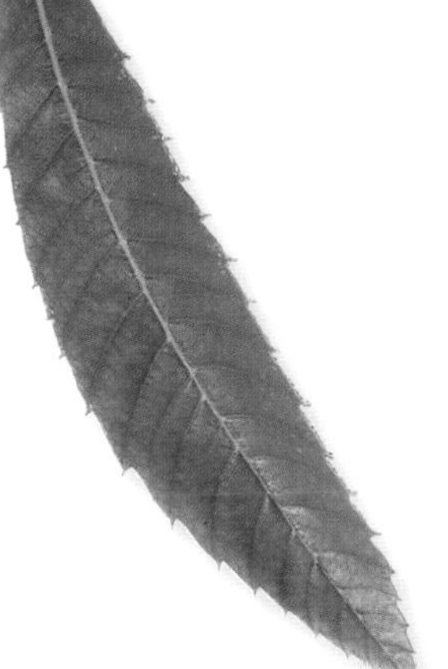

ABOVE *A leaflet and fruit of the edible chestnut tree, a remedy for anguish.*

PROFILE

- GOAL – Transformation; to widen the boundaries
- **Hornbeam is for the feeling Dr. Bach called the "dark night of the soul," when it feels that annihilation is all that will be left.**
- Associated symptoms may include sleep disturbance, hopelessness, and perhaps hidden despair.

DATA FILE

Use

Sweet Chestnut is for those moments when anguish is so great as to seem unbearable, when people feel that they have "come to the end of their tether," reached their limit, and are being stretched beyond endurance. When this happens things have to change. Sweet Chestnut helps to bring out hidden reserves, opening boundaries and expanding limits, which gives people the strength to grow.

Method

The boiling method *(see page 223)*

Centaurium erythraea

CENTAURY

A small pink flower of chalky soil. It is named after a centaur in Greek mythology, who cured himself from a poisoned arrow wound with centaury.

DATA FILE

Use

Centaury is for people who have an excessive desire to please and a willingness to serve. They can be taken for granted and exploited. Their will to help others is so strong that it undermines their individuality and they find it hard to say "no." They can become servants rather than helpers, and end up doing more than their fair share. This leads to frustration and a loss of self-confidence, appreciation, and expression. Their life becomes one of drudgery or self-martyrdom.

Method

The sun method *(see page 222)*

PROFILE

- GOAL – Service, in the widest sense
- **People who need Centaury lack will-power; they may be tired and exhausted. Inner frustration and anger may sap their inner strength.**
- The "weaker" partner in a co-dependent relationship may benefit from Centaury
- **Centaury helps balance the desire to serve by strengthening our will power and appreciation of ourselves. It helps us make a choice, to say "yes" or "no" from the heart.**

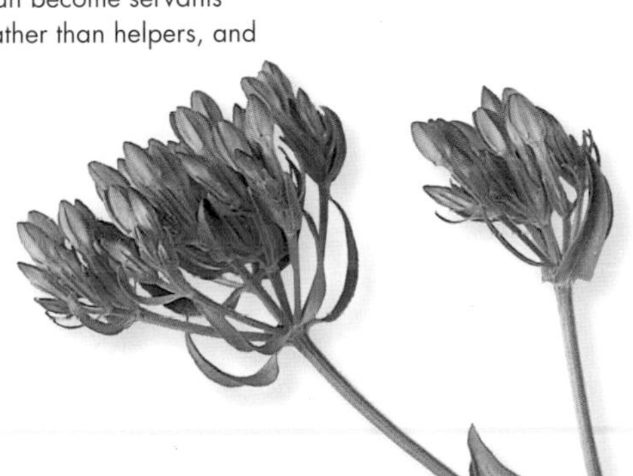

LEFT *The flowers of centaury, a plant which grows more readily in the wild than in cultivation.*

Ceratostigma willmottiana

CERATO

A small shrub with bright blue flowers which is often grown in gardens. It originally came from China and the Himalayas. Cerato is the only Bach Flower Remedy to be made from a cultivated plant.

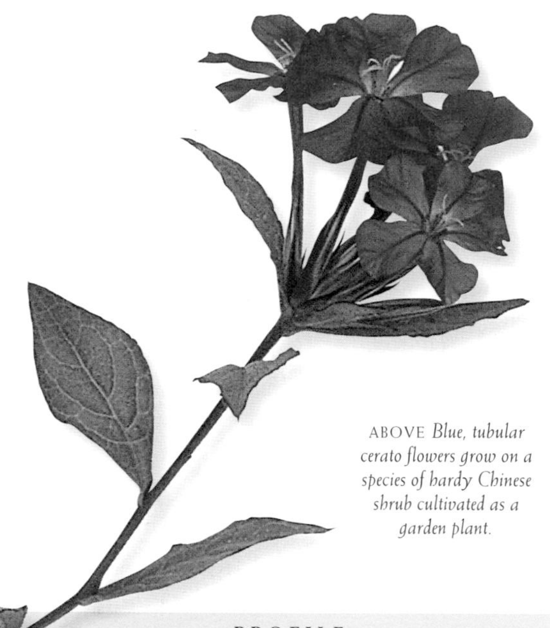

ABOVE *Blue, tubular cerato flowers grow on a species of hardy Chinese shrub cultivated as a garden plant.*

PROFILE

❧ GOAL – Inner confidence; to trust intuition
❧ **People who need Cerato may appear weak-willed and silly. They lack constancy, and may imitate others or become an ever-changing "fashion victim."**
❧ They may join cults or take up fads. ❧ **Cerato helps us to listen to advice from within, restores confidence, and strengthens our trust in ourselves to follow our path even if it runs contrary to the expectations of others.**

DATA FILE

Use

Cerato is for lack of trust in our own abilities and judgment. People who need Cerato are intelligent and curious, but they lack confidence in themselves, distrust their own intuition, and constantly seek the advice and approval of other people. They like to be seen to be doing the "right thing."

Method

The sun method *(see page 222)*

Chicorium intybus

CHICORY

A wayside plant with bright blue flowers. It is cultivated as a vegetable and blanched as a bitter plant to add to salads. The flowers close in the afternoon, and open again in the morning.

PROFILE

❧ GOAL – Love, free flowing and without strings
❧ **Those who need Chicory may be possessive and selfish. They may be fussy, nagging, and manipulative. They may be prone to illness if not "loved," or to hypochondria.** ❧ Chicory helps us to see love as a universal force, to give love selflessly and freely so that it may freely return to us.

DATA FILE

Use

Chicory is for those who see love as a transaction incurring duty, and as a method of control. They give love in order to receive it. Chicory types love and care publicly, even melodramatically, building up a stock of good works which they expect to be reciprocated, but love still does not flow their way.

Method

The sun method *(see page 222)*

ABOVE *The Chicory remedy is prepared from the pretty sky-blue flowers.*

BELOW *Chicory helps people to be selfless in love, which makes for more satisfying relationships.*

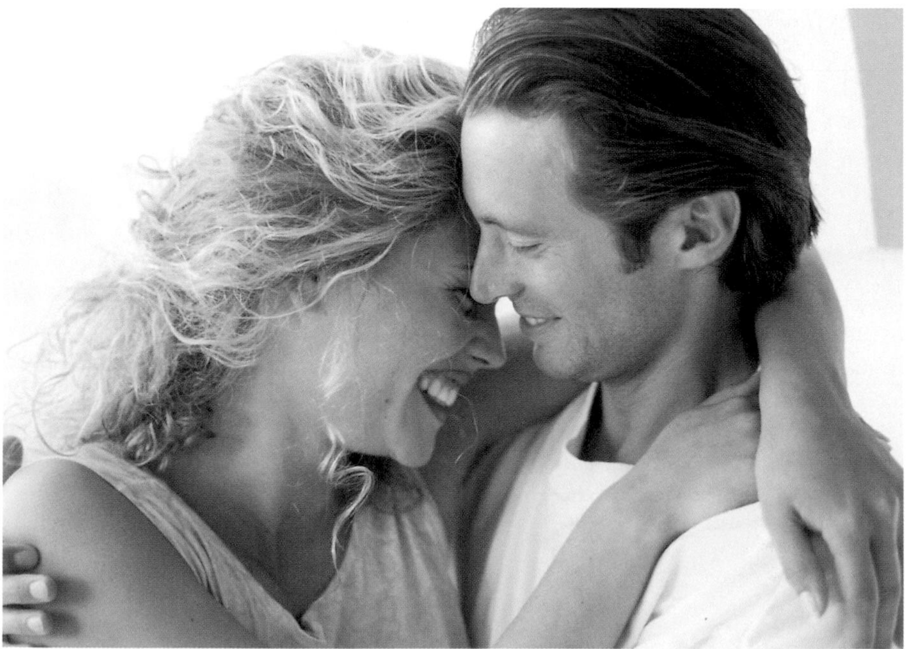

Clematis vitalba

CLEMATIS

The wild clematis is a rambling, perennial climber of woods and country hedges. Its common name is travelers' joy, and it bursts forth with a mass of beautiful flowers.

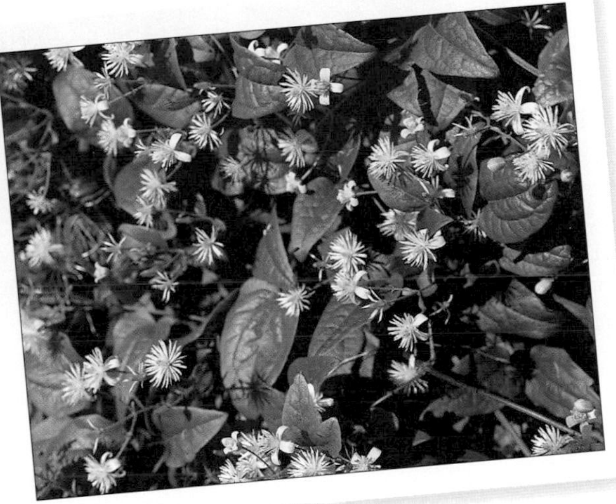

ABOVE *Wild clematis, travelers' joy or old man's beard is a poisonous plant and must be used carefully.*

DATA FILE

Use

For those who are dreamy and not fully awake. Sometimes they daydream or fantasize about a utopian future. Clematis people prefer to live in the mind or the spirit, rather than deal with contemporary issues and the mundane functions of everyday life. They tend to be airy and impractical individuals, drifting off into their own ideas, the typical "mad professor." They sometimes lead a sedentary life, are pale, and lack vitality and ambition. They are sensitive and sometimes need lots of sleep.

Method

The sun method *(see page 222)*

PROFILE

GOAL– Being awake and grounded in the body and in the present **People who need Clematis are dreamy, absent-minded, and lack interest in the present. They sometimes have a poor will to live. They may forget to eat, experience faintness and tiredness.**

If children resort to daydreaming as an escape, Clematis may be useful, although the child should be questioned to find the underlying cause.

PROFILE

GOAL– Mental balance and clarity; to read or speak clearly **People who need Bush Fuchsia may be nervous and stammer. Although intelligent, they are slow to learn. They may avoid situations which highlight this, or become shy.** They have difficulties with determining left and right, up and down. **Bush Fuchsia is specific for children with dyslexia or learning difficulties.** Bush Fuchsia aids concentration and confidence. **It is also useful when we are "stuck" in one mode of thinking, releasing energy to rebalance the mind.**

Epacris longiflora

BUSH FUCHSIA

A low, straggly shrub, bush fuschia flowers throughout the year with bright red, elongated, bell-like flowers hanging in a row from the stem. The leaves are small and heart-shaped. The plant needs full sun.

DATA FILE

Use

Bush Fuchsia is used to balance the hemispheres of the brain so that the rational left side and creative right side can be expressed with confidence. It is useful for all problems with learning difficulties, or translating marks from the page (words, symbols, music) into physical action. It boosts confidence when performing or speaking in public. Dyslexia and other learning disabilities, if not understood and addressed, can seriously affect self-worth and hinder the development of social skills.

Method

The sun method *(see page 222)*

BELOW *The long, hanging flowers of bush fuchsia adorn the shrub throughout the summer months.*

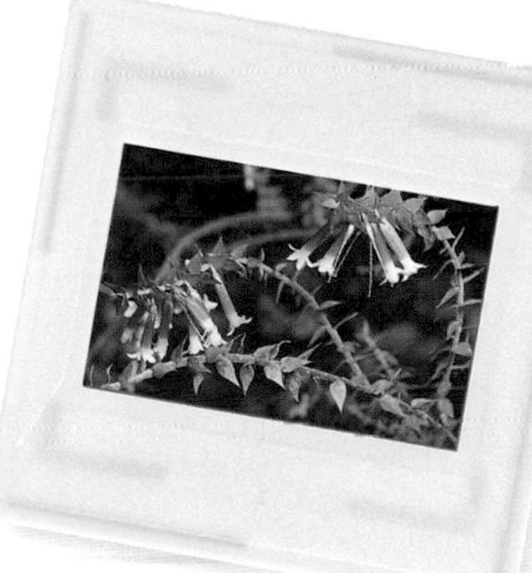

Fagus sylvatica

BEECH

The common beech tree grows to a majestic 100ft. (30m.), with a spread of 80ft. (25m.). The leaves take on rich yellow and orange hues in the fall.

DATA FILE

Use

Beech is for those who are being over-critical and intolerant, and according to Dr Bach, "for those who need to see beauty in all that surrounds them." Beech types have their own "way" and are very proud that they can cope. They think problems can be solved in their way, and are intolerant of those who cannot do this. They do not understand that everyone has different strengths and experiences. They think "cannot" means "will not," and therefore become irritable and short-tempered with others. They may also feel unappreciated.

Method

The boiling method *(see page 223)*

PROFILE

GOAL – Tolerance and empathy **People who need Beech may be lonely and isolated. Lack of understanding leads to narrow views and behavior.** Beech fills hearts with empathy and opens eyes to see beauty without judgment. It shows that we are individuals, with different ways of dealing with the world.

LEFT *The leaves and twigs of the common beech tree produce a remedy that can help those who are intolerant.*

Gentianella amarella

GENTIAN

Gentianella amerella flowers from late summer onward, with rich blue, violet to purple flowers. It likes dry, well-drained conditions, and sandy or chalky soils.

PROFILE

❧ GOAL – Courage to accept what is; encouragement to face the future positively ❧ **Gentian helps us to put setbacks and disappointments into perspective, and to once again display a positive attitude.**

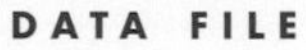

DATA FILE

Use

For despondency and mild depression due to circumstances. Gentian people are easily discouraged. When everything is going well they are happy, but they can be easily disheartened, and can slip back into a negative outlook. Doubt and lack of faith are important elements. Gentian restores the courage to recognize that life is not a competition and that there is no failure when trying our best.

Method

❦ The sun method *(see page 222)*

LEFT *The twisted purple flowers of this* Gentianella *species are similar to those of the honeysuckle.*

Grevillea buxifolia

GRAY SPIDER FLOWER

A common Australian evergreen, this shrub flowers for most of the year. It prefers acid soil and full sun.

DATA FILE

Use

Aspen and Mimulus are both for fear, but Gray Spider Flower is for extreme and intense feelings of terror, a blind panic which is immobilizing. The fear may be known or unknown, and it is associated with physical symptoms of inner terror which freeze the mind and body, and prevent thoughts moving forward. Gray Spider Flower frees the body and the mind to move, bringing faith that the terror will pass.

Method

❦ The sun method *(see page 222)*; pick the whole flower head at the end of the branch

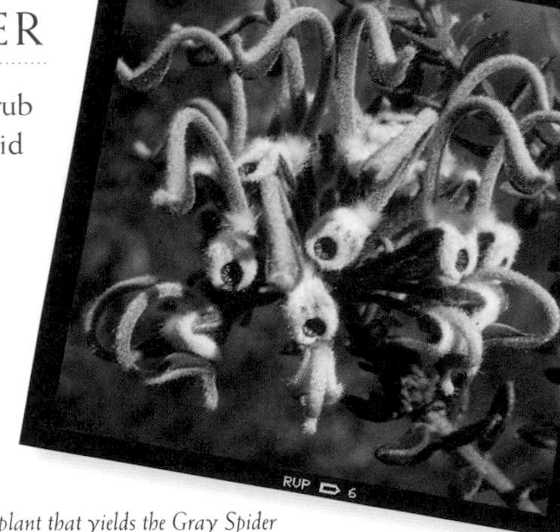

ABOVE *The plant that yields the Gray Spider Flower remedy is a tender evergreen that can be grown in sheltered areas outdoors in milder regions.*

PROFILE

❧ GOAL – Faith ❧ **For extreme, immobilizing terror of day or night; nightmares, disturbed sleep, or fear of sleep.** ❧ For shivering, pallor, palpitations, depression, and feelings of being psychically drained and exhausted. ❧ **Gray Spider Flower brings lightness, courage, and faith, the certainty that we are loved by the world.** ❧ It is ideal for children terrorized by bad dreams. ❧ **Take with Fringed Violet Flower for protection from fear of the supernatural and of psychic attack.**

Gossypium sturtianum

STURT DESERT ROSE

Sturt desert rose is a small shrub with mauve, hibiscus-like flowers which likes dry, stony ground. The flower remedy is good for feelings of worthlessness.

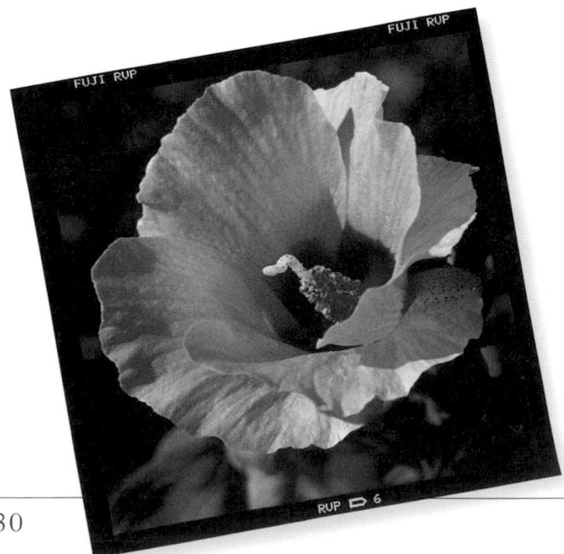

LEFT *Sturt desert rose is a delicate-looking, sun-loving plant that thrives in poor, dry soil and is a tough survivor.*

DATA FILE

Use

People who need Sturt Desert Rose are always apologizing for themselves and their actions. They blame themselves for everything, for things they should or should not have done, and feel guilt and remorse. They may have an acute sense of obligation and duty which is hard (or impossible) to live up to. Guilt and shame are both disabling emotions. Sturt Desert Rose enables self-acceptance, the understanding that we do what we can and must take responsibility (not blame) for the consequences. It enables reconciliation, allowing us to accept, forgive, and move on to pastures new.

Method

❦ The sun method *(see page 222)*

PROFILE

❧ GOAL– Self-acceptance, conciliation, communication true to self ❧ **For guilt, regret, remorse. People who need Sturt Desert Rose feel useless. They have low self-esteem and a sense of shame. They are characterized by self-criticism.** ❧ Associated symptoms include anxiety dreams, depression, especially of old hidden guilt. ❧ **Sturt Desert Rose facilitates self-acceptance, allowing forgiveness and healing.**

Helianthemum nummularium

ROCK ROSE

A low-growing, yellow-flowered plant found on chalky or gravely soils. Some varieties of rock rose are cultivated in rock gardens, but these are not suitable for use as flower remedies.

DATA FILE

Use

Rock Rose is one of the main ingredients of Rescue Remedy. It is to be taken in all cases of extreme fear, terror, panic, urgency, or danger. Rock Rose gives the courage to face life and death, frees the mind to act, bringing faith that the terror or panic will soon pass.

Method

- The sun method *(see page 222)*

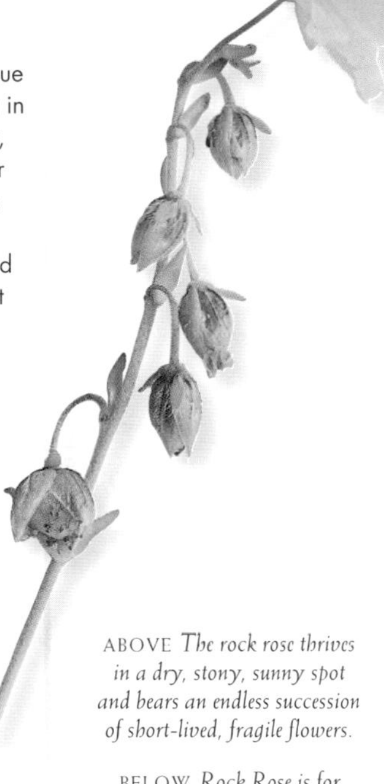

ABOVE *The rock rose thrives in a dry, stony, sunny spot and bears an endless succession of short-lived, fragile flowers.*

BELOW *Rock Rose is for people who suffer from extremes of panic or helplessness.*

PROFILE

GOAL– Personal courage **The person who needs Rock Rose experiences feelings of helplessness, terror, and blind panic.** Fear may cause palpitations, heart jitters, or panic attacks. **Rock Rose should be given for any perceived threat to the person, their self-image, or personal integrity.**

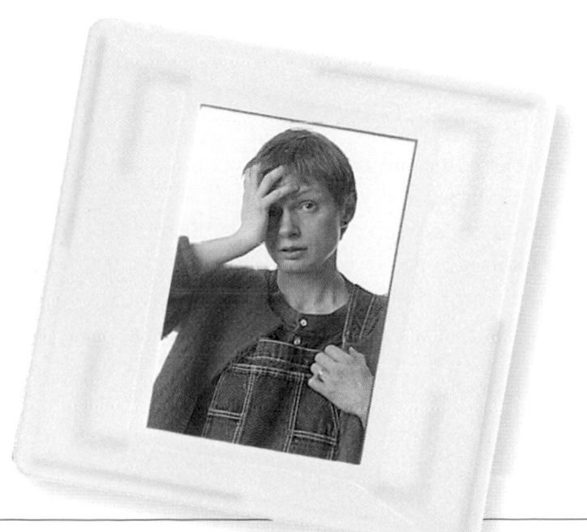

Hibbertia pendunculata

HIBBERTIA

A low, trailing plant of the open bush. The large, bright, and gleaming yellow flowers bloom in spring. It is frost-tender. The flower essence is good for those with a love of learning.

DATA FILE

Use

People who need Hibbertia love ideas and pursue knowledge at all costs. They may repress or deny their body and its needs, or have a rigid or dogmatic lifestyle. They continually read, attend lectures, courses, and workshops to improve themselves and gain status. They want to "know it all." They look deep within books, but never around at their surroundings. Their head is in the air and they are ungrounded. The search is ultimately unsatisfactory; knowledge grows from within and they must find themselves before they can change.

Method

- The sun method *(see page 222)*

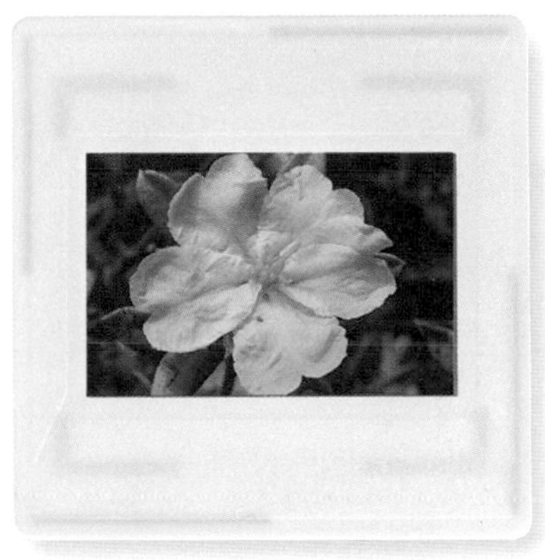

ABOVE RIGHT *With its bright yellow flowers and its preference for open spaces, Hibbertia encourages openness and confidence.*

RIGHT *Hibbertia is a good remedy for studious young people who may neglect the physical side of themselves.*

PROFILE

GOAL – Wisdom **For those who are intelligent, the "constant student," characterized by continual pursuit of knowledge for self-improvement or status, and love of "hidden knowledge." Such people may be fanatical or cult followers.** They may be neglectful of their body, or suffer sedentary and stress-related illnesses, indigestion, skin rashes, wasting or stiffness of muscles and joints. **Hibbertia encourages confidence and contentment. It links external knowledge with personal observations and physical needs, producing wisdom.**

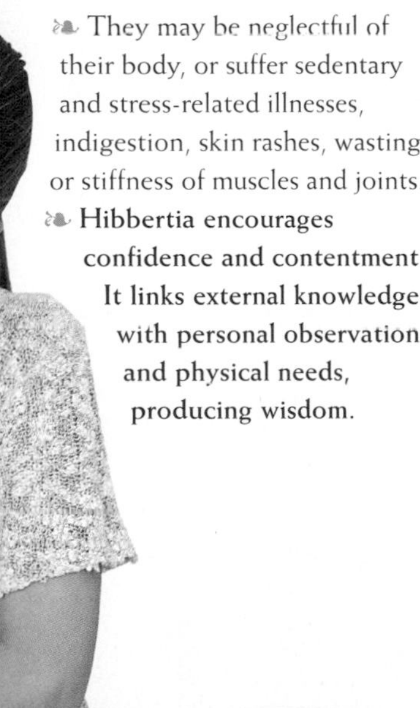

Hottonia palustris

WATER VIOLET

This is a delicate perennial plant with pale violet flowers and feathery leaves which is often found in ditches, as it grows submerged in water. The flowers appear above the water in summer.

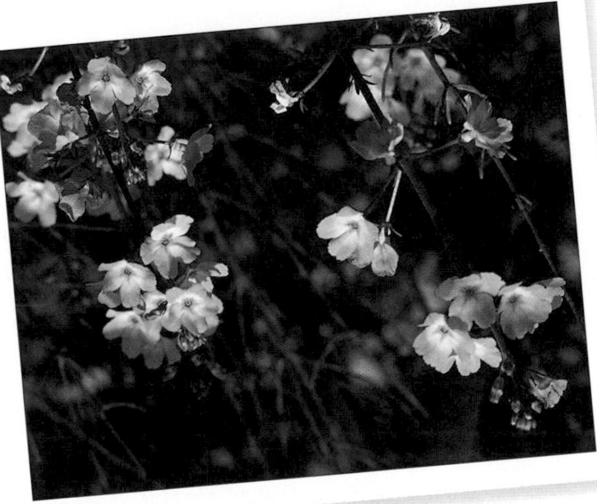

ABOVE *Water violets grow under water, and issue forth a delicate foam of lilac-colored flowers in early spring.*

DATA FILE

Use

Water Violet is for self-reliant people with an aloof, live-and-let-live attitude. They are quiet and spend much time alone, keeping others at a distance. When ill they keep to themselves and do not wish to be any "trouble" to those around them. They find it hard to share. In their isolation they may feel special, or chosen, a sensation which can distort their sense of belonging and self-worth. Water Violet gives the confidence to share – the strengths and weaknesses, the ups and downs, all of life's rich tapestry.

Method

The sun method *(see page 222)*

PROFILE

GOAL – Communication; sharing **The person needing Water Violet is reserved and self-contained. This can be seen as standoffish aloofness and pride, and thus lead to loneliness.** He or she may be solitary yet proud. **Water Violet allows us to acknowledge the inner self as a starting point from which to expand, communicate with the world, and share from the heart.**

Ilex aquifolium

HOLLY

Holly is a common evergreen tree, with spiky leaves and red berries. It is a powerful symbol of winter and is used in Christmas decorations. To produce berries on a female plant, a male plant needs to be grown nearby.

BELOW *The holly is not noted for its flowers, but these have an unmistakable and pervasive scent.*

DATA FILE

Use

Holly is for those who are attacked by feelings of hatred, envy, jealousy, suspicion, and revenge. The person who needs Holly has intense negative feelings. They also have other intense emotions, but they are too frightened to express these fully. The free flow of emotion and love is then blocked or expressed unclearly. This leads to tension, unclear communication, frustration, anger, and emotional outbursts.

Method

The boiling method *(see page 223)*

PROFILE

GOAL – Unconditional expression of affection and love. A useful affirmation might be: "I am opening my heart to express my love." **The negative emotions of the person who needs Holly may be spiteful and nagging, with intense feeling and outbursts of temper. They may be suspicious or mildly paranoid.** Useful for the "no!" negative states and temper tantrums of two-year-olds. **Holly allows us to recognize that these feelings are the negative expression of our caring interaction with others. It gives us the strength to open our hearts to the full flow of love.**

Juglans regia

WALNUT

A large, handsome, deciduous tree which is easily recognized by its popular edible nuts, walnut grows to about 50ft. (15m.) tall and is wide-spreading.

DATA FILE

Use

Walnut is for people who need to find constancy and protection from outside forces, those who need to move on and break links and old patterns with people and things. Walnut frees the person from interference, and gives protection so that it is possible to break inappropriate ties and pursue personal freedom. Walnut is useful for people on the brink of some major decision or change, for example children leaving home, the menopause, marriage, having babies.

Method

The boiling method *(see page 223)*

LEFT *The walnut fruit resembles the human brain and the remedy from the flowers is thought to strengthen and protect the mind.*

PROFILE

GOAL – Protection, sanctuary **Walnut is useful at any of the milestones of life: puberty, marriage, leaving home, change of job or country, etc.** People who have moved on but find old habits persistent can take Walnut to break links with the past. **Walnut is also useful for temporary distraction, or for domination by enthusiasm, or strong opinions of others.**

Impatiens glandulifera

IMPATIENS

A tall annual with large mauve flowers and exploding seed pods, Impatiens is common in damp places. It is sometimes called "touch me not," as the tightly coiled seed pods are apt to explode at the slightest touch.

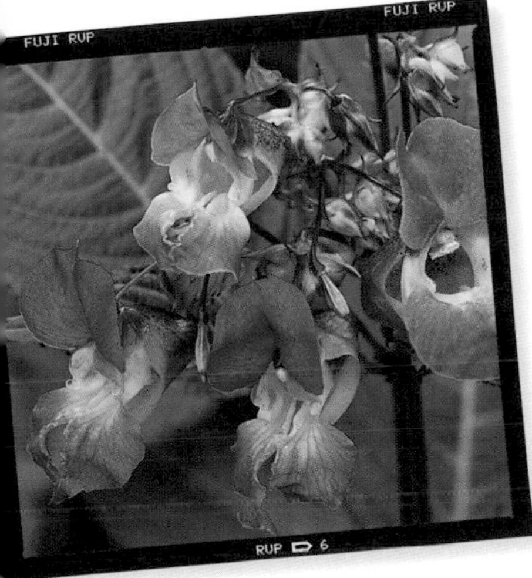

LEFT *Impatiens grows on the banks of streams and ditches, and its flowers nod gently in the breeze.*

PROFILE

❧ GOAL– Patience ❧ **Impatiens is for impatience and irritability at slowness, the desire to do everything quickly.** ❧ People who need Impatiens may fidget, find it hard to sit still, and therefore suffer from indigestion and nervous tension. ❧ **People who have learnt the lesson of Impatiens have patience, they are capable and decisive, knowing how to get things done and turn the pace of life to advantage.**

DATA FILE

Use

For those who are quick in thought and action, and who are always on the go. They know their mind and want things to be done at speed. They become irritable at hindrance, hesitation, and delay, and impatiently blame others. They can alienate people by being brusque and unsympathetic, speaking their mind quickly and without thought. They refuse to slow down even when illness overtakes them. They are truly in the "rat race." Impatiens restores acceptance of the natural pace of life, rather than fighting against it.

Method

The sun method *(see page 222)*

Larix decidua

LARCH

Larch is a tall conifer with needle-like leaves that are shed in the fall. Male and female flowers appear on the same tree in spring. It can grow to 100ft. (30m.) high, and the cones are small and erect.

PROFILE

❧ GOAL– Confidence ❧ **Larch can be used for any lack of confidence and self-esteem, for passivity and fear of trying, and for poor self-image and feelings of inferiority.** ❧ It is suitable for children starting a new school, and who feel they will not be as clever as the other children and so fear failure. ❧ **Feelings of worthlessness may hide deeper problems or a pattern of abuse. Other remedies may also be useful.** ❧ Larch strengthens confidence, and helps us appreciate our real worth and value our personal contribution to the planet.

ABOVE *The larch is the only cone-bearing tree to lose its leaves during the fall. Its timber has great strength.*

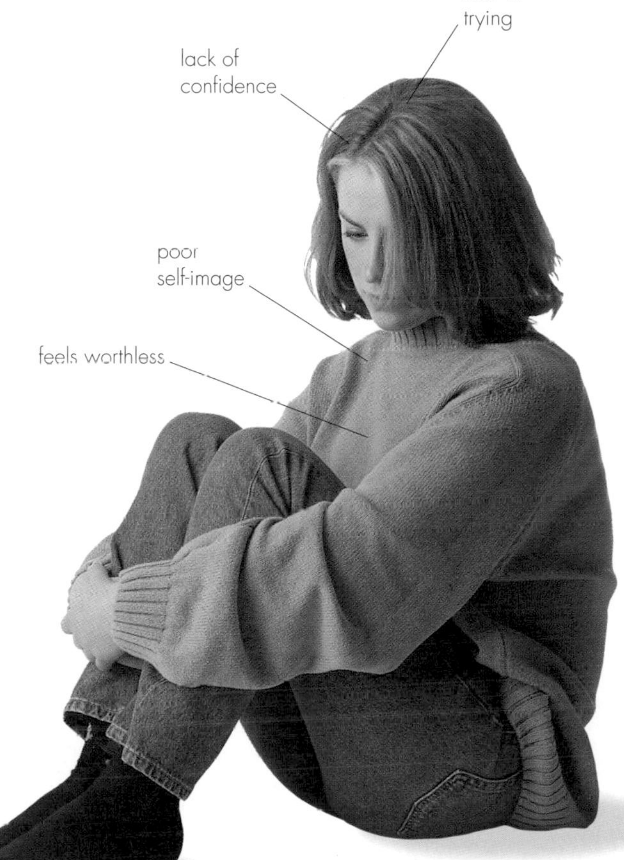

LEFT *The Larch remedy can help bring confidence and self-esteem, especially in teenage years.*

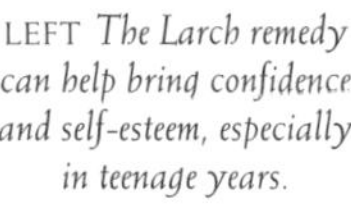

THERAPY CONNECTIONS

WALNUT

Traditional Home and Folk Remedies *p.92*

DATA FILE

Use

Larch is for those who lack confidence in themselves and fear failure, those who feel that they are not as capable as those around them. At times, lack of confidence may completely immobilize them and prevent them from even trying. They do not think that they are capable, or worthy of success. Feelings of total uselessness also can lead to great unhappiness, despair, and isolation. Larch increases confidence and strengthens personal will.

Method

The boiling method *(see page 223)*

Lonicera caprifolium

HONEYSUCKLE

Lonicera caprifolium is a strongly scented climber found in woods. The fragrance is sweet and long-lasting. The flowers are tubular and form a spreading head.

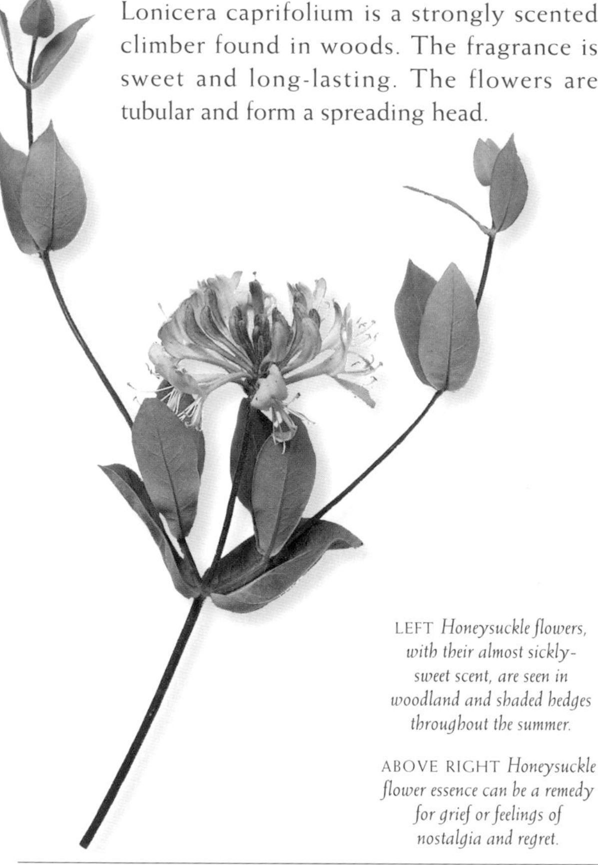

LEFT *Honeysuckle flowers, with their almost sickly-sweet scent, are seen in woodland and shaded hedges throughout the summer.*

ABOVE RIGHT *Honeysuckle flower essence can be a remedy for grief or feelings of nostalgia and regret.*

DATA FILE

Use

Honeysuckle is for those who dwell too much on memories of the past, on the "good old days," and who do not expect to experience such happiness and companionship again. The past seems rosy and familiar; the future seems dark, bleak, forbidding, and unknown. For nostalgia, a faraway sense of regret or loss, often tinged with pessimism. Nostalgia may be a temporary sensation, a fleeting regret, or it may be a pattern which prevents further joy and expression. Honeysuckle is appropriate for both.

Method

The boiling method *(see page 223)*

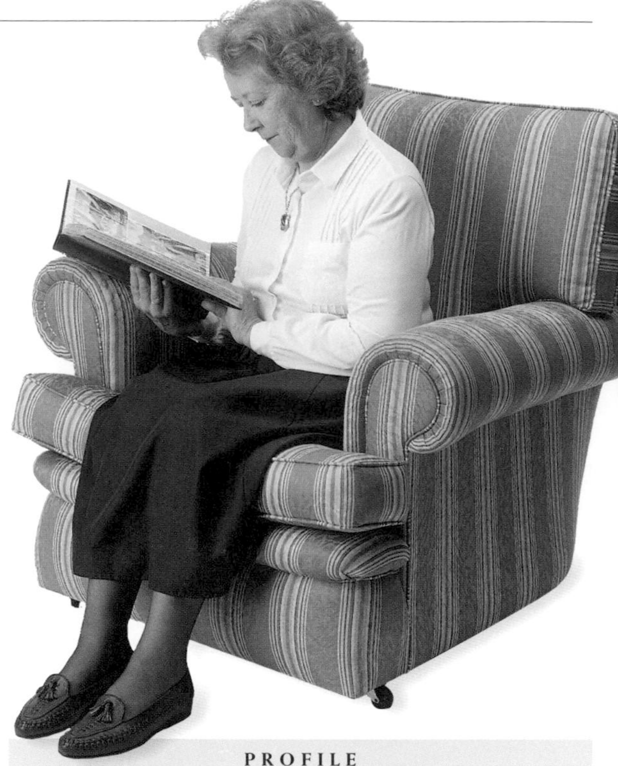

PROFILE

GOAL – To be completely "here" **A useful affirmation might be "I am here and now, growing from my past into a positive future."** Honeysuckle is for people who are not grounded in the present, who (for many reasons) are stuck in the past. **It is for homesickness or regrets.** It is also useful for grief and bereavement where these cause the person to dwell on the past. **Honeysuckle integrates past experiences and gives strength to face new challenges.**

Malus sylvestris

CRAB APPLE

The fruits yielded by this plant are small, yellow, and very acid. It grows in hedges and on waste ground. The crab apples make a piquant preserve. *Malus* provides a good show of color in the fall.

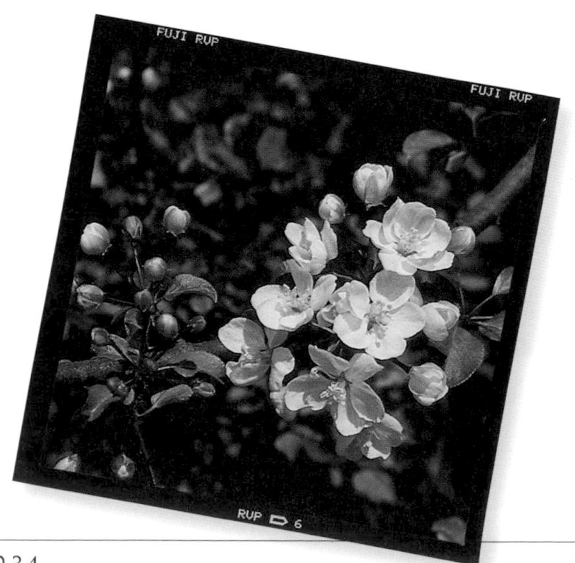

LEFT *The blossoms of the crab apple produce a fresh but bitter fruit that is also used to make country jellies and wines.*

PROFILE

GOAL – Cleaning and purification **Crab Apple is for people who feel unclean on any level. They may feel self-disgust or loathing and may hurt, punish, cut, or otherwise abuse themselves. They may have phobias or rituals around purity or cleanliness.** Crab Apple is also useful for spots and rashes on the face, so that they can be faced and the self accepted. **This remedy is a cleanser on all levels: physical, emotional, and spiritual.** It is also used to cleanse the body and spirit after contact with anything contagious or which feels unclean. **It may be added to baths or to skin creams.**

DATA FILE

Use

Crab Apple is a bitter acid fruit, useful for those who feel self-condemnation and disgust, in need of cleaning or detoxification. This may be a temporary feeling brought on by shame or remorse, or guilt over some act of which they are ashamed, or thoughts which are felt to be unclean. Crab Apple is also useful to encourage acceptance of spots or physical blemishes, and for a deep phobia or cleanliness fetish. It cleanses both the mind and body.

Method

The boiling method *(see page 223)*

Mimulus guttatus

MIMULUS

A pretty, water-loving plant common in damp places, Mimulus has rich yellow flowers in midsummer that resemble the snapdragon. It grows to 2ft. (60cm.)

DATA FILE

Use

Mimulus is for fear which can be identified, of known or worldly things. Aspen is also for fear, but for unknown fears. Mimulus should be taken for the everyday fears of pain, accidents, poverty, being alone, and misfortune. These understandable fears dominate responses, either prodding people into hasty action or freezing them into inaction. They are easily identified and faced, but underneath they are fed by insecurity and a negative attitude toward past experience. Mimulus is also for shy, timid people who tend to avoid social occasions and large crowds of people.

Method

The sun method *(see page 222)*

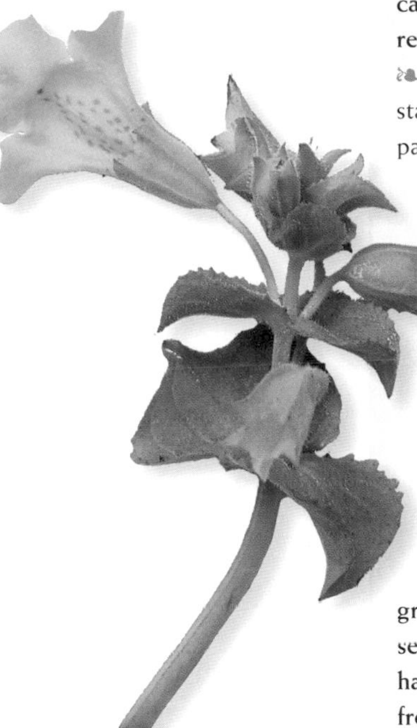

ABOVE *The mimulus or monkey plant is a bog plant, in need of shade, and cool, damp conditions.*

PROFILE

GOAL – Freedom; freedom from fear **For any fear which can be named. A trivial fear or phobia, if it can be named, will respond to Mimulus.** Fear can lead to stammering, palpitations, indigestion, sleeplessness, and troubled dreams. **Mimulus liberates us from fear and helps us to understand the rhythms and balances of everyday life, to grow beyond the limits set by fear, and to have the courage and freedom to respond in appropriate ways.**

Ornithogalum umbellatum

STAR OF BETHLEHEM

The delicate flowers of this wild lily are like six-pointed stars and bloom in late spring. *Ornithogalum umbellatum* is a spring-flowering bulb.

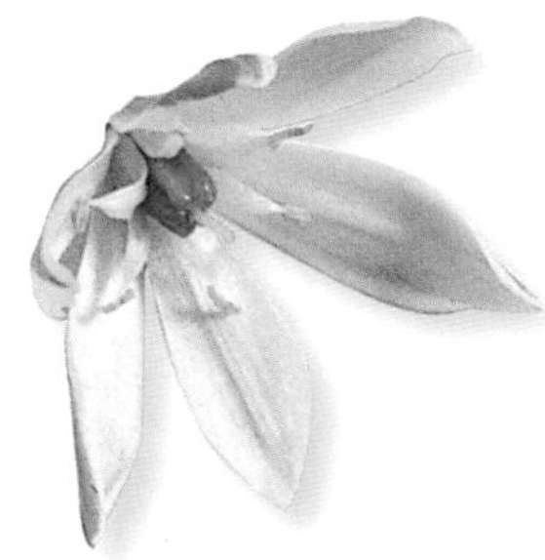

ABOVE *Star of Bethlehem grows wild in Asia and North Africa, and as far north as the U.K.*

PROFILE

GOAL – Peace and comfort **For shock, and its physical and emotional effects.** Long-repressed shock or trauma may lead to psychosomatic symptoms. **Star of Bethlehem neutralizes the effects of shock, so that the body and mind can again find equilibrium and comfort.**

DATA FILE

Use

Star of Bethlehem is used in Rescue Remedy to ameliorate the effects of shock – the shock of bad news, of loss, of an accident, even of being born. People "jump" with shock; waves ripple outward through the body, affecting every cell and tissue. Time is needed for everything to settle, to be comfortable in the body, but sometimes the trauma may be so extreme, or the shock unrealized or repressed, that the effects continue to resonate years later. Star of Bethlehem neutralizes the effects so that the body is able to harmonize.

Method

The boiling method *(see page 223)*

Olea europea

OLIVE

Olive is a small evergreen common in southern Europe. The fruits yield olive oil.

PROFILE

GOAL – Renewal and regeneration **For all exhaustion, physical, and mental tiredness after some effort or struggle.** Exhaustion can be so profound that life loses its interest and spark. **Olive helps restore vitality by helping people to relax and take a more balanced attitude toward life, making sure they allow themselves "quality" time for unwinding, rest, and spiritual renewal.**

DATA FILE

Use

For extreme fatigue of mind, body, or spirit after effort. People in need of Olive feel totally exhausted in every way. They feel that life is hard and without pleasure, that they have no more strength, and at times hardly know how they manage to keep going. They burn the candle at both ends, and become too tired even to think. They may depend on others for help. Olive helps people relax and switch off, so that the simple things of life – a warm bath, a walk in the sunshine, watching children, or sharing with friends – can refresh the spirit.

Method

The sun method *(see page 222)*

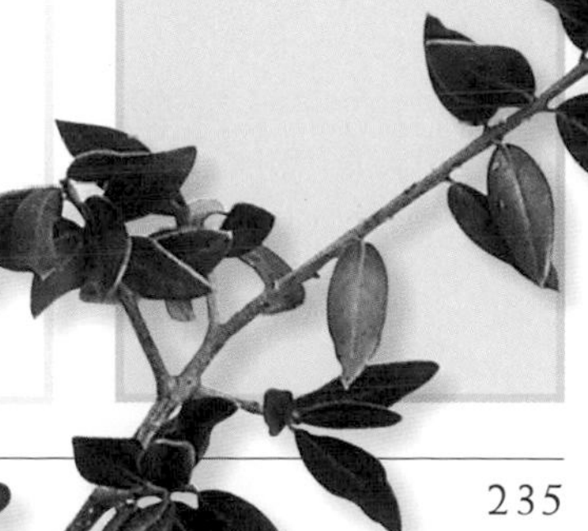

RIGHT *Olive oil has been used to soothe and heal for thousands of years, and the Olive remedy heals the spirit.*

THERAPY CONNECTIONS

OLIVE
Traditional Home and Folk Remedies *p.95*

APPLE
Traditional Home and Folk Remedies *p.94*

Pinus sylvestris

PINE

The Scotch pine is an evergreen tree often depicted in painting and song as the "lonesome pine." It has blue-green leaves and gray or reddish cones.

DATA FILE

Use

Pine is a very specific remedy for those who blame themselves and are suffering from self-reproach. Even when successful they are never content, and always feel that they could have done better. They blame themselves even when the fault is someone else's.

Method

The boiling method *(see page 223)*

ABOVE *The Scotch pine is a native of Europe and Asia that can grow to a great age.*

PROFILE

GOAL – Appropriate response; responsibility **For self-reproach and guilt, frequently groundless.** People who need Pine may carry the blame for the actions of others, and may apologize frequently and often needlessly. **Pine helps us understand that "responsibility" is the ability to respond. If we respond honestly and freely there is no need for blame and we can move on.**

Prunus cerasus

CHERRY PLUM

A small tree with red or yellow fruit, cherry plum is often grown as hedging and windbreaks. It flowers from early spring, with delicate pale pink flowers.

PROFILE

GOAL – Release; to let go of fear and to regain control of the emotions **People who need Cherry Plum may feel desperate, and fear they may hurt themselves and others. They may have bouts of hysteria.** Cherry Plum is useful for uncontrolled tantrums in children, when they are frightened by their own loss of temper. **Cherry Plum restores control and trust of the mind and emotions.**

DATA FILE

Use

Cherry Plum is for the fear of letting go or of losing control. The fearful thoughts may be of a suicidal, compulsive, or destructive nature. This mental pain and turmoil may happen during a period of great emotional or physical change, when the person is worn and stressed. Dr. Bach says it is "for fear of the mind being overstrained, of reason giving way, of doing fearful and dreaded things, not wished and known wrong, yet there comes the thought and impulse to do them."

Method

The boiling method *(see page 223)*

LEFT *The wild cherry plum is in flower almost before the arrival of spring. Flowering twigs are used for the remedy.*

Populus tremula

ASPEN

Aspen is a slender, silver-barked, deciduous tree. It grows to 30ft. (10m.), its almost circular leaves trembling in the slightest breeze.

THERAPY CONNECTIONS

PINE

Aromatherapy *p.166*

PROFILE

GOAL – Courage to face the unknown **The person who needs Aspen may feel frightened, a sense of dread, and that "something awful" may happen. This may be extreme enough to affect appetite, produce palpitations, and interrupt sleep patterns, bringing nightmares.** Aspen is suitable for the fears and nightmares of children where they cannot describe what they are frightened of. **Aspen brings reassurance that there is nothing to fear. It helps us to face the unknown with courage and trust.**

LEFT *Aspen is a type of poplar with gray-green leaves that flutter in the breeze. It also has cottony catkins.*

DATA FILE

Use

Dr. Bach says it is for "vague fear, for which there is no explanation or reason." The fear can be so deep that it is too frightening to express, and the sufferer feels burdened by doom, and inexplicable terror.

Method

The boiling method *(see page 223)*

Ptilotus atripicfolius

MULLA MULLA

A small plant from desert regions, mulla mulla responds to the weather, and sends out clusters of pink, long-lasting flowers when conditions are favorable. All but one of the many species of *Ptilotus* are exclusive to Australia.

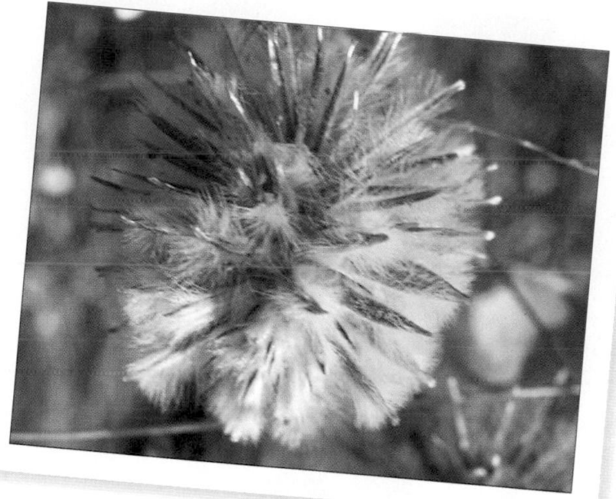

ABOVE *Like many desert plants, mulla mulla has stunning flowers, which seem to symbolize hope and life.*

DATA FILE

Use

For those suffering the effects of fire, heat, or radiation. In reality and symbolically, fire is profoundly powerful. In most traditions fire was a gift from the gods and had to be used with wisdom. Do we understand fire and use it wisely? Burning fossil fuels adds to the greenhouse effect and to the depletion of the ozone layer. Mulla Mulla helps the body recover from damage and protects it from harmful rays.

Method

- The sun method *(see page 222)*

PROFILE

❧ GOAL – Rejuvenation ❧ **People who need Mulla Mulla may have obvious burns, sunburn, or hot rashes. They may be suffering exhaustion from heat, or from working in over-hot conditions, or a hot climate.** ❧ Mulla Mulla helps them to be comfortable with the inner and outer manifestations of fire. ❧ **Mulla Mulla also protects from the damaging effects of heat, for example in laser treatment.**

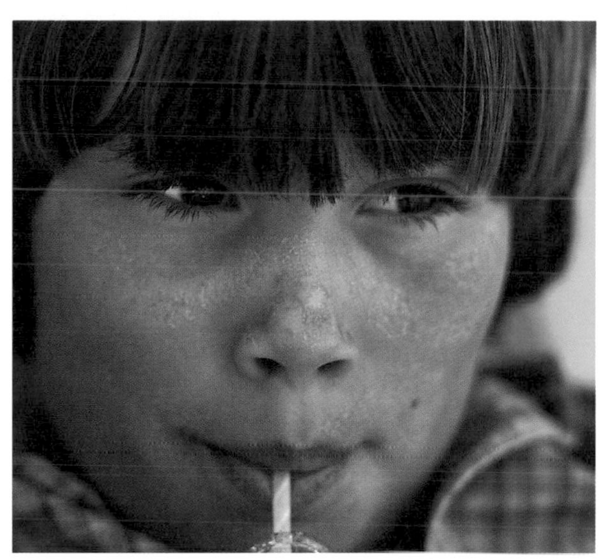

RIGHT *Mulla Mulla can help cool the effects of burns or heat exhaustion and over-exposure to the sun.*

Quercus robur

OAK

Quercus robur is the common oak. Most people recognize the acorns, but the flowers are less familiar. Male and female are borne on the same tree and appear from April onward.

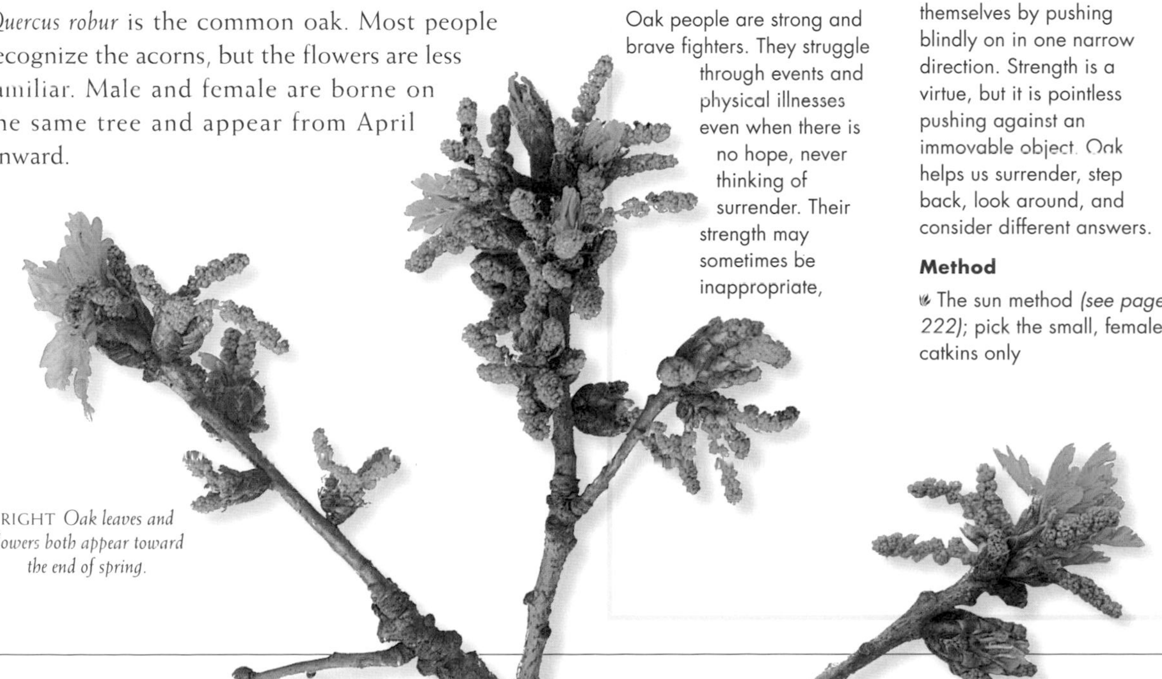

RIGHT *Oak leaves and flowers both appear toward the end of spring.*

DATA FILE

Use

Oak people are strong and brave fighters. They struggle through events and physical illnesses even when there is no hope, never thinking of surrender. Their strength may sometimes be inappropriate, and they can exhaust themselves by pushing blindly on in one narrow direction. Strength is a virtue, but it is pointless pushing against an immovable object. Oak helps us surrender, step back, look around, and consider different answers.

Method

- The sun method *(see page 222)*; pick the small, female catkins only

PROFILE

❧ GOAL – Adaptability and flexibility ❧ **Oak is for those who struggle on, never giving up.** ❧People who need Oak may overwork, and drive themselves relentlessly. ❧ **They can be obstinate, and, unless they rest or find another strategy, may exhaust themselves and break down.** ❧ Oak restores the true inner strength, which is flexible and adaptable.

Ricinocarpus pinifolius

WEDDING BUSH

Ricinocarpus pinifolius is a small bush with abundant, six-petalled white flowers. Male and female flowers grow on the same bush. The flowers were traditionally used for wedding decorations, giving the bush its name.

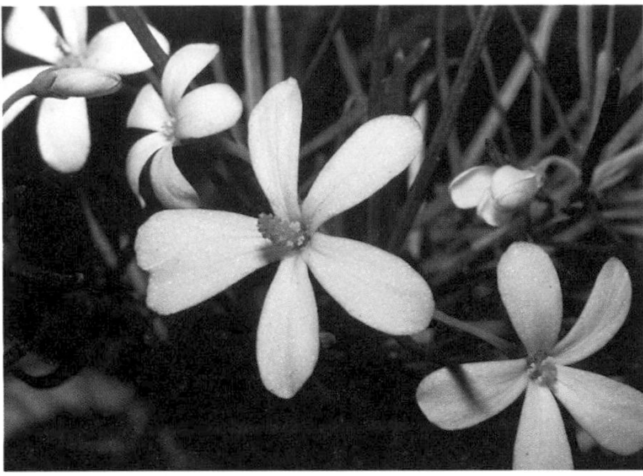

ABOVE *Just as the flowers of Wedding Bush make bridal bouquets, so the remedy keeps a sense of dedication alive.*

BELOW *Wedding Bush can help to bring a feeling of confidence to a relationship and an ability to see things through.*

DATA FILE

Use

Wedding Bush is like the glue which holds people together through thick and thin. It is for those who doubt their ability to commit or accept the responsibility of deep caring; for those with a pattern of starting but not finishing, moving on, and running away from the self in all aspects of life; for those who are an "emotional rolling stone." They may be in love with love (or the newness of love) and move from one affair to another, or they may have one job after another. Commitment is not just about long-term endurance, it is an attitude of mind involving self-worth. Wedding Bush reminds us of the privilege of being, and of our commitment to life.

Method

- The sun method *(see page 222)*; pick both male and female flowers

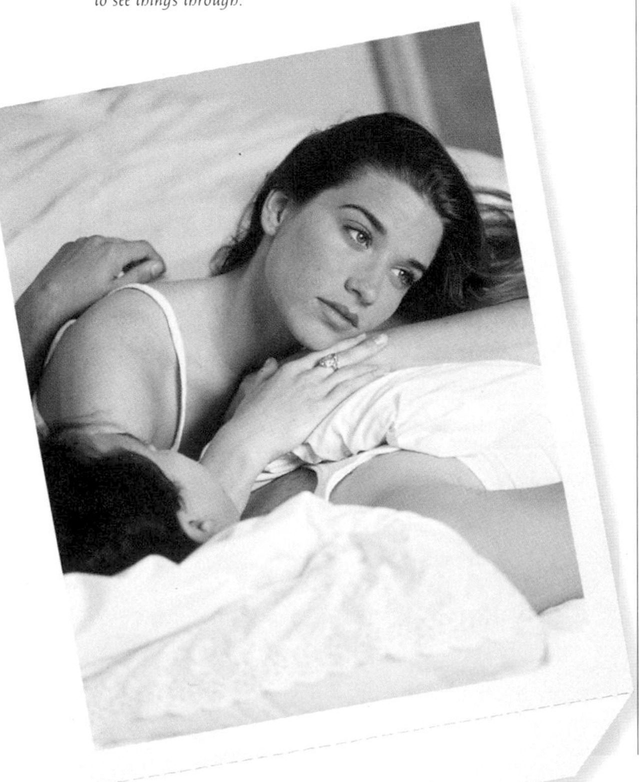

PROFILE

❧ GOAL – Commitment and dedication ❧ **For those who find commitment difficult and suffer indecision and procrastination.** ❧ For those with a pattern of starting but not finishing. ❧ **Wedding Bush encourages the confidence to commit, to feel the comfort rather than the burden of responsibility, to make a long-term dedication to life and its purpose.** ❧ Wedding Bush can also help us to carry through short-term jobs or commitments to a satisfying conclusion.

Rosa canina

WILD ROSE

The common wild rose, *Rosa canina* can be seen rambling over country hedges. The flowers appear in early summer, and vary in color from almost white to deep pink. The fruit, or rosehip, is a striking scarlet.

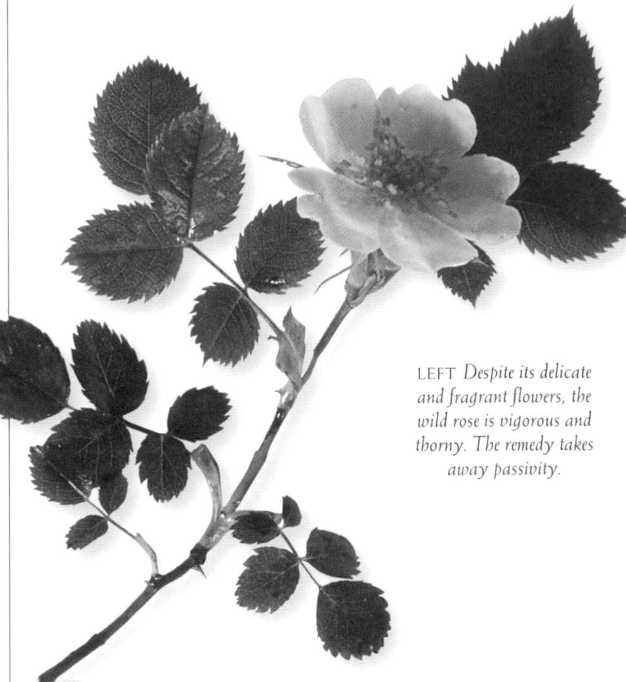

LEFT *Despite its delicate and fragrant flowers, the wild rose is vigorous and thorny. The remedy takes away passivity.*

DATA FILE

Use

Dr. Bach recommends Wild Rose for those who have become resigned to all that happens, for the fatalist. This person glides through life passively, taking it as it is, without motivation or expectation. He or she is apathetic about change and asks, "What is the use?". Such a person has given away his or her power and interest in life. Wild Rose stimulates this interest and an appreciation of life's color and joy. The remedy encourages action, and a purposeful pleasure in being and doing.

Method

- The boiling method *(see page 223)*

PROFILE

❧ GOAL – Interest in life; participation and action ❧ **People who need Wild Rose are fatalistic, resigned to events, and apathetic about change.** ❧ Wild Rose helps us to interact with all aspects of life and make an impact by creating our own unique and dynamic reality.

Salix alba var. vitellina

WILLOW

The willow is an attractive tree with thin, bright yellow twigs and long, narrow leaves. It is also known as the golden osier. The tree is often cut back hard to encourage the growth of strong, young shoots.

PROFILE

❧ GOAL – Maturity and natural balance ❧ **People who need Willow may be sulky and selfish, embittered with self-pity, and ungrateful for help.** ❧ They may experience psychosomatic illness, and tearfulness. ❧ **Willow helps us see that we create our own reality by focusing on different elements of our life. It encourages a more positive and mature attitude.** ❧ Willow may also be taken for a brief temporary embitterment

LEFT *Tall and graceful, with slender, silvery leaves, the willow is a water lover with supple, flexible branches.*

DATA FILE

Use

Willow is for people who find the bad things that happen to them hard to accept and are embittered. They take problems personally, and feel life has become a personal trial to endure, without hope or happiness. They blame the world when things go wrong. "It's not fair," they say, like a two-year-old child. Willow helps them see that with this self-pitying outlook they are creating their own oppression by continual negative thoughts.

Method

❧ The boiling method *(see page 223)*

Synapse arvensis

MUSTARD

The common wild mustard found growing in hedges and on waste ground has large yellow flowers that appear in early summer. This annual plant grows to about 2ft. (60cm.) and self-seeds readily.

ABOVE *The mustard used for this remedy is the yellow-flowered wild field mustard, also known as charlock.*

PROFILE

❧ GOAL – Hope and hopefulness ❧ **Mustard is for depression with no known cause, and for melancholia.** ❧ It is for people whose thoughts turn inward and whose life lacks light and pleasure. ❧ **Although these bouts of depression seem to come from nowhere, there may be a deeply hidden reason. If it happens frequently look for a cause. If there is a physiological or psychological root, seek professional assistance.** ❧ Mustard lightens our mood, giving us the faith and hope to carry on.

DATA FILE

Use

Mustard is used for dark clouds of gloom or deep, black depression that seems to come from nowhere. It is for the feeling of being under a cloud which blocks out the warming rays and optimism of the sun. It may lift just as suddenly as it arrived. While a person is under the dark cloud, it is hard for him or her to muster any feeling of happiness or hope. All clouds pass and Mustard restores hope and a sense of pleasure in living.

Method

❧ The boiling method *(see page 223)*

Scleranthus annuus

SCLERANTHUS

Scleranthus is a small, bushy, spreading plant with green flowers which grows to 4in. (10cm.) on sandy soils and in cornfields. The green flowers have no petals and grow at the forks and end of the stems.

PROFILE

❧ GOAL – Stability and balance ❧ **For people who are unable to decide between two things.** ❧ They are uncertain, indecisive, vacillate, and subject to erratic mood swings. ❧ **Scleranthus brings harmony, stability, and balance, allowing us to act decisively.**

DATA FILE

Use

For those who are unable to decide and who suffer much from hesitation and uncertainty. For confusion. People who need Scleranthus tend to be quiet and are not inclined to discuss their options with others. They need to learn to decide for themselves; it is important that they do so, but they cannot. Scleranthus gives the stability to listen to the inner self, and integrate the emotional and intellectual extremes (which sometimes seem contradictory) into balanced and sustained action.

Method

❧ The sun method *(see page 222)*

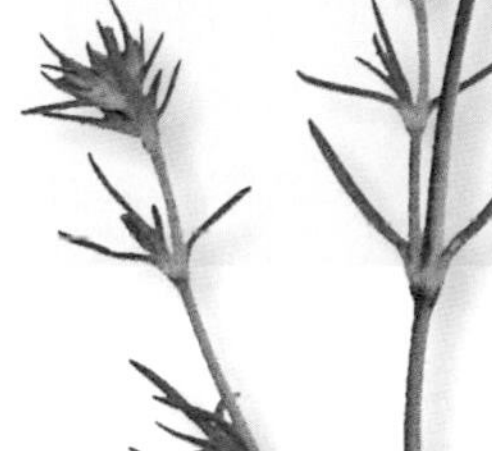

RIGHT *This branching annual plant has tiny green flowers from early spring to late summer.*

THERAPY CONNECTIONS

ROSE

Aromatherapy *p.168*

MUSTARD

Traditional Home and Folk Remedies *p.98*

Ayurveda *p.30*

WILLOW

Herbalism *p.129*

Telopea speciosissima

WARATAH

Waratah is the aboriginal word for beautiful. It is a shrub with magnificent red flowers packed together into a globe measuring 5in. (12cm.) across. It is a very striking plant.

PROFILE

❧ GOAL – To have the courage to be courageous
❧ **Waratah should be taken in times of crisis, emotional or physical. People who need it may feel unable to go on, trapped in a dark night of despair, even suicidal.** ❧ Physical signs may be exhaustion, interrupted or prolonged sleep, loss of the ability or interest to care for oneself. ❧ **Waratah reunites all aspects of the personality.** ❧ It also helps maintain personal integrity for coping with everyday challenges.

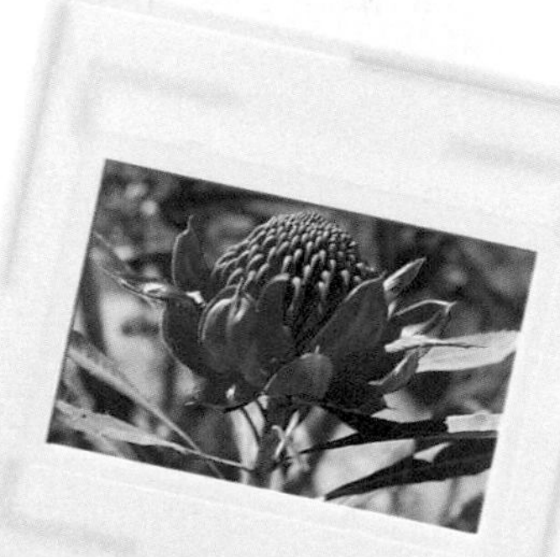

LEFT *With its stunning, globe-shaped flowers Waratah is a powerful remedy, bringing strength and confidence.*

DATA FILE

Use

Waratah is a very powerful and fast-acting remedy. It should be taken for despair, deep distress, and any emotional or physical crisis. The image of the globe of the flowers reflects how the remedy of Waratah brings everything in the personality together: strength, old and forgotten skills and lessons, trust, and love. It gives us the faith, and confidence to hold our head up in all weathers, to stand erect and just be ourselves – blooming, obvious, and beautiful.

Method

❧ The sun method
(see page 222)

Tetratheca ericifolia

BLACK-EYED SUSAN

This small scrubby plant of the Australian woodland is called "black-eyed" as the drooping, bell-like flowers have a core of black pollen-covered stamens surrounded by four mauve petals.

PROFILE

❧ GOAL – The "stand and stare" remedy; inner peace
❧ **People who need Black-eyed Susan are always "on the go." They hate waiting or delay, as they rush to accomplish things quickly.** ❧ Accompanying physical symptoms are irritability, poor digestion, restless sleep, and general tension and stress. They may also have nervous rashes. ❧ **Black-eyed Susan releases stress and helps us slow down and find the inner peace to "stand and stare," as in the lines of the poem, "What is this life if full of care/ We have no time to stand and stare."**

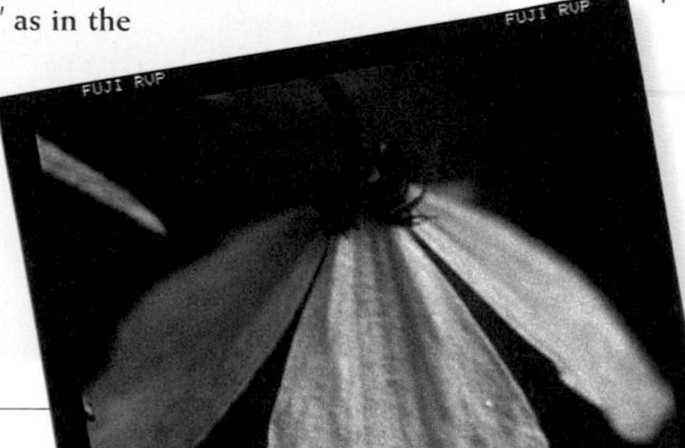

LEFT *Just as this plant's petals draw attention to the dark centers of the flowers, so the remedy can help people to focus on their inner core.*

DATA FILE

Use

Black-eyed Susan is for people who are always rushing and striving, for the workaholic who does not have time for him- or herself or the people around, and is expending all his or her energy at a fast rate. The flowers' petals protect the black center, so the remedy helps us turn inward, slow down, and pay attention to the inner rhythm.

Method

❧ The sun method
(see page 222)

Ulex europaeus

GORSE

Gorse is a bushy shrub with pea-like yellow flowers, which is abundant on poor, stony soils and heaths. It is almost leafless, but its green, spiny stems give it an evergreen appearance.

DATA FILE

Use

Gorse is for strong feelings of hopelessness and despair. People who need Gorse may seek help in order to please others, but underneath feel that nothing more can be done for them. They have lost the will to strive, perhaps in response to a life event, an accident, a medical diagnosis, or to a long-standing illness or fear. They are caught up in negativity, unwilling to try new avenues, and unwilling to hope. Gorse gives them the courage to try, building renewed hope, and giving the will to continue the fight toward recovery.

Method

❧ The sun method
(see page 222)

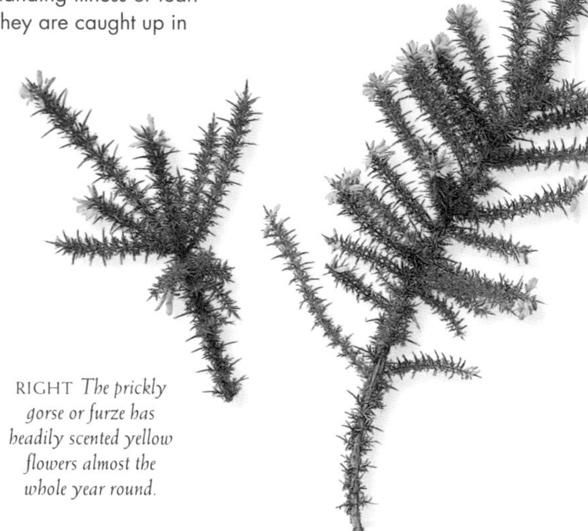

RIGHT *The prickly gorse or furze has headily scented yellow flowers almost the whole year round.*

PROFILE

❧ GOAL – Anything is possible; positive possibilities
❧ **Gorse is for hopelessness and despair when the person has decided to give up.** ❧ Gorse can help give people the heart to stay with a course of treatment. It is useful when a long period of retraining is necessary, for example after a stroke, loss of limbs, or a major accident, when the person feels that there is no use in trying. ❧ **Gorse helps open a door to possibilities, encourages an objective attitude, and strengthens the heart to face them.**

Ulmus procera

ELM

The magnificent English elm, once common in hedgerows and fields, is now, sadly, rare due to Dutch elm disease. It grows to a towering 120ft. (35m.) and spreads to 50ft. (15m.).

DATA FILE

Use

Elm is for temporary feelings of inadequacy. People who benefit from Elm do good work and are proud of themselves and their calling. They hope to do something important, and to be of service and benefit to all of humanity. They seek and aim for perfection. When this goal seems unattainable they can become overwhelmed. Elm is for brief faltering moments of despair and lack of confidence, when the task seems too much. Elm restores faith in ability, so that we do not strive for unattainable perfection, but instead appreciate the worth of our own actions.

Method

The boiling method *(see page 223)*

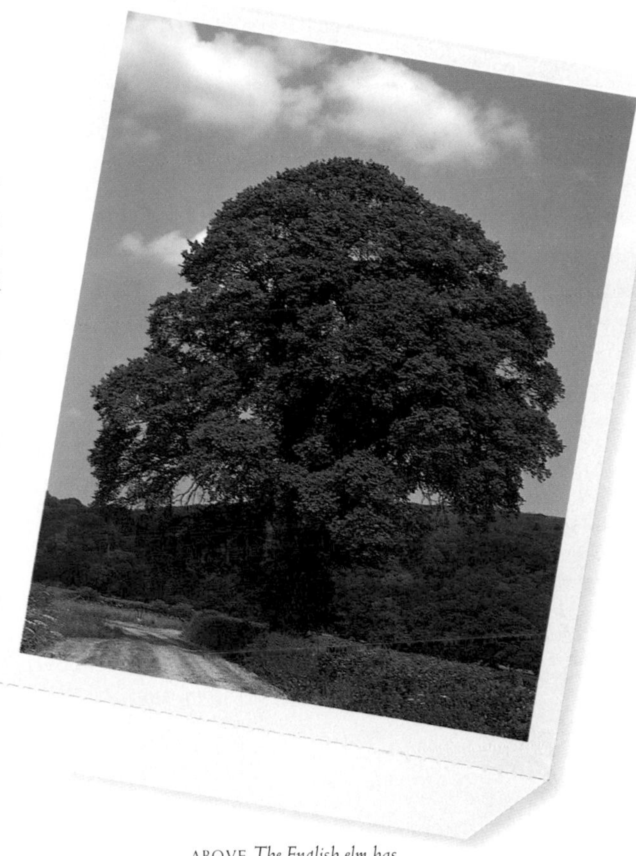

ABOVE *The English elm has clusters of small green flowers with long purple-pink stamens that appear before the leaves open.*

PROFILE

GOAL – Restores confidence. **People who need Elm are usually confident and capable, but are temporarily overwhelmed with the scope, weight, and burden of their work. They may be tired or feel exhausted, which can lead to mild depression.** Elm gives the strength to balance responsibilities with the practical needs of everyday reality and carry on.

(*See also* Larch.)

THERAPY CONNECTIONS

VERVAIN

Herbalism *p.138*

Verbena officinalis

VERVAIN

A common wayside perennial found in meadows, on the roadside, and in dry, sunny places, vervain bears many small, unscented lilac flowers.

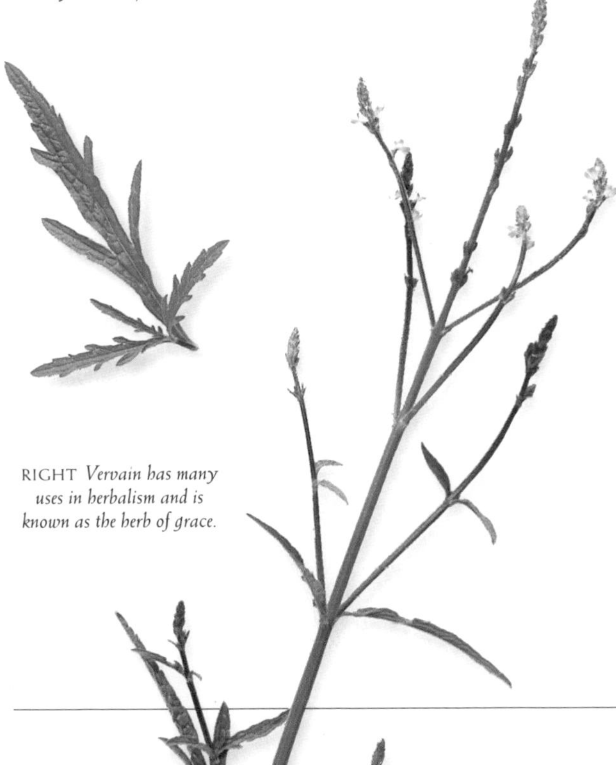

RIGHT *Vervain has many uses in herbalism and is known as the herb of grace.*

DATA FILE

Use

Vervain people have fixed ideas and principles. They are strong-willed and rarely change their views; they think they are right and obstinately maintain a stance, or fight on when others would have conceded. They are great doers and wish to convert all those around them. They strive with mental energy and will power, but the effort of trying to persuade others is extremely stressful, even exhausting. Vervain brings calm and the ability to relax a little and see the other point of view.

Method

The sun method *(see page 222)*

PROFILE

GOAL – Will; to relax and hear the will of the world **People who need Vervain are those whose activity is self-driven, often with overcommitment.** They may be overworked and experience stress-related illnesses, including anxiety, indigestion, insomnia, and sleep disorders. **Vervain brings calm and a space for reflection. It relieves stress and helps to bring the personal will into harmony with the world.**

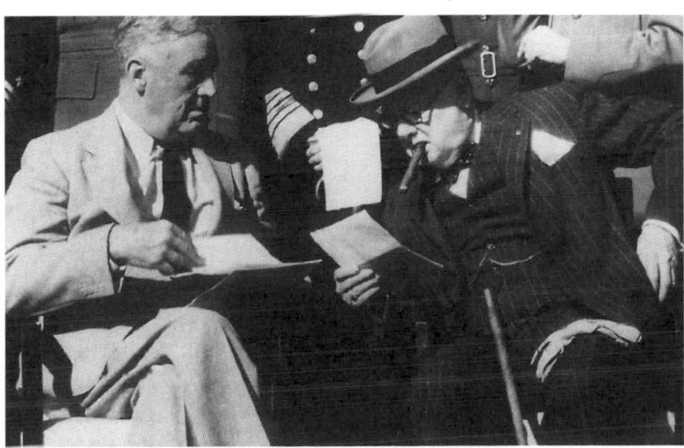

ABOVE *Vervain can be an aid to people who have to face stress and challenges.*

Vitis vinifera

VINE

The grape vine is a thick-trunked shrub, which climbs by means of tendrils. The flower clusters are small and green, and give way to the well-known fruit – green or purple berries.

DATA FILE

Use

Vine is for capable, confident, and successful people; for those who would be "king" (or "queen"). They believe they know best and that others would be happier if they followed. They can bully and dominate, disempowering others, and gaining authority at the expense of their confidence. Even in illness, from the sickbed, they can be ruthless and dominating, ordering their carers around. Vine encourages equality, and the respect each of us, as a fellow human being, is due.

Method

The sun method *(see page 222)*

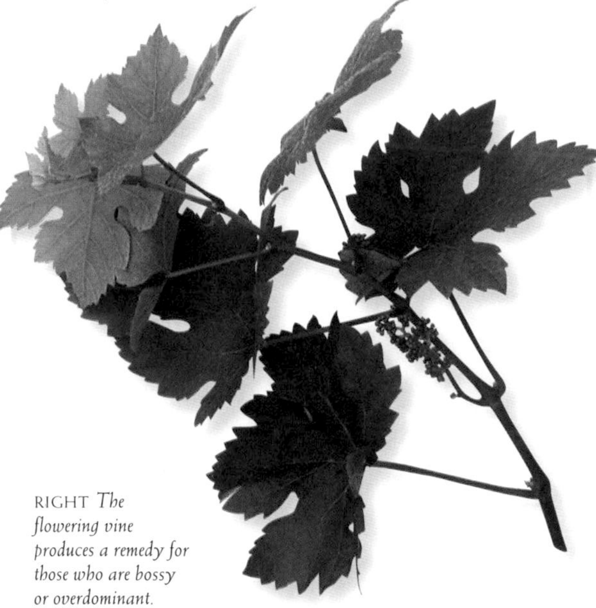

RIGHT *The flowering vine produces a remedy for those who are bossy or overdominant.*

PROFILE

GOAL – Power and natural authority; leadership by consent not through fear **Those who need Vine are dominating and bullying.** They can be cruel and callous through thoughtlessness. **They may also experience stress-related illnesses.** Vine allows us to stand back and let others express themselves, to respect the absolute authority of each person over their own inner life, and to acknowledge their personal choices.

Wahlenbergia spp.

BLUEBELL

This is a small perennial bluebell that is native to Australia. The small, blue, bell-like flowers appear in spring. *Wahlenbergia* thrives best in partial shade, and prefers a well-drained soil.

BELOW *A patch of wild Australian bluebells makes a breathtaking sight in spring.*

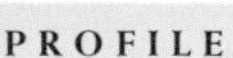

DATA FILE

Use

Bluebell is a remedy for the heart – it opens the heart to the flow of the universe. The heart may be closed through hurt, fear, or loneliness. People who need Bluebell are emotionally closed and fearful. They fear that love will run out and they will be left with nothing. They may be possessive and greedy, with objects representing love.

Method

The sun method *(see page 222)*

PROFILE

GOAL – Wholehearted abundance of love; sharing **People who need Bluebell are emotionally closed, and find it hard to share without keeping mental tally of all emotional transactions.** They are possessive, greedy, and possibly house-proud. Children will not share. **They may also have congestive and containing symptoms such as indigestion, cramps, constipation, or hemorrhoids.** Bluebell helps us own ourselves. The heart is like the magic wine flask in the fairy story. It never runs out. Each morning it is refilled to overflowing abundance.

BELOW *Bluebell remedy helps to conquer greed and possessiveness, and brings a will to love and share.*

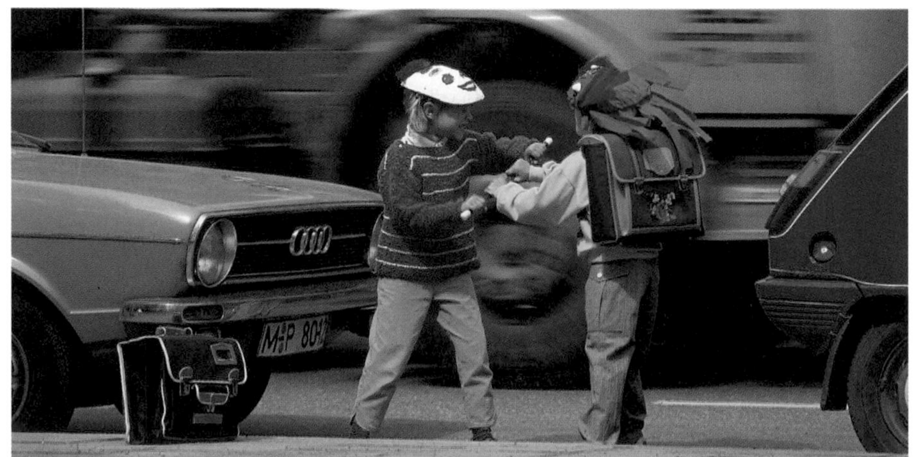

Wisteria sinensis

WISTERIA

Wisteria is a large, woody vine, originally from China. The flowers come before the leaves in spring, and hang in large drooping plumes of pale lilac and mauve. This climber can grow to 100ft. (30m.).

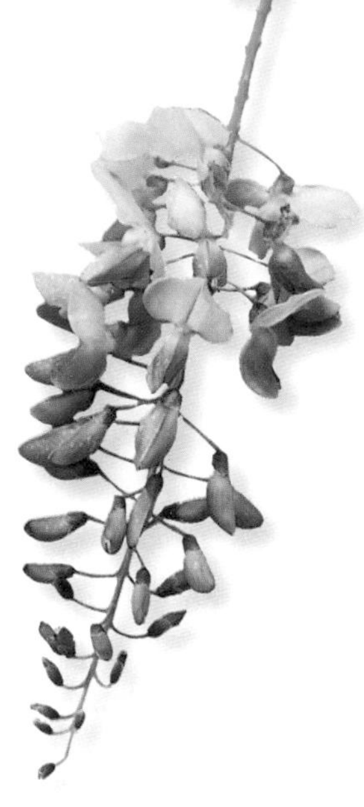

RIGHT *The soft gray racemes of wisteria have a gentle perfume which is found to be very soothing.*

DATA FILE

Use

In Western culture, sex and gender issues are sometimes seen as a matter of power and control. The term "war of the sexes" expresses this. Rape and sexual abuse frequently confirm this role and attitude to power. Wisteria helps people to overcome the inhibitions, blocks, and emotional conflicts produced by this dualistic attitude. It can help them to transcend the roles and to be comfortable with their sexuality. Wisteria can enable them to be open, express themselves, and experience the intimate power and passivity of the orgasm.

Method

- The sun method *(see page 222)*

PROFILE

❧ GOAL – To be comfortable with own sexuality, intimacy and trust ❧ **Women who need Wisteria may be frigid, cold, have a touch taboo, or not enjoy sex. They cannot "lose control" or give themselves.** ❧ Men who need Wisteria may be equally fearful and "role-bound," being macho or a "New Man," when they should let go and be themselves. ❧ **Associated symptoms may be genital herpes, warts, or pelvic congestion linked to a pattern or history of abuse, as well as very painful menstruation. If there is a history of abuse (in either sex), give other appropriate remedies.** ❧ Wisteria helps us experience intimacy and mutual trust.

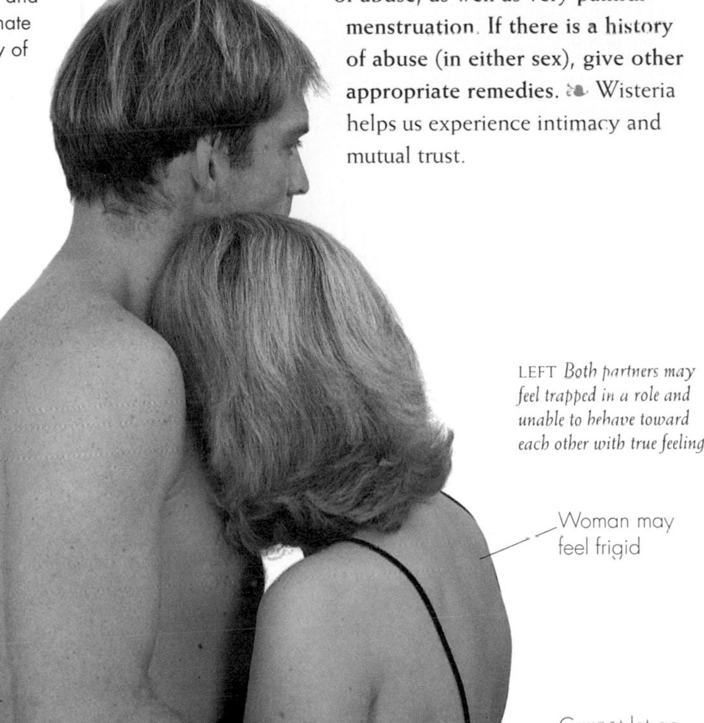

LEFT *Both partners may feel trapped in a role and unable to behave toward each other with true feeling.*

ROCK WATER

Water taken from a natural well or spring, preferably one with a traditional reputation for healing. There are many half-forgotten springs and wells. The water should be open and free-flowing. Choose a well or spring which is open to the air and sunshine, and is as natural as possible. Do not use water from a well dedicated to a saint, or within a church or shrine.

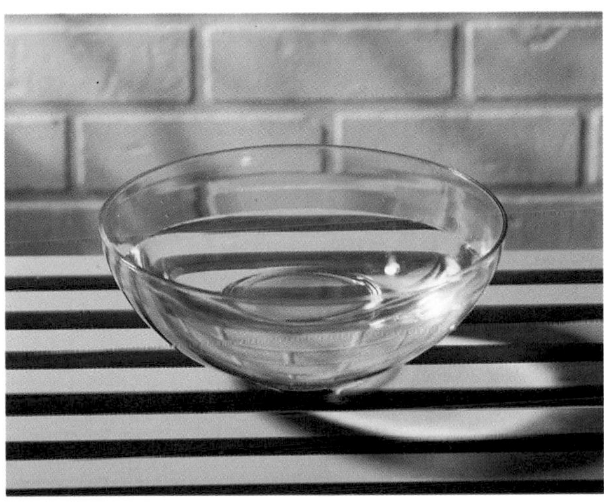

ABOVE *Pure, clear water, filtered by rock can encourage the spirit to flow.*

PROFILE

❧ GOAL – Harmony and discipline

❧ **People who need Rock Water may be rigid, narrow-minded, and very strict with themselves, to the point of self-denial.**

❧ They are perfectionists with exaggerated ideals, but unlike Vervain people they do not try to convert others. They are content to make themselves perfect.

❧ **Rock Water encourages flexibility in reaching goals which harmonize with the natural order of the world.**

DATA FILE

Use

Rock Water is for people who are very strict with themselves and unforgiving – like the rock. They practise self-discipline and deny themselves anything which might distract them from their goal. They have high ideals and are hard on themselves. True self-discipline does not involve denial. Denial is only necessary when the person is not acting from the heart and has a narrow view of his or her goal. Rock Water gives the flexibility of water, a pure spring flowing toward the sea.

Method

- The sun method *(see page 222)*

RESCUE REMEDY

Rescue Remedy can be bought as a liquid or as a cream. It is made from equal amounts of the five following essences:

- CHERRY PLUM – *for feelings of desperation*
- ROCK ROSE – *to ease terror, fear, or panic*
- IMPATIENS – *to soothe irritability and agitation*
- CLEMATIS – *to counteract the tendency to drift away from the present*
- STAR OF BETHLEHEM – *to address the mental and physical symptoms of shock*

Together, these flower essences make a safe mental sanctuary in which to recover. Carry Rescue Remedy with you for all emergencies.

CLEMATIS

STAR OF BETHLEHEM

IMPATIENS

ROCK ROSE

CHERRY PLUM

ABOVE *The five flowers whose essences are used to make up the Bach Flower Rescue Remedy.*

DATA FILE

Use

Rescue Remedy rebalances the body after any emotional or physical upset. It should be taken when a person feels in need of rescue, is unsettled, or is not quite in step with him or herself. This may be after a shock, an accident, an argument, a trying event like a divorce or separation, or any circumstance which has demanded supreme nervous effort. Rescue must take place before salvage and restoration.

Rescue Remedy speeds healing after surgery.

Use Rescue Remedy cream after sunburn, cuts, bruises, or damage from accidents.

Rescue Remedy can be added to any skin wash, douche, or compress if some element of rescue is needed. This method is also useful if nothing is allowed by mouth.

Rescue Remedy can also be given before a trying event, examination, court appearance, operation, hospital test, etc., to minimize the trauma. It is for all emergencies. Carry a small bottle with you.

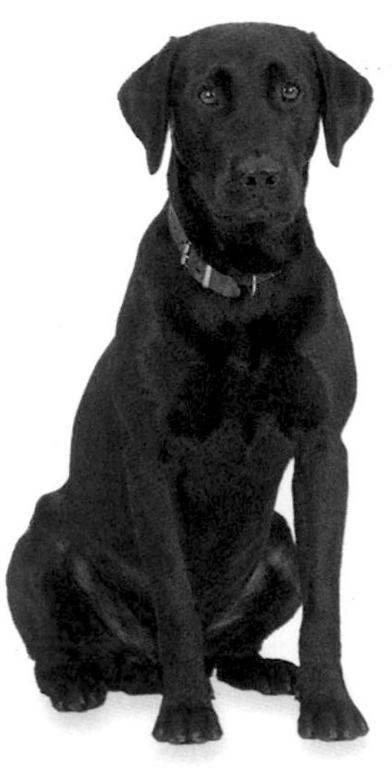

ABOVE *Even frightened or traumatized animals respond to treatment with Rescue Remedy.*

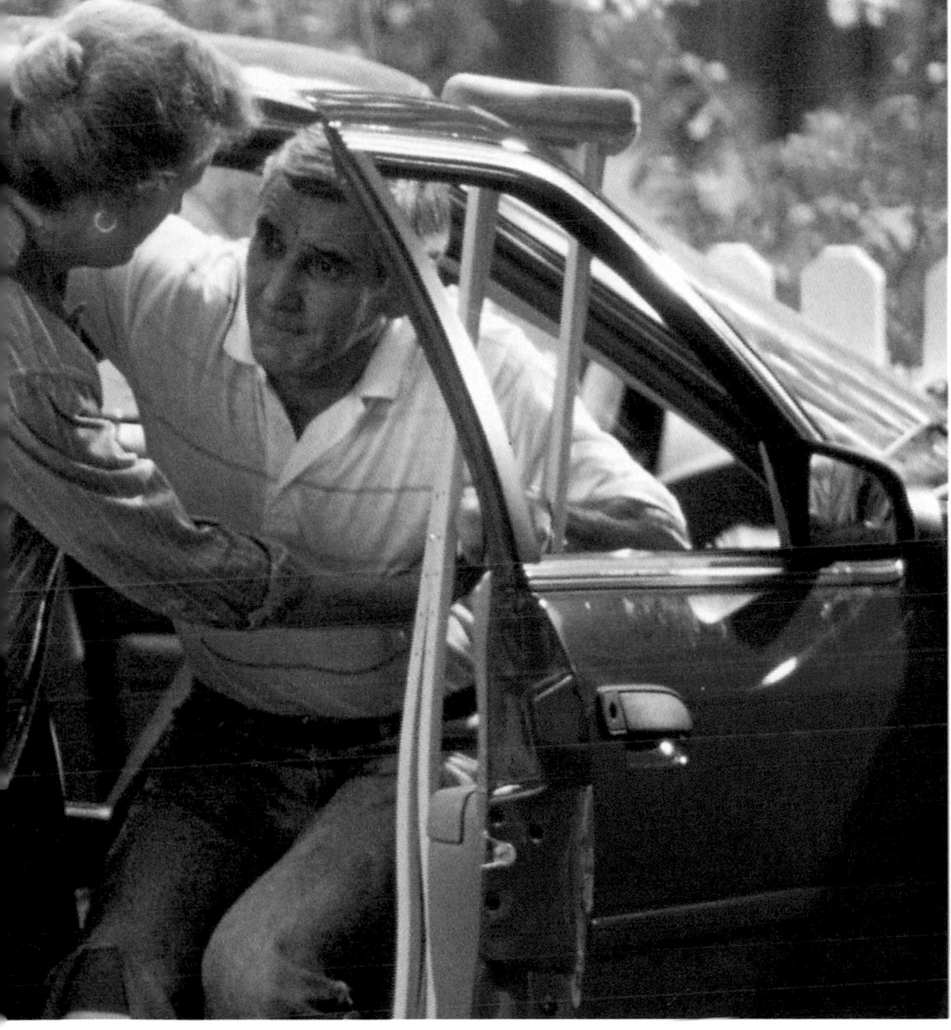

LEFT *Rescue Remedy can have a calming, stabilizing effect after an event such as a car crash.*

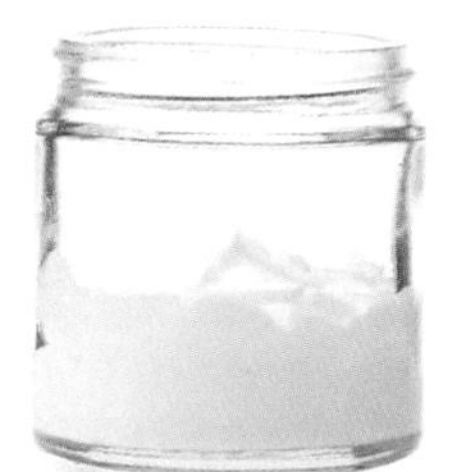

LEFT *A few drops of Rescue Remedy can be mixed into skin cream for external use.*

RECIPE

Home-made Rescue Remedy

Make a treatment bottle of Rescue Remedy by adding 2 drops of each constituent Bach Flower Remedy to a 1fl. oz. (30ml.) bottle of brandy.

A cream can be made at home by adding 4 drops of stock Rescue Remedy to a favorite skin cream or neutral base, then adding 2 drops of Crab Apple.

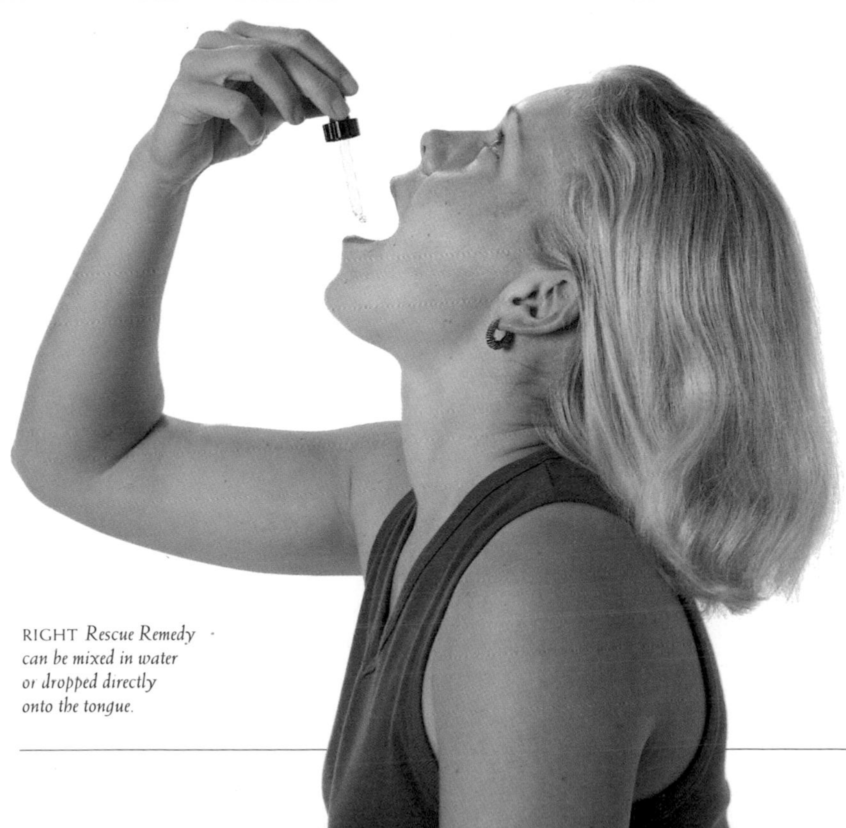

RIGHT *Rescue Remedy can be mixed in water or dropped directly onto the tongue.*

PROFILE

❧ GOAL– Rescue or salvation ❧ **Rescue Remedy is the only Bach Flower Remedy that is usually taken neat, straight from the stock bottle. Put 4 drops directly onto or under the tongue. Repeat dosage as often as needed.** ❧ Put 4 drops into a glass of water and sip throughout the day until you feel more settled. ❧ **Rescue Remedy is ideal for children and animals, and can be dropped into food or drinking water. A startled infant or baby can be reassured by putting 4 drops into the evening bath.** ❧ It can be given to plants and seedlings with success. ❧ **It is never too late to take Rescue Remedy. It will help overcome old and unspoken trauma if these are still upsetting you. But it is not a panacea, so once the immediate emotional crisis has calmed, look at the other remedies with a view to creating your own personal mix.**

VITAMINS AND MINERALS

Our understanding of vitamins and minerals – and other micronutrients, compounds, and elements – and their role in our body has improved dramatically over the last decades. We now know that "micronutrition" – or the vitamins, minerals, and other health-giving components of our food, such as amino acids, fiber, enzymes, and lipids – is crucial to life, and that by manipulating our nutritional intake, we can not only ensure good health and address ailments, but prevent illness and some of the degenerative effects of aging. Exciting new discoveries related to the nutrient components of our food mean that more than half of us are now taking supplementation in one form or another, convinced that diet itself – bearing in mind the stresses on our body and the polluted world in which we live – is inadequate to supply us with our nutritional needs.

ABOVE *More than 50 percent of the U.K. population now take some form of dietary supplement.*

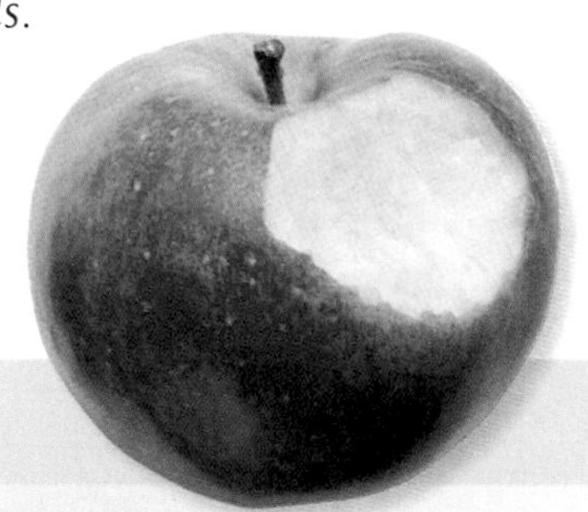

BELOW *Apples contain vitamin C, which helps combat infection and boost immunity.*

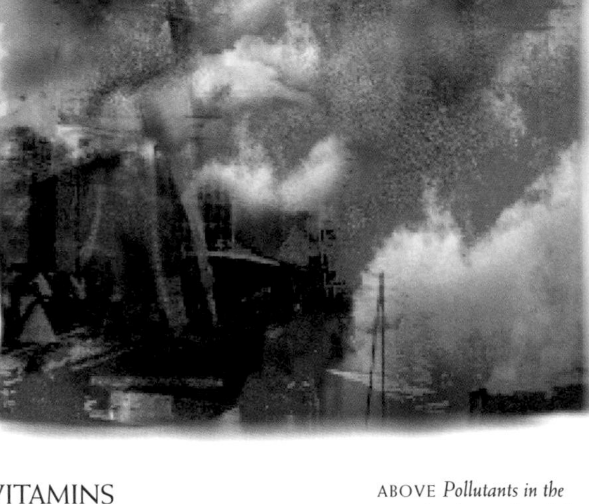

ABOVE *Pollutants in the atmosphere have a harmful effect on our health, making it even more important that we supplement our diet with vitamins and minerals.*

VITAMINS

Vitamins are a group of unrelated organic nutrients, which are essential to regulate the chemical processes that go on in the body – such as releasing the energy from food, maintaining strong bones, and controlling our hormonal activity. Ideally, vitamins are present in roughly the same quantity in various foods.

MINERALS

Minerals are inorganic chemical elements, which are necessary for many biochemical and physiological processes that go on in our bodies. Inorganic substances that are required in amounts greater than 100mg. per day are called minerals; those required in

A HISTORY OF NUTRITION

PREHISTORY

From the very earliest days of civilization, nutrition has formed the backbone of healthcare. Obtaining and eating food consumed most of early man's time, and food and herbs were our first medicine, used to treat a large number of conditions ranging from wounds and insect bites to infection. It became clear that food had powerful healing effects, and that a varied diet, rich in natural ingredients, was a prerequisite for good health. From that time, diet became a fundamental part of most therapies, and an integral element in almost all of the others.

18TH CENTURY

In the 18th century, English sailors were given lime or lemon juice in order to prevent scurvy, a disease caused by lack of vitamin C, which occurred as a result of long periods of time away at sea without fresh fruit or vegetables.

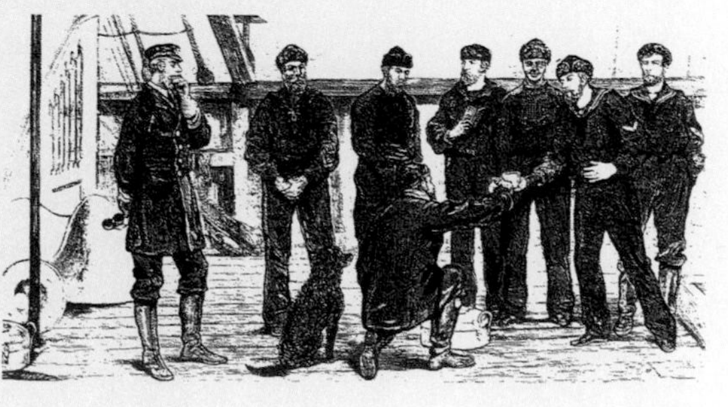

LEFT *From the 18th century English sailors ate limes as a protection against scurvy.*

19TH CENTURY

In the late 19th century, naturopaths drew attention to the use of food and its nutritional elements as medicine, a concept that was not new, but which had not been acknowledged as a therapy in its own right until that time. Naturopaths used nutrition and fasting to cleanse the body, and to encourage its ability to heal itself. As knowledge about food, its make-up, and the effects it has on our body became greater with the development of biochemistry, the first nutritional specialists undertook to treat specific ailments and symptoms with the components of food.

ABOVE *Since the 19th century, the nutritional components of food have been used as medicine.*

amounts less than 100mg. per day are called trace elements. Minerals are not necessarily present in foods – the quality of the soil and the geological conditions of the area in which they were grown play an important part in determining the mineral content of foods. Even a balanced diet may be lacking in essential minerals or trace elements because of the soil in which the various foodstuffs were grown.

There is evidence that "sub-clinical" deficiencies, in other words, a deficiency which is not extensive enough to be life-threatening or to produce large-scale symptoms, may be the cause of certain forms of cancer, heart disease, weight and skin problems, and a host of other health conditions.

AMINO ACIDS

An amino acid is any compound that contains an amino group and an acidic function. There are 20 amino acids necessary for the synthesis of proteins, which are essential for life. These 20 amino acids form the building blocks of all proteins and are involved in important biological processes, such as the formation of neurotransmitters in the brain. There are eight essential amino acids, which are:

- *phenylalanine*
- *valine*
- *threonine*
- *tryptophan*
- *isoleucine*
- *methionine*
- *lysine*
- *leucine*

The remaining 12 are called "nonessential," which means that they can usually be made by the body from other substances. In some conditions, however, nonessential amino acids are necessary, for example in cases of extreme illness or a very poor diet.

LIPIDS AND DERIVATIVES

Lipids are commonly called "fats," and while many fats are now known to be unhealthy, there are many that are essential to body processes and actually work to prevent the effects of "unhealthy" fats in our bodies. Many lipids and their derivatives are used to unclog arteries, work to retard the effects of aging, and to discourage heart disease and the build-up of cholesterol.

OTHER SUPPLEMENTS

There are a number of other food supplements that do not fall strictly within the definitions of vitamins, minerals, lipids, and amino acids. These include various elements that either have healing properties or are now known to be crucial to health.

NUTRITION TODAY

Nutrition has changed from a mainly physician-led dietary therapy, also called clinical nutrition, to a more profound theory of health based on treating the patient as a whole (holistic health), and looking for deficiencies that may be causing illness, which are specific to each individual.

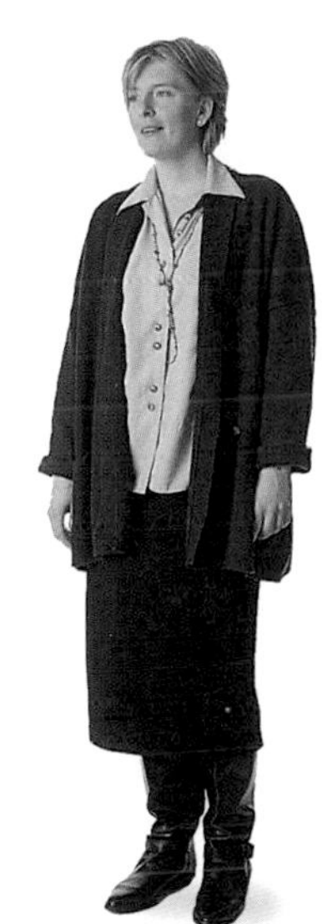

RIGHT *Many nutritionists now treat their patients holistically as a "whole being" composed of body, mind, and soul.*

20TH CENTURY

By the middle of the 20th century, scientists had put together a profile of proteins, carbohydrates, and fats, as well as vitamins and minerals, which were essential to life and to health. More than 40 nutrients were uncovered, including 13 vitamins. It was discovered that minerals were needed for body functions, and a new understanding of the body and its biochemistry fed the growing interest in the subject. In the 1960s, physicians began to treat patients with special diets and supplements, prescribed according to individual symptoms, problems, and needs, but while conventional medical physicians still discussed nutrition in terms of basic food groups, nutritionists were prescribing vitamins in megadoses.

Other elements and compounds were soon identified as necessary to human life, and we are now able to purchase and take substances like amino acids; bee pollen; lipids, such as evening primrose oil and cod liver oil; and seaweeds, acidophilus (healthy bacteria), and dietary enzymes.

ABOVE AND RIGHT *Conventional medical practioners discuss nutrition in terms of food groups, while nutritionists tend to prescribe vitamins in large doses.*

WHAT DO VITAMINS, MINERALS, AND OTHER ELEMENTS DO IN OUR BODIES?

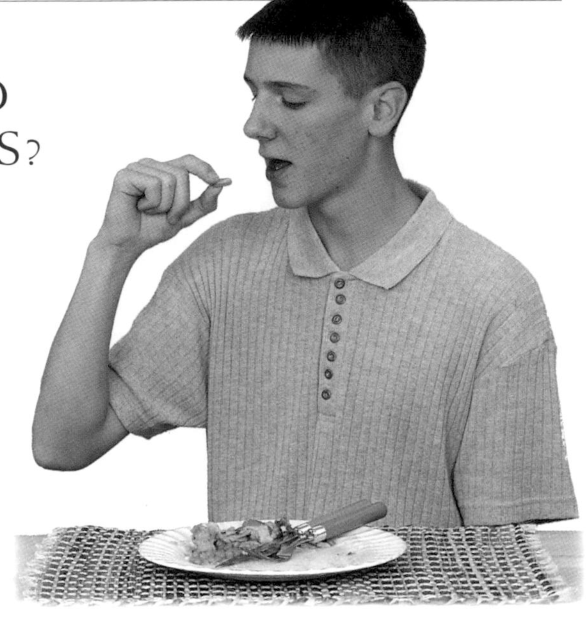

ABOVE *Most supplements are best taken on a full stomach, but read the label on the packet for precise information.*

SHOULD YOU TAKE SUPPLEMENTS?

Supplements are not a replacement for food, and most cannot be ingested without food. They cannot be taken in place of a good diet but their beneficial effects will be optimized if combined with a balanced intake of nutritious foods. People suffering from chronic conditions or who smoke or drink regularly may need to take supplements to ensure optimum health.

Micronutrients work in conjunction with one another, and taking large doses of any one supplement can upset the balance within the body. A good vitamin and mineral supplement will ensure that you are getting the correct amounts of each, according to the relationships between them. Extra supplements should only be taken on the advice of a registered nutritionist or medical practitioner. Where supplements are taken to discourage the course of illness – for example vitamin C for colds or flu – it is safe to take larger doses than usual. Read the packet for further information.

ABOVE *In some cases vitamin and mineral supplements should only be taken on the advice of a registered nutritionist.*

Vitamins, minerals, and other elements work together within the body to ensure that all processes can be carried out. When even one element is missing, the body becomes unbalanced and unable to work at its optimum level.

WHEN SHOULD SUPPLEMENTS BE TAKEN?

- The best time for taking most supplements is after meals, on a full stomach, although some vitamins and minerals work best on an empty stomach. Read the label on any supplement you plan to take to find out the best time to take it.
- Time-release formulas need to be taken with food, as their nutrients are slowly released over a number of hours. If there is not enough food to slow their passage through the body, they can pass the sites where they are normally absorbed before they have had a chance to release their nutrients.
- Take supplements evenly throughout the day for best effect.

WHEN TO SEE A PRACTITIONER

Most supplements can be taken safely without input from a nutritionist, but if you suffer from chronic health problems, or a specific ailment, it is best to seek expert advice. Amino acids and other elements should only be taken with the advice of a professional. A nutritionist will make sure that you are taking a balanced combination of nutrients that will work together to make you healthy. Remember that everyone's needs are different, based on overall health, diet, whether or not you smoke or drink, are pregnant, and other influences. It is sensible to ensure that you receive advice that is tailored specifically to your individual needs.

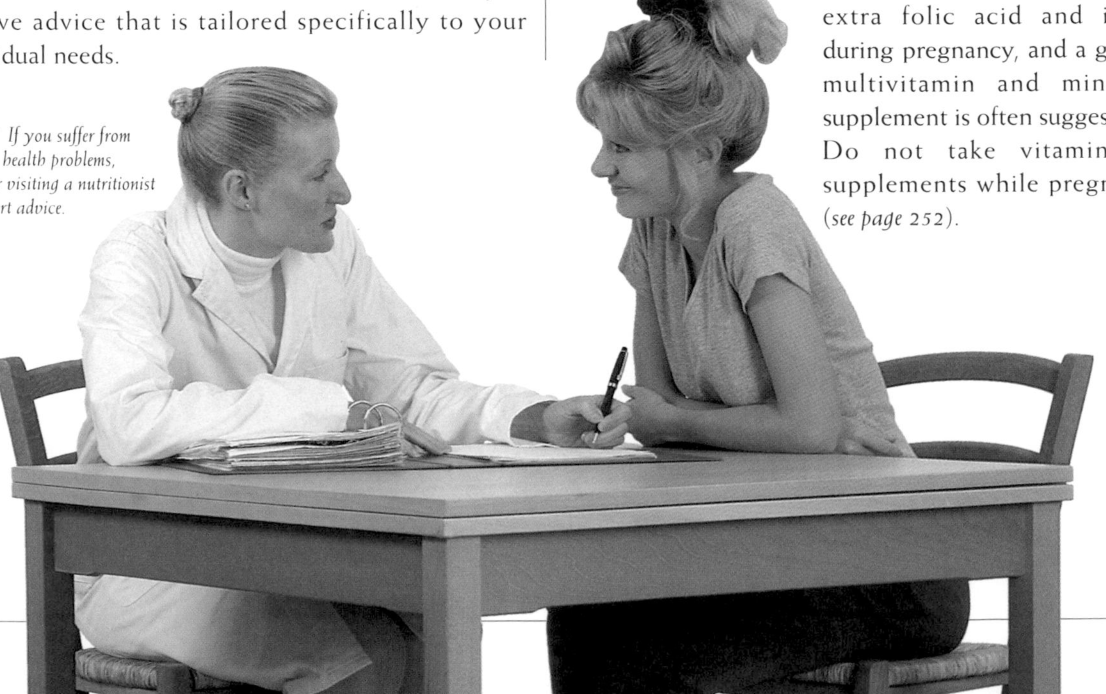

RIGHT *If you suffer from chronic health problems, consider visiting a nutritionist for expert advice.*

CHILDREN

Children need far lower doses than adults, and a healthy, organic diet should offer a large proportion of their nutritional needs. A good vitamin and mineral supplement will provide anything extra that is required, but if you feel your child needs further supplements, see a practitioner. If you are buying products yourself, read the label to ensure that the product is safe for children, and follow the advice carefully.

PREGNANCY

A growing baby puts heavy demands on your body when you are pregnant, and it is more important than ever to ensure that you have a good diet. Research has now proved that we need extra folic acid and iron during pregnancy, and a good multivitamin and mineral supplement is often suggested. Do not take vitamin A supplements while pregnant (*see page* 252).

A HEALTHY DIET

Our diet should be made up of complex carbohydrates (5–9 portions per day), fruits and vegetables (4–9 portions), proteins (3–5 portions), and fat (under 30g. per day is recommended for a healthy diet). But eating the right foods doesn't necessarily mean that you are getting enough nutrients. Refining and processing foods takes out much of the nutritional value, and pesticides and other agents used in the growing process place extra demands on our bodies. Before our food ever reaches the grocery store it may be nutritionally deficient. Therefore, take extra steps to preserve the nutritional content of your food whenever possible:

- Eat the skins of vegetables.
- Don't cut, wash, or soak fruit and vegetables until you are ready to eat them. Exposing their cut surfaces to air destroys many nutrients.
- Eat brown, unpolished rice and whole grains.
- Choose fresh fruit and vegetables first, but remember that nutritional value decreases with age. Frozen is a better option if you aren't going to eat the food immediately.
- Eat raw whenever possible, if cooking, use as little water as possible.
- If you do boil fruit or vegetables, use the water remaining after cooking in your sauces or gravy.
- Eat organic food whenever possible. It may be a little more expensive, but you can be sure that the food you are eating has not been processed, and has been grown without the use of pesticides and other chemicals.

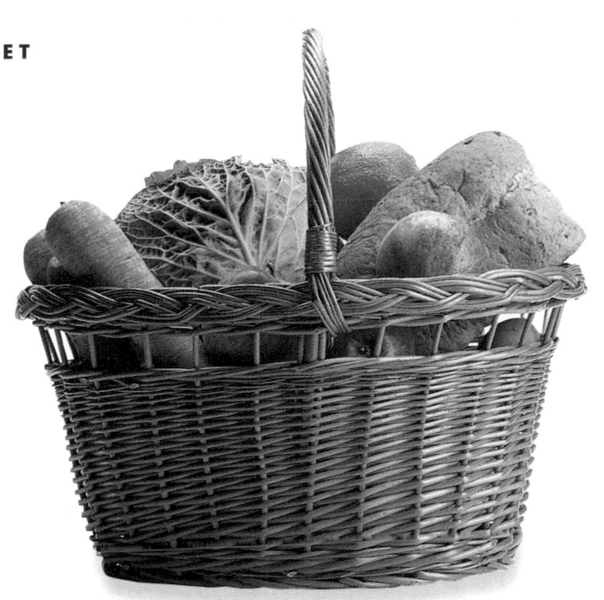

BELOW *Choose your daily dietary requirements from different groups of food – complex carbohydrates, fruit and vegetables, and fats and proteins.*

ABOVE *By the time our food reaches the grocery store it may have lost many of its valuable nutrients. Try to choose organic fruit and vegetables.*

FRESH FRUIT AND VEGETABLES

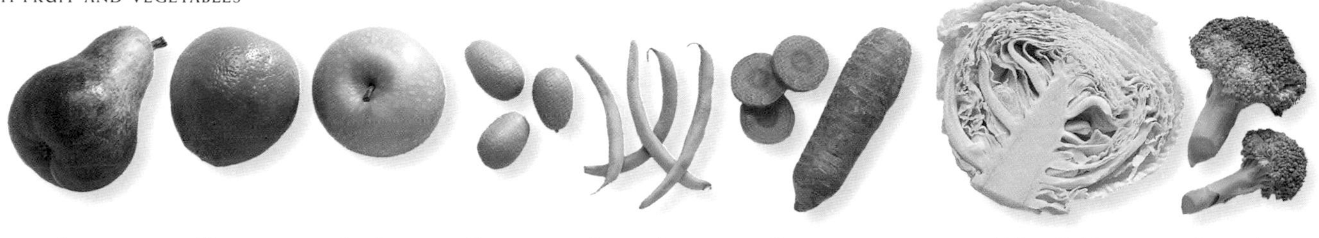

Pears · Oranges · Apples · Kumquats · Runner Beans · Carrots · White Cabbage · Broccoli

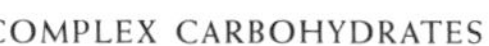

COMPLEX CARBOHYDRATES

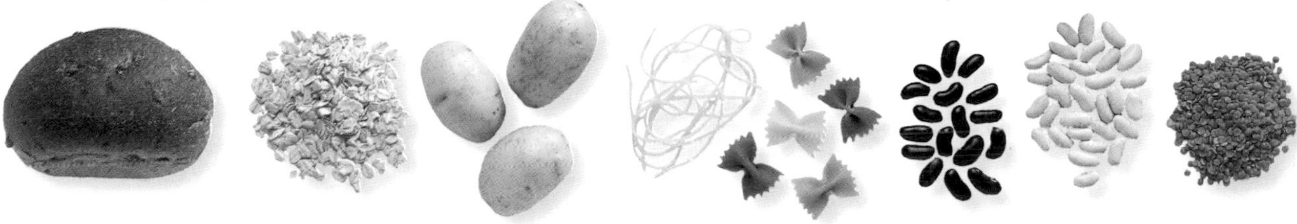

Wholemeal Bread · Oats · Potatoes · Pasta · Black beans · Haricot beans · Lentils

FATS AND PROTEINS

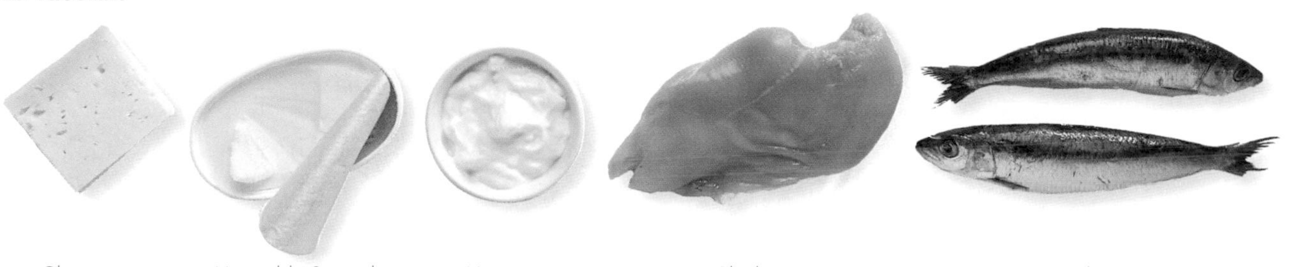

Cheese · Vegetable Spread · Yogurt · Chicken · Fish

SUPPLEMENT FORMS

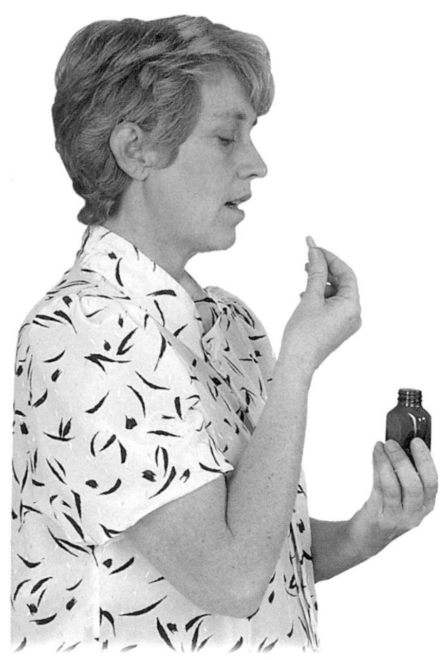

Most supplements come in a variety of forms, to allow for individual needs. They are also prepared with different quantities of the active ingredients, so read the label carefully to ensure that you are getting the correct quantity for your needs.

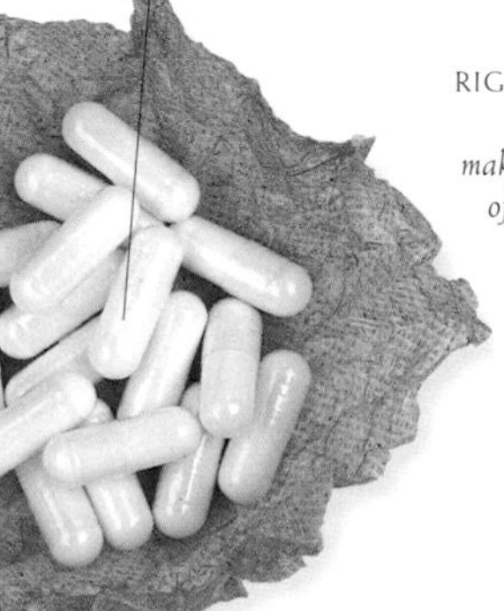

OIL CAPSULES

TABLETS

POWDER CAPSULES

ABOVE *Some supplements come in a variety of forms, allowing the individual to choose between powders, capsules, liquids, or tablets.*

WHICH SUPPLEMENT?

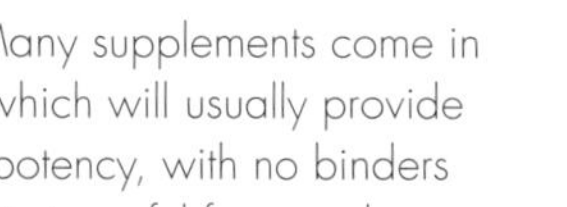

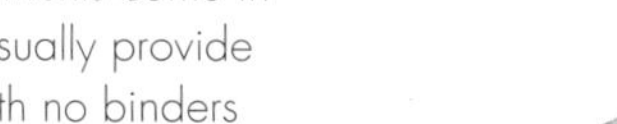

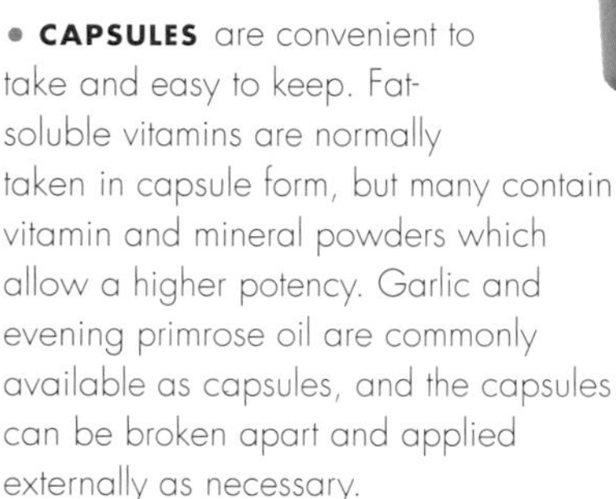

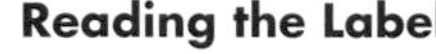

LEFT *If you find it too hard to swallow tablets, try taking a powder supplement sprinkled on yogurt.*

• **POWDERS** Many supplements come in powder form, which will usually provide you with extra potency, with no binders or additives. This is useful for people with allergies, or those who find it difficult to swallow a tablet. Powders are particularly useful for children – sprinkle a little powder in their breakfast juice, or stir it into some yogurt.

• **CAPSULES** are convenient to take and easy to keep. Fat-soluble vitamins are normally taken in capsule form, but many contain vitamin and mineral powders which allow a higher potency. Garlic and evening primrose oil are commonly available as capsules, and the capsules can be broken apart and applied externally as necessary.

• **LIQUIDS** are appropriate for people who have difficulty swallowing tablets or capsules. Many children's formulas come in liquid form for easy administration. Liquids can be mixed with food or stirred into drinks. Liquid supplements can also be applied externally.

• **TABLETS** Many supplements come in tablet form and these are the most practical for many people because they can be easily stored and they will keep for a long time. Check the label to see what is added to your tablets in the form of binders or fillers, which are added to preserve or bulk out the active ingredient.

Reading the Label

Supplements work in different ways, and you'll need to understand some of the key words that appear on the labels in order to choose which are most suitable for you.

Chelated is a term which appears on mineral supplements, and it means that the mineral is combined with amino acids to make assimilation more efficient. Most nutritionists recommend taking chelated minerals because they are 3 to 5 times more effective.

Time-release formulas are created with a process that allows them to be released into the body over an 8–10-hour period. These are particularly useful for water-soluble vitamins (*see pages 253–56*), any excess of which is excreted within 2 or 3 hours of taking the supplement. Time-release formulas are reputed to provide stable blood levels during the day and night.

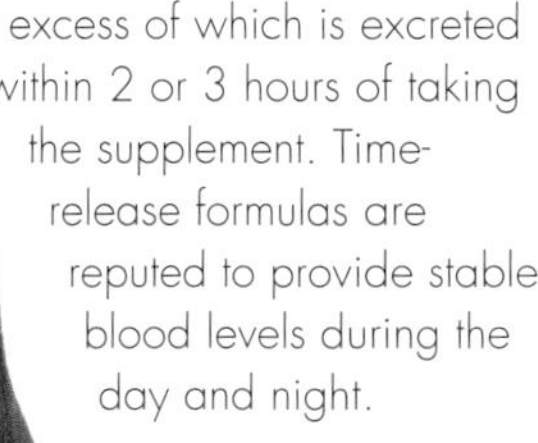

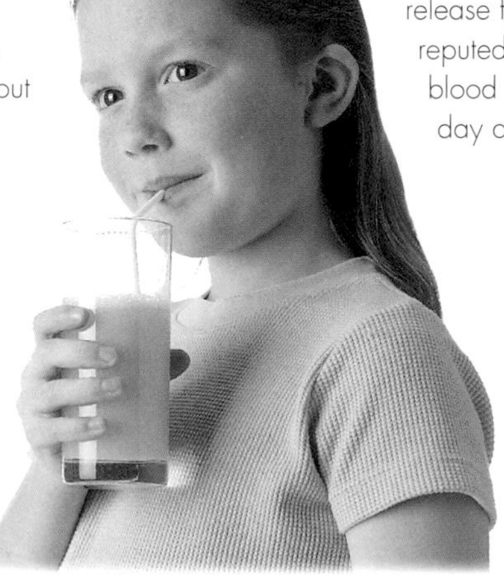

RIGHT *Liquid formulas can be added to fruit juices, making them a popular form of supplement for children.*

ANTIOXIDANTS

Much of the cell damage that occurs in disease is caused by highly destructive chemical groups known as free radicals. These are the products of oxidation, a process which occurs naturally in our body as we breathe. Today, because of the other elements in the air, there are more free radicals than ever. In small quantities free radicals can fight bacteria and viruses; in larger quantities they encourage the aging process and cause damage to our cells.

Fortunately, these can be combated by antioxidants – the ACE vitamins (vitamin A in the form of beta carotene, vitamin C, and vitamin E), and the minerals selenium and zinc, and to a lesser extent manganese and copper. Antioxidants protect other substances from oxidation. Many trials have shown that additional antioxidant vitamins – such as 2,000mg. of C and 400mg. of E daily – can significantly reduce the incidence of heart attacks, strokes, cataracts, and other diseases, and slow down the process of aging.

BELOW *Antioxidants, such as the ACE vitamins and zinc, can help combat cell damage caused by free radicals.*

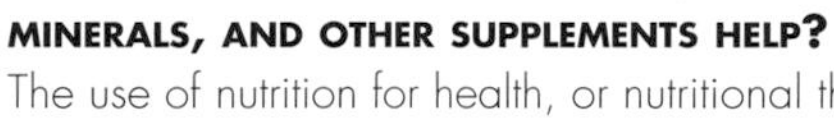

WHICH PROBLEMS CAN VITAMINS, MINERALS, AND OTHER SUPPLEMENTS HELP?

The use of nutrition for health, or nutritional therapy, can help with almost anything, since food is the basic fuel of all the chemical processes which take place in the body. Therefore, almost all ill health can have a basis in nutritional elements which are missing or insubstantial within the diet. Great success has been achieved treating conditions like rheumatism and arthritis, high blood pressure, fatigue, constipation, and other digestive disorders, the healing and recuperation processes following injury or surgery, skin problems, and many psychological and behavioral problems. Neuralgia, osteoporosis, PMS, post-natal illness, pregnancy problems, reduced immunities, stress, and viruses may respond to dietary treatment. In effect, however, all the systems in the body will be improved by a healthy diet. In a fit state you are much more likely to fight off infection and deal efficiently with any health problems or injury.

BELOW *Conditions such as rheumatism respond to dietary change, combined with vitamin and mineral supplements.*

BETA-CAROTENE

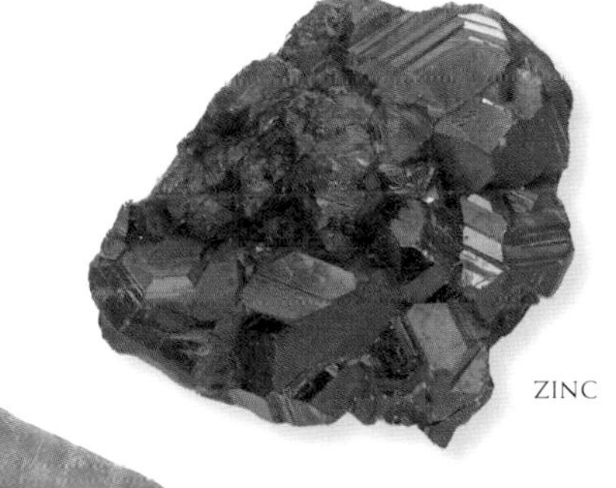

ZINC

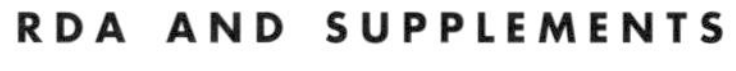

RDA AND SUPPLEMENTS

Governments around the world have provided guidelines for how much of each vitamin or mineral we need in our diets. These are called RDAs (recommended daily allowance) or RDIs (recommended daily intake) and they apply to healthy individuals with a good, balanced diet. These levels are "adequate" intake, and do not reflect new thinking on nutrition for optimal health and longevity. In other words, they are not therapeutic levels and they do not take into account the varying needs of the population. People with illnesses, a stressful lifestyle, or who are on medication, or eat a highly refined diet may need much more than the RDA.

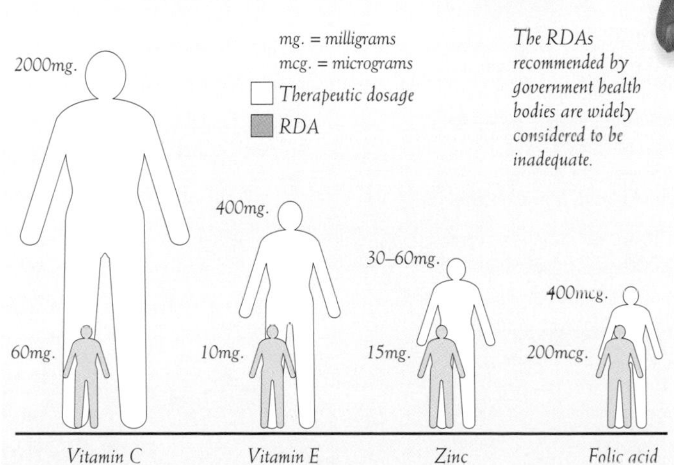

The RDAs recommended by government health bodies are widely considered to be inadequate.

VITAMIN A

U.S. RDA 3mg. E.U. RDA 800mcg.

Vitamin A is a fat-soluble vitamin that comes in two forms: retinol, which is found in animal products such as liver, eggs, butter, and cod liver oil; and beta-carotene, which our body converts into vitamin A when we need more. Beta-carotene is found in any brightly-colored fruits and vegetables.

Vitamin A was for many years called a "miracle" vitamin because of its effect on the immune system and growth. It is necessary for healthy skin and eyes, and allows us to see in the dark. Beta-carotene is an antioxidant (*see page 251*), and it has anti-carcinogenic properties.

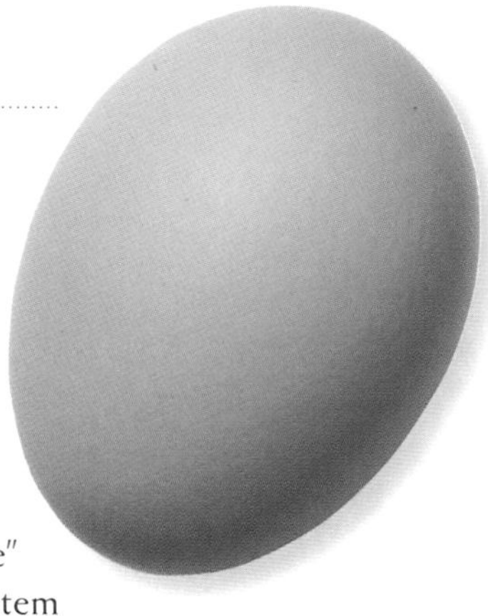

ABOVE *Retinol, one form of vitamin A, can be found in animal products such as eggs.*

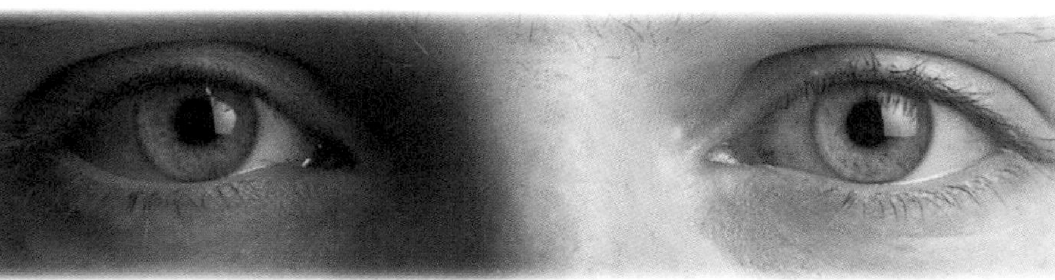

ABOVE *Vitamin A is necessary for good vision and helps prevent night blindness.*

BELOW LEFT *Carrots are a good source of beta-carotene, which our body converts into vitamin A when necessary.*

DATA FILE

Properties

- Anticarcinogenic.
- Prevents and treats skin disorders and aging of skin.
- Improves vision and prevents night blindness.
- Improves the body's ability to heal.
- Promotes the growth of strong bones, hair, teeth, skin, and gums.
- May help in the treatment of hyperthyroidism.

Best Sources

Vitamin A: cod liver oil, liver, kidney, eggs, and dairy produce.

Beta-carotene: carrots, tomatoes, watercress, broccoli, spinach, cantaloupe, apricots.

Dosage

- The RDA is a minium, and people with special needs (following illness, suffering from infections, with diabetes, for example) should have a higher level.
- Taken as vitamin A, up to 6,000mcg. is permissible if you are not pregnant.
- Taken as beta-carotene, 15mg. can be taken as a preventative measure against illness.

CAUTION

VITAMIN A AS RETINOL IS TOXIC AND SHOULD NOT BE TAKEN AT ALL AS A SUPPLEMENT BY PREGNANT WOMEN, AS IT CAN CAUSE BIRTH DEFECTS IN THE UNBORN CHILD.

B1 (THIAMINE)

U.S. RDA 1.2–1.5mg. E.U. RDA 1.4mg.

Thiamine is involved in all key metabolic processes in the nervous system, the heart, the blood cells, and the muscle. It is useful in the treatment of nervous disorders, and can protect against imbalances caused by alcoholism.

There are more cases of vitamin B1 deficiency than of any other nutritional element – this has been said to be due to a growth in alcoholism. Thiamine is found in all plant and animal foods, but good sources are whole grains, brown rice, seafood, and pulses.

DATA FILE

Properties

- Protects against imbalances caused by alcohol consumption.
- B1 may be useful in treating heart disease.
- May be beneficial in the treatment of neurological disease (particularly when caused by B1 deficiency).
- May help to treat anemia.
- May improve people's mental agility.
- May help to control diabetes which has been linked to deficiency.
- Useful in the treatment of herpes and infections.
- Helps to convert sugar to energy, in the muscles and the bones.

Best Sources

Pork, milk, eggs, whole grains, organ meats, brown rice, barley, seafood.

Dosage

- Heavy drinkers, smokers, pregnant women, or those taking the pill should increase normal dosage to up to 100–300mg. per day.
- Increase intake in stressful conditions. Will be most effective as part of a good B-complex supplement.

CAUTION

THIAMINE IS NONTOXIC, BUT IT IS RECOMMENDED THAT YOU DO NOT TAKE MORE THAN 400MG. DAILY.

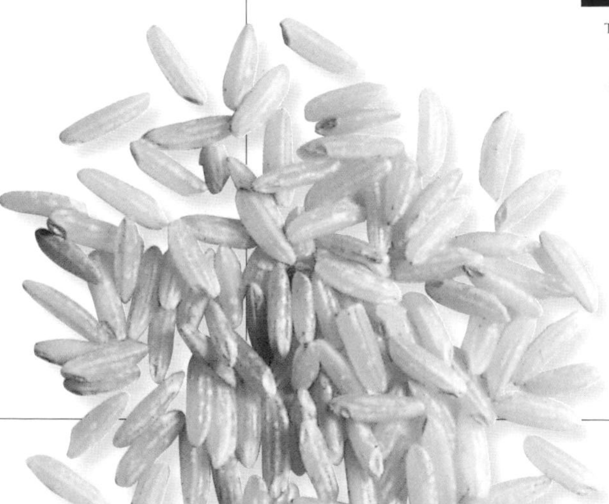

LEFT *Brown rice can help protect against imbalances caused by alcohol as it contains thiamine.*

B2 (RIBOFLAVIN)

U.S. RDA 1.7mg. E.U. RDA 1.6mg.

Riboflavin is a water-soluble member of the B-complex family of vitamins. It is crucial to the production of body energy and has antioxidant qualities. Riboflavin is not stored in any significant amount in the body, and deficiency is common.

Riboflavin is necessary for healthy skin, hair, and nails. Because it is destroyed by sunlight, it is recommended that you keep foods containing this vitamin in a dark, cool place. In particular, milk loses its riboflavin content after only two hours' exposure to sun.

BELOW *Dairy products, such as cheese, are one of the best sources of riboflavin. Intake should be increased during pregnancy and breast-feeding.*

CAUTION

RIBOFLAVIN IS NONTOXIC IN MOST DOSES, BUT IT IS RECOMMENDED THAT YOU DO NOT TAKE IN EXCESS OF 400MG. PER DAY UNLESS SUPERVISED BY A REGISTERED PRACTITIONER.

DATA FILE

Properties

- Works with enzymes to metabolize fats, protein, and carbohydrates.
- Aids vision.
- Promotes healthy skin, hair, and nails.
- Promotes healthy growth and reproductive function.
- Boosts athletic performance.
- Protects against cancer.
- Protects against anemia.

Best Sources

Milk, eggs, cheese, fortified breads and cereals, green leafy vegetables, fish.

Dosage

- Pregnancy, breast-feeding, taking the pill, and heavy drinking all call for an increased intake.
- Take as part of a B-complex supplement, and increase dosage in stressful situations. 100–300mg. is commonly suggested.

ABOVE *Avocado is a rich source of many vitamins, including niacin.*

CAUTION

IN HIGH DOSES, NIACIN MAY CAUSE DEPRESSION, LIVER MALFUNCTION, FLUSHING, AND HEADACHES.

AVOID DOSES LARGER THAN ABOUT 120MG. UNLESS YOU ARE UNDER THE SUPERVISION OF A REGISTERED PRACTITIONER.

B3 (NIACIN)

U.S. RDA 13–18mg. adults, 5–6mg. infants, 9–13mg. children under ten. E.U. RDA 15–18mg.

Niacin is one of the water-soluble B-complex vitamins, and it is essential for the synthesis of sex hormones and a healthy nervous system. Niacin may also be valuable in helping to prevent and treat schizophrenia, and in acting as a detoxicant, ridding the body of toxins, pollutants, and drugs.

Niacin takes the form of nicotinic acid and nicotinamide, and is a fairly recent addition to the family of B-complex vitamins, named as a vitamin only in 1937. Niacin has been shown to lower blood cholesterol and other body fats, and is useful in the prevention of heart disease. It may help to prevent diabetes.

DATA FILE

Properties

- Prevents and treats schizophrenia.
- Aids in cell respiration.
- Produces energy from sugar, fat, and protein.
- Maintains clear, healthy skin, nerves, tongue, and good digestion.
- May lower cholesterol and therefore protect against heart disease.
- Believed to be antioxidant.
- May prevent migraine headaches.
- Reduces blood pressure.
- May alleviate arthritis.

Best Sources

Meat, fish, wholegrain cereals, eggs, milk, cheese.

Dosage

- Large doses may be used therapeutically, but should be taken under the supervision of a physician or health practitioner.
- Doses of 20–100mg. of niacin, taken daily, may be beneficial. Best taken as part of a B-complex supplement.

BELOW *Eating foods rich in niacin, such as milk and wholegrain cereals, may lower cholesterol levels and protect against heart disease.*

B5 (PANTOTHENIC ACID)

U.S. RDA 10mg. E.U. RDA 6mg.

Pantothenic acid is a water-soluble member of the B-complex family of vitamins that helps maintain normal growth and the health of the nervous system. Pantothenic acid has become a popular supplement over the past decade for its ability to boost energy levels and improve immune response.

There is also evidence that pantothenic acid can lower cholesterol and protect against heart disease. Pantothenic acid is useful in reducing the effects of stress on the body, and is needed to convert choline into acetylcholine, which is necessary for brain functioning.

CAUTION

NO KNOWN TOXICITY, ALTHOUGH DOSES OF OVER 300MG. PER DAY SHOULD BE SUPERVISED BY A PRACTITIONER.

SOME PEOPLE REPORT STOMACH UPSETS AT DOSES HIGHER THAN 10G.

ABOVE *Pantothenic acid is an ideal supplement to take to boost the immune system.*

DATA FILE

Properties

- B5 encourages the healing of wounds.
- Helps the body in the production of energy.
- Reduces stress levels.
- Controls the metabolism of fat.
- Encourages functioning of the immune system.
- Prevents fatigue.
- Lowers cholesterol levels and so protects against heart disease.
- Prevents arthritis, and also treats it.
- May prevent hair loss and graying of hair.

Best Sources

Yeast, organ meats, eggs, brown rice, wholegrain cereals, molasses.

Dosage

- Best taken in B-complex formulas, up to 300mg. per day for therapeutic use.
- The normal dosage, which should help to prevent disease, is about 100mg. per day.

LEFT *An adequate intake of vitamin B5 will help to keep your hair in good condition.*

B6 (PYRIDOXINE)

U.S. RDA 2mg. E.U. RDA 1.6–2mg.

Pyridoxine is a water-soluble B-complex vitamin which is necessary for the production of antibodies and white blood cells. B6 is necessary for the absorption of vitamin B12. B6 is required for the functioning of more than 60 enzymes in the body and also for protein synthesis.

Of all the B vitamins, B6 is the most important for a healthy immune system, and it is thought to protect the body against some cancers. B6 is widely used for relieving the symptoms of PMS and menopause, and may cure some forms of infertility. This vitamin is also used to prevent skin inflammation, and maintain healthy teeth and gums.

DATA FILE

Properties

- Boosts immunity.
- Helps to control diabetes.
- B6 assimilates proteins and fats.
- Helps prevent skin and nervous disorders.
- Alleviates nausea.
- Treats symptoms of PMS and menopause.
- Reduces muscle cramps and spasms.
- Acts as a natural diuretic.
- Protects against cancer.

Best Sources

Meat, fish, milk, eggs, wholegrain cereals, vegetables.

Dosage

- Should always be taken as part of a B-complex supplement, and in equal amounts with B1 and B2.
- Time-release formulas are best because it lasts for only eight hours in the body.

CAUTION

VITAMIN B6 IS TOXIC IN HIGH DOSES, CAUSING SERIOUS NERVE DAMAGE WHEN TAKEN AT QUANTITIES OF MORE THAN 2G. PER DAY.

SOME PEOPLE REPORT SIDE-EFFECTS WITH DOSES AS LOW AS 100MG.

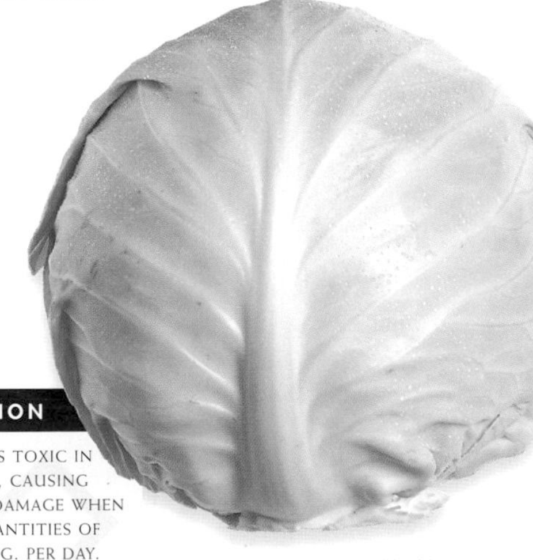

ABOVE *Vegetables like cabbage are one of the best sources of B6 and will help protect against cancer.*

B9 (FOLIC ACID)

U.S. RDA 400mcg. E.U. RDA 200–360mcg.

Folic acid is a water-soluble vitamin that forms part of the B-complex family. It is also known as vitamin Bc or vitamin B9. Low levels of folic acid may lead to anemia. Folic acid is essential for the division of body cells, and it is also necessary for the utilization of sugar and amino acids.

Recent findings indicate that folic acid can prevent some types of cancer and birth defects, and it is helpful in the treatment of heart disease. Most folic acid deficiency is the result of a poor diet, because it is abundant in foods such as leafy green vegetables, yeast, and liver. Taken from just before conception, and particularly in the first trimester of pregnancy, folic acid can help to prevent spina bifida.

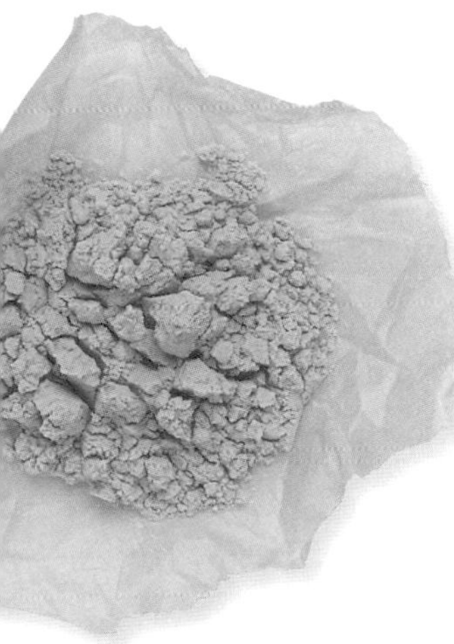

ABOVE *Folic acid is part of the B-complex family. It helps prevent some types of cancer.*

DATA FILE

Properties

- Improves lactation.
- May protect against cancer.
- Improves skin condition.
- Natural analgesic.
- Increases appetite in debilitated patients.
- Needed for metabolism of RNA and DNA.
- Helps form blood.
- Builds up babies' resistance to infection.
- Essential for transmission of genetic code.
- Prevents spina bifida.

Best Sources

Green leafy vegetables, wheat germ, nuts, eggs, bananas, oranges, and organ meats.

Dosage

- There are many people at risk of deficiency, including heavy drinkers, pregnant women, the elderly, and those on low-fat diets. Supplementation at 400–800mcg. is recommended for those at risk.
- It is best taken with a good multivitamin and mineral supplement.

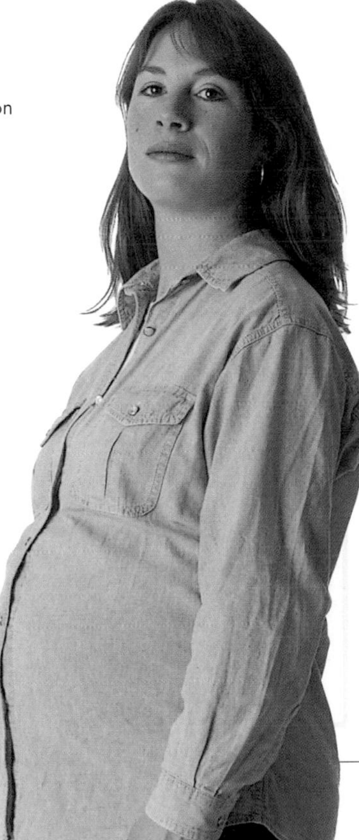

RIGHT *Recent scientific studies have shown that folic acid can help prevent birth defects such as spina bifida if taken prior to conception and during the first trimester.*

CAUTION

FOLIC ACID IS TOXIC IN LARGE DOSES AND CAN CAUSE SEVERE NEUROLOGICAL PROBLEMS.

HIGH DOSES MAY CAUSE INSOMNIA AND INTERFERE WITH THE ABSORPTION OF ZINC IN THE BODY.

B12 (COBALAMIN)

U.S. RDA 3mcg. E.U. RDA 2mcg.

Cobalamin is a water-soluble member of the B-complex vitamin family, and it is the only vitamin that contains essential minerals. B12 is essential for the healthy metabolism of nerve tissue, and deficiencies can cause brain damage and neurological disorders.

Vitamin B12 was once considered to be a "wonder drug" and was given by injection to rejuvenate. B12 may also reduce the risk of cancer and the severity of allergies, as well as boosting energy levels. Low levels of this vitamin result in anemia.

ABOVE LEFT *A deficiency of B12 can result in anemia.*

DATA FILE

Properties

- Needed for maintenance of the nervous system.
- Improves memory and concentration.
- Required to utilize fats, carbohydrates, and proteins.
- Increases energy.
- Promotes healthy growth in children.
- May protect against cancer.
- Protects against allergens and toxic elements.

Best Sources

Liver, beef, pork, eggs, cheese, fish, milk.

Dosage

- Dosages of 5–50mcg. should be adequate for most people; higher dosages should be supervised.
- Best taken as part of a B-complex supplement.

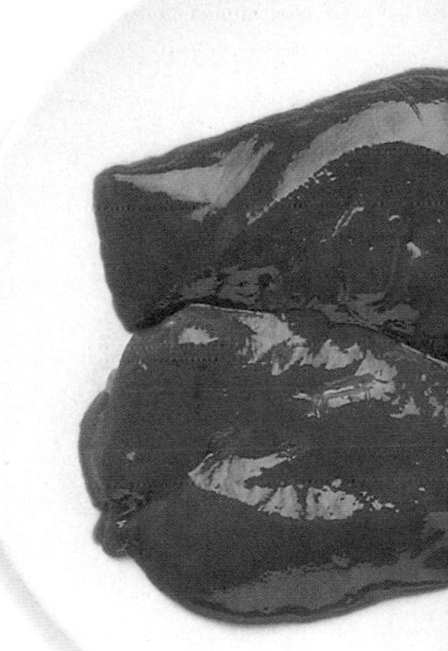

ABOVE *B12, necessary for proper maintenance of the nervous system, can be found in liver.*

CAUTION

ALTHOUGH VITAMIN B12 IS NOT CONSIDERED TO BE TOXIC, IT IS RECOMMENDED THAT YOU DO NOT TAKE MORE THAN 200MG. DAILY UNLESS YOU ARE UNDER THE SUPERVISION OF A REGISTERED PRACTITIONER.

Vitamin C

U.S. RDA 60mg. E.U. RDA 60mg.

Vitamin C is water soluble, which means that it is not stored by the body and we need to ensure that we get adequate amounts in our daily diet. More people take vitamin C than any other supplement, and yet studies show that a large percentage of the population have deficiencies.

Vitamin C is also known as ascorbic acid, and it is one of the most versatile of the vitamins we need to sustain life. It is one of the antioxidant vitamins (*see page 251*) and is believed to boost immunity, and to fight cancer and infection.

DATA FILE

Properties

- Reduces cholesterol and helps prevent heart disease.
- Speeds up the healing of wounds.
- Maintains healthy bones, teeth, and sex organs.
- Acts as a natural antihistamine.
- May help to overcome male infertility.
- Fights cancer.
- Boosts immunity and reduces the duration of colds and other viruses.
- Helps maintenance of good vision.
- Antioxidant.

Best Sources

Rosehips, blackcurrants, broccoli, citrus fruits, all fresh fruits and vegetables.

Dosage

- At least 60mg. per day is necessary for health, but more is required by smokers (25mg. is depleted with every cigarette), and people who are under stress, taking antibiotics, suffering from an infection, drink heavily, as well as after an accident or injury.
- Daily dosages of up to 1,500mg. per day appear to be safe, but take this in three doses, preferably with meals, and use a time-release formula.

BELOW *Rosehips are a good source of this important vitamin.*

ABOVE *Citrus fruits like oranges are rich in vitamin C.*

CAUTION

VITAMIN C MAY CAUSE KIDNEY STONES AND GOUT IN SOME INDIVIDUALS.

SOME PEOPLE SUFFER FROM DIARRHEA AND CRAMPS AT HIGH DOSAGES, ALTHOUGH THE VITAMIN IS CONSIDERED TO BE NONTOXIC AT EVEN VERY HIGH LEVELS.

Vitamin D

U.S. RDA 10mcg.
E.U. RDA 5mcg.

Vitamin D is a fat-soluble vitamin that is found in foods of animal origin and is known as the "sunshine" vitamin. Vitamin D can be produced in the skin from the energy of the sun, and it is not found in rich supply in any food.

ABOVE *The human body will manufacture vitamin D itself if the skin is exposed to sunlight.*

Vitamin D is important for calcium and phosphorus absorption, and helps to regulate calcium metabolism. Recent research suggests that it could have a role in protecting against some cancers and infectious diseases. Deficiency is caused by inadequate exposure to sunlight, and low consumption of foods containing vitamin D.

DATA FILE

Properties

- Protects against osteoporosis.
- May help in the treatment of psoriasis.
- Boosts immune system.
- May be useful in the treatment of cancer.
- Protects against cancer.
- Necessary for strong teeth and bones.

Best Sources

Animal produce, such as milk, eggs, oily fish, butter, cheese, cod liver oil.

Dosage

- Supplementation between 5–10mcg. is suggested for those at risk of deficiency.

CAUTION

VITAMIN D IS THE MOST TOXIC OF ALL THE VITAMINS, CAUSING NAUSEA, VOMITING, HEADACHE, AND DEPRESSION, AMONG OTHER PROBLEMS.

DO NOT TAKE IN EXCESS OF 10MCG. DAILY.

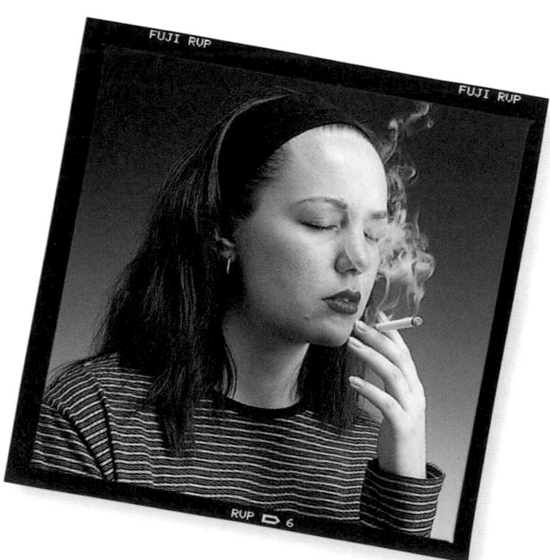

BELOW *It has been shown that smoking seriously hampers the body's ability to absorb vitamins.*

BELOW *Animal foods, such as oily fish, contain vitamin D, although sunlight, not food, is this vitamin's best source.*

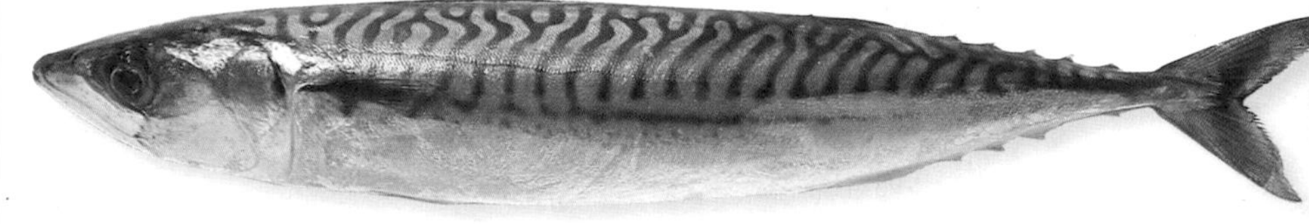

Vitamin E

U.S. RDA 20mg. E.U. RDA 10mg.

Vitamin E is fat soluble and one of the key antioxidant vitamins (*see page 251*). Its key function is as an anticoagulant, but its role in boosting the immune system and protecting against cardiovascular disease is becoming increasingly clear.

Apart from its crucial antioxidant value, vitamin E is important for the production of energy and the maintenance of health at every level. Unlike most fat-soluble vitamins, vitamin E is stored in the body for only a short period of time, and up to 75 percent of a daily dose is excreted in the feces.

DATA FILE

Properties

- Antioxidant, so helps to slow the process of aging.
- Protects against neurological disorders.
- Boosts immunity.
- Protects against cardiovascular disease.
- Alleviates fatigue.
- Accelerates healing, particularly of burns.
- Reduces the various symptoms of PMS.
- Treats skin problems and baldness.
- Helps prevent miscarriage.
- Acts as a natural diuretic.
- Prevents formation of thickened scars.

Best Sources

Wheat germ (fresh), soybeans, vegetable oils, broccoli, leafy green vegetables, whole grains, peanuts, eggs.

Dosage

- Available in many forms (the dry form is best for people with skin problems or oil intolerance).
- Daily dosage may be from 250–280mg., but you may be advised to take higher doses in some cases.

CAUTION

VITAMIN E IS NONTOXIC, EVEN IN HIGH DOSES, BUT IT IS SUGGESTED THAT YOU DO NOT TAKE IN EXCESS OF 350MG. UNLESS YOU ARE SUPERVISED BY A REGISTERED PRACTITIONER.

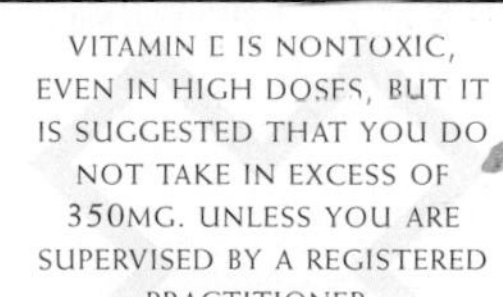

BELOW LEFT *One of the main antioxidant vitamins, vitamin E can be found in vegetable oils.*

BIOTIN (VITAMIN H)

U.S. RDA 300mcg. E.U. RDA 0.15mg.

Biotin is not a true vitamin, but it works with B-complex vitamins and is often called vitamin H, or co-enzyme R. Biotin is water soluble and is found in many common foods. It is essential for breaking down and metabolizing fats in the body.

Biotin is depleted in the body by alcohol, cooking or refining food, antibiotics, and when taken with raw egg whites, which contain avidin, a protein that prevents biotin absorption. Biotin works more effectively with vitamins B2, B6, B3, and A.

CAUTION

BIOTIN IS NONTOXIC, BUT IT IS SUGGESTED THAT YOU DO NOT TAKE IN EXCESS OF 300MG. UNLESS SUPERVISED BY A REGISTERED PRACTITIONER.

DATA FILE

Properties

- Prevents the hair from turning gray.
- Eases various muscular aches and pains.
- Treats eczema, dermatitis, and other skin conditions.
- Helps to prevent baldness.

Best Sources

Nuts, fruits, beef liver, egg yolks, milk, kidneys, unpolished rice, and brewer's yeast.

Dosage

- Biotin is normally included in most readily-available B-complex supplements.

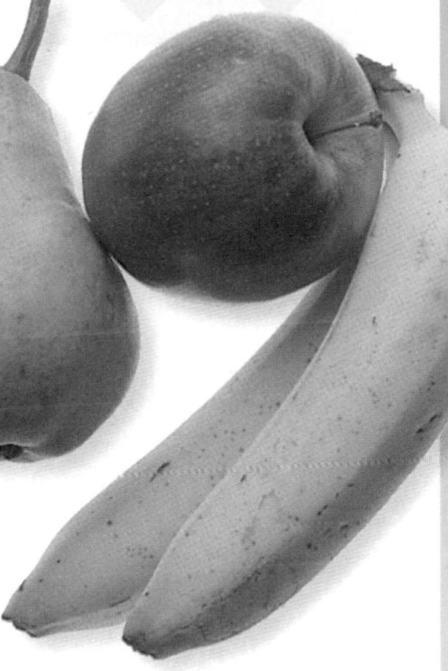

ABOVE *Found in fruits, biotin is essential for energy release from fats.*

Vitamin K

U.S. RDA none. E.U. RDA none.

The K vitamins are fat soluble, and are necessary for normal blood clotting. They are often used to treat the toxic effects of anticoagulant drops, such as Warfarin, and in people who have a poor ability to absorb fats.

Vitamin K occurs naturally in foods as vitamin K1, and is produced by intestinal bacteria as vitamin K2. Synthetic vitamin K is known as K3. Vitamin K1 injections are routinely given to newborn babies to prevent hemorrhage, but since a recent scare linked the vitamin with childhood leukemia it is now more often given as oral drops.

DATA FILE

Properties

- Controls blood clotting.

Best Sources

Cauliflower, spinach, peas, wholegrain cereals.

Dosage

- We need an estimated 500–1,000mcg. of vitamin K from our diet per day.

CAUTION

THERE ARE NO REPORTS OF TOXICITY, BUT BECAUSE OF THE POSSIBILITY THAT INJECTED VITAMIN K MAY BE RELATED TO CHILDHOOD LEUKEMIA, ORAL DROPS ARE SUGGESTED FOR NEWBORNS.

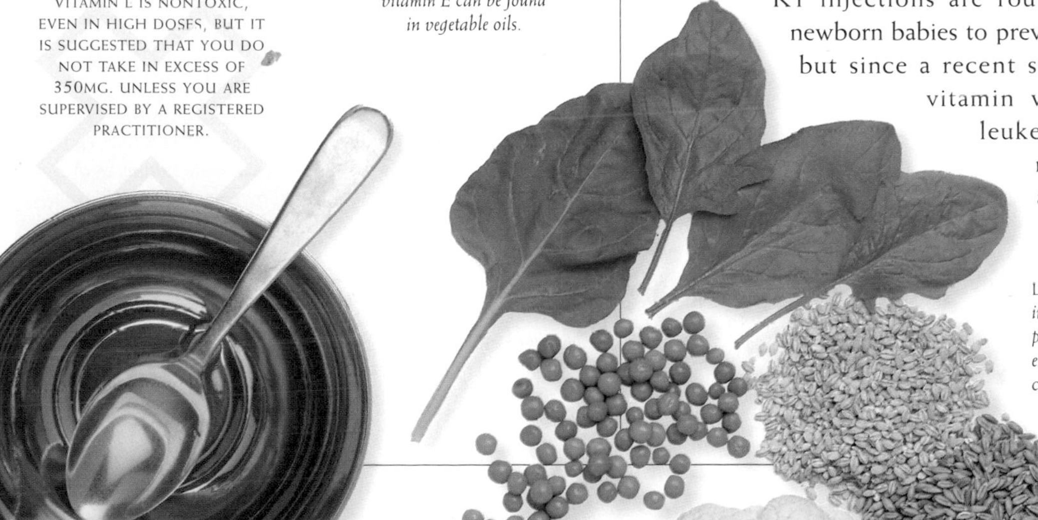

LEFT *Vitamin K, found in cauliflower, spinach, peas, and wholegrains, is essential for normal blood clotting.*

VITAMIN B BORON

U.S. RDA none. E.U. RDA none.

Boron is a trace mineral found in most plants, and it is essential for human health. Recent research has reported that boron added to the diet of post-menopausal women prevents calcium loss and bone demineralization – a revolutionary discovery for sufferers of osteoporosis.

It is also claimed that boron will raise testosterone levels and build muscle in men, and boron is therefore often used by athletes and bodybuilders. Boron is found in most fruit and vegetables, and does not appear in meat and meat products. Boron supplements are usually taken in the form of sodium borate.

DATA FILE

Properties

- Assists in the external treatment of bacterial and fungal infections.
- Helps to lower the incidence of arthritis.
- Prevents osteoporosis.
- Used to build muscles.

Best Sources

Root vegetables (such as potatoes, parsnips, and carrots) grown in soil that is rich in boron.

Dosage

- No RDA, but it is suggested that 3mg. should be taken daily to prevent osteoporosis.

CAUTION

BORON CAN BE TOXIC, WITH SYMPTOMS INCLUDING A RED RASH, VOMITING, DIARRHEA, REDUCED CIRCULATION, SHOCK, AND THEN COMA.

A FATAL DOSE IS 15–20G., 3–6G. IN CHILDREN. SYMPTOMS APPEAR AT ABOUT 100MG.

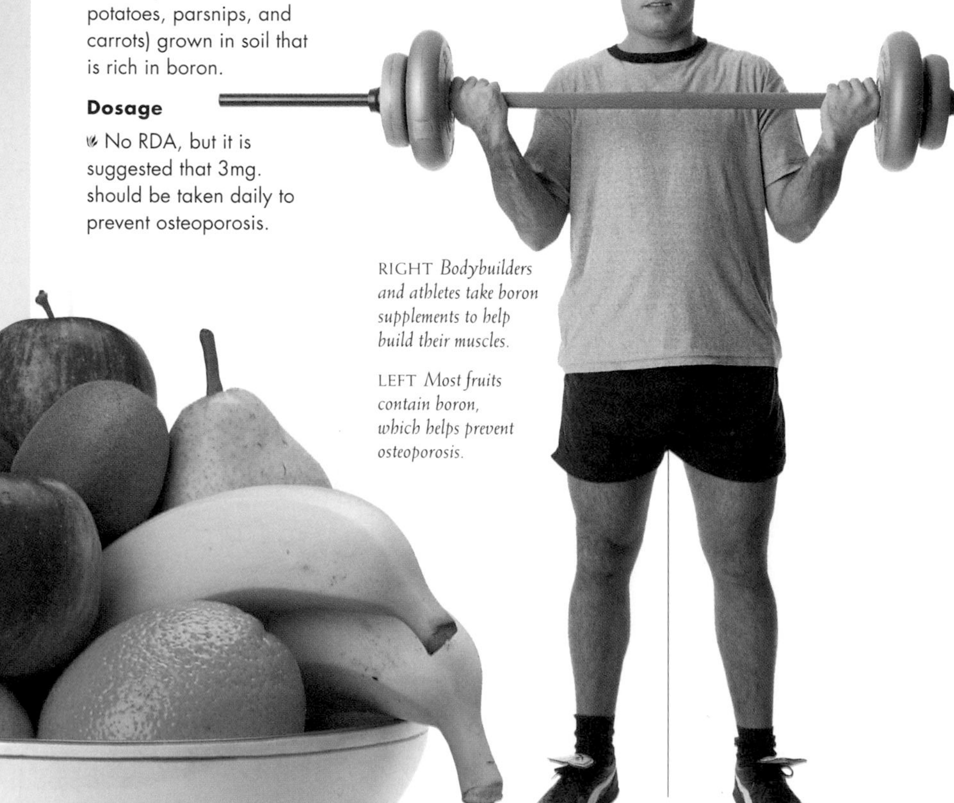

RIGHT *Bodybuilders and athletes take boron supplements to help build their muscles.*

LEFT *Most fruits contain boron, which helps prevent osteoporosis.*

Ca CALCIUM

U.S. RDA 800–1,200mg. E.U. RDA 800mg.

Calcium is an important mineral, and recent research shows that we get only about one-third of what we need for good health. Calcium is essential for human life – it makes up bones and teeth, and is crucial in the process of conducting messages along nerves. It ensures that our muscles contract, and that our hearts beat, and it is extremely important in the maintenance of the immune system, among other things.

There are many groups at risk of calcium deficiency – in particular the elderly – and because it is so important to body processes our bodies take what they need from our bones, which causes them to become thin and brittle. It is used therapeutically for allergies, depression, panic attacks, insomnia, and hyperactivity, and extra should be taken during pregnancy and while breast-feeding.

CAUTION

DOSES OVER 2,000MG. PER DAY MAY CAUSE HYPERCALCEMIA (CALCIUM DEPOSITS IN THE KIDNEYS), BUT SINCE EXCESS CALCIUM IS EXCRETED, IT IS UNLIKELY TO OCCUR UNLESS YOU ARE TAKING EXCESS QUANTITIES OF VITAMIN D ALONGSIDE.

RIGHT *All dairy products are rich in calcium, essential for healthy bones and teeth.*

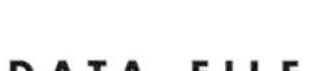

DATA FILE

Properties

- Prevents osteoporosis, and helps to treat the condition once symptoms manifest.
- Prevents cancer.
- Useful in the treatment of high blood pressure.
- Prevents heart disease.
- Useful in treating arthritis.
- Helps to keep skin healthy.
- Alleviates leg cramps.
- Encourages regular beating of the heart.
- Soothes insomnia.
- Helps the body to metabolize iron.
- Necessary for nerve-impulse transmission and muscular function.

Best Sources

Milk, cheese, dairy produce, leafy green vegetables, hard tap water, salmon, tinned fish, eggs, beans, nuts, tofu.

Dosage

- Experts recommend that calcium be taken in a good multivitamin and mineral supplement, although extra doses may be given up to 1,000mg. per day.
- More calcium is needed by women after the menopause, and while pregnant or breast-feeding.

Co COBALT

U.S. RDA none.
E.U. RDA none

Cobalt is an essential trace mineral. It is a constituent of vitamin B12. The amount of cobalt in the body is dependent on the amount of cobalt in the soil, and therefore in the food we eat. Most of us are not deficient in cobalt, although deficiency is much more common in vegetarians.

CAUTION

WHEN USED THERAPEUTICALLY, SIDE-EFFECTS OCCUR AT DOSES ABOVE 30MG.; THESE INCLUDE GOITER, HYPERTHYROIDISM, AND HEART FAILURE.

DATA FILE

Properties

Cobalt is able, with vitamin B12, to:

- Prevent pernicious anemia.
- Help in the production of red blood cells.
- Aid in the synthesis of DNA and choline.
- Encourage a healthy nervous system.
- Reduce blood pressure.
- Maintain myelin, the fatty sheath protecting the nerves.

Best Sources

Fresh leafy green vegetables, meat, liver, milk, oysters, clams.

Dosage

- Cobalt is rarely found in supplement form, but forms part of a good multivitamin and mineral supplement with the B-complex vitamins.
- An intake of 8mcg. daily appears to be adequate.
- Used therapeutically, side-effects occur at doses above 30mg. – hypothyroidism, goiter, and heart failure.

Cu COPPER

U.S. RDA 1.5–3mg. E.U. RDA 1.2mg.

Copper is an essential trace mineral, and is necessary for respiration – iron and copper are required for oxygen to be synthesized in red blood cells. Copper is also important for the production of collagen, which is responsible for the health of our bones, cartilage, and skin. Copper is also one of the antioxidant minerals (*see page 251*), which protect against free-radical damage. Arthritis sufferers report that copper bracelets reduce pain and inflammation associated with the condition, probably because traces of the mineral are absorbed by the skin and enter the bloodstream.

DATA FILE

Properties

- May prevent cancer.
- Protects against cardiovascular disease.
- Useful mineral in the treatment of arthritis.
- Boosts the immune system.
- Acts as an antioxidant.

Best Sources

Animal livers, shellfish, nuts, fruit, oysters, kidneys, and legumes.

Dosage

- Copper appears in good multivitamin and mineral supplements, and can be taken alone up to 3mg. daily.

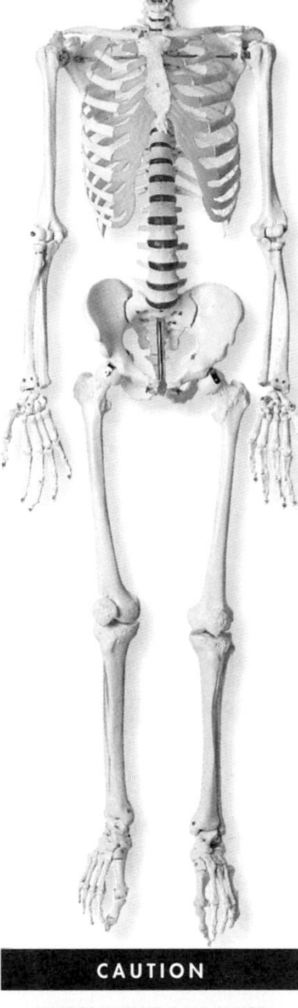

ABOVE RIGHT *Copper is important for collagen production, essential for healthy bones.*

CAUTION

EXCESS INTAKE CAN CAUSE VOMITING, DIARRHEA, MUSCULAR PAIN, AND DEMENTIA.

Cr CHROMIUM

U.S. RDA none. E.U. RDA none.

Chromium is a trace mineral that was discovered in the 1950s. It is an important regulator of blood sugar, and has been used successfully in the control and treatment of diabetes. It is involved in the metabolism of carbohydrates and fats, and is used in the production of insulin in the body.

High levels of sugars in the diet cause chromium to be excreted through the kidneys, so it is important to get enough in your diet if you eat sugary foods. The incidence of diabetes and heart disease decreases with increased levels of chromium in the body.

DATA FILE

Properties

- Aids in the control and production of insulin.
- Aids in the metabolism of carbohydrates and fats.
- Controls levels of cholesterol in the blood.
- Stimulates the synthesis of proteins in the body.
- Increases general resistance to infection.
- Suppresses hunger pains.

Best Sources

Wholegrain cereals, meat, cheese, brewer's yeast, molasses, egg yolk.

Dosage

- There is no RDA, but it is suggested that 25mcg. per day is adequate.
- If necessary, supplements of up to 200mcg. per day can be taken.

CAUTION

THERE IS NO EVIDENCE THAT CHROMIUM IS TOXIC, EVEN IN HIGH DOSES, SINCE ANY EXCESS IS EXCRETED. HOWEVER, IT IS SUGGESTED THAT YOU DO NOT TAKE MORE THAN 200MCG. DAILY UNLESS SUPERVISED BY A REGISTERED PRACTITIONER.

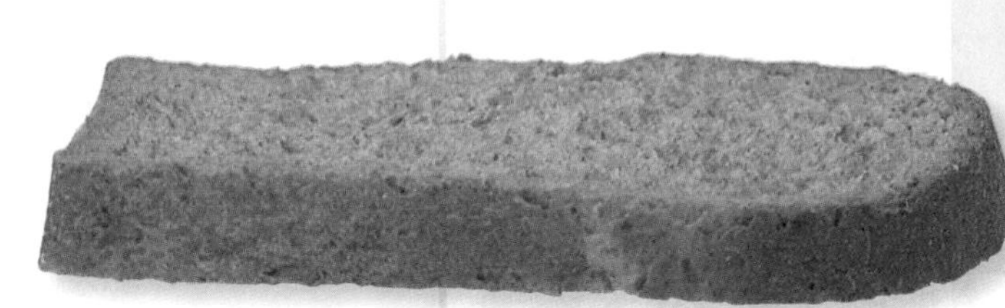

RIGHT *Eat wholegrain bread to ensure an adequate intake of chromium.*

F FLUORINE

U.S. RDA 1mg. fluoride, 3.6mg. sodium fluoride.
E.U. RDA none.

Fluorine is a trace mineral found naturally in soil, water, plants, and animal tissues. Its electrically charged form is "fluoride," which is how we usually refer to it. Although it has not yet been officially recognized as an essential nutrient, studies show that it is important in many processes, and may play a major role in the prevention of many 20th-century killers, like heart disease.

The major source of fluorine is drinking water, which is sometimes fluoridated, or has enough naturally occurring fluoride to make fluoridation unnecessary. Fluoride supplements should always be taken with calcium.

ABOVE *Fluoride can be found in many makes of toothpaste.*

DATA FILE

Properties

- Fluorine protects against dental caries.
- Protects against, and also treats, osteoporosis.
- It may help to prevent heart disease.
- May help to prevent calcification of organs and musculoskeletal structures.

Best Sources

Seafood, animal meat, fluoridated drinking water, and tea.

Dosage

- The major source is drinking water, and typical daily intake is 1–2mg.
- Tablets and drops are available from pharmacies, but should be limited to 1mg. daily in adults, and 0.25–0.5mg. for children.

CAUTION

AN EXCESS OF FLUORIDE CAUSES FLUOROSIS, CHARACTERIZED BY IRREGULAR PATCHES ON TOOTH ENAMEL, AND DEPRESSES THE APPETITE. EVENTUALLY THE SPINE CALCIFIES. FLUOROSIS IS RARE AND OCCURS AT LEVELS FAR ABOVE 10MG. PER DAY.

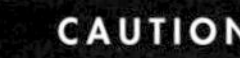

DO NOT SUPPLEMENT FLUORIDE WITHOUT THE ADVICE OF YOUR DENTIST.

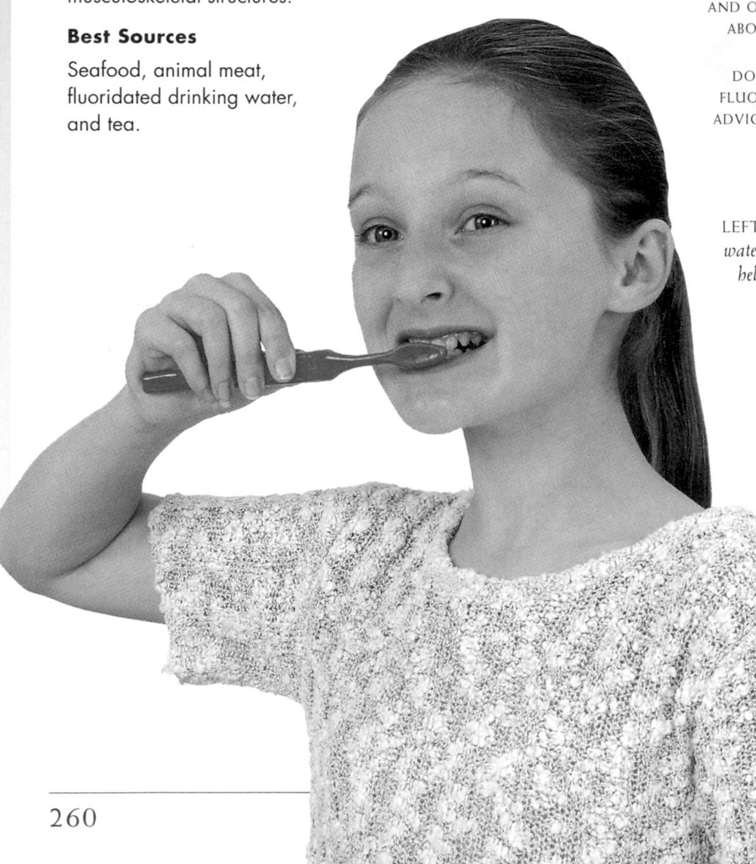

LEFT *Fluoride in drinking water and dental products helps to prevent dental cavities.*

Fe IRON

U.S. RDA 10–18mg., pregnant women 30mg.
E.U. RDA 14mg.

Iron is a trace mineral which is essential for human health. Iron-deficiency anemia, which is the condition most commonly associated with deficiency, was described by Egyptian physicists as long ago as 1500 B.C.E. Today, 10 percent of all women in the Western world suffer from iron-deficiency anemia.

We now know that iron is present in our bodies as hemoglobin, which is the red pigment of blood. Iron is required for muscle protein and is stored in the liver, spleen, bone marrow, and muscles. Efficient absorption of iron is highest in childhood, and reduces as we age. Our bodies need vitamin C in order to assimilate iron in an effective fashion.

CAUTION

EXCESS IRON CAN CAUSE CONSTIPATION, DIARRHEA, AND, RARELY, IN HIGH DOSES, DEATH.

BE VERY CAUTIOUS WHEN GIVING CHILDREN IRON SUPPLEMENTS – EVEN DOSES AS LITTLE AS 3G. CAN CAUSE DEATH.

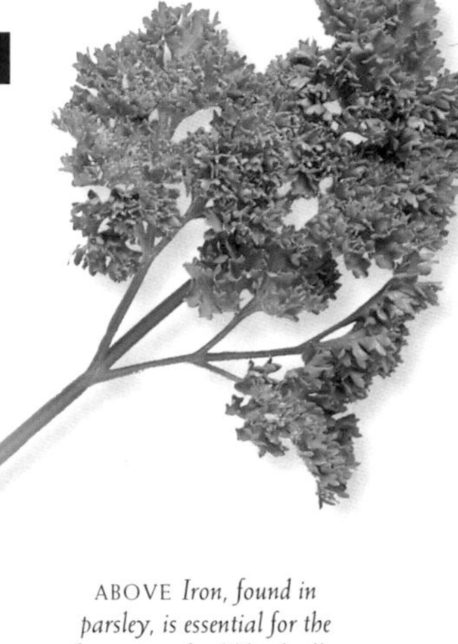

ABOVE *Iron, found in parsley, is essential for the formation of red blood cells.*

DATA FILE

Properties

- Improves physical performance.
- Anti-carcinogenic.
- Prevents learning problems in children.
- Prevents and cures iron-deficiency anemia.
- Improves immunity.
- Boosts energy levels.
- Encourages restful sleep and maintains energy levels.

Best Sources

Shellfish, brewer's yeast, wheat bran, offal, cocoa powder, dried fruit, cereals.

Dosage

- Pregnant, breast-feeding, and menstruating women, infants, children, athletes, and vegetarians may require increased levels of iron. Your general physician will prescribe iron supplements if they are necessary.
- Maximum dosage is around 15mg. daily, unless under medical supervision.

Ge GERMANIUM

U.S. RDA none. E.U. RDA none.

Germanium is a mineral which is abundant in the surface of the earth. Almost all foods commonly eaten contain some germanium. Some conditions have been reported to respond favorably to germanium given at therapeutic doses, including arthritis, angina, stroke, Raynauds disease, burns, and pain associated with cancer.

Germanium is believed to function by boosting the action of oxygen in generating energy. Because it maintains an equilibrium within the body, germanium is said to reduce high blood pressure, lower cholesterol levels, and generally to exert a good effect on the immune system. Germanium is now considered to be one of the antioxidant minerals (*see page 251*).

ABOVE *Although it is a useful mineral in the treatment of cancer, it is recommended that germanium supplement should only be taken with medical supervision.*

BELOW *The mineral germanium is found in almost all commonly eaten foods including garlic.*

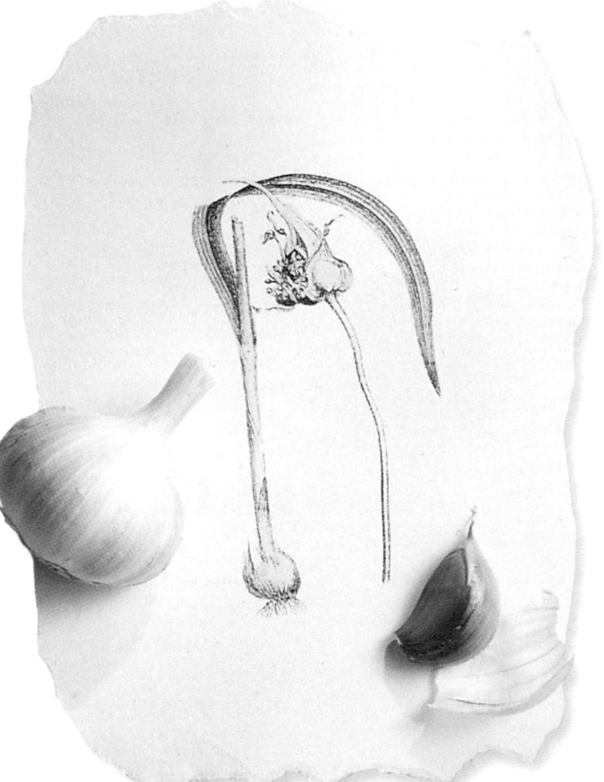

CAUTION

GERMANIUM IS SAFE UP TO QUITE A HIGH LEVEL, ALTHOUGH SKIN ERUPTIONS AND DIARRHEA HAVE BEEN REPORTED IN SOME PATIENTS TAKING THERAPEUTIC DOSES. ONLY USE THE SUPPLEMENT UNDER THE SUPERVISION OF A PHYSICIAN OR NUTRITIONIST.

DATA FILE

Properties

- Maintains the homeostasis in the body, and therefore may reduce high blood pressure and cholesterol levels.
- Germanium boosts the immune system.
- May be analgesic.
- May have antiviral, antibacterial, and antitumor activity.
- Useful as part of a cancer treatment program.
- Helps chronic Epstein-Barr virus syndrome.
- Useful in the treatment of HIV/AIDS.

Best Sources

Bran, whole wheat flour, vegetables, seeds, meats, dairy products.

Dosage

- Germanium supplementation is not recommended without a physician's supervision.

I IODINE

U.S. RDA 80–150mcg. E.U. RDA 150mcg.

Iodine is a mineral, which was first discovered in 1812 in kelp. Iodine was extracted and given its name because of its violet color. It occurs naturally and is a crucial constituent of the thyroid hormones, which monitor our energy levels.

Iodine deficiency is one of the key world health problems, and at least 200 million people suffer from conditions linked to inadequate iodine in the diet. Lack of iodine can cause goiter, underactive thyroid, cretinism, and can eventually lead to myxedema.

CAUTION

IODINE IS TOXIC IN HIGH DOSES AND MAY AGGRAVATE OR CAUSE ACNE. LARGE DOSES MAY INTERFERE WITH HORMONE ACTIVITY.

CRUCIFEROUS FOODS LIKE CABBAGE, BRUSSELS SPROUTS, CAULIFLOWER, AND BROCCOLI CONTAIN SUBSTANCES WHICH CAN CAUSE HYPOTHYROIDISM BY ANTAGONIZING IODINE. ANYONE WHO EATS LARGE QUANTITIES OF THESE VEGETABLES SHOULD CONSIDER AN IODINE SUPPLEMENT.

BELOW *Essential for the regulating of the thyroid gland, iodine is found in seafood.*

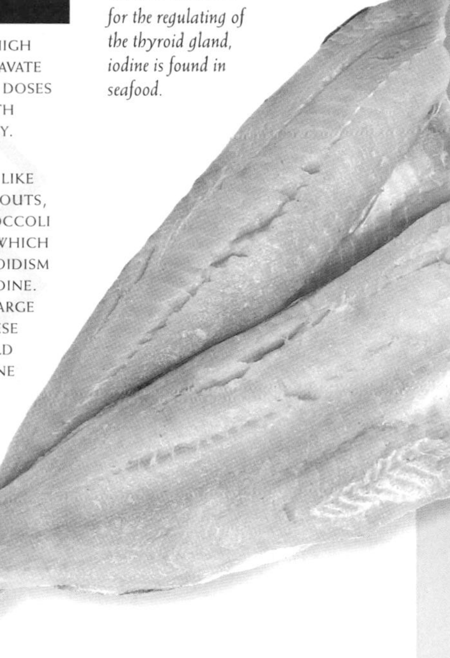

DATA FILE

Properties

- Determines the level of metabolism and energy in the body.
- Relieves the pain of fibrocystic breasts.
- Protects against the toxic effects of exposure to radioactive materials.
- Prevents goiter.
- Prevents thyroid disorders.
- Loosens mucus in the respiratory tract.
- Natural antiseptic.

Best Sources

Seafood and seaweed. Most table salt is fortified with iodine.

Dosage

- Iodine is best taken as potassium iodide.
- Take under the supervision of your physician or nutritionist.
- 150mcg. RDA iodine is adequate.

K POTASSIUM

U.S. RDA 3,500mg. E.U. RDA 3,500mg.

Potassium is one of the most important minerals in our body, working with sodium and chloride to form "electrolytes," the essential body salts that make up our body fluids. Potassium is crucial in order for the body to function. It plays a role in nerve conduction, the beating of the heart, energy production, the synthesis of nucleic acids and proteins, and the contraction of muscles.

Sweating can cause a loss of potassium, as do chronic diarrhea and diuretics. People taking certain drugs, including corticosteroids, high-dose penicillin, and laxatives, may suffer from potassium deficiency. Symptoms of this can include vomiting, abdominal distension, muscular weakness, loss of appetite, low blood pressure, and intense thirst.

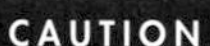

ABOVE *Dried fruits are a rich source of potassium, one of the most important minerals in our body.*

CAUTION

IN EXCESS (DOSES ABOVE 17G.), POTASSIUM MAY CAUSE MUSCULAR WEAKNESS AND MENTAL APATHY, EVENTUALLY STOPPING THE HEART.

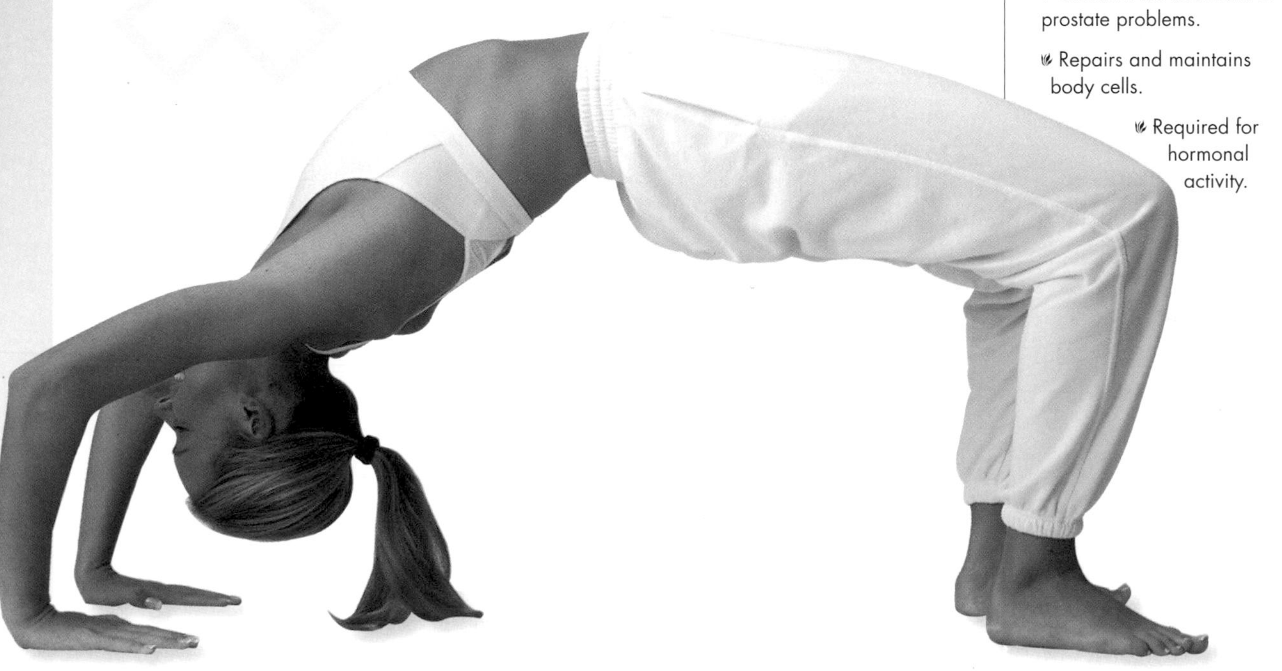

BELOW *To achieve athletic excellence, ensure that you have the recommended daily intake of potassium.*

DATA FILE

Properties

- Activates enzymes which control energy production.
- Prevents and treats high blood pressure.
- May help to protect against stroke.
- Improves athletic performance.
- May help treat and prevent cancer.
- Maintains water balance within cells.
- Stabilizes the internal structure of cells.
- Acts with sodium to conduct nerve impulses.

Best Sources

Fresh fruit and vegetables, particularly bananas.

Dosage

- Eat more fresh fruit and vegetables to increase potassium intake. Diuretic users and those in a hot climate may need up to 1.5g. in supplementary potassium daily.
- Take with zinc and magnesium for best effect.

ABOVE *Increase your intake of whole wheat bread to prevent magnesium deficiency.*

Mg MAGNESIUM

U.S. RDA 300–400mg. E.U. RDA 300mg.

Magnesium is a mineral that is absolutely essential for every biochemical process taking place in our bodies, including metabolism and the synthesis of nucleic acids and protein.

Magnesium deficiency is very common, particularly in the elderly, heavy drinkers, pregnant women, and regular, strenuous exercisers, and it has been proved that even a very slight deficiency can cause a disruption of the heartbeat. Other symptoms of magnesium deficiency include weakness, fatigue, vertigo, nervousness, muscle cramps, and hyperactivity in children.

DATA FILE

Properties

- Magnesium is necessary for many body functions, including energy production and cell replication.
- Essential for transmission of nerve impulses.
- Helps to prevent kidney stones and gallstones.
- Useful in the treatment of prostate problems.
- Repairs and maintains body cells.
- Required for hormonal activity.
- Required for most body processes, including production of energy.
- Useful in the treatment of high blood pressure.
- Protects against cardiovascular disease.
- Helps to treat the symptoms of PMS.

Best Sources

Brown rice, soybeans, nuts, brewer's yeast, whole wheat flour, legumes.

Dosage

- Dietary intake is thought to be inadequate in the average Western diet; supplements of 200–400mg. are recommended daily.

CAUTION

MAGNESIUM IS TOXIC TO PEOPLE WITH RENAL PROBLEMS OR ATRIOVENTRICULAR BLOCKS.

HIGH DOSES ARE BELIEVED TO CAUSE FLUSHING OF THE SKIN, THIRST, LOW BLOOD PRESSURE, AND LOSS OF REFLEXES IN SOME PEOPLE, ALTHOUGH THIS IS RARE.

Mn MANGANESE

U.S. RDA 2.5–7mg. E.U. RDA none.

Manganese is an essential trace element that is necessary for the normal functioning of the brain, and effective in the treatment of many nervous disorders, including Alzheimer's disease and schizophrenia. Deficiency is usually related to a poor diet – particularly one where there is a high intake of foods that are processed and refined.

Our understanding of Manganese is still incomplete, but it may prove to be one of the most important nutrients in human pathology. It appears likely that manganese is one of the antioxidant minerals (*see page 251*). There is some evidence that diseases such as diabetes, heart disease, and schizophrenia are linked to manganese deficiency.

DATA FILE

Properties

- Manganese maintains the healthy functioning of the nervous system.
- Necessary for female sex hormones.
- Necessary for the synthesis of the structural proteins of body cells.
- Necessary for normal bone structure.
- It is important in the formation of thyroxin in the thyroid gland.
- Necessary for the functioning of the brain.
- Used in the treatment of some nervous disorders.
- Necessary for metabolism of glucose.

Best Sources

Cereals, tea, green leaf vegetables, whole wheat bread, pulses, nuts.

Dosage

- 2–5 mg. is adequate, but doses up to 10mg. are thought to be safe.

CAUTION

TOXIC LEVELS ARE USUALLY QUITE RARE, BUT SYMPTOMS OF EXCESS MANGANESE MAY INCLUDE LETHARGY, INVOLUNTARY MOVEMENTS, POSTURE PROBLEMS, AND COMA.

BELOW LEFT *The trace element manganese, which can be found in pulses, is used in the treatment of some nervous disorders.*

Mo MOLYBDENUM

U.S. RDA 150–500mcg. E.U. RDA none.

Molybdenum is an essential trace element, and a vital part of the enzyme which is responsible for the utilization of iron in our bodies. Molybdenum may also be an antioxidant, and recent research indicates that it is necessary for optimum health.

Molybdenum can help to prevent anemia and is known to promote a feeling of well-being. A deficiency may result in dental caries, sexual impotence in men, and cancer of the gullet. Deficiency is usually the result of eating foods from molybdenum-deficient soils, or a diet that is high in refined and processed foods.

CAUTION

MOLYBDENUM IS TOXIC IN DOSES HIGHER THAN 10–15MG., WHICH CAUSE GOUT (A BUILD-UP OF URIC ACID AROUND THE JOINTS).

DATA FILE

Properties

- For utilization of iron, fats, carbohydrates; excretion of uric acid.
- Prevents impotence.
- Protects against cancer, anemia, dental caries.

Best Sources

Wheat, canned beans, wheat germ, liver, pulses, wholegrains, offal, eggs.

Dosage

- Optimal intake is not decided; 0.075–0.25mg. per day is adequate. Experts suggest 50–100mcg. per day as a preventive measure. Toxic in doses higher than 10-15mg., causing gout.

LEFT *Wheat is a good source of molybdenum. An adequate intake protects against cancer, anemia, and dental caries.*

P PHOSPHORUS

U.S. RDA 800–1,200mg. E.U. RDA 800mg.

Phosphorus is a mineral that is essential to the structure and function of the body. It is present in the body as phosphates, and in this form aids the process of bone mineralization and helps to create the structure of the bone.

Phosphorus is also essential for communication between cells, and for energy production. Phosphorus appears in many foods and deficiency is rare. Because of its role in strengthening our bones, we should eat twice as much calcium as phosphorus.

CAUTION

PHOSPHORUS CAN BE TOXIC AT DOSAGES OR INTAKE ABOVE 1G. PER DAY, IN SOME CASES CAUSING DIARRHEA, THE CALCIFICATION OF ORGANS AND SOFT TISSUES, AND MAKING THE BODY UNABLE TO ABSORB IRON, CALCIUM, MAGNESIUM, AND ZINC.

LEFT *Phosphorus, found in milk products, canned fish, and nuts, is essential for maintaining body functions.*

DATA FILE

Properties

- Forms bones and teeth.
- Produces energy.
- Cofactor for many enzymes and activates B-complex vitamins.
- Increases endurance, and fights fatigue.
- Forms RNA and DNA.

Best Sources

Yeast, dried milk and milk products, wheat germ, hard cheeses, canned fish, nuts, cereals, eggs.

Dosage

- Phosphorus deficiency usually accompanies deficiency in potassium, magnesium, and zinc, so take a supplement containing all four.
- Take under medical supervision only.

Se SELENIUM

U.S. RDA 50–100mcg.
E.U. RDA 10–75mcg.

Selenium is an essential trace element that has recently been recognized as one of the most important nutrients in our diet. It is an antioxidant (*see page 251*) and is vitally important in human metabolism. Selenium has been proved to provide protection against a number of cancers, and other diseases.

Selenium is necessary for the body's manufacture of proteins, and helps the liver to function efficiently. It also forms part of the male sperm, which means that deficiency can be linked to infertility in men. Other symptoms of deficiency include reduced immune activity, hair loss, and chest pains.

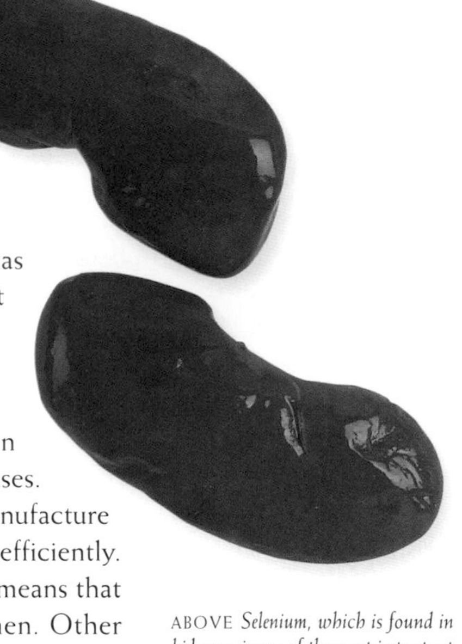

ABOVE *Selenium, which is found in kidneys, is one of the most important nutrients in our diet. It helps the liver to function effectively.*

CAUTION

SELENIUM CAN BE TOXIC IN VERY SMALL DOSES.

SYMPTOMS OF EXCESS INCLUDE BLACKENED FINGERNAILS AND A GARLIC-LIKE ODOR ON THE BREATH AND SKIN.

TAKE NO MORE THAN 500MCG. DAILY UNLESS SUPERVISED BY A REGISTERED PRACTITIONER.

DATA FILE

Properties

- Maintains healthy eyes and eyesight.
- Maintains good skin and healthy hair.
- Stimulates immune system.
- Prevents many cancers.
- Improves liver function.
- Protects against heart and circulatory diseases.
- May work to impede the aging process.
- Can detoxify alcohol, many drugs, smoking, and some fats.
- Increases male potency and sex drive.
- Useful addition to the treatment of arthritis.
- Alleviates hot flushes and symptoms of menopause.
- Helps treat dandruff.

Best Sources

Selenium is found in wheat germ, bran, tuna fish, onions, tomatoes, broccoli, kidney and whole wheat bread.

Dosage

- There is no RDA, but it has been suggested that men take 75mcg. of supplementary selenium and women take 60mcg.
- Selenium supplementation should be taken with 9–120mcg. of vitamin E to ensure that selenium works most efficiently.
- Dosages of 400–1,000mcg. have been used for immune stimulation, and for anticarcinogenic effects, but it is recommended that 50–200mcg. should be adequate to experience benefits.

RIGHT *Take vitamin E with selenium supplementation to ensure maximum benefit.*

Si SILICON

U.S. RDA none. E.U. RDA none.

Silicon is a trace element which is only just starting to be understood. It has been proved to be essential to animals, and it is thought that it is crucial to human life as well. Scientists believe that silicon plays some part in the make-up of our connective tissues, bones, skin, and fingernails.

Silicon is also known to play a role in preventing osteoporosis, by assisting the utilization of calcium within the bones. It also improves the strength of hair and nails by improving the production of keratin and collagen. Silicon is available as a supplement in the form of silicon dioxide. Silicea is a homeopathic remedy for disorders of the bones, joints, and skin.

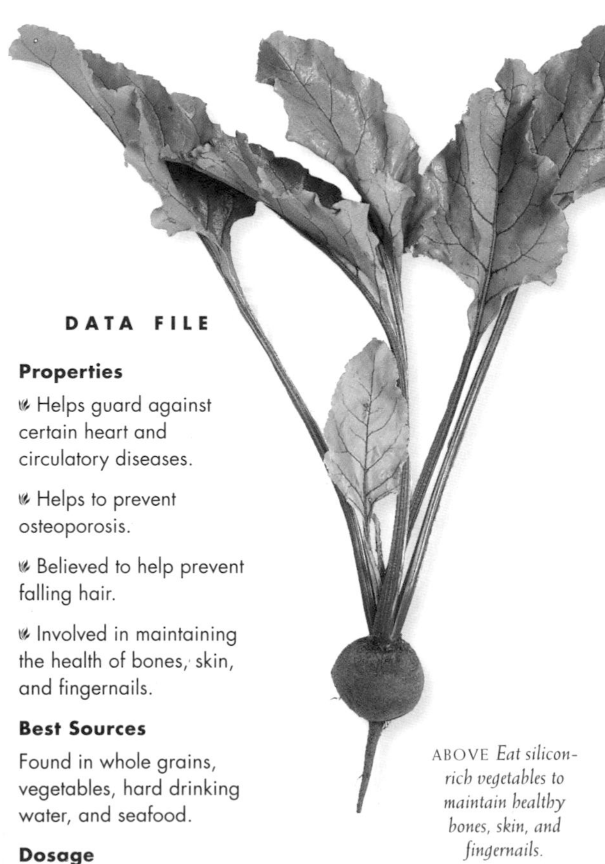

ABOVE *Eat silicon-rich vegetables to maintain healthy bones, skin, and fingernails.*

DATA FILE

Properties

- Helps guard against certain heart and circulatory diseases.
- Helps to prevent osteoporosis.
- Believed to help prevent falling hair.
- Involved in maintaining the health of bones, skin, and fingernails.

Best Sources

Found in whole grains, vegetables, hard drinking water, and seafood.

Dosage

- There is no official RDA, but we need 20–30mg. each day. Most of us get about 200mg. in our diet.

CAUTION

EXCESS SILICON CAN CAUSE KIDNEY STONES, BUT ONLY AT VERY HIGH DOSES.

V VANADIUM

U.S. RDA none. E.U. RDA none.

Vanadium is a trace mineral that has only recently been proved necessary for human life. At the turn of the 20th century, French physicians believed that vanadium was a miracle cure for a variety of illnesses, but it proved to be toxic at the levels they were prescribing, and it became less popular.

Today, it is believed that elevated levels of vanadium may cause manic depression, which is perhaps a clue to a little-understood disease. Normal doses are thought to reduce appetite, and to reduce blood fat and cholesterol levels.

DATA FILE

Properties

- Reduces high blood sugar by mimicking the effect of insulin on the cells.
- Prevents dental caries.
- Aids in the production of red blood cells.
- Encourages normal tissue growth and fat metabolism.
- Slows down cholesterol formation in blood vessels.
- Prevents heart disease and heart attacks.

Best Sources

Found in fish, parsley, radishes, strawberries, lettuce, and cucumber.

Dosage

- Vanadium supplements are not available, although some newer multivitamin and mineral supplements may contain low levels of it.

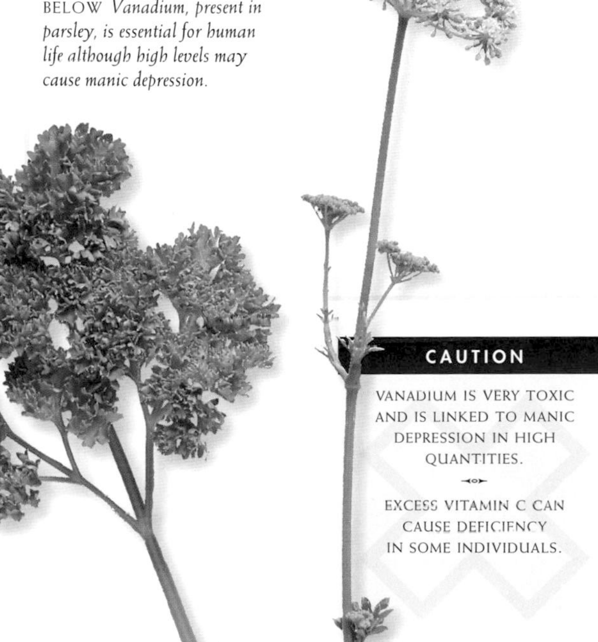

BELOW *Vanadium, present in parsley, is essential for human life although high levels may cause manic depression.*

CAUTION

VANADIUM IS VERY TOXIC AND IS LINKED TO MANIC DEPRESSION IN HIGH QUANTITIES.

EXCESS VITAMIN C CAN CAUSE DEFICIENCY IN SOME INDIVIDUALS.

Zn ZINC

U.S. RDA 15mg. E.U. RDA 15mg.

Zinc is one of the most important trace elements in our diet, and it is required for more than 200 enzyme activities within the body. It is the principal protector of the immune system, and is crucial for regulating our genetic information. Zinc is also vital for the structure and function of cell membranes.

Zinc is an antioxidant (*see page 251*) and can help to detoxify the body. A zinc deficiency can cause growth failure, infertility, impotence, and, in some cases, an impaired sense of taste. Eczema is commonly linked to zinc deficiency, and new research points to the fact that post-natal illness may be attributable to insufficient zinc in the diet. A weakened immune system and a poor ability to heal may also indicate deficiency.

ABOVE *A vital trace element in our diet, zinc is needed for over 200 enzyme functions in the human body.*

CAUTION

VERY HIGH DOSES (ABOVE 150MG. PER DAY) MAY CAUSE SOME NAUSEA, VOMITING, AND DIARRHEA.

DATA FILE

Properties

- Boosts the immune system.
- Prevents cancer.
- Prevents and treats colds.
- Maintains senses of taste, smell, and sight.
- May help to prevent age-related degenerative effects.
- Prevents hair loss.
- Treats acne and various other skin problems.
- Useful in treatment of rheumatoid arthritis.
- Prevents blindness associated with aging.
- Increases male potency and sex drive.
- Used to treat infertility.

Best Sources

Offal, meat, mushrooms, oysters, eggs, wholegrain products, brewer's yeast.

Dosage

- Take 15–30mg. daily, and increase copper and selenium intake if taking more zinc.

THERAPY CONNECTIONS

SILICON

Homeopathy *p.211*

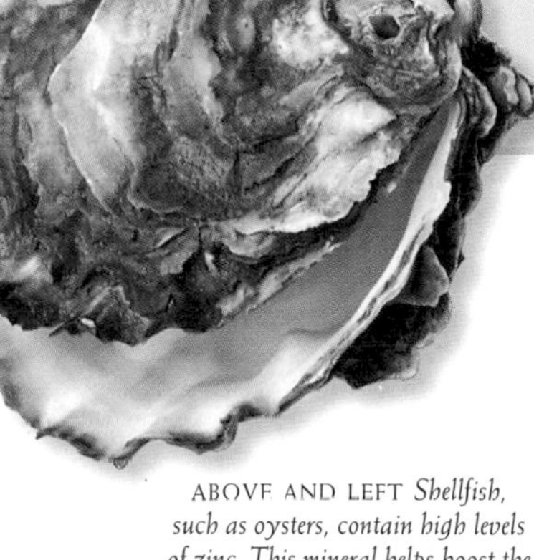

ABOVE AND LEFT *Shellfish, such as oysters, contain high levels of zinc. This mineral helps boost the immune system and is necessary for growth and development.*

AMINO ACIDS

L-ARGININE

L-arginine is one of the most important and most useful of the amino acids, with a significant role to play in the function of the muscles, growth, and healing, helping to regulate and support key components of the immune system. It is also extremely important for male fertility.

For adults, L-arginine is a nonessential amino acid, which means that it is capable of being synthesized in the body and it is therefore not essential that we get additional amounts in our daily diet. For children, however, L-arginine is essential.

CAUTION

TAKE ON AN EMPTY STOMACH, AND DO NOT TAKE IN EXCESS, WHICH COULD CAUSE MENTAL AND METABOLIC DISTURBANCES, AS WELL AS NAUSEA AND DIARRHEA.

PROLONGED HIGH DOSES MAY BE DANGEROUS TO CHILDREN, AND TO ANYONE WITH LIVER OR KIDNEY PROBLEMS.

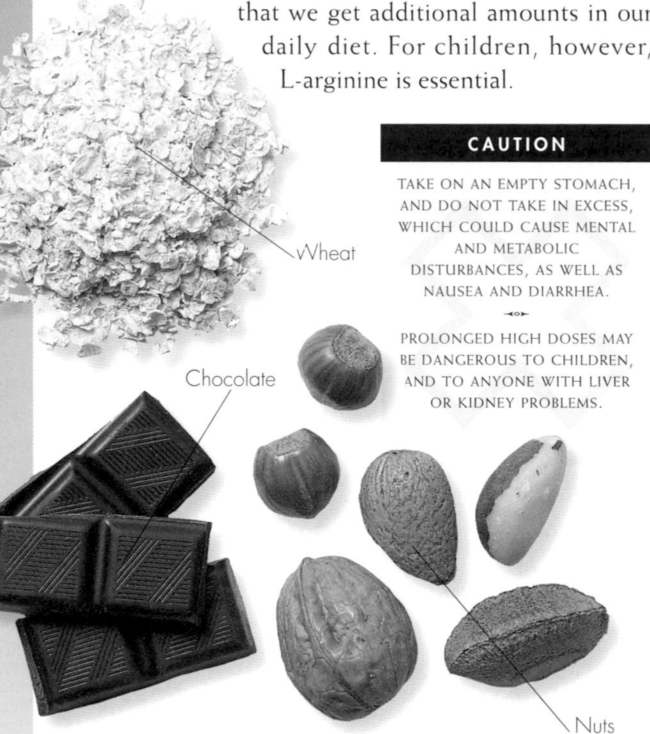

DATA FILE

Properties

- Boosts immunity.
- Inhibits the growth of a number of tumors.
- Builds muscle and burns fat, by stimulating the pituitary glands to increase growth hormone secretion.
- Helps to promote the healing of burns and other wounds.
- Helps to protect the liver and to detoxify harmful substances.
- Increases sperm count in men with a low count.

Best Sources

Raw cereals, chocolate, and nuts.

Dosage

The optimal intake is unknown, but doses up to 1.5g. appear to be safe. Take L-arginine with lysine, which inhibits herpes attacks in carriers.

LEFT *Found in chocolate, nuts, and cereals, L-arginine is one of the most important amino acids and is essential for young children.*

L-ASPARTIC ACID

L-aspartic acid is a nonessential amino acid which has been used for many years in the treatment of chronic fatigue. Studies confirm the efficiency of this amino acid in raising energy levels, and in helping to overcome the side-effects of drug withdrawal.

DATA FILE

Properties

- Disposes of ammonia, helping to protect the central nervous system.
- Helps treat fatigue.
- May improve stamina and endurance.

Dosage

- Supplements are available in 250–500mg. tablets; take 3 times daily with juice or water.

CAUTION

DO NOT TAKE WITH PROTEIN, SUCH AS MILK.

DO NOT TAKE MORE THAN 1G. WITHOUT THE SUPERVISION OF YOUR PHYSICIAN.

BELOW *L-aspartic acid has long been used to treat chronic fatigue.*

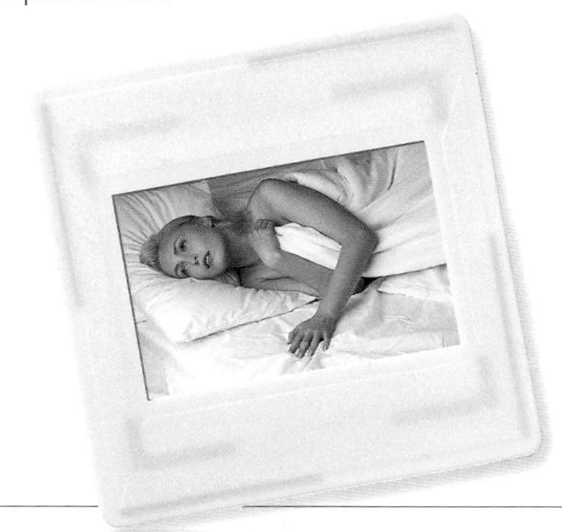

L-CYSTEINE

Cysteine contains sulfur, which is said to work as an antioxidant, protecting and preserving the cells in the body. It is also said to protect the body against pollutants, but much work has still to be done to understand the effects of this amino acid.

CAUTION

DIABETICS SHOULD NOT TAKE L-CYSTEINE SUPPLEMENTS UNLESS SUPERVISED BY A PHYSICIAN.

L-CYSTEINE MAY ALSO CAUSE KIDNEY STONES, BUT A HIGH VITAMIN C INTAKE SHOULD PREVENT THIS FROM OCCURRING.

BELOW *Eggs, meat, and dairy products all contain cysteine, which helps protect the body against free radicals.*

DATA FILE

Properties

- May protect against copper toxicity.
- Protects the body against damage by free radicals (*see page 251*).
- May help to reverse damage done by smoking and alcohol abuse.
- Offers protection against X-rays and nuclear radiation.
- May help to treat arthritis.
- Helps to repair DNA, thereby preventing the effects of aging.

Best Sources

Eggs, meat, dairy products, some cereals.

Dosage

- Take with vitamin C for best effect (three times as much vitamin C as L-cysteine). Doses up to 1g. are considered to be safe, but consult your physician first.

L-GLUTAMINE

L-glutamine is a derivative of glutamic acid, which is believed to help reduce cravings for alcohol. Studies are inconclusive as to the real benefits of taking this amino acid, and it is recommended that you do not take more than 1g. daily unless you are supervised by your physician.

DATA FILE

Properties

- Believed to help reduce craving for alcohol.
- May help to speed the healing of peptic ulcers.
- May help to counter attacks of depression.
- May energize the mind.
- May help to treat and prevent colitis.

Dosage

Up to 1g. daily is believed to be safe, but supplement only under the supervision of your physician.

L-HISTADINE

L-histadine is one of the lesser-known amino acids, and its role in our bodies is not yet fully understood. Research is ongoing into the possible effects of histadine supplementation.

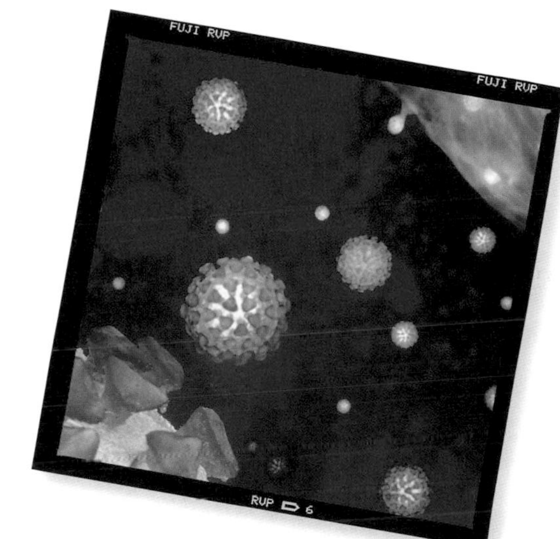

DATA FILE

Properties

- Used in the treatment of arthritis sufferers, who have an abnormally low level of this amino acid in their blood.
- May boost the activity of suppressor T-cells, which could be useful in the fight against HIV/AIDS and auto-immune conditions.

Dosage

Do not take more than 150mg. daily unless supervised by your physician.

LEFT *Research suggests that L-histadine may boost T-cell activity, which could make it important in HIV/AIDS treatment.*

GLYCINE

Glycine is considered to be the simplest of the amino acids, with a variety of properties which are still being studied by scientists.

CAUTION

IT IS RECOMMENDED THAT YOU DO NOT TAKE THIS AMINO ACID AS A SUPPLEMENT UNLESS SUPERVISED BY YOUR PHYSICIAN.

DATA FILE

Properties

- May help to treat low pituitary gland function.
- May be used in the treatment of spastic movement – particularly in patients suffering from multiple sclerosis.
- May help treat progressive muscular dystrophy.
- Used in the treatment of hypoglycemia, since it stimulates the release of glucagon, which mobilizes glycogen, which can then be released into the blood-stream as glucose.

Dosage

- Doses below 1g. are thought to be safe, but research is ongoing.

L-LYSINE

L-lysine is an essential amino acid, which means that it is necessary for life. It is needed for growth, tissue repair, and for the production of antibodies, hormones, and enzymes. Lysine should be obtained from eating foods such as fish, milk, cheese, and eggs, although it is possible to purchase lysine supplements.

CAUTION

NOT SUITABLE FOR CHILDREN.

DATA FILE

Properties

- Inhibits herpes – high doses are now believed to be effective in reducing the recurrence of outbreaks.
- May assist in building muscle mass.
- Helps to prevent fertility problems.
- Improves concentration.

Best Sources

Found in fish, milk, lima beans, meat, cheese, yeast, eggs, all proteins.

Dosage

- Up to 500mg. daily is believed to be safe.
- Some experts recommend 1,000mg. daily at mealtimes.
- It is usually advised that amino acids are taken on an empty stomach, with some juice or water.
- Take L-lysine with an equal quantity of arginine if an increase in muscle mass is the desired goal.

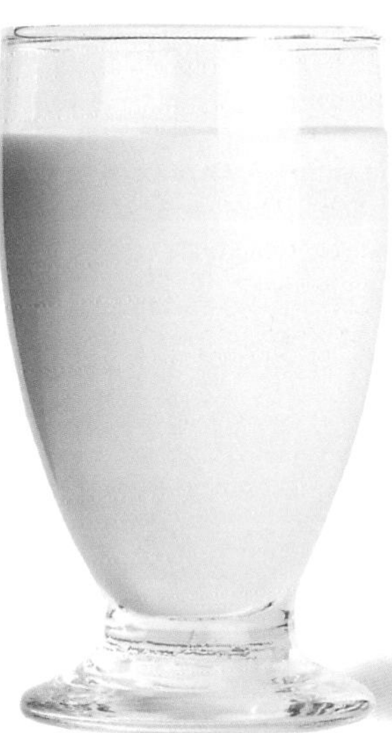

RIGHT *Milk is an ideal source of lysine, an essential amino acid that aids concentration and helps prevent fertility problems.*

L-METHIONINE

Methionine is a sulfur-containing amino acid that is very important in numerous processes in the body. Research shows that it may help to prevent clogging of the arteries by eliminating fatty substances.

BELOW *Eating methionine-rich foods, such as fish, milk, liver, and eggs, may help the body eliminate fatty substances in the blood.*

Eggs

Yogurt

Fish

Liver

DATA FILE

Properties

- May help to eliminate fatty substances from the blood, lowering the risk of heart attack.
- May help to regulate the nervous system.
- In conjunction with choline and folic acid, it may prevent some tumors.
- Necessary for the biosynthesis of taurine and cysteine.

Best Sources

Eggs, milk, liver, fish.

CAUTION

SUPPLEMENTATION IS NOT ADVISED, ALTHOUGH SOME PHYSICIANS MAY SUGGEST IT IN SPECIFIC CIRCUMSTANCES.

DL-PHENYLALANINE (DLPA)

DLPA is a form of the amino acid phenylalanine created from equal parts of D (synthetic) phenylalanine and L (natural) phenylalanine. DLPA has a unique role of activating and producing endorphins, which are the body's natural painkillers. Many people who do not respond to conventional painkillers respond successfully to DLPA, and its painkilling action increases over time. Do not confuse DLPA with L-phenylalanine.

DATA FILE

Properties

- A natural painkiller, useful for chronic pain and conditions like migraine, neuralgia, and leg cramps.
- Antidepressant.

Dosage

- Tablets are generally available in 375mg. doses, and can be taken up to six times daily (a maximum dose of 1.5g.).
- Higher doses should only be taken under the supervision of your physician. Take two or three times daily, before meals.

CAUTION

NOT SUITABLE FOR PREGNANT WOMEN OR FOR THOSE WHO SUFFER FROM PHENYLKETORNURIA (PKU).

IT MAY ELEVATE BLOOD PRESSURE, SO CHECK WITH YOUR PHYSICIAN IF YOU SUFFER FROM ANY CIRCULATORY DISORDER.

L-PHENYLALANINE

L-phenylalanine is an essential amino acid that is necessary for a number of biochemical processes, including the synthesis of neurotransmitters in the brain. It is said to promote sexual arousal and to release hormones that help to control appetite.

CAUTION

IF YOU SUFFER FROM SKIN CANCER, DO NOT TAKE L-PHENYLALANINE.

PEOPLE WITH HIGH BLOOD PRESSURE SHOULD ONLY TAKE SUPPLEMENTARY L-PHENYLALANINE UNDER THE SUPERVISION OF THEIR PHYSICIAN.

NOT SUITABLE FOR USE WITH MAOI ANTIDEPRESSANTS. PREGNANT WOMEN SHOULD NOT TAKE THIS AMINO ACID.

Almonds

Peanuts

Soybeans

Sesame seeds

DATA FILE

Properties

- May help to alleviate a bout of depression.
- May help to control addictive behavior.
- Encourages mental alertness.
- Promotes sexual arousal.
- Reduces hunger and cravings for food.

Best Sources

Found in proteins, cheese, almonds, peanuts, sesame seeds, and soybeans.

Dosage

- L-phenylalanine is usually available in 500mg. doses. Take on an empty stomach for best effect, and do not take with protein.

LEFT *Present in almonds, peanuts, soybeans, and sesame seeds, L-phenylalanine is said to control the appetite and alleviate depression.*

L-TRYPTOPHAN

This essential amino acid is used by the brain, along with several vitamins and minerals, to produce serotonin, a neurotransmitter. Serotonin, which regulates and induces sleep, is also said to reduce sensitivity to pain. It was one of the first amino acids to be produced for sale as a supplement, and it is useful as a natural sleeping aid.

DATA FILE

Properties

- May help to encourage sleep and to prevent jet lag.
- Reduces sensitivity to pain.
- Lessens a craving for alcohol.
- Natural antidepressant, and may help to reduce anxiety and panic attacks.

Best Sources

Cottage cheese, milk, meat, fish, turkey, bananas, protein sources.

Dosage

- Used to prevent panic attacks and depression, L-tryptophan should be taken between meals with juice or water (no proteins).
- To help induce sleep, take 500mg. along with vitamin B6, niacinamide, and magnesium an hour or so before bedtime.

CAUTION

THERE IS SOME EVIDENCE THAT IT MAY CAUSE LIVER PROBLEMS IN HIGH DOSES, AND ALTHOUGH STUDIES VARY, IT IS NOW BELIEVED THAT IT CAN BE TOXIC IN VERY HIGH DOSES. TAKE ONLY ON THE ADVICE OF YOUR PHYSICIAN.

L-TYROSINE

L-tyrosine is not an essential amino acid, which means that it is synthesized in the body. Tyrosine is involved with important neurotransmitters in the brain, and it is said to energize and help to relieve the effects of stress.

CAUTION

DO NOT TAKE TYROSINE IF YOU SUFFER FROM MIGRAINE HEADACHES, OR IF YOU TAKE MAOI ANTIDEPRESSANTS.

PEOPLE SUFFERING FROM HIGH BLOOD PRESSURE OR SKIN CANCER SHOULD NOT TAKE SUPPLEMENTARY TYROSINE WITHOUT THE APPROVAL OF A PHYSICIAN.

DATA FILE

Properties

- Helps to relieve stress, and encourages alertness and fewer physical symptoms of tension and stress.
- May act as an antidepressant.
- May be used to treat the emotional symptoms of PMS.
- May help to aid in the treatment of addiction to and withdrawal from cocaine and other addictive drugs.

Dosage

- Take with juice or water on an empty stomach (do not take with proteins, such as milk).
- Some experts suggest that it is more effective when taken in conjunction with up to 25mg. of vitamin B6.

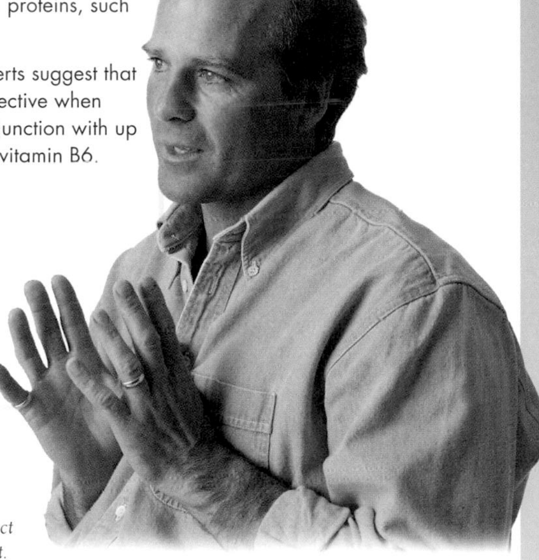

RIGHT *Tyrosine supplements may alleviate stress and act as an antidepressant.*

LIPIDS AND DERIVATIVES

FISH OILS

Fish oils contain two long-chain fatty acids called eicosopentaenoic acid (EPA) and docosahexaenoic acid (DHA) that affect the synthesis of prostaglandins, which have a regulatory effect on the body. There are numerous claims for fish oils, which are now believed to improve overall health and treat many health conditions.

CAUTION

FISH OILS MAY BE HARMFUL IN DIABETICS, CAUSING INCREASES IN BLOOD SUGAR AND A DECLINE IN INSULIN SECRETION.

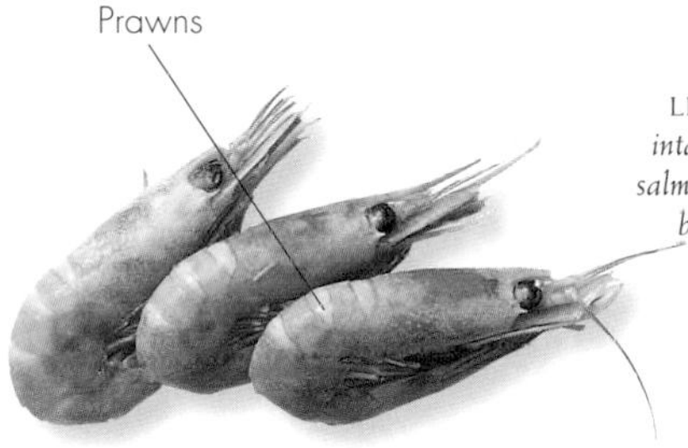

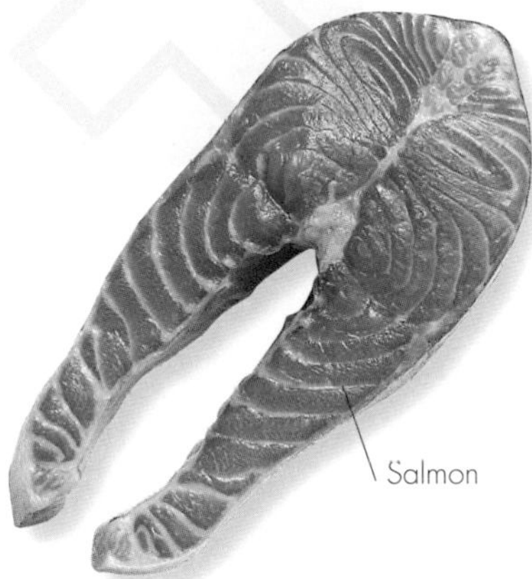

LEFT *Increase your intake of fish, such as salmon and prawns, to benefit from health-enhancing fish oils.*

DATA FILE

Properties

- May be useful in the treatment of kidney disease, and can counteract the effects of some immuno-suppressive drugs.
- May help to prevent cancer, in particular the onset of breast cancer.
- Stops progression of arthritis symptoms.
- May help to protect against high blood pressure.
- Helps to prevent cardiovascular disease.
- May help to prevent and treat psoriasis.

Best Sources

Fish, in particular herring, salmon, tuna, cod, prawns.

Dosage

- People suffering from arthritis or psoriasis can take up to 4g. daily, but for most people it is more appropriate to increase your intake of fish and seafood in order to achieve the benefits of the fish oils in their natural form.
- The maximum suggested dosage for supplements, taken without the supervision of your physician, is 900mg. per day.

EVENING PRIMROSE *(GLA)*

Native Americans were the first to recognize the potential of evening primrose oil as a healer, and they decocted (boiled) the seeds to make a liquid for healing wounds. Evening primrose oil is a rich source of gamma-linoleic acid, which is better known as GLA. The body makes GLA from essential fatty acids (EFAs). EFAs have numerous functions in the body, one of which is to manufacture hormone-like substances called "prostaglandins," which have very important effects on the body, such as toning blood vessels, balancing our water levels, and improving the action of the digestive system, and brain functioning. Prostaglandins also have a beneficial effect on the immune system.

CAUTION

DO NOT USE IF YOU SUFFER FROM TEMPORAL-LOBE EPILEPSY OR MANIC DEPRESSION.

BELOW *Evening primrose oil will help to keep your skin from becoming dehydrated.*

DATA FILE

Properties

- Reduces scaling and redness, prevents itching, and encourages healing in cases of eczema. Also used in the treatment of psoriasis.
- Discourages dry skin, and ensures that the cellular membranes that make up the skin are stable and strong. There is some evidence that the oil retards the aging process.
- Evening primrose oil may help to prevent MS, and appears to be particularly useful for children suffering from the condition.
- May help in cases of liver damage caused by alcohol (cirrhosis of the liver), hyperactivity in children, and cystic fibrosis.
- May have a stimulating effect on the body, encouraging it to convert fat into energy, which would make it an excellent treatment for obesity.
- Hormonal imbalances, perhaps causing conditions like PMS, and symptoms of the menopause may be eased by evening primrose oil, reducing symptoms of bloating, water retention, irritability, and depression.
- Reduces the inflammation of rheumatoid arthritis.
- Evening primrose may have an immunosuppressive effect on the body.

Dosage

- Evening primrose oil is most often taken in the form of capsules, but it is also available as an oil (sometimes flavored), and it can be applied to the skin to treat skin conditions.
- Take 500mg. each day for two months, and then for the 10 days preceding menstruation if you suffer from PMS. In menopause, 2,000–4,000mg. should be taken daily for four weeks, and then 500–1,000mg. daily thereafter.
- For asthma, take two 500mg. tablets three times daily for three to four months; then one tablet three times daily. If you are taking steroids, this treatment will not work because steroids interfere with evening primrose oil's action.

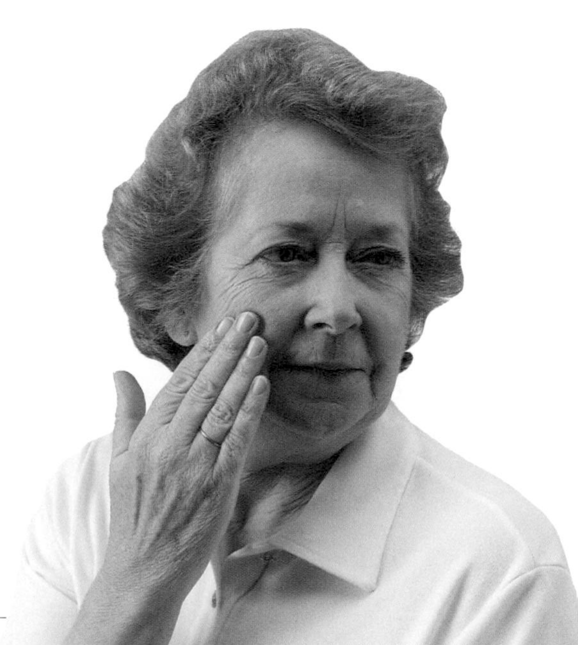

INOSITOL

Inositol is not a true vitamin, as it can be synthesized by the body, but it forms part of the B-complex family of vitamins, and is present in cereals and vegetables as phytic acid. There is a high concentration in the brain, stomach, spleen, liver, and heart.

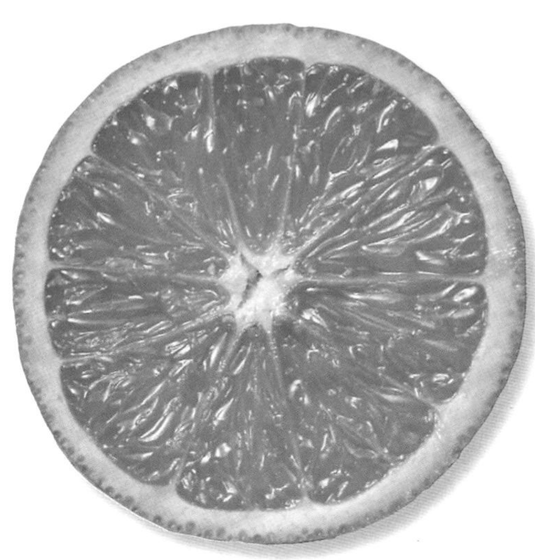

ABOVE *Citrus fruits are a valuable source of inositol, part of the B-complex vitamin family.*

DATA FILE

Properties

- Helps to dissolve fat.
- May help to prevent anxiety and tension.
- Ensures healthy hair and strong nails.
- Controls levels of cholesterol in the blood.
- Helps to encourage natural sleep.
- May help to treat schizophrenia and other nervous disorders.

Best Sources

Lethicin, liver, wheat germ, brown rice, citrus fruits, nuts, and cereals.

Dosage

- Natural sources are best, but if you are prescribed supplements, take in the form of myo-inositol to a maximum of 1,000mg. daily.

BELOW *To keep your nails in good condition, ensure that you have enough inositol in your diet.*

CAUTION

DIABETICS SHOULD ONLY TAKE INOSITOL UNDER THE SUPERVISION OF THEIR PHYSICIAN.

LECITHIN

Lecithin has for some time been a popular supplement, used for a variety of health conditions. It is comprised of choline, inositol, fatty acids, and phosphorus, and is available as a liquid or as dry granules. It is widely used in foods to maintain consistency, and is probably one of the only nutritious food additives.

CAUTION

IN SOME PEOPLE (IN LARGE QUANTITIES) MAY CAUSE DEPRESSION.

VERY HIGH DOSES MAY CAUSE NAUSEA, VOMITING, AND DIZZINESS.

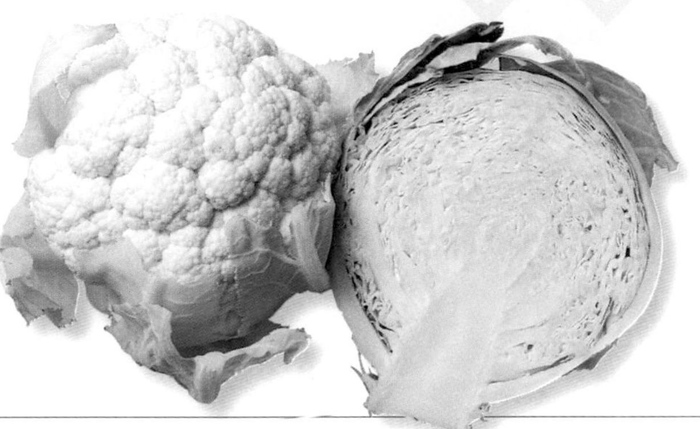

RIGHT *Increase your intake of lecithin-rich foods, such as cauliflower and cabbages to treat a wide variety of ailments.*

DATA FILE

Properties

- Protects against cardiovascular disease.
- Helps to reduce high blood pressure.
- Used to treat memory loss and conditions of the nervous system such as dementia and Alzheimer's.
- May help in the treatment of mental disorders such as manic depression.
- Lecithin has some action against viruses.
- May prevent and also treat gallstones.
- May help to treat viral hepatitis, repairing the membranes of the liver cells.

Best Sources

Found in egg yolks, soybeans, liver, meats, fish, cauliflower, and cabbage.

Dosage

- Doses of up to 1g. daily are acceptable, but see your physician to discuss your individual needs.
- Lecithin appears in a wide range of foods and it is probably best to increase your intake of these instead of supplementing.

OTHER SUPPLEMENTS

ACIDOPHILUS

Acidophilus (also known as *lactobacillus acidophilus*) is a source of friendly intestinal bacteria (flora). Healthy bacteria play an important role in our bodies, and unless they are continually supplied with some form of lactic acid or lactose (such as acidophilus) they can die, causing a host of health problems. Many physicians and health practitioners recommend taking acidophilus alongside oral antibiotics, which can cause diarrhea, destroy the healthy flora of the intestines, and lead to fungal infections. Acidophilus may also help to ensure vaginal health.

DATA FILE

Properties

- Keeps the intestines clean.
- Prevents yeast infections of the vagina.
- Aids the absorption of nutrients in food.
- Can eliminate bad breath (which has been caused by intestinal putrefaction).
- Can relieve and prevent constipation and flatulence.
- Can aid the treatment of acne and other skin troubles.
- Maintains intestinal health.

Best Sources

Natural, unflavored, "live" yogurt, sometimes known as "bio yogurt."

Dosage

- Acidophilus is not toxic and can be taken daily, with food, in unlimited amounts.

CAUTION

KEEP THE TABLETS IN THE REFRIGERATOR.

BEE AND FLOWER POLLEN

In flowering plants the pollen-producing spores are located in the stamens of flowers. Flower pollen is said to be purer than bee pollen. Bee pollen is found in the hives themselves. It is rich in protein and amino acids, and forms, with honey, the basic diet of all the bees in the hive, except for the queen (*see royal jelly, page 276*). Pollen has been used as medicine around the world for thousands of years.

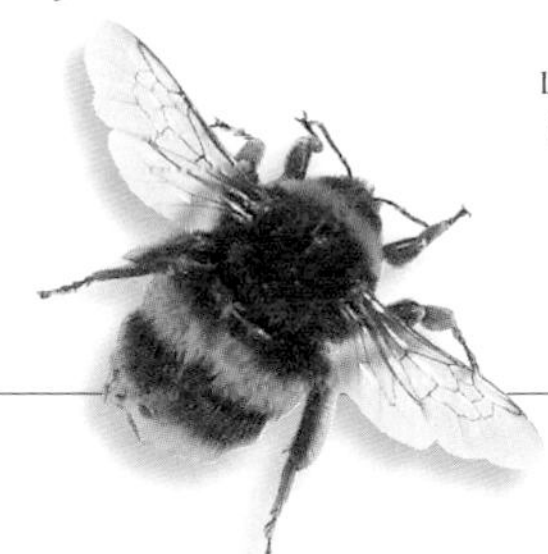

LEFT *Bee pollen is found in the hives of bees but it also present in small amounts in unpasteurized honey.*

DATA FILE

Properties

- Rich in both amino acids and protein.
- Helps to suppress appetite and cravings.
- May help to improve skin problems and retard the aging process.
- May help to treat problems of the prostate.
- Energizes the body.
- Regulates the bowels.
- May boost immunity and diminish allergies.

Best Sources

Unpasteurized honey contains small amounts of bee pollen.

Dosage

- 400mg. doses, taken daily, appear to be safe.
- Take pollen with food.

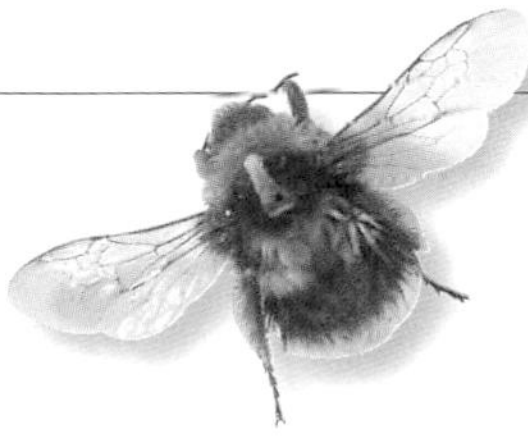

CAUTION

IF YOU SUFFER FROM HAY FEVER OR AN ALLERGY TO BEE STINGS, YOU MAY SUFFER A REACTION TO BEE POLLEN.

SEE YOUR PHYSICIAN OR PRACTITIONER BEFORE TAKING THIS SUPPLEMENT.

BIOFLAVONOIDS

Bioflavonoids were originally called vitamin P, and are also known as flavones. They accompany vitamin C in natural foods, and are responsible for the color in the leaves, flowers, and stems of food plants. Their primary job is to protect the capillaries, to keep them strong, and to prevent bleeding. Bioflavonoids are also anti-inflammatory. Many of the medicinally active substances of herbs are bioflavonoids.

DATA FILE

Properties

- Reduce bruising in susceptible individuals.
- Protect capillaries.
- Protect against cerebral and other hemorrhaging.
- Reduce bleeding during menstruation.
- Antioxidant (*see page 251*), and encourage the antioxidant qualities of vitamin C.
- Antiviral activity.
- Anti-inflammatory.
- Antiallergy.
- May help to cure colds.

Best Sources

Citrus fruits, apricots, cherries, green peppers, broccoli, lemons; the central white core of citrus fruits is the richest source.

Dosage

- Bioflavonoids are not toxic, and should be taken together with vitamin C for best effect.

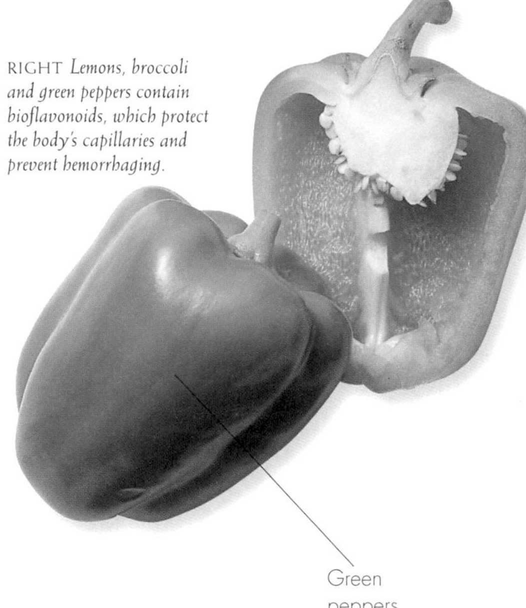

RIGHT *Lemons, broccoli and green peppers contain bioflavonoids, which protect the body's capillaries and prevent hemorrhaging.*

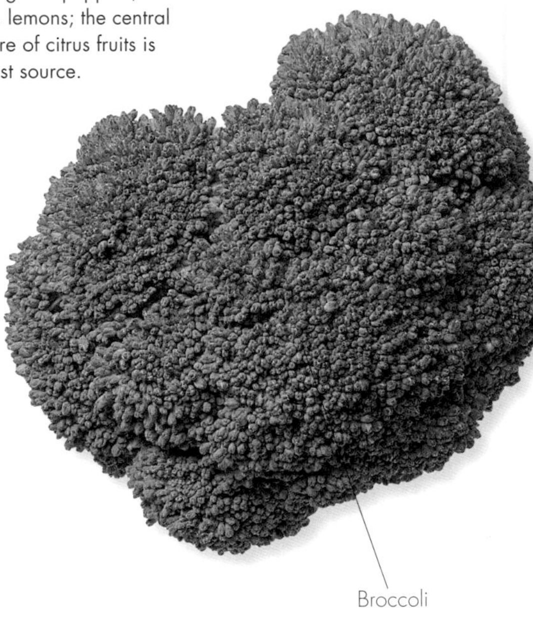

BREWER'S YEAST

Brewer's yeast is the same type of yeast that is used in the brewing process, and is quite different from the yeast that causes *Candida albicans*. It is a rich source of B-vitamins and amino acids, as well as some minerals, in particular chromium and selenium. It also contains naturally occurring nucleic acids (DNA and RNA), which are said to enhance the immune system, among other things.

CAUTION

BREWER'S YEAST IS NOT TOXIC AND CAN BE TAKEN DAILY WITHOUT ANY SIDE-EFFECTS.

SOME EXPERTS SUGGEST THAT IT MAY CAUSE YEAST INFECTIONS AND CHRONIC FATIGUE SYNDROME, BUT THIS HAS LARGELY BEEN DISCLAIMED.

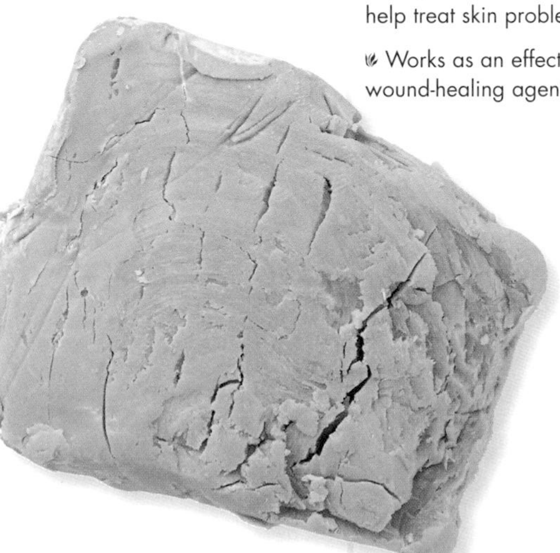

RIGHT *Brewer's yeast, which comes in powder or tablet form, contains B-vitamins and amino acids, as well as some minerals.*

DATA FILE

Properties

- May reduce wrinkling and help treat skin problems.
- Works as an effective wound-healing agent.
- Encourages the healing of burns.
- Rich source of B-vitamins, which can help to relieve stress and nervous disorders.
- Encourages the activity of the immune system.
- Increases energy.
- Used externally, to detoxify skin.

Dosage

- Brewer's yeast comes in tablets, and as a powder that can be sprinkled on food or drink.

CHARCOAL

Charcoal is a porous, solid product obtained when materials such as cellulose, wood, peat, bituminous coal, or bone are partially burned in the absence of air. Charcoal has always been popular for dealing with flatulence, bloating, and irritable bowel syndrome, by soaking up gas. Charcoal can be useful in the long-term management of kidney patients.

DATA FILE

Properties

- Reduces cholesterol in the blood.
- Reduces the risk of atherosclerosis.
- Absorbs gas and so acts as an antacid.
- Binds with cholesterol, toxins, and waste in the intestine, which has a cleansing effect.

Dosage

- Charcoal is available in tablet, powder, and capsule form.
- High doses (more than 50g. per day) should be supplemented with a well-balanced vitamin and mineral supplement.

CAUTION

ACTIVATED CHARCOAL CAN BIND WITH AND INACTIVATE SOME THERAPEUTIC DRUGS AND SUPPLEMENTAL NUTRIENTS, AND SHOULD BE TAKEN AT LEAST ONE HOUR BEFORE OR AFTER DRUGS OR SUPPLEMENTS ARE TAKEN.

IF YOU ARE ON PRESCRIPTION DRUGS, TAKE CHARCOAL ONLY WITH YOUR PHYSICIAN'S ADVICE.

BELOW *Charcoal is good for kidney problems, but only take it on your physician's advice.*

CO-ENZYME Q10

BELOW *Co-enzyme Q10 is an important substance for the efficient functioning of muscle cells.*

Co-enzyme Q10 is a vitamin-like substance found in all cells of the body. It is biologically important, since it forms part of the system across which electrons flow in the cells during the process of energy production. When there is a Q10 deficiency, the cell cannot function effectively, and the rate at which the muscle cells work is adversely affected.

DATA FILE

Properties

- Enhances immunity.
- Improves the heart-muscle metabolism.
- May help to prevent coronary inefficiency and heart failure.
- Anti-aging.
- Necessary for healthy functioning of the nervous system and the brain cells.

Best Sources

Meat (it is also made within the body).

Dosage

- 10mg., taken 3 times a day, has a therapeutic effect within the body.

CAUTION

CO-ENZYME Q10 IS FAT SOLUBLE, AND THEREFORE MAY BE TOXIC IN HIGH DOSES.

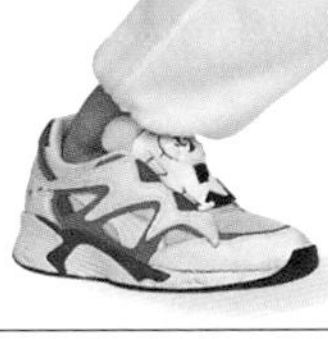

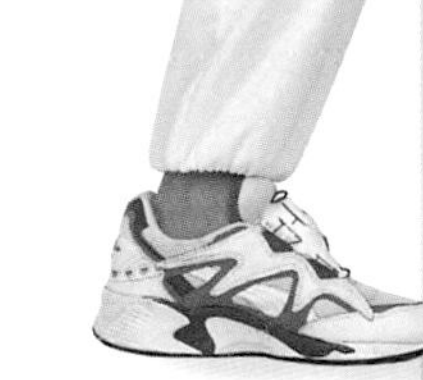

DHEA

Dehydroepiandrosterone (DHEA) is a hormone which we produce in our adrenal glands, and which also occurs naturally in the Mexican wild yam (potato). DHEA was for many years considered to be a cure-all, and indeed research has proved that it has invaluable therapeutic benefits, particularly in the prevention and treatment of cancer, but it is still very much under investigation and its many qualities have yet to be proven. It should be taken only if you have a known deficiency (less than 130mg/dl. in women and less than 180mg/dl. in men).

CAUTION

MANY SUPPLEMENTS THAT HAVE BEEN ANALYZED HAVE NO DHEA IN THEM, SO EXERCISE CAUTION WHEN CHOOSING A SUPPLEMENT.

DATA FILE

Properties

- Anticancer effects.
- Inhibits weight gain.
- May extend life span.
- DHEA is thought to have anti-aging effects.
- Works to reduce stress.
- Improves immunity.

Best Source

Mexican wild yam.

Dosage

- There is still some debate as to whether or not oral DHEA has any effect within the body, as in some studies it appears to be destroyed by the liver before it reaches the necessary tissues.
- See a registered practitioner for advice on supplementation.

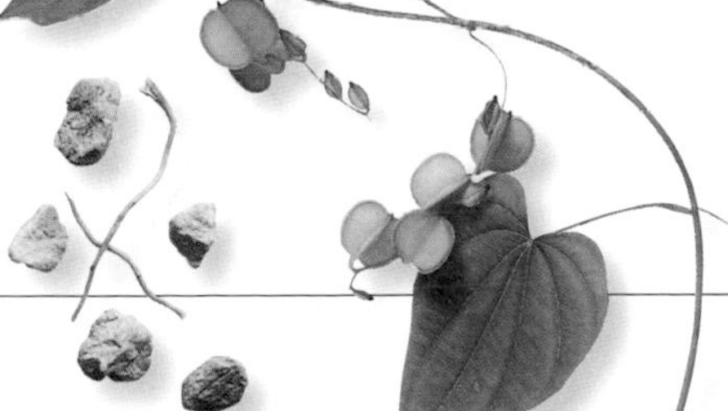

RIGHT *Mexican wild yam is the chief source of DHEA.*

DIETARY FIBER

Dietary fiber, also known as bulk and roughage, is an essential element in the diet even though it provides no nutrients. It consists of plant cellulose and other indigestible materials in foods, along with pectin and gum. The chewing it requires stimulates saliva flow, and the bulk it adds in the stomach and intestines during digestion provides more time for absorption of nutrients. A diet with sufficient fiber produces softer, bulkier stools, and helps to promote bowel regularity and avoid constipation and disorders such as diverticulosis.

CAUTION

A DIET OVERLY ABUNDANT IN DIETARY FIBER CAN CUT DOWN ON THE ABSORPTION OF IMPORTANT TRACE MINERALS DURING DIGESTION.

TAKE A GOOD MULTIVITAMIN AND MINERAL TABLET IF YOU INCREASE YOUR FIBER INTAKE SIGNIFICANTLY.

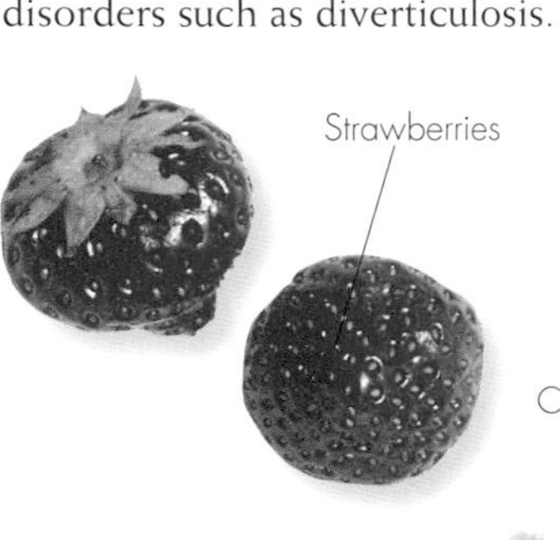

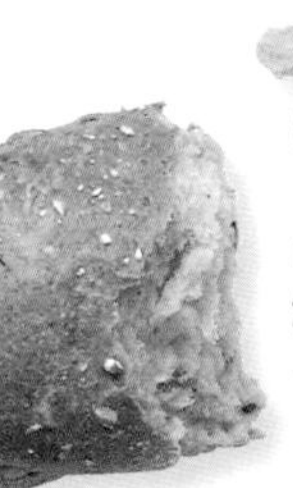

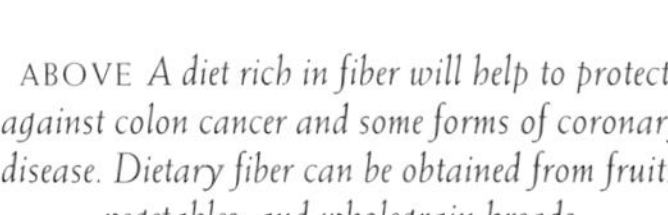

ABOVE *A diet rich in fiber will help to protect against colon cancer and some forms of coronary disease. Dietary fiber can be obtained from fruits, vegetables, and wholegrain breads.*

DATA FILE

Properties

- Reduces the production of cholesterol in the body.
- May protect against some coronary heart diseases.
- Helps to control diabetes.
- Helps to control weight.
- Can be used to treat certain intestinal disorders such as diverticulosis.
- Protects against cancers of the colon.

Best Sources

Fruit and vegetables, wholegrain breads and cereals, products made from nuts and legumes.

Dosage

- An intake of 20–60g. per day is ideal, and can be taken in the form of food, or as "soluble fiber," which is less likely to cause loose bowel movements.

GLANDULARS

Glandulars are concentrates of the hormonal glands, and have, over the past decade, been hailed as a wonder drug. Evidence does not, however, support these claims and many experts now discourage their use. The premise is that failing or aging glands can be rejuvenated by supplementation.

DATA FILE

Properties

- May improve sexual performance and libido.
- May help to build muscle.
- May help to control the spread of cancer.
- May help to treat hypoglycemia.
- May be used in the treatment of asthma.

Dosage

- Consult a registered practitioner before taking any glandulars.
- Do not take them at night, as they will cause insomnia.

CAUTION

GLANDULARS MAY CONTAIN MANY OF THE TOXINS LIVESTOCK ARE EXPOSED TO, SUCH AS ANTIBIOTICS, GROWTH HORMONES, PESTICIDES, HERBICIDES, AND FERTILIZERS.

ONLY TAKE THESE SUPPLEMENTS ON THE ADVICE OF A PHYSICIAN.

BELOW *Inhalers are most often used to treat asthma but glandulars have been said to help - only take them under medical supervision.*

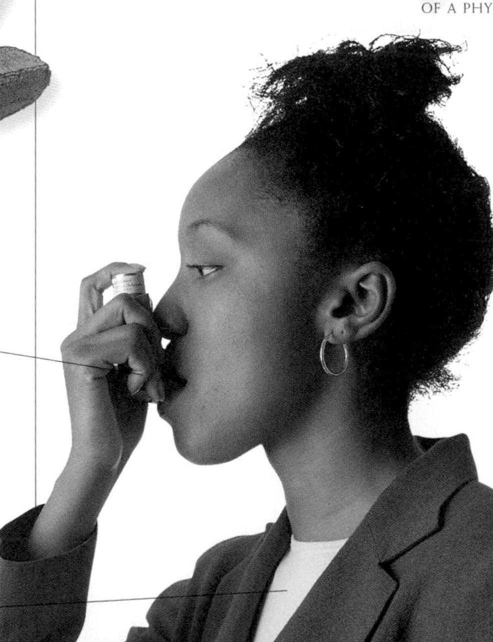

PABA

Para-aminobenzoic acid (PABA) is often grouped with the B-vitamins, and although it is water soluble, it is stored in the tissues and can be toxic at high doses. Freckles can sometimes be minimized by the use of sunscreen lotions containing para-aminobenzoic acid (PABA). PABA can be synthesized in the body, helps to form folic acid, and is important in the efficient utilization of protein.

CAUTION

HIGH DOSES CAN CAUSE NAUSEA, FEVER, SKIN RASH, AND DIARRHEA.

PABA MAY PROVE TOXIC TO THE LIVER IN HIGH DOSES.

DO NOT TAKE PABA IF YOU ARE USING ANY SULFONAMIDE ANTIBIOTICS.

ABOVE *Many sunscreens contain PABA as it helps shield the skin from harmful ultraviolet rays.*

DATA FILE

Properties

- Used for the treatment of Peyronie's disease.
- Shields the skin from the damage of ultraviolet rays.
- May rejuvenate skin.
- May help in the treatment of arthritis.
- May restore color to graying or white hair.
- Reduces the pain of burns (used externally).
- Keeps skin healthy and smooth, and helps to delay wrinkles (used externally).
- PABA is used in the treatment of eczema.

Best Sources

Liver, brewer's yeast, kidney, whole grains, rice, bran, and molasses.

Dosage

- Available in 30–1,000mg. strengths, and should be taken three times daily for best effect.
- Experts suggest that you do not take more than 30mg. daily because of side-effects (*see Caution*).
- Best taken in a good multivitamin supplement.
- Ointments are available for external use, and PABA is included in many sunscreen preparations.

PANGAMIC ACID

Also called vitamin B15, pangamic acid is not a vitamin in the strictest sense of the word, but it is a good antioxidant and some studies show promising results. Pangamic acid is water soluble, and it works much like vitamin E. It stimulates the carriage of oxygen to the blood from the lungs, and from the blood to the muscles and vital organs of the body. It also acts to detoxify poisons and free radicals, and to stimulate the "anti-stress" hormones.

CAUTION

THE FDA (FOOD AND DRUG ADMINISTRATION) IN THE U.S. HAS ATTEMPTED TO BAN THE SALE OF PANGAMIC ACID AS AN UNSAFE FOOD ADDITIVE, AND, APART FROM RUSSIAN STUDIES, THERE HAS BEEN LITTLE TO PROVE THE BENEFITS OF THE SUPPLEMENT. ONE STUDY SUGGESTS THAT IT MAY BE CARCINOGENIC.

DATA FILE

Properties

- Extends the life span of cells in the body.
- Helps to reduce a craving for alcohol.
- Encourages the body to deal efficiently with stress.
- Protects against pollution and cirrhosis of the liver.
- Helps synthesize protein.
- Helps angina and asthma.
- Lowers cholesterol levels.

Best Sources

Brewer's yeast, brown rice, whole grains, pumpkin seeds, sesame seeds.

Dosage

- Available in 50mg. capsules, and should be taken after the day's largest meal to avoid toxicity.
- Do not take more than 50mg. daily, and only supplement with the approval of your physician or registered practitioner.

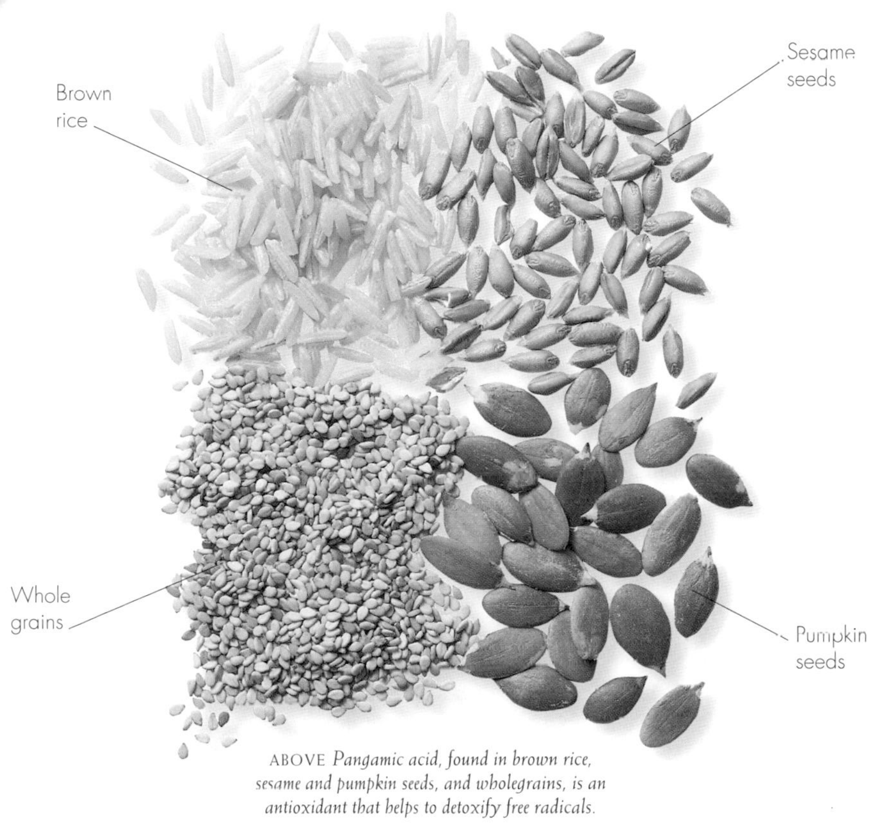

ABOVE *Pangamic acid, found in brown rice, sesame and pumpkin seeds, and wholegrains, is an antioxidant that helps to detoxify free radicals.*

PROPOLIS

Propolis is a sticky material collected by bees from buds or tree bark and used to seal the inside of the hive. It is a mixture of wax, resin, balsam oil, and pollen. It is said to act as an antibiotic and bactericide, and may be used to help wounds to heal. Propolis is rich in bioflavonoids.

CAUTION

BECAUSE THIS PRODUCT CONTAINS POLLEN, IT MAY CAUSE AN ALLERGIC REACTION IN SUSCEPTIBLE INDIVIDUALS.

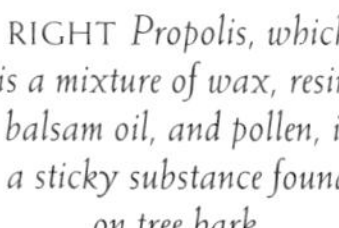

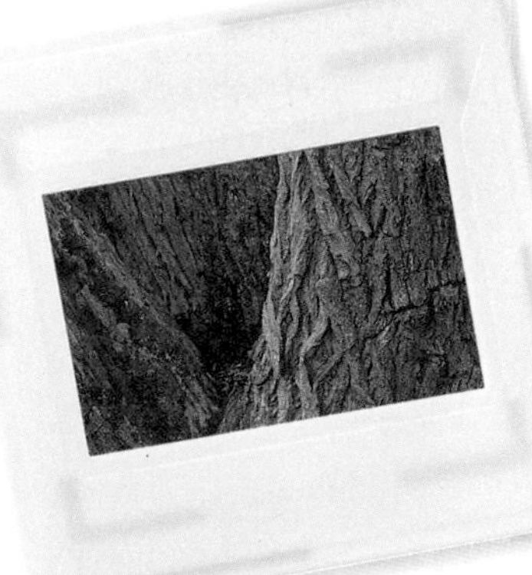

RIGHT *Propolis, which is a mixture of wax, resin, balsam oil, and pollen, is a sticky substance found on tree bark.*

DATA FILE

Properties

- Enhances immunity.
- Helps wounds to heal.
- Boosts energy.
- A natural anesthetic.
- Reduces cholesterol levels in the blood.
- Helps to reduce incidence and duration of colds.
- Natural antibiotic.

Dosage

- Propolis is available in tablet and liquid form, and does not appear to have any toxic levels.
- See your practitioner for details of suitable dosage.

SEAWEEDS

Seaweeds are not plants, but part of the Protista kingdom. They are better known as "algae," and there are four main types. Seaweeds appear in many foods, medicines, and cosmetics, and have been used therapeutically for thousands of years. Rich in iodine, they are used in the treatment of goiter.

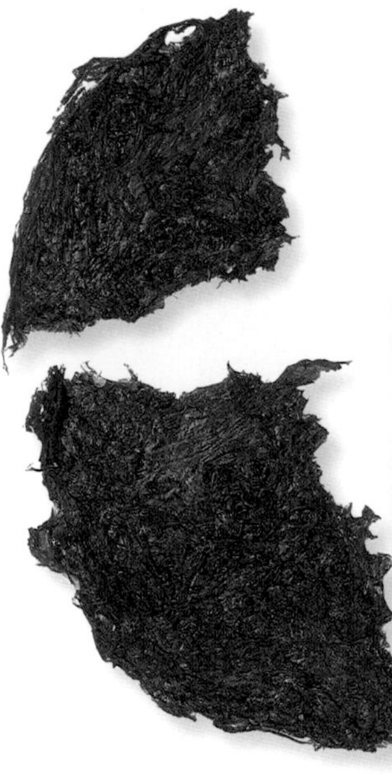

ABOVE *Seaweeds have been used in different cultures as a healing remedy and in cosmetics for centuries.*

BELOW *Seaweeds are an excellent source of protein, and should be included in your diet. They are also the richest natural source of iodine.*

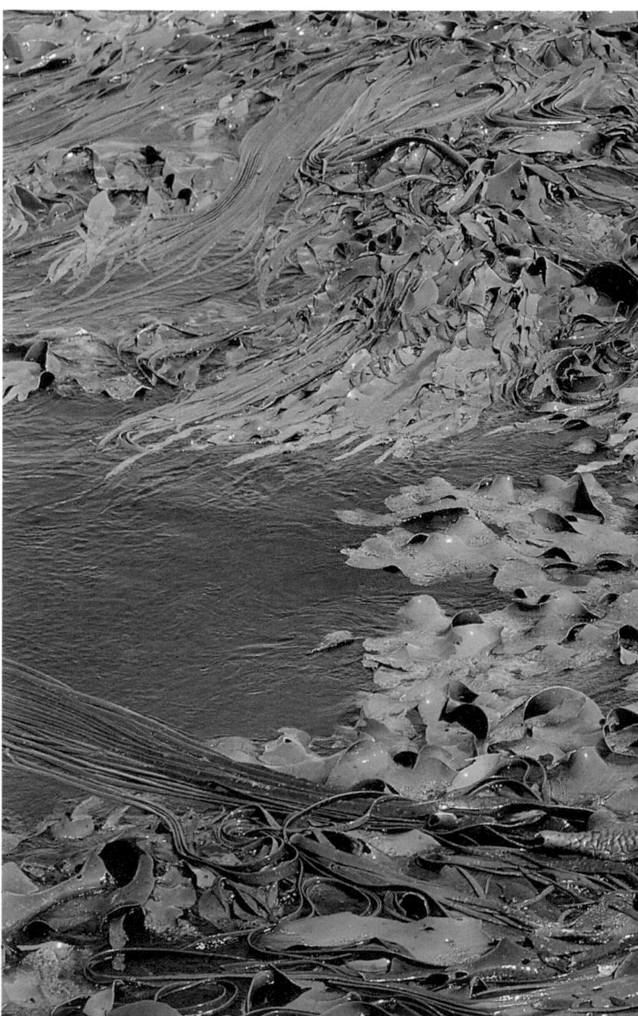

ROYAL JELLY

Royal jelly has been used for centuries for its health-giving and rejuvenating properties, and it is rich in vitamins, amino acids, and minerals. It is also the prime source of fatty acid, which is said to increase alertness and act as a natural tranquilizer (when necessary). Royal jelly is secreted by the salivary glands of the worker bees to feed and stimulate the growth and development of the queen bee.

DATA FILE

Properties

- Antibacterial.
- May prevent the development of leukemia.
- Has a yeast-inhibiting function, preventing conditions such as thrush and athlete's foot.
- Contains the male sex hormone testosterone, which may increase libido.
- Used to treat subfertility.
- May be useful in the treatment of ME and MD (muscular dystrophy).
- Helps to reduce allergies.
- Boosts the body's resistance to the harmful side-effects of chemotherapy and radiotherapy.
- Controls cholesterol levels.
- Boosts the immune system.
- Royal jelly is used in the treatment of skin problems, including eczema, psoriasis, and acne.
- Combined with pantothenic acid, royal jelly provides relief from the symptoms of arthritis.

Dosage

- Most tablets contain 100–500mg. of royal jelly.
- Optimum dosage is about 150mg. per day.
- Fresh is better, although more expensive.

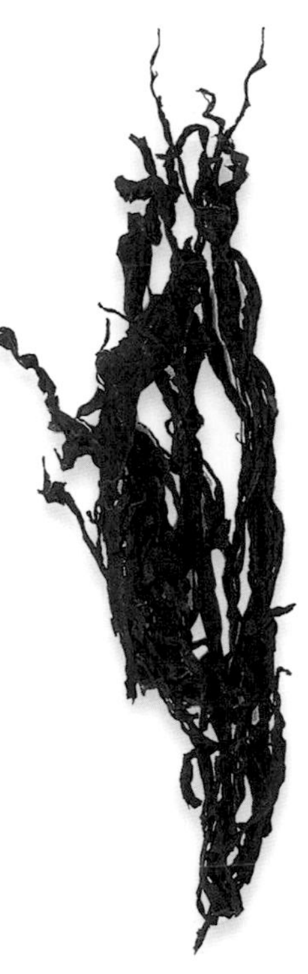

DATA FILE

Properties

- Antiviral activity.
- May prevent cancer.
- Used in the prevention and treatment of goiter.
- May help to reduce the effects of carcinogen, as well as radioactive material.
- Helps to counter the side-effects of radiotherapy and chemotherapy treatment.
- Natural antacid.
- Used in the treatment of intestinal disorders.
- Used in the treatment of exudative wounds.

Best Sources

Take seaweeds in their natural form, available from health food stores and many grocery stores (particularly oriental food stores).

Dosage

- There is no recommended dosage – consult a registered practitioner.

SPIRULINA

Spirulina are blue-green bacteria or algae, which are rich in GLA (gamma-linoleic acid, *see page* 270) and a wide variety of nutrients, including beta-carotene, inositol, calcium, vitamin E, magnesium, and phosphorus. In ancient times, spirulina was used as a staple food by the Aztecs of Mexico. It is now marketed in health food stores as a high-protein food supplement.

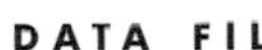

LEFT *Spirulina food supplements will help to keep your skin healthy and free of blemishes.*

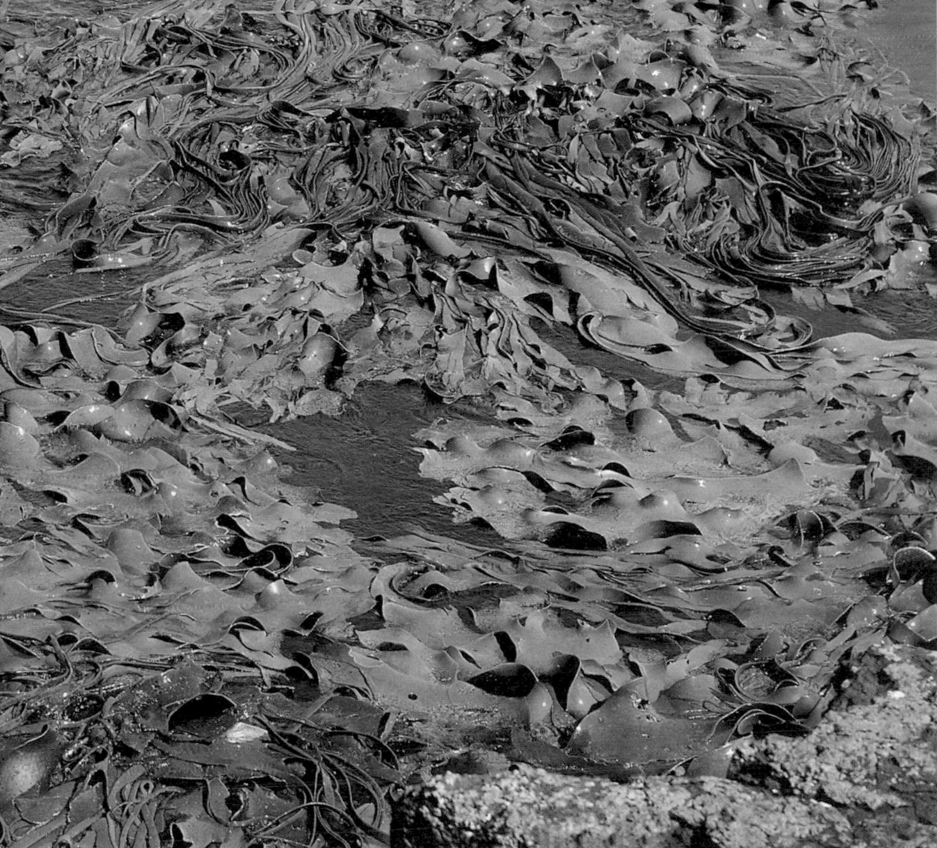

DATA FILE

Properties

- Rich in nutrients and high in protein (particularly useful for vegetarians).
- May suppress appetite.
- Maintains skin health and treats skin disorders.
- May contribute to healthy functioning of the intestines.
- General tonic properties.
- May be rejuvenating.
- Many spirulina have anti-cancer properties.

Best Sources

Fresh or freeze-dried spirulina.

Dosage

- There is no recommended dosage for spirulina – consult a registered practitioner.

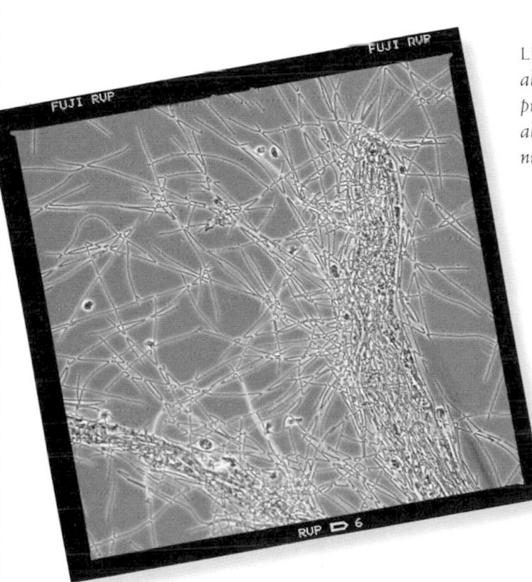

LEFT *Spirulina algae contain protein and are also rich in nutrients.*

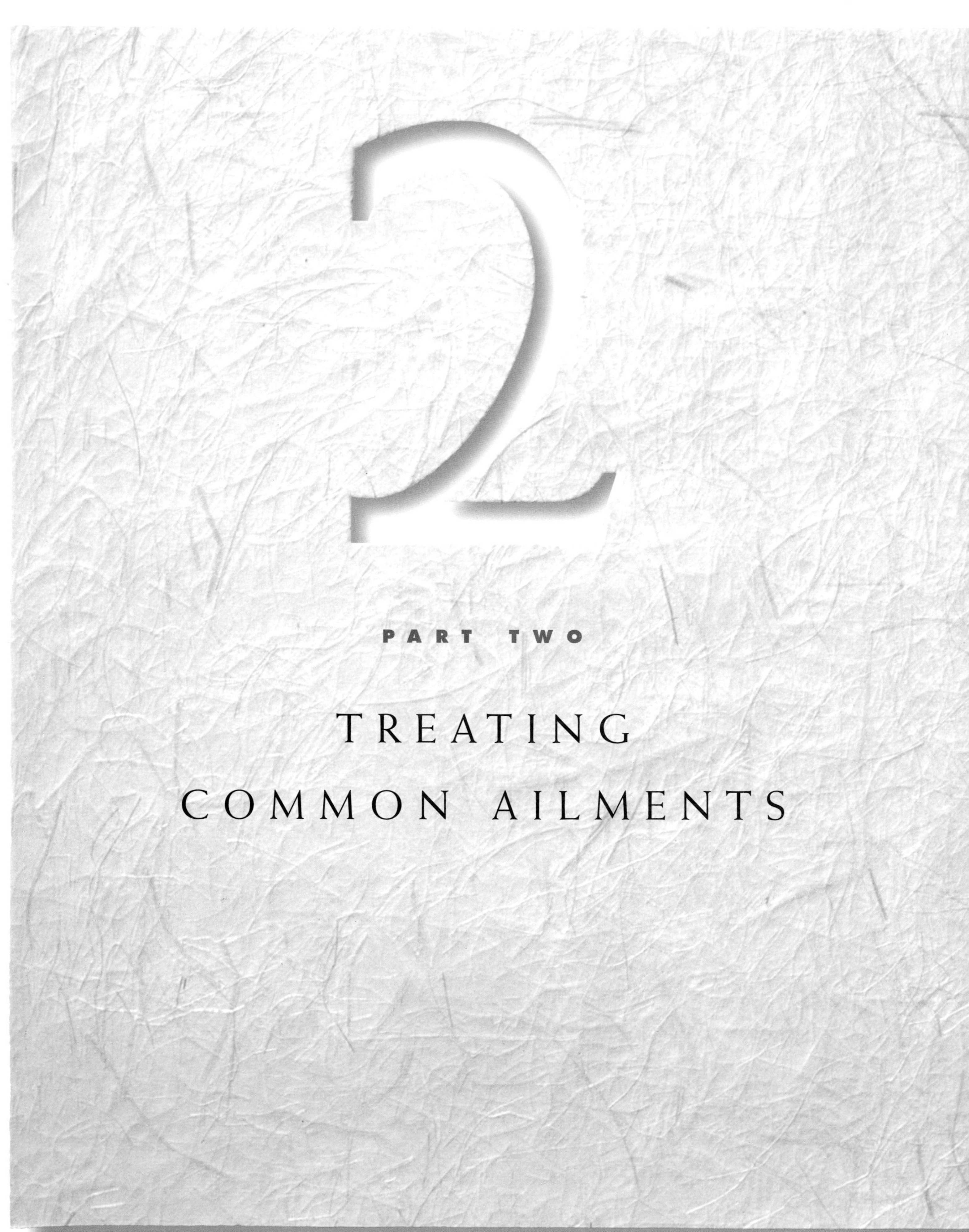

PART TWO

TREATING COMMON AILMENTS

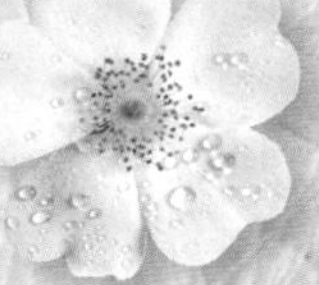

DISORDERS OF THE MIND AND EMOTIONS

Addictions

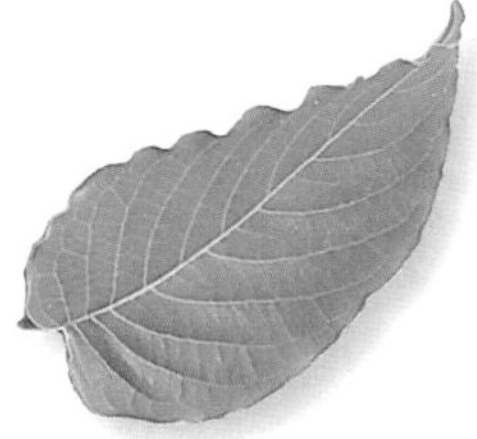

ABOVE *Add ylang ylang oil to the bath for its antidepressant qualities.*

An addiction is an overwhelming craving for or dependence on a substance, usually a drug, alcohol, or nicotine. The addiction may be limited to mental dependence, but it can become physiological if the way in which the body functions has changed through prolonged use of a substance. In such cases the addict will experience physical "withdrawal" symptoms without the substance in question.

Symptoms

• *loss of control over use of the drug or other substance* • *mood swings and irrational behavior* • *in drug addiction: – sore or red eyes with dilated or constricted pupils – irregular breathing – trembling hands – itchy or runny nose – nausea* • *drug withdrawal symptoms may include craving, depression, restlessness, yawning, sweating, abdominal pain, vomiting, diarrhea, loss of appetite, and suffering from gooseflesh*

DATA FILE

• Drugs with potential for misuse are narcotics, including morphine, opium, heroin, and methadone; depressants such as alcohol, barbiturates, and sedatives; stimulants such as cocaine and amphetamines; hallucinogenic drugs; and marijuana.

• Nicotine and caffeine can also be abused, and anabolic steroids and human growth hormone are often misused by athletes and bodybuilders seeking to increase muscle mass.

• True physical addiction is known to occur with the narcotics and depressants; psychological dependence, with or without physical symptoms, can develop from using many other prescription drugs, such as tranquilizers.

• Studies show that 50–80 percent of all alcoholics have a close relative who is an alcoholic. Some researchers therefore suggest that some alcoholics have an inherited physical predisposition to alcohol addiction.

• Alcoholism and alcohol abuse in the U.S. cost an estimated $98 billion and take 100,000 lives per year, according to the National Institute on Alcohol Abuse and Alcoholism.

• One-half of all traffic fatalities and one-third of all traffic injuries are related to the abuse of alcohol.

• One-third of all suicides and one-third of all mental health disorders are estimated to be associated with serious alcohol abuse.

• The relaxation smokers feel is because tobacco contains nicotine, an addictive alkaloid. A number of diseases have been directly linked to smoking, and in the U.S. alone tobacco use kills about 420,000 smokers each year.

• Every day about 3,500 Americans successfully quit smoking.

CAUTION

ADDICTIONS TO PHYSICAL SUBSTANCES SHOULD ALWAYS BE TREATED BY A REGISTERED PRACTITIONER.

DO NOT DISCONTINUE ANY PRESCRIPTION DRUGS UNLESS YOU ARE UNDER SUPERVISION.

LEFT *Alcohol causes a third of all mental disorders.*

TREATMENT

AYURVEDA
• This has proved very successful in treating addictions of all types, which it sees as fundamental imbalance within the body. Treatment will be tailored to your specific constitution and personal characteristics. *(See page 20.)*

CHINESE HERBALISM
• For alcoholism, heat would be cleared from the Lung and Liver, with watermelon or kudzu vine to detoxify Blood.
• Treatment would be specific for various other types of addiction.
• Strong green tea is used to cool the liver.

HERBALISM
• Oats will calm you down and help to strengthen your willpower. *(See page 117.)*
• Other herbs to calm the nervous system and reduce symptoms when you wish to withdraw from your addiction include skullcap and valerian. Drink daily as a tea. *(See pages 131 and 136.)*
• Cramp bark helps nervous tension and jitters. *(See page 138.)*

AROMATHERAPY
• Antidepressant oils include chamomile, clary sage, and ylang ylang. Use in the bath, and in a vaporizer by your bedside. A few drops on your clothing during the day will allow the effect to be maintained. *(See pages 146–71.)*

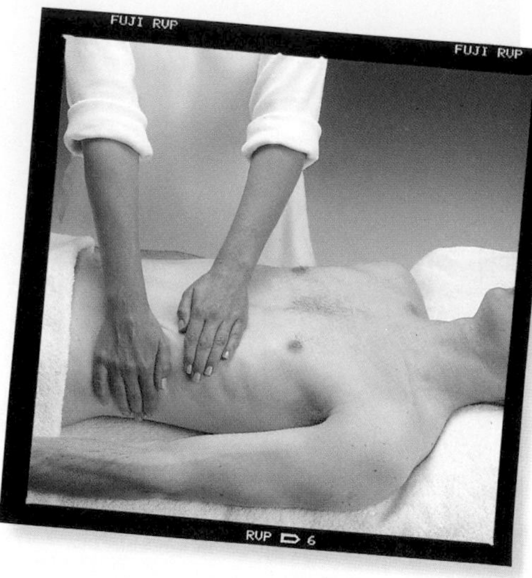

ABOVE *An aromatherapy massage encourages a positive attitude.*

• Massage with aromatherapy oil is extremely rewarding and a positive treatment. Try detoxifying oils such as juniper. *(See page 160.)*
• Aromatherapists suggest changing the oils used at regular intervals; although it is almost impossible to become physically addicted to an essential oil, you may come to regard it as a prop. *(See pages 146–71.)*
• Bergamot seems to be extremely useful in cases of food addiction. *(See page 153.)*

HOMEOPATHY
Homeopathic treatment would be constitutional, or tailored to your individual needs. Some useful addiction treatments are:
• Nux vomica, which helps to overcome a craving for smoking. *(See page 214.)*
• Kali phos., which strengthens the nervous system and may make it easier for a person to give up an addiction. *(See page 201.)*
• Arsenicum, for great anxiety, restlessness and fear of being alone. *(See page 182.)*
• Absinthium, when you feel depressed, disoriented, and dizzy.

FLOWER ESSENCES
• Crab Apple, for anyone who needs purification. *(See page 234.)*
• Gorse, when you are stuck in a negative pattern. *(See page 240.)*
• Mustard, for depression for no apparent reason. *(See page 239.)*
• Olive is particularly good for the recovery period. *(See page 235.)*

VITAMINS AND MINERALS
Treatment would ensure that there are no small nutritional deficiencies making you crave certain substances, and that deficiencies caused by addictions (such as vitamin B in alcoholics) are righted. Some amino acids may be used to create a specific physical effect, or act as a natural tranquilizer, which may help. Alcoholics are often deficient in GLA (gamma-linolenic acid), and it is recommended that you take evening primrose (a rich source) to help prevent mood swings. *(See page 270.)*

Obsessions and Compulsions

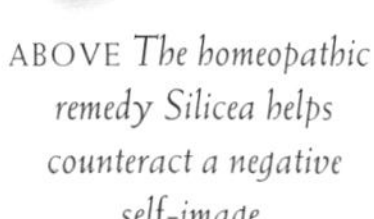

ABOVE *The homeopathic remedy Silicea helps counteract a negative self-image.*

An obsession is a persistent, recurring thought or idea, while a compulsion is an overwhelming drive to perform a particular act. When a person becomes dominated by these intrusions, despite knowing that they are irrational, he or she is said to be suffering from an obsessive-compulsive disorder. This may take the form of a hand-washing ritual, for example, or repeated checking that doors and windows are locked. The problem is often triggered by a stressful life event, but can also be due to subtle brain damage (usually the result of illnesses affecting the brain), especially when due to encephalitis. Obsessive-compulsive disorder is rare, although minor obsessional symptoms probably occur in about 15 percent of the population. At least two-thirds of all people who have obsessive compulsive disorder respond well to therapy. Symptoms may recur under stress but can usually be controlled.

SYMPTOMS

- *fear of contamination*
- *dermatitis caused by repeated washing*
- *inefficiency caused by repeated and meticulous checking*
- *aggressive thoughts and behavior*
- *depression may develop*

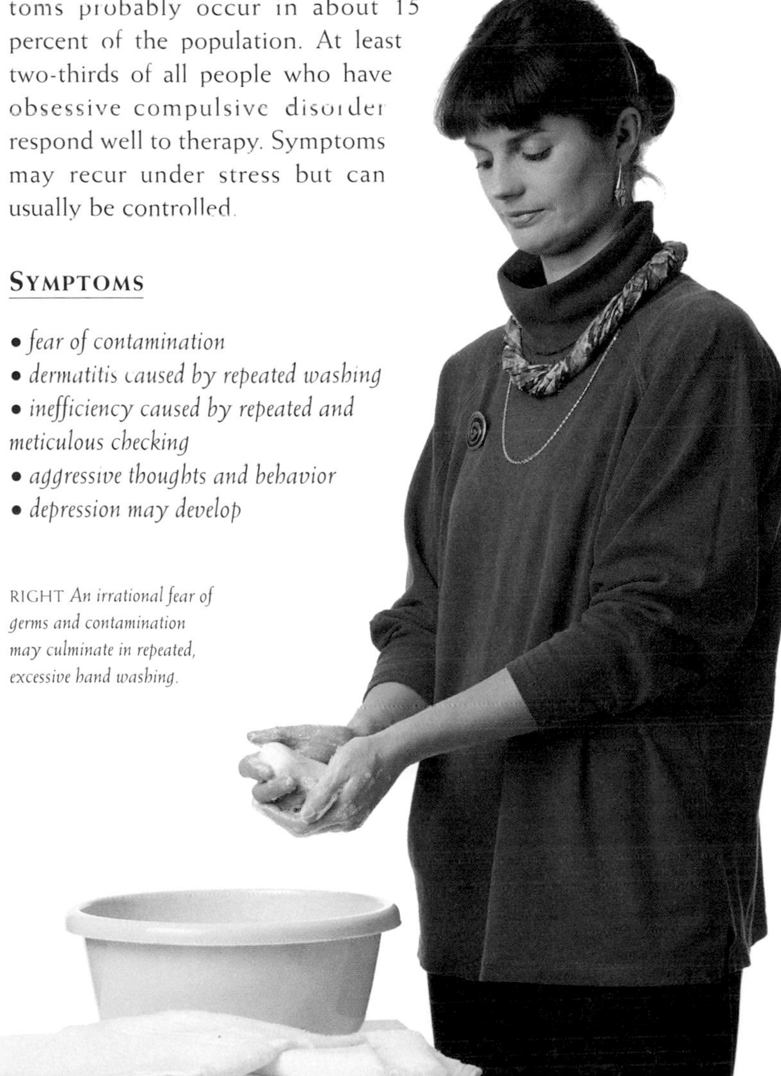

RIGHT *An irrational fear of germs and contamination may culminate in repeated, excessive hand washing.*

TREATMENT

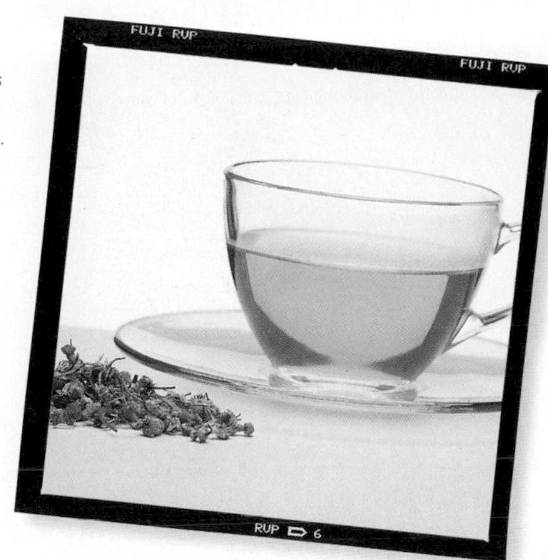

RIGHT *Certain herbs have beneficial effects on the nervous system. Take them in the form of an infusion.*

HERBALISM

- Drink certain infused herbs which act on the nervous system, including hops, valerian, vervain, chamomile, and passiflora. Taken on a regular basis, these herbs may help to ease tension and restrict various behavioral problems. *(See pages 119, 136, and 138.)*

AROMATHERAPY

- Relaxing oils, such as Roman chamomile or marjoram may help to achieve balance. Use regularly in the bath or on a burner in your room. *(See pages 150 and 165.)*
- Ylang ylang and clary sage may also help. *(See pages 169 and 148.)*

HOMEOPATHY

- Aurum is useful for feelings of worthlessness and overwhelming thoughts of death and dying. *(See page 184.)*
- Silicea for unshakable feelings of inadequacy, and an overwhelming urge to count small objects. *(See page 211.)*
- Take Anacardium when you feel that your mind is not your own and is being controlled by an external force. *(See page 179.)*

FLOWER ESSENCES

- Cherry Plum, for the fear of losing your mind, and to deal with irrational thoughts or behavior. *(See page 236.)*
- Crab Apple, for those who feel unclean or polluted on any level. *(See page 234.)*
- Vervain, for those who are strong-willed and need space for reflection. *(See page 241.)*
- White Chestnut, for an overactive mind, full of unwanted patterns of thought. *(See page 224.)*

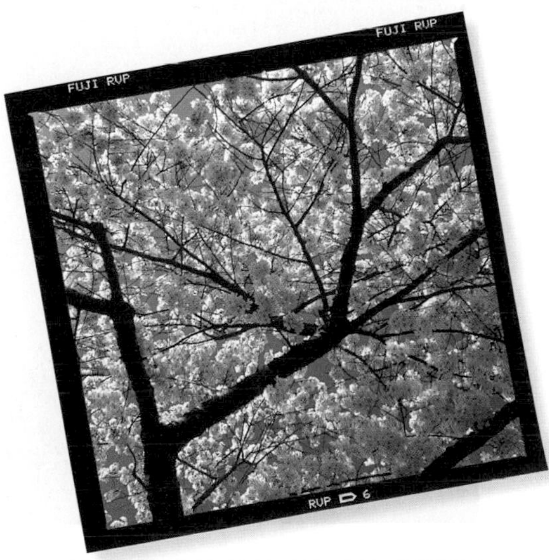

RIGHT *The flower remedy Cherry Plum helps quell illogical behavior patterns.*

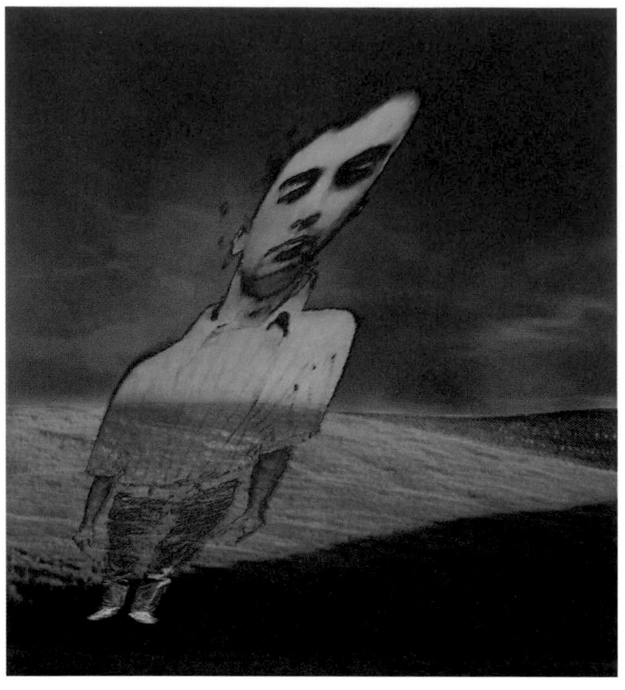

ABOVE *Phobias range from the manageable to the totally incapacitating.*

Phobias

A phobia is an irrational fear which the sufferer finds impossible to overcome. Some of the most common fears are claustrophobia (fear of enclosed spaces), agoraphobia (fear of open spaces), and acrophobia (fear of heights). A phobia can, however, relate to just about any object, person, or situation, and is probably caused by a subconscious reflex to avoid repeating an unpleasant experience. For the sufferer it may cause little more than mild embarrassment, or it may be totally debilitating and disruptive to everyday life. An estimated 10 percent of people in the U.K., and slightly more in the U.S., suffer from phobias of some description. Recent research indicates that most sufferers can cure themselves.

LEFT *Jasmine essential oil has a scent which calms an agitated mind.*

SYMPTOMS

• *rapid pulse* • *profuse sweating*
• *high blood pressure* • *trembling* • *nausea*

TREATMENT

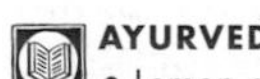

AYURVEDA

• Lemon or lime may be suggested for dizziness, and individual treatment would be prescribed according to your specific needs. *(See page 20.)*

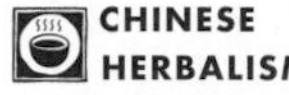

CHINESE HERBALISM

• A herbalist may suggest cooling herbs, and Gui Pi Wan, which addresses emotional problems.

• Ginseng, Chinese angelica and senega root may also be useful. *(See pages 56, 67, 70.)*

HERBALISM

• Valerian tea can help to reduce tension. Drink an infusion as required. *(See page 136.)*

AROMATHERAPY

Essential oils can be very useful in the treatment of phobias. The effect of certain smells can help to release tension and induce a feeling of calm. Some of the best oils to try are: bergamot, chamomile, clary sage, geranium, jasmine, juniper, lavender, marjoram, melissa, and ylang ylang, which are sedative. They can be used in the bath, in massage with a light carrier oil (such as sweet almond), or in a vaporizer. Carry a bottle of diluted oils with you – perhaps in a small sprayer – and apply them to the temples or pulse points in times of fear. *(See page 140.)*

ABOVE *Aconite is a homeopathic remedy for agoraphobia.*

HOMEOPATHY

There are dozens of homeopathic remedies which can be used to treat phobias, but they will be prescribed constitutionally, that is, the treatment would be tailored to your exact needs. Some to try may be:

• Arg. nit., for fear of heights. *(See page 181.)*
• Phosphorus, for fear of the dark. *(See page 208.)*
• Gelsemium, for fear of performing in public, when you feel weak at the knees. *(See page 195.)*
• Aconite, for agoraphobia, when you are terrified of dying or collapsing if you go out. *(See page 178.)*
• Arnica, for fears that are brought on by an accident. *(See page 182.)*
• Sulfur, when you need help and no other remedy seems to be indicated. *(See page 215.)*

FLOWER ESSENCES

Treatment would be based on your individual state of mind, but some of the following may help:

• Mimulus, for the everyday fears of known things, spiders, being late for work, flying, and being ill. *(See page 235.)*
• Aspen is for unknown fears, the vague and dark fears which hover and play on the imagination. *(See page 236.)*
• Rock Rose should be added when the fear is turning into terror and perhaps even panic. *(See page 231.)*
• Cherry Plum is for the fear that everything will fall apart. *(See page 236.)*
• Red Chestnut is for fear for another's safety. *(See page 224.)*
• The most important Bach Flower Remedy for fear, anxiety, and phobias, Rescue Remedy, is made up of five essences, Cherry Plum, Rock Rose, Impatiens, Clematis, and Star of Bethlehem. It works to treat fear, loneliness, despondency, and loss of focus. It rebalances the sufferer after an emotional upset and is particularly useful in panic attacks. Apply a few drops of the remedy to your tongue or pulse points. *(See page 244.)*

VITAMINS AND MINERALS

Vitamin B-complex and C are important for nerve functioning. Ensure that you eat regular meals, since low blood sugar can exacerbate the problem.

BELOW *Use an atomizer to apply your favorite essential oil at stressful moments.*

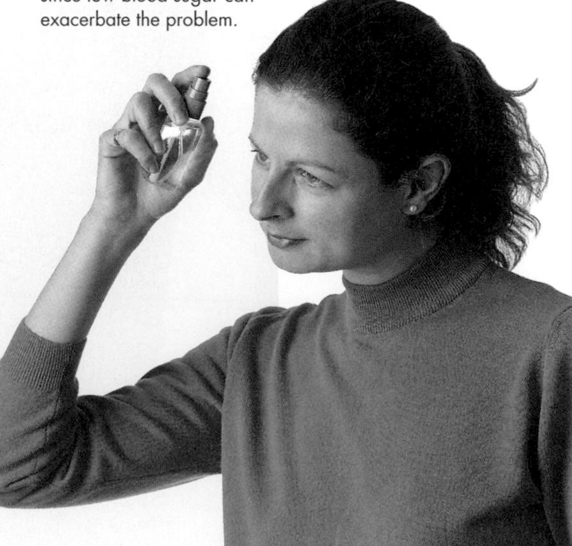

Depression

Depression is a prolonged feeling of unhappiness and despondency, often magnified by a major life event such as bereavement, divorce, or retirement. Many women experience depression after childbirth. Clinical depression is a genuine illness which overwhelms the sufferer so that he or she feels a hopelessness, dejection, and fear out of all proportion to any cause. Someone who is depressed may even contemplate or attempt suicide.

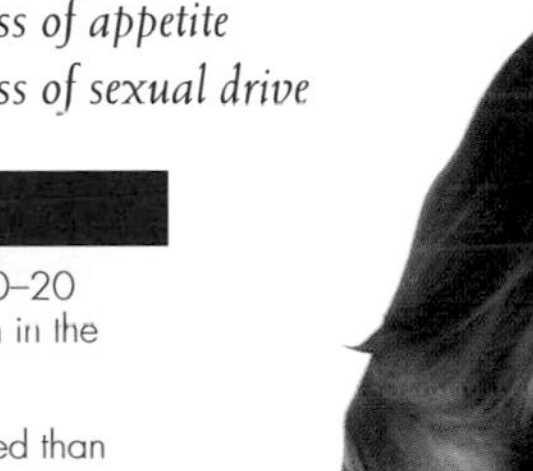

ABOVE *Chamomile essential oil has antidepressant qualities.*

Symptoms

- *slow speech* • *poor concentration* • *confusion and irritability* • *self-accusation and loss of self-esteem*
- *insomnia and early-morning waking*
- *a feeling of emptiness and despair*
- *loss of appetite*
- *loss of sexual drive*

DATA FILE

- Major depressions occur in 10–20 percent of the world's population in the course of a lifetime.
- Women are more often affected than men, by a 2:1 ratio.
- Relatives of patients with major depressive illnesses seem to be at some higher risk of becoming depressed, and about 2 percent of the population may have a chronic disorder known as a depressive personality.
- Unipolar depression consists of episodes that can recur several times in a person's life.
- Manic depression, or bipolar disorder, is a severe mental disorder involving manic episodes (characterized by an abnormally elevated or irritable mood, grandiosity, sleeplessness, extravagance, and a tendency toward irrational judgment) that are usually accompanied by episodes of depression (possibly including lethargy, a sense of worthlessness, lack of concentration, and guilt). Manic depression occurs in males and females equally, and is found more frequently in close relatives of people with the disorder.
- More than 8 billion people in the U.S. consult their general physician about treatment for depression.
- Up to 50 percent of people who suffer have a hereditary tendency.
- Seasonal affective disorder (SAD) is thought to be caused by a deficiency of corticotropin-releasing hormone.
- Cases of SAD are on the increase, and are thought to be partly due to increased stress levels.

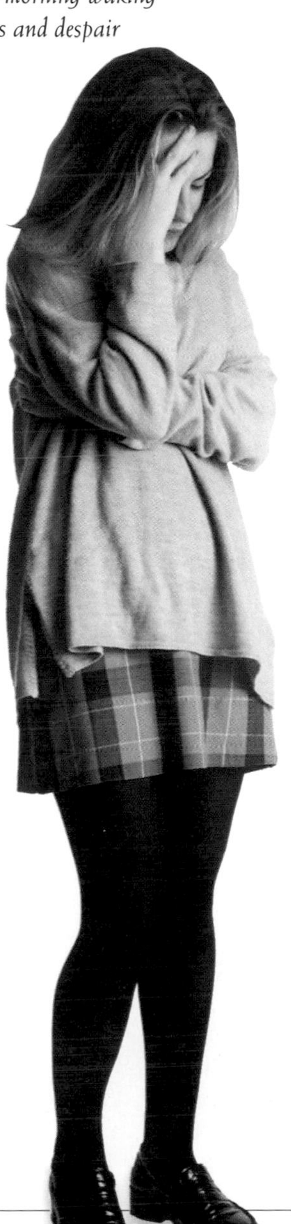

LEFT *Depression affects more women than men.*

TREATMENT

AYURVEDA

- Detoxification treatment would be followed by specific oral medication to balance the three doshas. Treatment is always individual. *(See page 20.)*

CHINESE HERBALISM

- Depression is believed to be caused by stagnation of the Liver qi, and may be treated with angelica, peony root, licorice, and thorowax root. *(See pages 56, 64, 67.)*

HERBALISM

- The best antidepressant and nervine (with a specific action for nerves) herbs include: balm, borage, limeflower, oats, rosemary, and vervain. These can be taken as herbal teas, added to the bath, or taken as tablets, or in tincture form (herbs suspended in alcohol). *(See page 104.)*

AROMATHERAPY

- There are a number of antidepressant oils, which can be used in the bath, in a vaporizer, on a light bulb and in massage. They include: neroli, jasmine, geranium, melissa, and rose.
- Ylang ylang, lavender, clary sage, and chamomile are sedative and antidepressant.

HOMEOPATHY

It will be necessary to see a homeopath to receive treatment that is suited to you, and which addresses the cause of your depression. Specific remedies include:

- Aurum, for feelings of worthlessness, suicidal feelings, and self-disgust. *(See page 184.)*
- Pulsatilla, for bursting into tears at the smallest slight. *(See page 209.)*
- Arsenicum, if you feel chilly, tired, restless, and obsessively tidy. *(See page 182.)*
- Ignatia, if depression has an external cause, such as bereavement. *(See page 200.)*

FLOWER ESSENCES

- Cherry Plum, for "fear of the mind being over strained, of doing dreaded things," and of being violent to oneself or others. *(See page 236.)*
- Agrimony, for deeply held emotional tensions which are hidden from others. *(See page 225.)*
- Gorse helps to combat feelings of hopelessness. *(See page 240.)*
- Gentian will help to improve a mild depression and despondency caused by a setback. *(See page 230.)*
- Mustard is for blacker and deeper feelings when there is no apparent cause. *(See page 239.)*
- Sweet Chestnut should be taken if you feel anguished and stretched beyond endurance. *(See page 227.)*

VITAMINS AND MINERALS

Depression which occurs just before menstruation (PMS) may be caused by a vitamin B6 deficiency; post-natal depression may be caused by a deficiency of vitamin B12, and folic acid. Nutritional supplements and allergy tests may be suggested by a practitioner. Ensure you have an adequate intake of vitamin C. Some therapists may recommend supplementing the amino acid tryptophan. *(See page 246.)*

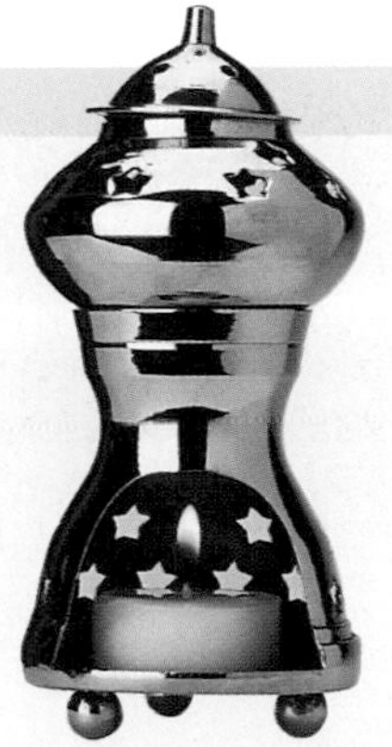

ABOVE *A vaporizer heats an essential oil to release its therapeutic qualities.*

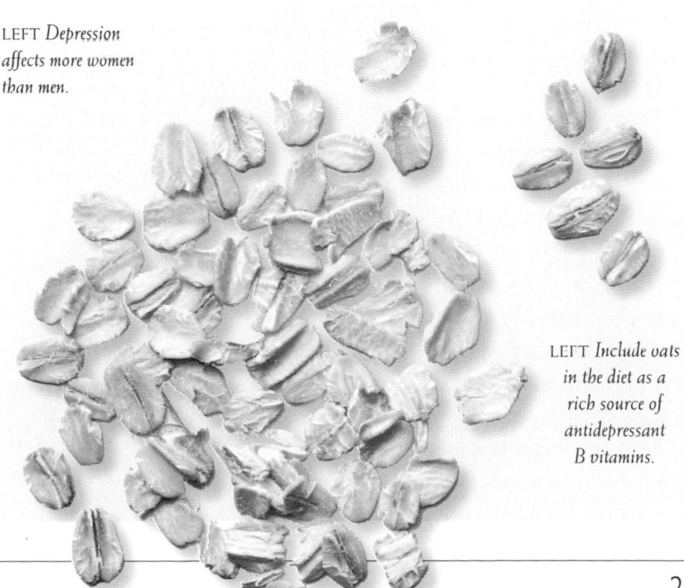

LEFT *Include oats in the diet as a rich source of antidepressant B vitamins.*

Stress

Each individual is able to cope with a different amount of stress in life, and while some seem to draw on endless reserves to keep going, others succumb. A certain amount of stress provides stimulation, but prolonged stress can cause mental and physical damage.

Most of us think of tense situations and worries as being the cause of stress. In reality, stresses are wide-ranging. They include environmental stresses, such as pollution, noise, housing problems, cold, or overheating; physical stresses, such as illnesses, injuries, an inadequate diet; and mental stresses, such as relationship problems, financial strains, bereavement; and job difficulties. All these factors affect the body, causing it to make a series of rapid physiological changes, called "adaptive responses," to deal with threatening or demanding situations.

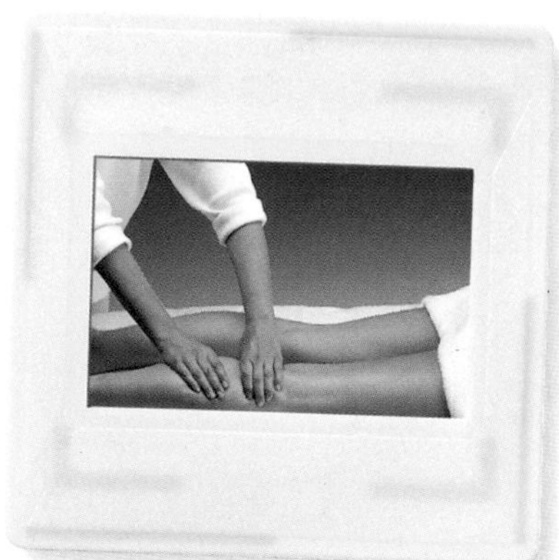

ABOVE *Human touch is very comforting and can be utilized in massage.*

In the first stage of stress, hormones are poured into the bloodstream. The pulse quickens, the lungs take in more oxygen to fuel the muscles, blood sugar increases to supply added energy, digestion slows, and perspiration increases. In the second stage of stress, the body begins to repair the damage caused by the first stage. If the stressful situation is resolved, the stress symptoms vanish. If the situation continues, however, exhaustion sets in, and the body's energy gives out. This stage may continue until vital organs are affected, and then disease or even death can result.

Symptoms

• *the increase in hormones such as adrenaline, noradrenaline, and corticosteroids in response to stress may cause the following: – increased breathing and heart rate – nausea – tense muscles* • *in the long term it is thought that stress can lead to: – insomnia – depression – high blood pressure – hair loss – allergies – ulcers – heart disease – digestive disorders – menstrual problems – palpitations – impotence and premature ejaculation*

DATA FILE

• Psychological stress results from perceived or anticipated threats. The stress may be acute, as in response to immediate danger, or chronic, as when an individual is experiencing an unhappy life situation. In either case, the body mechanisms are similar.

• Chronic physical illness is almost always accompanied by significant psychological effects.

• Long-lasting psychological stress, in turn, often leads to debilitating changes.

• Medical scientists divide people's behavior into two types, depending on their reactions to stress. People with type-A behavior react to stress with aggressiveness, competitiveness, and self-imposed pressure to get things done. Type-A behavior has been linked to increased rates of heart attack and other diseases. People with type-B behavior may be equally serious in their intentions, but are more patient, easygoing, and relaxed.

• Stress is a major factor in diseases whose physical symptoms are induced or aggravated by mental or emotional problems.

• Stress-related disorders comprise 50–80 percent of all illnesses, though stress may not be the only cause.

TREATMENT

AYURVEDA
• An Ayurvedic practitioner would prescribe supportive herbs, and use a balancing treatment specific to your needs. *(See page 20.)*

CHINESE HERBALISM
• Chinese medicine takes the view that it is not stress that causes illness, but how we deal with it. Herbs would be prescribed according to your specific needs, in order to support you throughout stressful periods, and tonify. *(See page 51.)*
• Treatment may be aimed particularly at the Kidneys, which have become exhausted through overwork, and to support the Blood and qi, which need to circulate harmoniously in the body. *(See page 50.)*

TRADITIONAL FOLK AND HOME REMEDIES
• Pumpkin seeds, which contain high quantities of zinc, iron and calcium, as well as B vitamins and proteins, which are necessary for brain function, will help you to deal with the effects of stress.
• Oats are vital for a healthy nervous system. In periods of stress, start the day with oatmeal, which will help to keep you calm, and prevent depression and general debility. *(See page 84.)*

HERBALISM
• Herbs that encourage relaxation and act as a tonic to the nervous system include balm, lavender, chamomile, passiflora and oats. These can be drunk as an infusion – as often as necessary when in a stressful situation. *(See pages 117 and 119.)*
• Ginseng is an excellent "adaptogenic" herb, which means that it lifts you when you are tired and relaxes you when you are stressed. It also works on the immune system and energizes. Some therapists recommend a daily dose at stressful times. *(See page 126.)*

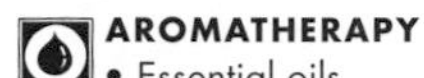

AROMATHERAPY
• Essential oils are excellent for stress reduction because many of them work on the nervous system and the brain to relax and soothe. *(See pages 146–71.)*
• Other oils are uplifting, which can be invaluable in times of serious stress. *(See pages 146–71.)*
• Massage with aromatherapy oils is very comforting – particularly the physical element of touch – and a few drops of essential oil in the bath can offer an opportunity to "wash away" the problems of the day while experiencing the benefits of the oil. Suitable oils include basil, chamomile, geranium, lavender, neroli, and rose. *(See pages 146–71.)*
• Oils which strengthen the adrenal system, which is weakened by stress, include rosemary, ginger, and lemongrass. *(See pages 146–71.)*

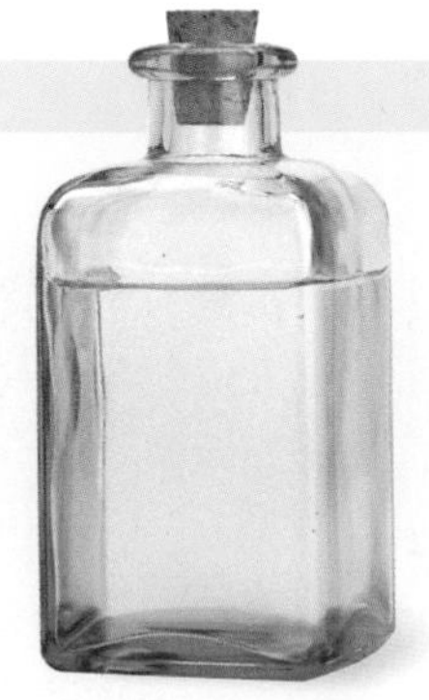

ABOVE *A massage blend which includes rosemary essential oil strengthens the adrenal system.*

VITAMINS AND MINERALS
Eating a good, balanced diet will make your body stronger and able to cope more efficiently with stress. B vitamins are often depleted by stress, so ensure that you are getting enough in your diet, or take a good supplement. There is some evidence that bee and flower pollen, available in tablets or in grains, can boost immunity and energize the body. Do not eat this if you are allergic to honey or bee stings. An amino acid called L-Tyrosine appears to energize and relieve stress, and studies show that people taking this supplement react better to stressful situations, staying more alert, less anxious, more efficient, and have fewer complaints about physical discomforts. Vitamin C is a great stress reliever, and boosts immunity, making you fitter and more healthy. *(See page 256.)*

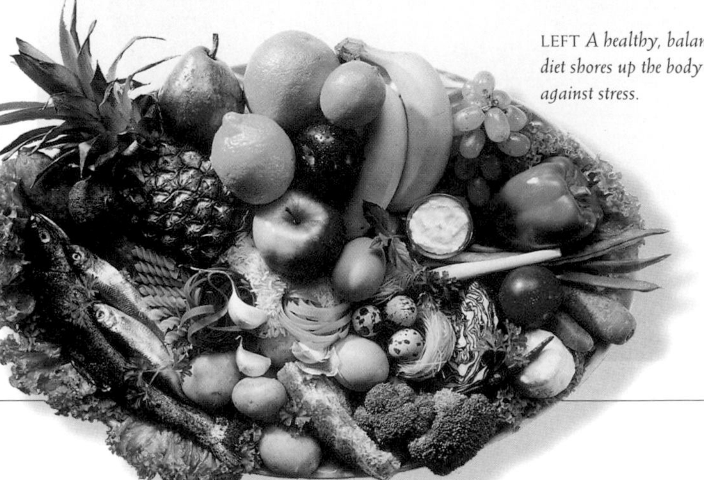

LEFT *A healthy, balanced diet shores up the body against stress.*

Anxiety

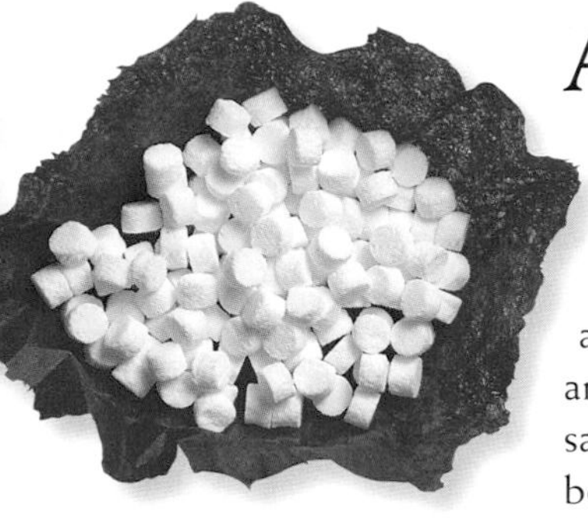

ABOVE *The homeopathic remedy Calcarea balances calcium levels in the body.*

Anxiety is a state of fear or apprehension in the face of threat or danger. It is a natural, healthy response since it allows the body to prepare itself (through adrenaline) to cope with the danger. Anxiety can, however, take a person over – a condition known as anxiety neurosis – and the person is then said to be in an anxiety state. This may be chronic anxiety, with a constant feeling of worry, associated with depression, or an acute anxiety attack, when the sufferer will be suddenly overwhelmed by fear and feelings of dread.

DATA FILE

- When we are faced with a frightening or threatening situation, our body goes into a "fight or flight" response, when adrenaline pours into the system and the body prepares itself for action. When no action follows, and nervous energy is not discharged, there is physiological confusion – otherwise known as a panic attack. Symptoms may include dizziness, visual disturbance, clammy hands, racing heart, dry mouth, and overbreathing.
- Up to 70 percent of people who have panic attacks end up seeing as many as ten physicians before being correctly diagnosed.
- Anxiety appears to affect twice as many women as men.
- Evidence exists that some people may be biochemically vulnerable to panic attacks.
- The National Center for Health Statistics reports that drugs for anxiety disorders are among the 20 drugs most frequently prescribed.
- In the U.K., a report by the Royal College of Psychiatrists stated that more than 9 million Britons will suffer from abnormal anxiety and fears at some point in their lives.
- Anxiety is an element of many psychological disorders, including phobias, panic attacks, obsessive-compulsive disorders, and post-traumatic stress disorder.

SYMPTOMS

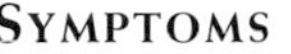

• dry mouth • sweaty palms • rapid pulse and palpitations • in anxiety neurosis: – breathlessness – headaches, general weakness, and fatigue – feeling of tightness in the chest – high blood pressure – abdominal pain and diarrhea – insomnia – loss of appetite

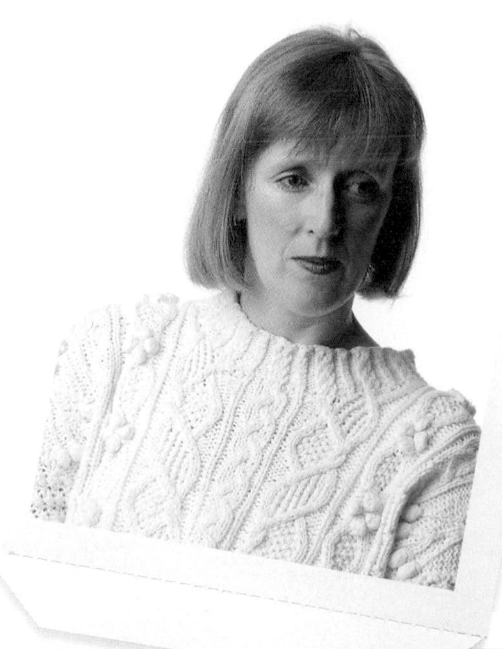

RIGHT *A persistent state of anxiety can sap energy and so self-perpetuate.*

TREATMENT

AYURVEDA

- An Ayurvedic medical practitioner would balance the tri-doshas, and use panchakarma for balancing the vátha. *(See page 20.)*

CHINESE HERBALISM

- A Chinese herbalist might suggest ginseng, Chinese angelica, and white peony root with thorowax root for relaxation. Treatment would be designed to strengthen the Spleen and enliven Liver qi. *(See pages 56 and 67.)*

TRADITIONAL FOLK AND HOME REMEDIES

- Oats contain thiamin and pantothenic acid, which act as gentle nerve tonics *(See page 84.)*

HERBALISM

- Herbal remedies would be used to calm the nervous system and to generally relax you.
- Skullcap and valerian are useful herbs, blended together for best effect. Drink this as a tea three times daily while suffering anxiety symptoms. *(See pages 131 and 136.)*
- Lady's slipper and lime blossom may also work to ease anxiety and tension. *(See page 134.)*

ABOVE *Make an infusion with 1–2 teaspoonsful of dried skullcap and boiling water.*

AROMATHERAPY

- A relaxing blend of essential oils of lavender, geranium, and bergamot in sweet almond oil or peach kernel oil may be used in the bath at times at great stress and anxiety. *(See pags 146–71.)*

HOMEOPATHY

Constitutional treatment will be appropriate for chronic conditions, and there are a number of remedies which will prove useful for relieving acute attacks. These include:

- Aconite, for dispelling a sudden panic attack. *(See page 178.)*
- Arsenicum may be useful if you feel insecure, restless, tired, and tend to fight anxiety by being obsessively tidy or really well organized. *(See page 182.)*
- Nat. mur. may be useful if you have a tendency to dwell on morbid topics and generally hate fuss. *(See page 206.)*
- Calcarea, if you fear for your sanity, forget things, and feel the cold. *(See page 186.)*
- Ignatia, if your anxiety follows the loss of a loved one or a specific, distressing event. *(See page 200.)*

FLOWER ESSENCES

- Remedies are prescribed according to the personal characteristics of the sufferer, and the cause and the nature of the anxiety.
- Try Elm for anxiety accompanying a feeling of being unable to cope, or Red Chestnut for anxiety over the welfare of others. *(See pages 241 and 224.)*
- Aspen, for anxiety for no apparent reason. *(See page 236.)*
- Rescue Remedy or Emergency Essence are useful during attacks. *(See page 244.)*

VITAMINS AND MINERALS

Increase your intake of B vitamins, which work on the nervous system, and avoid caffeine in any form. *(See pages 252–5.)*

Insecurity

Insecurity is a feeling that affects everybody at one time or another. It can be triggered by physical, social, financial, or emotional factors, and can often induce anxiety and its associated symptoms. Whatever the initial cause, when a person feels insecure that person's entire perception of his or her own competence and self-worth are thrown into question. Chronic insecurity, which can manifest itself as depression, shyness, lack of confidence, or an inability to form stable relationships, has less to do with external events than with unrealistic expectations and a poor self-image.

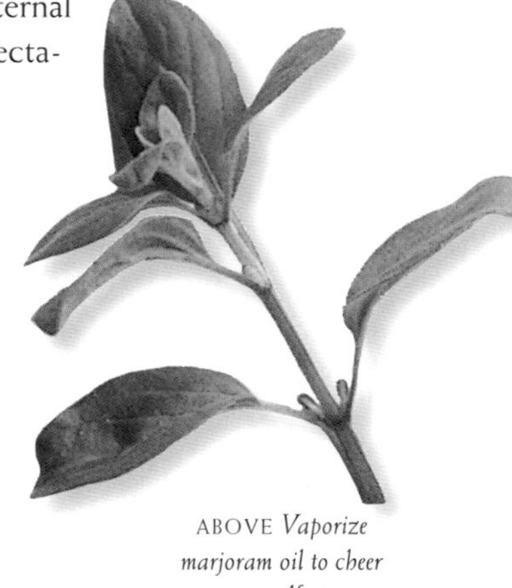

ABOVE *Vaporize marjoram oil to cheer yourself up.*

SYMPTOMS

- *dry mouth* • *sweaty palms*
- *rapid pulse and palpitations*
- *in anxiety neurosis: – breathlessness – headaches, general weakness, and fatigue – feeling of tightness in the chest – high blood pressure – abdominal pain and diarrhea – insomnia – loss of appetite*

TREATMENT

CHINESE HERBALISM
• Try herbs which work to balance the nervous system, including fleeceflower stem, poria, and wild jujube seeds. *(See pages 71 and 75.)*

HERBALISM
• Uplifting herbs such as rosemary, lavender, ginseng, damiana, or valerian. They can be drunk as infusions 3 times daily. *(See pages 125, 127, 135, and 136.)*

AROMATHERAPY
• Jasmine lifts the spirits and improves mental outlook – add a few drops to a vaporizer or your bath (not at bedtime). *(See page 161.)*
• Marjoram and thyme are cheering and can boost self-image. *(See pages 165 and 170.)*

HOMEOPATHY
• Aconite, for insecurity brought on by a traumatic experience. *(See page 178.)*
• Ignatia, for insecurity stemming from a particular cause, for example a bereavement. *(See page 200.)*
• Pulsatilla, if you feel tearful, worse for heat, and longing for company. *(See page 209.)*

FLOWER ESSENCES
• Mimulus is appropriate for fear and of known things, timidity and shyness. *(See page 235.)*
• Crab apple, for poor self-image. *(See page 234.)*
• Elm, for those who are usually confident but are experiencing a temporary crisis of confidence because they are overwhelmed by responsibility. *(See page 241.)*

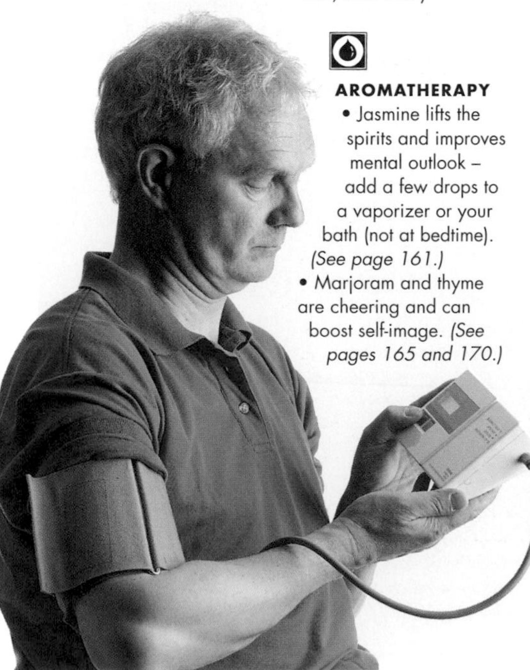

LEFT *Feelings of insecurity may trigger a rise in blood pressure.*

Memory Loss

A total or partial loss of memory is known as amnesia. It occurs as a result of either physical or mental disease (such as senile dementia), or physical trauma (such as a blow to the head or a fractured skull). The latter may induce a state of retrograde amnesia where the sufferer has no memory of the events immediately before the injury as well as those after. The period of amnesia in such cases is usually in proportion to the severity of the injury. Amnesia is caused by damage to, or disease of, brain regions concerned with memory function, and can also occur in some forms of psychiatric illness in which there is no apparent physical damage to the brain. Amnesia can very often be a complication of alcoholism, and can result from depression, anxiety, stress, poor nutrition, inadequate sleep, or lack of stimulation.

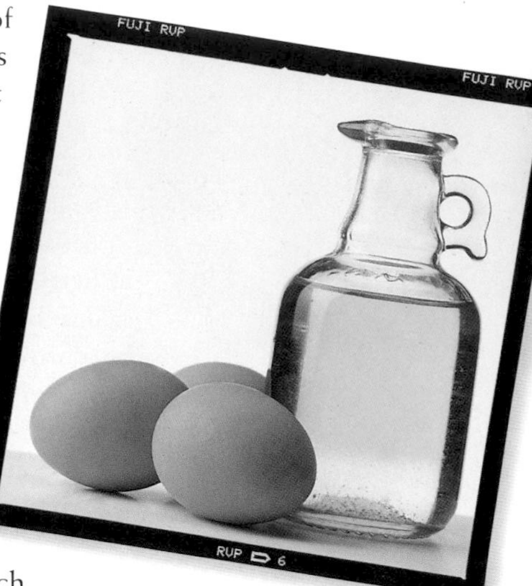

ABOVE *Sunflower oil and eggs contain lecithin which enhances functioning of the brain.*

TREATMENT

CHINESE HERBALISM
• Herbs to aid memory include fleeceflower root and black ginger seed. *(See page 71.)*
• Memory loss caused by stress or fatigue may be treated with Chinese wolfberry. *(See page 66.) (See also Anxiety, page 241.)*

HERBALISM
• Ginseng powder can act as a memory aid and general stimulant. *(See page 126.)*
• Add a small amount of gotu kola to your food or drink for several days, to revive your memory.
• Rosemary is said to comfort the brain and refresh the memory, and sage is also useful. *(See page 127.)*

HOMEOPATHY
Treatment would be constitutional, but the following may be of use:
• Anacardium when you are absent-minded because of an inner conflict. *(See page 179.)*
• Sulfur, for difficulty remembering words and names. *(See page 215.)*
• Calcarea, for wandering attention, particularly in the elderly. *(See page 186.)*
• Ignatia, for memory loss caused by a traumatic event or bereavement. *(See page 200.)*

FLOWER ESSENCES
• Star of Bethlehem, when memory is affected by an accident, bad news, or trauma. *(See page 235.)*

VITAMINS AND MINERALS
Your diet should be rich in B vitamins and protein, for amino acids are necessary for the brain to function efficiently. An amino acid supplement (containing all 22 acids) may be useful. Acetylcholine, which is formed in the body from lecithin, may help. Increase your intake of lecithin (found in sunflower oil and eggs) or take it as a supplement. *(See page 271.)*

Insomnia

A common complaint, insomnia is the inability to sleep or the disturbance of normal sleep patterns. It is difficult to qualify, because everyone has different sleep requirements, and sleeplessness is, in fact, a natural feature of aging. Insomnia is often caused by worry, emotional stress, and exhaustion. Other causes include pain; excess caffeine, alcohol and drugs; food allergy; or sleeping in a stuffy room. Insomnia can also be a symptom of depression.

RIGHT *To achieve a peaceful sleep, rest on a pillow containing dried lavender.*

DATA FILE

- In recent years, sleep-disorders medicine has become virtually a new branch of medicine, with centers for diagnosis and treatment now located throughout the U.S.
- 15–17 percent of the population suffer from sleep problems at some point.
- 50 percent of people who take sleeping pills for insomnia find the condition worsens.
- 200,000–400,000 car accidents each year are caused by drowsiness.
- Roughly speaking, 80 percent of our sleep is NREM (non-rapid eye movement) and 20 percent is REM (rapid eye movement). If you feel tired all the next day, you have probably not had enough NREM sleep; if you have problems with your memory, then inadequate REM sleep is to blame.
- Some 66 percent of people sleep for anything between 6.5 and 8.5 hours each night on a regular basis. Around 16 percent sleep for more than 8.5 hours every night and 18 percent for under 6.5 hours.
- Fatigue doesn't necessarily relate to the amount of sleep you have had. Doctors report that one of the most common problems they see in their surgeries on a daily basis is chronic fatigue – or TAT, tired all the time.
- Research now shows that some 80 percent of people complaining of being tired all the time (TAT) get adequate sleep, and that the problem lies in nutritional deficiencies which can be cleared up by improving the diet and taking a good multivitamin and mineral supplement.

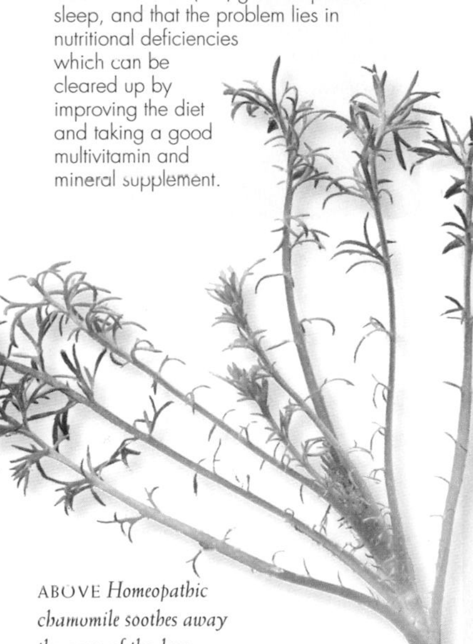

ABOVE *Homeopathic chamomile soothes away the cares of the day.*

SYMPTOMS

- *over-active mind causing difficulty in falling asleep*
- *nervousness and restlessness* • *nightmares once asleep*
- *irritability* • *mood swings involving hysterical behavior*
- *a fear of bedtime may eventually develop*

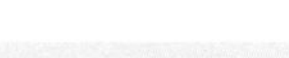

TREATMENT

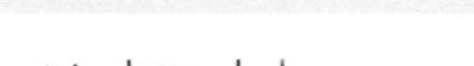

AYURVEDA

• Specific herbs to treat insomnia may include henbane, which is sedative.

CHINESE HERBALISM

• Useful herbs include hoelen, fleeceflower stem, and wild jujube. *(See pages 71 and 75.)*
• The herbalist may suggest that you sleep on a gypsum pillow.

TRADITIONAL FOLK AND HOME REMEDIES

• A hot foot-bath before bed helps relaxation by drawing blood away from the head. Add a little mustard powder to the water to increase the effect. *(See page 98.)*
• Lettuce is said to encourage sleep. Eat a large leaf about half an hour before bedtime.

HERBALISM

• A warm bath with a an infusion of chamomile, catnip, lavender, or limeflowers may be recommended. *(See pages 119 and 134.)*
• A cup of warm herb tea just before bed will soothe and help you to relax. Try chamomile, catnip, lemon balm, and limeflowers. *(See pages 119 and 134.)*
• Make a lavender pillow and place it under your usual pillow.

AROMATHERAPY

• A few drops of chamomile oil, clary sage, or lavender can be added to the bath. *(See pages 146–71.)*
• Try a gentle massage just before bedtime, with a few drops of chamomile, lavender, rose, or neroli blended into a light carrier oil. *(See pages 146–71.)*
• Place a few drops of lavender oil on your bedroom light bulb, just before bed, or place a few drops on a handkerchief and tie it to the bed. *(See page 161.)*

HOMEOPATHY

Remedies can be taken an hour before going to bed, for up to 14 days. Repeat the dose if you wake in the night and cannot get back to sleep. Insomnia is usually treated "constitutionally," so you may need to consult a registered homeopath for treatment. The following remedies may be helpful:
• Coffea, when your mind is overactive, and you are unable to switch off. *(See page 192.)*
• Nux vomica, when your sleeplessness is exacerbated by food or alcohol; you wake around 3 or 4A.M., then fall asleep just as it is time to get up; and consequently are irritable during the day. *(See page 214.)*
• Pulsatilla, when you are restless in the early hours of sleep, feeling uncomfortable, hot and then cold, are not thirsty and sleep with your arms above your head. *(See page 209.)*
• Arnica, when the bed feels too hard, and you are overtired, fidgety, and dream of being chased by animals. *(See page 182.)*
• Lycopodium, when your mind is active at bedtime, going over and over work done that day; you dream a lot, talk and laugh in your sleep, and then wake up at around 4A.M. *(See page 203.)*
• Arsenicum, for when you tend to wake between midnight and 2A.M., feeling restless, worried, and apprehensive. *(See page 182.)*
• Rhus tox., when you cannot sleep, are irritable, restless, and feel a need to walk about; especially if in pain. *(See page 210.)*

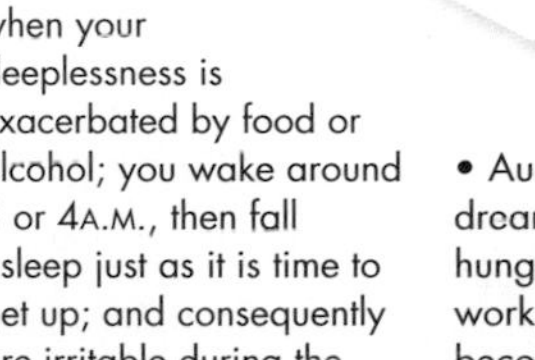

• Aurum, when you have dreams about dying, hunger, or problems at work, and consequently become depressed. *(See page 184.)*
• Aconite, when sleep problems are worse after shock or trauma; there is restlessness, nightmares, and fear of dying. *(See page 178.)*
• Chamomilla, when you are feeling irritable bedtime. *(See page 204.)*

FLOWER ESSENCES

• Worrying thoughts and mental arguments might respond to White Chestnut. *(See page 224.)*
• Indecision can be treated with Scleranthus. *(See page 239.)*
• Stress, strain, frustration, and inability to relax might respond to Vervain or Rock Water, Vine, Elm, Beech, or Impatiens could apply. *(See pages 229, 233, 241, 242, and 243.)*

VITAMINS AND MINERALS

Increase your intake of vitamins B, C, folic acid, zinc and calcium. Try a calcium supplement just before bedtime. *(See page 258.)*

DISORDERS OF THE BRAIN AND NERVES

MS (Multiple Sclerosis)

Multiple sclerosis is a chronic disease of the nervous system in which the protective sheaths that cover the nerves become inflamed and scarred, resulting in loss of nerve function. The initial attack is usually followed by recovery, but sufferers inevitably experience a cycle of remission (sometimes for years) and relapse with steadily increasing neurological damage and disability. The degree of improvement after each attack decreases and the physical disability is usually progressive. Eventually there may also be intellectual impairment. The cause of MS is unknown.

DATA FILE

- MS is not an inherited disease, but a predisposition may run in families.
- The cause remains unknown, but some researchers propose that it is an autoimmune disorder; others believe a viral infection may trigger the disease.
- MS is more common in temperate climates and is relatively rare in Asia and Africa, lending credibility to the theory that it might be related to diet or climate.
- U.S. cases are usually diagnosed from age 20 to 40.
- In most cases, MS follows a course of repeated remissions, with the symptoms returning with increased severity, over a period of years.
- Because of lack of persistent symptoms, many MS patients go for a number of years before being correctly diagnosed.
- The average life expectancy after onset is over 30 years, although some patients die within a few years of onset and others survive more than 50 years.

Symptoms

• limb weakness • visual deterioration, particularly in the center of the visual field • double vision • loss of sensation • staggering • impaired speech • facial paralysis

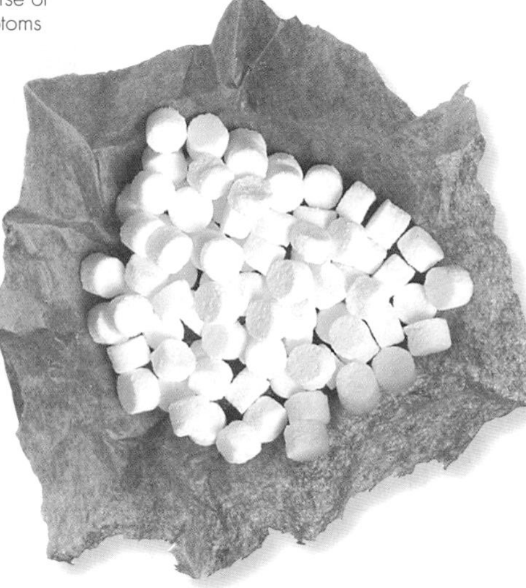

RIGHT *Potassium phosphate is the source for the homeopathic remedy Kali phosphoricum.*

TREATMENT

HOMEOPATHY Treatment is constitutional, but the following remedies may be useful while you are waiting for treatment:
- Tarantula, when movements of the hands, feet, and tongue are jerky. *(See page 215.)*
- Agaricus, for sharp, shooting pains, and weakness with shaking.
- Phosphorus, for exaggerated reflexes and a tendency to fainting. *(See page 208.)*
- Kali phos., for weakness in the back and legs, made worse by exercise, which causes overwhelming fatigue, pain, and even paralysis. *(See page 201.)*

FLOWER ESSENCES
- Rescue Remedy or Emergency Essence may help to ease the symptoms and control shaking and anxiety. *(See page 244.)*

VITAMINS AND MINERALS
- Eat plenty of foods that contain gamma-linoleic acid, which is found in sunflower and safflower oil, as well as evening primrose products. *(See page 270.)*
- Get plenty of vitamins B3, B6, B12, folic acid, C and E, and the minerals zinc and magnesium. *(See pages 253–57, 264 and 265.)*

Stroke

A stroke (cerebrovascular accident, or CVA) results from an interruption of the blood supply to any part of the brain. This may be caused by bleeding into or around the brain (cerebral hemorrhage), a clot which blocks an already damaged artery (cerebral thrombosis), or a small clot elsewhere in the bloodstream that eventually causes obstruction in an artery to the brain (cerebral embolism). Smoking, diabetes, high blood pressure, and atherosclerosis are all risk factors.

DATA FILE

- The effects of a stroke vary according to its cause and the part of the brain affected. The most serious (and often fatal) cause is cerebral hemorrhage, the first sign of which is a severe headache followed by: – paralysis down one side of the body – loss of vision to one side – fixed turning of the eyes to one side – possibly a seizure.
- The effects of cerebral thrombosis or embolism are similar to the above, but less serious, and recovery often follows.
- In the U.S. stroke is the third-ranking cause of death after heart disease and cancer, and about one-fourth of the neurologic patients in nursing homes are stroke victims.
- The death rate has declined by nearly 50 per cent since the late 1960s; in the early 1990s about 150,000 Americans of the 450,000 each year who suffered a new stroke died as a result.
- Stroke victims are generally elderly people with degeneration of blood vessels, but children and young adults also can have a stroke.
- More men than women are afflicted by a stroke.
- More people of African descent have strokes than any other race.
- Prior history of stroke increases the chance that you will have a repeat.
- Women using oral contraceptives are at greater risk of stroke.

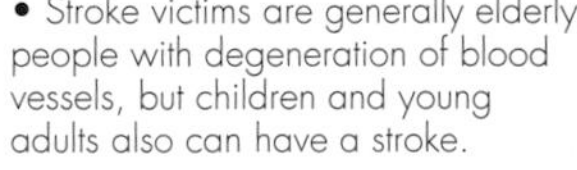

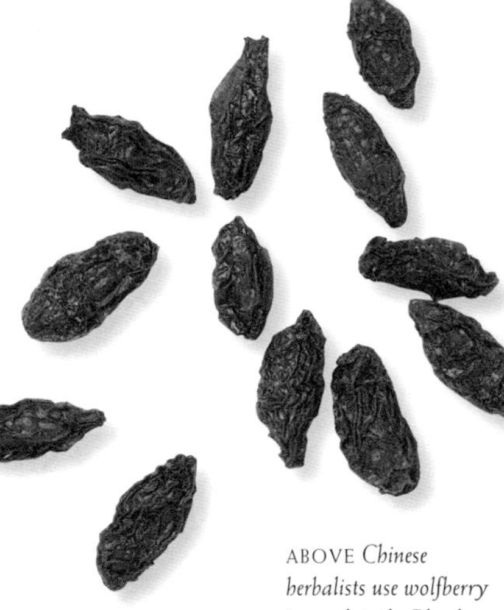

ABOVE *Chinese herbalists use wolfberry to regulate the Blood.*

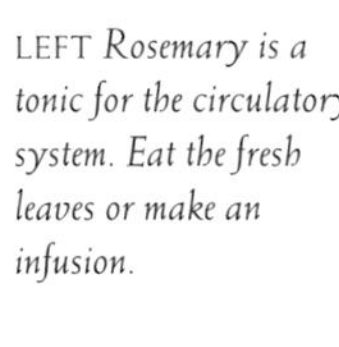

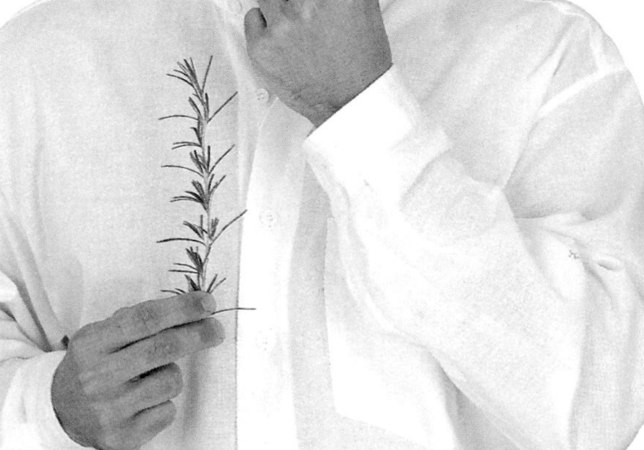

LEFT *Rosemary is a tonic for the circulatory system. Eat the fresh leaves or make an infusion.*

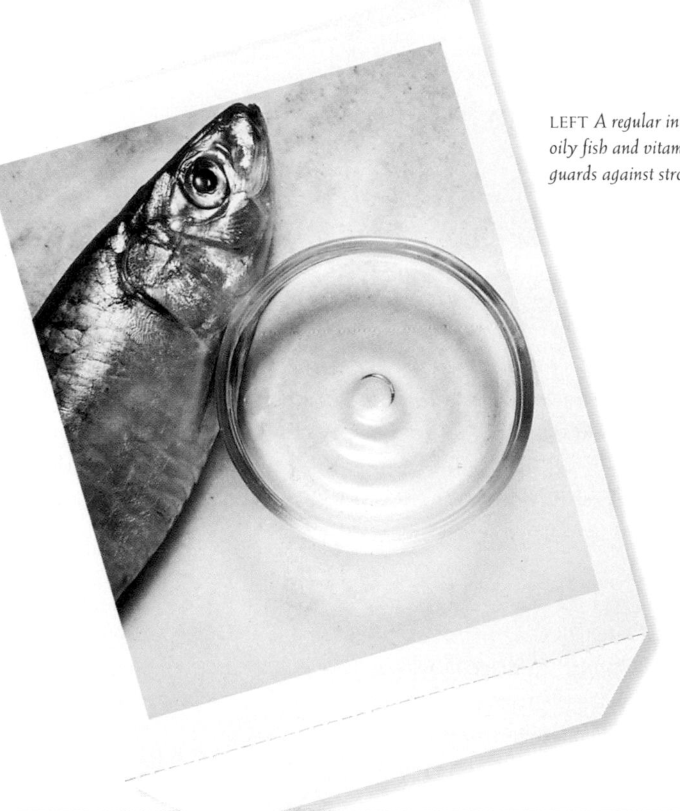

LEFT *A regular intake of oily fish and vitamin E guards against stroke.*

TREATMENT

HOMEOPATHY
Constitutional treatment from an experienced homeopath can aid recovery after a stroke. Changes in diet, exercise, and lifestyle will be recommended. There are also specific remedies which can be used while waiting for medical attention. These include:
- Belladonna, when the face is hot and flushed, with staring eyes. *(See page 183.)*
- Opium, when there is unconsciousness, and a blue face, and the patient is breathing heavily. *(See page 207.)*
- Nux mosch., for the first signs of an attack, often brought on by overindulgence.
- Aconite, for fear and panic. *(See page 178.)*

Following an attack:
- Aconite, immediately afterward and for the next 4 weeks. *(See page 178.)*
- Baryta, when there is physical and mental weakness after an attack, particularly in the elderly. *(See page 185.)*
- Aurum, for depression. *(See page 184.)*
- Gelsemium, when there is numbness, trembling, pain at the back of the head, and an inability to speak. *(See page 195.)*
- Lachesis for slow speech. *(See page 216.)*

FLOWER ESSENCES
- These remedies could play a part in helping to promote a more positive frame of mind in sufferers who are frightened, depressed, or affected by other negative attitudes.

VITAMINS AND MINERALS
- Prevention is easier than cure, and a good intake of oily fish and vitamin E with a wholefood diet is the best prevention against the small blood clots in the brain which are the cause of strokes. *(See page 257.)*
- Nutritional therapists use the herb ginkgo biloba after a stroke to improve the circulation in the brain and help to prevent further strokes.

HERBALISM
- Yarrow is recommended to improve circulation and tone the blood vessels. Drink an infusion 3 times daily. *(See page 112.)*
- Rosemary is useful and can be drunk or eaten fresh as soon as possible to improve the health of the circulatory system. *(See page 127.)*

CHINESE HERBALISM
- A Chinese herbalist is likely to offer herbs to regulate the Blood condition, such as peony bark and wolfberry. *(See pages 66 and 67.)*

AYURVEDA
- Ayurveda is a very popular method for rehabilitation of paralysis – special panchakarma therapy for vátha. *(See page 20.)*

Meningitis

The epidemic disease called cerebrospinal meningitis is caused by the meningococcus bacterium, an organism that inhabits the nose of healthy human carriers but that sometimes infects the blood and cerebrospinal fluid. The most common cause of bacterial meningitis is *Haemophilus influenzae* type b. Meningitis may result from head injuries and infections involving the eyes, ears, and nose; it can also be a complication of systemic disorders such as pneumonia and syphilis, both of which reach the brain via the bloodstream. Diagnosis is often made by lumbar puncture (spinal tap). A vaccine against *Haemophilus influenzae* type b was licensed for use in 1985. Children and immune-suppressed people are most susceptible.

CAUTION

MENINGITIS CAN LEAD TO SERIOUS BRAIN DAMAGE, BLINDNESS, DEAFNESS, OR EVEN DEATH URGENT MEDICAL ATTENTION IS REQUIRED IF MENINGITIS IS SUSPECTED.

Symptoms

• *viral meningitis: – headache, worse on bending – fever – nausea and vomiting – stiff neck – in severe cases there may also be muscle weakness, paralysis, impaired speech, double vision, and epileptic fits* • *bacterial (meningococcal) meningitis: – any/all of the above – a rash of red spots on the trunk of the body – drowsiness and eventually coma – convulsions and a characteristic high-pitched cry in babies and infants – in infants the fontanel on the top of the head may bulge and feel more tense than usual*

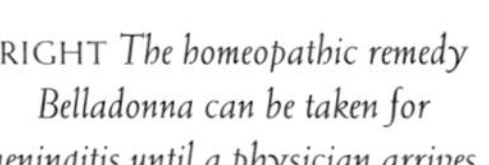

RIGHT *The homeopathic remedy Belladonna can be taken for meningitis until a physician arrives.*

TREATMENT

CHINESE HERBALISM
- A registered practitioner could treat this condition with herbal laxatives and anti-inflammatories, but treatment should be alongside conventional medical treatment.
- Herbs to boost the immune system following infection include ginseng. Treatment would address Deficient Blood and qi. Peony root and mulberry might be appropriate. *(See page 67.)*

HOMEOPATHY
Emergency remedies, to be taken every 10 minutes, until help arrives include:
- Arnica, for symptoms which arise after a head injury. *(See page 182.)*
- Aconite, for restlessness, fear and great thirst. *(See page 178.)*
- Bryonia, which treats a severe headache made worse by eye movement. *(See page 185.)*
- Belladonna, for staring eyes, delirium, and fever. *(See page 183.)*

FLOWER ESSENCES
- Take Rescue Remedy or Emergency Essence (apply to the temples or moisten the lips if the sufferer is not conscious) to calm and encourage the healing process. *(See page 244.)*

Encephalitis

Encephalitis is an inflammation of the brain tissue, usually caused by infection, but occasionally by poisoning. Primary encephalitis is caused by direct infection with viruses, which include herpes simplex, herpes zoster, or mosquito- and tick-borne viruses. Secondary encephalitis usually occurs as a complication of a viral infection such as mumps, measles, rubella, or chickenpox. The causative infection may enter the brain via the bloodstream. Many other infections involve only the surface membranes (*see Meningitis, page 289*), whereas others affect both meninges and brain, and cause meningoencephalitis. Encephalitis can be fatal within hours of onset, although many people make a full recovery even from serious attacks.

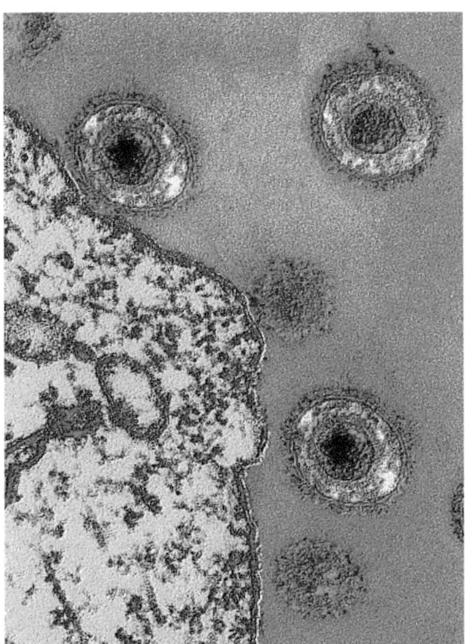

Symptoms

• in mild cases the symptoms are similar to those of other viral infections: – fever – headache – loss of appetite – lethargy and drowsiness • in more severe cases sufferers may experience: – double vision – mental confusion and impaired speech – stiff neck and back – epileptic fits – coma

LEFT *The chickenpox virus. Encephalitis may occur as a complication after infection by this virus.*

Treatment

HERBALISM
• Echinacea is antiviral, and can be taken alongside orthodox treatment, in order to boost the immune system and treat the infection. *(See page 120.)*
• Eat plenty of fresh garlic following the illness to speed recovery and treat the immune system. *(See page 113.)*
• Drink chamomile, catnip, or skullcap when you feel uncomfortable or restless. *(See pages 119 and 131.)*

AROMATHERAPY
• Essential oils of chamomile, lavender, peppermint, or tea tree can be dropped on a cold compress and used to bathe the forehead to soothe and encourage healing. *(See pages 146–71.)*

HOMEOPATHY
This condition is very serious and must be dealt with by a conventional doctor and treated as a medical emergency. While waiting for help, the following remedies may help:
• Belladonna, for a flushed face, delirium, and staring eyes. *(See page 183.)*
• Nux mosch., for drowsiness – especially in infants.
• Gelsemium, for dizziness, a tight band around the forehead, and weakness with trembling. *(See page 195.)*

VITAMINS AND MINERALS
• Take plenty of extra vitamin C and zinc, which will boost the immune system. *(See pages 256 and 265.)*

Parkinson's Disease

Parkinson's is a progressive disease in which degeneration of the nervous system, particularly the nerve cells in the brain, causes loss of control over voluntary movement. The damage is irreversible and the exact cause as yet unknown. It occurs most commonly among the elderly, and affects men more than women. Parkinson's involves the central gray matter of the brain (basal ganglia), resulting in deficiency of a neurotransmitter known as dopamine. The common form of this disease is caused by a premature degeneration of certain basal nuclei. Many centrally acting psychotropic drugs, manganese, other toxins, and anoxic cerebral damage may produce parkinsonian syndromes.

Symptoms

• difficulty in walking, tending to stoop and shuffle • involuntary head movements • stiffness of facial muscles, resulting in a fixed expression • stiffness of tongue muscles, causing impaired speech and dribbling • worsening of the tremor, making it impossible to write, use cutlery or drink from a cup • eventually there may be dementia

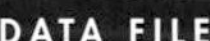

DATA FILE

• Onset of the disease is between the ages of 40 and 70.

• It can be induced by certain chemicals, such as one known as MPTP – a by-product of the street drug MPPP, a Demerol analogue – suggesting that parkinsonism might be environmental in origin.

• Parkinson's affects a half-million people annually in the U.S.

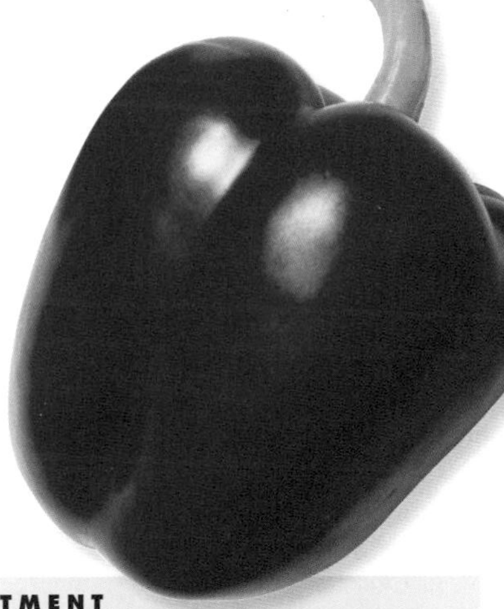

BELOW *Include foods rich in vitamin C, such as capsicum, in your diet to help the nervous system.*

Treatment

CHINESE HERBALISM
• The cause is believed to be Deficient Blood and Kidney Yang, and the following herbs might be useful: gastrodia tuber, peony root, peony buds, and wolfberry root. *(See pages 62, 66 and 67.)*

HERBALISM
• Herbs which work to boost the nervous system and brain function include ginseng, wild oats, which are calming and strengthening, astragalus and Chinese angelica, which also works to boost the immune system. *(See pages 115–7, and 126.)*

HOMEOPATHY
Treatment will be constitutional, under the supervision of an experienced homeopath. Specific remedies which are useful when symptoms are bad include:
• Hyoscyamus, for restless, twitching motions, and rude, suspicious, and jealous behavior. *(See page 198.)*
• Mercurius, for a sweet taste in the mouth, trembling hands, drooling, and sensitivity to heat and cold. *(See page 205.)*
• Gelsemium, for trembling and weakness affecting the tongue and eyes; and for a staggering gait. *(See page 195.)*
• Rhus tox., when there is stiffness and cramping made worse by damp and inactivity. *(See page 210.)*

VITAMINS AND MINERALS
• Take extra vitamin B6 and C to aid nervous function. *(See pages 254 and 256.)*

Epilepsy

Epilepsy is an indication of an abnormality in brain function. Generalized epilepsy (grand mal and petit mal) is the most common form and is caused by a great electrical discharge across the surface of the brain on both sides. Partial-seizure epilepsy (simple and complex) is confined to a localized area of the brain, often, but not always, the temporal lobe. The symptoms vary according to which area of the brain is affected.

ABOVE *Avoid certain aromatherapy oils, such as fennel.*

CAUTION

NEVER ATTEMPT TO OPEN THE MOUTH OR FORCE ANYTHING BETWEEN THE TEETH OF SOMEBODY WHO IS SUFFERING AN EPILEPTIC SEIZURE. LOOSEN THE PERSON'S CLOTHING AND ENSURE THAT HE OR SHE IS NOT IN ANY DANGER, AND THEN WAIT UNTIL THE SEIZURE HAS RUN ITS COURSE. PROLONGED, REPEATED GRAND MAL ATTACKS, WITH NO RECOVERY OF CONSCIOUSNESS, REQUIRE URGENT MEDICAL ATTENTION.

SYMPTOMS

• grand mal: – seizure may begin with a shout – loss of consciousness – foaming at the mouth – loss of bladder and bowel control – rhythmic contraction of all the body's muscles – the sufferer may end the seizure in a deep sleep • petit mal (particularly common among children): – momentary loss of consciousness – possibly jerky contractions of facial and finger muscles • simple partial seizure – hallucinations of smell, vision, or taste – twitching movements • complex partial seizure – as for simple partial seizure but with a feeling of fear and anger, and a period of unresponsiveness – the sufferer may behave in a robot-like way, and can be violent if interfered with

DATA FILE

- 1 in 100 people in the U.S. suffer from epilepsy.
- In 70 percent of cases the cause is unknown; genetic susceptibility may be a factor.
- In 75 percent of cases, epilepsy begins during the sufferer's childhood.
- When drugs fail to control seizures, surgery to remove the affected portion of the brain or to interrupt the pathways of seizure spread may be considered.
- For children who do not respond to other treatment, the ketogenic diet – high in fat, very low in carbohydrates – may be an option.

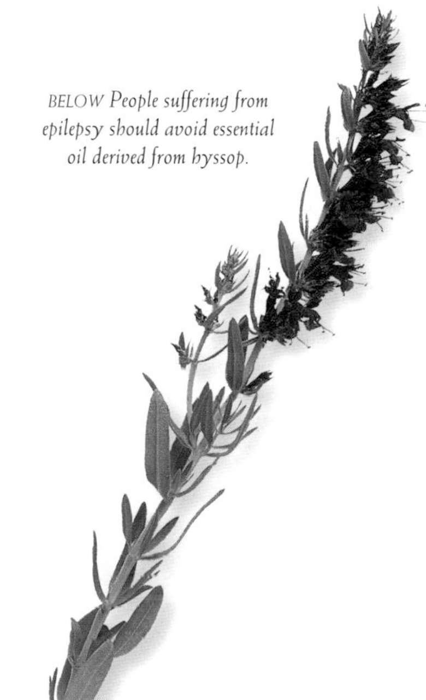

BELOW *People suffering from epilepsy should avoid essential oil derived from hyssop.*

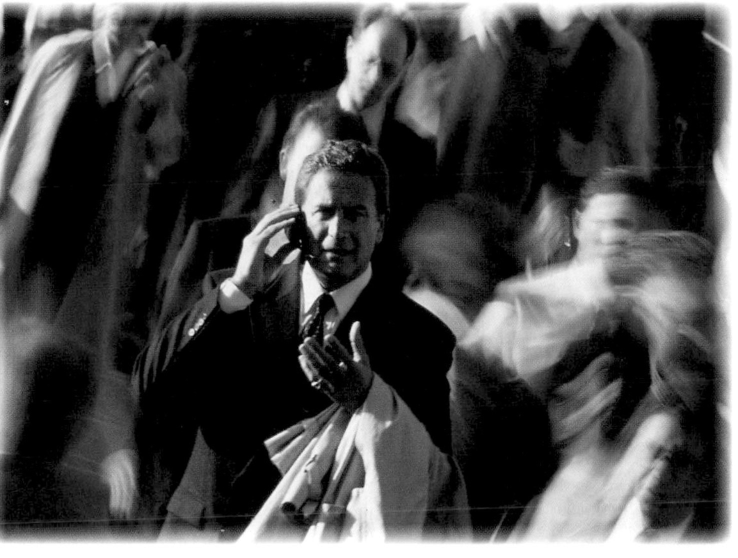

ABOVE *One percent of the U.S. population suffers from some form of epilepsy.*

TREATMENT

CHINESE HERBALISM
• The source of the problem is believed to be excess Heart mucus, internal Damp and stagnant qi or Blood. Sweet flag root and the juice of the young bamboo can prevent attacks in some cases.

HERBALISM
• Herbs to relax the central nervous system, including vervain and valerian, may be useful in reducing the frequency and severity of attacks. *(See pages 136 and 138.)*

AROMATHERAPY
• Studies show that extremely small doses of rosemary might be helpful in treating epilepsy, but this must only be done under the supervision of an aromatherapist with a medical qualification. *(See page 168.)*
• There are a number of oils to avoid if you have epilepsy, and these include sage, fennel, hyssop, and wormwood. *(See pages 146–71.)*

HOMEOPATHY
Remedies should be given as soon as the fit wears off.
• Chamomilla, for an attack brought on by an outburst of anger, characterized by one red cheek and greenish stools. *(See page 204.)*
• Ignatia, for a fit brought on by emotional upset. *(See page 200.)*
• Zinc, for fits brought on through illness, with fidgety, restless movements of the limbs and a bad temper.
• Aconite, for fits brought on by fright or fever. *(See page 178.)*
• Belladonna, when symptoms are made worse by jolting, and the sufferer is red-faced and staring. *(See page 183.)*

FLOWER ESSENCES
• Take a few drops of Emergency Essence or Rescue Remedy if you feel an attack coming on. This will calm you and may well abort an attack. *(See page 244.)*

VITAMINS AND MINERALS
• Extra vitamin B5, magnesium, calcium and zinc may help to prevent attacks. *(See pages 245, 258, 262, and 265.)*
• Vitamin D and B6 deficiency can prompt attacks. *(See pages 254 and 256.)*
• The amino acid taurine has been shown to control seizures.

Guillain-Barré Syndrome

Guillain-Barré syndrome is a specific type of neuropathy, or disruption of the nerves of the body. It is a serious disorder in which widespread inflammation of the nerves, caused by an immune problem, prevents normal nerve conduction. No cause is known, but an infectious agent, probably viral, is suspected. The disease often occurs one to three weeks after a mild gastrointestinal or respiratory infection. There has also been a noticeable incidence of the disease in certain recently inoculated patients. A vaccine used to combat the 1976–77 swine flu epidemic was implicated in several cases of Guillain-Barré syndrome.

ABOVE *Supplement your diet with a daily multivitamin and mineral tablet, to assist the nervous system.*

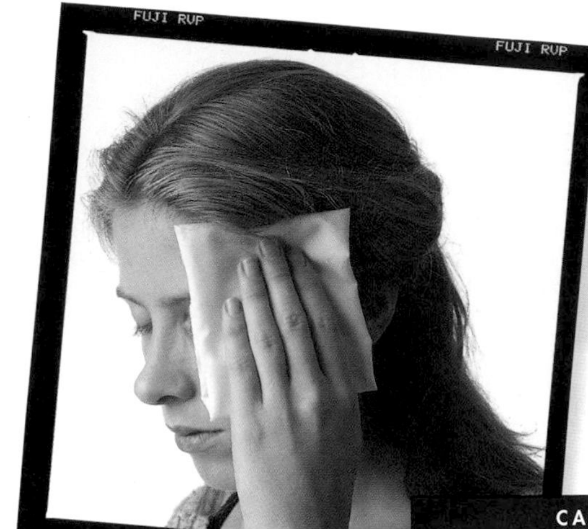

LEFT *A few drops of melissa oil on a cold compress, applied to the temples, will help.*

CAUTION

IF THE SUFFERER HAS ANY TROUBLE BREATHING, RING FOR AN AMBULANCE IMMEDIATELY.

Symptoms

• back pain • tingling in the limbs and muscular weakness • paralysis rapidly follows and may include the facial and respiratory muscles

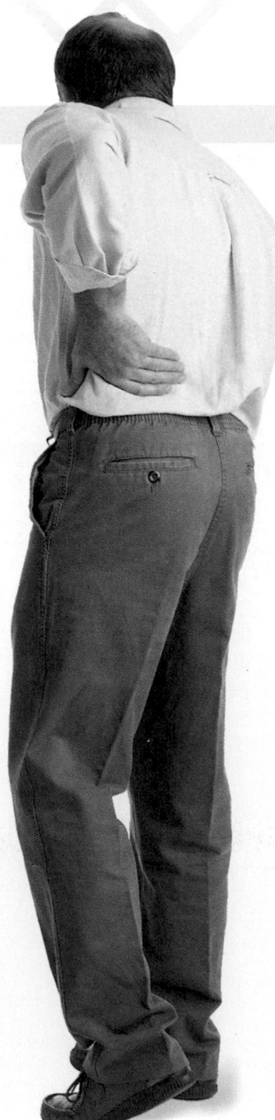

RIGHT *Back pain and muscular weakness can be a symptom of Guillain-Barré syndrome.*

TREATMENT

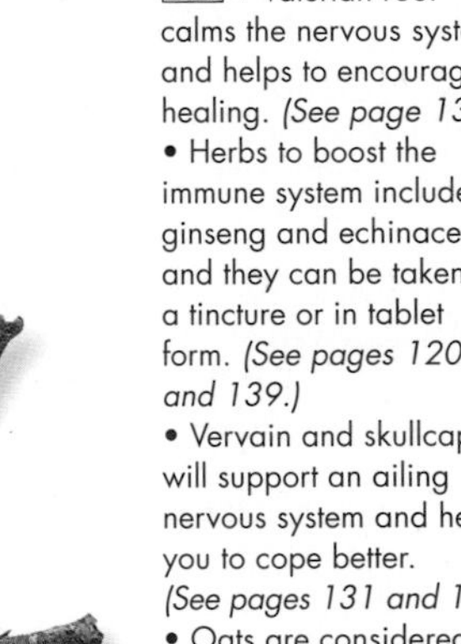

HERBALISM

• Valerian root calms the nervous system and helps to encourage healing. *(See page 136.)*
• Herbs to boost the immune system include ginseng and echinacea, and they can be taken as a tincture or in tablet form. *(See pages 120 and 139.)*
• Vervain and skullcap will support an ailing nervous system and help you to cope better. *(See pages 131 and 138.)*
• Oats are considered to be food for the nervous system, and are a general tonic. *(See page 117.)*

AROMATHERAPY

• The following oils are nervine, which means that they strengthen the nervous system, and they can be used alongside conventional drugs: chamomile, lavender, marjoram, melissa, and rosemary. Apply a few drops to a cold compress and hold over the temples. *(See pages 146–71.)*

HOMEOPATHY

Treatment must be constitutional, but specific remedies may help in the interim:
• Thuja, if symptoms begin after vaccination and the patient has no trouble breathing. *(See page 216.)*
• Aconite, if symptoms begin after a viral infection and there is no trouble breathing. *(See page 178.)*

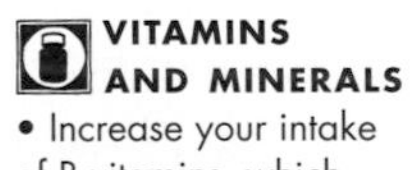

VITAMINS AND MINERALS

• Increase your intake of B vitamins, which aid the health of the nervous system. *(See pages 252–5.)*
• Nutritional deficiencies can disrupt the normal function of the nervous system, and extra vitamin E, along with most of the minerals and trace elements, including calcium, magnesium, zinc and manganese, are vital to normal brain function. Take a good vitamin and mineral supplement daily. *(See page 248.)*

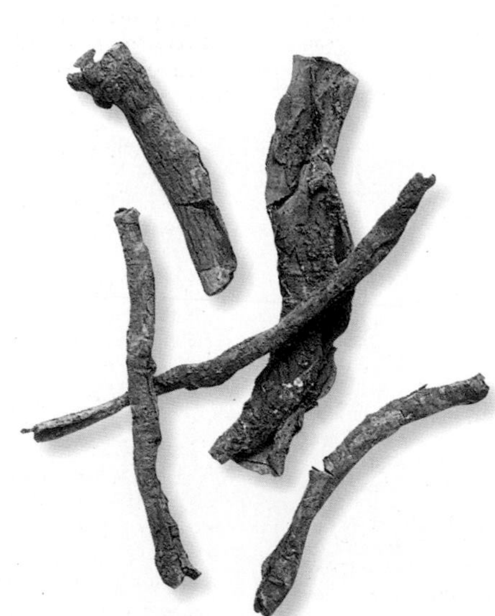

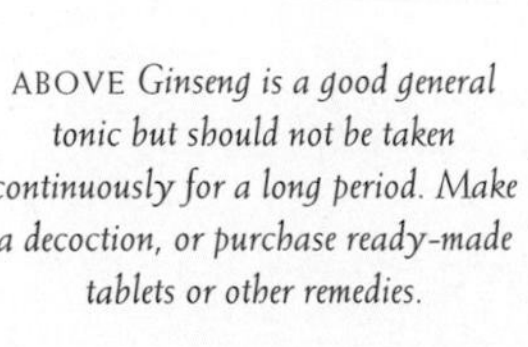

ABOVE *Ginseng is a good general tonic but should not be taken continuously for a long period. Make a decoction, or purchase ready-made tablets or other remedies.*

Shingles

Shingles is an extremely painful disease caused by the herpes zoster virus (which is also the chickenpox virus). Following an attack of chickenpox the virus remains dormant in the body. Many years later a drop in the efficiency of the immune system may cause reactivation of the virus, this time in the form of shingles, causing acute inflammation in the ganglia near the spinal cord.

DATA FILE

- Occurs most often in people over the age of 50 and may be activated through surgery or X-ray therapy to the spinal cord and its roots.
- In younger people, it is often associated with a weakening of the immune system.
- The pain, which can be disabling, may continue for a few months after the blisters heal.
- Shingles strikes 850,000 Americans each year.

Symptoms

• the first sign of shingles is sensitivity in the area to be affected, then pain • fever • sickness • a rash of small blisters develops on the fourth or fifth day; these turn yellow within a few days, form scabs, then drop off, sometimes leaving scars • in some cases there may be persistent pain for months or years (post-herpetic pain)

Avocados are rich in vitamins E, B, and C. Cabbage is a good source of vitamins C and A.
Rice provides B vitamins and carbohydrates.
Cheese is a good source of calcium.
Increase fruit intake for vitamin C.
Eat iron-rich foods such as liver and eggs.

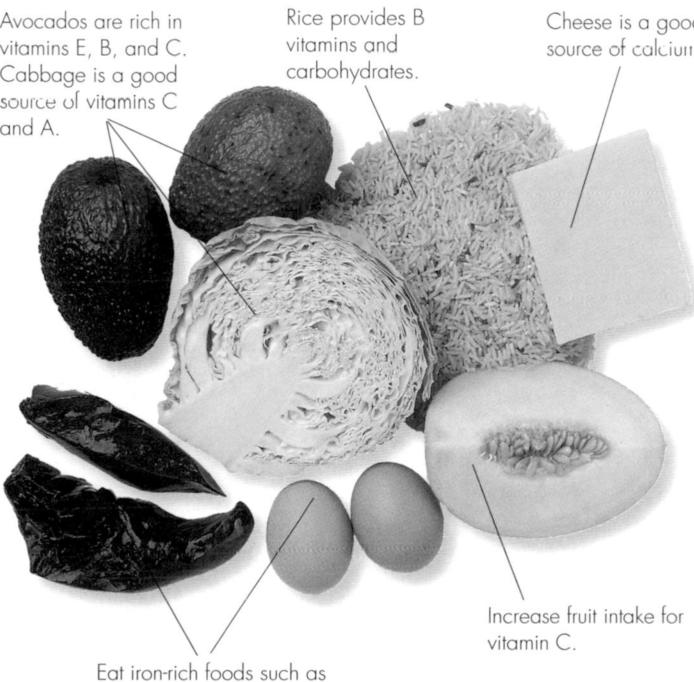

ABOVE *It is important to eat a balanced, nutritious diet, especially if it is suspected that a weakened immune system has caused shingles.*

CAUTION

SHINGLES OF THE FACE MAY AFFECT THE EYES AND SHOULD RECEIVE APPROPRIATE SPECIALIST MEDICAL ATTENTION.

TREATMENT

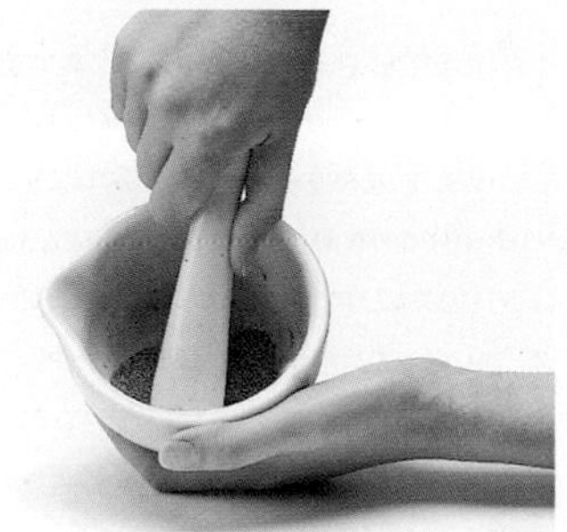

For treating the spots which develop, apply allspice paste. Grind cinnamon, cloves, and nutmeg in a pestle and mortar.

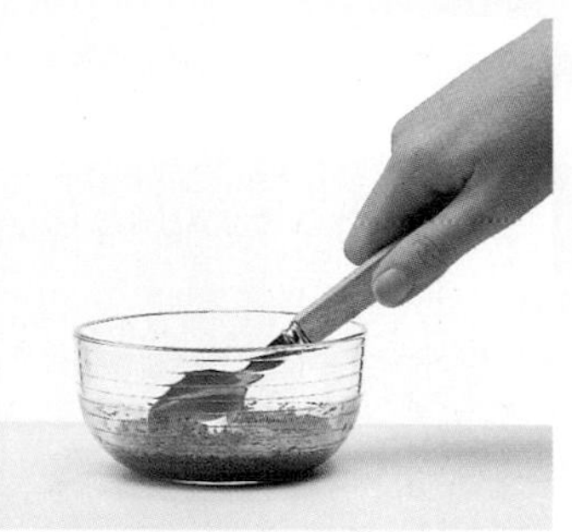

Add water to make a thick paste. Apply to spots to numb the pain. (You can also buy allspice as a pre-ground powder.)

HERBALISM

- Make an infusion of the following nervine herbs and drink three times daily: oats, skullcap, St. John's wort, and vervain. *(See pages 117, 124, 131, and 138.)*
- Diluted tinctures or cold infusion of marigold, plantain, and St. John's wort can be used to bathe the affected area. *(See pages 117, 124, 126.)*

AROMATHERAPY

- Essential oils can combine analgesics with antiviral properties, and can be applied as a compress, added to the bath, or massaged into the skin. Try combining two or more of bergamot, chamomile, geranium, eucalyptus, melissa, lavender, and tea tree. *(See pages 146–71.)*
- Dab the sores with lemon or geranium oil diluted in a little water. *(See pages 154 and 165.)*

CHINESE HERBALISM

- Treatment would address gall bladder heat and damp. Useful herbs include gentian and Oriental wormwood.

TRADITIONAL HOME AND FOLK REMEDIES

- Grind allspice and make a paste, then apply to the spots to relieve pain.
- Celery juice or celery tea can alleviate the pain and help to tone up the nervous system.
- Apply bruised juniper berries to the spots for effective pain relief.
- Fresh lemon can be cut and applied to the affected areas to relieve the pain. *(See page 87.)*

HOMEOPATHY

The following remedies can be taken every two hours for up to ten doses:

- Arsenicum, for burning pains which are worse between midnight and 2A.M., accompanied by skin eruptions and feeling restless, chilly, and anxious. *(See page 182.)*
- Lachesis, when the left side of the body is affected by swelling. *(See page 216.)*
- Rhus tox., for red, blistered, and itching skin which is improved with movement and warmth. *(See page 210.)*
- Fanunculus, for nerve pains and itching which are made worse by movement and eating.
- Sponge the blisters with a blend of Hypericum and Calendula tinctures, added to a little hot water. *(See pages 187 and 199.)*

VITAMINS AND MINERALS

- Eat plenty of foods that are rich in the B-complex vitamins, to aid nervous health. *(See pages 252–5.)*
- Increase your intake of vitamin C, and take a supplement of 1g. up to 4 times daily. *(See page 256.)*
- Supplementation with Vitamin E is now known to reduce the long-term symptoms associated with shingles. Take up to 1mg. daily, broken into 3 doses, with food. *(See page 257.)*
- Vitamin E oil, applied directly to the sores, will encourage healing. *(See page 257.)*
- An attack of shingles is a sign of general debility, and any of the treatments suggested for stress *(see page 284)* will help to tone up the system.

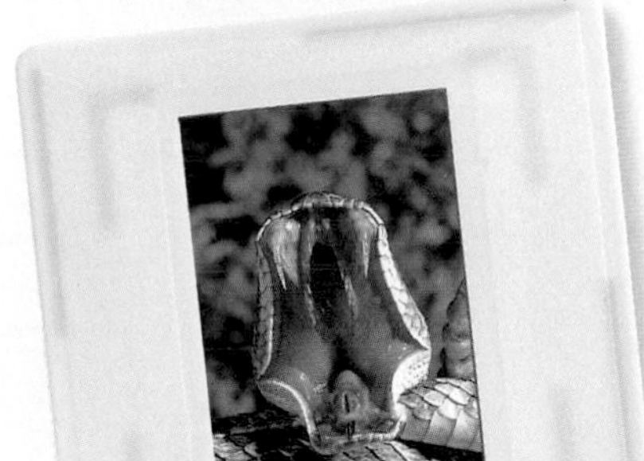

RIGHT *The homeopathic remedy Lachesis is made from the venom of the bushmaster snake.*

Neuralgia

Neuralgia is the term used to describe any pain originating in a nerve. If there is damage at any point along the route of a nerve, pain will then be referred to the area served by the affected nerve. Infection causing inflammation in a nerve can also cause neuralgia. The pain may be intermittent or continuous. Neuralgia has different causes, which give rise to certain specific types of neuralgic pain – trigeminal neuralgia, sciatica, post-herpetic neuralgia, and glossopharyngeal neuralgia.

DATA FILE

Specific types of neuralgia include:

- trigeminal neuralgia, in which the facial nerve is affected, causing severe one-sided facial pain.
- sciatica, in which spinal nerves are trapped between vertebrae, causing pain of varying severity in the back, sometimes extending down to the foot.
- Post-herpetic neuralgia, which causes a burning pain at the site of a previous attack of shingles.
- Glossopharyngeal neuralgia, in which pain is felt in the ear, the throat, and at the back of the tongue.

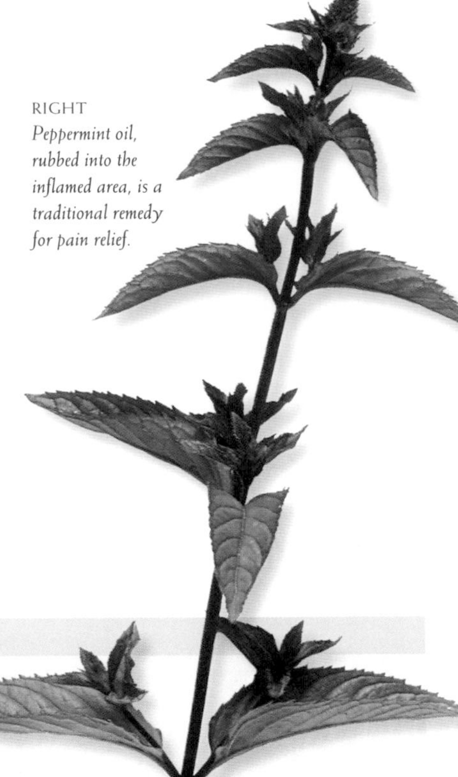

RIGHT *Peppermint oil, rubbed into the inflamed area, is a traditional remedy for pain relief.*

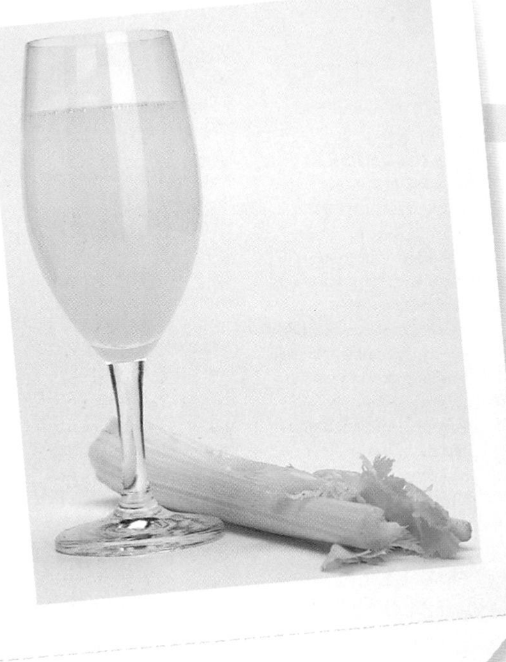

ABOVE *Celery juice relieves neuralgic pain. Make it by liquidizing fresh celery.*

TREATMENT

- Warm chamomile compresses applied to the affected area will ease inflammation and pain.
- Rub lemons on the affected area for pain relief. *(See page 87.)*
- Rub peppermint oil into the affected area.
- Clove oil can be used where pain is experienced inside the mouth. *(See page 90.)*

AROMATHERAPY

- Massage essential oil of eucalyptus, lavender, or chamomile into the affected area, or add the infused herbs to the bath. *(See pages 146–71.)*
- A compress of rosemary essential oil will improve the circulation in that area, which will encourage healing. *(See page 168.)*
- Blend one drop of mustard and pepper oils in some grapeseed oil, and massage into the affected area. *(See pages 146–71.)*

HOMEOPATHY

Treatment should be constitutional, and supervised by an experienced homeopath. Some of the following remedies may be helpful:

- Arsenicum, for an attack brought on by dry cold. You feel chilly, tired, restless, and have burning pains. *(See page 182.)*
- Lachesis, for pain that is worse after sleep. *(See page 216.)*
- Mag. phos., for pain that is relieved by applying heat and pressure. *(See page 204.)*
- Aconite, when symptoms come on suddenly, particularly after exposure to cold; the body feels congested and numb. *(See page 178.)*
- Colocynthis, for a neuralgia attack brought on by cold or damp, and which feels better for heat. *(See page 191.)*

VITAMINS AND MINERALS

- Vitamins B1, B2, and biotin help nerve health. *(See pages 252, 253, and 257.)*
- Take both extra vitamin E and chromium. *(See pages 257 and 259.)*

CHINESE HERBALISM

- Treatment would be aimed at addressing Wind, Damp and Heat which may have entered the meridians and are causing the illness. *(See page 50.)*
- Gentian and oriental wormwood may be useful.

TRADITIONAL HOME AND FOLK REMEDIES

- Celery juice or celery tea will help to ease the pain of neuralgia. *(See page 83.)*

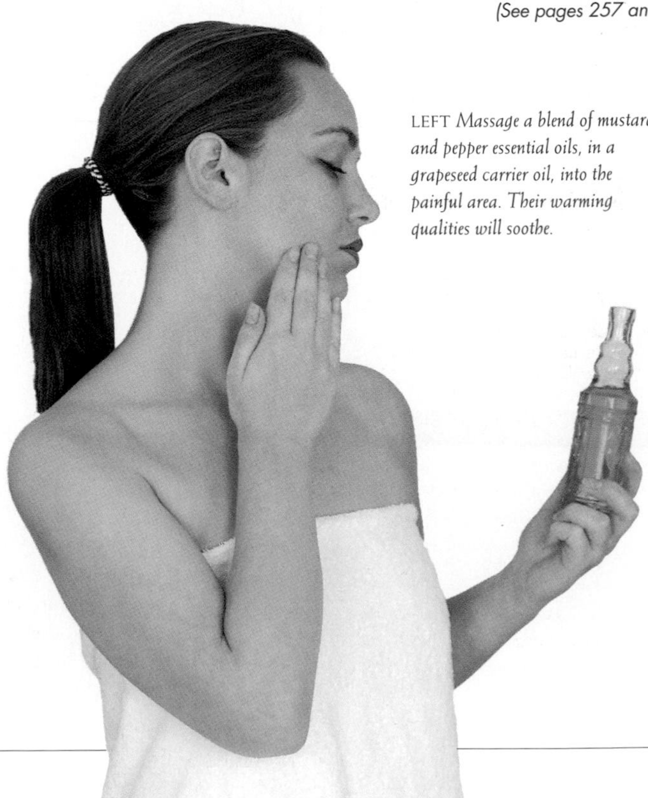

LEFT *Massage a blend of mustard and pepper essential oils, in a grapeseed carrier oil, into the painful area. Their warming qualities will soothe.*

Migraine

The classic feature of a migraine is a throbbing headache usually on one side of the head only. This is caused by the narrowing and dilating of the blood vessels in a part of one side of the brain. An attack may last for up to two days. There are two main types of migraine, common and the comparatively rare classical. Migraine can be hereditary, and may be triggered by many factors, including stress, hormonal changes (around menopause, menstruation, and occasionally pregnancy), oral contraceptives, and food that contains tyramine, an amino acid which affects the blood vessels. Foods rich in tyramine include bananas, cheese, chocolate, eggs, oranges, spinach, tomatoes, and wine. Other triggers include changes or extremes in temperature, lighting, or noise level. Migraine occurs in about 10 percent of the population, and is more common in women. Children may suffer from migraine, but this often manifests itself as an abdominal pain rather than a headache.

ABOVE *Eating a couple of feverfew leaves daily may stave off an attack of migraine.*

Symptoms

• *common migraine:- slowly developing severe headache, lasting from a few hours to two days – made worse by the smallest movement or noise – nausea and sometimes vomiting.* • *classical migraine:- headache preceded by an aura which generally takes the form a visual disturbance – this may consist of temporary loss of vision, focusing problems, blind spots, and flashing lights – possible speech problems – occasional weakness or temporary paralysis of the limbs or extremities – nausea and vomiting – sensitivity to light*

DATA FILE

• Some 16–18 million Americans suffer from migraine. Studies suggest that people who feel compelled to excel are especially susceptible to migraine.

• About 60 percent of all migraine sufferers are women, and most patients first develop symptoms between the ages of 10 and 30.

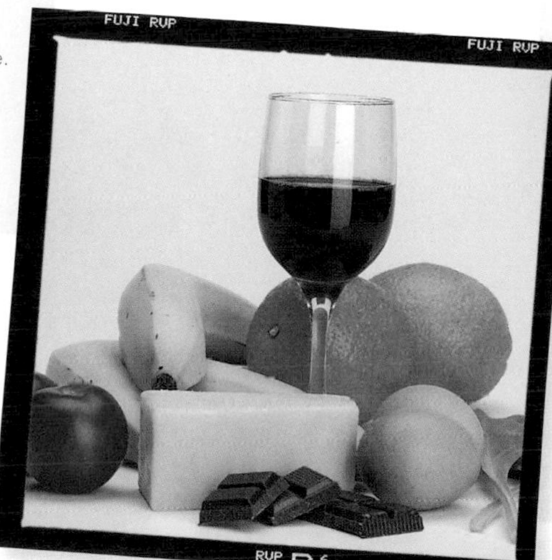

RIGHT *These foods contain tyramine, an amino acid which may trigger a migraine in some people.*

TREATMENT

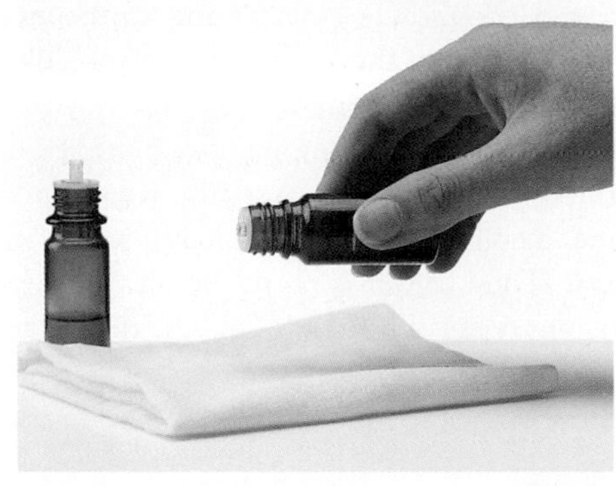

LEFT *Make a cool compress with a few drops each of lavender and peppermint essential oils on a damp cloth.*

AYURVEDA

• Treatment would be aimed at Ayurvedic oral formulas, and panchakarma shirovirechana. *(See page 20.)*

• Vilwadi lehya, an Ayurvedic product, can help with nausea.

CHINESE HERBALISM

• The cause is believed to be excess Liver qi stagnation, weakness in the stomach, and an imbalance of stomach and liver. Useful herbs include cassia tora and chrysanthemum.

HERBALISM

• Feverfew is an effective remedy for reducing the frequency of migraine. Take 2 or 3 small leaves between a little fresh bread, daily. Feverfew tablets are also available. *(See page 133.)*

• The following herbs can be infused for treating a mild attack of neuralgia: balm, meadowsweet, rosemary, and skullcap. *(See pages 121, 127, and 131.)*

• Apply a warm compress with Jamaican dogwood to the temples and forehead during an attack.

AROMATHERAPY

• Peppermint and lavender oils, applied to a cool compress, will help to relieve symptoms. *(See pages 161 and 164.)*

• Inhalations, baths, or massage of melissa, rosemary, or sweet marjoram can relieve the pain and shorten the duration of attacks. Used regularly, these methods can be preventive. *(See pages 146–71.)*

• A dab of lavender oil at the base of the nostrils can be used at the first signs of an attack. *(See page 161.)*

HOMEOPATHY

Treatment is constitutional, but the following remedies may be helpful in the event of an attack:

• Pulsatilla, for headache which is worse in the evening or during menstruation, and aggravated by rich, fatty foods; also for tearfulness. *(See page 209.)*

• Thuja, for a left-sided headache with the sensation of a nail being drilled into the skull. *(See page 216.)*

• Silicea, for pain that begins in the back of the head, settling above an eye. This is alleviated by wrapping the head. *(See page 211.)*

• Lycopodium, for pain that is worse on the right side of the body, painful temples and dizziness. *(See page 203.)*

• Nat. mur., for headache which is blinding and throbs, and which is worsened by warmth and movement, and where the attack is preceded by numbness around the mouth and nose. *(See page 206.)*

VITAMINS AND MINERALS

• Take extra vitamins B5, C, and E, and also evening primrose oil. *(See pages 254, 256, 257, and 270.)*

• Add fresh root ginger to food.

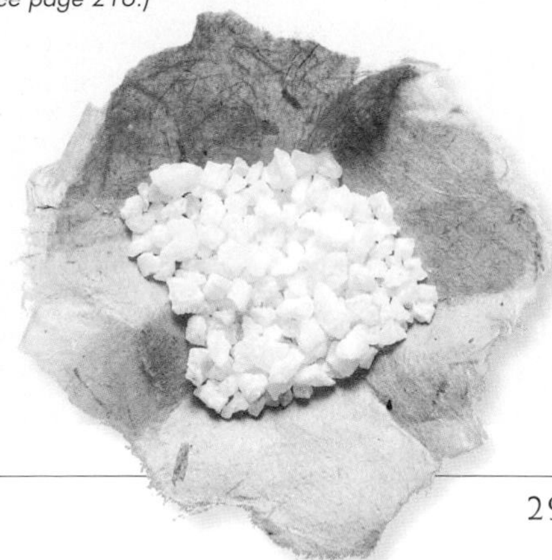

RIGHT *Nat. mur homeopathic remedy is common salt.*

Headache

Headaches are an extremely common complaint, and for the most part are due to muscular tension in the head, neck, or shoulders, or to congestion of the blood vessels supplying blood to the brain and muscles. In some cases a headache may be a symptom of a more serious underlying disorder, but often headaches are caused by stress, tiredness, poor posture, caffeine, alcohol, drugs, food allergy, eyestrain, sinusitis, or low blood sugar. They can also be the result of a head injury. There are many different types of headache and the degree and intensity of pain vary accordingly. It may occur in any part of the head, usually worsening towards the end of the day.

CAUTION

HEADACHES WITH ASSOCIATED FEATURES SUCH AS DOUBLE VISION, PROJECTILE VOMITING, WEAKNESS, PARALYSIS, VERTIGO, OR ONE-SIDED DEAFNESS REQUIRE URGENT MEDICAL ATTENTION.

Symptoms

• *sensation of a tight band around the head* • *a feeling of pressure at the top of the head* • *bursting or throbbing sensation* • *eye and neck pain* • *dizziness*

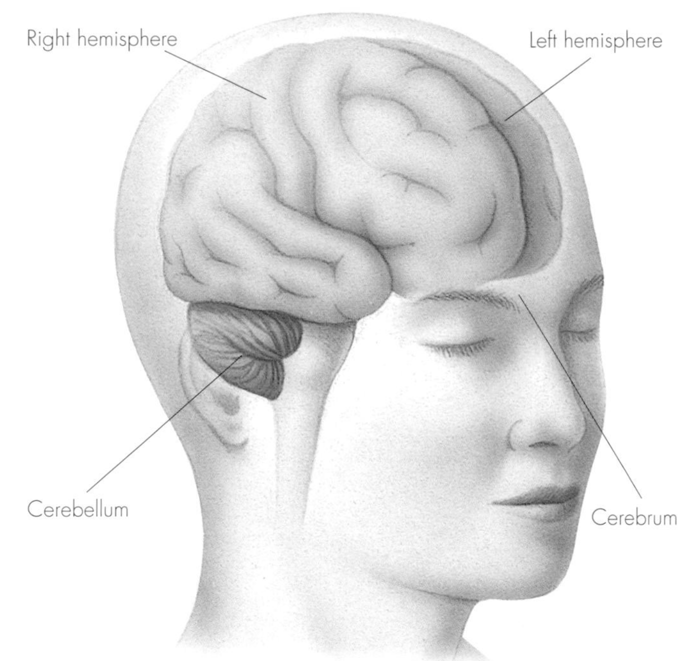

ABOVE *Headaches are very occasionally an indication of a serious disorder, such as a brain tumor.*

DATA FILE

- In the U.S., up to 50 million people every year seek medical advice about their headaches.
- $0.5 billion is spent on headache remedies annually.
- Almost 90 percent of all people seeking medical help for headaches suffer from tension-type headaches.
- Cluster headaches produce short, severe attacks of pain centered over one eye. They are so called because they occur in clusters, many times a day, for several months. Spontaneous remissions often take place, but the pain usually returns some months or years later.
- Cluster headaches are suffered most often by males.
- Researchers suspect that cluster headaches may be caused by a disorder in histamine metabolism, since they are usually accompanied by allergy symptoms such as tearing, nasal congestion, and a runny nose.

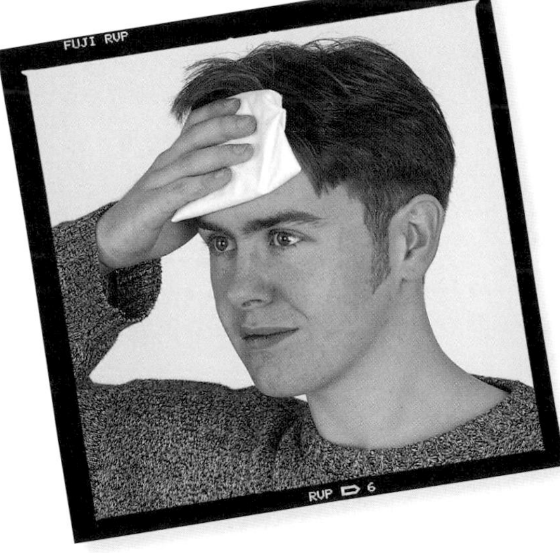

ABOVE *Heat 3 tablespoons of mustard oil, pour on to a cloth, and apply to the forehead to ease throbbing.*

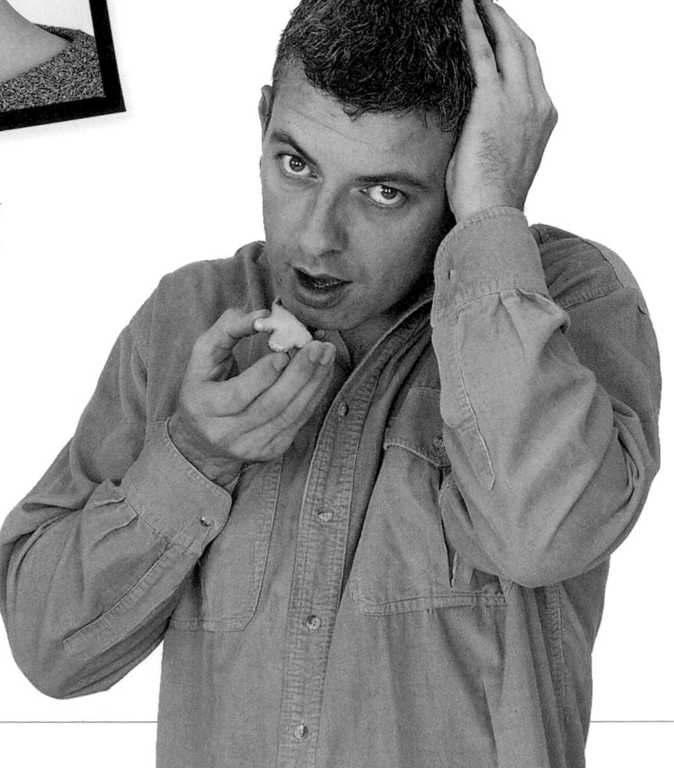

RIGHT *The Chinese trust ginger to relieve headaches. Chew a small piece of fresh root.*

TREATMENT

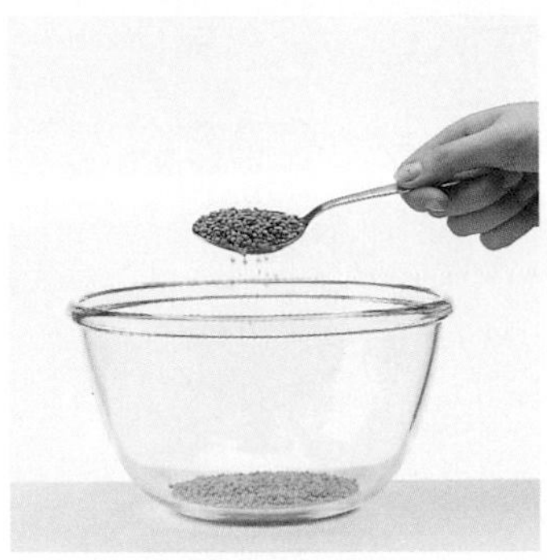

An Ayurvedic treatment for sinus-related headaches is the steam inhalation of coriander seeds. Put the coriander seeds into a small bowl.

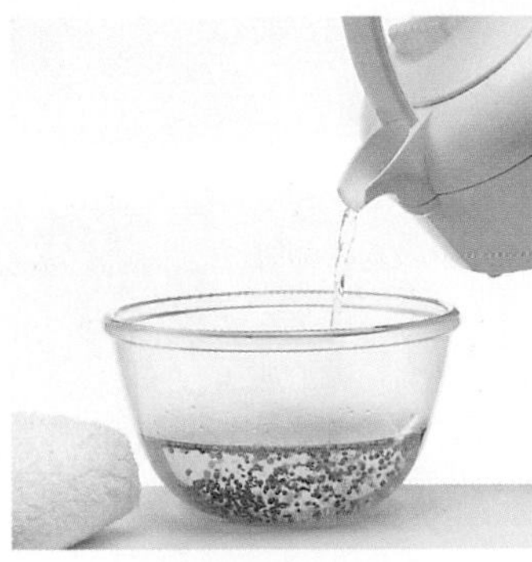

Pour on some boiling water, drape a towel over your head and the bowl, and inhale the steam. Coriander's active ingredient is a volatile oil.

AYURVEDA

• For headaches, heat 3 tablespoons of mustard oil, soak a cloth in the solution and apply to the forehead as required. *(See page 30.)*
• Coriander seeds, steeped for several minutes in boiling water, can be inhaled under a towel to relieve sinus-related headaches. *(See page 35.)*
• Asna vilwadi thaila is an oil, for external use, which relieves headaches.

CHINESE HERBALISM

• Traditional Chinese herbal medicine recommends ginger for headaches. Eat a small piece of fresh ginger root or make ginger tea from the fresh root or tea bags. If you prefer, mix a large pinch of powdered ginger into a glass of cool water and drink it, or try powdered ginger in capsules, available from health food stores.
• Ginseng is another favorite Chinese herbal remedy for headaches. *(See page 67.)*

TRADITIONAL HOME AND FOLK REMEDIES

• A ginger foot bath may ease the pain and warm the body.
• Chamomile tea soothes headache symptoms.
• A mustard foot bath is a traditional headache remedy. *(See page 98.)*
• A few grains of cayenne pepper, added to tea, ease a headache. *(See page 86.)*
• Fresh garlic bulbs, eaten in a salad, will clear headaches which have a feeling of congestion. *(See page 82.)*
• Parsley and peppermint teas will clear the head.

HERBALISM

• Sitting down with a relaxing cup of mild herbal tea is often good for a tension headache. Good choices are peppermint, spearmint, chamomile, rose hip, meadowsweet, or lemon balm. *(See pages 119, 121, and 125.)*
• Valerian root tea can also be helpful, but it may induce sleep – use it with caution. *(See page 136.)*
• Researchers are studying the benefits of the herb feverfew for treating chronic headaches and migraines. The leaves of this plant contain a substance that relaxes the blood vessels in your brain. Studies suggest that patients who eat a few fresh feverfew leaves or take an extract of the leaves every day have fewer and less severe migraines; the herb has no unpleasant side-effects. *(See page 133.)*

AROMATHERAPY

• The relaxing qualities of lavender oil make it a good treatment for a tension headache. This essential oil is very gentle, so you can massage a few drops of neat oil into your temples and the base of your neck. *(See page 161.)*
• Try mixing a drop or two of peppermint oil in a bowl of hot water and inhaling the steam, then lie down with a warm compress soaked in sweet marjoram oil on your forehead. *(See pages 164 and 165.)*
• Place a few drops of lavender oil at the base of your nostrils for almost instant pain relief. *(See page 161.)*
• Try taking a bath with relaxing oils such as chamomile or ylang ylang to soothe and relieve pain. *(See pages 146–71.)*

HOMEOPATHY

Most headaches would be dealt with constitutionally, that is, the treatment would be tailored to your individual needs. Other remedies to try include:
• Ignatia, for headaches caused by emotional stress. *(See page 200.)*
• Nux vomica, for headaches caused by overindulgence or stress. *(See page 214.)*
• Cimicifuga may be useful for pain caused by nervous muscular tension in the shoulders and neck. *(See page 190.)*
• Nux vomica or Pulsatilla are both useful in many cases of migraine. *(See pages 209 and 214.)*
• Aconite, for a sudden headache which feels worse for cold and is characterized by a tight band around the head. *(See page 178.)*
• Apis, for stinging, stabbing or burning headaches; when the body feels tender and sore. *(See page 180.)*
• Belladonna, for throbbing, drumming headaches with a flushed face. *(See page 183.)*
• Bryonia, for sharp, stabbing pain when the eyes are moved. *(See page 185.)*
• Hypericum, for a bursting, aching headache with a sensitive scalp. *(See page 199.)*
• Ruta, for a pressing headache caused by fatigue, and made worse by reading. *(See page 210.)*

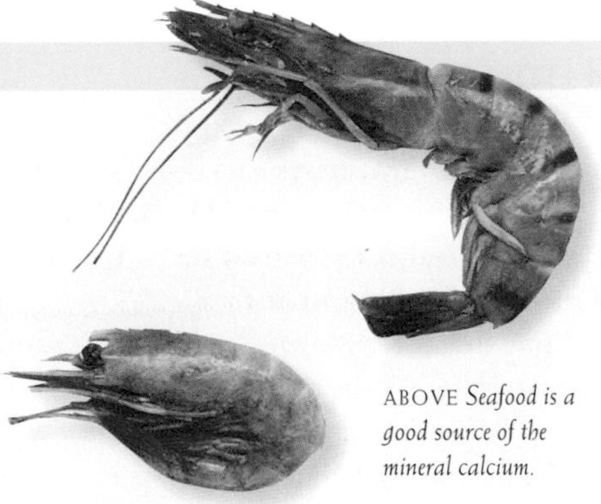

ABOVE *Seafood is a good source of the mineral calcium.*

VITAMINS AND MINERALS

• Frequent headaches could be a signal that you are low on some important vitamins and minerals. Low levels of niacin and vitamin B6 can cause headaches, for example, and all the B vitamins are needed to help combat stress and avoid tension headaches. Protein-rich foods such as chicken, fish, beans and peas, milk, cheese, nuts, and peanut butter are all good dietary sources of both niacin and vitamin B6. *(See page 253 and 254.)*
• The minerals calcium and magnesium work together to help prevent headaches, especially those related to a woman's menstrual cycle. Good sources of calcium are dairy products, tofu, dark green leafy vegetables such as kale or broccoli, and beans and peas. Magnesium is found in dark green leafy vegetables, nuts, bananas, wheat germ, seafood, and beans and peas. *(See page 258 and 262.)*
• If you can't eat some of these foods because they are headache triggers for you, taking a good daily multivitamin with minerals should provide enough of all the nutrients you need to help prevent headaches.

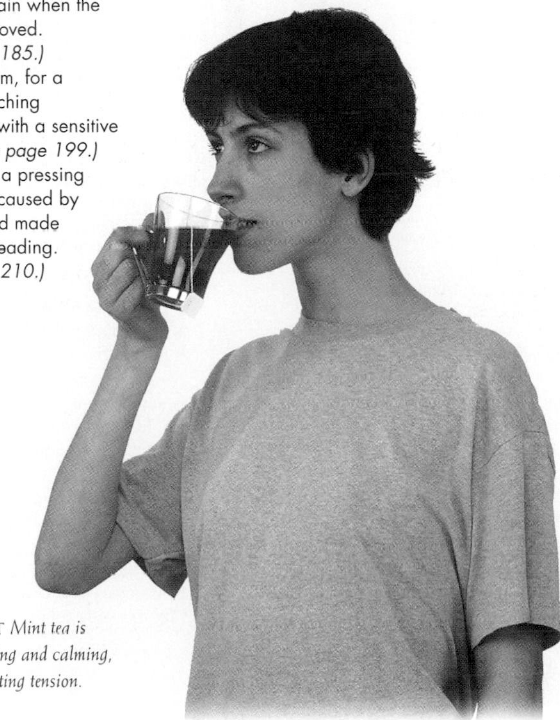

RIGHT *Mint tea is refreshing and calming, dissipating tension.*

Fainting

Fainting (or a vasovagal attack) is a brief loss of consciousness, usually brought on by strong emotion, shock, distress, or pain, and is most likely to occur in warm, crowded places. It is caused by a temporary shortage of blood supply to the brain, and there is also a slowing of the heart rate. A fainting episode acts, in fact, as a type of safety mechanism in that the fall restores the blood supply to the brain by gravity.

Symptoms

The characteristic loss of consciousness may be preceded by:
• yawning • sweating • nausea • deep, rapid breathing and a weak pulse • impaired vision • ringing in the ears • weakness and confusion

DATA FILE

• Fainting often occurs as a result of a vasovagal attack, in which overstimulation of the vagus nerve causes slowing of the heartbeat and a fall in blood pressure – which reduces the flow of blood to the brain. These attacks are commonly caused by pain, stress, shock, fear, or in a room with little oxygen. Other causes include prolonged coughing, straining to defecate or urinate, or blowing an instrument.

• Fainting may also result from postural hypotension (see page 299), which may occur when a person stands still for a long time, or suddenly stands up. This is common in the elderly, in sufferers of diabetes, and people taking high blood pressure medication or vasodilator drugs.

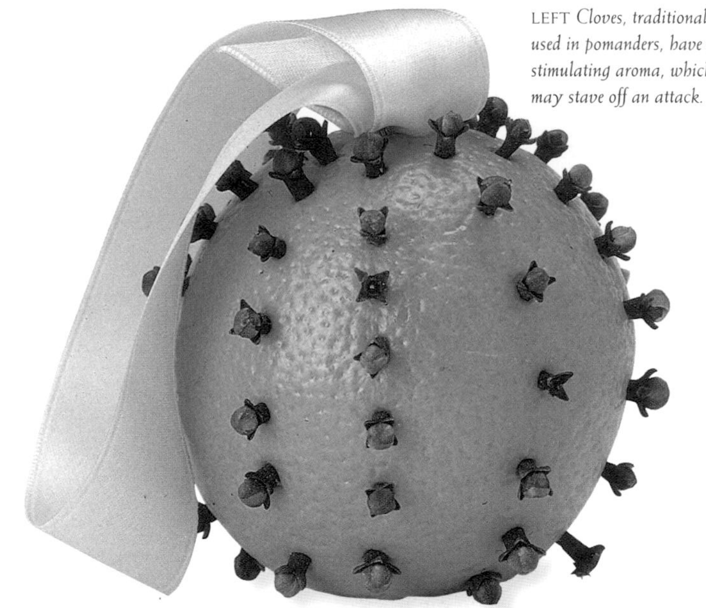

LEFT *Cloves, traditionally used in pomanders, have a stimulating aroma, which may stave off an attack.*

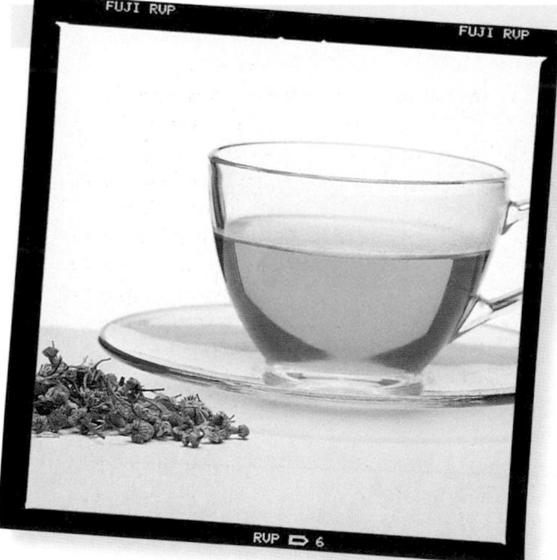

ABOVE *An infusion of ginger, cinnamon, and peppermint prevents fainting.*

TREATMENT

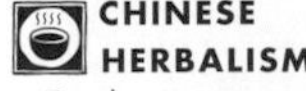

AYURVEDA The following Ayurvedic preparations will help to cure the condition: Aswagandharisthta, an oral tonic; Chandanadi thaila, an external oil; Kalyanaka ghritha, oral ghee. *(See page 20.)*

CHINESE HERBALISM
• Fresh ginger, cinnamon twigs, and peppermint would be useful, taken internally as an infusion or decoction, as required. *(See page 54.)*

TRADITIONAL HOME AND FOLK REMEDIES
• Eat fresh or grated apple when you start to feel faint; it is both restorative and calming. *(See page 94.)*
• Chew dried cloves, which are stimulating and can improve circulation. *(See page 90.)*

HERBALISM
• Small sips of ginger tea, or root ginger chewed, will help to restore, and prevent an attack. *(See page 139.)*
• Rosemary is stimulating, and taken regularly can prevent fainting spells. *(See page 127.)*
• A hot drink of honey and peppermint will help to prevent loss of consciousness. Drink when you first start to feel faint. *(See page 125.)*

AROMATHERAPY
• Hold a tissue with a few drops of peppermint or neroli oil, which can help when you feel faint or are in a state of shock. *(See pages 152 and 164.)*
• A few drops of rosemary oil, massaged into the temples, prevents loss of consciousness. *(See page 168.)*

HOMEOPATHY
Constitutional treatment is necessary if the condition is chronic, but specific remedies which can be taken every 5 minutes after or immediately before fainting (when the sensation of fainting begins) include:
• Veratrum, for fainting caused by anger.
• Coffea, for fainting brought on by excitement. *(See page 192.)*
• Ignatia, for fainting caused by an emotional shock or trauma. *(See page 200.)*
• Aconite, for fainting caused by fright and characterized by tension and pale, clammy skin. *(See page 178.)*
• Cocculus, for fainting caused by lack of sleep.
• Gelsemium, when you feel weak and shaky. *(See page 195.)*

FLOWER ESSENCES
• Rescue Remedy or Emergency Essence placed on the tongue or temples may help to prevent fainting. If you are prone to fainting, carry a bottle at all times and take at the first signs of weakness. *(See page 244.)*
• Clematis can be taken for the "far away" feeling that comes before an attack, to bring the mind back to present reality. *(See page 229.)*

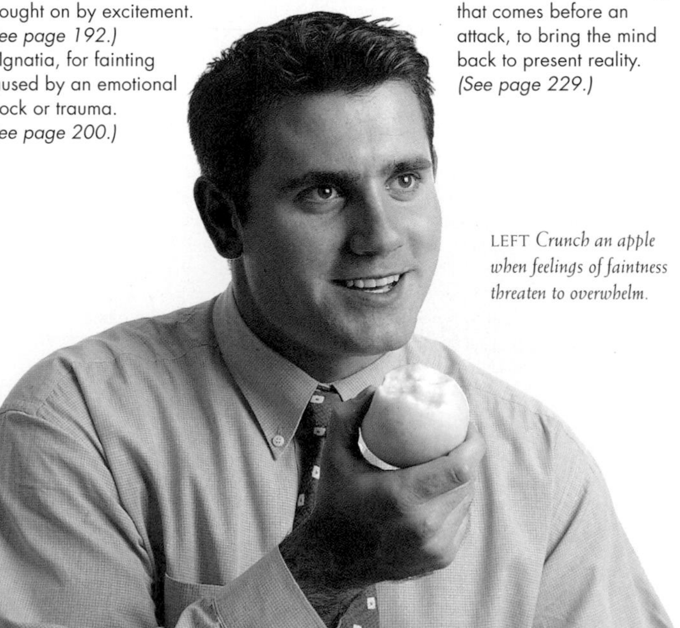

LEFT *Crunch an apple when feelings of faintness threaten to overwhelm.*

Dizziness

Dizziness is the sensation that everything around the sufferer is spinning, or that the brain is moving within the skull. In severe cases the sufferer may lose his or her balance and fall to the ground. Dizziness can be caused by a fault in the inner ear's balancing mechanism, or it may be due to a neurological disturbance. It can also be brought on by travel sickness, hyperventilation, anxiety, alcohol, drugs, and standing up suddenly from a sitting or lying position (postural hypotension). Postural hypotension is more common in the elderly and in people taking antihypertensive (high blood pressure) drugs.

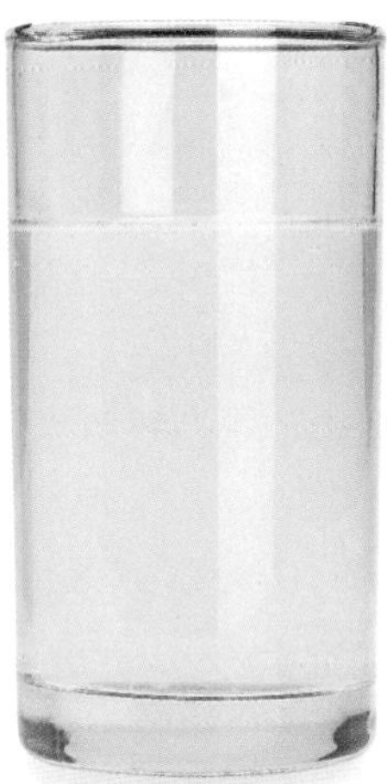

ABOVE *Ayurveda recommends drinking soda water with the juice of a lime or lemon.*

SYMPTOMS

- *spinning sensation* • *nausea* • *vomiting* • *pallor*
- *cold sweats*

CAUTION

SEVERE OR PROLONGED DIZZINESS SHOULD BE REPORTED TO YOUR PHYSICIAN.

BELOW *Ginger tea's stimulant qualities help to fend off an attack of dizziness.*

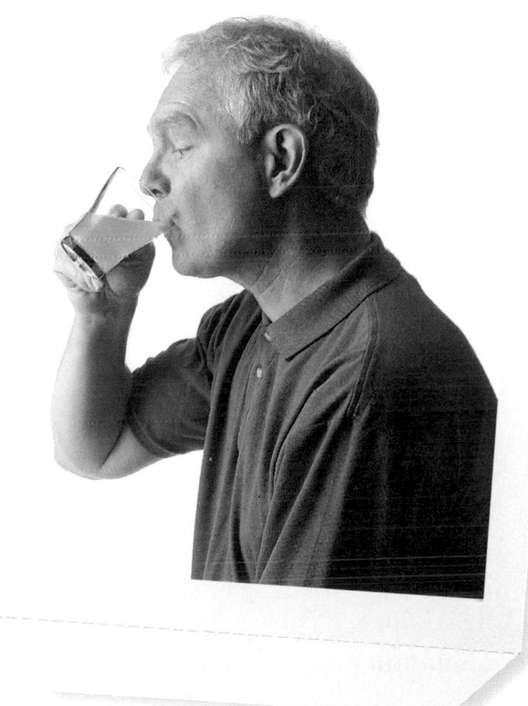

TREATMENT

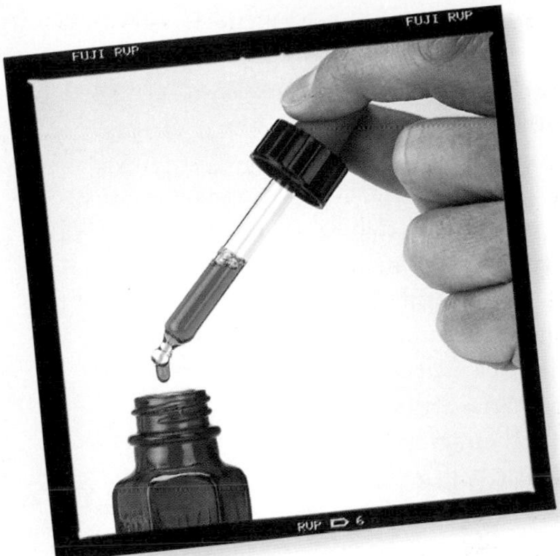

ABOVE *Rescue Remedy, made up of five flower essences, calms the patient and restores equilibrium.*

AYURVEDA

• Add the juice of a lime or lemon to half a glass of soda water and sip in small doses.

CHINESE HERBALISM

• Fresh ginger, cinnamon, and peppermint may help. *(See page 59.)*

• Mulberry can be used to nourish the blood.

HERBALISM

• Small sips of fresh ginger tea, made with root ginger, will help to ease the symptoms. *(See page 139.)*

• Teas of rock rose flowers or wild rose flowers, with a little honey, will be helpful.

HOMEOPATHY

• Gelsemium, for dizziness accompanied by a fit of trembling. *(See page 195.)*

• Nux vom., for when symptoms are made worse by flickering lights.

• Calcarea, when symptoms become worse after looking up. *(See page 186.)*

• Borax, for symptoms made worse by downward motion.

• Conium, when you feel worse lying down.

FLOWER ESSENCES

• If dizziness is associated with panic, stress, or anxiety, Emergency Essence or Rescue Remedy will be calming and restorative; take as required. *(See page 244.)*

VITAMINS AND MINERALS

• Take vitamins B2 and B3, and extra salt if you are sweating a great deal. *(See page 253.)*

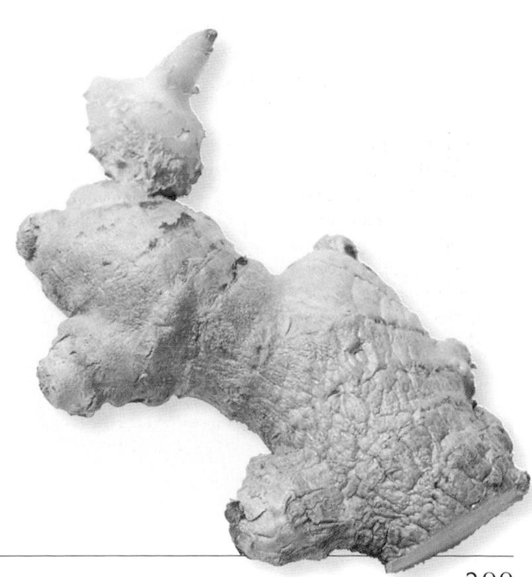

RIGHT *Peel fresh ginger thinly, to preserve the richest active properties which lie just under the skin.*

SKIN AND HAIR PROBLEMS

Dermatitis

Dermatitis is a very loose term (often used interchangeably with eczema) used to describe an inflammation of the skin from any cause. Exogenous dermatitis is caused by external factors (irritants such as washing powder), and tends to occur around infected wounds or ulcers. Endogenous forms are due to internal problems, including metabolic disorders. Scratching always aggravates dermatitis and may also cause infection. Types of dermatitis include: diaper rash, caused by the ammonia in urine; atopic dermatitis, complicated by allergies such as hay fever; infantile eczema; seborrheic dermatitis *(see Dandruff, page 306)*; dermatitis artefacta, caused by unnecessary scratching (it is self-inflicted and usually indicates an underlying emotional problem). The symptoms of dermatitis vary in severity and appearance according to the cause.

SYMPTOMS

• redness and blistering • swelling, weeping, and crusting of skin • itching with a strong impulse to scratch • burning sensation

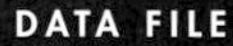

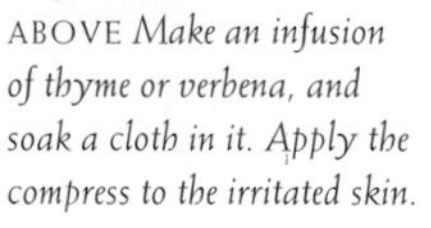

ABOVE *Make an infusion of thyme or verbena, and soak a cloth in it. Apply the compress to the irritated skin.*

DATA FILE

• Skin-contact dermatitis includes primary irritant dermatitis, allergic dermatitis, and photochemical dermatitis.

• Primary irritant dermatitis is the most common type and is caused by the direct toxicity of certain chemicals that come in contact with the skin.

• Allergic dermatitis involves the immune mechanism and requires prior sensitization of an individual to agents such as cosmetics, chemicals, plants, drugs, or costume jewelry.

• Photochemical dermatitis occurs when an individual with photosensitizing chemicals on his or her skin is exposed to light.

• Atopic dermatitis, or eczema, is a chronic inflammation that appears to run in families with a history of asthma and hay fever.

• Dermatitis can occur in single episodes, or may be chronic. Up to 90 percent of the U.S. population will suffer from dermatitis during their lifetime.

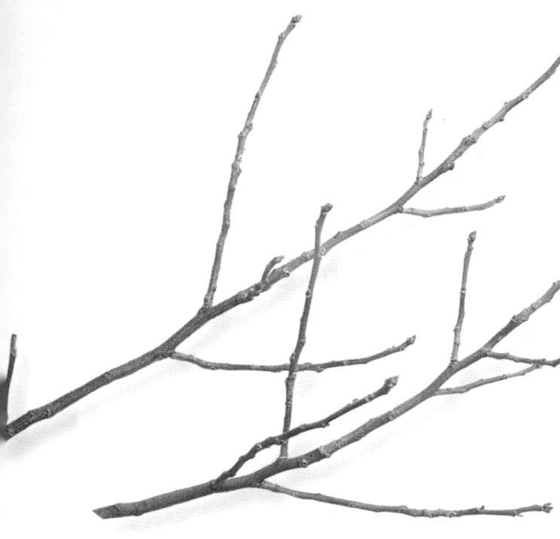

ABOVE *Rhus tox. is a homeopathic remedy for dermatitis which has erupted into blisters.*

TREATMENT

CHINESE HERBALISM

• Dittany bark and puncture vine fruit may help with itching.

TRADITIONAL HOME AND FOLK REMEDIES

• For dermatitis on the hands, rub them with the cold wet coffee grounds left after you have brewed a pot of coffee, to soothe.

HERBALISM

• Apply compresses of verbena or thyme tea to the area to soothe and cool. *(See page 135.)*

AROMATHERAPY

• Dilute and massage a few drops of aspic, cedarwood, niaouli, or chamomile into the affected area to ease itching. *(See pages 146–71.)*

• For contact dermatitis, calendula or chamomile oil. *(See pages 148 and 150.)*

HOMEOPATHY

• Sulfur, for when the skin feels as if it is burning, and becomes red, hot, and itchy. *(See page 215.)*

• Graphites, when the skin appears infected. *(See page 196.)*

• Petroleum, when there are deep cracks with a watery discharge.

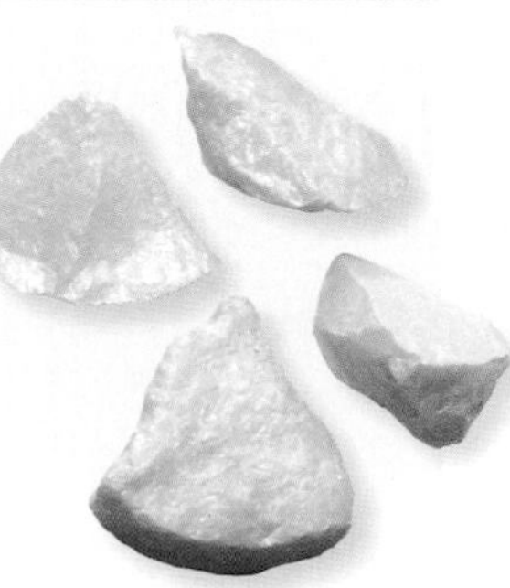

ABOVE *Homeopaths may prescribe Sulfur for a feeling of burning.*

• Urtica urens, for a nettle rash-type itchiness. *(See page 217.)*

• Rhus tox., for blisters that are worse at night and improve with warmth. *(See page 210.)*

FLOWER ESSENCES

• Crab Apple is the cleansing remedy. It works well when added to water for washing and baths. *(See page 234.)*

• Impatiens is very useful for people whose rashes are associated with feelings of irritability and impatience. Take internally or mix into a neutral cream. *(See page 233.)*

• Rescue Remedy, taken internally or used externally in a cream or wash, is useful for treating most skin problems. *(See page 244.)*

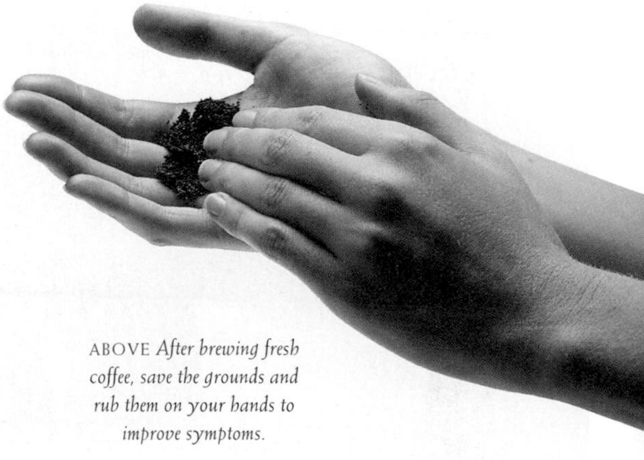

ABOVE *After brewing fresh coffee, save the grounds and rub them on your hands to improve symptoms.*

Eczema

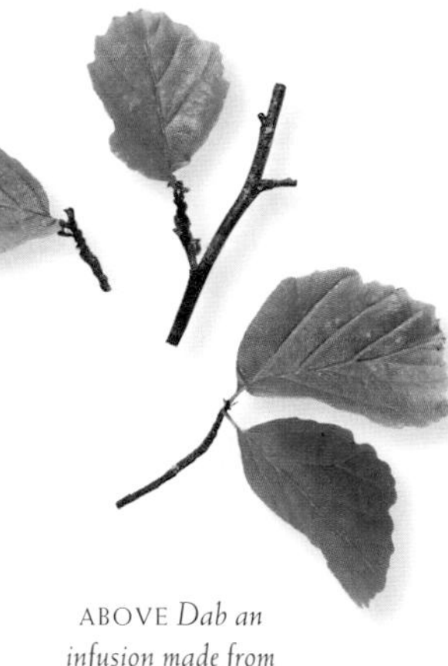

ABOVE *Dab an infusion made from witch hazel on the affected skin.*

Eczema (also called dermatitis) is an inflammation of the skin that causes itching and redness. It is a feature of many different skin disorders arising from many different causes. It can also be hereditary. Eczema is only infectious if it becomes secondarily infected. Types of eczema include: contact eczema (caused by allergens such as plants, metals, detergents, and chemical irritants); atopic eczema (associated with allergies such as hay fever); pomphylox eczema (triggered by emotional stress); and varicose eczema (occurring in the region of varicose veins).

SYMPTOMS

• red, scaly, cracked patches of skin, particularly on the hands, ears, feet, and legs • burning and itching with a strong urge to scratch, possibly leading to infection, particularly in children • small fluid-filled blisters which may burst to form sores

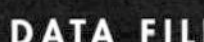
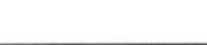

DATA FILE

- A person may contract eczema at any age and at any place on the body, but the ailment occurs chiefly on the ears, hands, feet, and legs.
- In infants, eczema is often caused by allergy to certain proteins in wheat, milk, and eggs.
- Emotional problems and severe mental stress are suspected of causing eczema in adults.
- Often, a family history of eczema exists, implying that heredity is also involved in some way.

BELOW *Sometimes eczema is brought on by stress. Massage helps to relax the sufferer.*

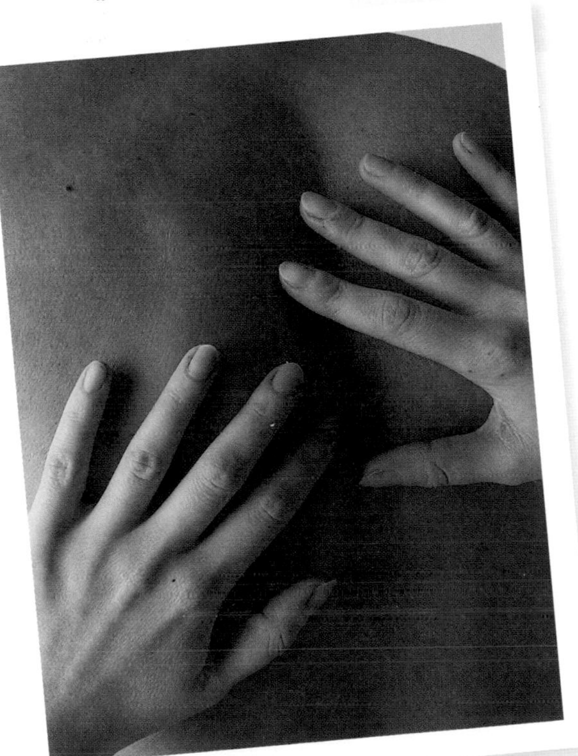

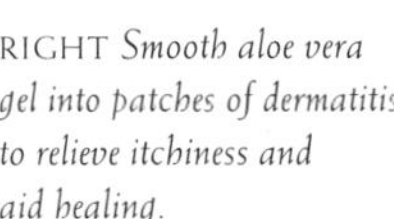
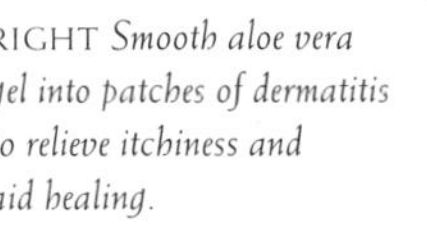

RIGHT *Smooth aloe vera gel into patches of dermatitis to relieve itchiness and aid healing.*

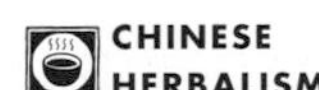

TREATMENT

AYURVEDA
- Cassia pods and aloe vera may be used. *(See pages 27 and 32.)*
- Treatment might consist of a number of related therapies, including herbalism, diet and lifestyle changes, cleansing routines, and treatment to balance the body systems so that they work more efficiently. *(See page 20.)*

CHINESE HERBALISM
- Chinese herbs will be prescribed according to the specific cause and symptoms of your eczema, but some possible herbs are: wormwood, peony root, and Chinese gentian. *(See page 67.)*
- Dittany bark and puncture vine fruit may help with itching

TRADITIONAL HOME AND FOLK REMEDIES
- An oatmeal bath will soothe irritation and reduce annoying itching. *(See page 84.)*
- Bathe sore patches with an infusion of witch hazel diluted in some warm water. *(See page 91.)*

HERBALISM
- Try drinking an infusion of burdock, chamomile, heartsease, marigold, and red clover, all of which are anti-inflammatory herbs. *(See pages 115, 117, and 119.)*
- Chickweed ointment can be applied directly to the affected area, and calendula oil may also be useful. *(See page 117.)*
- Blackberry leaf tea can be used topically.
- Aloe vera gel, from the leaf of the plant, will encourage healing. *(See page 114.)*

AROMATHERAPY
- A gentle massage with a blend of chamomile, lavender, and/or melissa essential oil in a little carrier oil can be used to treat eczema. *(See pages 146–71.)*
- Massage the affected areas with essential oils of chamomile, sage, geranium, and lavender, all blended together with a little carrier oil. *(See pages 146–71.)*

HOMEOPATHY
Eczema requires constitutional treatment, which means that treatment is tailored to your specific needs. The following remedies may be useful in the meantime:
- Sulfur, when the skin is burning, red, hot, and itchy. *(See page 215.)*
- Graphites, when the skin appears infected. *(See page 196.)*
- Petroleum, when there are deep cracks with a watery discharge
- Urtica urens, for a nettle rash-type itchiness. *(See page 217.)*
- Rhus tox., for blisters which are worse at night and improve with warmth. *(See page 210.)*

FLOWER ESSENCES
- Impatiens is very useful for people whose rashes are associated with feelings of irritability and impatience. Take internally or mix into a neutral cream. *(See page 233.)*
- Rescue Remedy, taken internally or used externally in a cream or wash, is useful for skin troubles. *(See page 244.)*

VITAMINS AND MINERALS
- Increase your intake of vitamin A, found in liver, eggs, butter, milk, and red and orange vegetables. *(See page 252.)*
- Take a B-complex supplement each day, and make sure your tablet contains good levels of niacin (B3), which is also found naturally in peanuts, meat, fish, and pulses. *(See page 253.)*
- Vitamin C and bioflavonoids (which are often contained in a good vitamin C supplement) act as a natural antihistamine. *(See pages 256 and 272.)*
- Evening primrose oil has been used successfully in the treatment of eczema, reducing itching and encouraging healing *(See page 270.)*

Psoriasis

Psoriasis is a common skin disorder which may affect any part of the body, but most often the elbows, knees, shins, scalp, and lower back. The characteristic bright pink or red plaques covered with silvery scaling are caused by a thickening of the outer skin layers. Psoriasis tends to run in families and usually begins in adolescence. Cold damp conditions, stress, anxiety, or an acute illness (such as tonsillitis) may all be triggers. There is also an association with arthritis of the fingers or toes. Psoriasis does not usually cause itching, nor is it contagious.

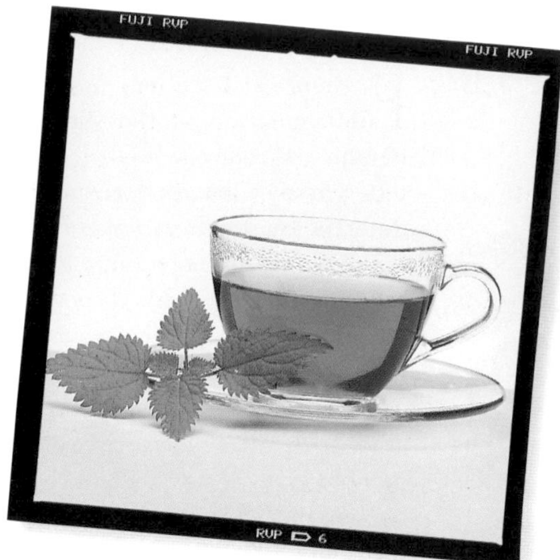

ABOVE *Sip nettle tea as a skin tonic. Nettles contain formic acid.*

Symptoms

• pain (rather than itching), with cracks appearing in the dry areas of the hands and feet • pustules on the palms of the hands or soles of the feet (pustular psoriasis) • glazed but not scaly plaques in moist areas of the body (flexural psoriasis) • distortion and pitting of the nails in some cases

TREATMENT

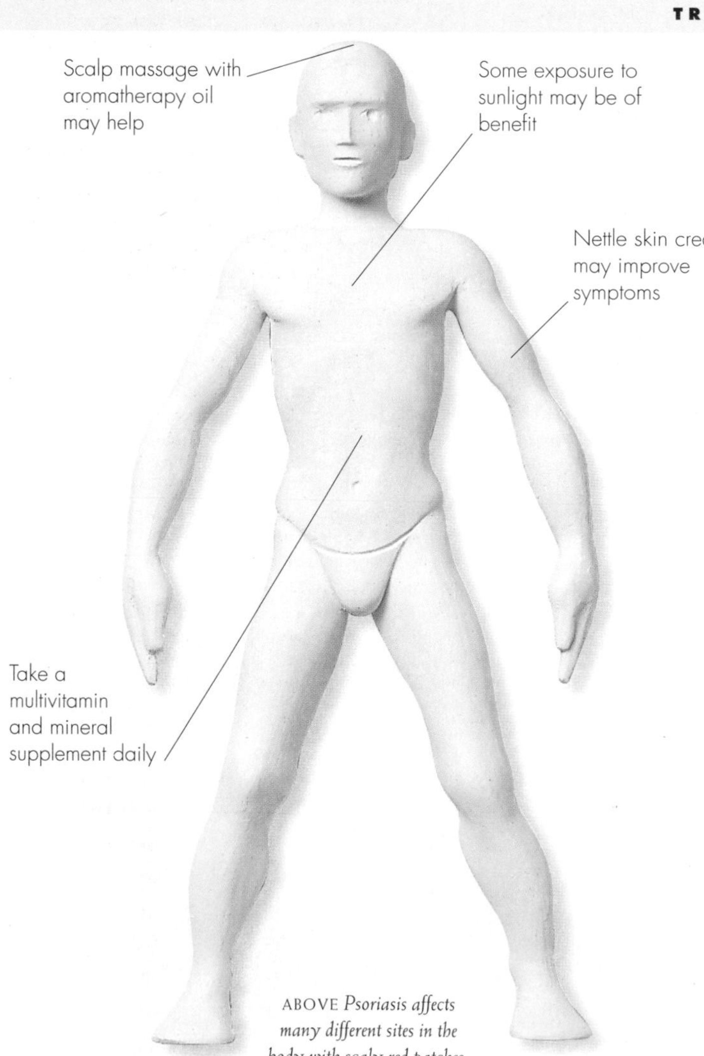

ABOVE *Psoriasis affects many different sites in the body with scaly red patches.*

CHINESE HERBALISM

• Dittany bark and puncture vine fruit may help with itching.

TRADITIONAL HOME AND FOLK REMEDIES

• Take at least 1 tablespoonful of olive oil a day and at least one raw vegetable salad. *(See page 95.)*

• Garlic is cleansing, and may ease the symptoms and prevent attacks. *(See page 82.)*

HERBALISM

• Licorice, for the inflammation of psoriasis. *(See page 122.)*

• Yarrow used twice weekly in bath water has proved beneficial in some cases. *(See page 112.)*

• Nettle tea and products based on nettles may be helpful. *(See page 137.)*

AROMATHERAPY

• Sedative and antidepressant oils such as lavender and chamomile can help to reduce the stress that exacerbates the condition. Use in the bath, massage, and skin creams. *(See pages 150 and 161.)*

• Bergamot essential oil, cajeput, and Roman chamomile can all be used as a beneficial massage oil. They may also be added to a bath, or placed in a vaporizer. *(See pages 146–71.)*

HOMEOPATHY

• Kali ars., for scaly skin aggravated by warmth.

• Arsenicum, for burning, hot areas, and feeling chilly and restless. *(See page 182.)*

• Graphites, for psoriasis that is worse behind the ears and weeping. *(See page 196.)*

• Sulfur, for patches that become worse after a bath and in heat. *(See page 215.)*

• Petroleum, when the condition is worse in winter.

FLOWER ESSENCES

• Impatiens is very useful for people whose rashes are associated with feelings of irritability and impatience. Take internally or mix into a neutral cream. *(See page 233.)*

• Rescue Remedy, taken internally or used externally in a cream or wash, treats most skin troubles. *(See page 244.)*

• Crab Apple is the cleansing remedy. It works well when added to water for washing and baths. *(See page 234.)*

VITAMINS AND MINERALS

• Increase your intake of vitamin A (as beta carotene), vitamin C, vitamin E, selenium, B-complex vitamins as part of a good multivitamin and mineral supplement, and also protein. *(See pages 252–57 and 264.)*

Urticaria

Urticaria is an allergic condition also known as hives or nettle rash. The rash of raised, whitish-yellow areas of skin surrounded by red inflammation is caused by the release of histamine into the tissues in response to triggers which may include heat, cold, sunlight, scabies, bites and stings, contact with plants, food additives, sensitivity to certain foods, and stress or anxiety. Acute urticaria typically develops very quickly, and usually disappears just as quickly; chronic urticaria is more persistent.

LEFT *The leaves of the aloe vera plant produce a gel which soothes a range of skin problems.*

Symptoms

• *rash of weals, especially on limbs and trunk* • *intense itching* • *swelling of the tongue and larynx may occur, possibly interfering with breathing* • *a feverish feeling* • *possibly nausea*

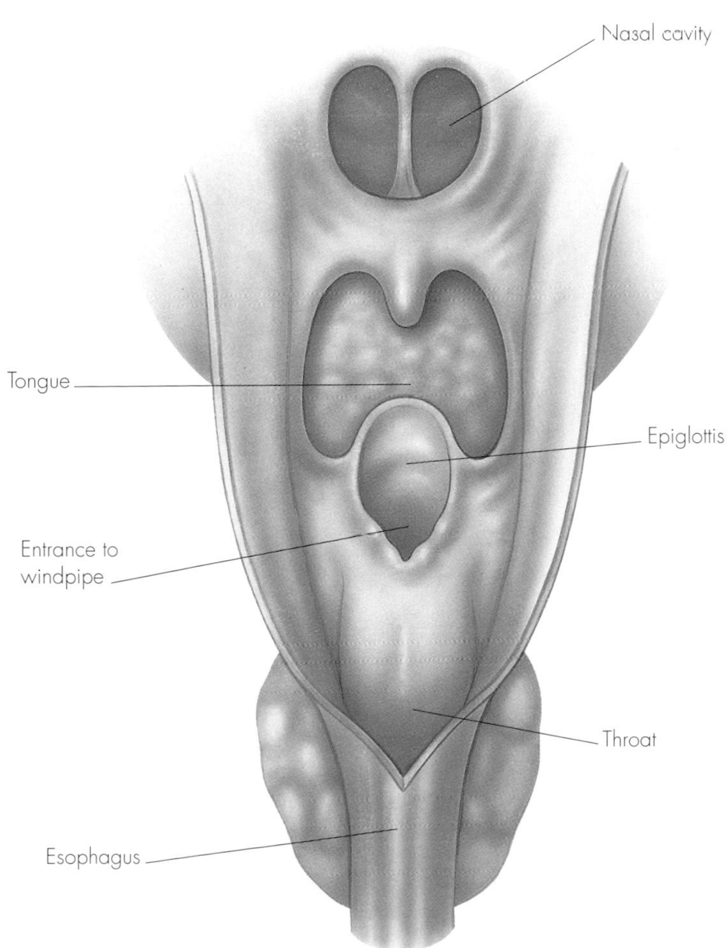

ABOVE *The larynx. Sometimes urticaria causes the tongue and larynx to swell, which may restrict breathing.*

TREATMENT

AYURVEDA

• Aloe vera can be used topically to soothe the rash. *(See page 27.)*

CHINESE HERBALISM

• The source of urticaria is considered to be Heat and Wind when red; and Heat, Cold and Wind for a cold white rash. Treatment may include chizomeotea or ledebouriella. *(See page 64.)*

TRADITIONAL HOME AND FOLK REMEDIES

• Add a few tablespoons of baking soda to the bath to relieve itching. *(See page 100.)*
• An oatmeal bath will soothe the rash. *(See page 84.)*
• Add a cupful of vinegar to the bath water to restore the balance of the skin. *(See page 102.)*

HERBALISM

• An infusion of chickweed and chamomile can be used to bathe the affected area. *(See page 119.)*
• Balm and heartsease can be drunk 3 times daily to soothe and reduce inflammation.
• For urticaria brought on by anxiety and stress, drink an infusion of valerian twice daily. *(See page 136.)*
• Urtica urens cream will soothe and promote healing.

AROMATHERAPY

• A warm bath with essential oil of chamomile or melissa will soothe the skin and help to prevent stress-related attacks. *(See pages 150 and 163.)*

HOMEOPATHY

• Apis, for burning and swelling, particularly of the lips and eyelids. *(See page 180.)*
• Urtica, for a rash that feels like stinging nettles, and is worse when touched or after it has been scratched. *(See page 217.)*
• Nat. mur., for chronic urticaria exacerbated by stress. *(See page 206.)*
• Rhus tox., for burning, itching, and blisters. *(See page 210.)*
• Sulfur, for relief of red, itchy, puffy skin, which is made worse by heat. *(See page 215.)*
• Arsenicum, for symptoms accompanied by restlessness and anxiety. *(See page 182.)*

FLOWER ESSENCES

• Impatiens is very useful for people whose rashes are associated with feelings of irritability and impatience. Take internally or mix into a neutral cream. *(See page 233.)*

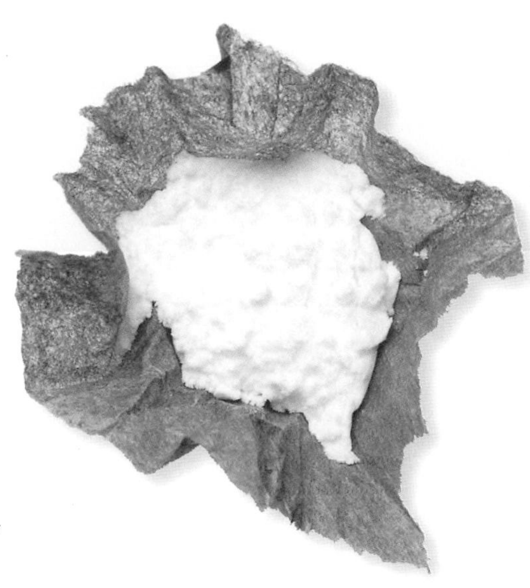

RIGHT *Sprinkle a few tablespoonsful of baking soda into your bathwater to temper the itching.*

Prickly Heat

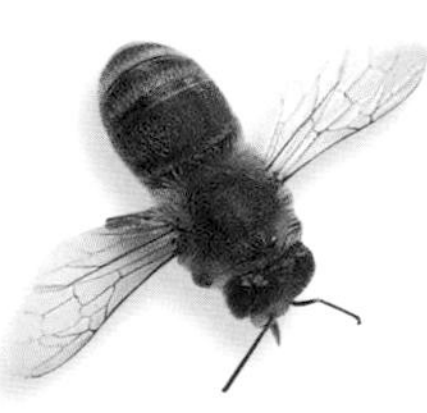

ABOVE *The honey bee is the source of the homeopathic remedy Apis.*

Prickly heat, or heat rash, occurs as a result of sweat duct blockage (probably due to excessive dampness of the skin) in particularly hot and humid weather. It produces a rash of red spots on the face and/or body, which usually disappears within hours of the sufferer moving into the shade, or his or her acclimatization. Occasionally, however, it may develop into patches of eczema. Children, the elderly and the obese are all particularly susceptible.

TREATMENT

HERBALISM • Chickweed infusions can be made into cool compresses and applied to the affected area. Chickweed ointment can be applied as needed.

AROMATHERAPY • Add a few drops of lavender and sandalwood oils to a little calendula oil, and massage into the affected area. *(See pages 146–71.)*

HOMEOPATHY • Apis, taken every 2 hours for up to 10 doses. *(See page 180.)*
• Merc. Sol. can be used as a preventive measure. *(See page 213.)*

FLOWER ESSENCES
• Impatiens is very useful for itching. Take internally or mix into a neutral cream. *(See page 233.)*
• Rescue Remedy, taken internally or applied externally in a cream or wash, helps most skin troubles. *(See page 244.)*

VITAMINS AND MINERALS
• Take plenty of vitamin C, which will help to discourage itching and the rash. *(See page 256.)*

SYMPTOMS

• a constant prickling or itching sensation • tiny blisters may form in severe cases as a result of salt crystals forming in the sweat gland ducts

BELOW *Citrus fruit is a good source of vitamin C, needed to alleviate skin problems.*

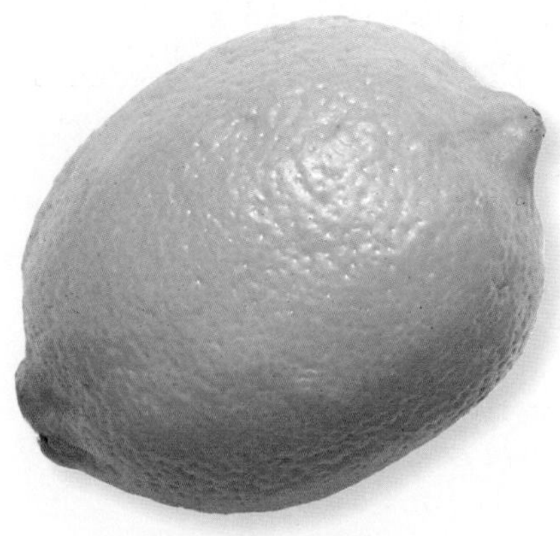

Perspiration

Perspiration is generally stimulated by heat and is the body's way of regulating temperature. Excessive sweating (or hyperhidrosis) is caused by overactive sweat glands. It may be confined to specific areas such as the palms of the hands, armpits, groin and feet, or it may occur all over the body. When perspiration exceeds the bounds of what is considered normal, it may be due to an overactive thyroid gland, the menopause, prolonged fever, or stress or other psychological factors.

SYMPTOMS

• an unpleasant body odor may occur if perspiration comes into contact with bacteria on the skin • in severe cases the skin in affected areas may become damp and damaged

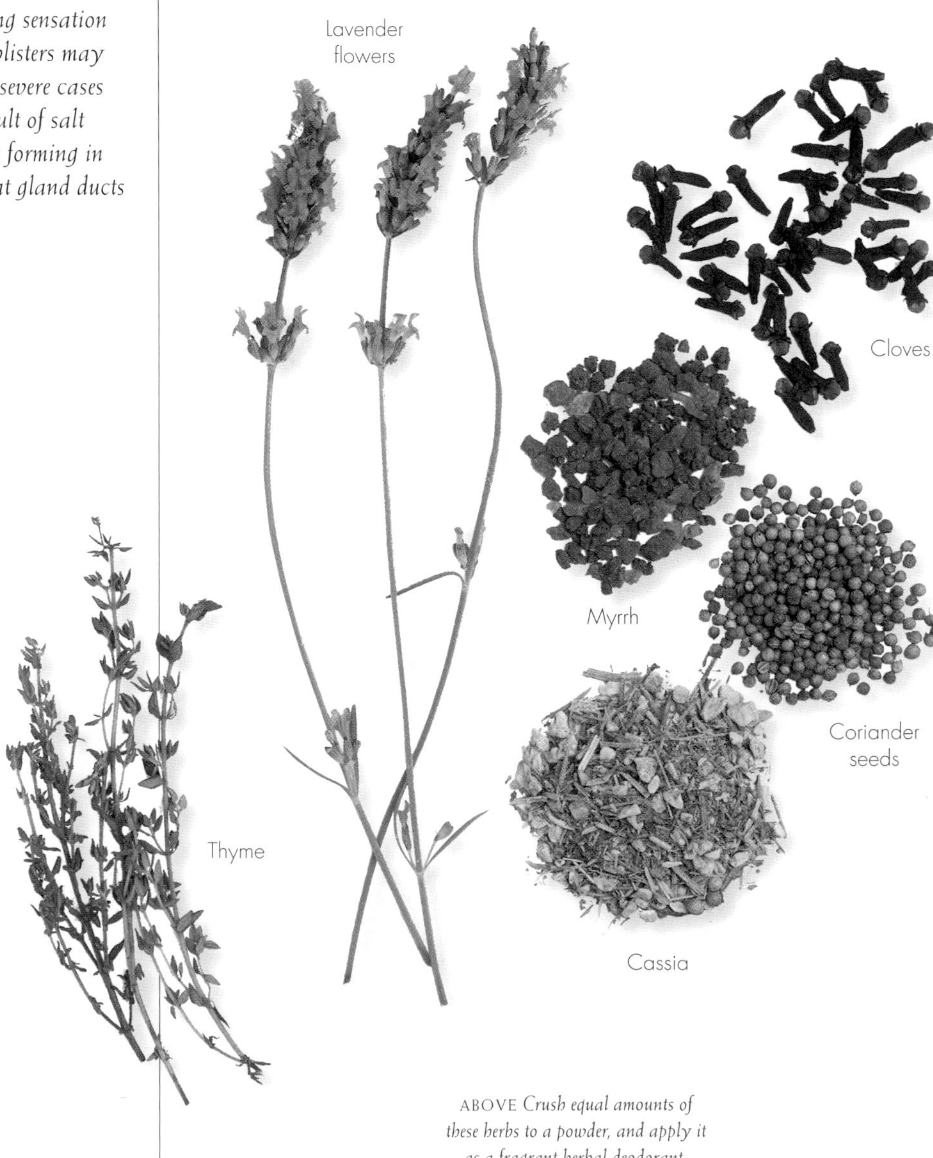

ABOVE *Crush equal amounts of these herbs to a powder, and apply it as a fragrant herbal deodorant.*

TREATMENT

CHINESE HERBALISM
• Excess sweating is thought to be caused by a deficiency of qi or yin. *(See page 49.)*
• For yin deficiency, use gray lily turf root, cork tree bark, and peony. *(See pages 67 and 68.)*
• Try ledebouriella and astragalus for deficient qi. *(See pages 57 and 64.)*

HERBALISM
• Marigold infusion can be drunk to produce a perspiration increase, when necessary. *(See page 117.)*
• A herbal deodorant would include cloves, myrrh, coriander seeds, cassia, lavender flowers, and thyme, in equal amounts and ground into a powder. Use in the bath, or under the arms. This may cause a rash in sensitive people. *(See page 135.)*

AROMATHERAPY
• Cypress oil is astringent and refreshing, and can be massaged into the feet for excess perspiration, or combined with lavender oil in a light massage oil and massaged under the arms. *(See page 156.)*
• Oils with deodorizing properties are bergamot, clary sage, eucalyptus, lavender, neroli, petitgrain, and rosewood. *(See pages 146–71.)*
• Detoxifying oils include fennel, garlic, juniper, and rose. *(See pages 146–71.)*
• Basil, chamomile, juniper, peppermint, and tea tree oils promote sweating, if there is a lack of it. *(See pages 146–71.)*

HOMEOPATHY
Constitutional treatment is most appropriate, but the following may help:
• Lycopodium, for smelly perspiration, worse on feet and under arms. *(See page 203.)*
• Mercurius, for smelly sweat. *(See page 205.)*
• Sulfur, for sweating on the head, with morning diarrhea. *(See page 215.)*
• Calcarea, for sour sweat. The sufferer is likely to be overweight, and feels cold and clammy. *(See page 186.)*
• Silicea, for sweaty, smelly feet in a thin person. *(See page 211.)*
• Aethusa, for insufficient perspiration production.

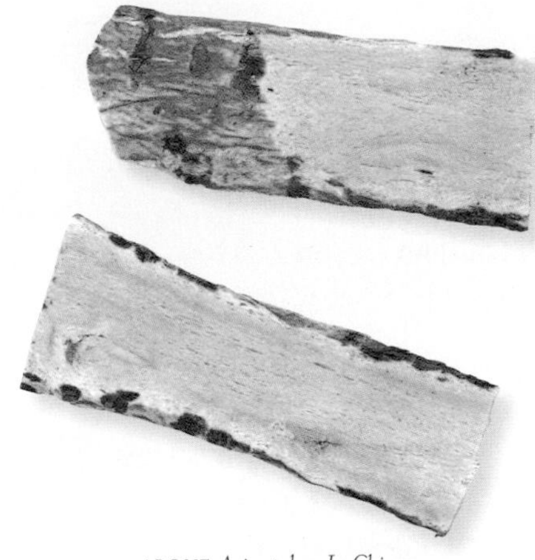

ABOVE *Astragalus. In Chinese medicine, depleted qi causes health problems. Astragalus restores qi.*

RIGHT *To help stop sweaty feet, rub a little cypress oil into the skin.*

Bruising

(See under Heart, Blood, and Circulation, page 354.)

Sunburn

Sunburn occurs on exposure to bright sunlight and is caused by the effects of ultraviolet light. It is most likely to affect people with pale complexions or those who are unused to being in the sun.

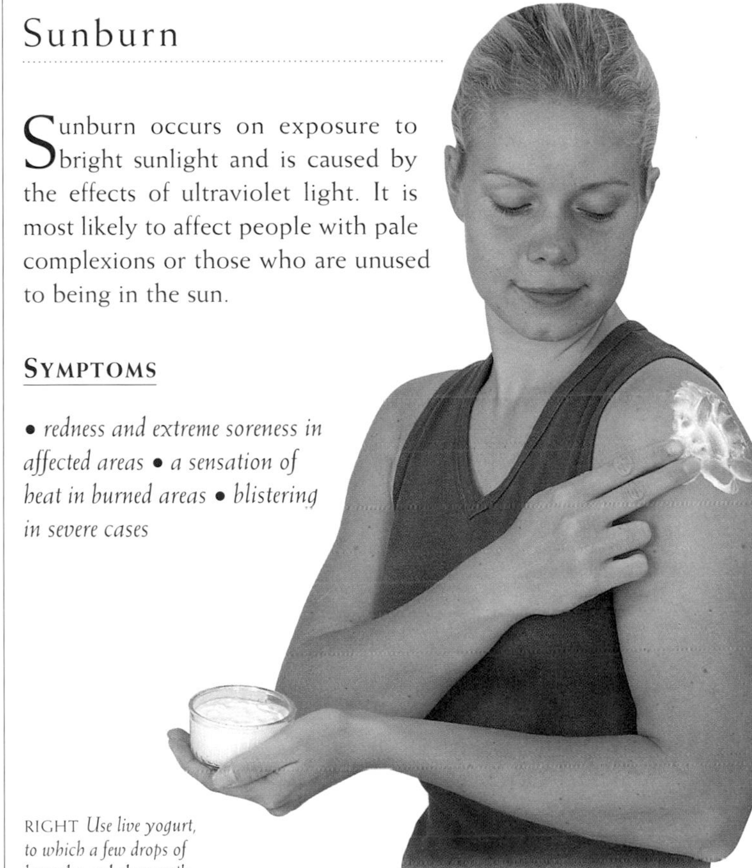

RIGHT *Use live yogurt, to which a few drops of lavender and chamomile oils have been added.*

Symptoms

• *redness and extreme soreness in affected areas* • *a sensation of heat in burned areas* • *blistering in severe cases*

TREATMENT

AYURVEDA
• Aloe vera can be used on burned areas to soothe and to heal. *(See page 27.)*

HERBALISM
• Urtica urens ointment eases the pain and helps to prevent skin damage.

AROMATHERAPY
• Add a few drops of lavender and chamomile oils to a tub of live yogurt, and apply to affected areas to soothe, encourage healing, and reduce inflammation. *(See pages 146–71.)*

HOMEOPATHY
• Merc. Sol. can be used to prevent and treat sunburn. *(See page 213.)*

FLOWER ESSENCES
• Rescue Remedy cream heals damaged tissue and reduces the discomfort. *(See page 244.)*

VITAMINS AND MINERALS
• Rub a little vitamin E oil into the affected area, soon after the burning, to help the healing process and prevent peels and scarring. *(See page 257.)*

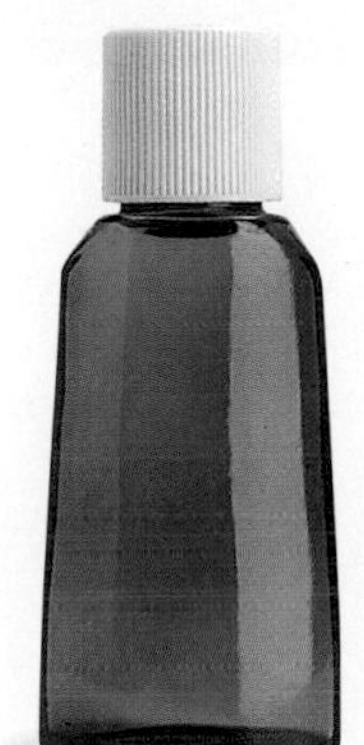

LEFT *Vitamin E oil encourages the sunburned skin to repair itself. Rub it in as an aftersun treatment.*

Warts

A wart is a small, hard growth, usually brown or flesh-colored, on the skin. It may be caused by any one of 30 strains of the human papilloma virus. Warts are highly contagious, but not dangerous, and can occur more frequently when the immune system is compromised.

DATA FILE

- The common wart, verruca vulgaris, may occur anywhere on the body.
- Verruca plana is a round, yellowish, flat-topped wart found mainly on the backs of the hands.
- Verruca filiformis is a long, thin wart found on the eyelids, armpits, and neck.
- The venereal wart, a pink, cauliflower-like growth, is found on the genitals (sexually transmitted).
- The plantar wart (or verruca) is a flat wart on the sole of the foot which may be forced into the thick skin of that area.

TREATMENT

TRADITIONAL HOME AND FOLK REMEDIES

- Rub fresh lemon into the wart daily, and keep moist (with a plaster), paring back any hardened skin. *(See page 87.)*
- Rub fresh garlic into the wart to fight the fungal infection, and eat lots of garlic to boost immunity. *(See page 82.)*
- Mix castor oil and baking powder into a paste, and apply at night with a plaster, leaving it exposed during the day.

HERBALISM

- Squeeze the fresh sap of a dandelion stalk on to the wart every day until it disappears. *(See page 134.)*
- Milkwort can be mashed and applied directly to the wart.

AROMATHERAPY

- Apply a little lemon oil directly to the wart; continue treatment until the wart disappears. *(See page 154.)*
- When the wart disappears, add a few drops of lavender oil to vitamin E oil and apply to the area for a week, to encourage healing and prevent scarring and further infection. *(See page 161.)*
- Overall body massage with rosemary, juniper, or geranium will help to strengthen the immune system. *(See pages 146–71.)*

HOMEOPATHY

- Thuja, for soft, fleshy warts that ooze and bleed. *(See page 216.)*
- Causticum, for warts on the face or fingertips, and painful verrucas. *(See page 189.)*
- Dulcamara, for hard, smooth, fleshy warts on the back of hands. *(See page 213.)*
- Kali mur., for warts growing on the hands.
- Nat. carb., for weeping warts on the toes.
- Antimonium, for horny warts caused by or associated with a callus. *(See page 179.)*

CAUTION

GENITAL WARTS MUST BE TREATED IN AN STD OR GU (GENITOURINARY) CLINIC, AND TREATMENT CAN BE COMPLEMENTED BY HEALING REMEDIES, BUT ONLY UNDER THE CARE OF A REGISTERED PRACTITIONER.

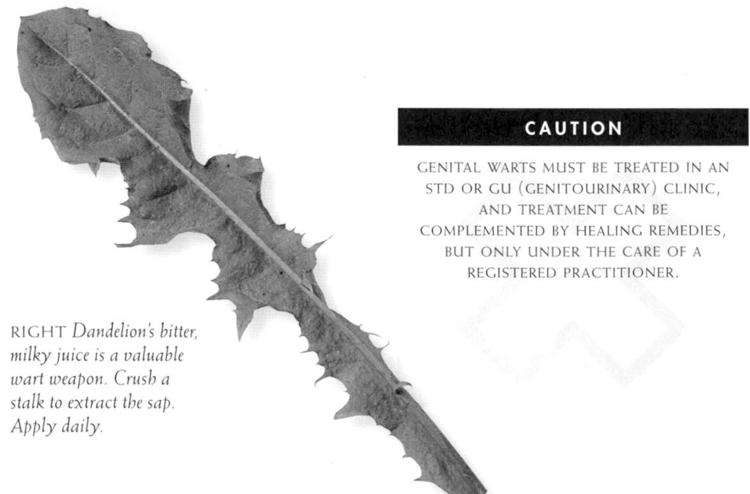

RIGHT *Dandelion's bitter, milky juice is a valuable wart weapon. Crush a stalk to extract the sap. Apply daily.*

Dandruff

Dandruff occurs when the fine cells of the outer layer of skin on the scalp are shed at a faster rate than normal, causing the characteristic flakes of dead skin. This is caused by a disorder of the sebaceous glands. If too little sebum is secreted the hair is dry and dandruff appears as white flakes; if too much sebum is produced the hair is greasy, and the dandruff yellow. The flakes are usually most obvious after brushing or combing the hair, which loosens them. Certain types of seborrheic dermatitis are also responsible for dandruff, which will cause inflammation and itchiness in addition to flaking.

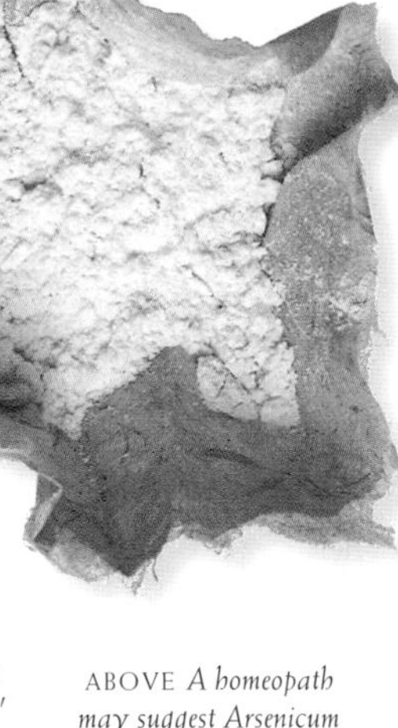

ABOVE *A homeopath may suggest Arsenicum if the scalp is sensitive and feels dry.*

TREATMENT

HERBALISM

- Improve circulation to the scalp. Rosemary is the herb of choice, taken internally as a tea and used as an application. *(See page 127.)*
- For dry hair, rub rosemary-infused oil into the scalp before washing. *(See page 127.)*
- For greasy hair, add rosemary vinegar or a few drops of rosemary essential oil to the rinsing water. *(See page 127.)*
- Take a combination of the herbs burdock, kelp, and heartsease internally to improve the general condition of the scalp. *(See pages115 and 122.)*

AROMATHERAPY

- Rosemary, cedarwood, tea tree, or patchouli can be massaged into the scalp, added to unscented shampoos, and used in the final rinse when washing your hair. *(See pages 146–71.)*
- Dilute lavender oil in a little almond or coconut oil and massage into the scalp to eliminate dandruff. *(See pages 146–71.)*

HOMEOPATHY

Constitutional treatment may be useful, but the following remedies may help:

- Arsenicum, for a dry, sensitive, hot scalp with bare patches of skin. *(See page 182.)*
- Nat. mur., for a white crust around the hairline, and greasy hair. *(See page 206.)*
- Fluoric acid, for flaky scalp and hair loss.
- Graphites, for a moist scalp with smelly crusting. *(See page 196.)*
- Sulfur, for thick dandruff which is itchier at night. *(See page 215.)*
- Sepia, for moist, greasy scalp, which is sensitive around the ears. *(See page 212.)*

VITAMINS AND MINERALS

- Increase your intake of selenium, vitamin E, vitamin C, B-complex vitamins, and zinc. *(See pages 252–57, 264, and 265.)*

Hair Loss

It is normal to shed about 150 hairs a day, but sometimes this number may be increased by various stresses on the body. Hereditary hair loss is known as alopecia. It affects men far more than women and tends to be a feature of aging, starting with a receding at the temples or forehead, which gradually progresses (though rarely ending in total baldness). Other causes of hair loss include severe illness with high fever, pregnancy and childbirth, shock, stress, damage to the skin (from burns, infection, radiation, chemical injury), skin cancer, chemotherapy, excess of vitamin A, hypothyroidism, and syphilis.

LEFT *If you suffer from hair loss try drinking sage tea as it stimulates growth.*

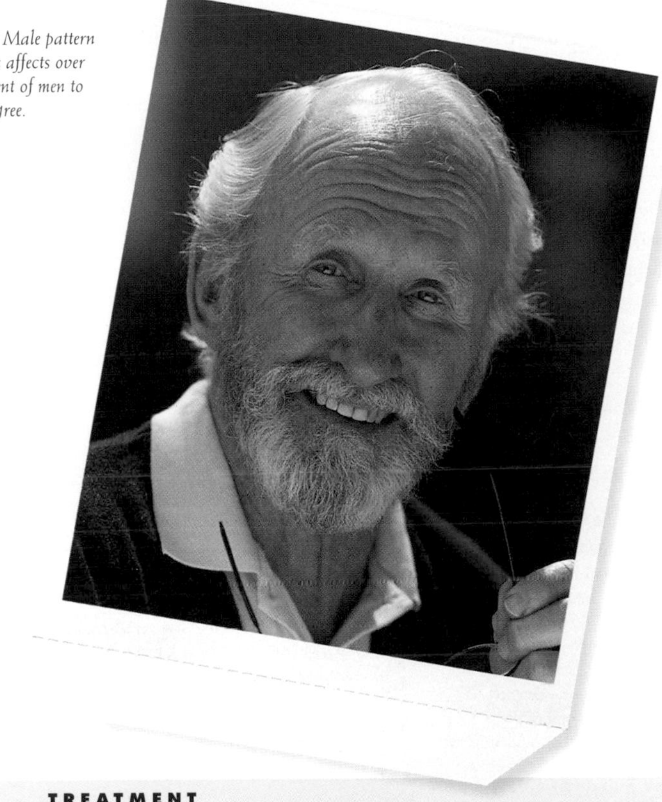

RIGHT *Male pattern baldness affects over 80 percent of men to some degree.*

DATA FILE

- Baldness, or alopecia, is total or partial loss of scalp hair. The condition may be temporary or permanent.
- The most common type of alopecia is pattern baldness, a hereditary trait that is expressed more often in males than in females because it depends on the influence of the male hormone testosterone.
- Pattern baldness in males extends until only a sparse growth of hair remains on the back and sides of the head. Up to 86 percent of men in the U.S. will experience some pattern balding.
- In women, baldness usually extends until only a sparse growth remains across the crown.
- Premature baldness may partly result from an imbalance of sex hormones.
- Sudden temporary hair loss sometimes occurs as a result of typhoid fever, flu, pneumonia, or stress.
- Gradual thinning of the hair may be caused by severe nutritional deficiency, tuberculosis, cancer, and disorders of the thyroid gland or pituitary gland.
- Temporary baldness may also be caused by exposure to nuclear radiation or X-rays, or by the internal use of certain anticancer drugs.

TREATMENT

CHINESE HERBALISM

- Shou Wu Pian nourishes Liver Blood, Kidney qi and jing. It is commonly used in China to keep hair from graying.
- Hair loss is attributed to Deficient Liver and Kidneys, and specific herbs to address this include wolfberry, mulberry, and fleeceflower root. *(See pages 66 and 71.)*

TRADITIONAL HOME AND FOLK REMEDIES

- Sage tea, drunk and applied externally, will stimulate hair growth.
- Nettle tea helps to cleanse the system, and encourages the growth of hair.

HERBALISM

- Improve circulation to the head with daily intake of rosemary tea and shoulder stands. *(See page 127.)*
- Massage the scalp with infused oil of fenugreek or ginger. *(See page 139.)*
- Rinse with nettle vinegar. *(See page 137.)*

AROMATHERAPY

- Lavender, rosemary, sage, cedarwood, patchouli, or ylang ylang can be massaged into the scalp and added to mild unfragranced shampoos. *(See pages 146–71.)*

HOMEOPATHY

- Lycopodium, for hair loss after childbirth. *(See page 203.)*
- Aurum, for hair loss with headaches and boils breaking out on the scalp. *(See page 184.)*
- Phosphoric acid, for hair loss after grief, and with exhaustion.
- Arnica, for hair loss starting after injury. *(See page 182.)*
- Selenium, for painful scalp and loss of body hair along with hair on head.
- Sepia, for hair loss related to the menopause and childbirth. *(See page 212.)*

VITAMINS AND MINERALS

- Increase your intake of vitamin B-complex (high-dosage tablet, twice daily), choline, inositol, calcium, magnesium, vitamins and minerals in a good supplement. *(See pages 252–5, 258, 262, and 270.)*

BELOW *Make sage tea by pouring a cup of boiling water on 1-2 teaspoonsful of leaves.*

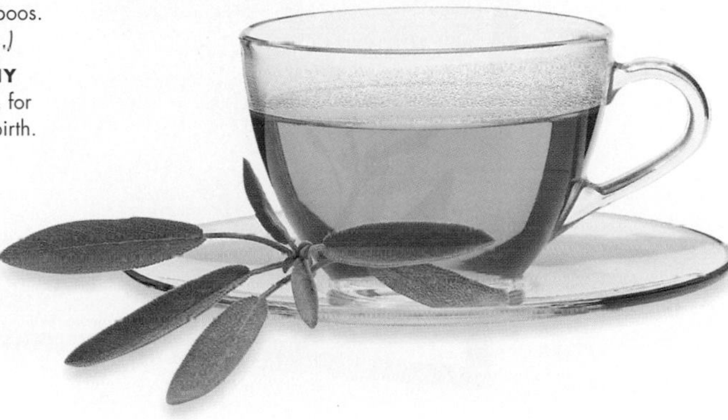

Boils

A boil is a swollen, pus-filled area occurring on the site of an infected hair follicle. The staphylococcus bacterium is usually responsible, but other causes may include eczema, scabies, diabetes, poor personal hygiene, or obesity. A boil begins as a painful red lump, then hardens and forms a yellow head. The most common areas for boils to appear are the back of the neck, the groin, and the armpits. A boil on an eyelash is known as a stye, and where a group of adjacent hair follicles are affected the resultant boil is known as a carbuncle.

Symptoms

• burning, throbbing sensation in and around the affected area • sensitivity to the slightest touch once pus has formed

TREATMENT

TRADITIONAL HOME AND FOLK REMEDIES
- Apply a warm poultice made with figs or honey to the affected area. *(See pages 90 and 101.)*
- Soak a sterile cloth with hot thyme tea and hold it over the boil for a time.
- A hot cabbage leaf poultice, applied to the area, will help to draw out the infection. *(See page 85.)*
- Eat plenty of garlic if you are prone to boils; garlic is cleansing and chronic boils indicate that you may have a high level of toxins in your body. *(See page 82.)*

HERBALISM
- Drink infusions of thyme or red clover 3 times daily during attacks. *(See page 135.)*
- Drink echinacea 2 or 3 times daily to boost the immune system and purify the blood. *(See page 120.)*

AROMATHERAPY
- A warm compress with essential oil of chamomile, lemon, lavender, or thyme will help to bring the boil out. *(See pages 146–71.)*

HOMEOPATHY
- Belladonna, for red, tender, new boils. *(See page 183.)*
- Hep. sulf., for boils that are sensitive and weep easily. This will also bring the boil to a head. *(See page 198.)*
- Gunpowder, for weeping but not painful boils.
- Arsenicum, for burning skin aggravated by heat. *(See page 182.)*

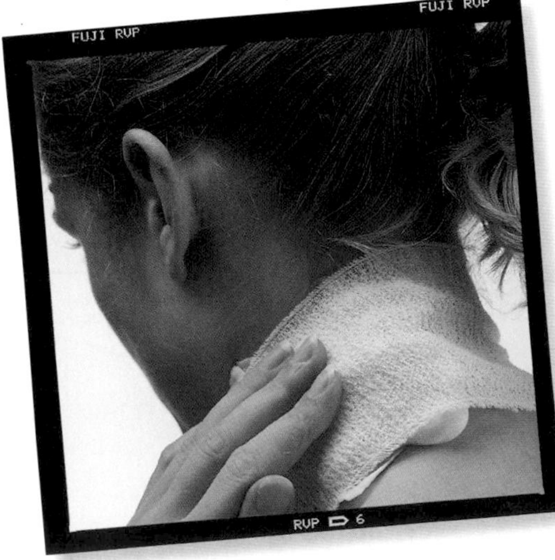

RIGHT *A warm poultice, made with mashed figs, will relieve pain and bring the boil to a head.*

Cold Sores

Cold sores are painful fluid-filled blisters which crust over after bursting. They usually appear on the mouth and around the lips or nose, sometimes in clusters. They are caused by viral infection (herpes simplex). The virus is harbored by most people, most of the time, but is most likely to cause problems when the immune system is compromised, dealing with other viral infections (such as a cold), or when one is run down. Cold sores are highly contagious.

ABOVE *A healthy diet prevents many health problems by keeping the immune system at optimum efficiency.*

CAUTION

COLD SORES ARE INFECTIOUS – WASH HANDS CAREFULLY AFTER APPLYING ANY LOTION, AND USE A PERSONAL TOWEL.

Symptoms

• pain and soreness from the characteristic crusting blister
• cracking and weeping may occur, particularly if sores are in the corners of the mouth

TREATMENT

HERBALISM
- St. John's wort tincture, applied immediately, should prevent development of a sore. *(See page 124.)*
- Once the cold sore is established, myrrh tincture can be applied sparingly to help dry it up.

AROMATHERAPY
- Bergamot, eucalyptus, and tea tree oils will help to treat the blisters, and should be applied at the first sign of a sore. *(See pages 146–71.)*
- Lavender oil will help to heal blisters that erupt. *(See page 161.)*

HOMEOPATHY
Constitutional treatment is best, but the following remedies may help:
- Nat. mur., for deep cracks in the lower lip, dry mouth, and puffy burning cold sores. *(See page 206.)*
- Rhus tox., for mouth and chin sores, and ulcers at the corner of the mouth. *(See page 210.)*
- Sempervivum, for ulcers in the mouth, and bleeding gums; and when the condition is worse at night.
- Capsicum, for cracks at the corners of the mouth, pale lips, a rash on the chin, blisters on the tongue, and bad breath.

VITAMINS AND MINERALS
Cold sores tend to crop up when you feel run down, so it is important that you eat healthily and ensure that you get plenty of the following nutrients, which boost immunity:
- Wholegrain cereals like brown rice and wholewheat bread, fruit, pulses (beans and lentils), a few nuts and seeds for their vital oils.
- A daily multivitamin and multimineral preparation – especially one containing high amounts of the antioxidant nutrients – acts to boost immune activity. *(See page 251.)*
- Vitamin C stimulates immunity and is antiviral as well as being antifungal. *(See page 256.)*
- Acidophilus will encourage the healthy bacteria in your gut, which will help to fight off infections and infestations. *(See page 271.)*
- Zinc stimulates the immune system, and acts as an antiviral and antifungal agent. *(See page 265.)*

Abscess

An abscess is a pocket of pus which may occur in any bacterially infected area of the body. White blood cells are sent by the body's defense system to attack the bacteria in question and they do so by engulfing them, thereby creating the pus-filled swelling. Dental abscesses (usually around the root of a tooth) are particularly common.

Symptoms

- *swelling, pain, and discomfort in the affected area* • *the abscess and surrounding area may feel hot to the touch*
- *fever* • *nausea*
- *sweating*

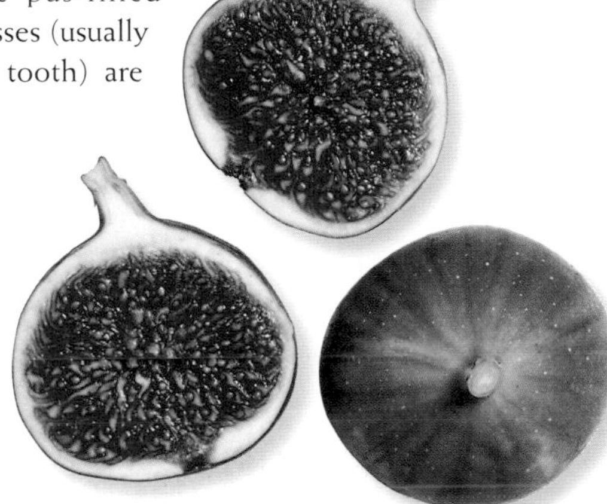

ABOVE and RIGHT *Figs are mentioned in the Bible as a treatment used by Hezekiah.*

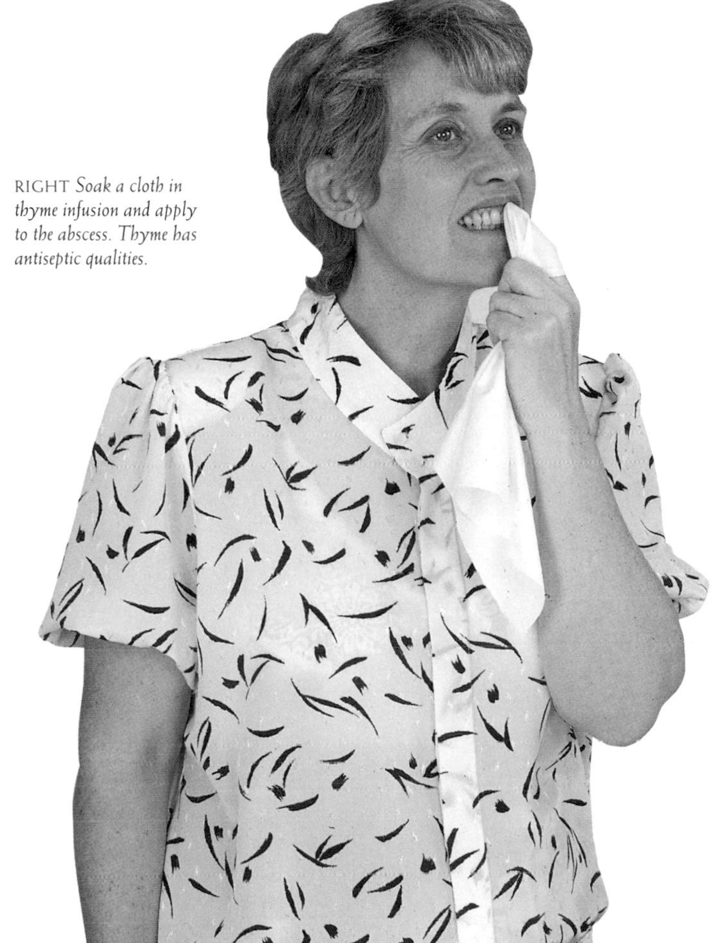

RIGHT *Soak a cloth in thyme infusion and apply to the abscess. Thyme has antiseptic qualities.*

TREATMENT

AYURVEDA
- Kalanchoe may be useful.

CHINESE HERBALISM
- Treatment would address Heat and Fire poison in the Blood.
- Externally, use peony flowers or rhubarb ointment. *(See pages 67 and 73.)*
- Internally, violet, wild chrysanthemum, dandelion, and golden thread are useful. *(See page 61.)*

TRADITIONAL HOME AND FOLK REMEDIES
- Apply a warm fig or honey poultice to the abscess. *(See pages 90 and 101.)*
- Soak a sterile cloth with hot thyme tea and apply.
- A hot poultice, made with cabbage leaves, will help to draw out infection. *(See page 85.)*

HERBALISM
- Drink infusions of thyme or red clover 3 times daily during attacks. *(See page 135.)*
- Drink echinacea 2 or 3 times daily to boost the immune system and purify the blood. *(See page 120.)*

AROMATHERAPY
- A warm compress with essential oil of chamomile, lemon, lavender, or thyme will help to bring the abscess out. *(See pages 146–71.)*

HOMEOPATHY
- Hep. sulf., for an abscess which is tender, causing sharp pain. *(See page 198.)*
- Belladonna, for early stages, where there is tenderness and throbbing pain. *(See page 183.)*
- Silicea, for a slow-forming abscess, with swelling, which does not appear to come to a head. *(See page 211.)*
- Mercurius, for the early stages, if perspiration is smelly and you are irritable. *(See page 205.)*

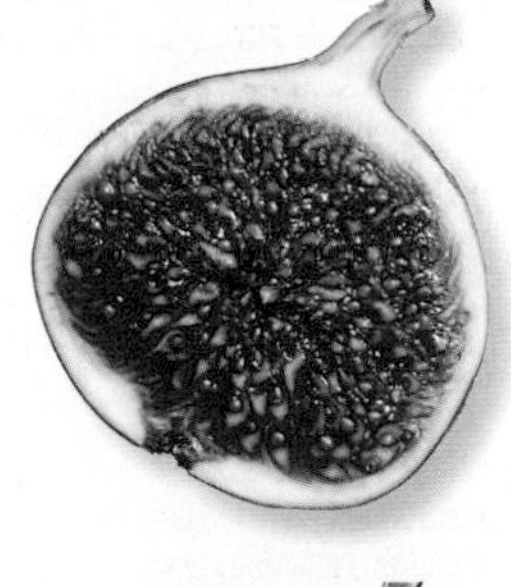

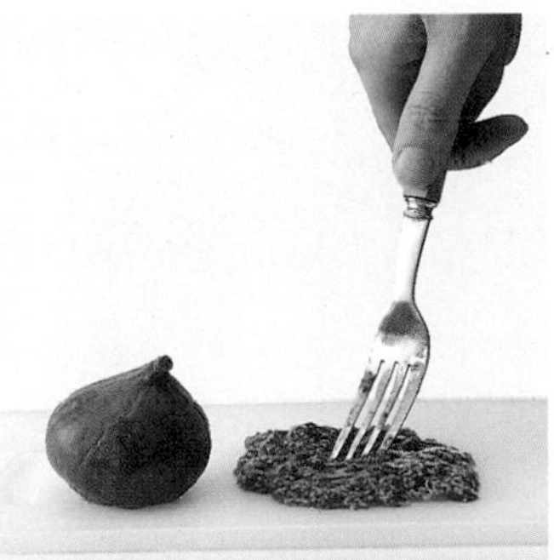

To make a warm fig poultice, you can use either lightly roasted fresh figs, or dried figs. Split the fig and mash up the soft, pulpy interior. This can be warmed by adding a little boiling water.

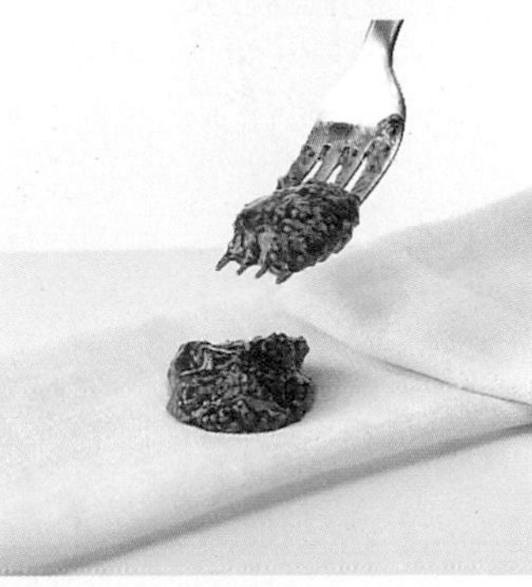

Place the mixture on a clean piece of cloth. Use either linen, gauze or cotton. The whole compress can then be warmed by placing on a hot water bottle. (This is also useful to warm it up again after it cools.) Apply to the skin

Acne

Acne is a skin disorder most common among adolescents. It is caused by the hormonal changes at puberty, which lead to an increase in the activity of the sebaceous (oil-producing) glands. Sebaceous glands secrete through pores and hair follicles – which are most abundant on the face and scalp – a fatty lubricant known as sebum. Acne occurs when the pores become clogged with sebum. Blackheads – external plugs formed of sebum and dead cells – may be invaded by bacteria, which cause pus-filled inflammations, or pimples. The overlying skin may become stretched to the point of rupture, resulting in lesions and, in prolonged severe cases, eventual scarring. Sweating can aggravate acne, as do some oral contraceptives, lack of sunlight, poor skin hygiene, face creams, cosmetics, and exercise.

Symptoms

• red, inflamed spots • spots may become inflamed and infected, in which case they are extremely painful

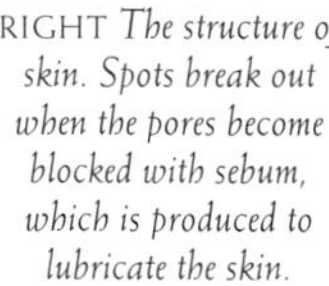

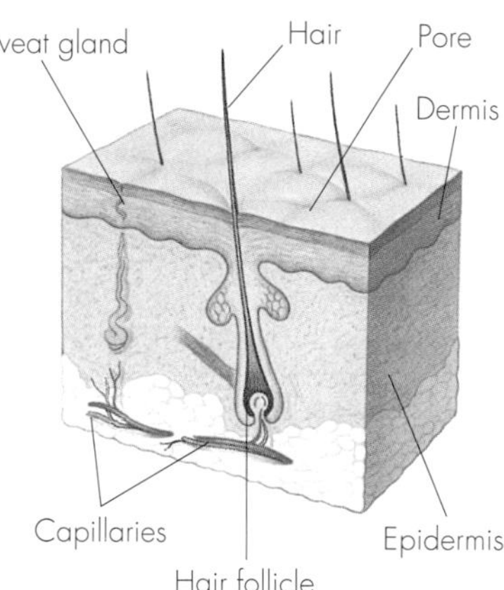

RIGHT *The structure of skin. Spots break out when the pores become blocked with sebum, which is produced to lubricate the skin.*

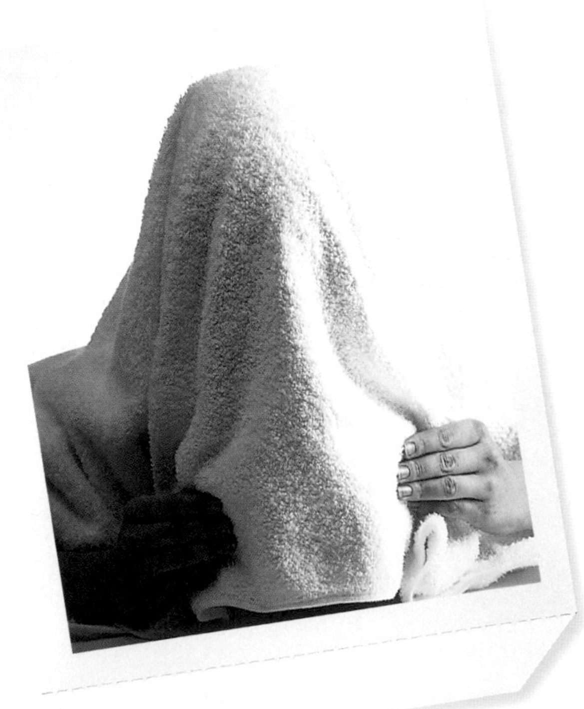

LEFT *Try steaming the face with a herbal infusion. Put chickweed, elderflower, and marigold in a bowl, and pour on boiling water.*

DATA FILE

• Males are more often affected than females, and the condition is not confined to adolescence.

• The exact cause of acne is not known, but it is believed to be related both to genetic predisposition and to the increased hormonal activity that occurs during puberty.

• In a reaction comparable to allergy, certain foods may increase irritation in susceptible persons.

• Acne affects more than 60 percent of the population of the U.S.

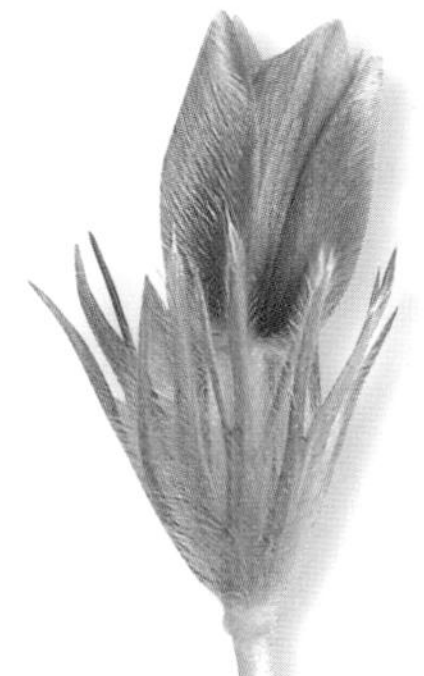

RIGHT *Pulsatilla is often prescribed by homeopaths for complaints starting in adolescence.*

TREATMENT

CHINESE HERBALISM

• Cai Feng Zhen Zhu an Chuang Wan/Margarite acne pills. This is an excellent remedy for acne. It contains Pearl.

• Treatments to clear excess Heat in the Blood and Stomach include chrysanthemum, dandelion, and honeysuckle, with cucumber and watermelon juice applied externally. *(See page 65.)*

HERBALISM

• A facial steam with chickweed, elderflower, and marigold may be useful for soothing and drawing out infection. *(See pages 117 and 130.)*

• Take echinacea, burdock root, cleavers, or yellow dock, sipped 3 times daily as a decoction, to cleanse the system and fight infection. *(See pages 115, 120, and 128.)*

• Massage comfrey ointment into any old spots to reduce scarring. *(See page 132.)*

HOMEOPATHY

Treatment should be constitutional, but the following remedies may help:

• Silicea, when there is scarring. *(See page 211.)*

• Ant. tart., for pus-filled pimples. *(See page 179.)*

• Sulfur, for chronic acne, with rough hard skin, and proneness to diarrhea. *(See page 215.)*

• Kali brom., for itchy spots, accompanied by unpleasant dreams.

• Hep. sulf., for large spots resembling boils. *(See page 198.)*

• Pulsatilla, when the spots are aggravated by rich, fatty foods; and if the sufferer dislikes stuffy rooms and is often tearful. *(See page 209.)*

FLOWER ESSENCES

• Gorse is useful for people who have given up hope of finding a cure. *(See page 240.)*

VITAMINS AND MINERALS

• Try a multivitamin and mineral supplement which is low in iodine. *(See page 261.)*

• Increase intake of vitamin E, vitamin A (as retinol, see Vitamin A, caution, page 252), zinc. *(See pages 252, 257, and 265.)*

• Eliminate processed foods.

Impetigo

Impetigo is a highly contagious skin infection caused by bacteria such as streptococci and staphylococci . Infection may follow a break in the skin or occur secondarily to dermatitis, insect bites, and fungus infections. The skin reddens and small, fluid-filled blisters appear on the surface. The blisters tend to burst, leaving moist, weeping areas underneath. The released fluid dries to leave honey-colored crusts on the skin. The infected area may spread at the edges, or another patch may develop nearby. In severe cases there may be swelling of the lymph nodes in the face or neck, accompanied by fever. Itching is common and scratching can spread the infection. It usually first appears around the mouth and nose, but can spread rapidly if other parts of the body are touched after touching a blister. It can be passed on to others by direct contact or by sharing towels. Impetigo occurs most commonly (although not exclusively) in children, particularly in hot, humid climates. Severe attacks are often attributed to poor standards of personal hygiene.

Symptoms

• *reddening of affected areas* • *small fluid-filled blisters which often burst and weep, then dry out to form a yellow crust* • *itching* • *very rarely a kidney inflammation or blood poisoning may develop*

TREATMENT

TRADITIONAL HOME AND FOLK REMEDIES
• Dab the area with cider vinegar, as often as possible throughout the day. *(See page 102.)*
• Clean the area with fresh cabbage juice 2 or 3 times daily. *(See page 85.)*
• Honey is a strong antibiotic and can be applied directly to the sores, and taken internally to boost the immune system. *(See page 101.)*

HERBALISM
• Heartsease can be taken internally or used as a wash to treat impetigo; it is both softening and drying, and can soothe the skin.

AROMATHERAPY
• A few drops of tea tree oil, applied neat to the affected area, will encourage healing and prevent the infection from spreading; it also has immuno-stimulant properties to help your body fight infection. *(See page 162.)*

HOMEOPATHY
• Antimonium, for blisters cropping up around the nostrils and mouth. *(See page 179.)*
• Arsenicum, for blisters and feelings of exhaustion and restlessness. *(See page 182.)*
• Croton, for blisters around the scrotum.

VITAMINS AND MINERALS
• Vitamin A is necessary for healthy skin. *(See page 252.)*
• Ensure that you get enough of the B-complex vitamins in your diet. *(See pages 252–5.)*
• Vitamin C will help the body to fight infection. *(See page 256.)*

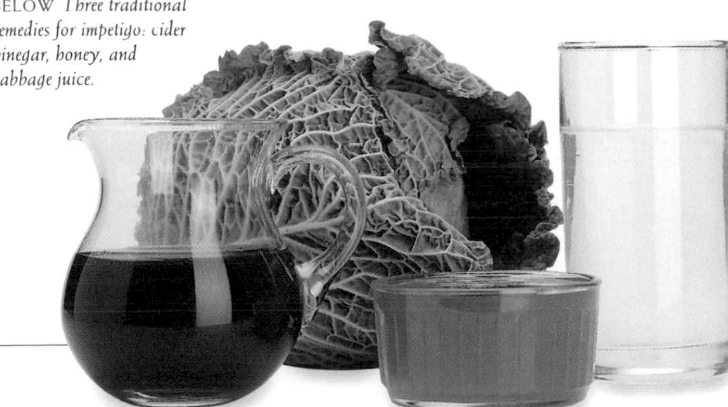

BELOW *Three traditional remedies for impetigo: cider vinegar, honey, and cabbage juice.*

Nail Problems

The nail forms a shield at the end of the fingers and toes. The nail itself is colorless and transparent, but appears pink because of the blood vessels lying under the skin. The end of the nail is white because of air beneath it. The crescent or moon, also called the lunule, located near the root of the nail, appears white because it does not firmly adhere to the connective tissue. The nail plate consists of dead, cornified cells. Nails grow from between 1/500–1/20in. (0.05–1.2mm.) per week. If the nail is lost, it takes approximately seven months to grow out fully.

Fingernails grow faster than toenails, and nails of individual fingers of the same hand grow at different rates. Growth increases during the summer, and is slower in cold climates, and sometimes during illness.

Nails are vulnerable areas and subject to several possible problems *(see Data File)*.

ABOVE *A rosemary oil blend can be massaged into the base of the nails to help improve circulation.*

DATA FILE

• Onycholysis – detachment of the nail from its bed. This may occur as a result of a collection of blood (a hematoma) forming underneath it, most commonly caused by injury. Other possible causes of onycholysis include psoriasis, thyrotoxicosis, and fungus infection. Complete shedding of the nail can lead to a cessation of nail growth.

• Paronychia – an infection of the soft tissue around the nail. It is usually the result of repeated minor injury, causing pain, swelling, and inflammation. Pus may sometimes appear at the nail edge.

• Horizontal ridges – these usually indicate an infection in the skin around the nail.

• Nail thickening – a feature of psoriasis and fungus infection.

• Nail-biting – an anxiety- or boredom-related habit which, in severe cases, may cause damage to the cuticles and even infection.

TREATMENT

CHINESE HERBALISM
• Brittle nails are attributed to the kidneys, and watermelon and nori (seaweed) would be advised.

AROMATHERAPY
• Add a little rosemary oil to a light carrier oil and massage into the base of the finger and toenails to improve circulation to the area. *(See page 168.)*
• Use tea tree oil on the affected area for bacterial or fungal infections. *(See page 162.)*

HOMEOPATHY
• Antimonium, for brittle, horny nails. *(See page 179.)*
• Thuja, for brittle nails with a red base. Also for ingrown toenails. *(See page 216.)*
• Graphites, for thick, deformed, brittle, painful, or crumbling nails. *(See page 196.)*
• Silicea, for deformed nails with white spots. *(See page 211.)*
• Belladonna, for the early stages of infection (yeast or bacterial). *(See page 183.)*

VITAMINS AND MINERALS
• Take zinc, vitamin C, and vitamin B-complex for fungal infections. *(See pages 252–56 and 265.)*
• White spots are often a sign of a deficiency of zinc or vitamin A. *(See pages 252 and 265.)*
• Deformed nails can be caused by deficiency of vitamins A, B-complex, and C, calcium, magnesium, zinc, and essential fatty acids. *(See pages 252–56, 258, 262, and 265.)*
• Iron deficiency can lead to nail problems; increase your iron intake. *(See page 260.)*
• Fungal infections can be improved by eating live yogurt each day, or taking acidophilus supplements. *(See page 271.)*

Edema

Edema is swelling or puffiness of tissues due to fluid retention. It is an obvious physical symptom of a number of disorders including kidney disease, heart failure, and cirrhosis of the liver. Edema may also occur as a result of injury (where the injured blood vessels are made more water-permeable) and changes in hormonal levels (before menstruation, during pregnancy, or through the use of oral contraceptives).

ABOVE *Evening primrose oil contains gamma-linoleic acid, which is a highly unsaturated fatty acid.*

Symptoms

- *edema may be accompanied by weight gain and breathing difficulties*

TREATMENT

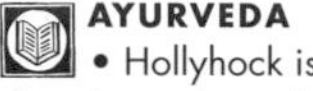

AYURVEDA
- Hollyhock is a diuretic, and may help ease the condition.

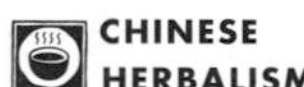

CHINESE HERBALISM
- The problem is thought to be due to excess water and Kidney Deficiency; useful herbs for treatment include ginseng, water plantain, poria, cinnamon twigs, and ephedra. *(See pages 59, 67, and 71.)*
- Wu Ling San pills tonify the Spleen Yang to move water and resolve edema, particularly edema of the lower abdomen.
- Jin Gui Shen Qi Wan tonifies the Kidney Yang to resolve edema, particularly of the lower legs.
- In practice, the latter two may be applicable in any particular case.

TRADITIONAL HOME AND FOLK REMEDIES
- Evening primrose oil, taken in capsule form daily, can help to prevent water retention.
- Swelling can be relieved by eating plenty of fresh apples. *(See page 94.)*
- Celery is also a good diuretic, and acts on the kidneys to encourage their action. *(See page 83.)*
- Eat fresh grapes to prevent bloating.

HERBALISM
- Yarrow, dandelion, and uva ursi are natural diuretics, and they can be drunk three times daily, as required. *(See page 112.)*

AROMATHERAPY
- Essential oils of rosemary, lavender, and geranium will help to reduce bloating and discourage depression. *(See pages 146–71.)*
- Rub a little cedarwood, fennel, rosemary, or sandalwood oils, blended in a light carrier oil, into the areas most affected, or in a whole body massage to have an overall diuretic effect. *(See pages 146–71.)*

HOMEOPATHY
- Arsenicum, when the feet and ankles are swollen, and you feel restless and chilly. *(See page 182.)*
- Apis, for swelling accompanying inflammation, with stinging pains that become worse in heat. *(See page 180.)*
- Nat. mur., for swelling in hot weather or in hot rooms. *(See page 206.)*

LEFT *Grapes have a cleansing action, and will prevent bloating. They are also rich in vitamin C.*

Scabies

Scabies is an infestation of the skin by the mite *Sarcoptes scabiei*, or itch mite. The mites burrow in the skin to lay eggs, particularly in the sides of the fingers, the elbows, groin, buttocks, nipples, and penis. The newly hatched mites reach adulthood within 14 days, and they, in turn, mate on the skin, thus perpetuating the infestation. Scabies is extremely infectious and can be transmitted by direct or indirect contact.

Symptoms

- *intense itching, particularly at night* • *a rash, which may become infected as a result of scratching*

CAUTION

DO NOT GIVE SULFUR TO ANYONE SUFFERING FROM ECZEMA WITHOUT THE SUPERVISION OF A HOMEOPATH.

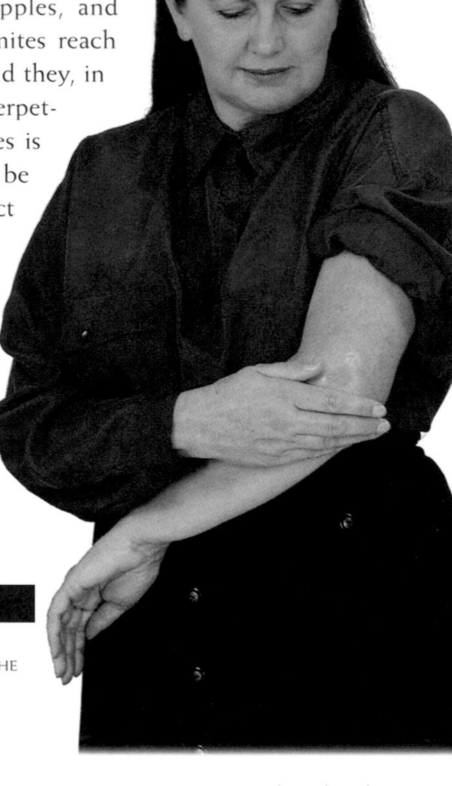

ABOVE *Rub neat lavender oil into the infestation as an initial measure, to help control the itching.*

TREATMENT

AROMATHERAPY
- Use tea tree or lavender oil on the sores, to heal and prevent itching and inflammation. *(See page 162.)*
- Rub the whole body with neat lavender oil, and then make a solution of lavender, aspic, and juniper in 4 teaspoons of vodka, and use that daily until symptoms improve. *(See page 161.)*

HOMEOPATHY
- Try Sulfur, given every 10 hours for 3 or 4 days, for the infected or anyone who has been in contact with someone infected. *(See page 215.)*
- Psorinum, derived from the scabies mite, may be useful.

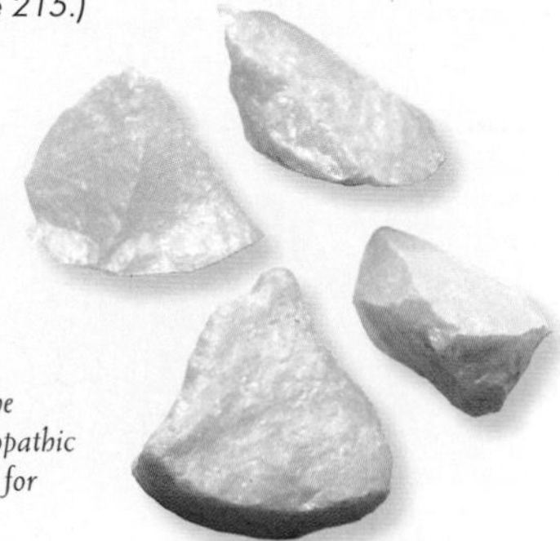

RIGHT *Sulfur is the source for the homeopathic remedy Sulfur, used for skin eruptions.*

Cellulite

Cellulite, believed to be accumulations of fat under the skin, is recognizable by its characteristic orange peel look. The uneven appearance results from the thickened fat cells, fluids, and toxins. It is far more prevalent among women than men, and is thought to have some links with female hormones. Possible triggers are poor circulation, alcohol, refined sugars, and caffeine, which contribute to the build-up of toxins in the body. Cellulite is not generally recognized as a medical condition by many doctors. Persistent, unsightly fat is often a deposit for toxins, either environmental or dietary. Exercise, skin brushing, massage, and eating as many organic and as few processed foods as possible may help.

Symptoms

• areas of skin with a dimpled orange peel appearance which may be slightly tender • these patches occur predominantly on the buttocks, hips, thighs, and upper arms

CAUTION

DO NOT USE JUNIPER BERRIES IN HERBAL PREPARATIONS IF YOU HAVE DIABETES, FOR THEY LOWER THE BLOOD SUGAR. DO NOT EAT FRESH PARSLEY IN PREGNANCY.

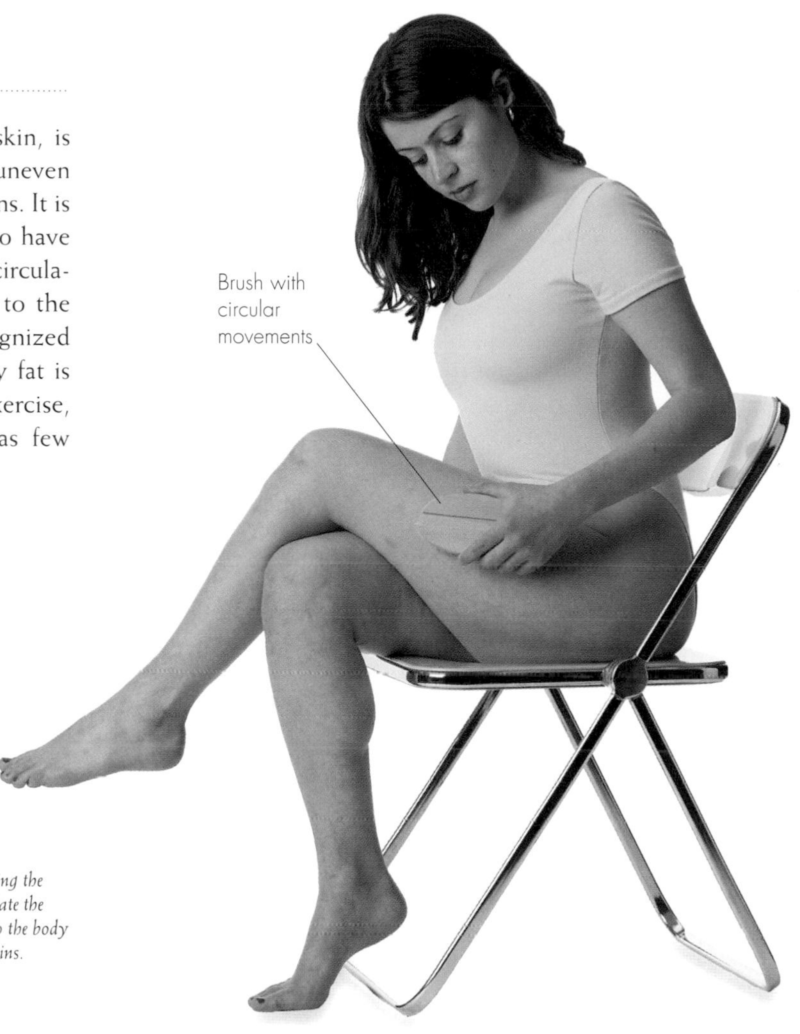

RIGHT *Brushing the skin will stimulate the system and help the body to flush out toxins.*

TREATMENT

Parsley is a diuretic; it is also high in vitamin C
Fresh ginger stimulates body processes such as circulation
Juniper's volatile oil helps cleanse the system

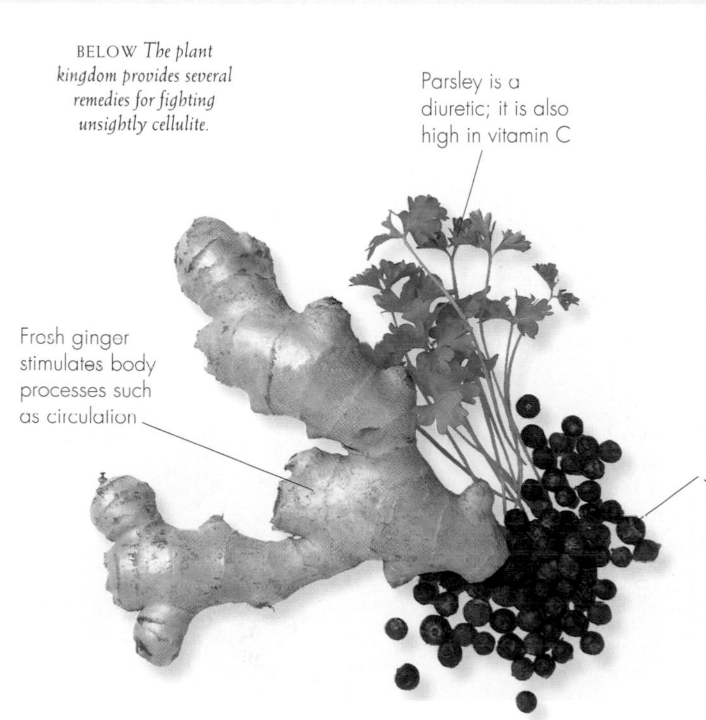

BELOW *The plant kingdom provides several remedies for fighting unsightly cellulite.*

TRADITIONAL HOME AND FOLK REMEDIES

• Eat fresh parsley, which is a good detoxificant and diuretic.

HERBALISM

• Massage with juniper-infused oil and take a cleansing tea with herbs such as marigold. *(See page 117.)*

• Fresh ginger improves circulation in the body; drink an infusion, or chew fresh ginger daily to help reduce the condition. *(See page 139.)*

• Juniper berries are cleansing and detoxifying, and chewing them can help prevent and treat cellulite.

AROMATHERAPY

• A blend of geranium and rosemary or grapefruit, juniper or cypress used in massage and skin lotion, or add to the bath and use a loofa to stimulate the tissues. *(See pages 146–71.)*

• Rose oil soothes tissues, and affects the liver function, to encourage cleansing. It also strengthen the veins, which helps circulation. Add a little to the bath, or massage some into the area. *(See page 168.)*

VITAMINS AND MINERALS

• Avoid cigarettes, caffeine, alcohol, and other toxins, which are believed to build up in the body, and drink plenty of fresh water to flush the system.

Corns and Calluses

A callus is a hardened and thickened area of skin occurring as a result of constant friction. The skin cells respond to the friction by reproducing, which results in the characteristic hardening of skin. Calluses generally appear on the fingers and toes, knees, palms of the hands, and soles of the feet. When a callus on a toe joint becomes painful, it is known as a corn. The pain is caused by pressure on nerve endings. Soft corns can appear between the toes. Manual laborers are prone to calluses, which can be permanent, while ill-fitting shoes and high heels can be responsible for calluses on the feet or corns.

LEFT *Garlic was a traditional antiseptic treatment for dispersing hard swellings.*

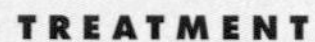

TREATMENT

AYURVEDA
• Place your feet in a basin with 4 tablespoons of mustard seeds and some boiling water to soothe. *(See page 30.)*

TRADITIONAL HOME AND FOLK REMEDIES
• Corns can be softened and treated by painting them with fresh lemon juice or vinegar. *(See page 87.)*
• Apply compresses of fresh garlic to the area. *(See page 82.)*

AROMATHERAPY
• Tea tree is a good oil for skin problems, and has mild analgesic and anti-inflammatory properties, which will help to ease the discomfort of corns and calluses. *(See page 162.)*
• Pare the thickening skin away, and apply an emollient cream with rose oil. *(See page 168.)*

HOMEOPATHY
• Antimonium is the most effective remedy. *(See page 179.)*

VITAMINS AND MINERALS
• Increased intake of vitamins A and E can help to encourage the health of the skin. *(See pages 252 and 257.)*

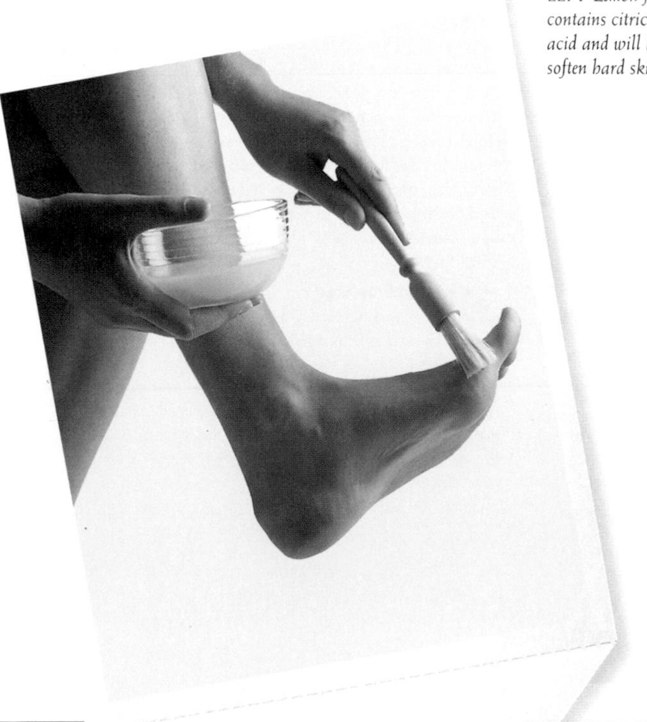

LEFT *Lemon juice contains citric acid and will help soften hard skin.*

Athlete's Foot

Athlete's foot (or tinea pedis) is a fungal infection which attacks the warm, moist areas between the toes, most commonly between the fourth and fifth toes. It is highly infectious, spreading through close physical contact, notoriously in the changing facilities at public swimming baths. Once acquired, athlete's foot is very persistent. It usually affects people with particularly sweaty feet, and those whose personal hygiene is inadequate.

SYMPTOMS

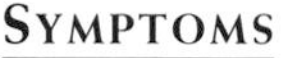

- *discomfort and itching in the affected area*
- *painful cracks in the skin* • *peeling skin* • *blisters*
- *dry and scaly or damp and blistered skin*
- *unpleasant odor*
- *in severe cases the toenails may crumble*

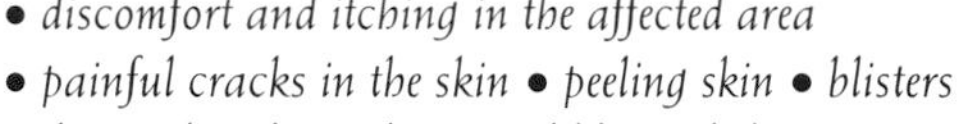

RIGHT *Live yogurt is antifungal, and will help soothe itchy skin. Use it every day.*

TREATMENT

HERBALISM
• Echinacea, marigold, and myrrh tinctures, which are antifungal, can be dabbed on the affected area as often as required. *(See pages 117 and 120)*

AROMATHERAPY
• A foot bath with tea tree oil, eucalyptus, patchouli, myrrh, and/or lavender is effective as all the oils are soothing and antifungal. Also add to unscented skin lotion. *(See pages 146–71.)*

HOMEOPATHY
• Treatment would be constitutional to boost the immune system, but Silicea might be useful. *(See page 211.)*

VITAMINS AND MINERALS
• Take extra vitamin C and zinc, to boost immune activity and help fight infection. *(See pages 256 and 265.)*
• Apply a little live yogurt to the area daily, for its antifungal properties.
• Take acidophilus tablets daily to help restore natural bacteria in the body which help to fight fungal infections. *(See page 271.)*

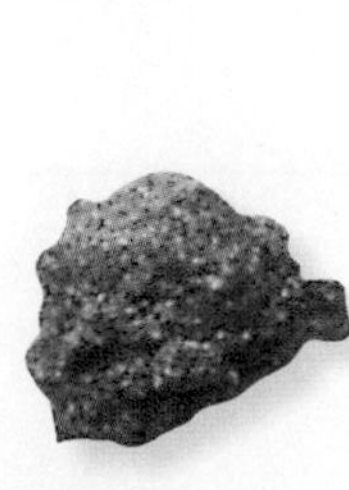

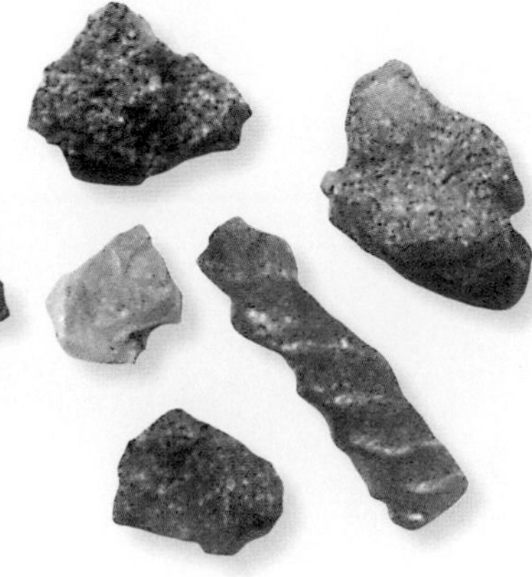

RIGHT *Myrrh essential oil is extracted from resin produced by the trunk of a tree,* Commiphora myrrh. *It is used to make a soothing and antifungal foot bath.*

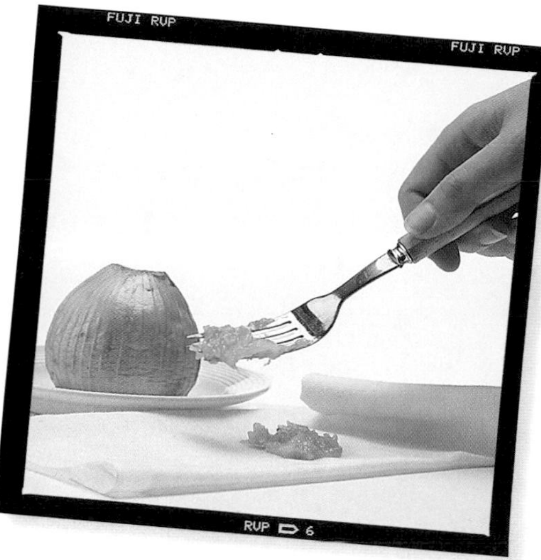

LEFT *Mash a roasted onion and make into a poultice. It will help chilblains to heal.*

Chilblains

A chilblain is a circular, raised, red swelling appearing on the fingers or toes during cold weather. It is caused by the narrowing of small arteries in the cold, which restricts the flow of blood. This leads to tissue damage in the area concerned from shortage of oxygen and glucose fuel, and bacteria may also accumulate there.

Symptoms

- *pain and itching in the area of skin affected* • *swelling and redness*

TREATMENT

CHINESE HERBALISM

- Treatment would be aimed at Deficient Yang qi, and useful herbs include cinnamon twigs, red sage, angelica, dried ginger, and aconite root. *(See pages 56 and 59.)*

TRADITIONAL HOME AND FOLK REMEDIES

- Ginger, taken internally as a tea, or chewed (the root), or externally (in the bath) will warm the body, and both prevent and treat chilblains.
- A roasted onion poultice can be applied to chilblains to draw the heat to the surface and encourage healing. *(See page 82.)*
- A poultice of mustard can be applied to chilblains to warm the area. *(See page 98.)*

HERBALISM

- Nettle tea, and creams and ointments can be applied to the affected area. Drink an infusion of nettle. *(See page 137.)*
- Improve the general circulation of the body by taking rosemary tea with a pinch of cayenne. *(See pages 118 and 127.)*
- Rub a hot oil made with cayenne, pepper or mustard over the chilblain. Do not apply this if the skin is broken; use marigold ointment instead. *(See pages 117 and 118.)*
- When chilblains have caused the skin to break, apply calendula ointment to promote healing. *(See page 117.)*

AROMATHERAPY

- Lemon, lavender, chamomile, cypress, peppermint, or black pepper essential oil can be used in massage, in a bath or foot bath, or dabbed on the affected area. *(See pages 146–71.)*

HOMEOPATHY

- Agaricus, for chilblains that burn and itch and are not relieved by cold compresses.
- Petroleum, for burning, itching chilblains worsened by damp.
- Calcarea, when the chilblains are worse in cold weather, and the patient feels chilly and prone to head sweats. *(See page 186.)*
- Pulsatilla, for chilblains that are most painful when the limbs hang down, and which are worsened by warmth. *(See page 209.)*

VITAMINS AND MINERALS

- Eat plenty of garlic, and brewer's yeast, which will encourage the healthy functioning of the circulatory system.
- Increase your intake of oily fish.
- Vitamins C and E will encourage the healthy functioning of the circulatory system. *(See pages 256 and 257.)*
- Vitamin E oil, applied to burst chilblains, will help prevent scarring and encourage healing. *(See page 257.)*

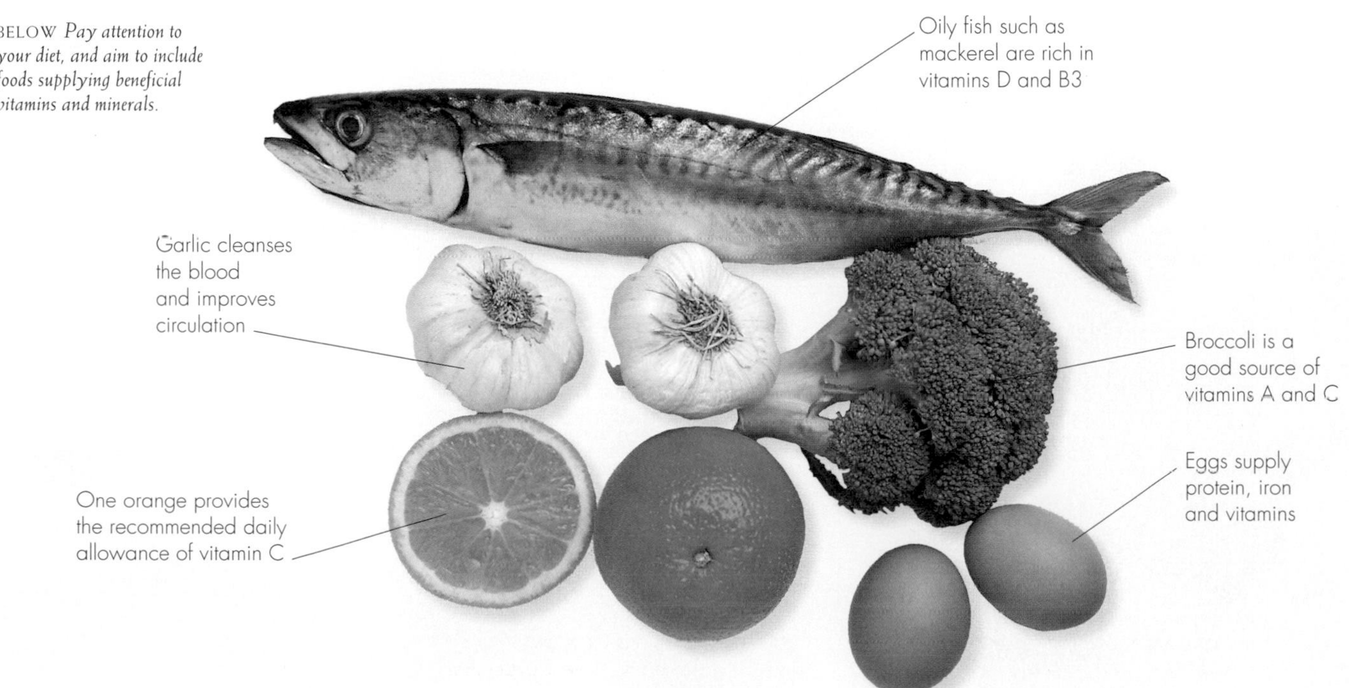

BELOW *Pay attention to your diet, and aim to include foods supplying beneficial vitamins and minerals.*

EYE PROBLEMS

Glaucoma

Glaucoma results from the pressure of fluid in the eyeball becoming too high. This causes compression and obstruction of the blood vessels which feed the optic nerve, resulting in optic nerve fiber damage and visual disturbances. Untreated, glaucoma leads to blindness, but is usually only found if looked for, say through routine checks. It tends to run in families, and its incidence increases with age.

SYMPTOMS

• acute glaucoma: – painful, red eye, hard and tender to touch, possibly with dilated pupil – misting of vision, then severe visual impairment – nausea and/or vomiting – possibly abdominal pain • a warning sign of acute glaucoma may be a sub-acute attack, usually at night. There will be: – visual disturbances such as seeing concentric rings around lights – fogginess of vision – dull aching pain in the eye • chronic simple glaucoma: – slow but progressive loss of peripheral vision which can go unnoticed until the damage is irreversible – loss of central vision follows

TREATMENT

HOMEOPATHY
• Belladonna is the prime remedy, and it can be taken every 15 minutes, for up to 10 or 12 doses, as soon as you experience symptoms. This is suitable for chronic simple glaucoma only. *(See page 183.)*

FLOWER ESSENCES
• When symptoms begin, take Rescue Remedy or Emergency Essence, which will calm you and help you to deal with the pain. *(See page 244.)*

VITAMINS AND MINERALS
• Avoid excessive quantities of protein in your diet, which can exacerbate or contribute to glaucoma.
• Ensure you have an adequate intake of vitamins A, B1, B12, C, and the minerals chromium and zinc, which can contribute to the health of the eyes. *(See pages 252, 255, 256, 259, and 265.)*

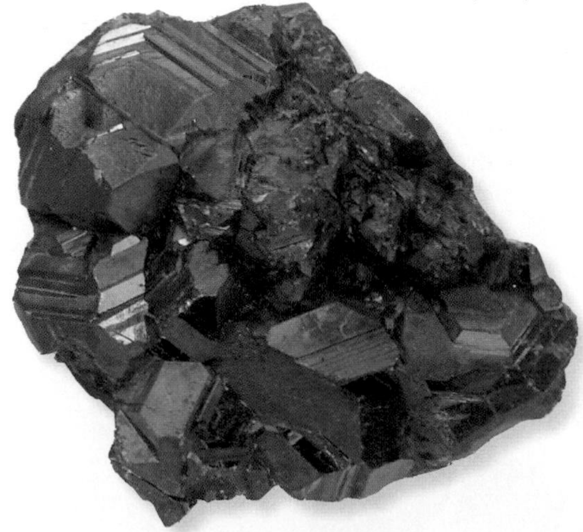

ABOVE *Vital for the protection of cell membranes, zinc can help maintain healthy eyes.*

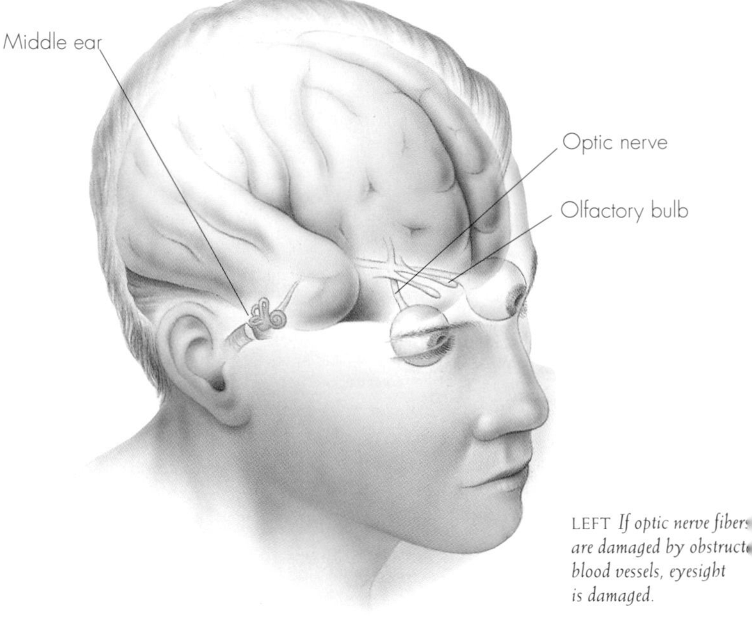

LEFT *If optic nerve fibers are damaged by obstructed blood vessels, eyesight is damaged.*

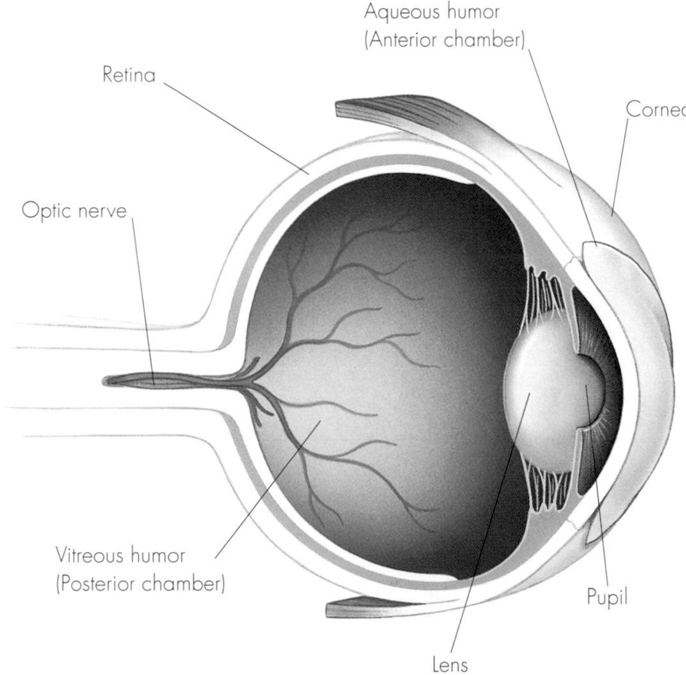

ABOVE *The eyeball is filled with fluid: if its pressure becomes too high, loss of vision ensues.*

CAUTION

SYMPTOMS OF ACUTE OR SUB-ACUTE GLAUCOMA REQUIRE URGENT MEDICAL ATTENTION.

Cataract

A cataract is an opacification of the edges of the lens of the eye which has spread inward to reach the part of the lens that is directly behind the pupil. It is caused by a coagulation of the proteins of the lens. Cataracts are often hereditary or a part of aging, but may also be a feature of Down's syndrome, diabetes, nutritional deficiencies, severe skin problems, or long-term use of steroids. Radiation or injury to the eye can also cause cataracts, and they may be present at birth as a result of German measles during pregnancy.

Symptoms

• loss of image clarity and blurring, with progressively less and less perception of detail; a person with a fully formed cataract may only be able to distinguish the presence of light and the direction from which it is coming • a change in the perception of colors • scattering of light rays caused by the opacity of the lens, which can make night driving difficult or even dangerous

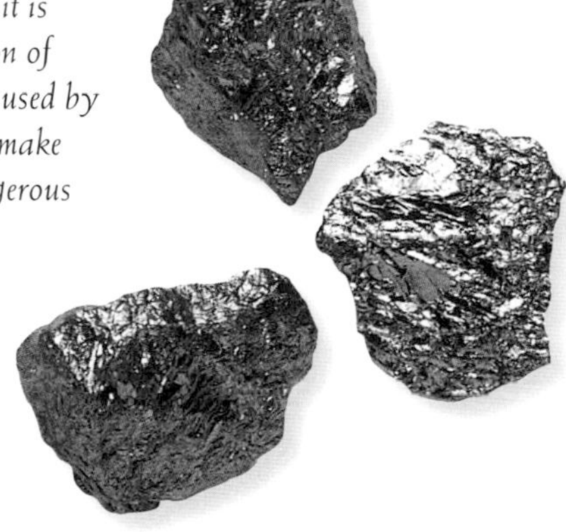

RIGHT *Silicea is prepared from silicon, found in quartz, flint, and sandstone.*

TREATMENT

CHINESE HERBALISM
• Treatment would address weak Liver and Kidneys resulting from Deficient Blood. Herbal remedies might include wolfberry, chrysanthemum flowers, dendronbrum, rumania.

HOMEOPATHY
See a homeopath for constitutional treatment, or if the following remedies fail to work after about two months. Specific remedies, which can be taken 3 times daily for up to a week, and then twice daily thereafter include:
• Silicea, if your cataract has begun to affect your sight. *(See page 211.)*
• Phosphorus, for a misting sensation. *(See page 208.)*
• Calcarea, when circular lines are evident on the lens. *(See page 186.)*

VITAMINS AND MINERALS
• Increase your intake of antioxidants, including vitamins A, C, and E, and also selenium, which prevent the growth of cataracts in the eyes. *(See pages 252, 256, 257, and 264.)*
• Bioflavonoids will also help in prevention and treatment, and these can be taken separately or in conjunction with vitamin C. *(See pages 256 and 272.)*

Black Eye

A "black eye" (known medically as a periorbital hematoma) is the result of blood being released from veins in the eyelids and surrounding area into the tissues around the eye. This produces the characteristic blackish-blue bruising. It is usually caused by a blow to the eye. The bruising can last from a few days to a month, and will go through several color changes, usually ending in pale yellow before fading completely.

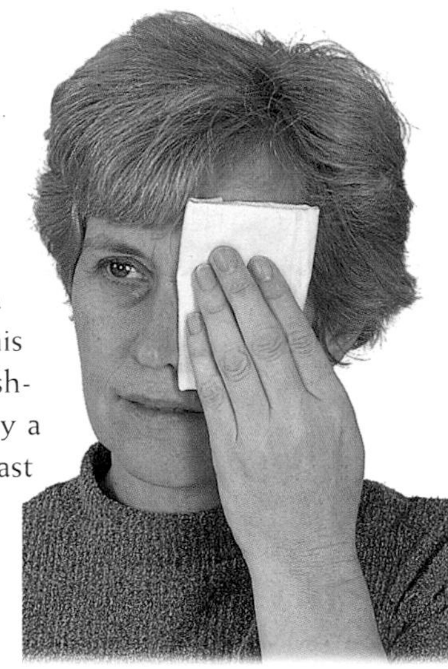

ABOVE *For a black eye, infuse lavender leaves and wrap in a handkerchief.*

Symptoms

• soreness in and around the eye • pain on pressure • in severe cases there could be swelling, which may make it difficult to open the eye

TREATMENT

HERBALISM
• Make an infusion of fresh lavender leaves, and wrap it in a fine handkerchief. Place it on the bruised area when the leaves have cooled.

TRADITIONAL HOME AND FOLK REMEDIES
• Bruise caraway seeds, and heat them with hot, soft bread. Cool slightly and apply to the bruised area.
• A cool witch hazel compress can be applied to the area to encourage healing. *(See page 91.)*
• Place a cold compress on the area, which will reduce swelling and allow fluid to circulate, which will facilitate healing.

AROMATHERAPY
• A few drops of calendula, lavender, and marjoram oil can be placed on a cool cloth and applied to the bruise. Avoid the eyelids and the corner of the eye. *(See pages 146–71.)*

HOMEOPATHY
• Arnica should be taken as soon as possible after the injury, and continued until the bruising disappears. Follow this with Ledum, which will disperse the swelling. *(See page 182.)*
• Aconite is useful in the initial stages, following the blow or trauma to the area. *(See page 178.)*

FLOWER ESSENCES
• Use Rescue Remedy or Emergency Essence cream and lightly dab over the affected area to help the healing process. *(See page 244.)*
• Rescue Remedy or Emergency Essence can be taken internally after the trauma to help you cope with pain and encourage healing. *(See page 244.)*

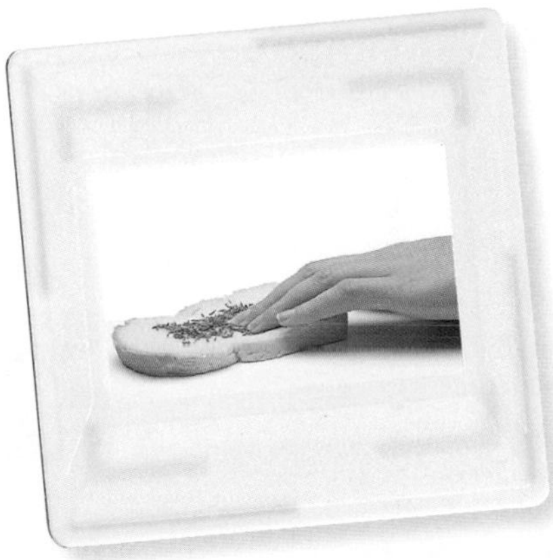

LEFT *Bruise caraway seeds in a pestle and mortar, and spread on soft bread. Heat, and apply to the area.*

Conjunctivitis

Conjunctivitis is an inflammation of the conjunctiva (the mucous membrane that covers the outer layer of the eyeball and lines the eyelids). It is generally caused by either viral or bacterial infection, or by an allergic reaction to substances such as pollen, cosmetics, and solutions used for contact lenses. Either one or both eyes may be affected. Viral conjunctivitis is a common ailment which sometimes occurs in epidemic proportions, spreading rapidly.

ABOVE *Drink sage infusion to invigorate the immune system.*

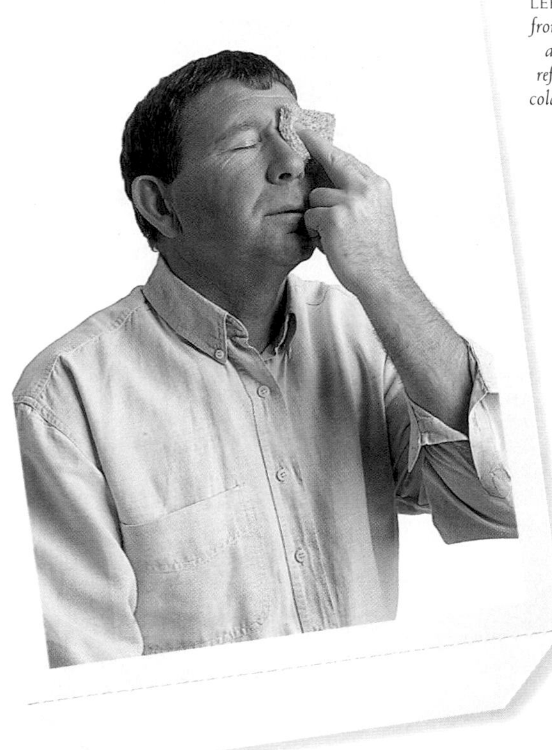

LEFT *Cut the crusts from a slice of bread and put it in the refrigerator. When cold, hold to the eye.*

SYMPTOMS

• redness and soreness with irritation, dryness, and grittiness of the eyes • possibly slightly blurred vision • bacterial conjunctivitis produces a yellow discharge which hardens during sleep, causing stickiness in and around the eye • viral conjunctivitis produces only minimal discharge • swollen and puffy eyelids in allergic conjunctivitis, but no discharge

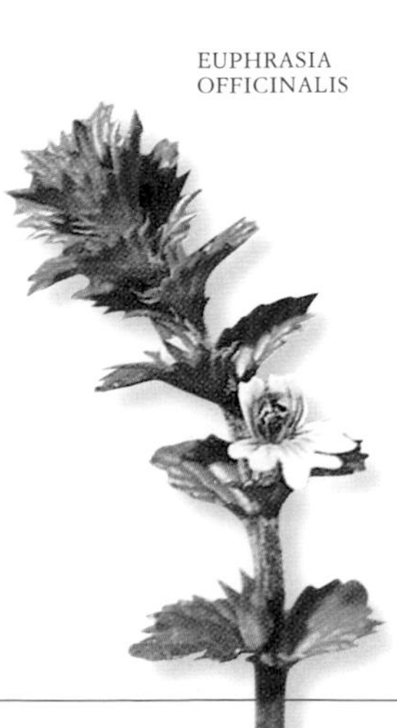

EUPHRASIA OFFICINALIS

TREATMENT

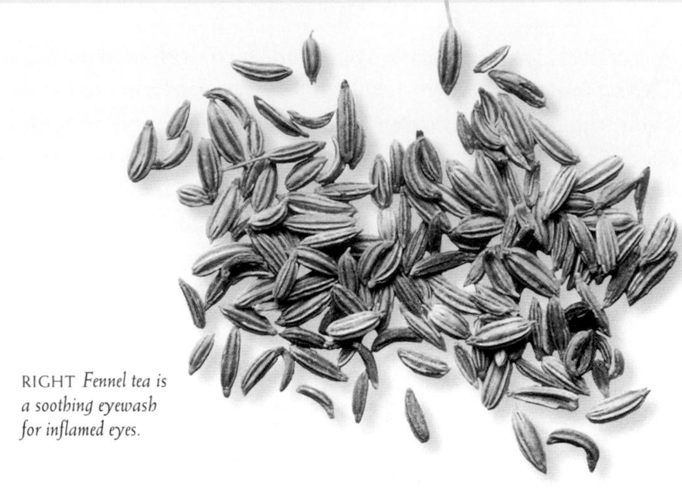

RIGHT *Fennel tea is a soothing eyewash for inflamed eyes.*

AYURVEDA
• Treatment would consist of panchakarma treatment (detoxification), and nasya, together with inhalations and an eyewash. Treatment would be specific to your needs. *(See page 20.)*

CHINESE HERBALISM
• The source of the problem is believed to be Wind Heat in the Liver meridians, and herbal treatment might include bamboo leaves, violets, and chrysanthemum flowers. Boil these together, strain, and use the cool water to bathe the eyes.

TRADITIONAL HOME AND FOLK REMEDIES
• Apply cold bread to closed eyes to reduce the inflammation of conjunctivitis, and soothe itching. *(See page 101.)*
• Boil fennel seeds to make an eyewash for conjunctivitis and sore, inflamed eyes.
• Honey water can be used to cleanse the eye; it acts to destroy any infection, soothe, and encourage healing. *(See page 101.)*

HERBALISM
• Infusions of the following herbs can be taken internally to ease the condition: echinacea (which boosts the immune system and acts as a natural antibiotic), eyebright, golden seal, sage. *(See pages 120 and 129.)*
• Infusions of chamomile, elderflower, eyebright, and golden seal can be applied externally. A tincture of some of these herbs can also be used to make an eyewash. *(See pages 119 and 130.)*

AROMATHERAPY
• Make a warm compress with a few drops of lavender, chamomile, or rose oil, and apply to the affected area to encourage healing and draw out infection. *(See pages 146–71.)*

HOMEOPATHY
• Euphrasia is suitable for burning, itchy eyes. *(See page 194.)*
• One or two drops of Euphrasia tincture can also be used to bathe the eyes. *(See page 194.)*
• Pulsatilla can be used when there is mucus collecting in the corner of the eyes. *(See page 209.)*
• Hep. sulf. will be useful to draw out infection. *(See page 198.)*

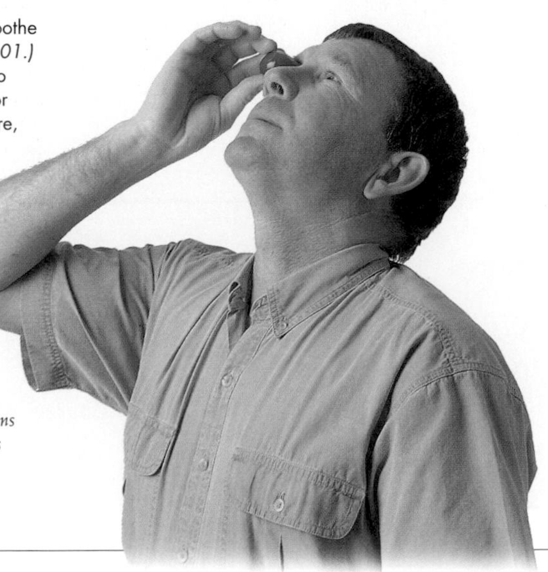

RIGHT *Herbal infusions make good eyewashes for curing soreness.*

Stye

A stye is an abscess occurring around the root of an eyelash, usually caused by staphylococcal bacteria. A collection of pus at the base of the eyelash produces the characteristic small, yellow head. Styes usually last for around seven days, but the infection may spread to adjacent follicles. They tend to occur when general resistance is low.

SYMPTOMS

• *redness, soreness, and swelling* • *pain and sometimes irritation*

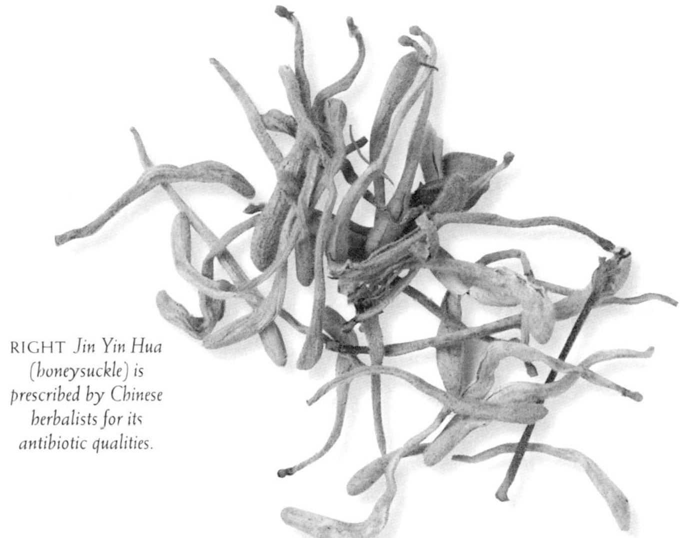

RIGHT *Jin Yin Hua (honeysuckle) is prescribed by Chinese herbalists for its antibiotic qualities.*

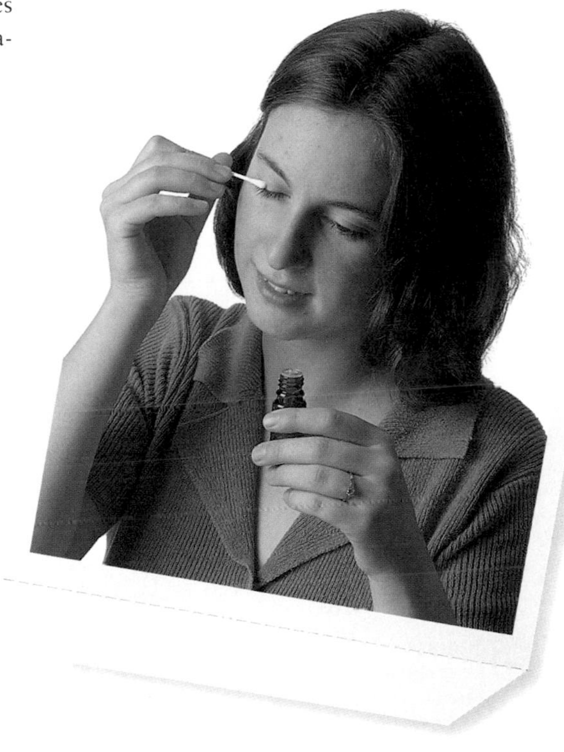

LEFT *Dab a stye with tea tree oil to utilize its bactericidal properties.*

TREATMENT

CHINESE HERBALISM
• Anti-inflammatory herbs, and herbs to detoxify and boost the immune system will be appropriate, including the preparation Jin Yin Hua, which acts as an antibiotic to help fight the bacterial infection. *(See page 65.)*

TRADITIONAL HOME AND FOLK REMEDIES
• A warm bread poultice applied directly to the stye will help bring out the infection. *(See page 101.)*

HERBALISM
• Echinacea and poke root will boost the immune system, which is particularly useful if you suffer from recurrent styes. *(See page 120.)*
• Chamomile or eyebright can help to reduce swelling. *(See page 119.)*
• Marigold tincture can be applied directly to the stye, and taken internally to boost the immune system. *(See page 117.)*

AROMATHERAPY
• A drop of lavender or tea tree oil, on a cotton swab, can be dabbed at the base of the stye. Take care not to let it enter your eyes. *(See pages 146–71.)*

HOMEOPATHY
Recurrent styes should be treated constitutionally, and your homeopath will take steps to improve your overall immune response.
• Pulsatilla, in the first instance. *(See page 209.)*
• If this does not work, try Staphisagria, every hour, for up to 10 doses.

CAUTION

RECURRENT EPISODES OF STYES MAY BE AN INDICATION OF DIABETES AND SHOULD THEREFORE BE INVESTIGATED.

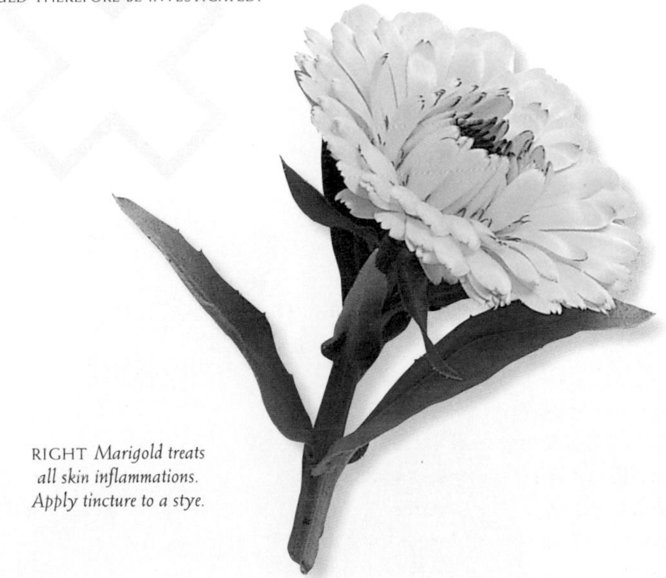

RIGHT *Marigold treats all skin inflammations. Apply tincture to a stye.*

Eyestrain

Eyestrain is used to describe any discomfort or distress related to the eyes or seeing. It is not, however, a medical term. The body's response to visual difficulty is to contract the muscles around the eye, and it is this that may cause the sensation of strain. Prolonged and constant use of a VDU system, intense periods of reading, wearing incorrectly prescribed glasses, and working in bad light can all lead to eyestrain, but these things do not necessarily damage the eyes as is popularly believed.

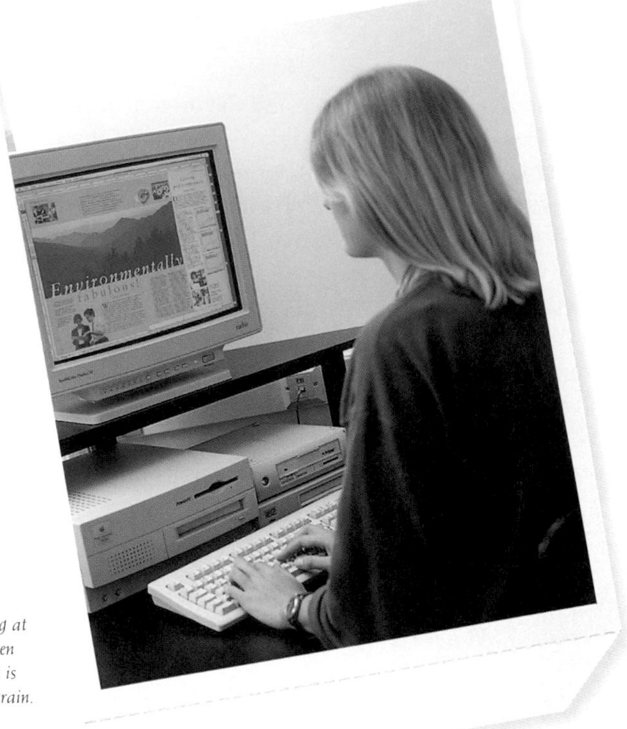

RIGHT *Staring at a computer screen for long periods is a cause of eyestrain.*

Symptoms

• feeling of tightness around the eyes • focusing difficulties • recurrent headaches, particularly across the forehead and behind the eyes

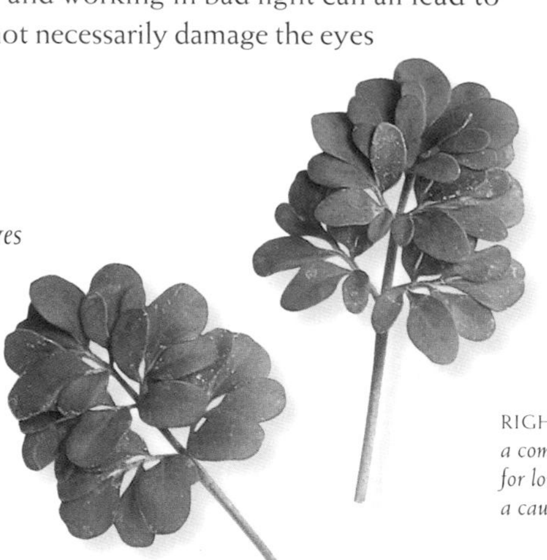

RIGHT *Rue, itself an antispasmodic, is the source of Ruta, a homeopathic remedy sometimes prescribed for eyestrain.*

TREATMENT

TRADITIONAL FOLK AND HOME REMEDIES

• A slice of cucumber over tired, strained eyes is invigorating and soothing. *(See page 89.)*

• Drink fresh lemon juice, which is restorative. *(See page 87.)*

• Roast an apple and apply the pulp to the eye area to relieve inflamed or tired eyes. *(See page 94.)*

• The ancient Greeks used fresh white cabbage juice, mixed with a small amount of honey, to relieve sore or inflamed eyes. *(See page 85.)*

CHINESE HERBALISM

• Chinese practitioners believe that eye problems may be due to exhausted Blood, and the following herbs may be useful: wolfberry, mulberry, chrysanthemum flowers, and cassia seed. *(See page 66.)*

HERBALISM

• Cool compresses of chickweed, eyebright, or marigold should be placed over the eyes and left for 10–15 minutes. *(See page 117.)*

AROMATHERAPY

• A few drops of fennel oil, on a cool compress laid over the eye area, will soothe puffy, inflamed eyes. *(See page 159.)*

• Add 1 drop of lemon or rose aromatherapy oil to 2 tablespoons of carrier oil, and massage into the temples and the bony areas around the eyes (avoid the immediate eye area). *(See pages 146–71.)*

HOMEOPATHY

The following remedies can be taken up to 4 times per day for a week. If the symptoms persist, see your homeopath.

• Ruta, when eyes feel strained after reading for long periods; also good for a burning sensation. *(See page 210.)*

• Arnica, for tired eyes resulting from long periods of driving and looking into the distance. *(See page 182.)*

• Nat. mur., when eyes are painful on looking up, down, or sideways. *(See page 206.)*

VITAMINS AND MINERALS

• Vitamin A and vitamin B12 are useful if you suffer from periodic or chronic eyestrain. *(See pages 252 and 255.)*

RIGHT *Massage the bony areas around the eyes with an aromatherapy oil blend.*

BELOW *Natrum mur. is a tissue salt and works on the body's cells.*

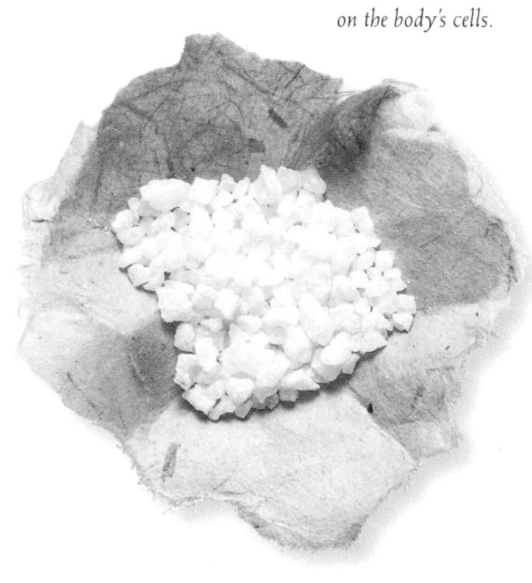

Squint

A squint (or strabismus) is a condition in which only one eye focuses on an object of interest. In a divergent squint the other eye looks outward, while in a convergent squint it looks inward. A squint in children may be caused by congenital hypermetropia (long-sightedness), or physical defects in the cornea, lens, retina, nerves, and muscles of the eye. Acquired in adulthood, a squint is usually indicative of an underlying disease elsewhere in the body (possibly encephalitis, meningitis, septicemia, syphilis, or various brain disorders).

LEFT *Gelsemium remedy, first made in 1862 from the false jasmine plant, may help a squint.*

Symptoms

- *in addition to the characteristic squint appearance adults may also experience double vision*

CAUTION

IF YOU BEGIN TO EXPERIENCE DOUBLE VISION, SEE YOUR PHYSICIAN.

TREATMENT

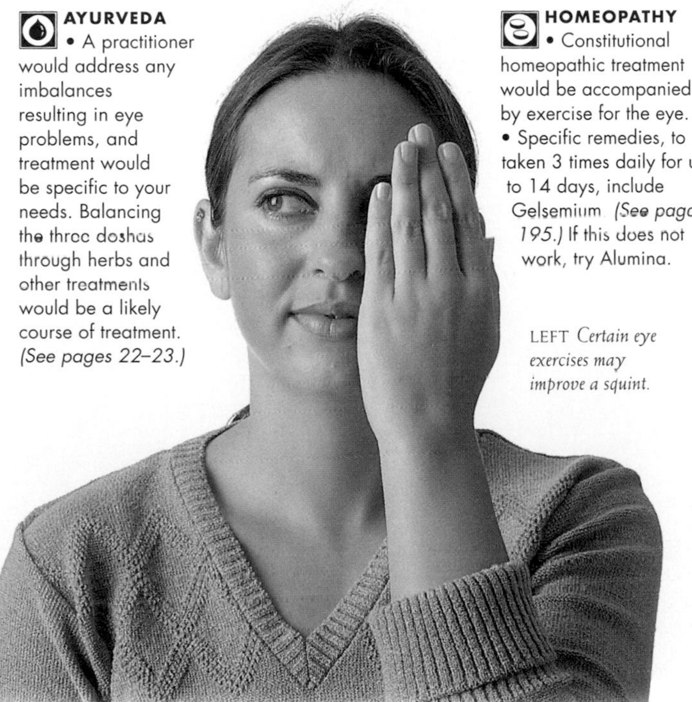

AYURVEDA
- A practitioner would address any imbalances resulting in eye problems, and treatment would be specific to your needs. Balancing the three doshas through herbs and other treatments would be a likely course of treatment. *(See pages 22–23.)*

HOMEOPATHY
- Constitutional homeopathic treatment would be accompanied by exercise for the eye.
- Specific remedies, to be taken 3 times daily for up to 14 days, include Gelsemium. *(See page 195.)* If this does not work, try Alumina.

LEFT *Certain eye exercises may improve a squint.*

Twitching Eyelids

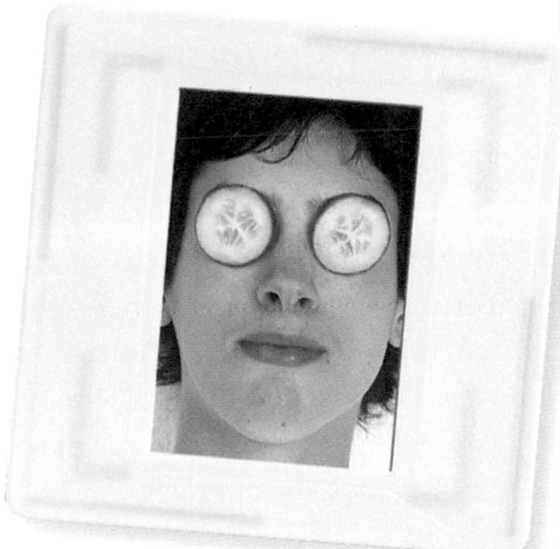

ABOVE *Cucumber is cooling and refreshing for irritated eyes.*

Twitching (fasciculation) of the eyelids is caused by a brief, involuntary contraction of the flat muscle around the eye. It is a very common phenomenon and is only a cause for concern if it is very persistent, as it may then be an indication of nerve disease. A twitch or tic commonly affecting adults is blepharospasm, in which there is spasmodic closure of one or both eyes. This is usually a feature of psychological disturbance and may be associated with other bodily tics.

TREATMENT

TRADITIONAL HOME AND FOLK REMEDIES
- Place a slice of cucumber on the eyes to soothe and reduce irritation. *(See page 89.)*

HERBALISM
- Because most twitches are caused by tension or tiredness, relaxing herbs would be prescribed, including chamomile, lavender, and vervain. Drink as infusions. *(See pages 119 and 138.)*

AROMATHERAPY
- A few drops of lavender or marjoram oil added to the bath will relax and rejuvenate. *(See pages 161 and 165.)*
- Try a few drops of chamomile or rose oil on a cool compress, placed over the eye area, and massage a drop in a light carrier oil into the muscles surrounding the eye area. Avoid the immediate eye area. *(See pages 150 and 168.)*

HOMEOPATHY
Constitutional treatment would be most appropriate, but the following remedies can be taken every 4 hours for up to 6 doses:
- Pulsatilla, for twitching accompanied by inflammation of the eye. *(See page 209.)*
- Codeinum, for twitching eyelids.

FLOWER ESSENCES
- Vervain is useful for those whose overenthusiasm is putting them under stress. *(See page 241.)*
- Hornbeam, for exhaustion and the feeling of being in a rut. *(See page 227.)*
- Impatiens, for irritability and a rushed lifestyle. *(See page 233.)*

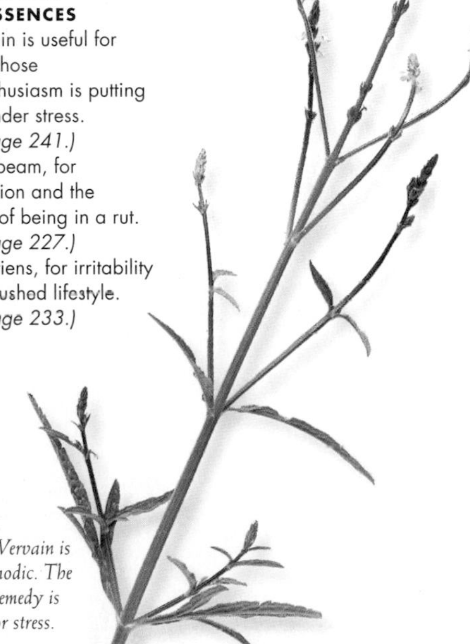

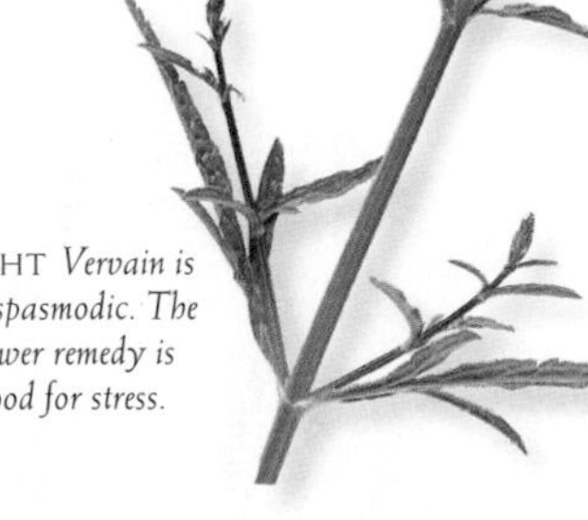

RIGHT *Vervain is antispasmodic. The flower remedy is good for stress.*

EAR PROBLEMS

Tinnitus

Tinnitus is a hissing, buzzing, whistling, or ringing sound experienced in the ear (one or both). It is usually continuous, but the sufferer's awareness of it is intermittent. Tinnitus is related to damage to the hair cells of the inner ear. Persistent tinnitus is usually associated with a degree of hearing loss, and can be triggered by explosions or prolonged loud noise. It may also be a symptom of colds and flu, ear infections and excessive ear wax, brain or head injuries, Ménière's disease, and otosclerosis.

DATA FILE

- The ringing, roaring, clicking, or hissing sounds heard with tinnitus are actually warning signs of such things as infection, Ménière's disease, and otosclerosis. They may also be caused by hard masses of wax in the ear; a stuffy nose; such drugs as quinine, antibiotics, aspirin, and alcohol; and excessive smoking.
- Sensorineural hearing loss is often accompanied by ear noise, or tinnitus. Because the inner ear has no pain fibers, damage is not accompanied by pain.
- More people lose hearing today than in past years; the average pop concert or stereo headset can impair hearing in less than a half-hour.
- About 30 percent of adults over 65 have hearing loss, and as much as one-third of cases are associated with exposure to loud noise.

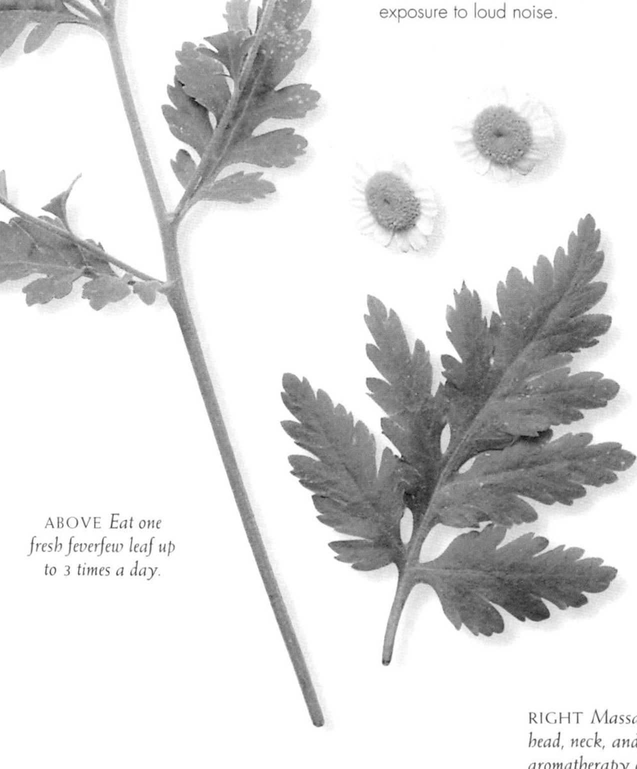

ABOVE *Eat one fresh feverfew leaf up to 3 times a day.*

TREATMENT

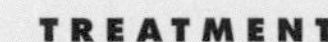

CHINESE HERBALISM
- A herbalist might treat a Blood Deficiency, and use the following herbs: Shu di Huang and Tu Su Zi, which are commonly used in the treatment of tinnitus. *(See pages 62 and 73.)*

HERBALISM
- For tinnitus caused by blood congestion or pressure in the head, try black cohosh. Use 10–30 drops of tincture diluted in water, and drink it as often as necessary.
- Feverfew is effective for tinnitus, and taken daily may prevent attacks. *(See page 133.)*
- Tinnitus caused by poor circulation or high blood pressure may respond to treatment with hawthorn. *(See page 119.)*

AROMATHERAPY
- Use oils which increase the circulation, including rosemary, cypress, lemon, and rose. Massage of the head, neck, and chest using these oils may help, as will one or more in a blend heated in a vaporizer or burner. *(See pages 146–71.)*

HOMEOPATHY
Treatment should be constitutional, but some remedies which may help include:
- Salicylic acid, for roaring in the ears, dizziness, and deafness.
- China sulf., for any buzzing, hissing, or singing sounds in the ears.
- Kali iod., for ringing in the ears and no other obvious symptoms.

VITAMINS AND MINERALS
- Try increasing the following nutrients in your diet: magnesium, potassium, and manganese. Deficiency of these has been linked with tinnitus. *(See pages 262 and 263.)*
- Eat plenty of food rich in vitamins A and C, and bioflavonoids, which are very good for circulation. *(See pages 252 and 256.)*

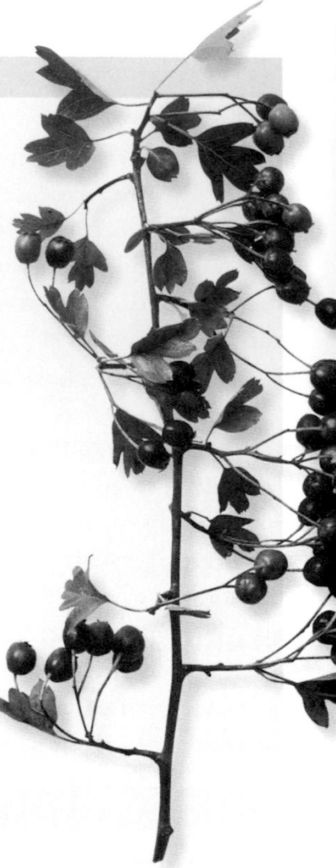

ABOVE *Hawthorn is a tonic for the circulatory system, which may help some cases.*

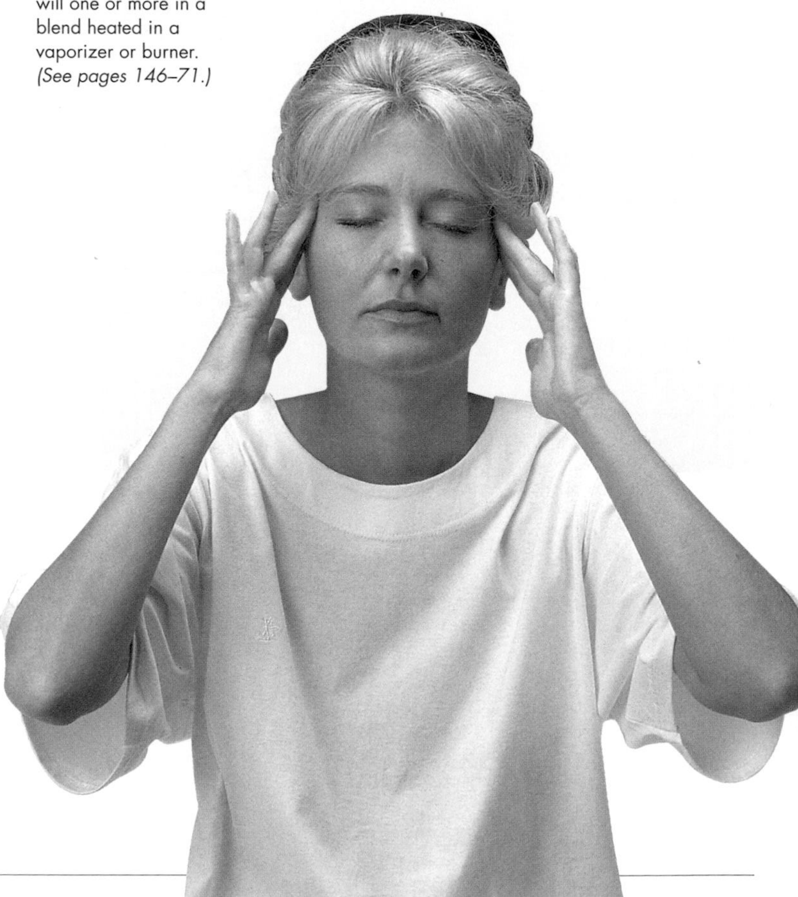

RIGHT *Massage the head, neck, and chest with aromatherapy oils that increase circulation.*

Middle Ear Infection (Otitis Media)

ABOVE *Children are prone to infections of the middle ear.*

The most common ear infections are middle ear infections (otitis media). The middle ear is located behind the eardrum and connected to the throat by the Eustachian tube. Bacteria may therefore travel to the middle ear from the throat when infections occur there, or they may also enter through a perforation in the eardrum. The eardrum may be perforated, or ruptured, by shattering blasts or sharp objects, as well as by infection. Very loud noises, a change in pressure (such as when flying), and violent sneezing while suffering an ear infection may also, in some cases, cause perforation.

Young children, with shorter and straighter Eustachian tubes than adults, are especially prone to middle ear infections. The tendency is also apparently inherited. Chronic infections may also be associated with allergies, tuberculosis, measles, and other diseases.

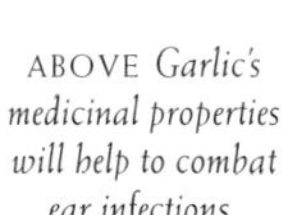

ABOVE *Garlic's medicinal properties will help to combat ear infections.*

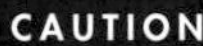

CAUTION

ALWAYS CONSULT YOUR PHYSICIAN IF THE EAR DRUM "BURSTS" OR PERFORATES, AS IT CAN LEAD TO SERIOUS COMPLICATIONS, INCLUDING DEAFNESS AND, IN SOME CASES, MENINGITIS.

Symptoms

• *intense pain* • *fever* • *in severe cases pressure in the middle ear builds up to such an extent that the eardrum perforates in order to release the discharge; this may lead to external ear infection and a degree of temporary or permanent hearing loss*

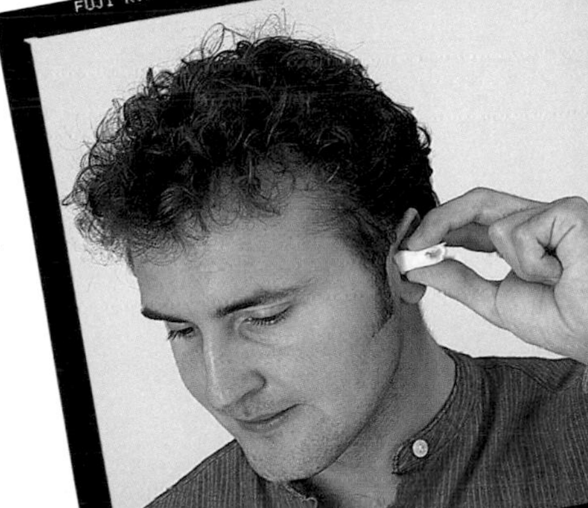

RIGHT *Wrap a piece of garlic in gauze, warm it, and insert into the ear canal.*

TREATMENT

AYURVEDA
• Purified and concentrated extracts of garlic might be used to control and treat infection. *(See page 26.)*
• Panchakarma would be appropriate. *(See page 22.)*

TRADITIONAL HOME AND FOLK REMEDIES
• Peel the skin from a bud of garlic, and cut to fit the outside of the ear canal. Wrap in a piece of gauze, heat gently, and insert into the canal. *(See page 82.)*

HERBALISM
• Mullein oil is a traditional herbal treatment. Place a few dropS on a cotton ball and gently place in the ear canal. *(See page 137.)*
• Anti-inflammatory and antibacterial herbs include chamomile, echinacea, golden rod, and golden seal, and they can be taken internally or infused and dropped into the ear canal. *(See pages 119 and 120.)*
• Steep yarrow and pour the warm liquid into the ear canal to soothe and reduce infection. *(See page112.)*

AROMATHERAPY
• Massage a blend of anti-infectious oils around the ear and down the neck. Suitable oils include lavender, chamomile, and tea tree. *(See pages 146–71.)*
• Mix a drop of clove oil in a little grapeseed carrier oil and massage around the neck and ear. *(See pages 146–71.)*

HOMEOPATHY
Chronic ear infections should be treated constitutionally. Acute attacks may respond to the following, taken every half-hour for up to 10 doses.
• Hep. sulf. may be useful for infection accompanied by sharp pain. *(See page 198.)*
• Belladonna, for a throbbing earache with redness around the ear, accompanied by fever. *(See page 183.)*
• Aconite, for an attack which comes on suddenly, particularly after exposure to cold. *(See page 178.)*
• Pulsatilla, when there is pain, as if the eardrum is being pushed out. *(See page 209.)*

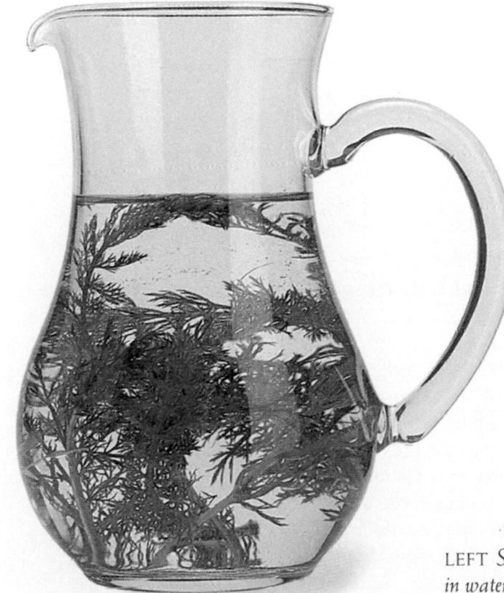

LEFT *Steep yarrow leaves in water, and pour the warm liquid into the ear.*

Outer Ear Infection (Otitis externa)

An inflammation or infection of the outer ear can cause severe pain, possibly a discharge, and impaired hearing. Such symptoms may be due to a number of factors, such as infection by fungi or bacteria, or a foreign body in the ear. Boils or abscesses lead to a build-up of pus which causes severe pain in the ear.

DATA FILE

Reasons for infection include:

- Boils often result from infection by Staphylococcus bacteria. Infection often occurs through a break in the skin caused by scratching an itch, or may enter the ear from polluted water. Boils are painful, the ear may swell, and infection may spread to the inner ear.
- Fungus infections are sometimes called "swimmer's ear" because the dampness is favorable to fungal growth.
- Damage from constant probing of the ear may lead to bacterial or fungal infection or inflammation.
- An allergic reaction to a foreign body can cause an ear infection.

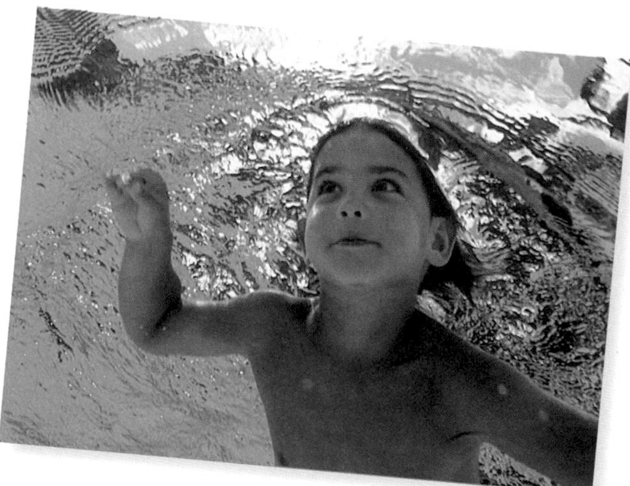

BELOW *Regular swimmers may be more likely to suffer outer ear infections, particularly if the water is not clean.*

TREATMENT

TRADITIONAL HOME AND FOLK REMEDIES

- A roasted onion can be applied to the outer ear canal (hot) to draw out infection and to ease the pain. *(See page 82.)*
- A bread poultice *(see Earache, page 326)* will reduce inflammation and pain. *(See page 101.)*
- Warm a little garlic oil, saturate a cotton bud, and place in the ear canal to draw out infection. *(See page 82.)*

HERBALISM

- Mullein oil will reduce external pain and encourage healing. St. John's wort oil exerts a similar beneficial effect. *(See pages 124 and 137.)*
- Wash the ear canal with a warm infusion of herbs such as chamomile, elderflower, or golden seal, which are antiseptic. *(See pages 119 and 130.)*

AROMATHERAPY

- Apply a little tea tree oil to the end of a cotton bud and gently swab the outer ear canal, and the ear itself. *(See page 162.)*
- Warm some marjoram oil in grapeseed oil, massage around the ear and dab a few drops into the ear canal. Apply a little more to a cotton ball and insert into the ear and leave overnight. This will reduce pain and encourage healing. *(See pages 146–71.)*

HOMEOPATHY

- Belladonna, for pain and redness. *(See page 183.)*
- Mercurius, when there is a smelly discharge. *(See page 205.)*
- Aconite, for an acute infection characterized by sharp shooting pains. *(See page 178.)*

FLOWER ESSENCES

- Take Rescue Remedy or Emergency Essence to ease symptoms and induce calm. *(See page 244.)*

Labyrinthitis (Otitis interna)

Labyrinthitis (otitis interna) is an inflammation of the part of the inner ear responsible for balance (the labyrinth). A viral infection is usually the cause of labyrinthitis (possibly in the course of mumps or flu), although it may be the result of infection spreading through the bone from middle ear infection. Infection may also reach the inner ear (via the bloodstream) from somewhere else in the body. Less commonly, a bacterial labyrinthitis results from a head injury. In labyrinthitis, inflammation of the fluid-filled chambers (labyrinth) of the inner ear causes disruption of the individual's sense of balance. As well as vertigo, labyrinthitis may cause nausea, vomiting, nystagmus (abnormal, jerky movements of the eyes), tinnitus, and hearing loss.

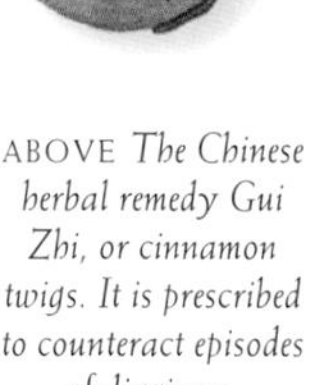

ABOVE *The Chinese herbal remedy Gui Zhi, or cinnamon twigs. It is prescribed to counteract episodes of dizziness.*

CAUTION

UNTREATED BACTERIAL LABYRINTHITIS MAY LEAD TO PERMANENT DEAFNESS, OR SPREAD TO CAUSE MENINGITIS.

SYMPTOMS

• a spinning sensation • unsteadiness, faintness, and possibly falling • nausea and vomiting • partial deafness • ringing or hissing in the ears (see Tinnitus, page 322)

TREATMENT

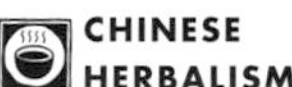

CHINESE HERBALISM

- Fresh ginger, cinnamon twigs, and peppermint will help with the dizziness. *(See page 59.)*
- Mulberry can be taken to nourish the Blood.

HERBALISM

- Treatment to boost the immune system, including echinacea, would be appropriate. *(See page 120.)*
- Ginger root, candied or chewed raw, will help to ease the nausea. *(See page 139.)*
- Try Chinese angelica, which can restore energy, stimulate white blood cells and the formation of antibodies to fight infection. *(See page 115.)*
- Licorice helps recovery, stimulating formation and efficiency of white blood cells and antibodies. *(See page 122.)*

HOMEOPATHY

- Conium, for dizziness which worsens when lying down.
- Belladonna, for a feeling of fullness in the ear, worsened by moving around. *(See page 183.)*
- Nat. mur., for symptoms accompanied by a headache and sometimes by constipation. *(See page 206.)*
- Phosphorus, when dizziness is made worse by looking down. *(See page 208.)*
- Gelsemium, when you feel weak and trembling. *(See page 195.)*
- Calcarea, when an attack of dizziness is made worse by looking up. *(See page 186.)*

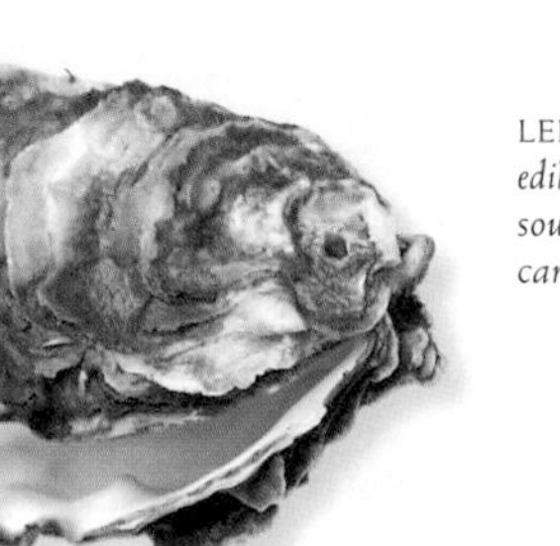

LEFT *The European edible oyster is the source for Calcarea carbonica.*

Glue Ear

Glue ear is a persistent condition in children in which there is a build-up of sticky fluid in the middle ear. It may be caused by chronic nose or throat infection, but can also be due to allergies or exposure to draughts. It may also be associated with chronically enlarged tonsils and adenoids, causing Eustachian tube obstruction. Glue ear does not cause any pain but does impair normal hearing. This in turn can lead to other problems, such as falling behind in class, since hearing is essential for speech development and learning.

CAUTION

SEVERE INATTENTION AMONG CHILDREN UNDER TWO YEARS COULD WELL BE DUE TO PARTIAL DEAFNESS CAUSED BY GLUE EAR. IT IS ESSENTIAL THAT THIS IS INVESTIGATED IN ORDER TO AVOID LONG-TERM SPEECH, COMPREHENSION, AND INTELLECTUAL IMPAIRMENT.

Symptoms

- *hearing impairment*

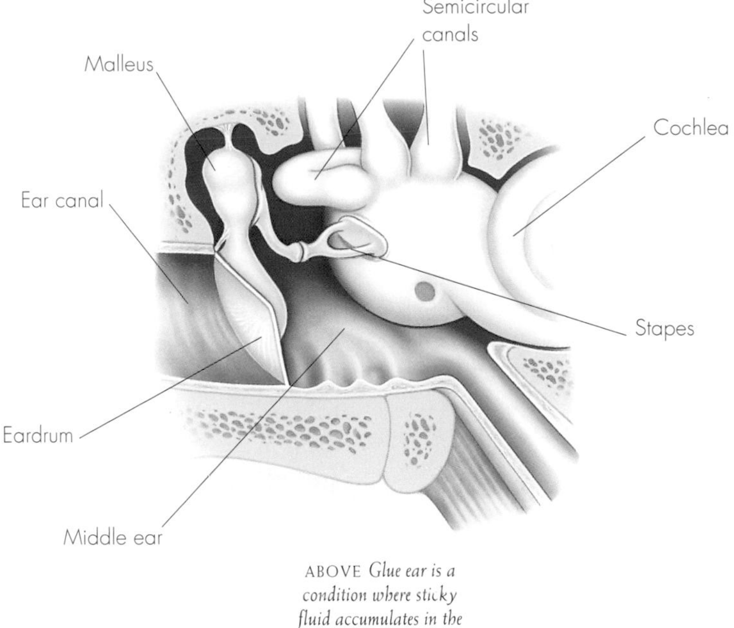

ABOVE *Glue ear is a condition where sticky fluid accumulates in the middle ear.*

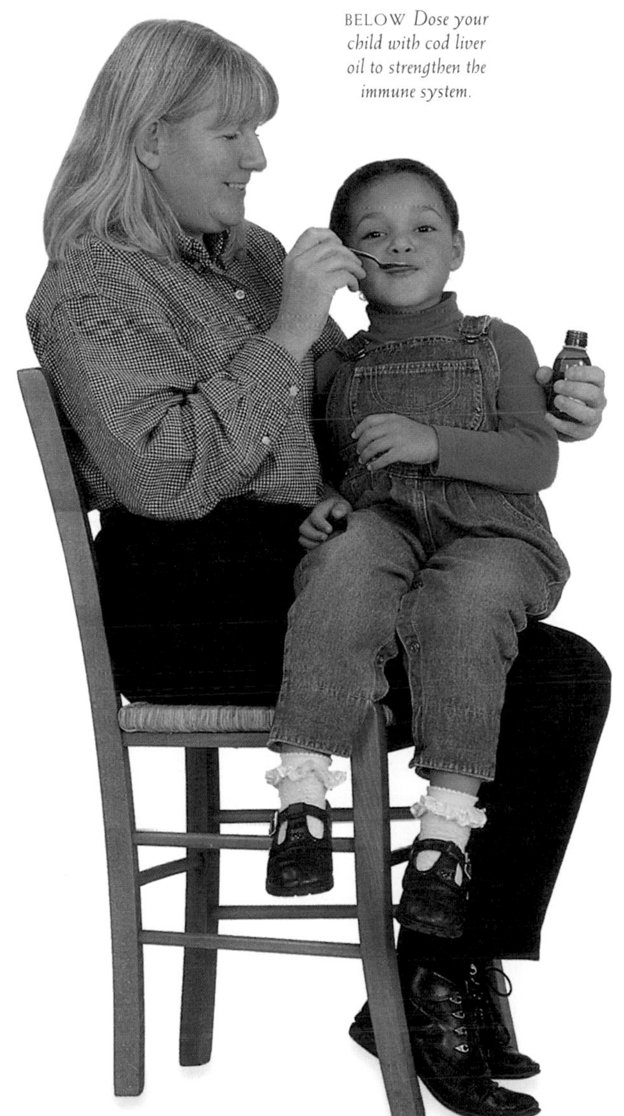

BELOW *Dose your child with cod liver oil to strengthen the immune system.*

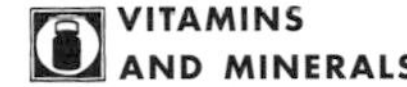

TREATMENT

CHINESE HERBALISM
- Herbs to reduce inflammation and mucus (phlegm) would be Sheng di Huang or Chinese senega root/Polygala. *(See pages 70 and 72.)*

TRADITIONAL HOME AND FOLK REMEDIES
- Drink lemon and honey or cider vinegar to clear the mucus and to strengthen the immune system. *(See pages 87, 101, and 102.)*

HERBALISM
- Clean away discharge with a warm infusion of herbs such as chamomile or golden seal, which are antiseptic. *(See page 119.)*
- Herbal remedies to boost the immune system include chamomile, echinacea, peppermint, and wild indigo. *(See pages 120 and 125.)*
- Herbs to help clear the catarrh include elderflowers, euphrasia, golden rod, and hyssop. *(See page 130.)*
- Herbs which are able to reduce catarrh include golden rod, ground ivy, and elderflower. *(See page 130.)*

AROMATHERAPY
- Dilute essential oils of lavender, chamomile, eucalyptus, or rosewood in a light carrier oil. Warm and massage around the ear and neck. *(See pages 146–71.)*

HOMEOPATHY
- Kali mur., when there are cracking sounds in the affected ear, accompanied by swollen glands in the neck.
- Lycopodium, when there is deafness and a roaring sound is experienced in the affected ear. *(See page 203.)*
- Pulsatilla, for a full feeling in the ear, and weepiness. *(See page 209.)*
- Mercurius, when there is thick, smelly discharge. *(See page 205.)*

VITAMINS AND MINERALS
- Chronic infection can be caused by a build-up of catarrh *(see page 329)*. Reduce consumption of dairy produce and any other possible allergens, including wheat.
- Take cod liver oil and vitamin C to give a boost to the immune system. *(See page 256.)*

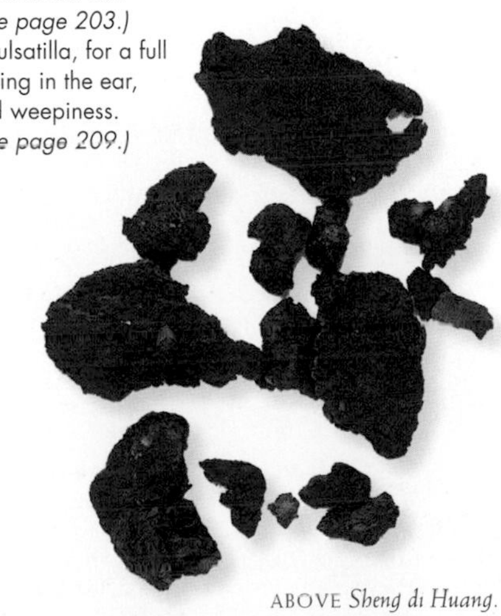

ABOVE *Sheng di Huang. In Chinese medicine this is a cooling herb, prescribed to relieve Heat.*

Earache

Earache is particularly common among children. It is usually (but not always) caused by a change in pressure in the middle ear as a result of a failure in the ear's pressure-equalizing mechanism. The failure occurs when the flow of air to and from the middle ear is impeded by a blockage in the Eustachian tube. The other most frequent causes of earache are acute infection of the middle ear or the ear canal *(see pages 323 and 324)*.

Pain in the ear area may be a feature of problems in other nearby parts of the body, such as the teeth, jaw, throat or neck.

DATA FILE

Earache may be a feature of:

- enlarged adenoids causing Eustachian tube blockage
- infection of the middle ear in which the obstruction in the Eustachian tube interferes with fluid drainage
- a boil or infection by viruses, bacteria or fungi in the external ear passage
- teething in babies, and dental decay
- sinusitis

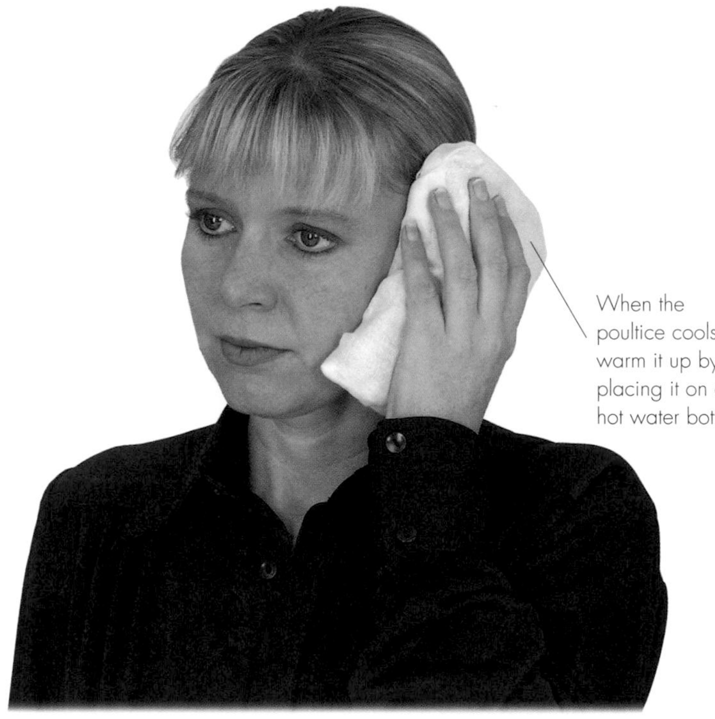

When the poultice cools, warm it up by placing it on a hot water bottle

RIGHT *A warm poultice of ginger or roasted onion will help earache.*

TREATMENT

TRADITIONAL HOME AND FOLK REMEDIES

- Warm a slice of bread with the crusts removed, and pound it with a handful of bruised caraway seeds. Add some hot brandy to make a paste, and apply as a hot poultice to reduce inflammation of the ear. (See page 101.)
- Crush and simmer root ginger and make a poultice to apply to the affected ear.
- Roast an onion, and then apply it hot (take care – test first) to the ear for relief of pain and control of discharge. (See page 82.)

HERBALISM

- Apply a little St. John's wort oil to the area, and massage in gently. (See page 124.)
- Massage a little warmed olive oil, with a few drops of chamomile or elderflower tincture, around the ear, and use a dropper to insert a little into the affected canal. (See pages 119 and 130.)

AROMATHERAPY

- Make a hot compress, to apply directly to the ears and neck to ease the pain, using diluted chamomile, eucalyptus, lavender, or rosewood oils. (*See pages* 146–71.)

HOMEOPATHY

- Chamomilla, for severe pain and need of comfort. (See page 204.)
- Pulsatilla, if the pain feels like the eardrum is being pushed out, and you feel weepy. (See page 209.)
- Hep. sulf., for throbbing pain made better by a warm compress. (See page 198.)
- Belladonna, for throbbing pain that is improved by application of a cold compress. (See page 183.)
- Aconite, for an earache that comes on suddenly. (See page 178.)

FLOWER ESSENCES

- Emergency Essence or Rescue Remedy can be applied to the temples or taken internally to soothe and reduce any panic. (See page 244.)

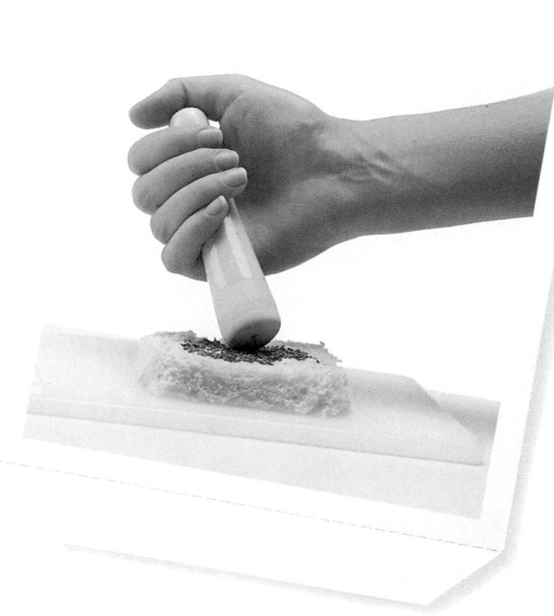

ABOVE *Make a poultice paste by pounding caraway seeds on a slice of bread, and moistening with hot brandy.*

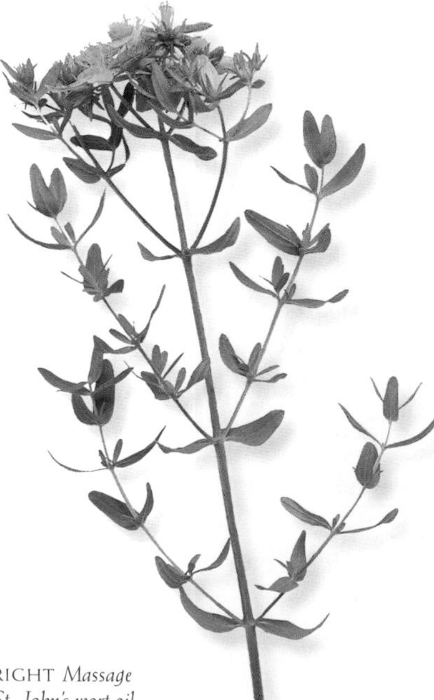

RIGHT *Massage St. John's wort oil into the ear area.*

Ear Wax

Ear wax is a sticky, fatty secretion produced by the glands in the outer ear to protect the eardrum by trapping dust and small objects. Normal soft wax is disposed of naturally by the ear, but hard or dried wax accumulates. An excess of ear wax obstructs the ear canal, and the blockage may be worsened by swimming or bathing since the wax absorbs water.

Symptoms

- *a sensation of fullness or aching in the ear*
- *partial hearing loss caused by inflammation in the ear canal*

TREATMENT

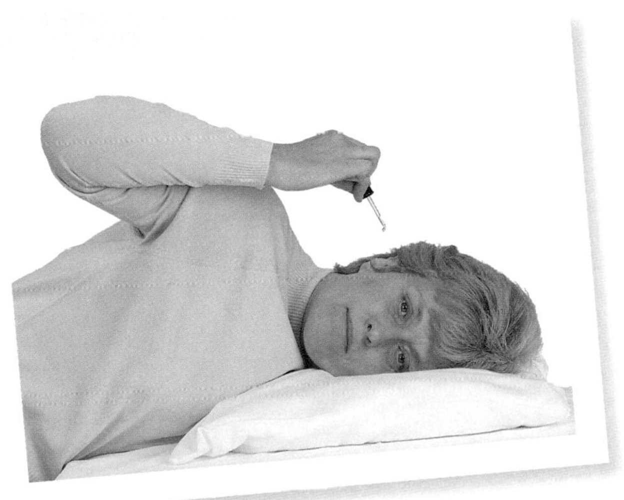

ABOVE *To use an ear dropper, lie with the head on a pillow. This allows the oil to penetrate the ear canal.*

CHINESE HERBALISM
- Drop a little warmed almond oil into the ear to soften the wax, making it easier to remove.

TRADITIONAL HOME AND FOLK REMEDIES
- A little warmed garlic oil, dropped into the ear, will soften the wax and occasionally dislodge it. *(See page 82.)*
- Use an ear candle (available from health stores) to heat and draw out excess wax.

HERBALISM
- Make a warm infusion of chamomile, elderflowers, or marigold, or put a few drops of the tincture into some warm water. Using a dropper, place the liquid in the ear canal and stop with a cotton ball. Repeat several nights running until the wax has softened and is absorbed by the cotton. *(See pages 117, 119, and 130.)*

AROMATHERAPY
- Put a few drops of warm chamomile oil, blended in a light carrier oil, into the ear canal and block gently with a cotton ball. Repeat until wax has softened. *(See page 150.)*

HOMEOPATHY
- Causticum, when there is a build-up of wax with some related loss of hearing. *(See page 189.)*

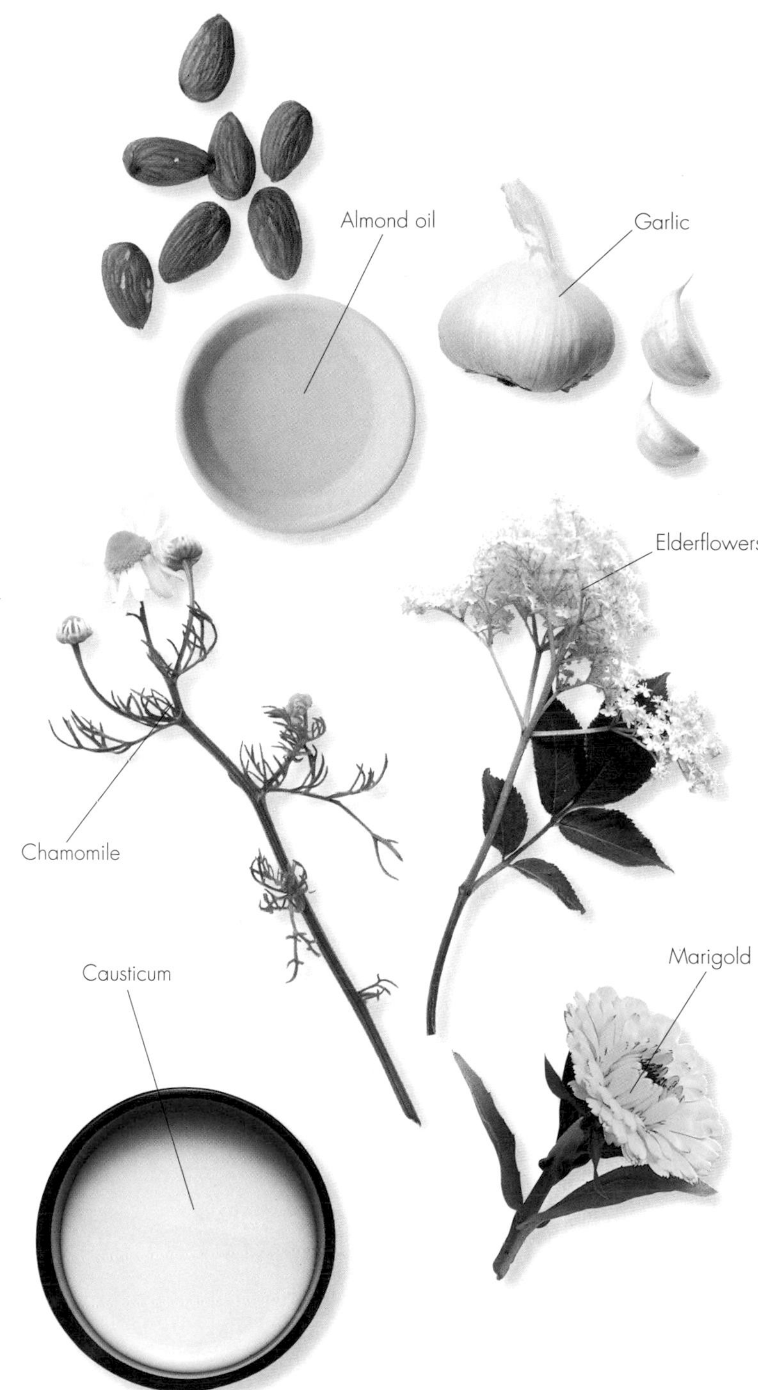

ABOVE *Sources of treatment in some of the major healing remedies: almonds and their oil (Chinese), garlic (traditional home remedies), elderflower and marigold (herbalism), slaked lime (source of Causticum in homeopathy), chamomile (source of chamomile oil in aromatherapy).*

CAUTION

CONSTANT PRODDING OR CLEANING OF THE EAR CAN LEAD TO EXCESSIVE EAR WAX PRODUCTION.

NASAL PROBLEMS

Sinusitis

Sinusitis is an inflammation of the sinuses – the air-filled cavities located in the bones around the nose. When this occurs the lining of the sinuses swells, causing a blockage in the channel that drains them. A build-up of mucus discharge results, creating intense pressure and pain. Sinusitis usually develops as a complication of a viral infection such as a cold, but pollution or tobacco can also be triggers. Severe symptoms should be referred to your physician.

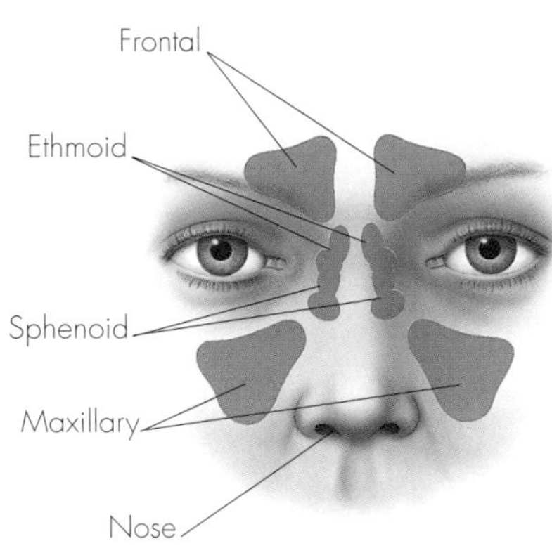

ABOVE *The sinus cavities within the skull are lined with mucous membrane. Inflammation of this membrane can be very painful.*

DATA FILE

- More than 50 percent of cases are caused by bacterial infection.
- In one U.S. study, 50 percent of sufferers had an immune-system problem.
- 10 percent of all cases are caused by dental problems.
- The proximity of the paranasal sinuses to the brain makes sinus infections potentially dangerous.
- Inflammation of the sinuses may develop from an allergy or from bacteria introduced through the nasal channels, causing an infection accompanied by pain and tenderness.
- Chronic sinusitis may result from either form or a combination of both.
- Maxillary sinusitis can result from a cold or can be caused by swimming in contaminated water.
- Rarely, extraction of a molar tooth will break the floor of the maxillary sinus, leaving an opening for bacteria to enter and cause infection.
- Frontal and ethmoid sinusitis share symptoms of localized headache, surface tenderness, and, occasionally, swelling of the eyelids.
- Sphenoid sinusitis can cause blurred vision because of the proximity of this sinus to the optic nerves.

SYMPTOMS

• nasal congestion with thick, stretchy mucus • nosebleeds and sneezing • loss of sense of smell • headache with a sensation of pressure in and around the head • severe pain around the eyes and cheeks (particularly on bending down), sometimes feeling like toothache

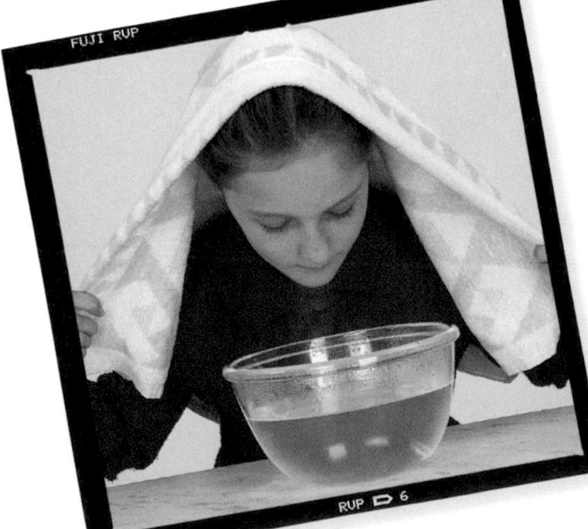

RIGHT *Steam inhalation can quickly bring relief to sinusitis in many cases. There are several herbs and plant oils that can be added to the water.*

TREATMENT

AYURVEDA
- Treatment will involve the elimination of kapha with nasya (inhalation of oils). Herbal treatment may be prescribed, including coriander for sinus problems and related headaches. Detoxification will be appropriate. *(See page 20.)*

CHINESE HERBALISM
- Bi Yan Pian pills are very good for sinusitis, especially with sticky yellow nasal discharge, which is hard to get out.
- A herbal prescription of Cang er Zi San, when there is lots of green nasal discharge, headache and pain.
- Xin Yi San, when there is lots of clear or white nasal discharge, nasal congestion, and pain.
- Peppermint, honeysuckle, tangerine peel, and zanthium fruit may all be useful. *(See pages 59 and 65.)*

TRADITIONAL HOME AND FOLK REMEDIES
- Peppermint is antispasmodic and decongestant. Infuse some fresh or dried leaves in a bowl of boiling water, and inhale the steam.
- Combine the juice of a fresh peeled and pulped horseradish root with the juice of two or three lemons, and take a half-teaspoon between meals. Use for several months until the mucus in the sinus clears. *(See pages 84 and 87.)*

HERBALISM
- Elderflower is excellent for catarrh and sinusitis. Drink an infusion as required to reduce symptoms and encourage healing. *(See page 130.)*
- Drink an infusion of golden seal every two hours during an acute attack.

AROMATHERAPY
- Try steam inhalations of lavender, eucalyptus, and tea tree, which are anticatarrhal and antibacterial. Lavender in particular will act as an anti-inflammatory and ease any painful symptoms. *(See pages 146–71.)*

HOMEOPATHY
- Kali bich. is the main remedy, particularly for thick, sticky mucus that accumulates in the throat, and which is difficult to clear. *(See page 200.)*
- Try Hep. sulf. if Kali bich. does not help. *(See page 198.)*
- Pulsatilla, for sinusitis accompanied by weepiness and pain above the eyes. *(See page 209.)*

VITAMINS AND MINERALS
- Many cases are caused by food allergy or intolerance. See a practitioner if you suspect this is the cause.

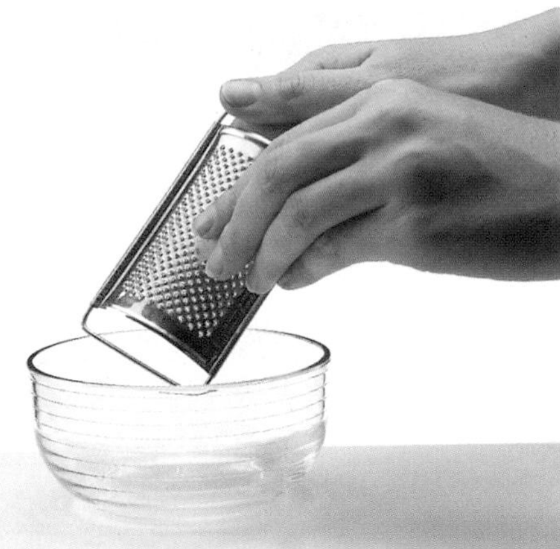

LEFT *Grate a freshly peeled horseradish root to a pulp and combine this with lemon juice. Taken between meals, it will help to clear the sinuses.*

CAUTION

GOLDEN SEAL IS NOT APPROPRIATE FOR PEOPLE WITH HIGH BLOOD PRESSURE, OR FOR PREGNANT WOMEN.

Catarrh

Catarrh is the term used to describe the overproduction of thick phlegm by the mucous membranes of the air passages to the lungs, the larynx, the nose, and sinuses. Cells which produce and secrete a watery mucus are present in the mucous membranes, which line the passages, and they are composed of large, thin-walled veins whose blood supply serves to warm incoming air. Inflammation of the membranes as a result of a cold or flu is the usual cause, but other triggers include smoking, inhalation of dust, chronic sinusitis, upper respiratory tract infection, and allergy. A series of colds in close succession may lead to chronic catarrh. Complementary therapists believe that chronic catarrh that is not obviously due to viral or bacterial infection, allergy, chemical irritants, or dry air, all of which irritate or inflame the mucous membranes, is a symptom of general toxicity of the body – catarrh is the body's attempt to rid itself of toxins that are not being adequately dealt with by the liver, or properly excreted by the kidneys, bowels, and skin.

Nasal cavity

Pharynx

Larynx

LEFT *In catarrh there is an excess of mucus in the nose and throat, caused by a cold or other illness, or in allergic reactions.*

Symptoms

• blocked, possibly painful nose, or excessively runny nose • cough with phlegm • earache • ulcers may develop on the septum (the bone that separates the nostrils) • possibly nosebleeds

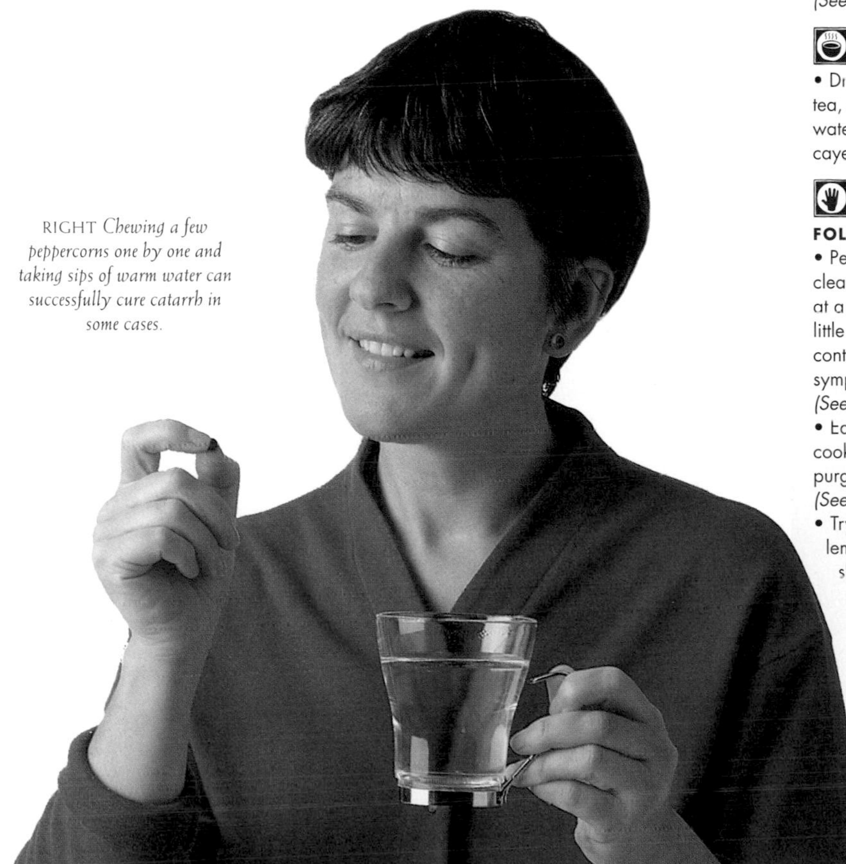

RIGHT *Chewing a few peppercorns one by one and taking sips of warm water can successfully cure catarrh in some cases.*

TREATMENT

AYURVEDA

• Coriander can help to relieve sinus problems and prevent the build-up of catarrh. Brown the seeds and boil them in water with root ginger. Boil until the liquid is reduced and drink (with a little honey) as required. *(See page 35.)*

CHINESE HERBALISM

• Drink ginger or sage tea, and drink onion water with a pinch of cayenne pepper.

TRADITIONAL HOME AND FOLK REMEDIES

• Peppercorns will help to clear catarrh. Chew one at a time, followed by a little hot water, and continue until the symptoms have gone. *(See page 97.)*

• Eating either raw or cooked onions helps to purge stubborn catarrh. *(See page 82.)*

• Try a drop of fresh lemon in each nostril – slightly painful, but enormously powerful! *(See page 87.)*

• Mustard powder can be added to a foot bath to help decongest nasal passages and clear catarrh. *(See page 98.)*

HERBALISM

• Herbs such as golden rod, elderflower, and eyebright are anti-catarrhal and astringent. When catarrh is accompanied by infection, supplement with echinacea and garlic. *(See pages 113, 120, and 130.)*

• Poke root is a good tonic and acts to prevent and reduce catarrh.

AROMATHERAPY

• Thyme and eucalyptus oils may be inhaled to ease symptoms, and it is a good idea to keep niaouli by the bed, as it can help you to sleep. *(See pages 146–71.)*

• Many oils are decongestant and expectorant, including chamomile, hyssop, mint, niaouli, pine, and clary sage. Rub into the chest and temples in a light carrier oil, or place several drops in a bowl of boiling water and inhale. *(See pages 146–71.)*

HOMEOPATHY

Chronic catarrh should be treated constitutionally, but the following remedies may be helpful:

• Arsenicum for thick, yellow discharge which makes the nose and the surrounding area sore. *(See page 182.)*

• Pulsatilla, for yellow or green catarrh that is not painful, accompanied by feelings of weepiness. *(See page 209.)*

• Nat. mur., for catarrh resembling raw egg white, with a dry nose and the loss of taste and smell. *(See page 206.)*

• Calcarea, for yellow and smelly catarrh. *(See page 186.)*

• Sulfur, when there are dry scabs inside the nose, causing bleeding, and when the nose is stuffier indoors than outdoors. *(See page 215.)*

VITAMINS AND MINERALS

• Increase your intake of vitamin C and zinc, which help to reduce symptoms. *(See pages 256 and 265.)*

• If you are prone to chronic catarrh, cut down on intake of dairy produce, which may exacerbate the condition. *(See pages 249.)*

• It may also be caused by over-consumption of sugar and too many refined carbohydrates.

• Ensure that your home is free of dust and avoid smoking.

Hay Fever

Hay fever (also known as allergic rhinitis) is an allergic reaction to airborne irritants such as grass, tree, or flower pollens. These allergens (and others including dust, animal fur, feathers, spores, plants, and chemicals) trigger a reaction which causes swelling of the nasal membrane and the production of the antibodies which release histamine. It is this chemical substance that is responsible for the characteristic allergic symptoms.

Symptoms

• runny nose, congestion, and sneezing • red, itchy eyes • sore throat • wheezing, which can develop into asthma

DATA FILE

• The timing of the symptoms will depend on the type of pollen at fault: February to May, with a peak in April, for tree pollen; June to July for grass pollen; and July to August for weeds such as nettles, golden rod, and mugwort. In the autumn, spores and mould are likely to cause hay fever.

• At least 22 million Americans suffer from hay fever in some form.

• Most cases involve some dermatitis (in the form of urticaria or hives), and temporary asthma is common during the hay fever seasons in susceptible people.

• German researchers have found that three bananas contain enough magnesium to quell a hay fever attack.

• Babies born in the spring, when pollen is in the air, are more likely to develop hay fever later in life.

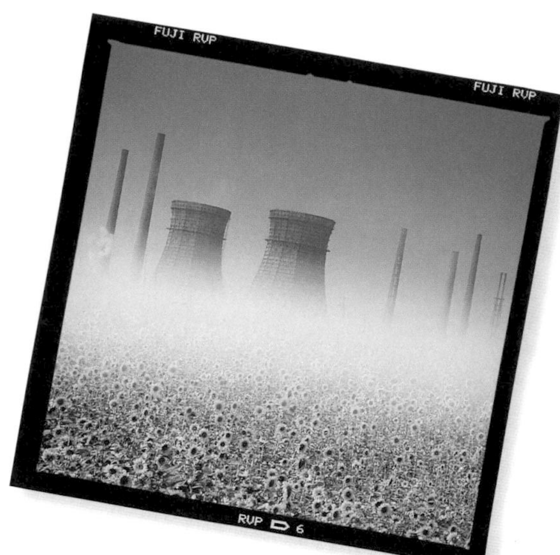

RIGHT *Susceptibility to hay fever will increase near to sources of airborne irritants such as flower pollen and emissions from factory sites and power stations.*

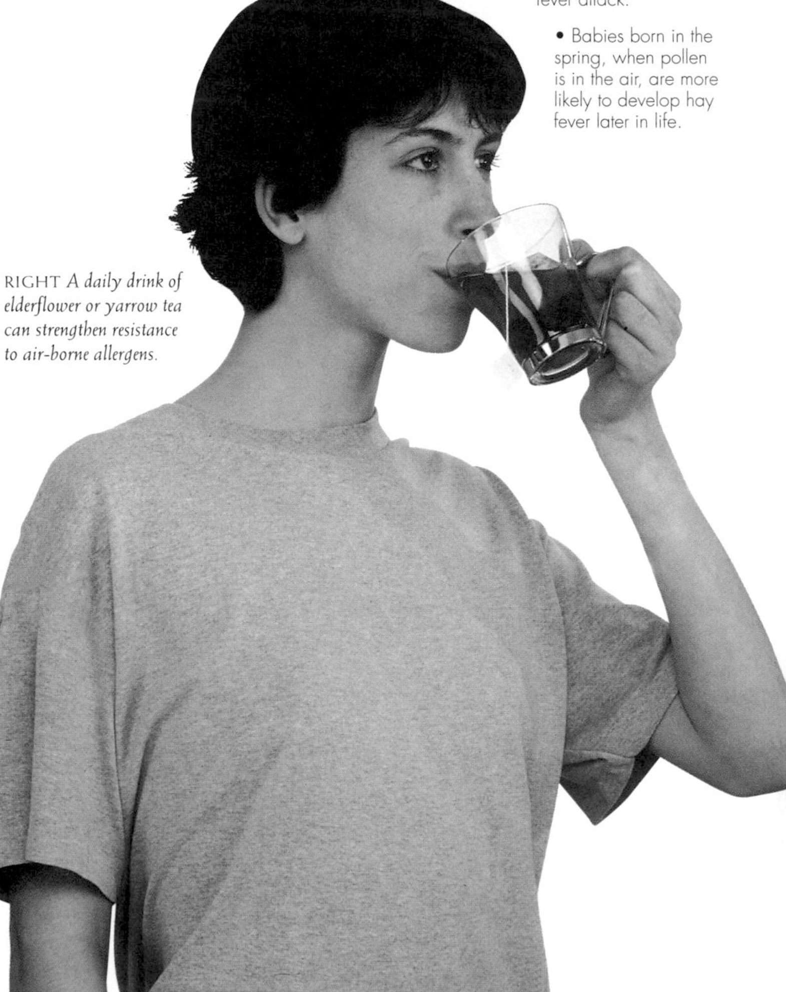

RIGHT *A daily drink of elderflower or yarrow tea can strengthen resistance to air-borne allergens.*

TREATMENT

CHINESE HERBALISM
• Bi Yan Pian/Nose inflammation pills, for Wind Cold or Wind Heat to the face; sneezing, itchy eyes, facial congestion and sinus pain, acute and chronic rhinitis, and nasal allergies.
• A herbal prescription of Yu Ping Feng San/Jade screen helps prevent hay fever, and guards against allergies.
• Cang er Zi Tang/Xanthium powder, for allergic rhinitis with a thickened yellow catarrh or a blocked nose.

TRADITIONAL HOME AND FOLK REMEDIES
• A teaspoon of local honey, before and during the season, helps many people. *(See page 101.)*
• Eat plenty of fresh garlic to boost the immune system, and to act as an anticatarrhal agent. *(See page 82.)*

HERBALISM
• Strengthen resistance with a tea of elderflowers and yarrow for some weeks before the pollen season starts. *(See pages 112 and 130.)*
• Soothe itchy eyes with an elderflower, eyebright, or chamomile compress. Eyebright tea or capsules will relieve symptoms.

AROMATHERAPY
• Chamomile in the bath and in massage will help to ease symptoms. *(See page 150.)*
• Steam or dry inhalations of lavender and/or eucalyptus can help for sneezing and runny nose. Also use in the bath. *(See pages 159 and 161.)*
• Melissa may soothe and calm the allergic reaction. *(See page 163.)*

HOMEOPATHY
Hay fever can be deep-seated and take some time to cure, and treatment should be constitutional. However, there are preventive remedies, including the following:
• Allium, for hay fever where the sufferer has a burning nasal discharge. *(See page 178.)*
• Sabadilla, for hay fever with a sore throat.
• Arsenicum, when there is a constant need to sneeze. *(See page 182.)*
• Euphrasia, when the eyes are itching and red. *(See page 194.)*

FLOWER ESSENCES
• Rescue Remedy or Emergency Essence will help to ease symptoms during an attack, and help to produce a more positive frame of mind. *(See page 244.)*

VITAMINS AND MINERALS
• Vitamin C combined with bioflavonoids will act as a natural antihistamine to control symptoms. *(See pages 256 and 272.)*
• Taking extra pantothenic acid may help to relieve hay fever symptoms. *(See page 254.)*
• Bee pollen can help prevent allergies when taken for several weeks before the hay fever season. *(See page 27.)*
• Royal jelly is also a useful hay fever treatment. *(See page 276.)*

BELOW *Unfortunately, many people can be allergic to their own pets.*

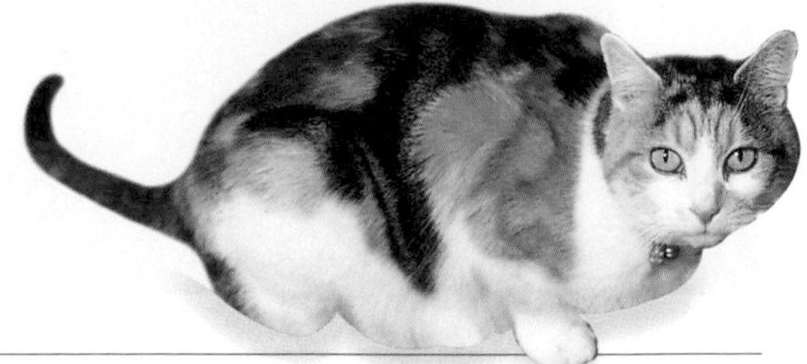

Disturbed Sense of Smell

The olfactory nerves in the nose have many hair-like nerve fibers or smell receptors. When we sniff, a waft of air passes over the receptors, allowing us to identify a smell. Loss of the sense of smell (or "anosmia"), whether temporary or permanent, can be severely debilitating and in some instances dangerous – if it fails to alert us to the presence of gas or smoke, for example. It may occur as a result of: head injury in which damage is sustained to the twigs of the olfactory nerve; colds or flu.

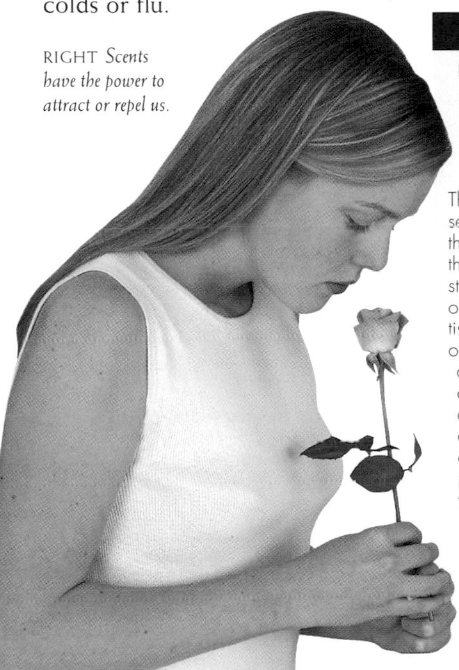

RIGHT *Scents have the power to attract or repel us.*

DATA FILE

Despite the close association, taste and smell are distinct. In the case of taste, chemicals that evoke sweet, sour, bitter, and salty sensations stimulate taste bud receptors located in the throat and on the tongue and palate. This stimulation triggers nerve cells to send signals to the brain stem, located in the base of the brain. Odors register in the brain when airborne chemicals stimulate receptors located on the olfactory epithelium, a small patch of tissue positioned high in the nose. The olfactory system is vitally important in determining food flavors. During chewing and swallowing, odor-laden air is forced from the rear of the oral cavity to the olfactory receptors, evoking many flavor sensations that people usually associate with taste but which are almost completely dependent on the sense of smell. If you pinch your nose while swallowing food, the flow of air to the olfactory receptors is prevented, resulting in a decrease or elimination of the perception of the food's taste.

TREATMENT

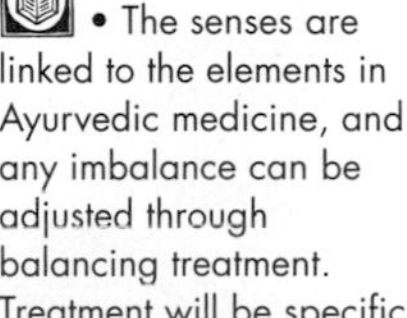

AYURVEDA
• The senses are linked to the elements in Ayurvedic medicine, and any imbalance can be adjusted through balancing treatment. Treatment will be specific to the patient's needs. *(See page 20.)*

HOMEOPATHY
Treatment will be constitutional, but the following remedies may be useful:
• Ignatia, for sensitivity to tobacco smoke. *(See page 200.)*
• Graphites, for sensitivity to flower scents. *(See page 196.)*
• Carbolic acid, when all smells are overpowering.
• Belladonna, for a sudden smell of rotten eggs. *(See page 183.)*

VITAMINS AND MINERALS
• A zinc deficiency can cause problems with your sense of smell – ensure that you have an adequate dietary intake, or take a daily supplement of zinc. *(See page 265.)*

CAUTION

VERY RARELY, CANCER PATIENTS REPORT SPECIFIC SMELL AND TASTE CHANGES. IF YOU DEVELOP AN ACUTE SENSE OF SMELL SUDDENLY, SEE YOUR PHYSICIAN.

Nosebleeds

Nosebleeds are very common, resulting either from persistent probing, an injury, infection of the mucous membrane, or from drying and crusting. Injury or infection which damages the moist lining of the nose can quite easily rupture tiny local blood vessels and cause bleeding; more often, bleeding occurs for no apparent reason. There is some association between nosebleeds and high alcohol intake.

RIGHT *Lavender oil applied on a cotton bud will encourage healing.*

TREATMENT

TRADITIONAL HOME AND FOLK REMEDIES
• Lemon is a natural styptic. Place a drop in the offending nostril, on the end of a cotton bud. *(See page 87.)*

AROMATHERAPY
• A drop of lavender oil, placed in the nostril on a cotton bud, will encourage healing and help to staunch the flow of blood. *(See page 161.)*

HOMEOPATHY
• Aconite, for a sudden nosebleed. *(See page178.)*
• Arnica, for a nosebleed brought on by injury or bruising. *(See page 182.)*
• Phosphorus, for a nosebleed brought on by blowing the nose violently. *(See page 208.)*
• Rhus tox., for nosebleeds after strenuous exercise. *(See page 210.)*
• Lachesis, for nosebleeds occurring in hot weather. *(See page 216.)*

FLOWER ESSENCES
• Rescue Remedy or Emergency Essence will help in cases of emotional distress, and a few drops diluted in water and placed in the nostril may help to encourage the healing process. *(See page 244.)*

CAUTION

NOSEBLEEDS WHICH DO NOT STOP WITHIN A COUPLE OF HOURS SHOULD BE CHECKED BY A PHYSICIAN. DO NOT STEM THE BLEEDING TOO QUICKLY IN THOSE SUFFERING FROM HIGH BLOOD PRESSURE – ALLOW THE BLEEDING TO CONTINUE FOR 10 MINUTES BEFORE TAKING ACTION.

CONTRARY TO POPULAR MYTH, NOSEBLEEDS ARE NOT ALWAYS A SIGN OF HIGH BLOOD PRESSURE, BUT IF YOU ARE OVER 40, OR SUSPECT HIGH BLOOD PRESSURE, SEE YOUR PHYSICIAN.

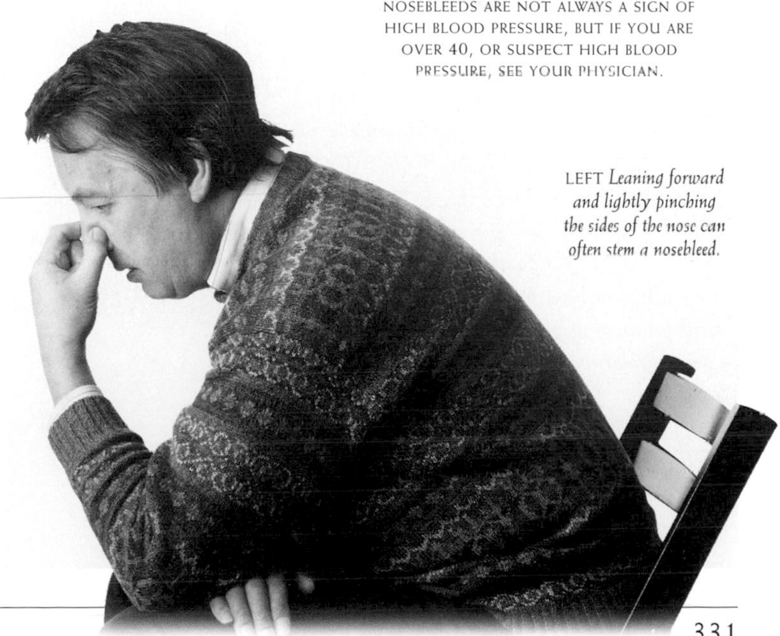

LEFT *Leaning forward and lightly pinching the sides of the nose can often stem a nosebleed.*

DENTAL PROBLEMS

Gingivitis

Gingivitis is inflammation of the gums. It may sometimes occur as a result of infection or ill-fitting dentures, but most usually it is caused by an accumulation of plaque and impacted food around and under the gums. Left untreated, gingivitis may lead to loosening of the affected tooth (periodontitis) through damage to the membrane securing it. It is a very common problem, particularly during pregnancy. Gingivitis may also result from systemic disorders such as vitamin C deficiency (scurvy) and endocrine disturbances (diabetes mellitus). Prevention and treatment include good oral hygiene and control or correction of local and systemic factors. The incidence of gingivitis appears to increase with age; at the age of 10, 15 percent of the U.S. population suffer; by the age of 50, more than 50 percent have gingivitis. A blood test can now detect gum disease six months before symptoms set in.

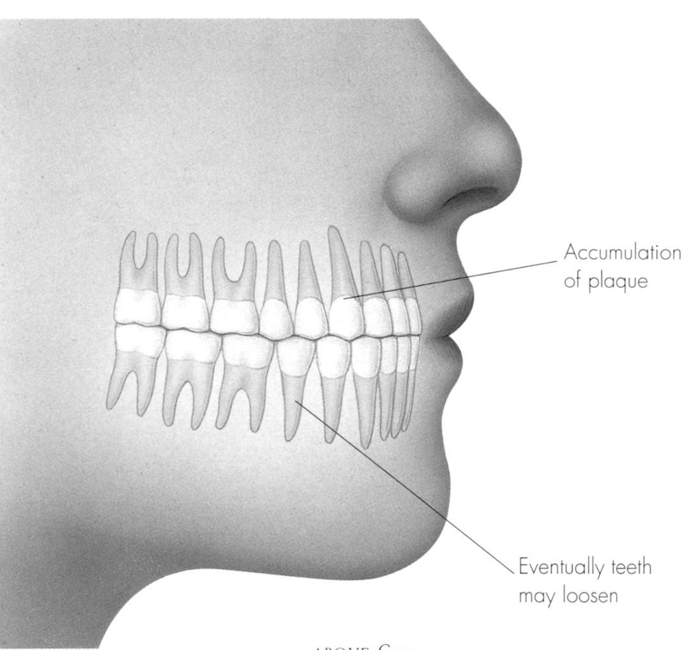

ABOVE *Gum inflammation can lead to periodontitis if not treated, and this causes the teeth to loosen and fall out.*

Symptoms

• swollen and tender gums which bleed easily after brushing • halitosis (bad breath) if areas of tissue death occur • possibly earache from referred pain

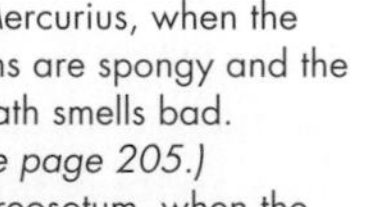

TREATMENT

TRADITIONAL HOME AND FOLK REMEDIES

• Peach pit tea is useful for mouth infections. Rinse your mouth with the hot tea three times a day.

HERBALISM

• Depending on the problem, some herbs, such as myrrh, are highly astringent and antiseptic, and may be useful locally. Other treatments may be used internally to increase the patient's resistance.
• Golden seal can make an effective poultice, and will treat any infection.
• Comfrey mouthwash will help to heal mouth abrasions, and reduce swelling and bleeding. *(See page 132.)*

HOMEOPATHY

Gingivitis may be treated homeopathically. One of the following specific remedies may be taken every 4 hours for up to 3 days:

• Mercurius, when the gums are spongy and the breath smells bad. *(See page 205.)*
• Kreosotum, when the gums are red, inflamed, and swollen, and bleed easily, with the roots of the teeth exposed.
• Nat. mur., when gums bleed easily, there are ulcers and a taste of pus in the mouth, accompanied by sensitive teeth. *(See page 206.)*
• Phosphorus, for gums which bleed easily when touched, gaps between teeth and gums. *(See page 208.)*
• Silicea, for painful, swollen gums, very sensitive to cold, and which bleed easily. *(See page 211.)*
• Abscesses generally seem to respond well to Hep. sulf., Belladonna, Silicea, or Mercurius. *(See pages 183, 198, 205, and 211.)*

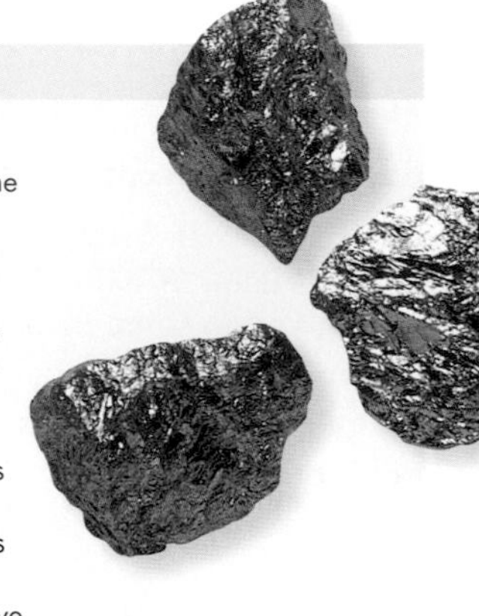

ABOVE *Silica, source of the homeopathic remedy Silicea which can be an effective treatment.*

VITAMINS AND MINERALS

• Apart from a visit to a dental hygienist, followed by daily brushing and flossing, a healthy diet will promote healthy gums.
• Vitamin C is important for the production of collagen. Most tissues in the body are made from this. *(See page 256.)*
• Co-enzyme Q10 supplements have been found beneficial in some cases of gum disease.

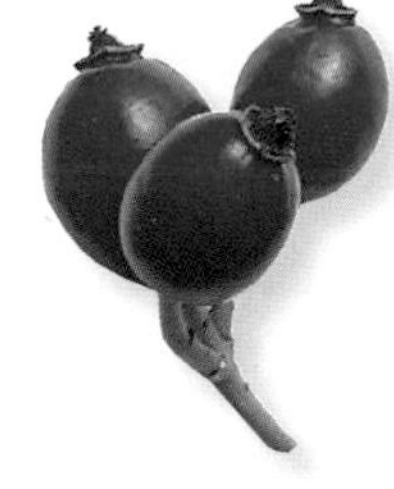

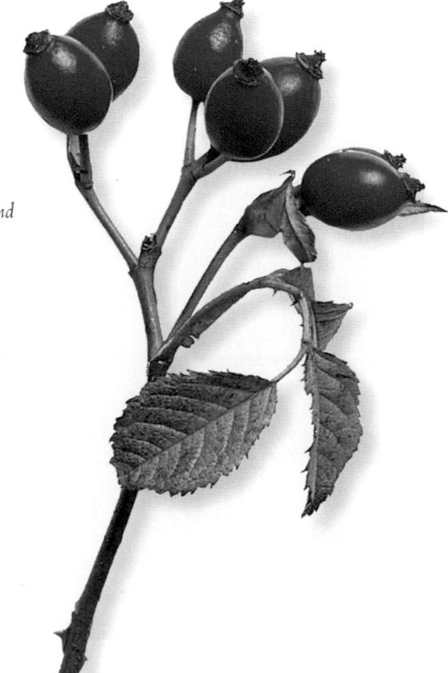

RIGHT AND LEFT *Rosehips and oranges are an excellent source of vitamin C which is required to maintain healthy gums. Included in the diet they can prevent vitamin C deficiency, one of the factors that can lead to gingivitis.*

Toothache

Aching or pain in a tooth is generally a result of tooth decay (or "caries"). When the hard enamel of the tooth is damaged, this allows infecting organisms to enter the tooth, which results in inflammation and pain. If a tooth is sensitive to heat, cold, or sweet things, or gives pain lasting for more than a few minutes, nerves in the tooth may be inflamed due to advanced decay. If pain is absent, except when you bite, your tooth or filling may be broken. In either case, it is recommended that you see your dentist within 48 hours. Toothache after a filling is not unusual, on contact with cold air or drinks, but if the pain persists and the tooth becomes sensitive to heat as well, a return visit will be necessary.

RIGHT *Cayenne pepper, a temporary remedy for toothache and sore gums.*

TREATMENT

AYURVEDA

- Crush a clove of garlic and apply to the tooth. *(See page 26.)*
- Dip a small cotton ball into cinnamon oil and apply to the affected area. *(See page 34.)*

CHINESE HERBALISM

- Treatment would address Heat in the Stomach, and decayed or damaged teeth.
- Gypsum and ginseng might be used to relieve heat. *(See page 67.)*

HERBALISM

- A herbalist might recommend tinctures of echinacea or myrrh to encourage healing and reduce the risk of infection. *(See page 120.)*
- Cayenne can act as a local anesthetic for painful teeth and gums. *(See page 118.)*
- Fennel may be applied to the cheek in the form of a poultice, which will reduce inflammation and ease symptoms. *(See page 121.)*

AROMATHERAPY

- Peppermint or clove oils can be applied directly to the area to act as a natural analgesic. *(See pages 146–71.)*
- Oil of coriander will reduce inflammation and pain. *(See page 156.)*
- Rub a little lavender oil on to the face and jaw to ease pain and distress. *(See page 161.)*

HOMEOPATHY

- Chamomilla, when there is unbearable pain, made worse by cold air, or warm food and drinks. *(See page 204.)*
- Mercurius, for tender spongy gums which bleed easily, and when there is great thirst and shooting pains. *(See page 205.)*
- Apis, when gums feel tight and swollen, and the toothache burns and stings. *(See page 180.)*
- Staphisagria, for severe toothache made worse by cold air, food, and pressure, and where the cheeks are red and swollen.
- Plantago, for nervy teeth, aggravated by cold air and pressure, but which are better on eating.
- Belladonna, for throbbing pain and a dry mouth. *(See page 187.)*
- Aconite, when pain comes on quickly. *(See page 178.)*
- Arnica, for pain after a filling or an extraction. *(See page 182.)*

FLOWER ESSENCES

- Rescue Remedy or Emergency Essence can be applied to the affected area, and taken internally to reduce pain and encourage healing. *(See page 244.)*

DATA FILE

Dental caries is a bacterially-caused destruction of the enamel and dentine of the tooth. If untreated, it leads to an infection of the dental pulp and an abscess of the apex of the tooth. The bacteria produce both acid and enzymes to break down the tooth. Sweet foods that stick to the tooth increase the activity of the bacteria. Saliva tends to protect against caries, so decreased saliva flow usually increases caries. Tooth shape and hereditary factors also determine susceptibility to the disease.

CAUTION

TOOTHACHE IS AN INDICATION OF AN UNDERLYING PROBLEM, WHICH SHOULD BE INVESTIGATED BY A DENTIST IMMEDIATELY.

Tooth Abscess

In cases of badly neglected decay infection may gain access to the root canal of the affected tooth or teeth. Inflammation of the tissues around the root causes tissue destruction and the collection of pus, forming an abscess. A tooth abscess may spread sideways under the gum to form what is known as a gumboil, which may open, giving relief from pain. Plaque re-forms within 24–48 hours of brushing, so regular brushing is essential to prevent decay. Some research shows that allergy sufferers – whose immune activity is heightened – have fewer cases of tooth decay. Periodontal disease is the second most common infectious ailment in the U.S.

SYMPTOMS

• intense pain, which may be intermittent, or continuous and throbbing • increased pain on biting or chewing • swelling and inflammation of the surrounding gum • in severe cases there may be fever

TREATMENT

TRADITIONAL HOME AND FOLK REMEDIES

- Break the large ridges of a cabbage, heat gently, and apply to the abscessed tooth. *(See page 85.)*
- Split a fig and heat it. Apply to the abscessed tooth. *(See page 90.)*
- Rinse your mouth with apple cider vinegar to reduce inflammation and infection. *(See page 102.)*
- Chew fresh sage leaves or garlic, for antiseptic effect. *(See page 82.)*

HERBALISM

- Comfrey mouthwash or ointment will help to heal and draw out the infection. *(See page 132.)*
- Clove oil will reduce inflammation and ease the pain.
- A hot garlic compress, applied to the area, will help to draw out infection and encourage healing. *(See page 113.)*
- A tincture of myrrh can be used as an antiseptic and healing mouthwash.

AROMATHERAPY

- Dab on some clove oil, or suck a clove, for its analgesic and antiseptic properties.
- Make a gargle containing a few drops of antiseptic oils, such as chamomile, clove, lemongrass, or niaouli. *(See pages 146–71.)*

HOMEOPATHY

- Mercurius, where there is copious saliva and the gums are spongy. *(See page 205.)*
- Gunpowder, for the discharge of pus from boils on the gums.
- Hypericum and Calendula, used in solution as a mouthwash. *(See page 199.)*
- Belladonna, at the first hint of an abscess. *(See page 183.)*
- Hep. sulf., when the abscess is in place. *(See page 198.)*

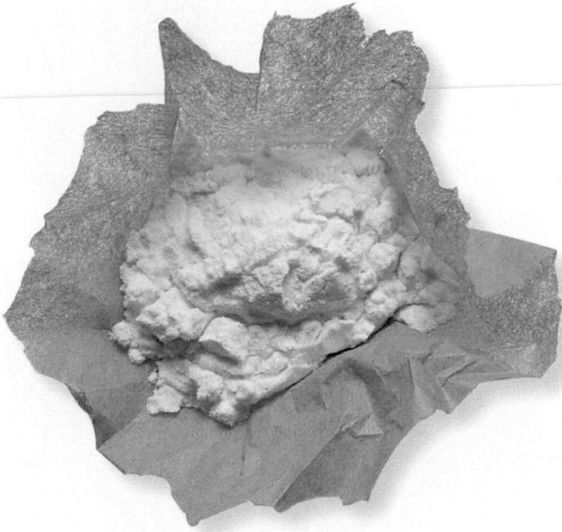

BELOW *Sulfur, the source for Hep. sulf., which is a homeopathic remedy for toothache with an abscess.*

Dental Discomfort (following treatment)

Discomfort following dental treatment is usually caused by injury (perhaps to a nerve) or bruising around the tooth that has been worked on. This may occur immediately after treatment, or pain may follow initial discomfort after an anesthetic has worn off. There may also be some blood loss. Persistent pain following treatment may signal infection.

RIGHT *Arnica root, a source of the homeopathic remedy Arnica which can be used after dental treatment.*

TREATMENT

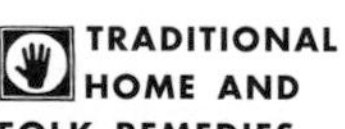

TRADITIONAL HOME AND FOLK REMEDIES
• Oil of clove or macerated cloves can be applied to the area to prevent infection, reduce the inflammation and prevent discomfort. *(See page 90.)*

HOMEOPATHY
• Arnica should be taken immediately after treatment, every hour for up to 10 doses. *(See page 182.)*
• Ruta, for infections after teeth have been removed. *(See page 210.)*
• Phosphorus, for bleeding after a tooth has been extracted. Take every 10 minutes for 1 hour. *(See page 208.)*
• Hypericum, for pain occurring after treatment. *(See page 199.)*
• Ledum, for pain after an injection. *(See page 202.)*

FLOWER ESSENCES
• Rescue Remedy or Emergency Essence will help to reduce the effects of trauma, and encourage the healing process. *(See page 244.)*

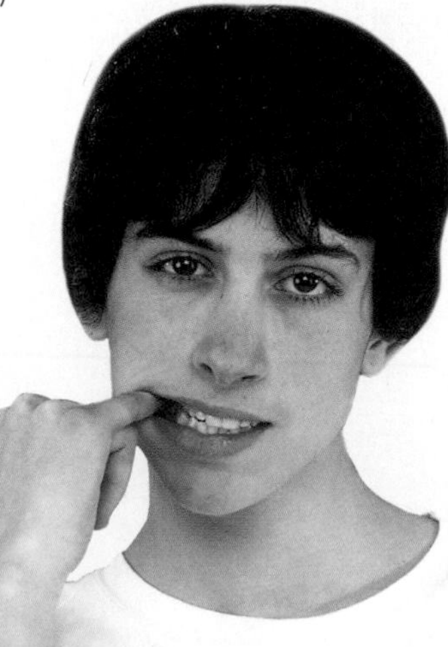

LEFT *Oil of cloves can be gently applied to the painful area inside the mouth.*

Grinding of Teeth

Habitual grinding or clenching of the teeth is known as bruxism. It is usually performed unconsciously, but is audible to others. It is common among children and the elderly, and often occurs during sleep. In severe cases the enamel of the teeth may be worn away. There may be some links with anxiety and with alcohol consumption.

TREATMENT

AYURVEDA
• An Ayurvedic medical practitioner would balance the tri-doshas, and use panchakarma for balancing the vátha. *(See page 22.)*

CHINESE HERBALISM
• A Chinese herbalist might suggest ginseng, Chinese angelica, and white peony root with thorowax root for relaxation. Treatment would be designed to strengthen the Spleen and enliven Liver qi. *(See pages 56 and 67.)*

TRADITIONAL HOME AND FOLK REMEDIES
• Oats contain thiamine and pantothenic acid, which are gentle nerve tonics. *(See page 84.)*

HERBALISM
• Herbal remedies would be used to calm the nervous system and to relax you. Skullcap and valerian are useful herbs, blended together for best effect. Drink this as a tea 3 times daily while suffering the symptoms. *(See pages 131 and 136.)*
• Lady's slipper and limeflowers may ease anxiety and tension that may exacerbate the condition. *(See page 134.)*

AROMATHERAPY
• A relaxing blend of essential oils of lavender, geranium, and bergamot in sweet almond oil or peach kernel oil may be added to the bath to calm nerves and prevent attacks. *(See pages 146–71.)*

HOMEOPATHY
Constitutional treatment will be appropriate if there are emotional causes, but some of the following remedies may be useful:
• Arsenicum, for grinding of teeth during sleep, especially between midnight and 2 or 3A.M. *(See page 182.)*
• Zinc, when the gums bleed and teeth become loose.
• Phytolacca, when there is an overwhelming urge to clench the teeth.

FLOWER ESSENCES
• Remedies would be useful if there is an emotional cause underlying the condition. *(See page 244.)*
• Elm, for anxiety accompanying a feeling of being unable to cope. *(See page 241.)*
• Red chestnut, for anxiety over the welfare of others. *(See page 224.)*
• Aspen, for anxiety for no apparent reason. *(See page 236.)*

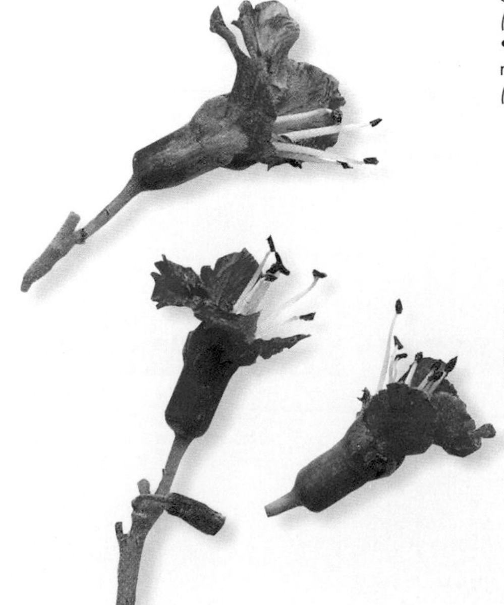

LEFT *Red chestnut is one of the flower essences that may help with the emotional causes of tooth grinding.*

Fear of Dental Treatment

Fear of dental treatment (dental phobia) is an extremely common phenomenon – some studies show that nearly 80 percent of the U.S. population suffer some feelings of fear about dental treatment. Full-scale phobia is one of the most common types of phobia in both the U.K. and the U.S. Sufferers develop intense feelings of anxiety and panic from an association between dentists and pain and discomfort, despite the fact that modern dental technology has eliminated much of the pain of treatment. Both adults and children may be affected (children are particularly vulnerable if they sense that their parents are frightened).

Most modern dentists are aware of the nervousness affecting many people, and may offer home visits or sedation, anesthetics, hypnosis, and other forms of relaxation. Relaxation for Living, in the U.K., has produced a pamphlet called "Don't Dread the Dentist", with tips for overcoming dental phobia. (*See also Phobias, page* 282.)

RIGHT *Aconite leaves, the source for Aconite, a homeopathic remedy for acute fear.*

Symptoms

- *rapid pulse* • *profuse sweating*
- *high blood pressure* • *trembling*
- *nausea*

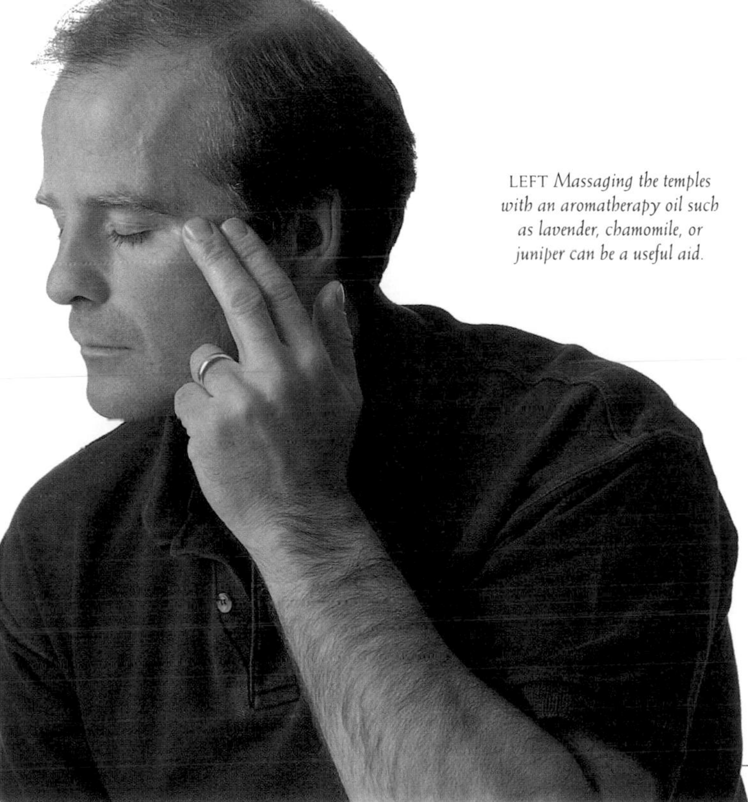

LEFT *Massaging the temples with an aromatherapy oil such as lavender, chamomile, or juniper can be a useful aid.*

TREATMENT

AYURVEDA
- Lemon or lime may be suggested for dizziness, and individual treatment would be prescribed according to your specific needs. *(See page 20.)*

CHINESE HERBALISM
- A herbalist may prescribe cooling herbs, and Gui Pi Wan, to help with emotional problems.
- Ginseng and Chinese angelica and senega root may also be useful. *(See pages 56, 67 and 70.)*

HERBALISM
- Valerian tea can help to reduce tension. Drink an infusion as required. *(See page 136.)*

AROMATHERAPY
- The effect of certain smells can help to release tension and induce a feeling of calm. Some of the best oils to try are bergamot, chamomile, clary sage, geranium, jasmine, juniper, lavender, marjoram, melissa, and ylang ylang, which are sedative. They can be used in the bath, in massage with a light carrier oil (such as sweet almond), or in a vaporizer. Carry a bottle of diluted oils with you and apply to the temples or pulse points before dental treatment. *(See pages 146–71.)*

HOMEOPATHY
- Aconite, for intense fear. Take before and after treatment. *(See page 178.)*
- Gelsemium, for shaking and weak legs and knees, and overall apprehension. *(See page 195.)*
- Chamomilla, for a child who throws a tantrum about seeing the dentist. *(See page 204.)*

FLOWER ESSENCES
- Mimulus, for fear of known things. Make a personal remedy, and take a few drops every time you think of the dentist. Take hourly before going for treatment. *(See page 235.)*
- Rescue Remedy or Emergency Essence will help to reduce feelings of fear and panic. Take hourly before treatment, and also during treatment. *(See page 244.)*

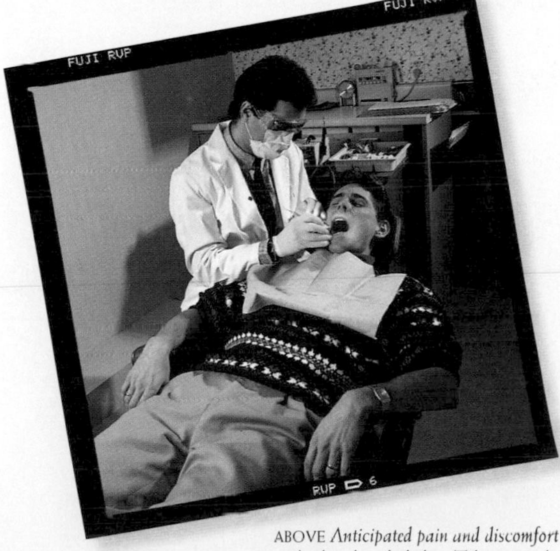

ABOVE *Anticipated pain and discomfort can lead to dental phobia. Taking remedies to overcome feelings of fear, tension, and apprehension can help.*

MOUTH AND THROAT PROBLEMS

Sore Throat

A sore throat (or pharyngitis) is an inflammation of the pharynx – the area of the throat between the back of the nose and the beginning of the trachea and vocal cords. It is usually caused by infection, which can be viral or bacterial in origin. A sore throat is a feature of illnesses such as tonsillitis and may also signal the onset of glandular fever, flu, or scarlet fever. If scarlet fever is not treated with antibiotics it may lead to rheumatic flu or kidney failure. Inflammation of the throat can also be caused by heavy smoking or drinking, abuse of gargles or mouthwashes, general vitamin deficiency, or food allergy; it can also be a symptom of blood disorders such as anemia. A sore throat will usually resolve itself in a few days, but infection, accompanied by high fever and malaise, may take up to three weeks. Streptococcal sore throat, or strep throat, is an inflammation of the throat and tonsils caused by bacteria and is the most common type of strep infection. Onset is usually sudden and is accompanied by pain, redness, and swelling in throat tissues, pus on the tonsils, fever, headache, and malaise. If left untreated, strep throat can lead to rheumatic fever.

SYMPTOMS

• *boarseness and thirst* • *pain, causing difficulty in swallowing* • *possibly a burning sensation* • *slight fever* • *enlarged and tender lymph nodes in the neck* • *possibly earache*

CAUTION

DO NOT TAKE GOLDEN SEAL WHILE PREGNANT.

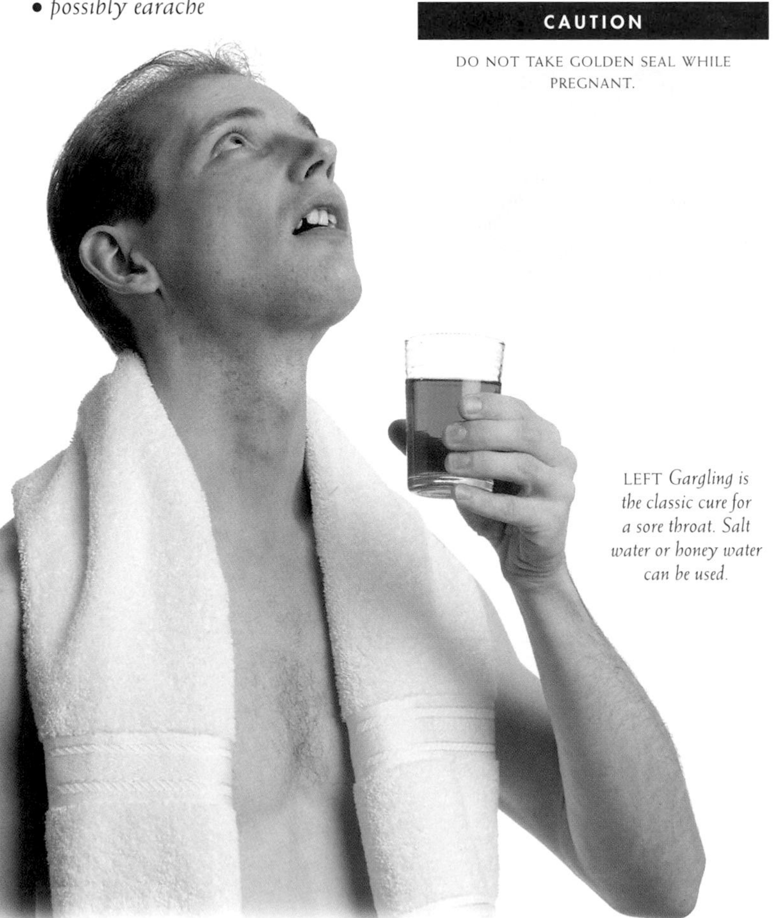

LEFT *Gargling is the classic cure for a sore throat. Salt water or honey water can be used.*

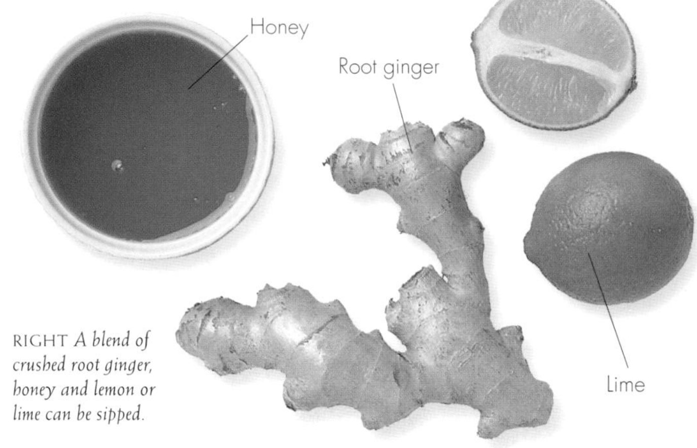

RIGHT *A blend of crushed root ginger, honey and lemon or lime can be sipped.*

TREATMENT

AYURVEDA
• Dasamoola rasayna, an oral syrup, will treat a sore throat.
• Crush a piece of root ginger to extract the juice, and add to a tablespoon of honey and 3 tablespoons of lime. Sip 4 times a day.
(See page 47.)

CHINESE HERBALISM
• Yin Qiao Jie du Pian pills, for a sore throat accompanied by flu symptoms, swollen lymph nodes, and headaches.
• Sang Ju Gan Mao Pian or Sang Ju Yin Pian, for a sore throat with symptoms of cold.
• Liu Wei di Huang Wan, for Kidney Yin-Deficient sore throat. Also for chronic dry sore throat, with hot palms and soles, and night sweats.
• Honeysuckle tea may be useful. *(See page 65.)*

TRADITIONAL HOME AND FOLK REMEDIES
• Gargle with salt water to ease symptoms and reduce inflammation.
(See page 103.)
• Apply an apple cider vinegar compress to the throat to ease symptoms.
(See page 102.)
• Gargle with honey water, which acts to encourage healing and deal with infection.
(See page 101.)
• White cabbage juice is anti-inflammatory and will draw out infection.
(See page 85.)
• A hot honey and lemon drink will reduce symptoms and encourage healing. *(See pages 87 and 101.)*

HERBALISM
• Eat fresh garlic whenever possible, to absorb its antibacterial and antiviral properties.
(See page 113.)
• A gargle of red sage will help to soothe a sore throat. *(See page 129.)*
• Golden seal powder, added to a cup of hot water, can be infused and drunk as required.
• Tincture of calendula can be added to a cup of boiled water for a mouthwash to encourage healing and treat infection. *(See page 117.)*
• Burdock or comfrey teas will ease the pain. *(See pages 115 and 132.)*

AROMATHERAPY
• A steam inhalation of benzoin, lavender, or thyme will ease the discomfort and help to treat the infection.
(See pages 146–71.)
• Massage a little lavender oil, blended in a light carrier oil, into the neck. *(See page 161.)*
• Dab the throat with diluted tea tree oil on a cotton bud – it is analgesic and fights infection, which will help to ease symptoms and treat the cause.
(See page 162.)

HOMEOPATHY
• Belladonna, for sore throat accompanied by a red face and fever.
(See page 183.)
• Gelsemium, when swallowing is painful, with weakness, exhaustion, pain in the neck and ears.
(See page 195.)
• Apis, when the pain is worse on the right side of the body, and improves after cold drinks.
(See page 180.)
• Lachesis, when pain is worse on the left side, there is a feeling of constriction, and pain is worse when swallowing saliva but better when swallowing food.
(See page 216.)
• Aconite, for a sore throat that comes on suddenly, with a burning throat and swollen tonsils.
(See page 178.)

VITAMINS AND MINERALS
• Increase vitamin C intake. *(See page 256.)*
• Suck a zinc lozenge.
(See page 265.)

Tonsillitis

Tonsillitis is an inflammation of the tonsils located at the back of the throat. It is generally due to either viral or bacterial infection (often by the streptococcal bacteria), and causes swelling and redness of the tonsils, possibly with white or yellow spots of pus. The adenoids may also become inflamed and infected. Tonsillitis can occur at any time but is particularly common during childhood. In rare cases complications such as quinsy (an abscess behind the tonsil), kidney inflammation, or rheumatic fever may develop.

Symptoms

- *swelling and tenderness of the lymph nodes in the neck* • *sore throat with pain on swallowing* • *headache, earache, and general weakness and malaise* • *fever* • *bad breath*
- *constipation*

DATA FILE

- Tonsillitis is more common in children than in adults.
- Tonsillitis usually develops suddenly as a result of a streptococcal infection but may also be caused by a viral infection.
- In chronic tonsillitis the tonsils tend to flare up in episodes of acute infection, causing scarring that makes them difficult to treat in subsequent attacks.

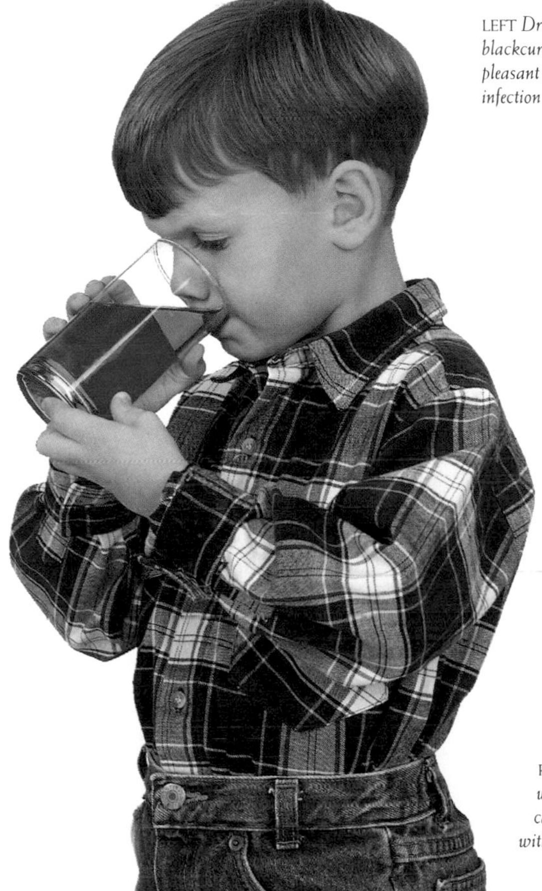

LEFT *Drinking hot blackcurrant juice is a pleasant way to treat the infection causing tonsillitis.*

TREATMENT

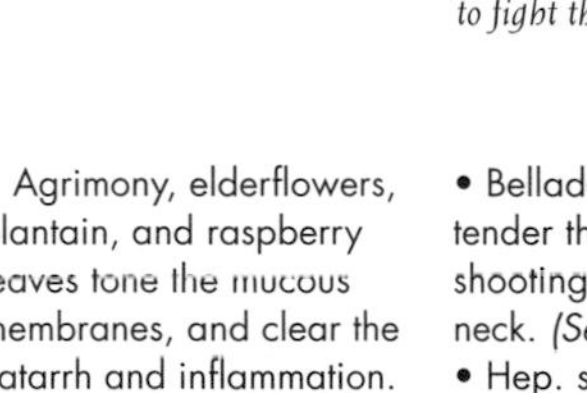

ABOVE *Applying tea tree oil direct to the tonsils can help to fight the infection.*

AYURVEDA

- Apply a cloth with mustard oil to the forehead to ease the pain and reduce fever. *(See page 30.)*
- Root ginger can be chewed, and mixed with honey and lemon to make a soothing drink. *(See page 47.)*

CHINESE HERBALISM

- Treatment would be aimed at Fire, Poison, Wind, and Heat. Avoid spicy food and drink honeysuckle tea. *(See page 65.)*

TRADITIONAL HOME AND FOLK REMEDIES

- Blackcurrant tea or juice (hot) will treat infection and relieve the sore throat.
- Drink plenty of hot honey and lemon or honey and apple cider vinegar to fight infection and boost immunity. *(See pages 87, 101, and 102.)*

HERBALISM

- A red sage gargle will address infection and reduce symptoms. *(See page 129.)*
- Herbs to boost the immune system include echinacea, garlic, myrrh, sage, and wild indigo. *(See pages 113, 129, and 130.)*
- Cleavers, marigold, and poke root will help the lymphatic system. *(See page 117.)*
- Herbs to reduce fever by inducing sweating are chamomile, elderflowers, yarrow, and limeflowers. *(See pages 112, 119, 130, and 134.)*
- Agrimony, elderflowers, plantain, and raspberry leaves tone the mucous membranes, and clear the catarrh and inflammation. *(See pages 112, 126, 128, and 130.)*
- Herbs to soothe painful tonsils include comfrey, marshmallow, and mullein. *(See pages 114, 132, and 137.)*

AROMATHERAPY

- Thyme oil is a powerful antiseptic and has a local anesthetic effect to reduce the discomfort. Use in a vaporizer, and add to a light carrier oil and massage into the neck. *(See page 170.)*
- Lavender and benzoin can be added to a cup of cooled, boiled water and gargled. *(See pages 161 and 170.)*
- Tea tree oil, applied neat to the tonsils on the end of a cotton bud, fights infection and discomfort. *(See page 162.)*

HOMEOPATHY

Chronic tonsillitis must be treated constitutionally, but for acute conditions try:

- Belladonna, for a sore, tender throat, with shooting pains and a stiff neck. *(See page 183.)*
- Hep. sulf., for a feeling that there is a fishbone caught in the throat, and when pain is alleviated by warm drinks, the breath is foul, and there is yellow pus. *(See page 198.)*
- Lycopodium, for a throat sore on the right side, and where the tongue is dry and puffy but not coated, the throat is better after cold drinks, and worse between 4 and 8A.M. or P.M. *(See page 203.)*
- Mercurius, when the throat is dark red, swollen, and sore, and worse on the right side, and when the breath smells and there are hot sweats. *(See page 205.)*
- Phytolacca, for a rough, constricted, hot throat, with red, swollen tonsils and pain extending to the ears. The throat is worse on the right side and with heat.

VITAMINS AND MINERALS

- Cod liver oil tablets, along with vitamin C and garlic, will speed up the healing process. *(See page 256.)*

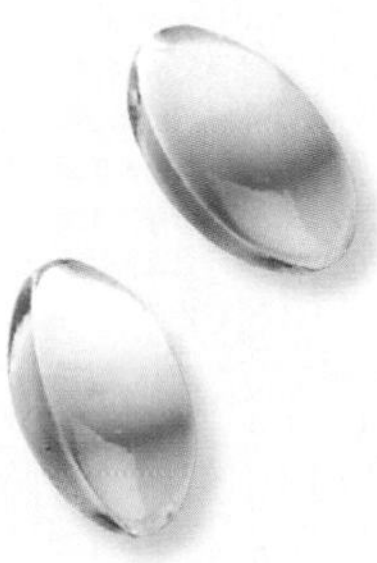

RIGHT *Cod liver oil, which can be taken in capsule form, can help with the healing process.*

Laryngitis

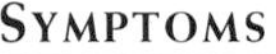

Laryngitis is an inflammation of the voice box (the larynx) in which the larynx and vocal cords become swollen and sore, distorting the vocal apparatus. Acute laryngitis is usually a complication of a sore throat, cold, or other upper respiratory tract infection, and should last for only a few days. It can also be an allergic reaction to inhaled pollen. Chronic laryngitis is more persistent and may be caused by long-term irritation from smoking, overuse of the voice, or excessive coughing. It can be an occupational hazard for singers and teachers.

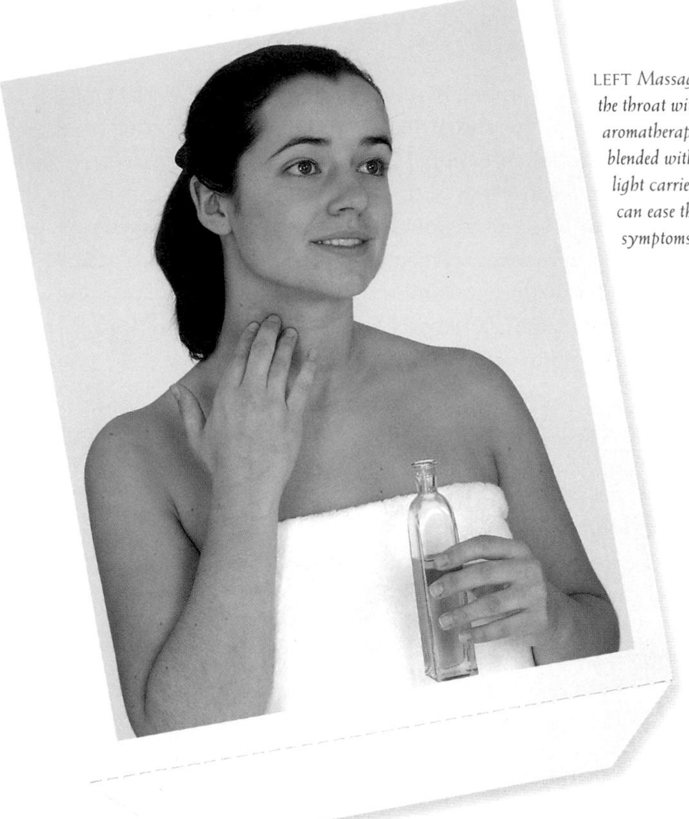

LEFT *Massaging the throat with aromatherapy oils blended with a light carrier oil can ease the symptoms.*

Symptoms

- *the throat is inflamed and mucus-coated in acute laryngitis*
- *the larynx is dry and inflamed in chronic laryngitis*
- *hoarseness*
- *difficulty in raising the voice above a whisper*
- *dry, irritating cough*

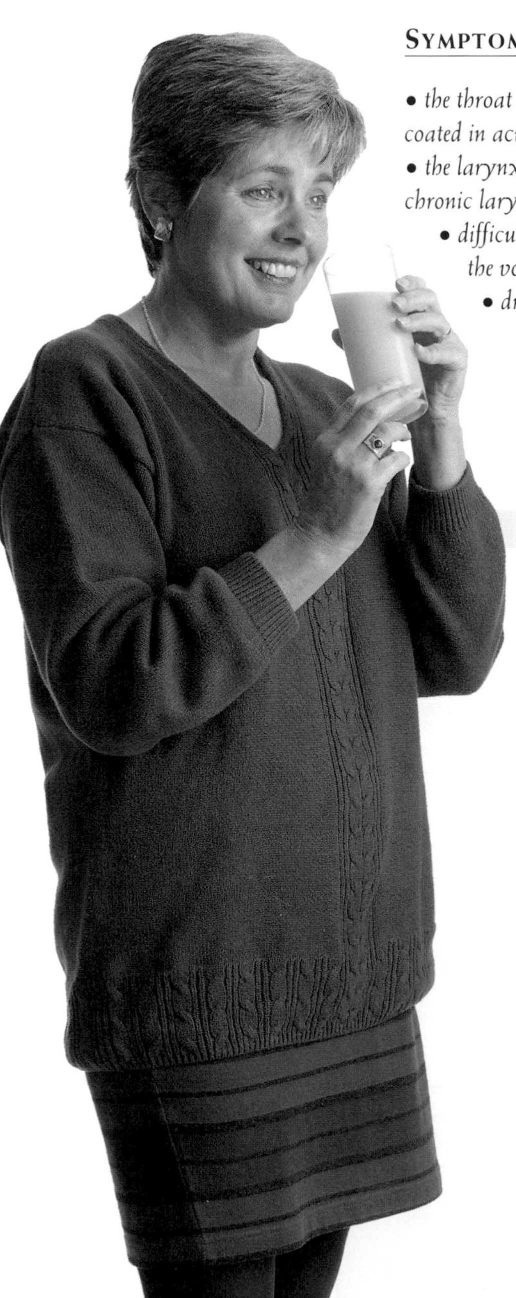

LEFT *Plenty of vitamin C is required in the diet to combat infection. Drinking freshly pressed orange juice can help.*

TREATMENT

AYURVEDA

• Hollyhock is useful for throat inflammation.

CHINESE HERBALISM

• Treatment would address poisoned Heat in the lungs, and the following herbs may be appropriate: peppermint, honeysuckle flowers, mulberry, lily, and licorice. *(See pages 64 and 65.)*

TRADITIONAL HOME AND FOLK REMEDIES

• Drink a glass of honey and lemon or honey and apple cider vinegar in hot water as required to reduce any inflammation and infection, and encourage healing. *(See pages 87, 101, and 102.)*

RIGHT *A glass of warm lemon and honey is a tried and tested home treatment.*

HERBALISM

• Drink an infusion of red sage, or gargle, to reduce inflammation. *(See page 129.)*

• Echinacea both treats and prevents laryngitis – drink infusion 3 times daily. *(See page 120.)*

AROMATHERAPY

• Gargle with a drop of geranium, pepper, rosemary, or tea tree oil in a glass of boiled water, as required, to prevent and treat inflammation and infection. *(See pages 146–71.)*

• Massage the throat area with a drop of lavender or tea tree oil in a light carrier oil. *(See pages 161 and 162.)*

• Try a steam inhalation of sandalwood or thyme to ease inflammation and reduce infection. *(See pages 169 and 170.)*

HOMEOPATHY

Treatment would be constitutional, but some of the following remedies may help:

• Aconite, when symptoms come on suddenly, and there is restlessness and anxiety. *(See page 178.)*

• Spongia, for a dry, barking cough – particularly useful for croup. *(See page 213.)*

• Lachesis, for chronic laryngitis, particularly if you talk a great deal. *(See page 216.)*

• Hep. sulf., when symptoms are worse in the morning and after exposure to cold; symptoms are accompanied by a loose cough and a choking feeling. *(See page 198.)*

• Apis, where the problem has been caused or exacerbated by allergy, and there is redness and swelling. *(See page 180.)*

• Ignatia, when the condition sets in after a trauma of some sort. *(See page 200.)*

• Baryta carb., when you lose your voice often, without any obvious cause. *(See page 185.)*

VITAMINS AND MINERALS

• Eat a diet rich in vitamin C to increase resistance to infection. *(See page 256.)*

• Avoid alcohol.

Oral Thrush

Oral thrush is a fungal infection which appears as raised creamy spots on the lining of the mouth, lips, and throat. The Candida albicans fungus occurs naturally in the mouth and other moist, warm areas of the body, but if excessive growth is allowed to take place infection can result. This may occur if the bacteria that usually keep it in check are themselves under attack by antibiotics, or if the immune system is compromised for any other reason. Oral thrush is most common in the young and elderly, and in people who wear dentures. Women also appear to be more susceptible than men.

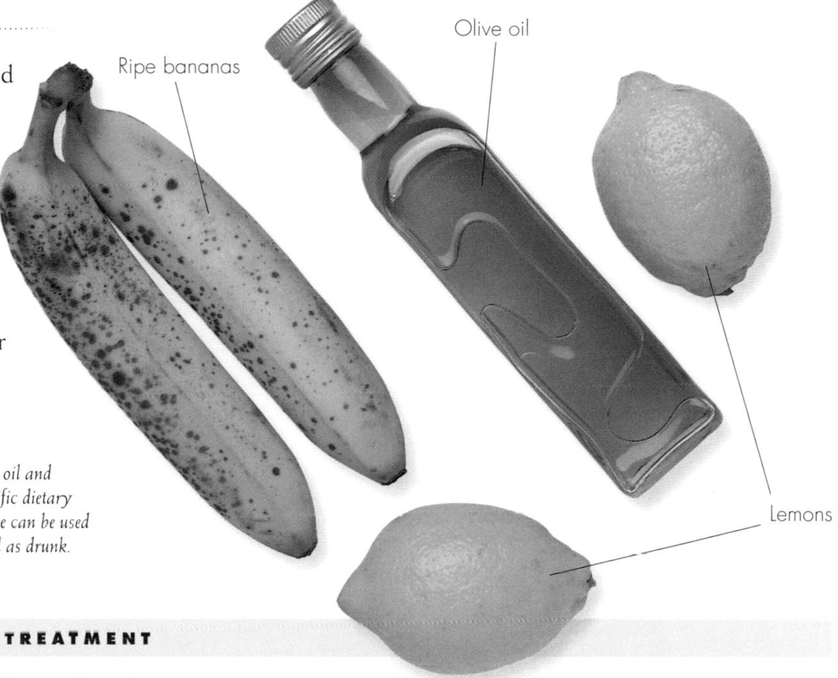

RIGHT *Olive oil and bananas are specific dietary aids, and lemon juice can be used externally as well as drunk.*

Symptoms

- *pain, soreness, and irritation in the affected area*
- *raised creamy spots in the mouth*

TREATMENT

CHINESE HERBALISM
- Gentian and Oriental wormwood may be prescribed to treat fungal infections of the mouth.

TRADITIONAL HOME AND FOLK REMEDIES
- Eat fresh live yogurt, and dab on to the affected patches, as required. *(See page 93.)*
- Olive oil prevents yeast becoming fungus in the body, and should be drunk or used in cooking, as often as possible. *(See page 95.)*
- Rub raw garlic on to the affected areas, and incorporate plenty of raw garlic into your diet. *(See page 82.)*
- Lemon will help to soothe discomfort and encourage healing. Drink a cup of hot lemon and honey in water 3 times daily. *(See page 87.)*

HERBALISM
- Aloe vera mouthwash has an antifungal effect. *(See page 114.)*
- Barberry prevents the growth of fungus, and stimulates the immune system. Take 3 times daily.
- Caprylic acid is a good antifungal agent. Take 3 capsules with each meal.
- Chew fresh juniper berries to reduce inflammation and attack the Candida fungus.

AROMATHERAPY
- Add a few drops of myrrh, tea tree, or lavender oil to a cup of boiled water and rinse the mouth several times daily to destroy fungal infection. *(See pages 146–71.)*

HOMEOPATHY
Constitutional treatment to boost immunity will be offered, but the following remedies may also be useful:
- Capsicum, when patches are hot and sore and worse after cold drinks.
- Borax, at first symptoms.
- Arsenicum, for thrush associated with mouth ulcers and which occurs when you are run down. *(See page 182.)*
- Mercurius, when your tongue is hot and trembling, and you have more saliva than usual. *(See page 205.)*

VITAMINS AND MINERALS
- Take acidophilus tablets, and eat plenty of ripe bananas to encourage the growth of healthy bacteria in the body, which will reduce the severity of attacks and act to prevent them. *(See page 271.)*

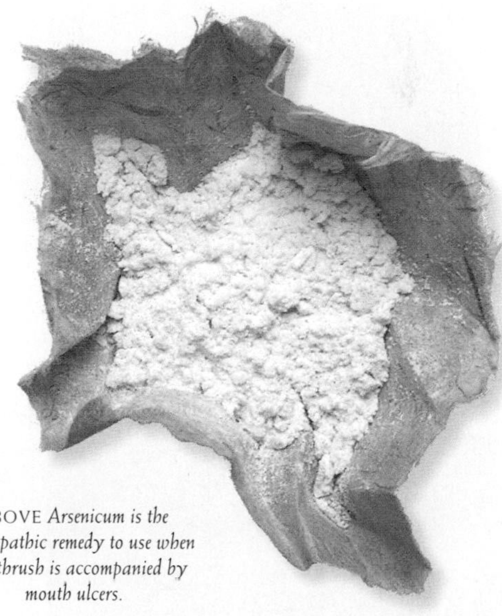

ABOVE *Arsenicum is the homeopathic remedy to use when oral thrush is accompanied by mouth ulcers.*

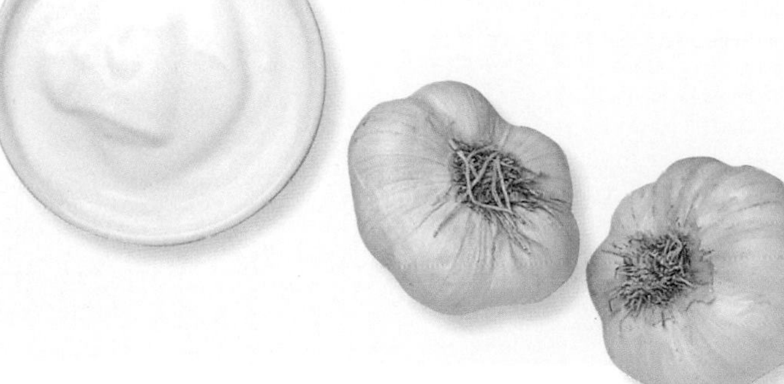

RIGHT *Yogurt and garlic and both beneficial. They can be applied to the sore area and added to the diet.*

Mouth Ulcers

Mouth ulcers are white, gray, or yellow open sores with an outer ring of red inflammation, and occur when the mucous membrane or skin surface becomes pitted, resulting from an erosion or disintegration of the tissues. They appear on the inside of the lips, cheeks, or floor of the mouth, and may occur as a result of aggressive tooth brushing, ill-fitting dentures, accidentally biting the side of the mouth, or eating very hot food. They can also be triggered by stress or being run down, and can be a feature of Crohn's disease, ulcerative colitis, and coeliac disease, or food allergy. Women may be particularly prone to mouth ulcers around menstruation. In children, contact with the herpes simplex virus that causes cold sores may manifest itself as mouth ulcers. Mouth ulcers are common, affecting one in five U.S. adults.

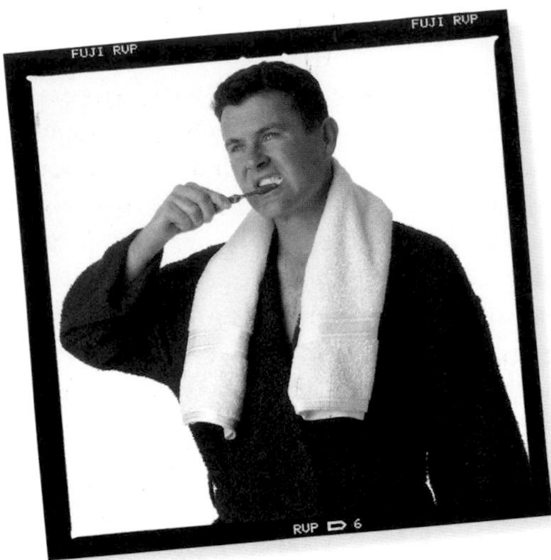

ABOVE *Mouth ulcers can occur as a result of brushing the teeth too vigorously.*

SYMPTOMS

• *pain and stinging in affected area, particularly when eating acidic or spicy foods* • *dry mouth*

TREATMENT

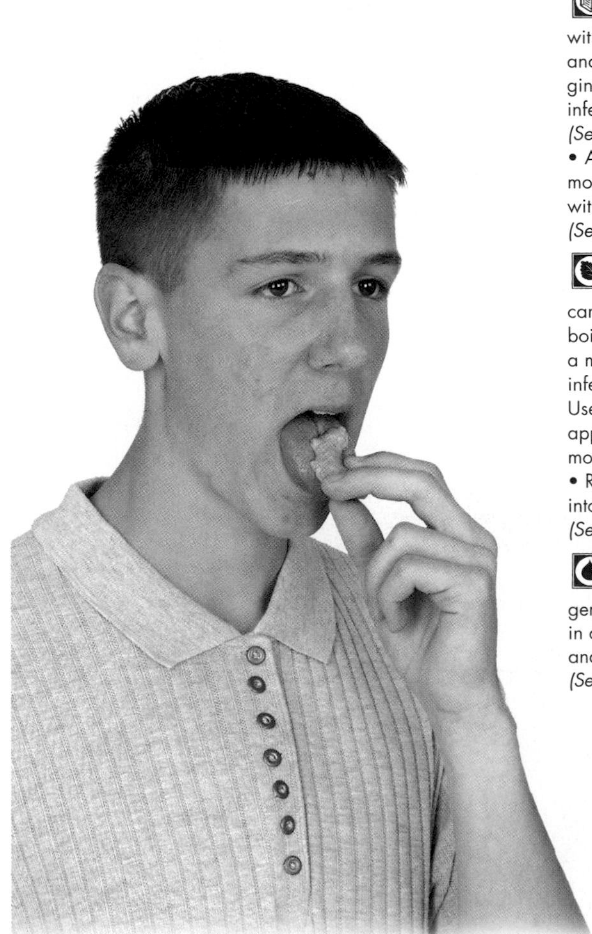

LEFT *Rubbing the tongue with a piece of fresh ginger root is good for some infections of the mouth.*

AYURVEDA

• Rub the tongue with a piece of ginger, and chew fresh root ginger to treat fungal infections of the mouth. *(See page 47.)*

• Aloe vera is useful for mouth ulcers associated with the herpes virus. *(See page 27.)*

HERBALISM

• Tincture of myrrh can be added to a cup of boiled water and used as a mouth rinse to destroy infection or infestation. Use the tincture neat and apply to sores in the mouth with a cotton bud.

• Rub a little aloe vera gel into the affected area. *(See page 114.)*

AROMATHERAPY

• Mix a drop of geranium and lavender oil in a cup of boiled water and gargle as required. *(See pages 161 and 165.)*

HOMEOPATHY

• Arsenicum, when ulcers are on the edges of the tongue, with burning pains. *(See page 182.)*

• Mercurius, for ulcers that erupt on the palate or tongue, and which are yellow and spongy. *(See page 205.)*

• Kali bich., for ulcers that feel thick and firm, and sting. *(See page 200.)*

VITAMINS AND MINERALS

• Take supplements of vitamin A, E, and B2. *(See pages 252, 253, and 257.)*

• Vitamin E oil can be applied directly to the ulcers. *(See page 257.)*

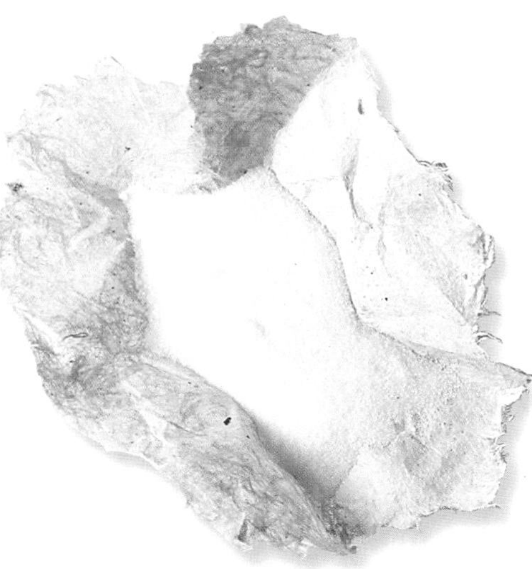

ABOVE *Use the homeopathic remedy Kali bich. when ulcers feel thick and firm, and sting.*

Bad Breath

Bad breath (or halitosis) is often caused by accumulated food debris as a result of poor dental hygiene, smoking, and alcohol consumption. It may be accompanied by dribbling during sleep and a yellowish, thickly coated tongue. Bad breath can also be a symptom of many disorders including gingivitis, tonsillitis, sinusitis, oral thrush, diabetes, acute bronchitis, liver failure, cancer of the mouth, throat, larynx, lungs, or esophagus, chronic gastritis, underproduction of saliva, and constipation.

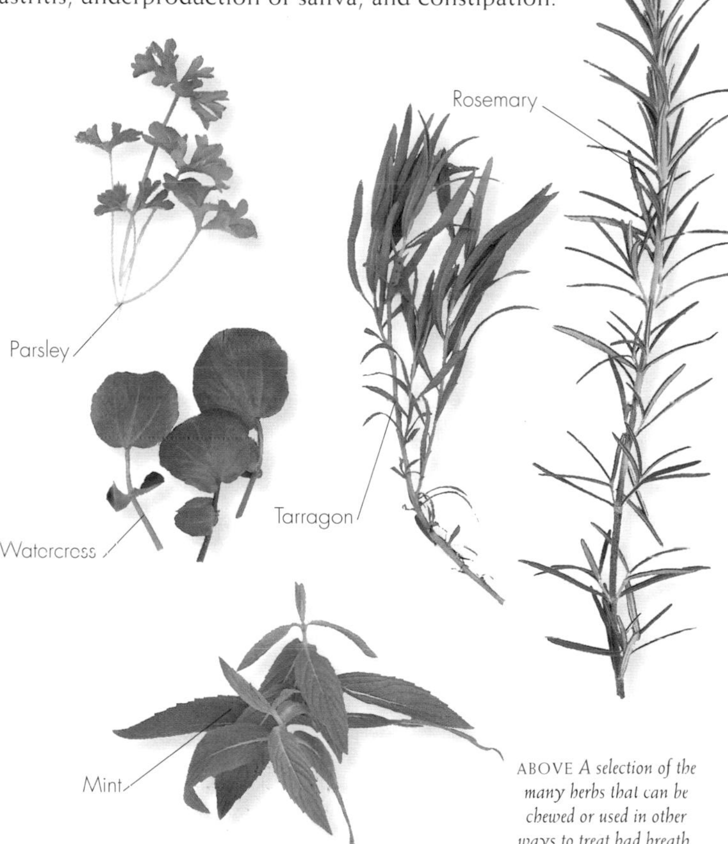

ABOVE *A selection of the many herbs that can be chewed or used in other ways to treat bad breath.*

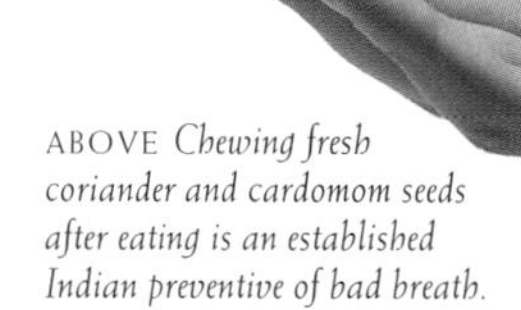

ABOVE *Chewing fresh coriander and cardomom seeds after eating is an established Indian preventive of bad breath.*

TREATMENT

AYURVEDA
- Chew fresh coriander or cardamom seeds after meals – they will act as a digestive and discourage bad breath. *(See pages 35, 38.)*

CHINESE HERBALISM
- Treatment would be aimed at stomach damp heat, using golden thread, peppermint tea, giant hyssop, and radish seeds. *(See page 54 and 61.)*

TRADITIONAL HOME AND FOLK REMEDIES
- Drink a combination of fresh carrot, celery, watercress, and cucumber juice with some paprika. *(See pages 83, 86, 89, and 94.)*

HERBALISM
- Chew fresh rosemary leaves, or make a mouthwash with a pinch of cloves, cinnamon, anise seed, and rosemary. Steep in a cup of sherry for a week, and then strain. Use daily as required. *(See page 127.)*
- Chew fresh watercress, which is rich in chlorophyll and vitamin C.
- Chew walnut bark and rub it on the gums, then gargle with lemon water.
- Chew fresh parsley, thyme, mint, or tarragon. *(See page 135.)*

AROMATHERAPY
- Add a drop of myrrh essential oil to a cup of cool, boiled water, and rinse the mouth daily. *(See page 155.)*
- Thyme or fennel oil will be equally effective. *(See pages 159 and 170.)*

HOMEOPATHY
- Nux vomica, for breath that smells sour, particularly after meals or drinking alcohol. *(See page 214.)*
- Petroselinium, for breath that smells of onions.
- Nitric acid for bad breath with loose teeth and mouth ulcers.
- Pulsatilla for bad breath after eating fatty foods, and which is accompanied by a dry mouth and no thirst. *(See page 209.)*
- Mercurius, for breath that smells, with copious saliva and a yellow, furry tongue. *(See page 205.)*

VITAMINS AND MINERALS
- Store your toothbrush in grapefruit seed extract to destroy bacteria and other germs which may be encouraging bad breath.

Cold Sores

Cold sores are fluid-filled blisters which crust over after bursting. They usually appear on the mouth and around the lips, sometimes in clusters. They are caused by viral infection (herpes simplex). Most of us are exposed to the herpes simplex virus by the age of five, and can carry an immunity to it. In children who do not successfully fight off the virus, cold sores are manifested as painful mouth ulcers, which appear when the sufferer is run down, or when the immune system is depressed or overstressed. Once you succumb to the virus, you may carry it for the rest of your life, and attacks may be triggered by extremes of weather, or by being run down. In some women, cold sores are worse, or appear more often, during menstruation. There is some evidence that cold sores may be linked to atherosclerosis. Cold sores are highly contagious. *(See under Skin and Hair, page 308.)*

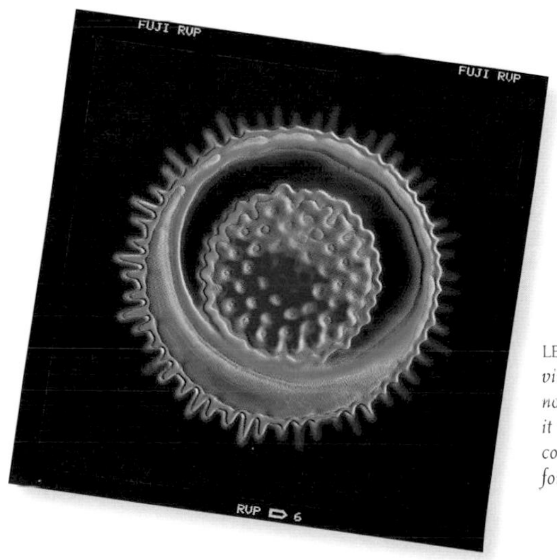

LEFT *The herpes simplex virus. If immunity is not acquired to this virus, it may manifest itself as cold sores periodically for life.*

LUNG AND RESPIRATORY DISORDERS

Tuberculosis

More commonly known as TB, tuberculosis is an infectious disease caused by three species of bacteria. The infecting bacteria enter the body through the digestive tract (often in unpasteurized milk from infected cows), or may be spread by person-to-person droplet infection. The lungs are usually the first organs to be affected, but the lymph nodes, the skin, and bones are all possible targets. The disease is most common in areas where poor housing, diet, and sanitation are predisposing factors, or where the immune system is compromised (as in HIV/AIDS). Once established, TB can cause complications such as tuberculosis pleurisy and tuberculosis meningitis. In its latent phase, the disease causes a lesion at the infected site which leaves a characteristic scar but no associated symptoms. If the lesion does not heal, then progressive pulmonary tuberculosis (consumption) develops, causing symptoms in its active phase.

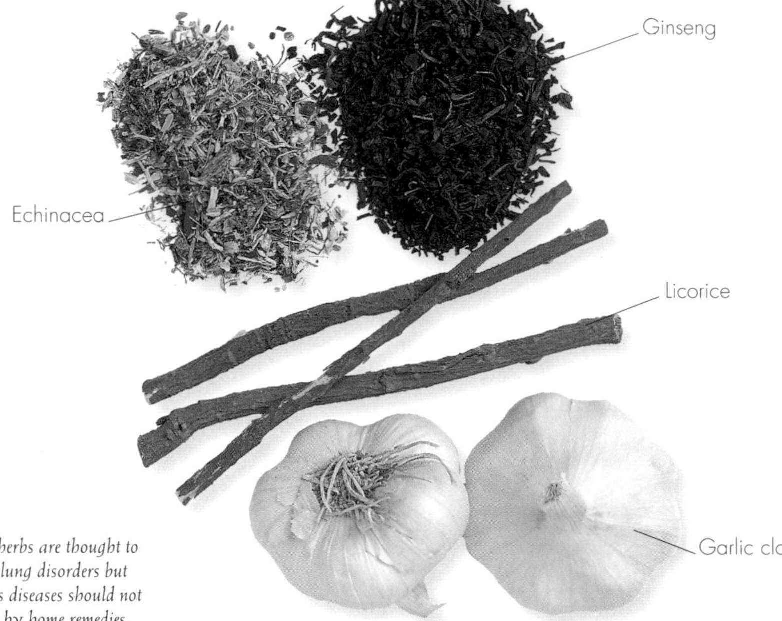

ABOVE *Several herbs are thought to help in cases of lung disorders but potentially serious diseases should not be treated solely by home remedies.*

SYMPTOMS

- *loss of appetite* • *fever* • *persistent cough with blood-stained mucus*
- *night sweats* • *fatigue*
- *marked weight loss*

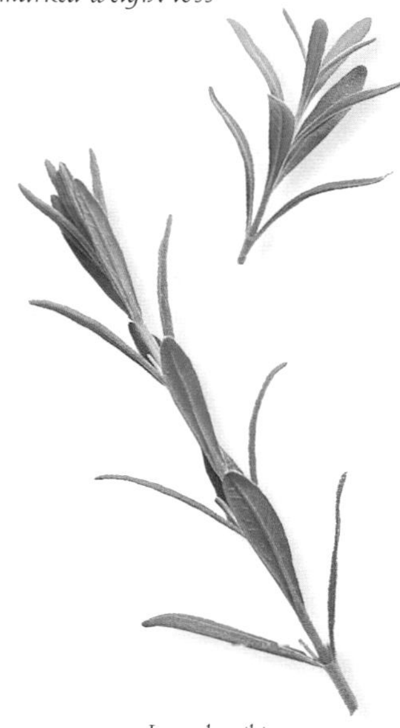

ABOVE *Lavender oil is one of the antibacterial oils that can help to prevent infections.*

CAUTION

IF TB IS SUSPECTED, SEE YOUR PHYSICIAN IMMEDIATELY.

TREATMENT

AYURVEDA
• Stramonium will help with bronchial spasm and congestion.

HERBALISM
Herbs to boost the immune system would be most appropriate:
• Licorice helps recovery, stimulating formation and efficiency of white blood cells and antibodies.
• Garlic helps to prevent many infections, including those which have become immune to antibiotics. *(See page 113.)*
• Echinacea is widely used for chronic and acute infections, cleansing the blood and lymphatic system, stimulating the production of white blood cells and antibodies. *(See page 120.)*
• Ginseng can boost immunity, as well as stimulating white blood cell production and aiding recovery after illness. *(See page 126.)*

AROMATHERAPY
• Anti-infectious oils which can be used in a vaporizer include: garlic, tea tree, and lavender. *(See pages 146–71.)*
• Use antibacterial oils to prevent further infection, such as juniper, rosemary, bergamot, or eucalyptus. *(See pages 146–71.)*

HOMEOPATHY
The following remedies may help alongside conventional treatment, or alone under the guidance of an experienced homeopath:
• Baccillinum, for fever and weight loss.
• Arsenicum, for exhaustion, chilliness, and a thirst for small sips of water. *(See page 182.)*
• Calcarea, for weakness, fever, cold hands and feet. *(See page 186.)*

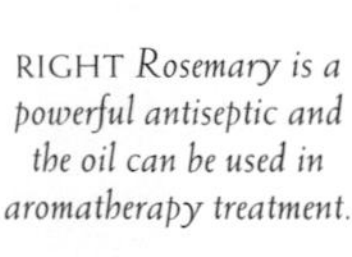

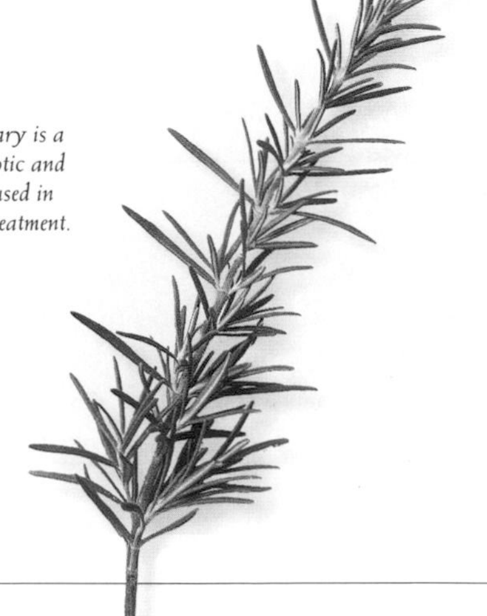

RIGHT *Rosemary is a powerful antiseptic and the oil can be used in aromatherapy treatment.*

DATA FILE

- The bacilli can remain dormant for years before becoming active.
- The disease is not spread through a single exposure to infected droplets, but by extended contact with someone who is infected.
- In the mid-1980s there was a resurgence of tuberculosis in the U.S., first noticed among prison populations and in AIDS patients.
- The further spread of TB may in part be related to crowded urban living conditions.
- Since the mid-1980s, a drug-resistant strain has spread, in part because some patients do not follow the long-term treatment regimen once they feel better.
- TB may also be acquired by drinking unpasteurized animal milk.
- A vaccine known as BCG (Bacille Calmette-Guerin), prepared from a living but weakened strain of bacilli, confers some protection against tuberculosis.
- Most at risk in the U.S. are Mexican, African, South American, and Asian immigrants, American men between the ages of 25 and 44, drug and alcohol users, anyone with a weakened immune system, and residents in institutions.
- Experts say that up to 90 percent of the U.S. population have encountered the bacteria, but most are able to fight off the infection.
- The U.S. Lung Association estimates that approximately 14 in 100,000 are affected by TB.
- One tubercule bacillus can replicate itself billions of times in one month.

Pneumonia

Pneumonia is an infection of the lung caused by bacteria or viruses entering the lungs via the upper respiratory tract, leading to inflammation of the lung tissue. There are two main types of the disease: bronchopneumonia, which is usually confined to areas of tissue surrounding the bronchi, and lobar pneumonia, which affects a whole lobe (or more) of the lung. Pneumonia begins with irritation of lung tissue. The walls of air sacs (alveoli) swell or are destroyed, and plasma, red blood cells, and white blood cells from lung capillaries fill the alveolar spaces. The portion of the lung involved becomes relatively solid and basically is rendered temporarily nonfunctional.

Symptoms

• *rapid, shallow breathing* • *chest pain* • *sore throat and headache* • *cough with mucus and possibly blood* • *fever, sweating, and attacks of shivering*

CAUTION

SEEK URGENT MEDICAL ATTENTION IF PNEUMONIA IS SUSPECTED – IT CAN BE FATAL AMONG THE ELDERLY OR VERY YOUNG, OR PEOPLE ALREADY ILL FROM OTHER CAUSES, SUCH AS STROKE OR HIV/AIDS.

DATA FILE

• Viruses are believed to cause about half of all types of pneumonia.

• The most common form of bacterial pneumonia is caused by Pneumococcus. Staphylococcus, Bacteroides, or Klebsiella.

• Primary atypical pneumonia is a special type of pneumonia that occurs frequently in children and young adults, caused by the micro-organism Mycoplasma pneumoniae.

• Pneumocystis carinii causes pneumonia in those with depressed immune systems and is commonly associated with AIDS.

• Children under one, and people over 60, diabetics, smokers, and alcoholics are most at risk of infection.

• There are over 2 million cases in the U.S. each year.

• Between 40,000–70,000 people die of pneumonia in the U.S. every year.

• Positive diagnosis can only be made with X-ray.

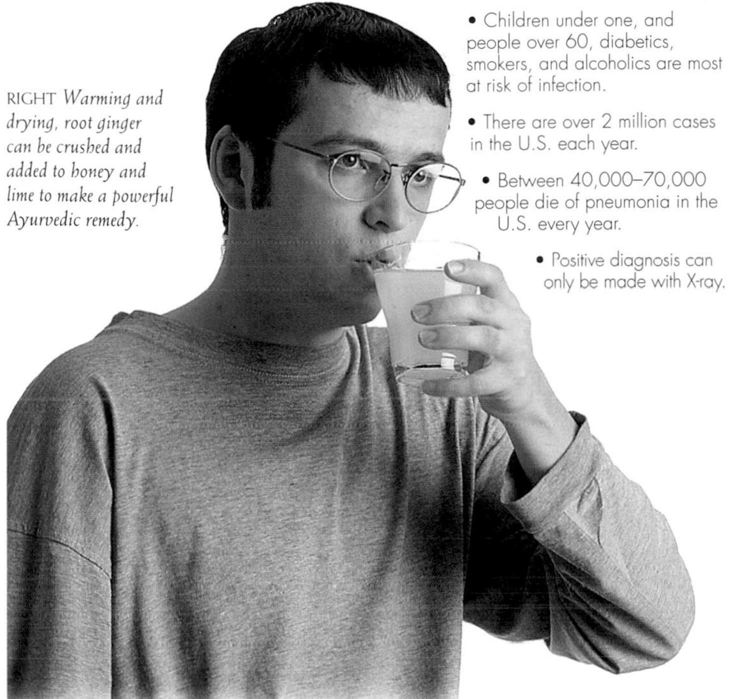

RIGHT *Warming and drying, root ginger can be crushed and added to honey and lime to make a powerful Ayurvedic remedy.*

TREATMENT

AYURVEDA
• Heat mustard oil and apply as a compress to the head to reduce fever. *(See page 30.)*
• Crush root ginger, add to a little honey and lime, and drink as required. *(See page 47.)*

CHINESE HERBALISM
• The problem is believed to be Mucus and Heat in the Lungs, and can be treated with peach kernel, skullcap, and fritillary bulb. *(See pages 63, 72, and 74.)*

HERBALISM
• Try an infusion of coltsfoot, which soothes coughs and helps to fight infections, particularly respiratory infections.
• Raw garlic and onions will help to expel phlegm and fight infection. *(See page 113.)*
• Drink an infusion of boneset to clear congestion and relieve aches and pains.
• Fenugreek with lemon and honey will help to bring down fever and deal with any infection.
• Ginseng is a great all-round restorer and will help to bring down body temperature and fight infection. *(See page 126.)*

AROMATHERAPY
• A steam inhalation of eucalyptus and tea tree will aid breathing, open the lungs, and help fight infection. *(See pages 159 and 162.)*
• A massage of niaouli or cajeput can be used to fight infection and ease symptoms, but this should not be used when there is fever. *(See pages 162 and 163.)*

HOMEOPATHY
Constitutional treatment is necessary after and during the illness, but the following remedies may help in a case of mild pneumonia:
• Aconite, for sudden onset with anxiety and fever. *(See page 178.)*
• Bryonia, for sharp chest pains which are made worse by moving about. *(See page 185.)*
• Sanguinaria, for pneumonia after flu, with right lung affected and accompanied by rust-colored phlegm.
• Phosphorus, for rust-colored phlegm, weakness, trembling, and a thirst for cold drinks. *(See page 208.)*

VITAMINS AND MINERALS
• Include plenty of fluids and foods rich in vitamin C and zinc, which will encourage the immune system. *(See pages 256 and 265.)*

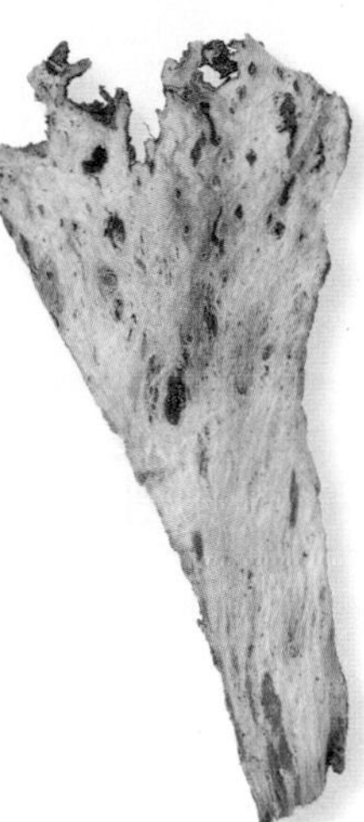

ABOVE *Skullcap, one of the "Three Yellows" of Chinese herbalism used to clear severe infections with signs of Heat.*

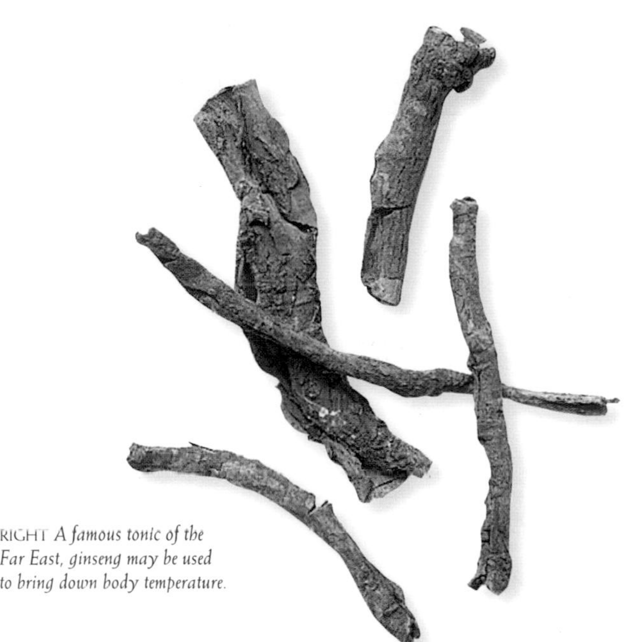

RIGHT *A famous tonic of the Far East, ginseng may be used to bring down body temperature.*

Asthma

Asthma is a condition in which the muscles of the bronchi (the air tubes of the lung) contract in spasm, obstructing the flow of air and making breathing out, in particular, very difficult. Asthma is becoming increasingly common, especially among children, and may be triggered by a number of factors, including allergens (such as house dust or pets), pollution, infection, emotional trauma, or physical exertion. Asthma is divided into two categories: intrinsic, for which there is no identifiable cause for attacks, and extrinsic, which is caused by something, usually inhaled, that triggers an attack.

In many asthma patients, inflammation of the lining of the airways leads to increased sensitivity to a variety of environmental triggers that can cause narrowing of the airways, resulting in obstruction of airflow and breathing difficulty. In some patients, the mucus glands in the airways produce excessive thick mucus, further obstructing airflow.

An asthma attack may be brief or last for several days. Typically, an attack begins within minutes after exposure to a triggering agent. Some patients have only occasional or "seasonal" symptoms, while others have daily symptoms.

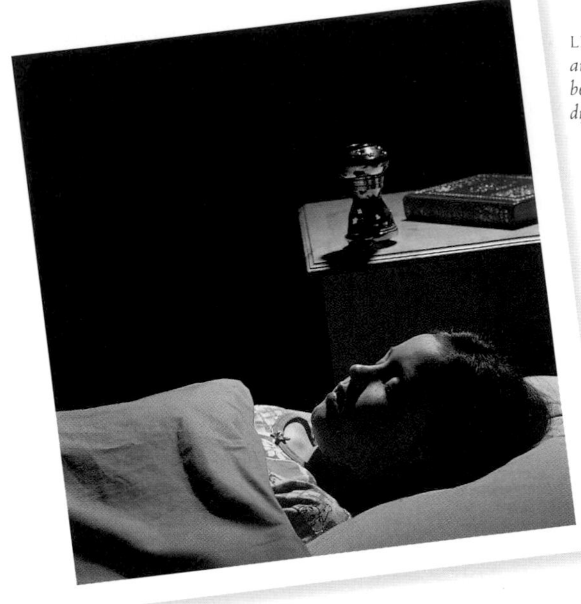

LEFT *Antispasmodic aromatherapy oils can be inhaled from a diffuser.*

Symptoms

• difficulty in breathing • an increase in pulse rate • wheezing, especially on breathing out • a persistent dry cough • a sensation of tightness around the chest

DATA FILE

- The prevalence of asthma is only about 1 or 2 percent worldwide, but in the U.S. asthma affects about 6 percent of children.
- In the U.S. asthma affects 1 in 20 adults, affecting over 7 million adults and 3 million children, or roughly 4 percent of the population.
- Children under 16 and adults over 65 are most commonly affected.
- The incidence of hospitalization for children suffering from asthma and asthma-related illness has increased by 500 percent over the last 30 years.
- The incidence of asthma in the U.K. population has increased 30 times over the last 30 years.
- Asthma is on the increase in the Western world, and although orthodox medicine can control all the worst symptoms, there is no sign of a cure being found.
- Drinking caffeine is said to open the airways and reduce symptoms by one-third in asthma sufferers.

CAUTION

A PROLONGED ATTACK OF SEVERE ASTHMA THAT DOES NOT RESPOND TO SIMPLE REMEDIES REQUIRES IMMEDIATE MEDICAL ATTENTION.

IF A COUGH LASTS FOR MORE THAN 10 DAYS, OR IS ACCOMPANIED BY FEVER, DIFFICULT BREATHING, BLUE LIPS, DROWSINESS, OR DIFFICULTY IN SPEAKING, CONTACT YOUR PHYSICIAN.

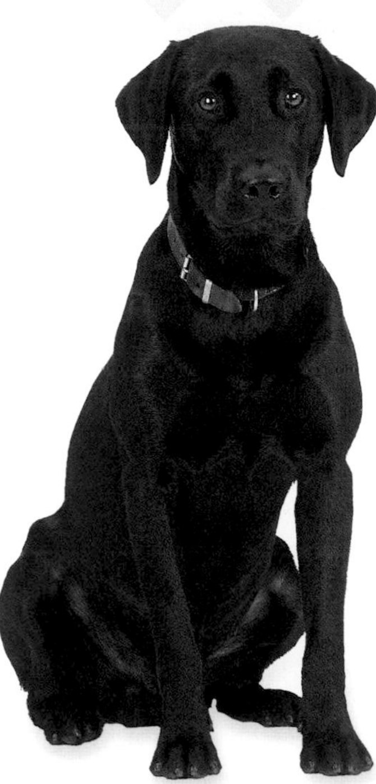

ABOVE *Asthma sufferers may find attacks are brought on by encounters with the family pet.*

TREATMENT

AYURVEDA
- Common ginger and stramonium may be used to treat asthma. *(See page 47.)*

CHINESE HERBALISM
- The cause of the illness is considered to be Phlegm produced by weakness of the Spleen and Kidneys. Almond and ephedra may be prescribed to open the Lungs.

HERBALISM
- Any of the herbs suggested for stress *(see page 284)* will help you to relax, which should decrease the incidence of attacks.
- Elecampane can be infused to treat asthma. Drink daily if you are prone to attacks.
- During a mild attack, grindelia, hyssop, wild cherry bark, and motherwort will help. *(See page 124.)*
- Turmeric has a bronchodilatory effect, and it can be sipped sprinkled in a cup of warm water.

AROMATHERAPY
- A steam inhalation of chamomile, eucalyptus, or lavender essential oils can be taken during an attack and immediately afterwards to ease panic and to help open the airways. *(See pages 146– 71.)*
- Pine oil in the bath or a vaporizer will reduce the incidence of attacks. *(See page 166.)*
- Bergamot, clary sage, neroli, chamomile, and rose are antispasmodic, as well as being relaxant, and they will be particularly useful for attacks brought on by stress. *(See pages 146–71.)*

HOMEOPATHY

Chronic asthma must be treated constitutionally, but the following remedies can be used for mild attacks, while waiting for medical attention:
- Ipecac., for wheezy children who cough until they vomit up a little mucus. *(See page 189.)*
- Arsenicum, for waking between midnight and 2A.M., accompanied by difficult breathing. *(See page 182.)*
- Bryonia, for asthma at the end of a cold, with a hard, dry cough. *(See page 185.)*
- Nat. sulf., for asthma in damp weather, with a loose cough and yellowish mucus. *(See page 207.)*
- Lachesis, for asthma that starts in spring or autumn, or at the menopause. *(See page 216.)*

FLOWER ESSENCES
- Take Rescue Remedy when you feel symptoms coming on. This will ease symptoms and prevent a full-blown attack. *(See page 244.)*

VITAMINS AND MINERALS
- Increase your intake of vitamin B6, which is said to reduce the frequency and severity of attacks. *(See page 254.)*

Coughs

Coughs are necessary to expel foreign bodies and mucus from the trachea and airways of the lungs. Coughing is a symptom rather than an illness, and can indicate sinusitis, croup, bronchitis, pneumonia, flu, viruses, the early stages of measles, asthma, whooping cough, or an excess of catarrh from the nose or sinuses, due to irritation or infection.

A dry cough may be caused by mucus from infections or colds, chemicals in the atmosphere, a foreign object or nervousness which constricts the throat. A loose, wetter cough is caused by inflammation of the bronchial tubes produced by an infection or allergy. A constant nighttime cough, or one which recurs with each cold and is hard to get rid of, may indicate asthma.

DATA FILE

Various terms describe the type of cough:

- An acute cough starts suddenly, and is usually resolved within a day or two.
- A chronic cough persists, sometimes for many weeks.
- A productive cough brings up lots of catarrh or mucus.
- A nonproductive cough brings up very little or no mucus, and usually sounds harsh and hard.

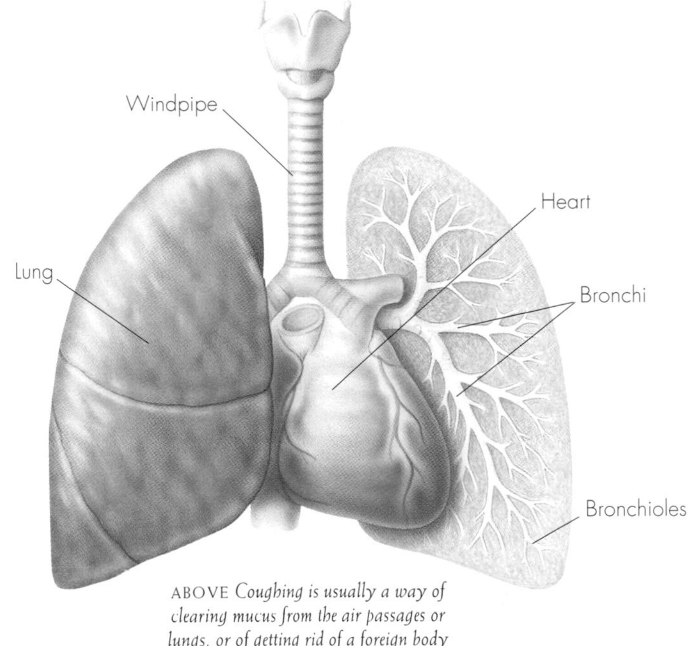

ABOVE *Coughing is usually a way of clearing mucus from the air passages or lungs, or of getting rid of a foreign body in the respiratory tract.*

TREATMENT

AYURVEDA

- Brown 4 tablespoons of coriander seeds in a frying pan, then boil with 4 cups of water, with 4 slices of root ginger. Reduce to 2 cups of liquid, strain, and drink. *(See page 35.)*
- Other herbs to consider are sunflower, henbane, and stramonium.

TRADITIONAL HOME AND FOLK REMEDIES

- A tincture of garlic (place several garlic cloves in brandy and leave for 2 or 3 weeks, then strain) or garlic syrup (tincture, or fresh garlic mixed with a little honey) will help the body to fight infection. It also works to cleanse the blood. *(See page 82.)*
- Ginseng in hot herbal tea warms the body and eases symptoms.
- Honey and lemon will ease coughs and encourage healing. *(See pages 87 and 101.)*
- Mustard powder, mixed with a little water, can be made into a poultice and applied to the chest area. *(See page 98.)*
- Apply a warm roasted onion poultice to the chest, or drink a warm onion broth to cleanse and reduce congestion. *(See page 82.)*

LEFT *Tincture of garlic is made by steeping garlic cloves in a jar of brandy.*

HERBALISM

- Peppermint tea can be drunk to soothe. *(See page 125.)*
- Add lightly macerated licorice root sticks to your herbal drink to ease. *(See page 122.)*
- Aniseed, marshmallow, and wild cherry bark are useful for unproductive, irritating coughs. *(See page 114.)*
- Use golden seal, plantain, and thyme if infection is present. *(See pages 126 and 135.)*

AROMATHERAPY

- Inhale the steam from a few drops of eucalyptus oil in boiling water, as it is expectorant and decongestant. *(See page 159.)*
- Pine oil, in a vaporizer, will ease coughing and act to restore the lungs. *(See page 166.)*
- Massage frankincense or sandalwood into the chest and back. *(See pages 147 and 169.)*
- Essential oil of myrrh reduces mucus and phlegm. *(See page 155.)*

HOMEOPATHY

- Pulsatilla, for a loose, wet, rattling cough, which is worse in the morning and when in bed at night. *(See page 209.)*
- Ant. tart. is especially useful for elderly people who suffer from persistent rattling cough, and are full of loose mucus but cannot seem to bring it up. *(See page 179.)*
- Rumex, for a very tickly cough, when cold air irritates the nose and throat.
- Bryonia, for a dry cough where the chest feels sore from coughing. *(See page 185.)*
- Phosphorous, for a tickling cough in delicate people with weak chests. *(See page 208.)*
- Drosera, for a violent tickly cough with retching and pain in the ribs. *(See page 193.)*
- Chamomilla, for a dry, irritating cough with wheezing, and which is worse at night and makes you feel irritable. *(See page 204.)*

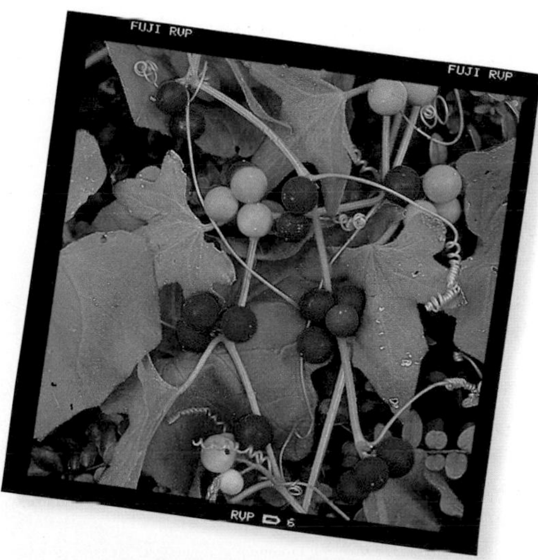

ABOVE *Bryony, the source of the homeopathic remedy Bryonia, useful for a dry cough with a sore chest.*

CAUTION

IF A COUGH LASTS FOR MORE THAN 10 DAYS, OR IS ACCOMPANIED BY FEVER, DIFFICULT BREATHING, BLUE LIPS, DROWSINESS OR DIFFICULTY SPEAKING, CONTACT YOUR PHYSICIAN.

Flu

More properly known as influenza, flu is a viral disease of the upper respiratory tract, spread by the contaminated droplets (via coughing and sneezing) of other sufferers. The three main types of flu are caused by three different viruses – A, B, and C. Type C, once caught, confers immunity. Types A and B, however, are constantly mutating so that our bodies cannot build up resistance against them. Incubation of the virus is generally one or two days, during which time it is infectious, and therefore notoriously impossible to contain.

ABOVE *High fever and aching limbs can be relieved by taking fenugreek mixed with lemon and honey.*

DATA FILE

- When new strains of influenza virus arise, they spread rapidly around the world, infecting millions of people and causing many deaths.
- Flu victims 50 years old or older, children, and immune-deficient people are at risk of developing pneumonia and other secondary infections.
- Over the age of 65, pneumonia and flu are the fifth leading cause of death.
- The disease is produced by any one of three types of Orthomyxovirus virus (A, B, and C), of which there are many strains.
- Vaccines have been developed that have been found to be 70–90 percent effective for at least six months against either A or B types, and a genetically engineered live-virus vaccine is under development.
- Vaccination is considered especially important for older people, patients with cardiac or respiratory diseases, and pregnant women.
- The incidence of infection is highest among school-age children, partly because of their lack of previous exposure to various strains.
- Approximately every ten years, influenza pandemics have been caused by new strains of type-A virus.
- Epidemics, or regional outbreaks, have appeared every 2 to 3 years for influenza A, and every 4 to 5 years for influenza B.

SYMPTOMS

• high fever, possibly accompanied by shivering • sore throat, and possibly a dry, unproductive cough • runny nose and sneezing • breathlessness and general weakness • headache, stiff and aching joints, and muscular pain • nausea and loss of appetite • possibly insomnia and depression

TREATMENT

AYURVEDA

- Heat mustard oil and apply as a compress to the head to reduce fever. *(See page 30.)*
- Crush root ginger, add to a little honey and lime, and drink as required. *(See page 47.)*
- Bitter orange, sunflower, and coriander may be useful in treating flu. *(See pages 35, 40.)*

TRADITIONAL HOME AND FOLK REMEDIES

- Some warmed apple juice (preferably fresh) can ease the fever. *(See page 94.)*
- Barley water is a traditional remedy for high fever – particularly one caused by infection and inflammation. *(See page 92.)*
- Ginseng powder can be added to herbal teas to restore.
- Drink hot lemon and honey in a cup of warm water to ease inflammation and fever. *(See pages 87 and 101.)*
- Gargle with lemon juice to kill germs and help to stop the spread of the virus. *(See page 87.)*

HERBALISM

- Drink an infusion of boneset to relieve aches and pains and clear congestion.
- Fenugreek with lemon and honey will help to bring down fever and soothe aching limbs.
- Ginseng is a great all-round restorer and will help to bring down body temperature to normal. *(See page 126.)*
- Use wormwood, sage, and licorice to prevent flu. *(See pages 122 and 129.)*

AROMATHERAPY

- Gargle with tea tree oil to prevent the spread of infection. *(See page 162.)*
- Use a eucalyptus or peppermint inhalation to unblock sinuses and the chest. *(See pages 159 and 164.)*
- Massage tea tree and geranium oil into the chest and head to reduce symptoms and fight infection. *(See pages 162 and 165.)*
- Oils which act to bring down fever include bergamot, chamomile, melissa, and tea tree. *(See pages 146–71.)*

HOMEOPATHY

- Gelsemium, for occasions when muscular weakness, aching, and heaviness predominate. *(See page 195.)*
- Rhus tox., for flu that starts after getting wet, where there is a lot of aching in joints rather than muscles. Accompanied by restlessness and inability to get comfortable. *(See page 210.)*
- Bryonia, for a bad headache and dry cough, with a desire to lie quite still. *(See page 185.)*
- Eupatorium perfoliatum, for intense aching in the back and limbs, together with shivery chills.
- Arsenicum, when you feel debilitated, often with loss of fluids, and with accompanying watery diarrhea and sometimes vomiting. *(See page 182.)*
- Baptisia, for gastric flu, when you feel very "wiped out," and your body feels bruised, or scattered around the bed; also with sudden bouts of diarrhea or vomiting. *(See page 184.)*

VITAMINS AND MINERALS

- Eat plenty of foods rich in vitamin C, bioflavonoids and zinc, which will encourage healing, help to fight infection, and boost the action of the immune system. *(See pages 256, 272, and 265.)*
- Royal jelly acts as a tonic and an antiviral agent. *(See page 276.)*

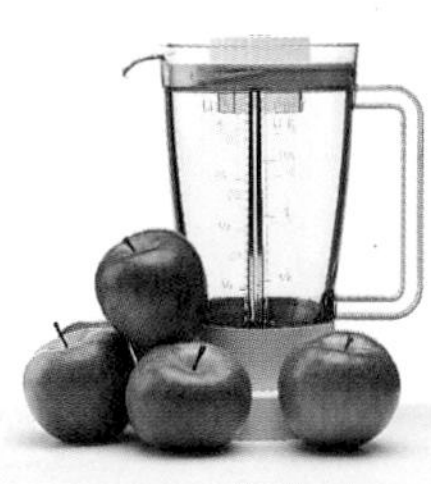

ABOVE *Freshly made apple juice is a good home remedy, providing vitamin C to help to combat infection. Using a juice extractor enables this to be made quickly and easily.*

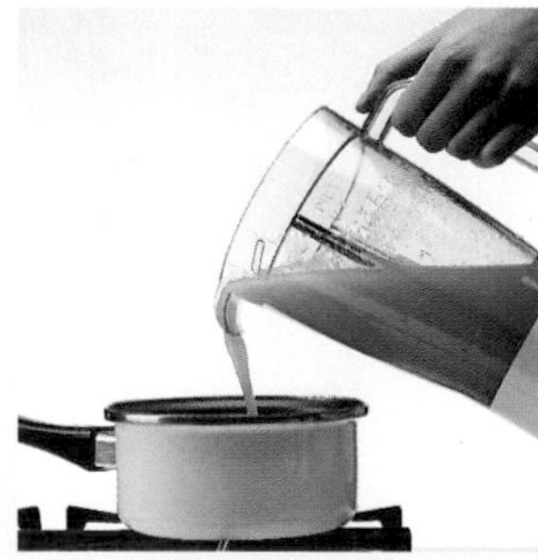

ABOVE *The apple juice can be poured into a pan and gently warmed, but it must not be boiled or overheated or the vitamin content will be severely reduced.*

LEFT *Flu is characterized by a high fever with a runny nose and sneezing.*

Emphysema

Emphysema is a progressive disease in which the tiny air sacs in the lungs (alveoli) break down, reducing the area available for gas exchange. This means that insufficient oxygen reaches the vital organs, and too much carbon dioxide enters the bloodstream. Emphysema is particularly common among heavy smokers and sufferers of asthma and chronic bronchitis. Industrial pollutants may also be a cause, as well as hereditary factors.

The exact cause of pulmonary emphysema is unknown. Cigarette smoking is closely associated with the disease, and in some cases a genetic link is suspected, in that a significant number of people with emphysema lack a gene that controls the liver's production of a protein called alpha-1 antitrypsin, or AAT. Emphysema rarely occurs before the age of 40, and women appear to be less prone, although with the increase in the numbers of women smoking this may change.

Symptoms

• breathlessness, especially on exertion • a cough producing sputum • the chest may become barrel-shaped as the disease progresses • a blue tinge to the skin (cyanosis) • respiratory failure may eventually occur

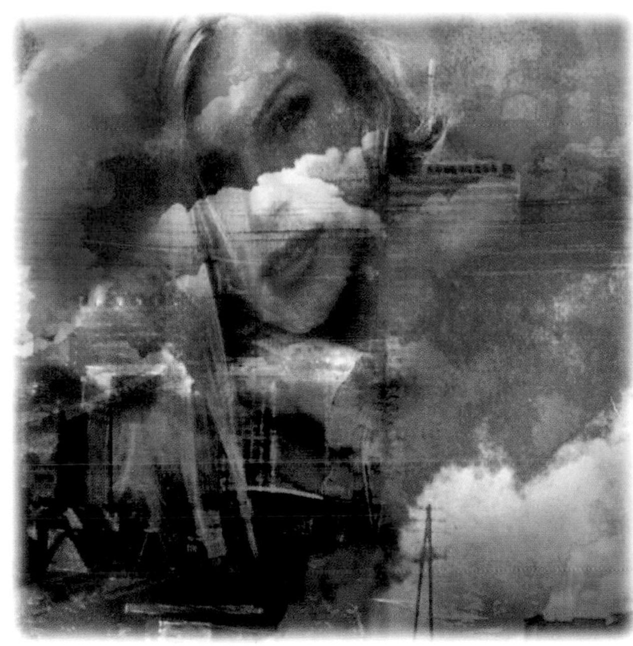

ABOVE *The exact causes of this disease are not known, but smoking and breathing polluted air are two major contributors.*

TREATMENT

AYURVEDA
• Boil 2 or 3 cloves of garlic in 2 cups of water until tender. Crush into the water and drink to relieve chest pain. *(See page 26.)*
• Stramonium may be useful.

HERBALISM
• Peppermint tea will soothe inflammation and help to open lungs. *(See page 125.)*
• Slippery elm bark soothes the chest and lungs, and can be added to any herbal tea. *(See page 136.)*

AROMATHERAPY
• Massage oils of cedarwood, peppermint, or eucalyptus into the chest daily, to open lungs and reduce coughing. *(See pages 146–71.)*
• Make an inhalation of eucalyptus, and use as required to expel phlegm. *(See page 159.)*

HOMEOPATHY
• Emphysema cannot be cured, but the symptoms can be alleviated and the condition arrested by constitutional treatment.
• See coughs *(page 345)*, bronchitis *(page 349)*, and asthma *(page 344)* for remedies that fit specific symptoms.

LEFT *Garlic cloves can be boiled in water for an Ayurvedic remedy.*

Garlic bulb

Garlic clove

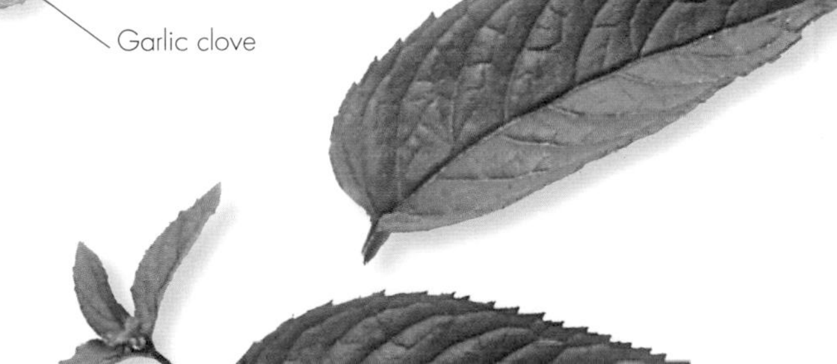

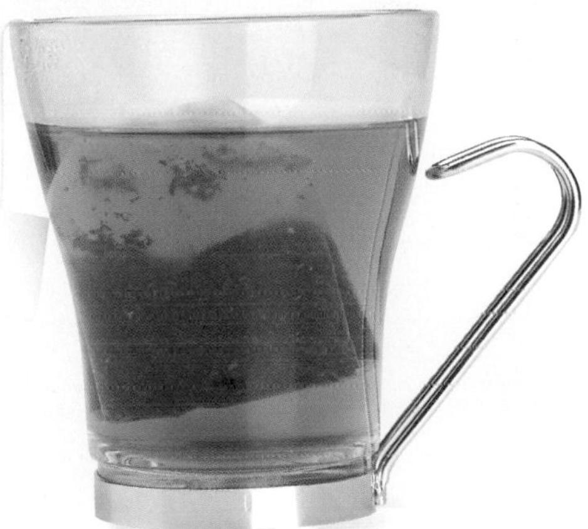

LEFT and RIGHT *Peppermint leaves can be used to make a soothing tea.*

Pleurisy

Pleurisy (or pleuritis) is an infection, viral or bacterial in origin, caused by an inflammation of the pleura – the sac-like membrane surrounding the lungs. The two layers of the inflamed pleura rub together to cause the characteristic creaking noise in the chest that makes diagnosis so easy. A surplus of pleural fluid may also be produced by the inflammation, causing a pleural effusion which can be detected on physical examination. In a very few cases, pleurisy may be an indication of more serious diseases such as lung cancer or pulmonary embolism, while chronic pleurisy may be a symptom of tuberculosis. Before the advent of antibiotics, pleurisy was a life-threatening condition and one of the most common causes of death, particularly in children. Today, the condition is usually easily diagnosed and treated in the early stages.

Symptoms

- *stabbing pain, usually at a particular point in inhalation or on coughing*

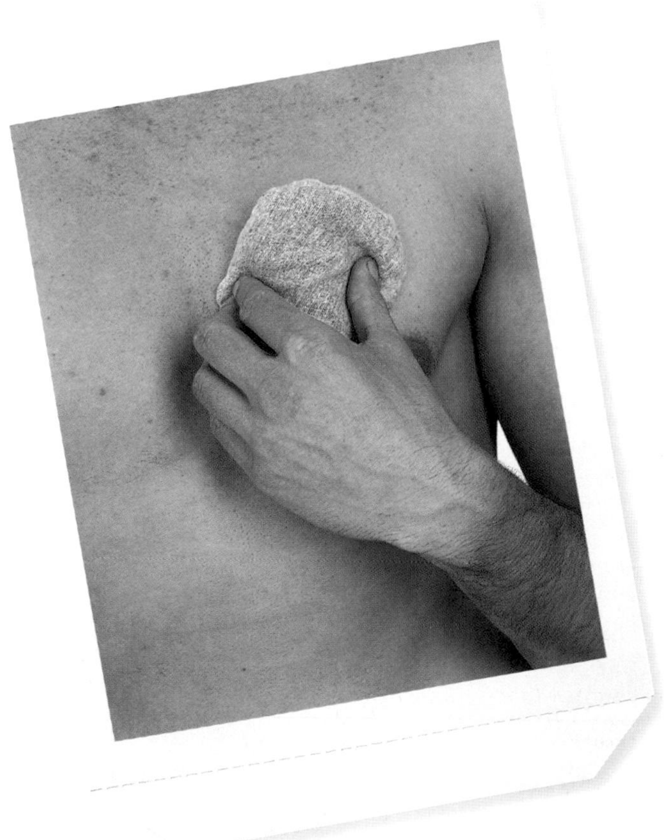

ABOVE *An inflammation of the pleura causes a sharp, stabbing pain in the chest. Apply a leaf tea compress to relieve symptoms.*

CAUTION

IF YOU DO NOT FEEL BETTER AFTER A DAY (TAKING DOSES EVERY HOUR), SEE YOUR PHYSICIAN.

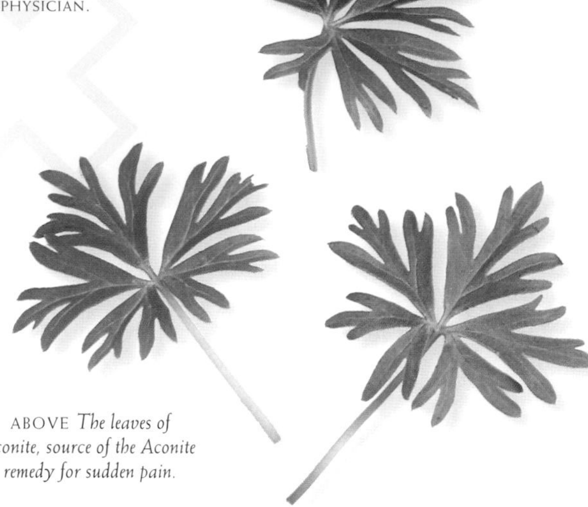

ABOVE *The leaves of aconite, source of the Aconite remedy for sudden pain.*

TREATMENT

TRADITIONAL HOME AND FOLK REMEDIES

- Apple cider vinegar compresses will reduce inflammation and encourage healing. *(See page 102.)*

HERBALISM

- Comfrey root or leaf tea compresses can be applied to the chest to ease inflammation. *(See page 132.)*
- Wrap a bruised wet plantain leaf across the chest to soothe symptoms. *(See page 126.)*
- Combine a handful of sage leaves and corn silk to strengthen the kidneys and expel water from the system. *(See page 129.)*

AROMATHERAPY

- The following anti-inflammatory oils can be used in gentle massage of the chest and back, or in the bath or an inhaler to encourage healing: bergamot, calendula, chamomile, myrrh. *(See pages 146–71.)*
- Lavender can be sniffed during an attack to calm you and help fight infection. *(See page 161.)*

HOMEOPATHY

During an acute attack, the following remedies may be useful:

- Aconite, for a sudden sharp pain, usually after exposure to cold wind. *(See page 178.)*
- Cantharis, for breathlessness and burning pains with mild fever and a dry cough. *(See page 188.)*
- Belladonna, for sudden pain and a hot flushed face accompanied by thirst. *(See page 183.)*
- Hep. sulf., for slower recovery, with fluid on the lungs. *(See page 198.)*
- Bryonia, for pain that is made worse by movement, and which is accompanied by thirst and general irritability. *(See page 185.)*
- Sulfur, for sharp, cutting pains that are made worse by movement. *(See page 215.)*

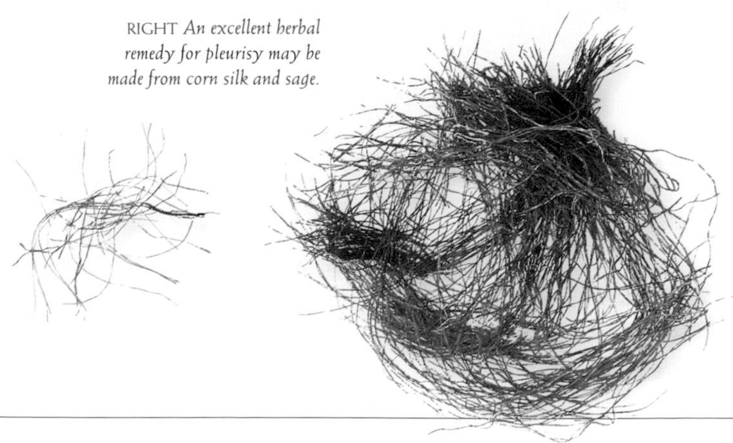

RIGHT *An excellent herbal remedy for pleurisy may be made from corn silk and sage.*

Bronchitis

Bronchitis is an inflammation of the lining of the bronchi (the air tubes of the lungs). Acute bronchitis in which mucus infected with bacteria is expelled from the lungs often follows a viral illness such as a cold or flu. Smoking and a damp, dusty, or foggy atmosphere can lead to chronic bronchitis resulting from long-term irritation of the air passages.

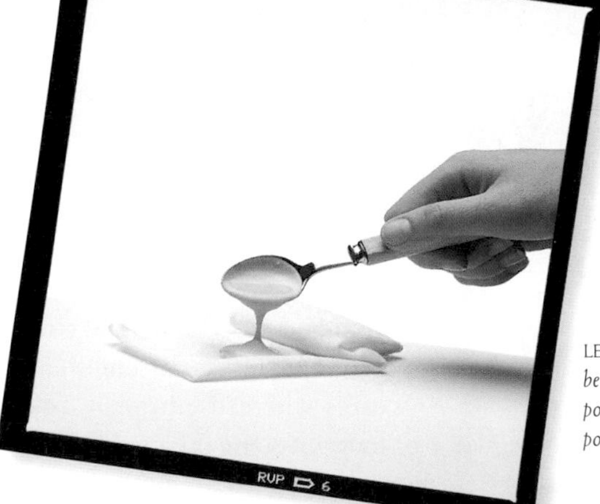

LEFT *Chest congestion may be relieved by applying a poultice of mustard seed powder and water.*

Symptoms

ABOVE *Mustard powder can be used to make a warming poultice for the chest.*

• a cough, dry at first but with gradually increasing sputum • possibly chest pain • fever • shortness of breath and wheezing • in cases of chronic bronchitis symptoms may begin in winter, but then persist throughout the year

DATA FILE

- Smokers are 50 times more susceptible to bronchitis.
- Male sufferers outnumber female sufferers by ten to one.
- Ayurvedic breathing exercises, and yoga, generally assist breathing and shortness of breath.
- Acute bronchitis is usually caused by infection by one of the many viruses that cause the common cold or influenza, and is frequently associated with measles.
- Acute chemical bronchitis may be caused by the inhalation of irritating fumes, such as smoke, chlorine, ammonia, and ozone.
- Chronic bronchitis results from prolonged irritation of the bronchial membrane, causing coughing and the excessive secretion of mucus for extended periods. By far the most common cause of chronic bronchitis is cigarette smoking, but air pollution, industrial fumes, and dust are also recognized lung irritants.

CAUTION

IF YOUR TEMPERATURE RISES ABOVE 39 DEGREES, OR IF YOU COUGH BLOOD, CALL YOUR PHYSICIAN.

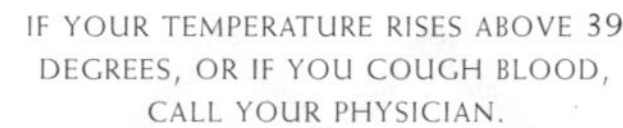

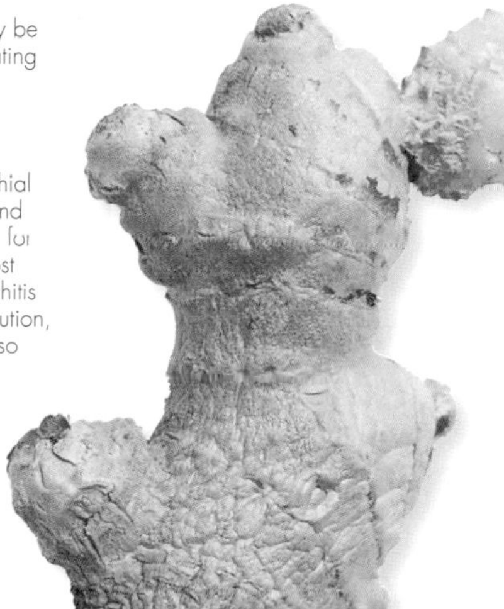

RIGHT *Ginger root is a warming treatment, and in Ayurveda it is mixed with honey and lime juice to make a curative drink.*

TREATMENT

AYURVEDA
- Heat mustard oil and apply as a compress to the head to reduce fever. *(See page 30.)*
- Crush root ginger, add to a little honey and lime, and drink as required. *(See page 47.)*
- Hollyhock may be appropriate, as well as bitter orange and stramonium.

CHINESE HERBALISM
- The source is believed to be external Wind, Cold, or Heat in cases of acute bronchitis, and internal Deficient Spleen or Lung, or internal Mucus for chronic bronchitis.
- Acute conditions will respond to fritillary bulb, plantain seed, and balloon flower root. *(See pages 63 and 69.)*
- Chronic conditions would respond to honeysuckle flowers, mulberry leaves, gardenia fruit. *(See page 65.)*

TRADITIONAL HOME AND FOLK REMEDIES
- Honey and lemon work to fight infection and ease coughs. *(See pages 87 and 101.)*
- Combine mustard seed powder and water to make a poultice to decongest the chest. *(See page 98.)*
- Onions will soothe inflamed membranes and induce perspiration. *(See page 82.)*

HERBALISM
- Anise diluted in a small amount of water soothes a hacking cough.
- Wild cherry bark extract added to any herbal drink relieves coughing.
- Coltsfoot can be added to licorice and honey to alleviate coughs.
- Rub garlic oil into the chest to fight infection and encourage healing. *(See page 113.)*
- Drink ginseng in hot water, as it will help to eliminate infection and ease coughing fits. *(See page 126.)*
- Peppermint tea will soothe the cough and help to bring out the infection. *(See page 125.)*

AROMATHERAPY
- Oils to help clear the congestion include eucalyptus and thyme, which can be inhaled as required. *(See pages 159 and 170.)*
- Ginger oil can be diluted and rubbed into the chest for chronic bronchitis, to dispel mucus. *(See page 171.)*
- Juniper, myrrh, and rosemary will help to prevent mucus, and act to detoxify the body. *(See pages 146–71.)*

HOMEOPATHY
The following remedies can be offered for acute bronchitis; chronic bronchitis must be treated constitutionally:
- Pulsatilla, for symptoms that are worse in stuffy rooms, and for a cough which is dry at night and loose in the morning. *(See page 209.)*
- Ipecac., for nausea, vomiting, and suffocation feelings. *(See page 189.)*
- Bryonia, for a dry, stabbing cough accompanied by a headache and great thirst. *(See page 185.)*
- Phosphorus, for a tight, tickly cough, when you are pale, anxious, and thirsty for cold water. *(See page 208.)*
- Aconite, for sudden onset bronchitis, with a dry cough and chills. *(See page 178.)*

VITAMINS AND MINERALS
- Increase your intake of vitamins B, C, and A, and zinc. *(See pages 252–5, 256 and 265.)*

Tracheitis

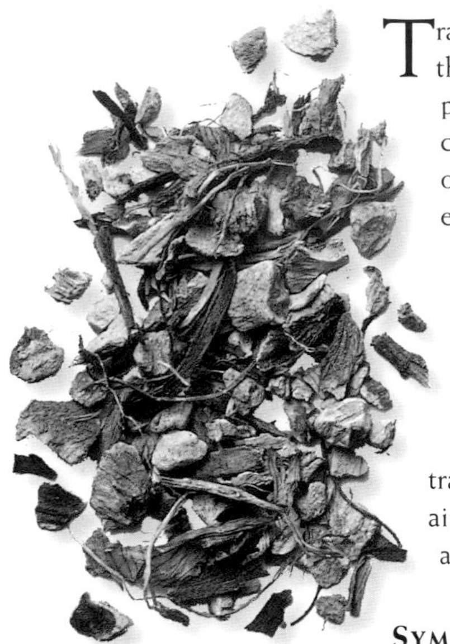

ABOVE *Rumex is the homeopathic treatment for certain types of sore throat.*

Tracheitis is an acute inflammation of the lining of the trachea (windpipe). It is usually viral in origin but can sometimes be bacterial. It is often associated with an infection elsewhere in the upper respiratory tract, such as bronchitis or influenza. Tracheitis is the most common cause of painful attacks of croup in young children. In cases where the bronchi of the lungs become infected (laryngotracheobronchitis), the walls of the airway swell, which can lead to asphyxia in small children.

Symptoms

• *pain in the upper part of the chest* • *soreness behind the breastbone* • *hoarseness* • *wheezing* • *a painful dry cough*

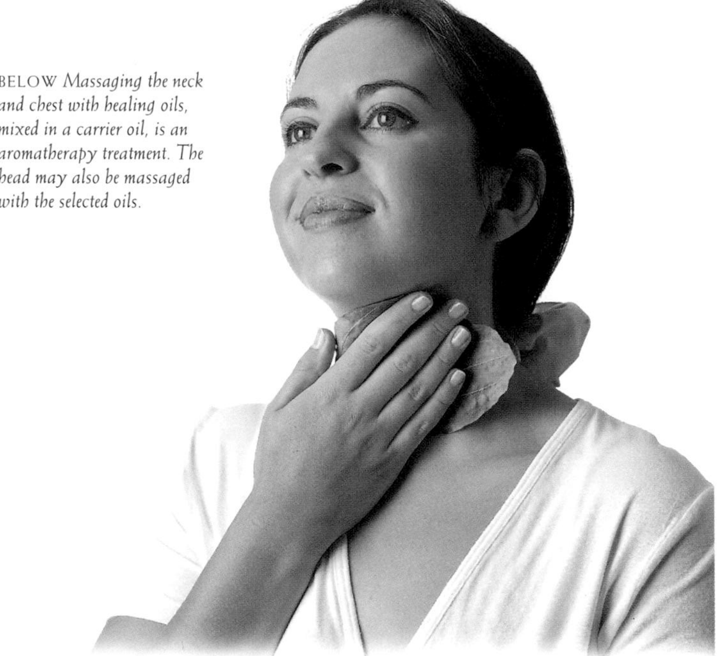

BELOW *Massaging the neck and chest with healing oils, mixed in a carrier oil, is an aromatherapy treatment. The head may also be massaged with the selected oils.*

TREATMENT

AYURVEDA
• Hollyhock may be useful for throat irritation.

HERBALISM
• Comfrey root or leaf tea compresses on the throat and neck will help ease inflammation. *(See page 132.)*
• Wrap a bruised, wet plantain leaf across the throat to soothe symptoms. *(See page 126.)*

AROMATHERAPY
• Anti-inflammatory oils can be used in gentle massage of the chest, neck, and head, or in the bath or an inhaler to encourage healing. Try bergamot, calendula, chamomile, and myrrh. *(See pages 146–71.)*

HOMEOPATHY
• Rumex, for a raw feeling in the throat, a tickly cough, and where the throat is sore to the touch.
• Stannum, when there is sweet yellow phlegm and pain after coughing.
• Bryonia, when pain is made worse by talking, smoke, and warm rooms. *(See page 185.)*
• Phosphorus, for a hacking cough, thirst for cold drinks, and a raw feeling. *(See page 208.)*
• Kali bich., for sticky phlegm that is difficult to expel. *(See page 200.)*

VITAMINS AND MINERALS
• Take extra vitamin C and zinc to boost the immune system. *(See pages 256 and 265.)*

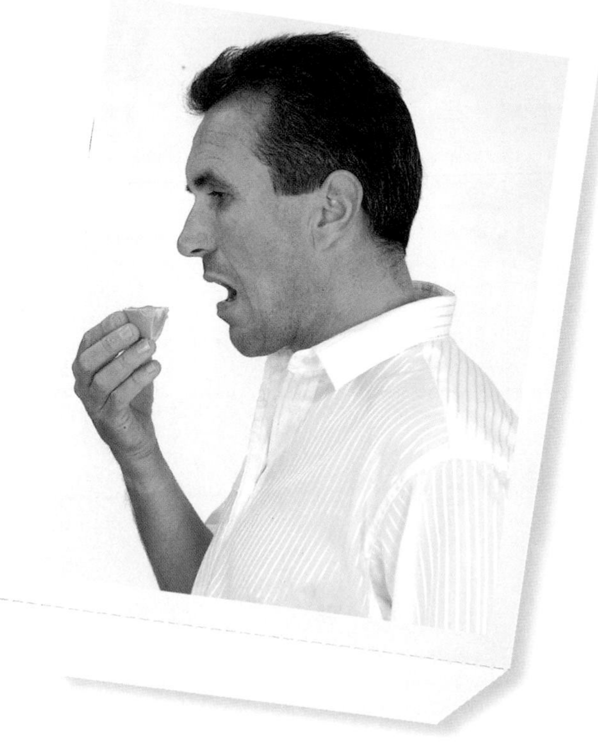

RIGHT *Boosting the immune system by taking extra vitamin C in the form of oranges will help fight infections, such as tracheitis, and prevent further occurrences.*

Hyperventilation

Hyperventilation is the term used to describe the act of breathing more quickly and deeply than normal, and which causes excessive loss of carbon dioxide from the blood. This can lead to alkalosis (an increase in blood alkalinity). It can occur at high altitudes, as a result of heavy exercise, during panic attacks, or as a response to poisoning (as in an aspirin overdose). Hyperventilation associated with uncontrolled diabetes or with kidney failure represents the body's efforts to eliminate excess carbon dioxide in dealing with acidosis. Chronic hyperventilation is association with a combination of fatigue and over-arousal (lack of sleep, plus stress, for instance); it may also stem from organic problems in the brain, or in the lungs themselves. Acute attacks are usually a reaction to emotional or physical trauma.

SYMPTOMS

- *a feeling of not getting enough air* • *the muscles of the forearms and calves may go into spasm, causing involuntary bending and extension of the wrists and ankles*

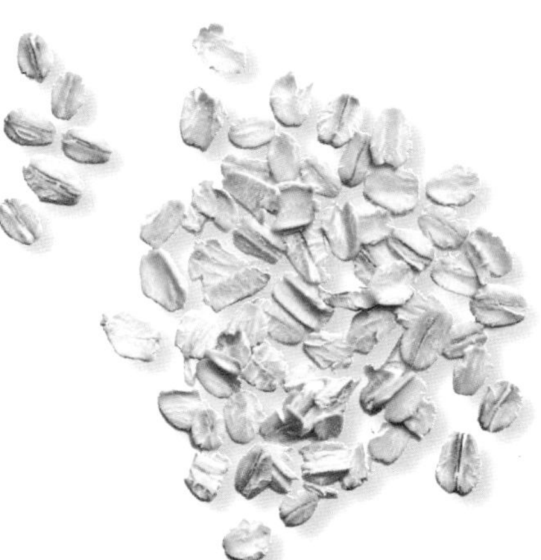

ABOVE *Oats contain a gentle nerve tonic and eating them regularly can be of great help for people who suffer panic attacks.*

RIGHT *Physical trauma, even being overactive and overaggressive in sport, can lead to hyperventilation.*

TREATMENT

AYURVEDA

- An Ayurvedic medical practitioner would balance the tri-doshas, and use panchakarma for balancing the vátha. *(See page 22.)*

CHINESE HERBALISM

- A Chinese herbalist might suggest ginseng, Chinese angelica, and white peony root with thorowax root for relaxation. Treatment would be designed to strengthen the Spleen and enliven Liver. *(See pages 56 and 67.)*

TRADITIONAL HOME AND FOLK REMEDIES

- Oats contain thiamine and pantothenic acid, which act as gentle nerve tonics. *(See page 84.)*

HERBALISM

- Herbal remedies would be used to calm the nervous system and to relax you. Skullcap and valerian are useful herbs, blended together for best effect. Drink this as a tea three times daily while suffering symptoms. *(See pages 131 and 136.)*
- Lady's slipper and limeflowers may also work to ease factors which may be causing the condition. *(See page 134.)*

AROMATHERAPY

- A relaxing blend of essential oils of lavender, geranium, and bergamot in sweet almond oil or peach kernel oil may be used in the bath at times of great stress and anxiety. *(See pages 146–71.)*

HOMEOPATHY

- Take Aconite every 5 minutes for up to six doses in an acute attack. *(See page 178.)*
- Constitutional treatment will be necessary for chronic conditions.

FLOWER ESSENCES

- Rescue Remedy or Emergency Essence will help to calm you in an attack. *(See page 244.)*
- Elm, for an attack linked to anxiety accompanying a feeling of being unable to cope. *(See page 241.)*
- Aspen, for an attack caused by anxiety for no apparent reason. *(See page 236.)*

VITAMINS AND MINERALS

- Increase your intake of B vitamins, which work on the nervous system. *(See pages 252–5.)*
- Avoid caffeine in any form.

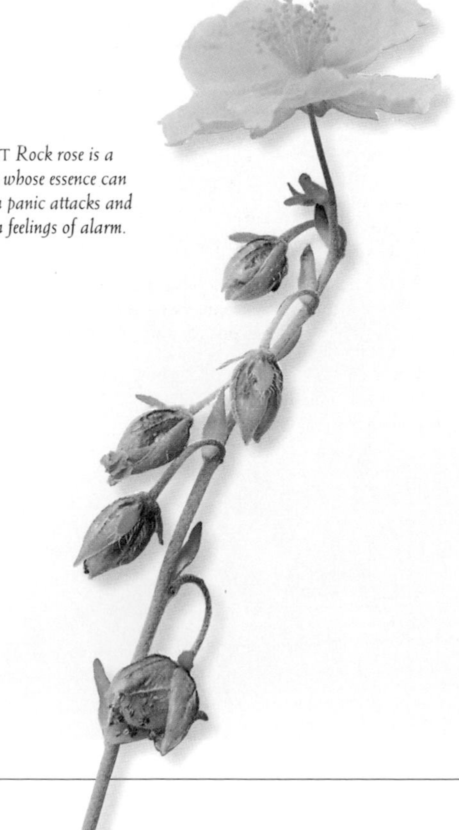

RIGHT *Rock rose is a flower whose essence can help in panic attacks and sudden feelings of alarm.*

Hiccups

A hiccup is a common irritation of the diaphragmatic nerves which causes involuntary inhalation of air. A lowering of the diaphragm and the sudden closure of the vocal cords result in the characteristic hiccup sound. Hiccups may be brought on by indigestion and drinking carbonated drinks, and can also occur during pregnancy and as a result of alcoholism. Most attacks last only a few minutes, usually with a brief interval in between attacks. Frequent, prolonged attacks of hiccups, which are extremely rare, may lead to severe exhaustion.

CAUTION

WHILE HICCUPS ARE USUALLY QUITE INNOCUOUS, THEY MAY BE A FEATURE OF MORE SERIOUS DISORDERS SUCH AS PLEURISY, HIATUS HERNIA, AND PNEUMONIA.

Symptoms

- *prolonged episodes of hiccups may be accompanied by chest pain*
- *if persistent, hiccups can eventually be extremely exhausting*

TREATMENT

CHINESE HERBALISM

- The cause is thought to be Heat, Cold, or Food Stagnation. Berilla stems, rhubarb, and ginger will be used to treat hiccups. *(See page 73.)*

TRADITIONAL HOME AND FOLK REMEDIES

- Squirt some lemon juice to the back of your throat, or suck a piece of fresh lemon. *(See page 87.)*
- Give babies a sip of water with honey. *(See page 101.)*

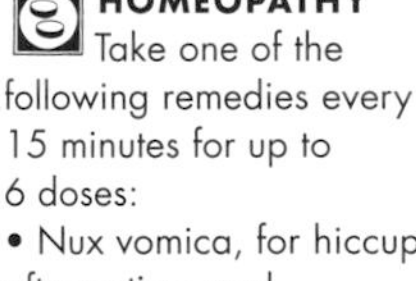

HOMEOPATHY

Take one of the following remedies every 15 minutes for up to 6 doses:

- Nux vomica, for hiccups after eating, and accompanied by belching. *(See page 214.)*
- Arsenicum, for hiccups which are worse after cold drinks and accompanied by a chilly feeling. *(See page 182.)*
- Ignatia, when hiccups come on after emotional upset, eating, drinking, or smoking. *(See page 200.)*
- Mag. phos., for a sore chest and retching. *(See page 204.)*
- Cicuta, for violent, noisy hiccups.

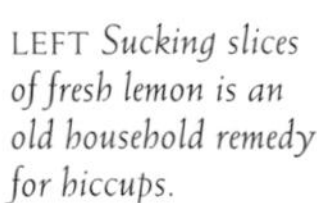

LEFT *Sucking slices of fresh lemon is an old household remedy for hiccups.*

Common Cold

The common cold is an infection of the upper respiratory tract which may be caused by any one of up to 200 strains of virus. These are spread either by inhaling droplets coughed or sneezed by others, or, more probably, by direct hand-to-hand contact with sufferers. When infection occurs, the walls of the respiratory tract swell and produce excess mucus, giving rise to the typical cold symptoms of stuffy or runny nose, throat discomfort, malaise, and occasional coughing. Colds can produce fevers of up to 39°C (102°F) in infants and children, but such fevers in adults indicate that the infection is probably influenza. The incubation period is from 1–3 days, after which symptoms occur, and most colds run their course in 3–10 days. Infants and elderly people are susceptible to complications such as sinusitis, ear inflammations, and pneumonia.

ABOVE *Ayurvedic medicine has a cold preparation derived from sunflowers, which is warming to the system.*

In conventional medicine, colds are treated with rest and fluids, in addition to antihistamines, decongestants, and cough medicines, as needed. Aspirin is recommended only when symptoms are severe, because it increases viral shedding and makes the sufferer more contagious. Vaccines are of little use in prevention because so many kinds of viruses are involved. Research suggests that interferon (a protein produced by animal cells when they are invaded by viruses, which is released into the bloodstream or intercellular fluid to induce healthy cells to manufacture an enzyme that counters the infection) could prevent the spread of colds and may prove useful to people at high risk of complications.

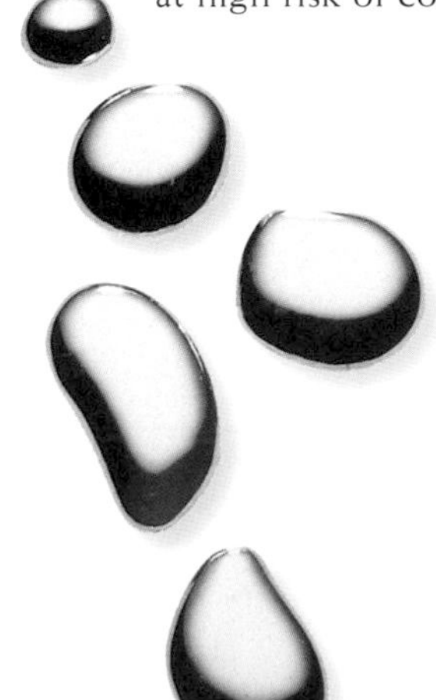

Symptoms

- *sneezing and runny nose* • *mild fever* • *headache* • *coughing and a burning or sore throat* • *catarrh*

LEFT *Mercury or quicksilver is the source of a homeopathic remedy used when the cold starts with a sore throat and affects the glands.*

TREATMENT

AYURVEDA

• Brown 4 tablespoons of coriander seeds in a frying pan, then boil with 4 cups of water, with 4 slices of root ginger. Reduce to 2 cups of liquid, strain, and drink. *(See page 35.)*

• Sunflower may be useful. *(See page 40.)*

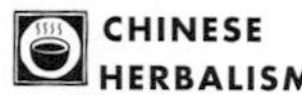

CHINESE HERBALISM

• Plantain seed, peppermint, mulberry, honeysuckle, and skullcap may be prescribed to address weakness of the Lung, Cold, and Wind. *(See pages 65 and 74.)*

TRADITIONAL HOME AND FOLK REMEDIES

• Barley water with lemon and honey will encourage healing and shorten the duration of a cold. *(See page 92.)*

• Cinnamon is an excellent warming herb, and can be added to food and drinks, or as an oil to a vaporizer, to treat and prevent colds and flu.

• Fresh garlic, eaten daily, will discourage the onset of a cold. Garlic will also work to reduce fever. *(See page 82.)*

• Honey, eaten fresh or added to herbal teas, will encourage healing and prevent secondary infections occurring. *(See page 101.)*

• Steep lemons in hot water, and a little honey; drink regularly in the cold season, or during a cold, to restore yourself and prevent infection. This will also treat coughs. *(See pages 87 and 101.)*

• A mustard poultice on the chest or mustard added to a foot bath will act as a decongestant. *(See page 98.)*

HERBALISM

• Ginger promotes perspiration and helps soothe the throat. *(See page 139.)*

• The herb echinacea will encourage immune response, and acts as a natural antibiotic. *(See page 120.)*

• Peppermint helps to reduce the symptoms of a cold. *(See page 125.)*

• Ginseng powder, added to any warming herbal tea, will boost the immune system and help the body to fight the infection. *(See page 126.)*

AROMATHERAPY

• Tea tree and lemon oils help to fight infection. Massage, in a light carrier oil, into the chest and head, or place in the bath or a burner. *(See pages 146–71.)*

• Lavender oil in the bath will help you sleep, to aid recovery – particularly good if there is a cough. *(See page 161.)*

• Eucalyptus oil can kill bacteria and soothe inflamed mucous membranes. *(See page 159.)*

HOMEOPATHY

• Aconite, in the first stage of a cold. *(See page 178.)*

• Belladonna, for colds with a high temperature and great thirst. *(See page 183.)*

• Mercurius, for colds that begin with a sore throat, with swollen glands. *(See page 205.)*

• Gelsemium, for flu-like symptoms, weakness, and achiness. *(See page 195.)*

• Allium, for streaming nose and eyes where the discharge makes the nose red raw. *(See page 178.)*

• Pulsatilla, for runny nose with thick, yellow or green mucus. *(See page 209.)*

• Nat. mur., for colds with a crop of cold sores; sneezing and watery eyes. *(See page 206.)*

• Dulcamara, when the nose is stuffed up with catarrh in rainy or windy weather. *(See page 213.)*

• Bryonia, if you feel like a bear with a sore head. *(See page 185.)*

VITAMINS AND MINERALS

• Citrus fruit is rich in vitamin C, which will help the body to fight infection. *(See page 256.)*

• Zinc is known to reduce the duration of a cold; suck a zinc lozenge at the first signs. *(See page 265.)*

• Royal jelly acts as a tonic and an antiviral agent. *(See page 276.)*

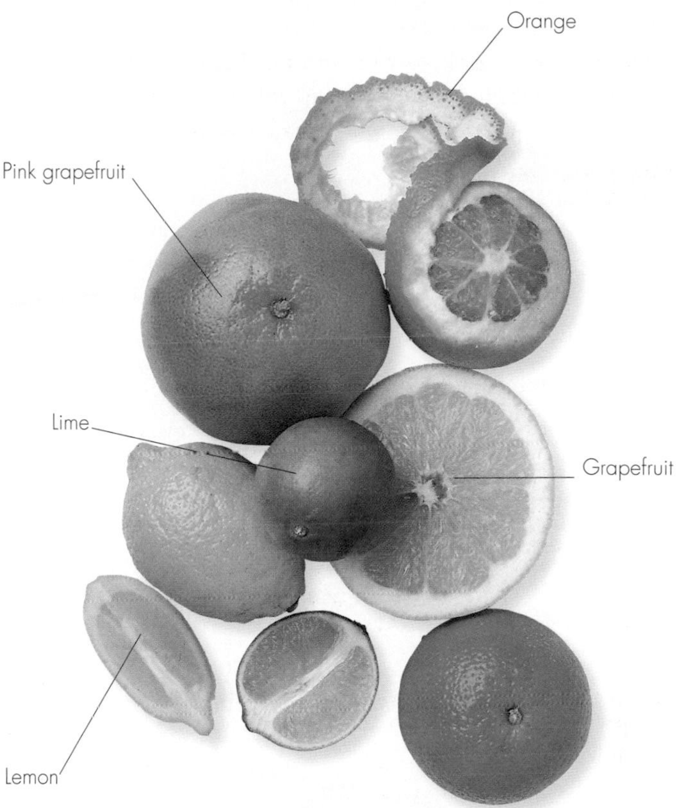

ABOVE *Citrus fruits are the favorite natural remedy for a cold. They are the perfect source of vitamin C, which helps the body to fight infection.*

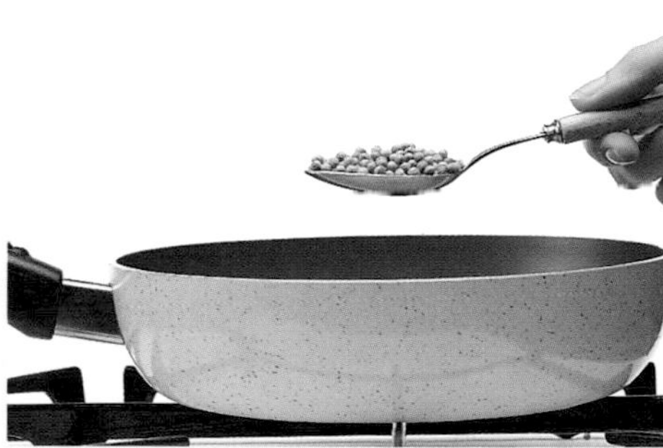

Both ginger and coriander are useful in treating colds. To make a decoction, brown 4 tablespoons of coriander seeds.

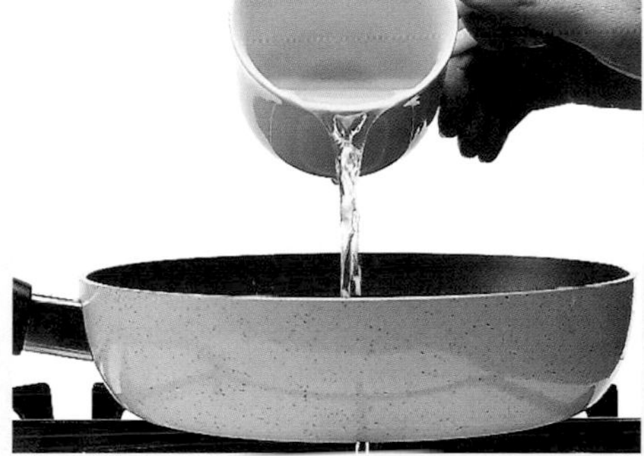

Once the seeds are browned, add 4 cups of water and bring to the boil.

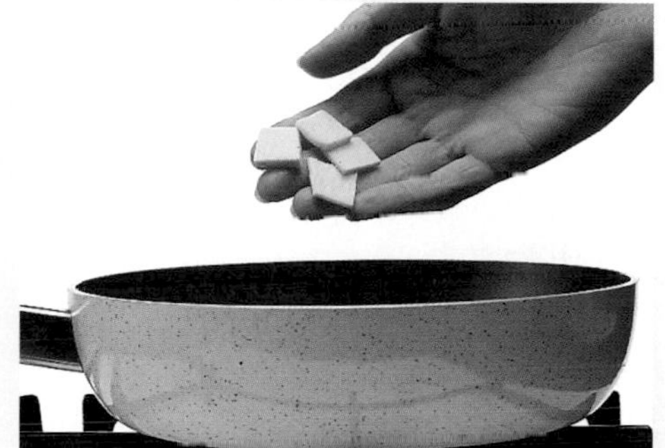

Add 4 slices of root ginger and reduce the liquid to 2 cups and strain. Drink to reduce a fever.

HEART, BLOOD, AND CIRCULATORY DISORDERS

High Blood Pressure

Blood pressure is the force with which the blood presses against the arterial walls as it circulates. In a person with high blood pressure, or hypertension, this force is greater than normal and causes the arterial walls to narrow and thicken, putting extra strain on the heart. Blood pressure fluctuates even in healthy individuals. It tends to increase with physical activity, excitement, fear, or emotional stress, but such elevations are usually transient. Most physicians will not make the diagnosis of hypertension unless the pressure is high on at least three separate occasions. Obesity, alcohol and sugar intake, and hereditary and ethnic factors all contribute, as will diabetes, kidney disease, and pregnancy. It is usually only when the secondary complications – damage to the arteries, brain, eyes, or elsewhere in the body – have developed that symptoms occur, by which time the condition is serious.

DATA FILE

- In the U.S. at least 50 million people have hypertension.
- Hypertension is usually described as being a systolic pressure greater than 139, or a diastolic pressure greater than 89, or both. The World Health Organization defines it as being consistently above 160mm. Hg. systolic, and 95mm. Hg. diastolic.
- In the U.K. high blood pressure is extremely common, affecting 10–20 percent of the adult population.
- High blood pressure is more frequent and more severe in African Americans than in the white U.S. population, and in both races in the south-eastern United States than in the rest of the nation.
- It is uncommon but not unheard of in children and adolescents.
- In young adulthood and early middle age, high blood pressure occurs more frequently in men than in women; thereafter the reverse is true.
- Hypertension occurs worldwide and is most prevalent in Japan and northern China.
- In societies that consume little or no salt the incidence of hypertension is extremely low.

SYMPTOMS

- *mild hypertension has no symptoms*
- *severe hypertension: – headaches – shortness of breath – visual disturbances – giddiness*

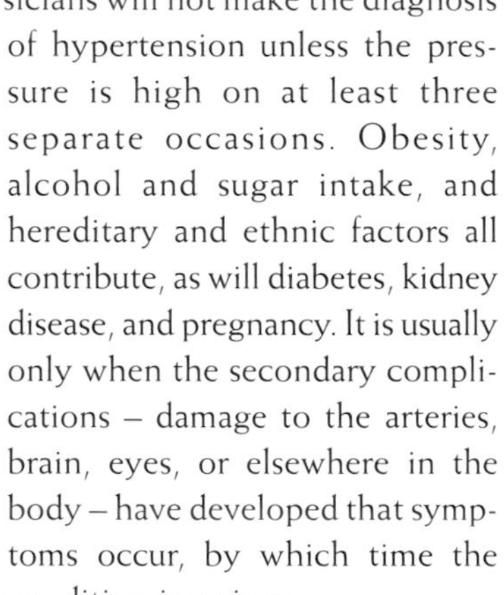

LEFT *Garlic is one of the most healing plants known to humankind. It has been shown to lower blood pressure, so if you suffer from hypertension eat plenty of raw garlic.*

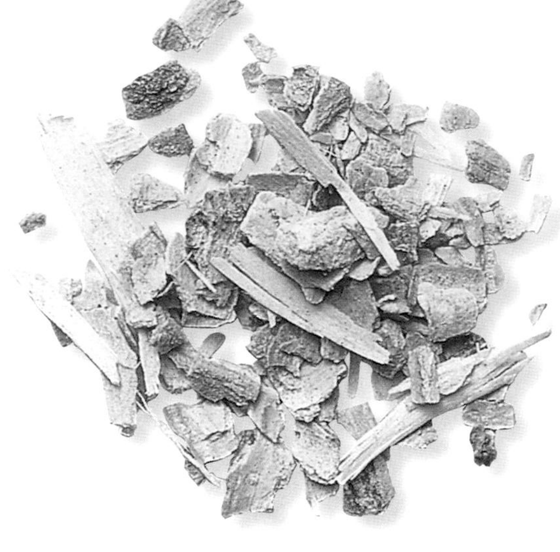

LEFT *Cramp bark is a useful herbal remedy for high blood pressure as it helps the arteries to dilate.*

TREATMENT

AYURVEDA
- The Ayurvedic products Dashamoola and Sarpaganda are used for treating high blood pressure.

CHINESE HERBALISM
- Internal Wind is believed to be the cause, and treatment will calm Liver Yang and Blood Wind. The herbs used might include chrysanthemum flowers, peony root, astragalus. *(See page 67.)*

TRADITIONAL HOME AND FOLK REMEDIES
- Eat plenty of fresh raw garlic, which acts as a tonic to the circulatory system and maintains its health. *(See page 82.)*

HERBALISM
- Hawthorn berries, infused, are a good heart tonic. *(See page 119.)*
- Cramp bark can be used to encourage the arteries to dilate. *(See page 138.)*
- Limeflowers and yarrow are also useful in the treatment of high blood pressure. *(See pages 112 and 134.)*

AROMATHERAPY
- Lavender will soothe and relax. *(See page 161.)*
- Regular massage with oils of lavender, marjoram, and ylang ylang can have a beneficial effect. *(See pages 146–71.)*

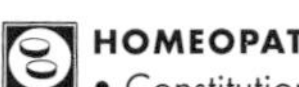

HOMEOPATHY
- Constitutional treatment is appropriate.

VITAMINS AND MINERALS
- Increase your intake of dietary fiber, and of potassium, calcium, and magnesium, which have a balancing effect on the circulation and encourage the action of the heart. *(See pages 258 and 262.)*

CAUTION

ROUTINE BLOOD PRESSURE CHECKS SHOULD BE UNDERTAKEN BY EVERYONE AS A MATTER OF COURSE. SUSTAINED HIGH BLOOD PRESSURE CAN CAUSE SEVERE DAMAGE TO THE HEART, KIDNEYS, AND EYES, AND SHOULD NOT BE IGNORED. DO NOT TAKE HERBAL REMEDIES WHILE TAKING CONVENTIONAL MEDICATION WITHOUT CONSULTING YOUR PHYSICIAN.

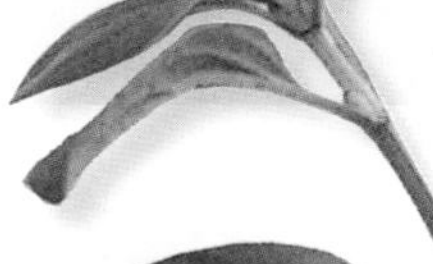

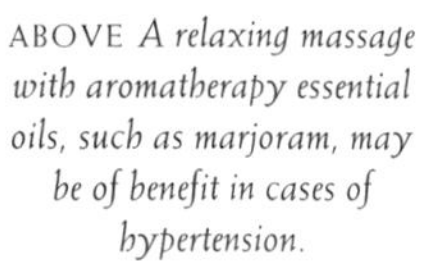

ABOVE *A relaxing massage with aromatherapy essential oils, such as marjoram, may be of benefit in cases of hypertension.*

Low Blood Pressure

Low blood pressure, or hypotension, is an abrupt fall in blood pressure due possibly to the heart's failure to maintain it or to severe loss of fluid from the circulation. It is perhaps most commonly noticed on standing up suddenly from a sitting or prone position, but can also result from severe hemorrhage, burns, gastroenteritis, or dehydration.

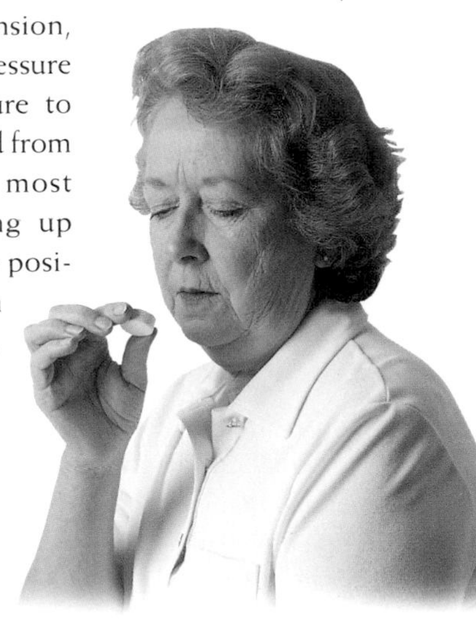

ABOVE *Many homeopathic treatments, such as Ignatia or Aconite, are excellent remedies for hypotension.*

Symptoms

- *fainting (due to the blood volume circulating being insufficient to supply the brain and lungs); older people in particular and those taking drugs against hypertension may experience fainting episodes, accompanied by paleness, a weak pulse, and dilated pupils*

DATA FILE

Blood pressure is conventionally written as two numbers, systolic pressure over diastolic pressure. Systolic pressure is the maximum blood pressure that occurs during the contraction of the heart; diastolic pressure is the lowest pressure measured during the interbeat period. The medically acceptable upper limit for blood pressure in an adult has been lowered in recent years and is now considered to be 140/90mm. Hg.

TREATMENT

CHINESE HERBALISM

- Treatment would be aimed at Deficient qi in the Blood and Heart. Ginseng and Chinese angelica might be used. *(See pages 56 and 67.)*

HERBALISM

- Broom is useful for treating low blood pressure, as it tones the arteries.
- Ginger, hawthorn tops, and rosemary will also be useful as they are stimulating and work to encourage circulation. *(See pages 119, 127, and 139.)*

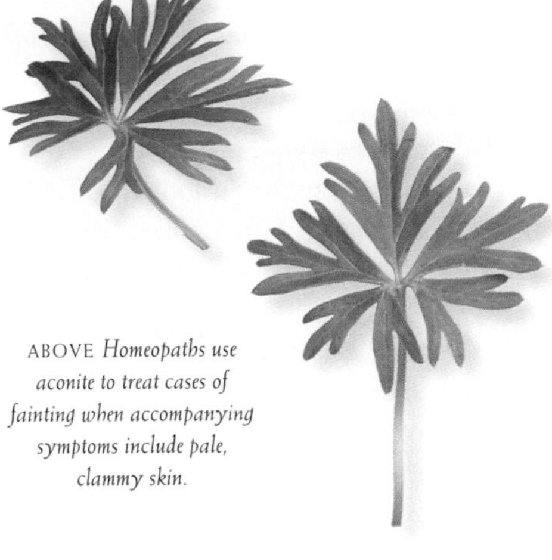

ABOVE *Homeopaths use aconite to treat cases of fainting when accompanying symptoms include pale, clammy skin.*

AROMATHERAPY

- Regular massage with oils of black pepper, lemon, sage, or rosemary, which stimulate and warm, will be useful. *(See pages 146–71.)*

HOMEOPATHY

Treatment would be constitutional, but the following remedies may help if you feel a tendency to faint:

- Veratrum, for fainting caused by anger.
- Coffea, for fainting brought on by excitement. *(See page 192.)*
- Ignatia, for fainting caused by an emotional shock or trauma. *(See page 200.)*
- Aconite, for fainting caused by fright, and characterized by tension and pale, clammy skin. *(See page 178.)*
- Cocculus, when caused by lack of sleep.
- Gelsemium, when you feel weak and shaky. *(See page 195.)*

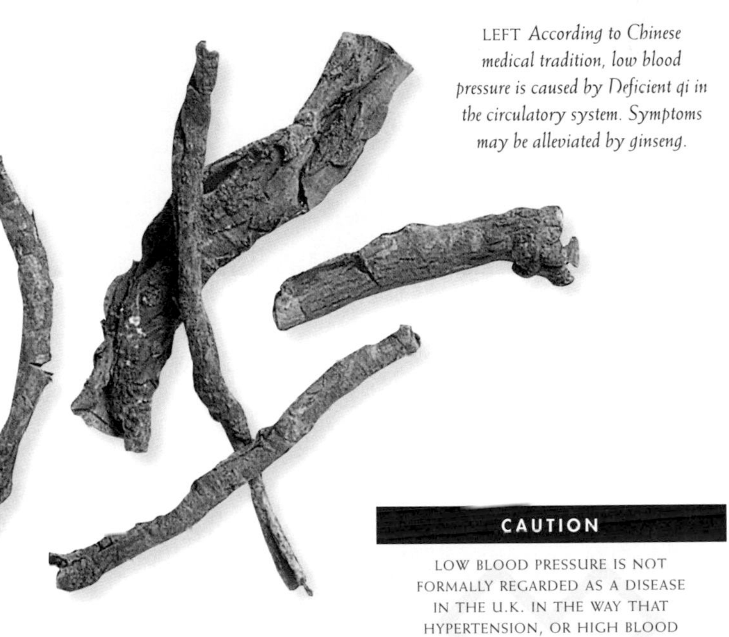

LEFT *According to Chinese medical tradition, low blood pressure is caused by Deficient qi in the circulatory system. Symptoms may be alleviated by ginseng.*

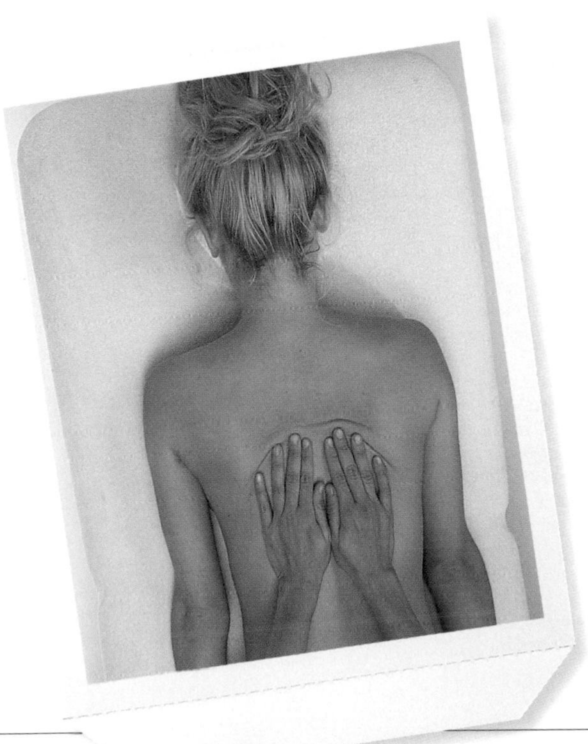

LEFT *Regular massage with stimulating essential oils such as black pepper, lemon or sage, may help regulate blood pressure.*

CAUTION

LOW BLOOD PRESSURE IS NOT FORMALLY REGARDED AS A DISEASE IN THE U.K. IN THE WAY THAT HYPERTENSION, OR HIGH BLOOD PRESSURE, IS. GENUINE HYPOTENSION CAN, HOWEVER, BE FATAL, AND MUST BE GIVEN URGENT MEDICAL ATTENTION.

Leukemia

Leukemia is the name given to a group of serious diseases in which certain white blood cells reproduce arbitrarily, replacing and interfering with the blood's normal components. Untreated, this disorder will lead to a fatal shortage of red blood cells, bleeding, or infection. Leukemia can be classified into two main groups – acute and chronic. Acute leukemia is rapid in onset, affecting children in particular, while chronic leukemia is slower in onset, with a much greater life expectancy for sufferers.

DATA FILE

- Acute and chronic leukemias, together with the other types of tumors of the blood, bone cells (myelomas), and lymph tissue (lymphomas), cause about 10 percent of all cancer deaths and about 50 percent of all cancer deaths in children and adults less than 30 years old.
- Lymphoblastic leukemia is more common in children, with 50 cases per 1 million of the population occuring between the ages of two and four.
- In the U.K. there are 10 cases per million of the population up to the age of 75, then 50 cases per million thereafter.
- When untreated, acute leukemia is fatal in one to two years and often fatal within about six months of onset.

Symptoms

• *acute leukemias are most common in children and are characterized by: – general aching and tiredness – susceptibility to infection – bleeding gums – sore throat – swelling of glands in the neck, groin, and armpits – appetite and weight loss – severe anemia* • *chronic leukemias are characterized by: – slow onset of fatigue – gradual enlargement of the spleen until it is so big as to cause a dragging sensation and pain in the upper left abdomen – gradual weight loss – nosebleeds – painful and prolonged erections in men – fever and night sweats*

TREATMENT

AROMATHERAPY
• Essential oils can be very supportive, but massage must not be used if you are suffering from leukemia. Add a few drops of niaouli or bergamot to the bath, or place in a vaporizer. *(See pages 153 and 163.)*

HOMEOPATHY
• Chronic and acute leukemia are given constitutional treatment, to help the body to cope with the effects of conventional medication.

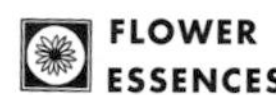

FLOWER ESSENCES
• Remedies are very useful in helping with accompanying negative feelings.
• Mimulus, for fear and concern. *(See page 235.)*
• Rescue Remedy or Emergency Essence, for trauma and shock. *See page 244.)*
• Agrimony, for hiding true feelings of distress behind a cheerful face. *(See page 225.)*
• Elm, for times when the pressures of responsibility seem overwhelming. *(See page 241.)*

CAUTION

A PRECISE MEDICAL DIAGNOSIS OF THE TYPE OF WHITE BLOOD CELL INVOLVED MUST BE MADE IN ORDER TO TREAT THE DISEASE EFFECTIVELY SINCE DIFFERENT CELLS CALL FOR DIFFERENT TREATMENTS.

LEFT *Flower essence therapists recommend Agrimony in cases where patients hide their true feelings behind a facade of great cheeriness.*

Enlarged Spleen

The spleen is located on the left side of the body below the ribs and is responsible for removing dead blood cells from the blood. It varies in size and weight according to the amount of blood it contains in storage and its immune functions. In adult humans the spleen functions both as an immunologically active organ and as a filter for white and red blood cells. All of the blood in the human body passes through the spleen approximately every 90 minutes. Slight enlargement of the spleen is normal during and after digestion, and the size of the spleen in adults usually ranges from 3 ½–8oz. (100–250g.). Abnormal enlargement, or splenomegaly, may occur in the course of a number of diseases, including: malaria, typhoid, hemolytic anemia, leukemia, Hodgkin's disease, glandular fever, septicemia, and syphilis. An enlarged spleen becomes firmer and can easily be felt on physical examination.

ABOVE *Oak, the source of Quercus. It is used homeopathically to treat an enlarged spleen.*

CAUTION

AN ENLARGED SPLEEN IS FAR MORE LIKELY TO RUPTURE THAN A NORMAL, HEALTHY SPLEEN. IN THE EVENT OF A RUPTURE, THE MAIN DANGER IS FROM SEVERE HEMORRHAGE, WHICH CAN BE FATAL IF IT IS NOT TREATED IMMEDIATELY.

Symptoms

• *symptoms will vary according to the cause of enlargement, but the general area of the spleen will be very tender*

TREATMENT

HERBALISM
Any of the herbs that help the immune action will be useful, including the following:
• Licorice can enhance recovery, stimulating white blood cell and antibody formation and efficiency. *(See page 122.)*
• Garlic helps to prevent infections of all kinds, including those which have become resistant to a dose of antibiotics. *(See page 113.)*
• Echinacea is widely used to treat chronic and acute infections, cleansing the blood and lymphatic system, and stimulating production of white blood cells and antibodies. *(See page 120.)*
• Ginseng can boost immunity and encourage the body to deal efficiently with stress, as well as stimulating white blood cell production and aiding recovery after illness. *(See page 126.)*

HOMEOPATHY
Treatment would be constitutional, but the following may help, depending on the cause:
• Quercus, for an enlarged spleen associated with cirrhosis of the liver, and swollen ankles.
• Nat. mur., for a swollen spleen with constipation, salt cravings, and oversensitive reactions. *(See page 206.)*

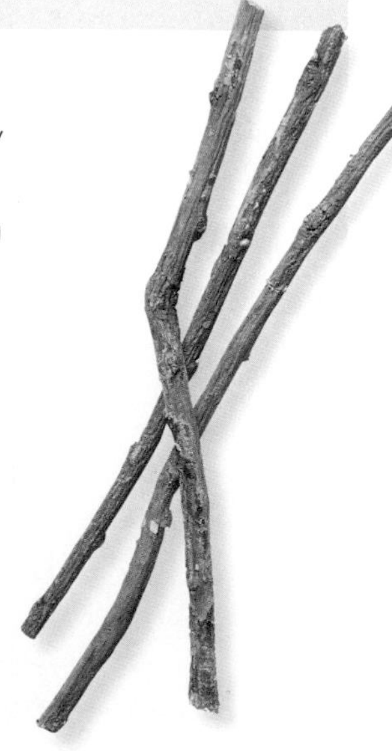

ABOVE *Licorice, which stimulates the formation of white blood cells, will help the immune system to recover from an enlarged spleen.*

Anemia

Anemia is a deficiency of hemoglobin – the chemical that carries oxygen – in the red cells of the blood. The most common cause of anemia is iron deficiency resulting from excessive blood loss (through trauma, surgery, childbirth, or heavy menstrual bleeding), poor diet, or failure to absorb iron from food. Other causes of anemia include: excessive destruction of red blood cells (hemolytic anemia); vitamin B12 deficiency (pernicious anemia); and the inherited disorders of sickle cell anemia and thalassemia.

DATA FILE

- Of all sufferers, 20 percent are women, and 50 percent are children.
- The most common type of anemia is iron deficiency anemia, most often resulting from chronic blood loss; also from lack of iron in the diet, impaired absorption of iron from the intestine, or an increased need for iron, as occurs during pregnancy.
- Iron is an essential component of the hemoglobin, which carries oxygen to the tissues in chemical combination with its iron atoms.
- Pernicious anemia is a chronic inherited disease of middle-aged and older people in which the stomach fails to produce a factor needed for the absorption of vitamin B12, which is essential for mature red blood cells.
- Aplastic anemia is the result of the failure of bone marrow cells to manufacture mature red cells. It is usually caused by toxic chemicals (for example, benzene) or by radiation.

Symptoms

- *weakness and fatigue*
- *breathlessness on minimal exertion*
- *pale skin and lips* • *headaches, dizziness, and possibly fainting in severe cases* • *in pernicious anemia there may be: – nosebleeds – a sore tongue – "pins and needles" in the hands and feet*

CAUTION

IRON DEFICIENCY IN POST-MENOPAUSAL WOMEN AND IN MEN SHOULD ALWAYS BE INVESTIGATED.

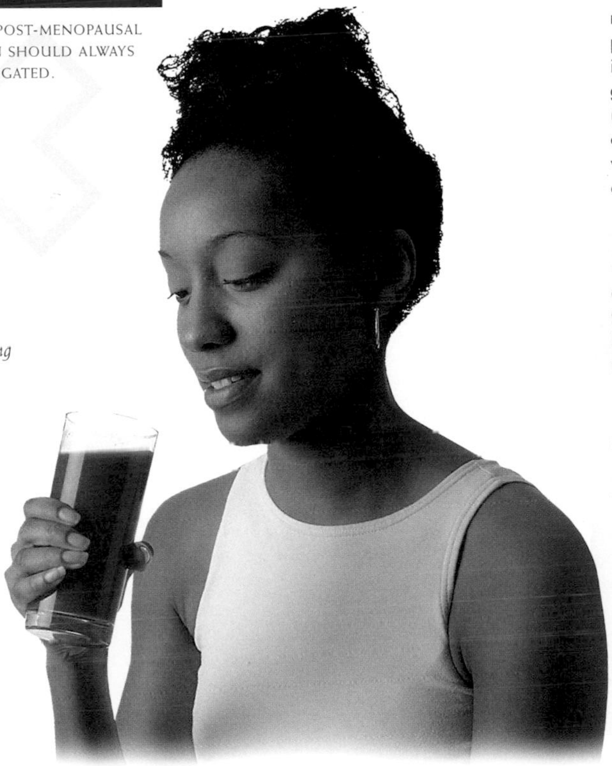

RIGHT *If you are suffering from anemia try drinking carrot juice, a traditional remedy for iron deficiency.*

TREATMENT

Anemia sufferers will benefit greatly from eating watercress.
Eggs are a good source of iron.
A portion of oats a day will help combat anemia.
Pumpkin seeds contain measurable amounts of iron.

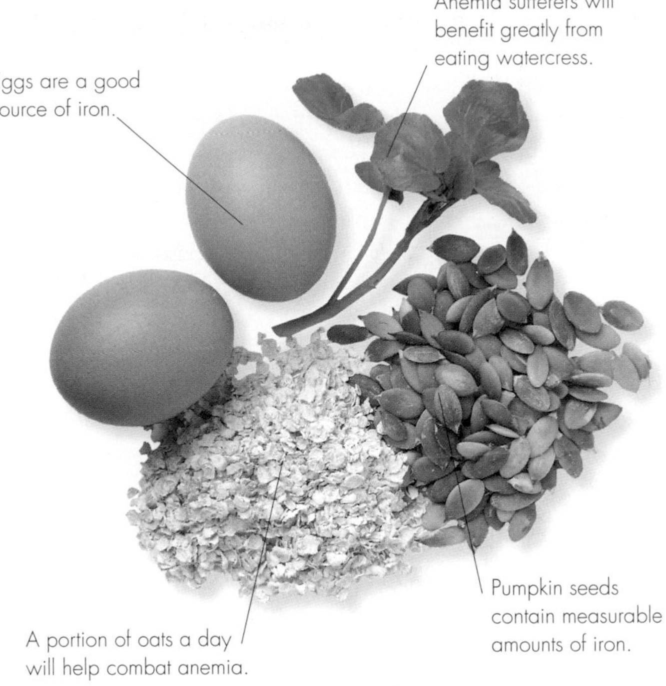

ABOVE *Eating foods rich in iron will help the hemoglobin levels in your blood to rise.*

AYURVEDA
- There are a number of Ayurvedic products available, including Kalyanaka ghritha (oral ghee), Kishor (oral pills) and Avipathi choorna (oral powder), which would complement a treatment program.

CHINESE HERBALISM
- The cause would be attributed to a Spleen not transforming qi, and Gui Pi Wan (return spleen tablets) would be useful.

TRADITIONAL HOME AND FOLK REMEDIES
- Nettle tea is rich in iron; drink daily.
- Beet and carrot juice may be drunk to treat the condition. *(See page 89.)*

HERBALISM
- Chinese angelica root may be helpful. Take as tincture, decoction, or tea. *(See page 115.)*
- Alfalfa, dandelion root, nettles, watercress, and yellow dock are rich in iron. *(See pages 128, 134, and 137.)*

AROMATHERAPY
- Lavender essential oil is helpful where the anemia is associated with palpitations and dizzy spells. *(See page 161.)*
- Massage with Roman chamomile essential oil. *(See page 150.)*

HOMEOPATHY
- Ferr. phos. helps assimilation of iron from food. *(See page 194.)*
- Nat. mur., for anemia with constipation, headache, and a tendency to cold sores *(See page 206.)*
- Calc. phos., for anemia during a growth spurt, and irritability. *(See page 186.)*
- Picric acid, for anemia with mental overload.

VITAMINS AND MINERALS
- Iron-rich foods include oats, egg yolks, pumpkin seeds, and watercress. *(See page 260.)*
- Calcium, copper, vitamin C, and B vitamins must be present for the body to assimilate iron; ensure you have a sufficient intake in your diet. *(See pages 252–5, 256, 258, and 259.)*
- Vegetarians should take extra vitamin B12. *(See page 255.)*
- Avoid drinking tea at mealtimes as this makes iron absorption less efficient

Angina

Angina (known medically as *angina pectoris*) is chest pain caused by a narrowing of the arteries, with the result that the blood supply to the heart muscle is not enough to meet its demands for oxygen and nutrients. The pain most commonly occurs after physical exertion, a heavy meal, cold weather, or various other circumstances requiring the heart to work harder. Groups likely to be susceptible to angina include smokers, diabetics, and the overweight.

ABOVE *Hawthorn is a good herbal tonic for angina and may be taken with most orthodox drugs (except dioxin).*

SYMPTOMS

• severe pain in the chest, often spreading up to the neck and down the left arm • a feeling of tightness in the chest • there may also be pain between the shoulder blades

DATA FILE

• Cardiovascular disease has been a major health problem in the U.S. for years and is the leading cause of death.

• Nearly 1 million people die each year of cardiovascular disease.

• The death rate from cardiovascular diseases has declined since the mid-1970s, due to modification of risk factors for disease, and improvements in diagnosis and treatment.

• At first, angina may only be evident during periods of exercise or emotional stress, resolving when the activity ceases. Later, it may occur even at rest.

• An estimated 50 million Americans have cardiovascular disease and are unaware of it.

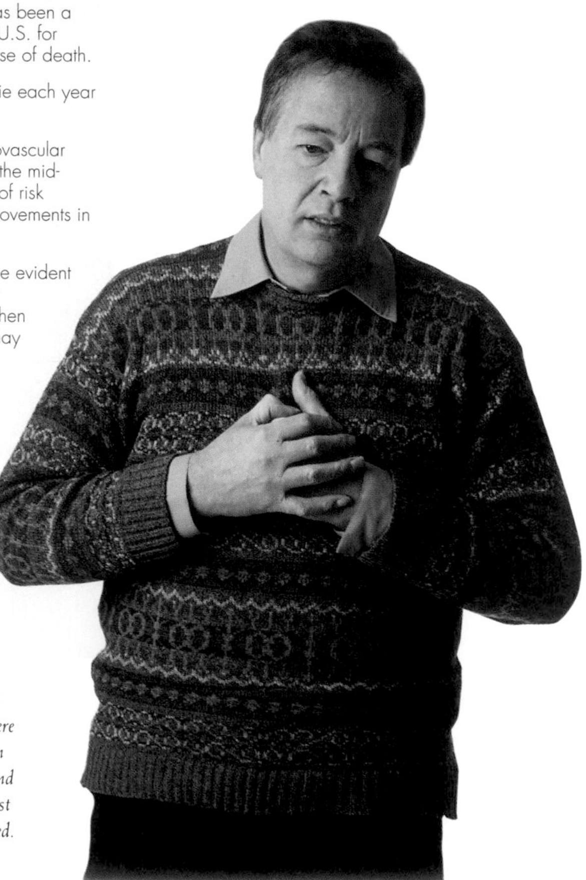

RIGHT *Angina is characterized by severe chest pain that often spreads to the neck and the left arm. The chest will also be constricted.*

TREATMENT

CHINESE HERBALISM

• Treatment would be aimed at stagnant qi in the Blood and Heart. Herbs used may include safflower, cinnamon twigs, red sage root, peony root, and macrosten onion bulb. *(See pages 58, 59, and 67.)*

HERBALISM

• Hawthorn berries, made into an infusion, are a good tonic for the heart. *(See page 119.)*

• Motherwort is useful for the treatment of angina. Sip a motherwort decoction 3 times daily. *(See page 124.)*

• Balm and limeflowers are tonics for the heart and the circulatory system, and regular infusions will help ensure their healthy functioning. *(See page 134.)*

HOMEOPATHY

Treatment would be constitutional, but the following remedies may help in mild attacks:

• Cactus, for a constricted chest and consequent trouble breathing.

• Lilium, for a bursting feeling in the heart, with palpitations and some pain in the right arm.

• Naja, for an irregular pulse, accompanied by anxiety and fearfulness.

• Glonoinum, for a fluttering heart, a sensation of blood rushing, difficulty breathing, and faintness, which are made worse by heat. *(See page 196.)*

VITAMINS AND MINERALS

• Increase your intake of dietary fiber and oily fish (such as sardines, herring, salmon, and mackerel).

• Raw garlic aids the functioning of the circulatory system, and helps treat the condition.

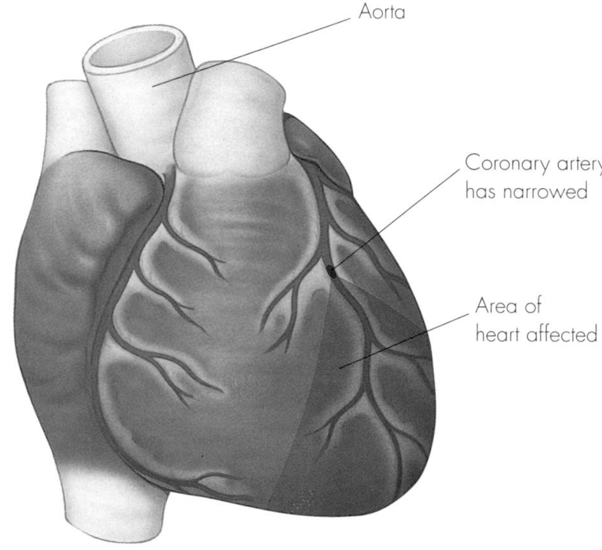

ABOVE *Angina occurs when the muscular wall of the heart becomes short of oxygen.*

CAUTION

PROLONGED OR MORE SEVERE CASES OF ANGINA CAN BE A PRECURSOR TO A HEART ATTACK AND SHOULD RECEIVE URGENT MEDICAL ATTENTION.

Palpitations

The average heart beats about 72 times a minute and pumps about 3,6000 gallons (13,640l.) of blood a day. During exercise, the pumping action automatically increases three- or fourfold, in response to the tissues' demand for increased oxygen. Palpitation refers to a fast or irregular heartbeat. Palpitations are quite common and usually harmless, often brought on by physical exertion or fright. Frequent or prolonged palpitations, however, may be an indication of heart disease, particularly if accompanied by dizziness, fainting, or chest pain. The sensation of a "missed" beat is due to a premature ectopic beat followed by a compensatory gap before the next beat. This can be induced by anxiety or stimulants such as caffeine and nicotine.

Symptoms

- *pounding in the chest following exercise*
- *uncomfortable awareness of a rapid heart rate when anxious*

TREATMENT

CHINESE HERBALISM
- Treatment would be aimed at addressing a Heart Blood deficiency, and may include the use of asparagus root and wild jujube seed. *(See page 75.)*

HERBALISM
- Motherwort, drunk as an infusion, may help if palpitations are linked to anxiety or stress. *(See page 124.)*
- Broom, limeflowers, mistletoe, and valerian are useful herbs for treating palpitations. *(See pages 134 and 136.)*

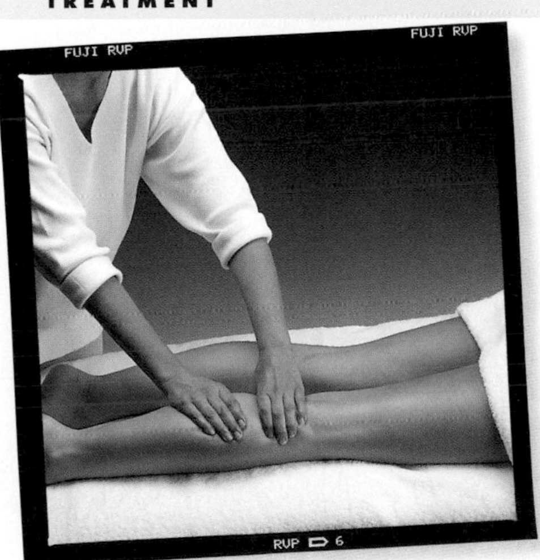

ABOVE *Soothing essential oils, such as ylang ylang or mandarin, may be used in aromatherapy massage to calm palpitations.*

AROMATHERAPY
- If your palpitations are linked to emotional causes, calming oils such as ylang ylang, marjoram, lavender, and mandarin will help. Place a few drops in the bath, or use in regular massage. Carry a bottle with you, and sniff in times of distress. *(See pages 146–71.)*
- Peppermint, aniseed, lavender, melissa, rosemary, and neroli essential oils can be used separately or combined in a good massage oil to treat palpitations. *(See pages 146–71.)*

HOMEOPATHY
- Nux vomica, when palpitations are brought on by overindulgence. *(See page 214.)*
- Nat. mur., for strong palpitations and chest constriction, made worse by heat. *(See page 206.)*
- Cactus, for violent palpitations which are worse before menstruation, with dizziness, shortness of breath, and flatulence.
- Pulsatilla, when palpitations are brought on by heat or rich fatty foods. *(See page 209.)*
- Lachesis, for fainting, a constricted feeling, and anxiety. *(See page 216.)*

FLOWER ESSENCES
- Rescue Remedy or Emergency Essence will help to calm panic and anxiety associated with the onset of palpitations. *(See page 244.)*

Gangrene

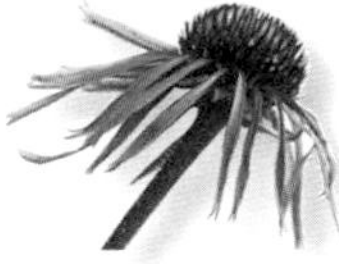

ABOVE
The Echinacea species is used to make a homeopathic remedy for persistent, festering, septic wounds.

Gangrene is the decay and eventual death of tissue as a result of inadequate blood supply. This may be caused by injury, burns, frostbite, or by disorders such as atherosclerosis, embolism, thrombosis, and diabetes. Excessive smoking can also lead to gangrene.

Symptoms

- *if the affected area is not infected, it will typically be dry, and brown or black in color*
- *if bacteria have entered the affected tissue, festering occurs, leading to "wet" gangrene*
- *infection of the affected area by one of the clostridia family of gas-producing soil bacteria leads to "gas" gangrene. This is characterized by swelling of the tissues, particularly the muscles, which spreads rapidly to healthy tissues; discoloration; and severe illness*
- *antibiotics can sometimes prevent gangrene from spreading*

CAUTION

TREATMENT IS URGENT, AND YOU SHOULD BE SEEN BY YOUR PHYSICIAN.

TREATMENT

HOMEOPATHY
The following symptoms can be used on an emergency basis, for up to 10 doses:
- Echinacea, when the wound turns septic and also smells foul.
- Euphorbia, for wet gangrene in a chronic ulcer.
- Lachesis, for pain which is worse after sleeping, and when the affected area is blue or purple. *(See page 216.)*
- Arsenicum, when the skin is ulcerated, cold makes the pain worse, and you feel restless. *(See page 182.)*

VITAMINS AND MINERALS
- Vitamin E taken orally and applied to the wound or gangrenous area will promote healing. *(See page 257.)*

BELOW *Vitamin E will promote healing. It can be taken by mouth or applied externally.*

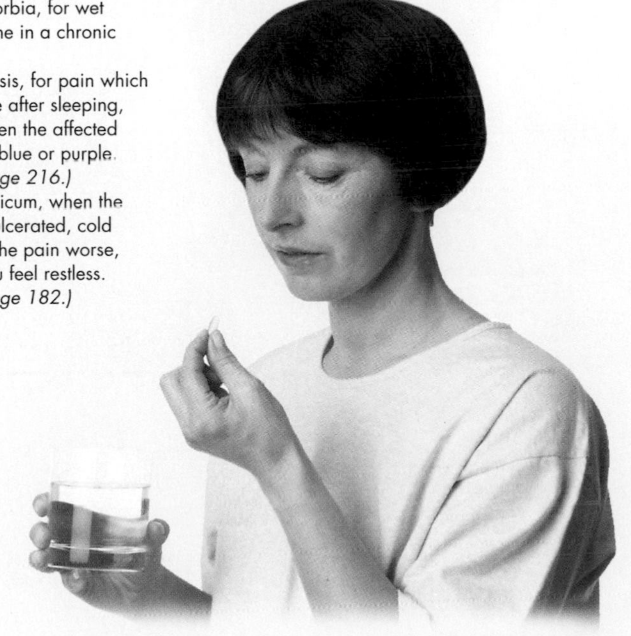

Atherosclerosis

Atherosclerosis is a degenerative disease of the arteries in which a fatty patch (atheroma) consisting mainly of cholesterol builds up on the wall of an artery. This eventually hardens and partially blocks the artery, causing the formation of a blood clot behind it. It is a progressive condition, generally worsening with age, and is most dangerous when the arteries supplying blood to the heart and brain are affected. Contributing factors to the development of atherosclerosis include smoking, high blood pressure, high blood cholesterol, heredity, and diabetes.

DATA FILE

Atherosclerosis can lead to:

- heart attack and angina, where the coronary arteries (supplying the heart) are affected
- stroke, where the carotid arteries (supplying the brain) are affected
- severe pain in the legs on walking when the femoral arteries (supplying the legs) are affected
- severe anemia

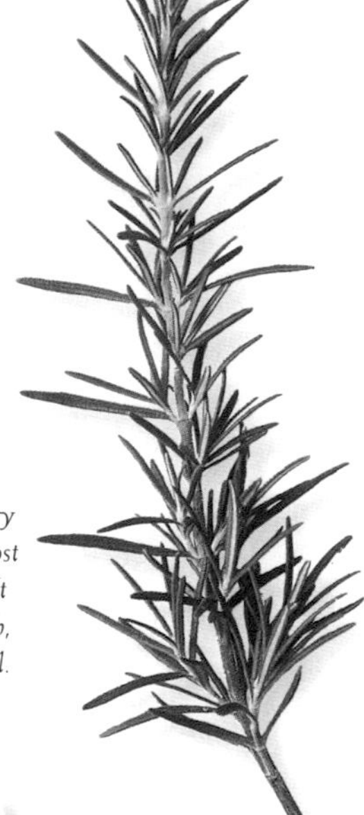

RIGHT *Rosemary can be used to boost the circulation. It can be taken fresh, dried, or as an oil.*

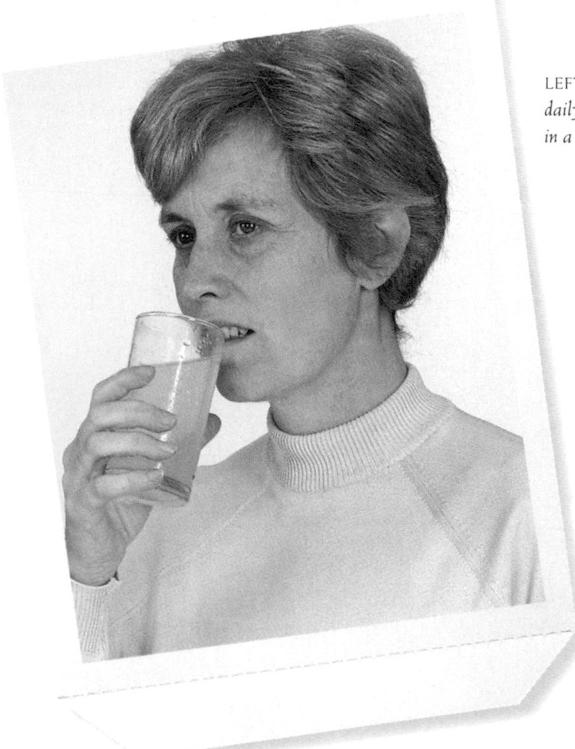

LEFT *Drink barley water daily to keep your heart in a healthy condition.*

TREATMENT

TRADITIONAL HOME AND FOLK REMEDIES

- Increase your intake of olive oil, which breaks down cholesterol and fatty deposits in the blood. *(See page 95.)*
- Drink barley water daily to ensure that your heart is healthy. *(See page 92.)*
- Garlic, onions, and yogurt all have a beneficial effect on the heart. *(See pages 82 and 93.)*

HERBALISM

- Lavender oil helps to regulate the heart and may prevent heart attack. Use the herb in the bath, or the oil in a vaporizer or gentle massage.
- Rosemary – fresh, dried, or as an oil – can be used to stimulate the circulatory system. *(See page 127.)*
- Hawthorn berries and tops, and limeflowers are both useful herbs for arterial diseases. *(See pages 119 and 134.)*

AROMATHERAPY

- Regular massage with juniper and lemon can help to break down fatty deposits in the body. *(See pages 154 and 160.)*

HOMEOPATHY

- Baryta carb., if you suffer from high blood pressure and palpitations. *(See page 185.)*
- Phosphorus, for treating fainting spells, salt cravings, and nervousness. *(See page 208.)*
- Glonoinum, for tight congested headache and pounding arteries. *(See page 196.)*
- Vanadium, for fainting, dizziness, liver problems, feeling that the heart is being compressed.

VITAMINS AND MINERALS

- Increase your intake of dietary fiber, and reduce your intake of salt and sugar.
- Increase your intake of foods with bioflavonoids, to improve artery health. *(See page 272.)*

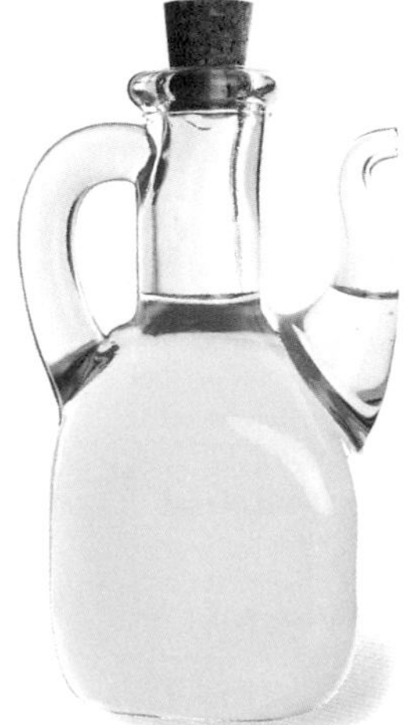

RIGHT *Scientific studies have proved that consumption of olive oil lowers cholesterol levels in the blood.*

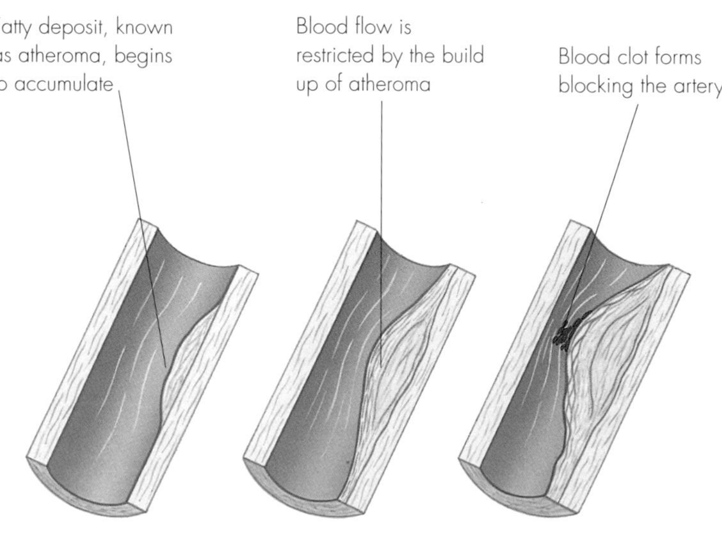

ABOVE *Atherosclerosis occurs when fatty deposits build up in the wall of an artery, restricting blood flow, and leading to the formation of a blood clot.*

Aneurysm

An aneurysm is a swelling or bulge in the wall of an artery that can vary in shape, size, and cause. A potentially fatal complication is rupture of the vessel, resulting in massive hemorrhage. It may occur in the main artery, the aorta, as a result of weakness in the muscular wall, possibly through atherosclerosis, syphilis, or a congenital defect. It can eventually rupture, causing fatal internal bleeding. It can also develop in the left ventricle of the heart (ventricular aneurysm) following a heart attack, and can lead to heart failure or an embolism. Aneurysms can also occur in the blood vessels of the brain. These are often congenital.

DATA FILE

There are many different types of aneurysms:

- Arterial aneurysms may be due to atherosclerosis, trauma, infectious injury, or a congenital defect. They occur most often in elderly people.
- Aortic aneurysms usually occur in the abdominal portion of the aorta, generally below the arteries leading to the kidney.
- A relatively common type of aneurysm – giant aneurysms – cause a hemorrhage in the brain.
- Defects in eye arteries may result in multiple aneurysms of the retina.
- Dissecting aneurysms, also called aortic dissection, begin suddenly as a tear in the inner vessel lining followed by entry of blood.
- A ventricular aneurysm may occur following a heart attack. Scar tissue forms over the dead heart cells and creates a patch over the weakened area, which may then bulge when the heart contracts.

Symptoms

• severe headaches • painful spine from the pressure of the swelling in the aorta, which can also cause: – a cough – voice loss – and difficulty in swallowing • in a dissecting aneurysm the wall of the affected artery splits, forcing blood between the layers

BELOW *Oily fish, such as mackerel, contain fatty acids that are believed to be a valuable protection against cardiovascular disease.*

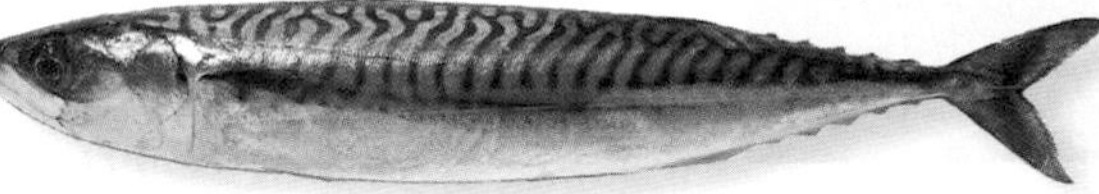

TREATMENT

AROMATHERAPY
- Oils like chamomile and cypress will bring about the contraction of the capillaries. Use in the bath or in a vaporizer. *(See page 150.)*

HOMEOPATHY
- For a burst aneurysm, ring for emergency help and take aconite every 5 minutes until help arrives. *(See page 178.)*

Constitutional treatment is appropriate for a developing aneurysm, but the following treatments will help until you receive treatment:

- Baryta carb., for raised blood pressure, palpitations, possible atherosclerosis, and pallor. *(See page 185.)*
- Lycopodium, for aneurysm of the aorta, where symptoms worsen between 4 and 8P.M. *(See page 203.)*
- Kali iod., for bone pain, which is worse at night and when in warmth.

VITAMINS AND MINERALS
- Eat plenty of garlic and brewer's yeast, which will encourage the healthy functioning of the circulatory system. *(See page 272.)*
- Increase your intake of oily fish.
- Vitamins C and E will encourage the healthy functioning of the circulatory system. *(See pages 256 and 257.)*

Varicose Veins

Varicose veins are swollen and twisted veins, most commonly found in the legs but also in the rectum (where they are known as hemorrhoids), the scrotum, and the esophagus. The swelling is caused by a weakness in the valves of the veins, which leads to increased pressure on the vein walls. This can be the result of deep vein thrombosis, obesity, pregnancy, prolonged sitting or standing, constipation, prolapse, or it may be hereditary.

ABOVE *Raw beetroot is said to help varicose veins and should be eaten daily for its value as a powerful tonic.*

Symptoms

• extremely sore, swollen, and tender veins • swelling of the legs • bruising and discoloration • burning sensation • aching calves • irritated and flaky skin • ulcers • in severe cases, a vein may rupture and bleed

TREATMENT

CHINESE HERBALISM
- The source of the problem is bad circulation, stagnant qi, and stagnant Blood, and the following herbs would be used: angelica, cinnamon twigs, and astragalus; honey might be used externally. *(See pages 56, 57, and 59.)*

TRADITIONAL HOME AND FOLK REMEDIES
- Raw beetroot should be eaten daily, for its healing and strengthening action.
- A mustard poultice, may help to encourage circulation in the area. *(See page 98.)*

HERBALISM
- Calendula oil, or marigold tea as a compress can be applied. *(See page 117.)*
- Herbs to repair and tone the veins include hawthorn berries, horse chestnut, prickly ash and yarrow – all of which can be infused and drunk. *(See pages 112 and 119.)*

AROMATHERAPY
- Rosemary oil, blended with a light carrier oil, can be massaged into the legs. *(See page 68.)*
- Essential oils of juniper and lavender can be diluted and massaged into the surrounding area, or used in the bath. *(See pages 160 and 161.)*

HOMEOPATHY
- Hamamelis, for bruised, sore veins, and piles. *(See page 197.)*
- Carb. veg., for mottled and marbled skin. *(See page 188.)*
- Pulsatilla, especially during pregnancy, and if warmth makes symptoms worse. *(See page 209.)*
- Ferr. phos., for pale legs that redden easily, but are better on walking. *(See page 194.)*

VITAMINS AND MINERALS
- Increase your intake of vitamins E and C, and bioflavonoids, which improve blood vessel health. *(See pages 257, 256 and 272.)*
- Increase your intake of dietary fiber, which will prevent constipation.
- Rutin helps to keep the vein walls in good shape.

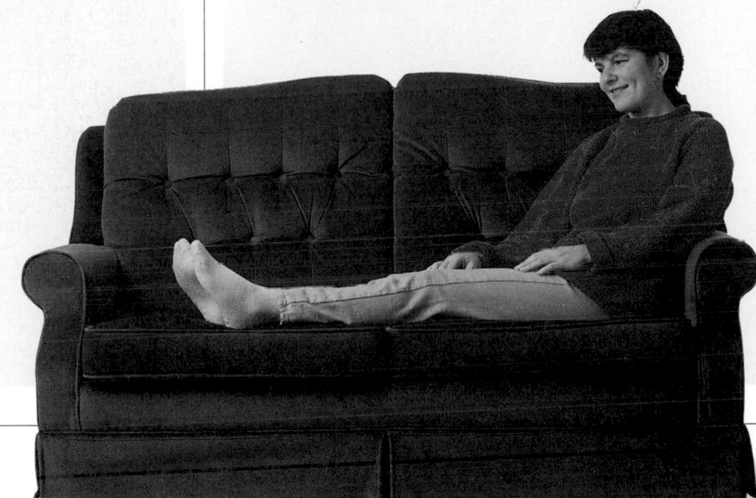

LEFT *Poor circulation, often the cause of varicose veins, may be improved by elevating the legs.*

Raynaud's Disease

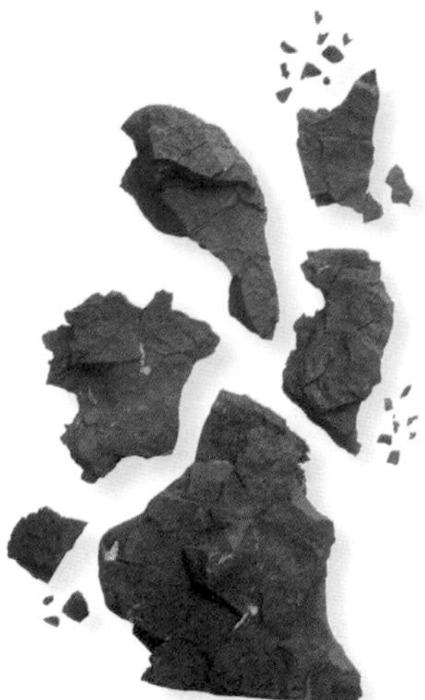

ABOVE *The homeopathic remedy Carbo vegitabilis is used to treat conditions where the symptom picture is characterized by icy mottled skin.*

Raynaud's disease is a disorder in which the arteries of the fingers and (less often) the toes go into spasm on exposure to cold. Raynaud's disease is more common in women than men, and its onset usually occurs in young adulthood. It affects mainly young women, has no known cause, and is rarely serious. Raynaud's phenomenon, however, caused by disease or occupational hazard, is more problematic: inflammation of the arteries of the fingers and toes occurs, sometimes leading to the formation of a blood clot.

Symptoms

• tingling sensation, burning, and numbness in fingers or toes • affected areas turn white, then blue, then red • painful ulcers or even tissue death (gangrene) can occur in cases where the disease persists for years

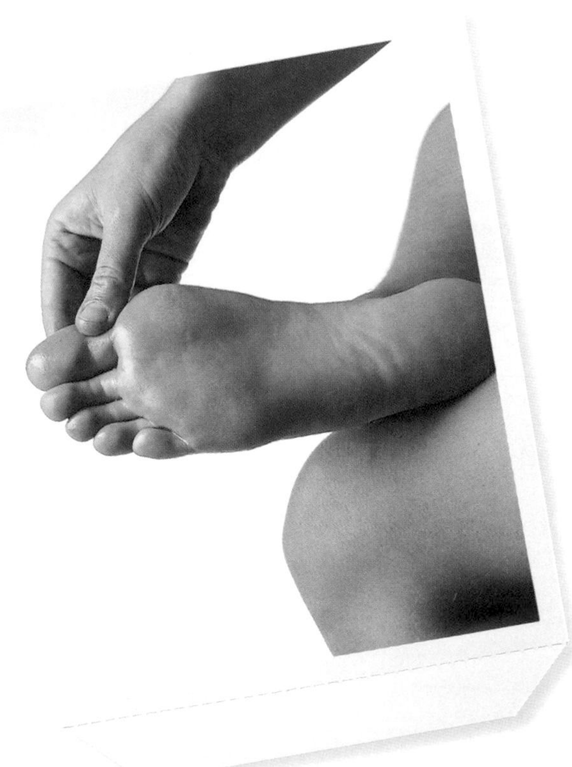

ABOVE *In Ayurvedic medicine, hands and feet are massaged with warm mustard and sesame oils to stimulate the circulation.*

TREATMENT

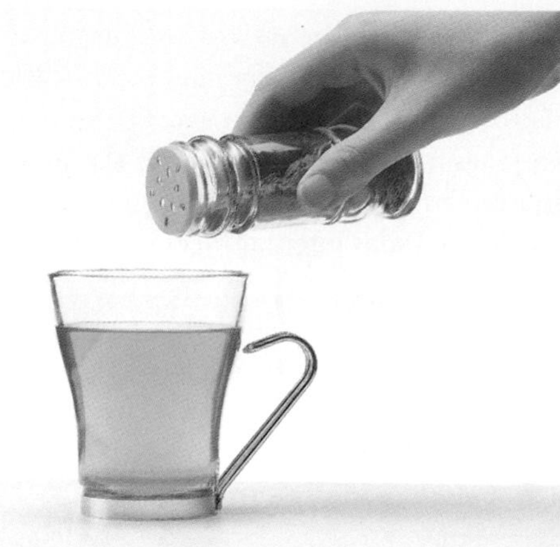

ABOVE *Herbalists add cayenne pepper to herbal tea to treat conditions when there is poor circulation.*

AYURVEDA

• Massage hands and feet with a mixture of warm mustard and sesame seed oils. *(See page 30.)*

CHINESE HERBALISM

• Cinnamon twigs and Chinese angelica may be useful. *(See pages 56 and 59.)*

HERBALISM

• Cayenne pepper can be added to any herbal tea to stimulate the circulation and warm the body. *(See page 118.)*

• Fresh ginger can be chewed, and the juices swallowed, to improve circulation and act as a tonic to the heart. *(See page 139.)*

AROMATHERAPY

• Rubefacient oils such as black pepper, lemon, and rosemary can be massaged into the affected area to increase circulation and warmth. *(See pages 146–71.)*

HOMEOPATHY

Constitutional treatment is advised, but the following may help:

• Carb. veg., for icy, mottled-looking skin. *(See page 188.)*

• Lachesis, for blue or purple skin, worse after sleep. *(See page 216.)*

• Pulsatilla, for symptoms that are made worse by heat or hanging the limb. *(See page 209.)*

• Arsenicum, for swelling, burning and itching made worse by exposure to cold. *(See page 182.)*

• Cactus, for icy cold, swollen hands and feet.

• Secale, for burning sensation in fingers or toes.

VITAMINS AND MINERALS

• Increase your intake of iron, and ensure that you take plenty of foods rich in vitamin C alongside, which helps the absorption of iron. *(See pages 260 and 256.)*

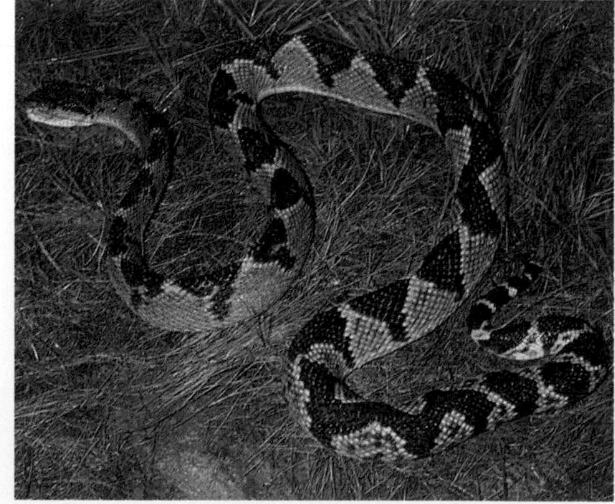

ABOVE *Lachesis is prepared from the bushmaster snake. It is used to treat complaints where there is mottled, purplish skin.*

Bruising

Bruising (or ecchymosis) results from the release of blood from the capillaries into the tissues under the skin. The characteristic bluish-black mark on the skin lightens in color and eventually fades as the blood is absorbed by the tissues and carried away. Bruising usually occurs as a result of an injury, but can occasionally be spontaneous and an indication of an allergic reaction, or more serious diseases such as leukemia and hemophilia.

Symptoms

- *pain on pressure*
- *in severe cases, pain on attempting to move the affected area*

CAUTION

A CASE OF BRUISING WITHOUT ANY OBVIOUS CAUSE REQUIRES MEDICAL INVESTIGATION AS IT MAY BE AN OUTWARD SYMPTOM OF A MORE SERIOUS CONDITION.

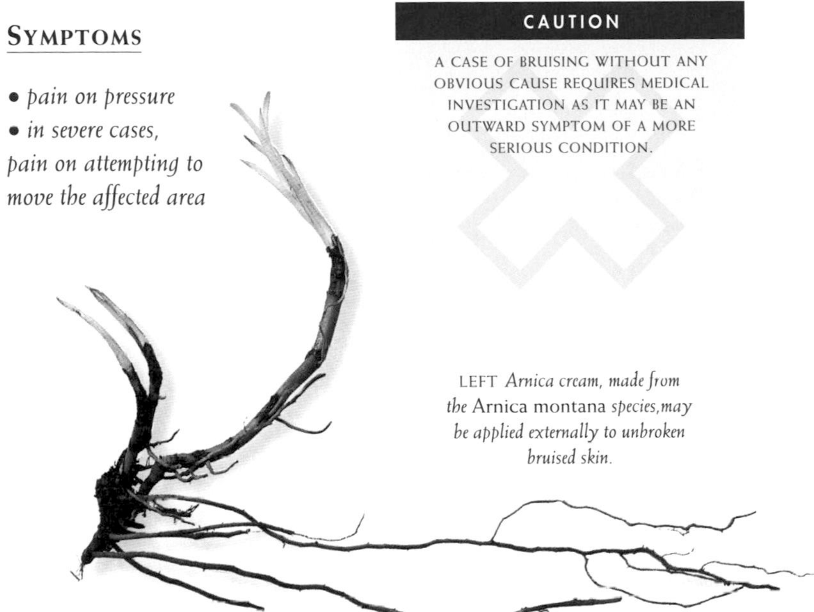

LEFT *Arnica cream, made from the* Arnica montana *species, may be applied externally to unbroken bruised skin.*

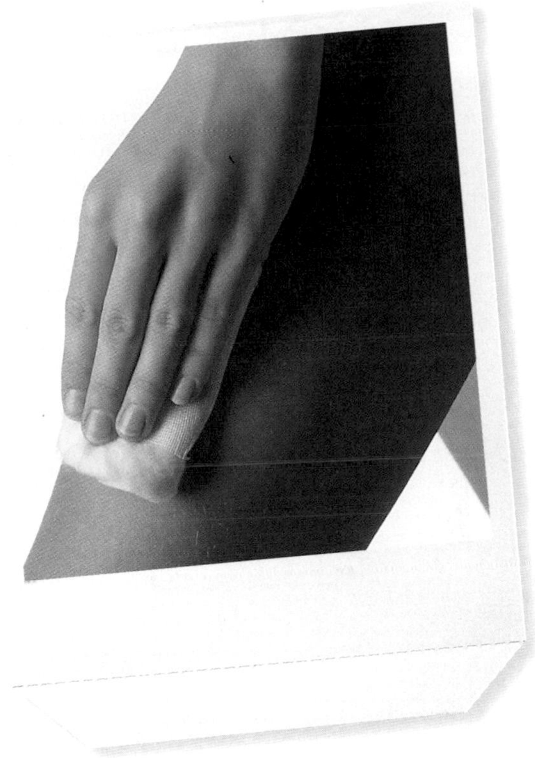

ABOVE *Apply a cold vinegar compress to relieve bruises and swelling.*

TREATMENT

TRADITIONAL HOME AND FOLK REMEDIES

- Macerated and heated cabbage leaves can be applied to the affected area. *(See page 87.)*
- A mustard poultice or black pepper oil draws the blood away from the bruise. *(See pages 97 and 98.)*
- A vinegar compress can be used for all bruises or swelling. Avoid the eye area. *(See page 102.)*
- Witch hazel tincture can be used to relieve swellings and bruises. Apply to a cool compress. *(See page 91.)*
- Use roasted onions in a poultice to help heal bruising. *(See page 82.)*

HERBALISM

- Bathe the area in witch hazel, which disperses the blood and encourages healing. *(See page 123.)*

HOMEOPATHY

- Arnica, where there is bruising due to trauma or injury. *(See page 182.)*
- Hamamelis, for bruising with broken skin, or due to poor circulation. *(See page 197.)*
- Ruta. grav., for bruising that feels as if it is in the bone. *(See page 210.)*
- Hypericum, when bruising involves nerve endings, such as fingers and toes. *(See page 199.)*
- Homeopathic remedy and tincture of Calendula will ease symptoms. *(See page 187.)*

FLOWER ESSENCES

- Rescue Remedy can be applied to the bruised area, to encourage healing and prevent the negative effects of trauma. *(See page 244.)*
- Crushed agrimony roots and leaves can be used as a compress for bruises or taken internally. *(See page 225.)*
- Comfrey is exceptional for healing, and can be applied as a compress or poultice on the bruise.
- Daisy is also known as bruisewort; bruise the leaves and flowers and add them to wheat germ oil.
- Crushed yarrow can be placed on fresh cuts or bruises.

VITAMINS AND MINERALS

- Increase your intake of vitamin C and bioflavonoids, to help the health of the capillaries. *(See pages 256 and 272.)*
- Zinc strengthens the integrity of the capillaries. *(See page 265.)*

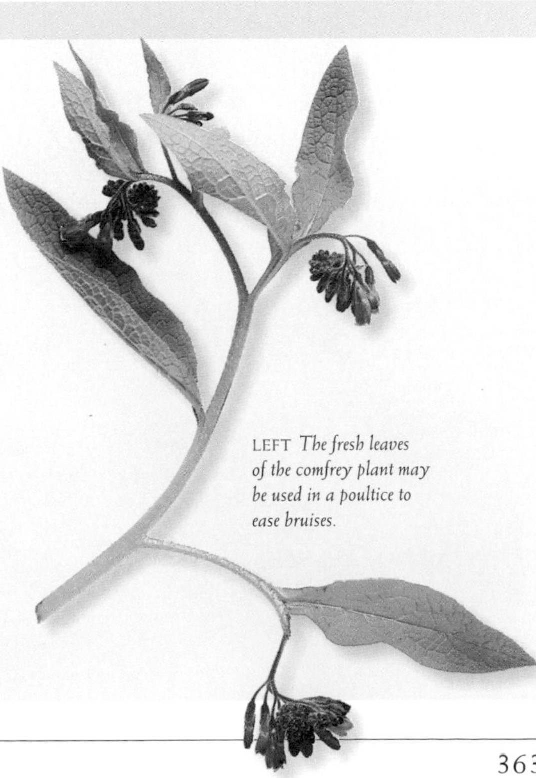

LEFT *The fresh leaves of the comfrey plant may be used in a poultice to ease bruises.*

DISORDERS OF THE DIGESTIVE SYSTEM

Nausea and Vomiting

ABOVE *Nausea may be relieved by chewing a piece of crystallized ginger.*

Nausea (a feeling of sickness) and vomiting are symptoms of various disorders, which include gastroenteritis, inner ear infection, migraine, excessive food or alcohol intake, hiatus hernia, pancreatitis, indigestion, food poisoning, gallstones, or liver disease. They may also be caused by hormonal changes in pregnancy and menstruation, travel, or by certain smells and sights. Nausea may be accompanied by a feeling of faintness and dizziness. Vomiting is usually preceded by nausea, and may be accompanied by sweating, excessive salivation, and a slowing of the heart rate. A constant feeling of nausea with no vomiting, but with a headache and abdominal pain, is most likely to be stress- or anxiety-related.

CAUTION

IF NAUSEA OR VOMITING ARE ACCOMPANIED BY SEVERE PAIN LASTING FOR MORE THAN ONE HOUR, OR IF VOMIT IS BLOOD-STAINED, SEEK URGENT MEDICAL ADVICE.

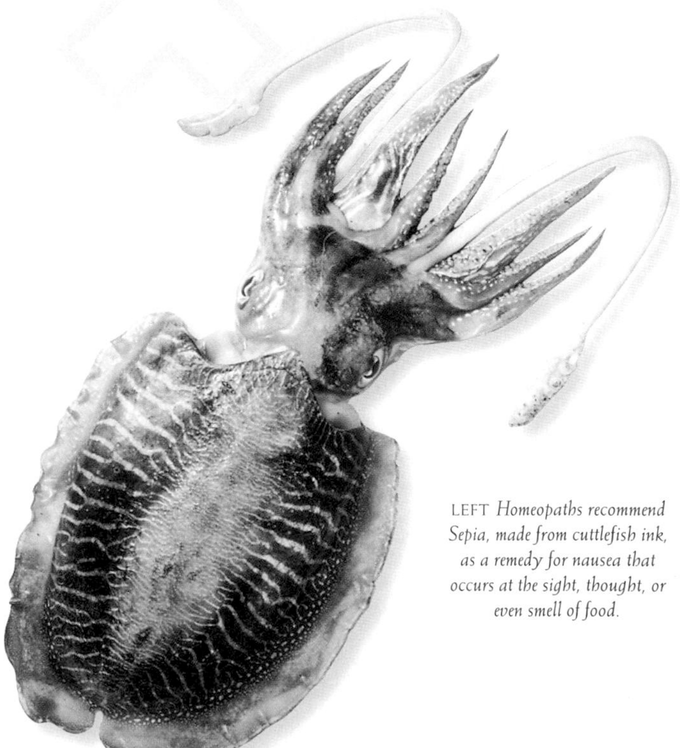

LEFT *Homeopaths recommend Sepia, made from cuttlefish ink, as a remedy for nausea that occurs at the sight, thought, or even smell of food.*

TREATMENT

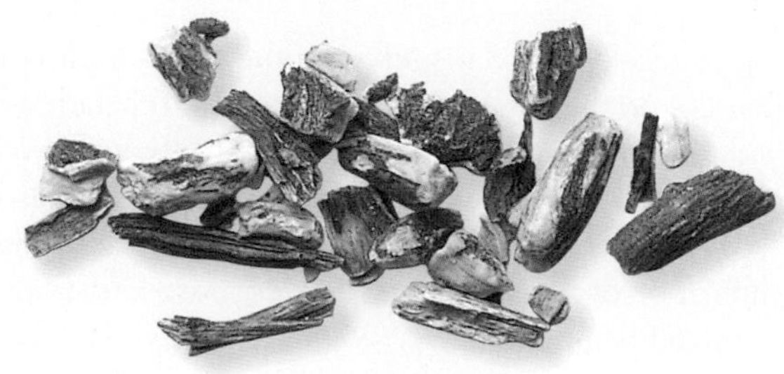

ABOVE *Dandelion root is a liver stimulant and tonic. Drink dandelion coffee when nausea may be a result of liver problems.*

CHINESE HERBALISM

- Treatment would be aimed at ascending Stomach qi, and useful herbs may include root ginger, Ren Dan, Shen Chu Cha, Xiang Sha Yang Wei Pian, or Bu Zhong Yi Qi Wan.
- Er Chen Wan pills, a classical formula to dissolve Phlegm, resolve Spleen Damp and harmonize the center (digestive organs), as well as symptoms brought on by food retention in the Stomach.

HERBALISM

- Drinking ginger tea or chewing a piece of crystallized ginger warms the stomach and allays cold nausea. This can be used for relief of sickness in pregnancy or during travel. *(See page 139.)*
- Persistent nausea may indicate liver trouble: seek advice. Take decoction or coffee made of dandelion root. *(See page 134.)*

HOMEOPATHY

- Sepia, when you feel nauseous at the thought or smell of food, but feel better for eating. *(See page 212.)*
- Nux vomica, when nausea is made better by vomiting, and may be caused by overindulgence. *(See page 214.)*
- Lactic acid, when there is profuse salivation and a history of anemia.
- Tabacum, for nausea and vomiting relieved by uncovering the abdomen.
- Arsenicum, when nausea and vomiting are accompanied by diarrhea, and symptoms are worse between midnight and 2A.M. *(See page 182.)*
- Phosphorus, for cravings for cold water, which is then vomited, with blood in the vomit and burning pains in the stomach. *(See page 208.)*
- Pulsatilla, for vomiting after rich, fatty food, with some tearfulness. *(See page 209.)*
- Arnica, when vomiting follows a head injury. *(See page 182.)*
- Aconite, when vomiting and severe pain last for more than one hour, and are not relieved by vomiting. *(See page 178.)*

FLOWER ESSENCES

- Rescue Remedy or Emergency Essence will be useful for prolonged or distressing vomiting; it will help to reduce panic and calm the mind and body. *(See page 244.)*

VITAMINS AND MINERALS

- Take vitamin B6 for morning sickness (consult your doctor first) and for travel sickness. It is appropriate for children if given in half-doses. *(See page 254.)*

BELOW *Star of Bethlehem, as one of the five ingredients of Bach's Rescue Remedy, is used to treat cases of prolonged or distressed nausea.*

Jaundice

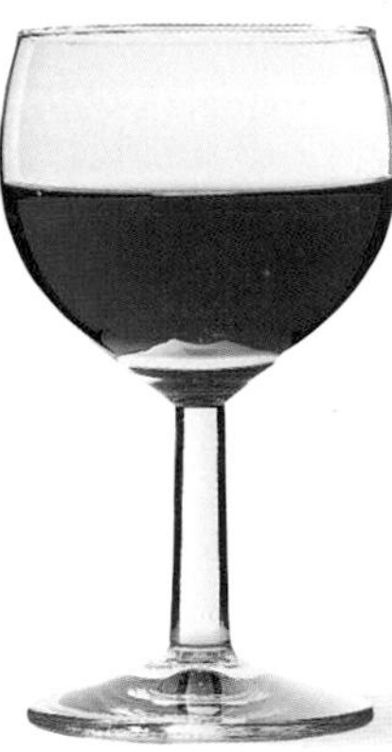

ABOVE *Avoid drinking alcohol if you have jaundice.*

Jaundice refers to a yellowing of the whites of the eyes and of the skin caused by bilirubin – a natural coloring substance. Under normal circumstances, bilirubin is released by red blood cells and passed to the intestine in bile, via the liver. If the liver is diseased, however, or if there is bile duct blockage, it accumulates in the blood, causing the characteristic yellow staining of tissue.

Newborn infants frequently develop mild jaundice, which lasts several days until a normal excess of red blood cells is destroyed. This condition is not normally considered to be serious. Erythroblastosis fetalis, a serious form of jaundice in infants, generally is due to a Rh factor incompatibility. Adolescents and young adults who have a viral inflammation of the liver often develop jaundice; jaundice in middle-aged adults is commonly due to gallstones. In older adults jaundice may signal cancer of the liver or the bile ducts. It is often the first symptom of liver damage in alcoholics.

Symptoms

- *yellowing of the skin and the whites of the eyes*
- *darkened urine* • *pale-colored stools*

CAUTION

JAUNDICE IS NOT A DISEASE IN ITSELF, BUT IS AN INDICATION OF AN UNDERLYING DISORDER SUCH AS HEPATITIS, GALLSTONES, HEMOLYTIC ANEMIA, CIRRHOSIS OF THE LIVER, PANCREATITIS, OR PANCREATIC CANCER. THE CAUSE OF JAUNDICE SHOULD ALWAYS BE INVESTIGATED IMMEDIATELY.

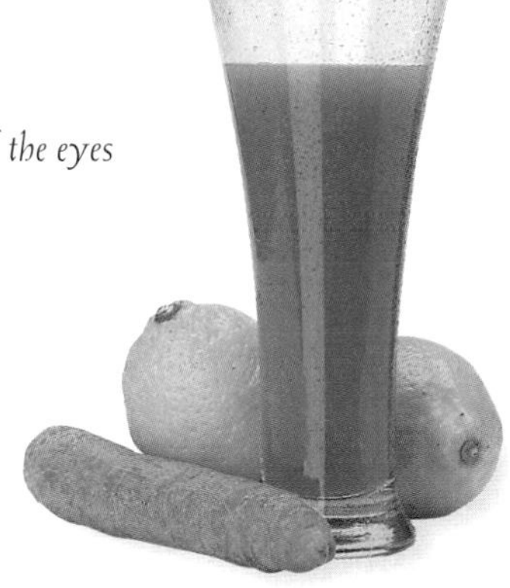

ABOVE *A daily drink of carrot and lemon juice will help relieve jaundice.*

TREATMENT

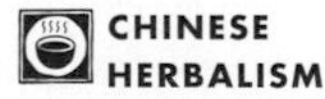

CHINESE HERBALISM
• Treatment would be aimed at Dampness in the Gall Bladder and Liver, and useful herbs may include gardenia fruit, oriental wormwood, and the bark of the cork tree. *(See page 68.)*

HERBALISM
• Any of the following herbs can be used to tonify the liver: golden seal, verbena, barberry, blue flag, dandelion, and wild yam. *(See pages 120 and 133.)*

AROMATHERAPY
• Oils that strengthen the liver include chamomile, cypress, lemon, peppermint, rosemary, and thyme. Use one or a blend of these oils in massage, or in a vaporizer in your room. *(See pages 146–71.)*

HOMEOPATHY
• Constitutional treatment would accord with the cause of the jaundice.
• Crotalus is appropriate for jaundice caused by hemolytic anemia.

VITAMINS AND MINERALS
• Drink fresh carrot and lemon juice daily.
• Avoid alcohol and caffeine.
• Eat plenty of fresh fruit and vegetables, as well as whole grains and cereals.

Hiatus Hernia

A hiatus hernia occurs when part of the stomach slides up through the esophageal opening in the diaphragm into the chest. As a result of this the stomach's contents regurgitate into the esophagus, which may cause damage and inflammation (esophagitis). The underlying cause of hiatus hernia is unknown, but this common condition tends to occur more often in obese people (and especially in women in later middle age), and in those who smoke. In some cases it is present at birth.

Symptoms

• *severe heartburn (a burning pain behind the breastbone) that worsens on bending, straining, and lying down* • *if esophagitis occurs there may be associated symptoms of acid in the mouth, difficulty in swallowing, and ulceration*

RIGHT *A hiatus hernia is characterized by severe heartburn that becomes more painful if you bend forward or lie down.*

TREATMENT

CHINESE HERBALISM
• Treatment would be individual, but there are a number of herbs which will restore the balance. *(See pages 48–75.)*

HOMEOPATHY
• Constitutional treatment would be suggested, but the remedies for indigestion will be appropriate. *(See page 368.)*
• Calc. fluor., a tissue salt, will help elasticity.

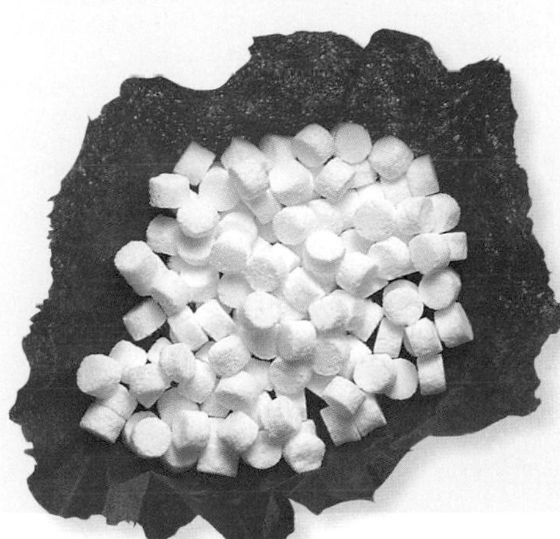

LEFT *The homeopathic remedy Calc. fluor. will help maintain tissue elasticity and so may be a useful treatment for a hiatus hernia.*

Appendicitis

The appendix is 1–8in. (2–20cm.) long, about as thick as a pencil, and hollow. It consists mostly of lymphoid tissue, like the tonsils and adenoids, and is easily invaded by micro-organisms. One out of every 15 people develops appendicitis, the inflammation of an infected appendix. This is a medical emergency that usually requires the surgical removal of the appendix. For many years the appendix was regarded as a vestigial organ with no function in the human body, but it is now thought to be one of the sites where immune responses are initiated. Appendicitis is particularly common in adolescents and young adults.

Symptoms

- *pain and tenderness beginning in the center of the abdomen, then moving to the right and down towards the groin*
- *possibly nausea and vomiting*
- *fever*

CAUTION

PERFORATION OF THE APPENDIX CAN LEAD TO PERITONITIS – A SERIOUS, POTENTIALLY FATAL INFLAMMATION OF THE MEMBRANE LINING THE ABDOMINAL CAVITY.

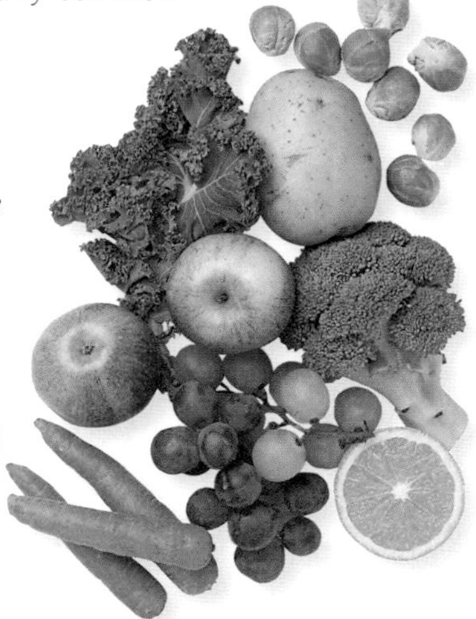

ABOVE *To avoid constipation make sure you eat plenty of fresh fruit and vegetables.*

TREATMENT

HERBALISM
- Treatment is aimed at preventing the condition in people who have a "grumbling" appendix, with inflammation and recurring abdominal pain. The following herbs will help to resolve inflammation and irritation: agrimony, chamomile, echinacea, licorice, and wild yam. These can be combined or taken separately, up to 3 times a day. *(See pages 112–139)*

HOMEOPATHY
Urgent medical treatment will be required, but the following remedies can be offered, every 15 minutes, while waiting for help:
- Lachesis, for cutting, tearing pains, a distended abdomen and irritability. *(See page 216.)*
- Bryonia, for intense pain over the appendix area. *(See page 185.)*
- Belladonna, for pain that is made worse by movement, accompanied by a red, flushed face. *(See page 183.)*

After an operation, the following remedies help:
- Arnica, to prevent bruising and encourage healing. *(See page 182.)*
- Phosphorus, to relieve nausea caused by the effects of the anesthetic. *(See page 208.)*

FLOWER ESSENCES
- Rescue Remedy or Emergency Essence can be given while waiting for help, to calm and reduce anxiety. *(See page 244.)*

VITAMINS AND MINERALS
- Eat plenty of fresh fruits and vegetables, and avoid getting constipated.
- Never use laxative preparations, which will aggravate the condition.

Gastroenteritis

Gastroenteritis is an acute inflammation of the stomach and intestine, causing violent upset. It may be due to bowel organisms such as salmonella or other bacterial toxins or viruses that may contaminate food or water; food intolerance; or excessive alcohol intake. The symptoms and their severity will vary according to the cause. It can also be a side effect of certain drugs. Gastroenteritis is most serious in the elderly and in babies because of the danger of dehydration through vomiting and diarrhea.

Symptoms

- *fever* • *abdominal pain* • *nausea and vomiting* *diarrhea* • *in severe cases there may be shock and collapse*

TREATMENT

TRADITIONAL HOME AND FOLK REMEDIES
- Very ripe bananas will ease nausea, act as a gentle constipant, and help to restore the healthy bacteria in the intestines.
- Live yogurt, taken by the teaspoon throughout the day, can help to restore bacteria to the stomach and digestive tracts. *(See page 93.)*
- Honey is a natural antibiotic and anti-inflammatory. Mix a few teaspoonfuls in a cup of warm water and sip. Freeze into ice cubes if you find hot drinks difficult to manage. *(See page 101.)*

HERBALISM
- Make an infusion of comfrey root and meadowsweet to treat the infection and relieve the associated symptoms. *(See pages 121 and 132.)*
- Arrowroot or slippery elm tea can be sipped during the worst symptoms to soothe the digestive tract, and afterwards to help restore bowel health. *(See page 136.)*

AROMATHERAPY
- Massage chamomile and geranium essential oils into the abdomen to bring relief from pain and discomfort. *(See pages 150 and 165.)*

HOMEOPATHY
The following remedies can be taken hourly, as required:
- Arsenicum, for burning abdominal pains, accompanied by great thirst. *(See page 182.)*
- Pulsatilla, for symptoms which are worse at night, and tearfulness. *(See page 209.)*
- Baptisia, if a salmonella infection is suspected – stools dark, bloody, and smelly, nearly liquid. *(See page 184.)*
- Mercurius for diarrhea, where there is blood and mucus in the stools. *(See page 205.)*
- Phosphorus, for a burning sensation when stools are passed, with vomiting and cravings for cold water, which is then vomited. *(See page 208.)*
- Sulfur for burning diarrhea which is at its worst around 5a.m., with a red, itchy anus. *(See page 215.)*

VITAMINS AND MINERALS
- Take acidophilus to restore the healthy flora in the intestines, which will help to fight infection. *(See page 271.)*

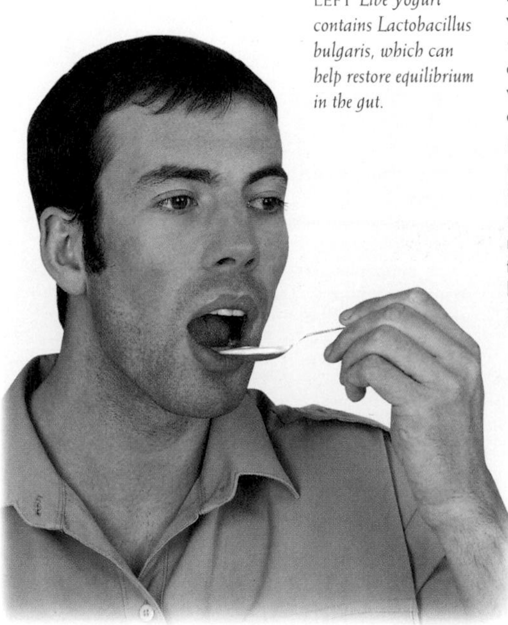

LEFT *Live yogurt contains Lactobacillus bulgaris, which can help restore equilibrium in the gut.*

DATA FILE

- 2 million people in the U.S. suffer from food poisoning each year.
- The most common type of food poisoning, accounting for nearly 70 percent of cases, is due to Salmonella typhimurium, a bacterium commonly found in meat, eggs, and milk.
- The Staphylococcus bacteria, another type of food poisoning, multiply rapidly at room temperature and are usually transmitted by careless food handling; workers may sneeze or cough on food, or may have infected pimples or wounds on the hands or face and transmit the bacteria to the food.
- If food contaminated by the bacterium Clostridium botulinum is improperly canned or bottled the bacteria are able to produce a toxin, which produces the disease botulism. The mortality rate can be as high as 65 percent.
- Diarrhea and vomiting may result from infection by the protozoan Entamoeba histolytica, acquired by eating uncooked vegetables or drinking contaminated water (amoebic dysentery).
- Certain rare strains of the bacteria Escherichia coli can cause food poisoning in young children, the elderly, and people with impaired immune systems. E. coli, normally found in the intestines and fecal matter of humans and animals, can survive in meat if the meat is not cooked past 155°F.

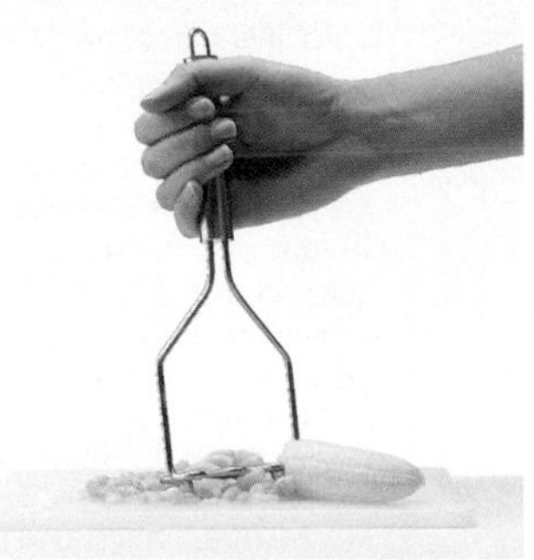

ABOVE *Bananas are easily digestible and will ease the discomfort of diarrhea. They are best eaten ripe and may be mashed to ease digestion.*

CAUTION

IF SYMPTOMS PERSIST FOR MORE THAN 48 HOURS, OR ARE ACCOMPANIED BY SEVERE PAIN, CALL FOR EMERGENCY HELP.

Peptic Ulcer

Peptic ulcers occur most commonly in the duodenum, near the junction with the stomach, and in the stomach wall. They usually occur singly as round or oval wounds. The erosions are usually shallow, but can penetrate the entire wall, leading to hemorrhage and possibly death. When gastric juices (consisting of hydrochloric acid, mucus, and a digestive enzyme called pepsin) act upon the walls of the digestive tract, a peptic ulcer results. Peptic ulcers tend to become chronic.

The peptic ulcer develops when there is imbalance between the normal "aggressive" factors, the acid-peptic secretions, and the normal "resistance" factors, such as mucus and rapid cellular replacement. Physical and mental stress are thought to be triggers, as are hereditary factors, smoking, excessive alcohol intake, and non-steroidal anti-inflammatory drugs (NSAIDs). Gastric (stomach) ulcers affect both men and women, usually over the age of 40, while duodenal ulcers are more common in men. Ulcers in the lower esophagus are relatively rare and are usually associated with hiatus hernia (see page 365) and esophagitis. Peptic ulcers affect approximately 10 percent of the U.S. population. Duodenal ulcers are two to three times more common than gastric ulcers, and people with blood group O are more likely to get them.

ABOVE *Coriander is given in Ayurvedic medicine for peptic ulcers.*

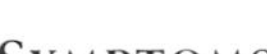

Symptoms

- *gastric ulcers: a gnawing, burning pain, which is worse during or after eating, nausea, and vomiting* • *duodenal ulcers: intermittent upper abdominal pain characteristically relieved by eating, pain usually begins around mid-morning and sufferers are often woken up by it at night* • *peptic ulcers: may bleed, causing blood in vomit and dark, blackish stools; occasionally a peptic ulcer perforates, causing severe pain and shock*

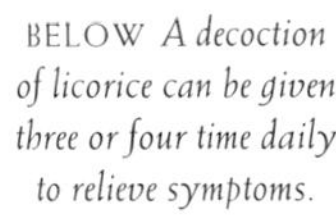

BELOW *A decoction of licorice can be given three or four time daily to relieve symptoms.*

TREATMENT

AYURVEDA
- Suitable herbs which might be suggested include bitter orange, coriander, and kalanchoe. *(See page 35.)*

CHINESE HERBALISM
- Treatment would be aimed at unblocking stagnant Stomach qi, excess Heat, and a weak Spleen. Suitable herbs may include dandelion, ginseng, and corydalis tuber. *(See page 67.)*

HERBALISM
- Licorice has a soothing effect on the stomach and the mucous membranes, and a decoction can be drunk three or four times each day to ease symptoms. *(See page 122.)*
- A decoction of marshmallow root is healing. *(See page 114.)*
- Comfrey or slippery elm may also be of help. *(See pages 119 and 136.)*

AROMATHERAPY
- Oils of chamomile, frankincense, geranium, and marjoram can be diluted and massaged into the abdomen. *(See pages 146–71.)*

HOMEOPATHY
Treatment would be constitutional, but the following remedies may be appropriate:
- Nux vomica, for pain which is worse after eating. *(See page 214.)*
- Anacardium, when pain is relieved by eating. *(See page 179.)*
- Kali bich., for pain in a small, distinct position in the stomach area. *(See page 200.)*
- Phosphorus, for burning pains and vomiting which are better for cold drinks. *(See page 208.)*
- Bryonia, for a feeling of a stone in the stomach and sensitivity to touch. *(See page 185.)*

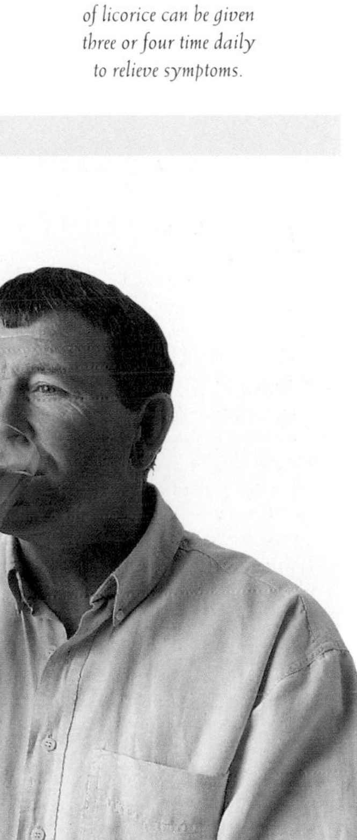

Indigestion

Indigestion (or dyspepsia) is a general term which usually refers to abdominal discomfort, nausea, heartburn (burning sensation or pain behind the breastbone), hiccups, and flatulence. Indigestion refers to discomfort in the upper abdomen – gastric distress – often brought on by eating too much, by eating too quickly, or by eating very rich, spicy, or fatty foods. Nervous indigestion is a common effect of stress. Indigestion is also commonly caused by excessive smoking, excessive alcohol or caffeine consumption, pregnancy, or anxiety. It can also be a feature of several diseases, including esophagitis (inflammation of the lining of the esophagus), gastroenteritis (see page 366), peptic ulcer (see page 367), and gallstones (see page 369).

Symptoms

• *abdominal discomfort* • *nausea* • *heartburn (burning sensation or pain behind the breastbone)* • *hiccups* • *flatulence*

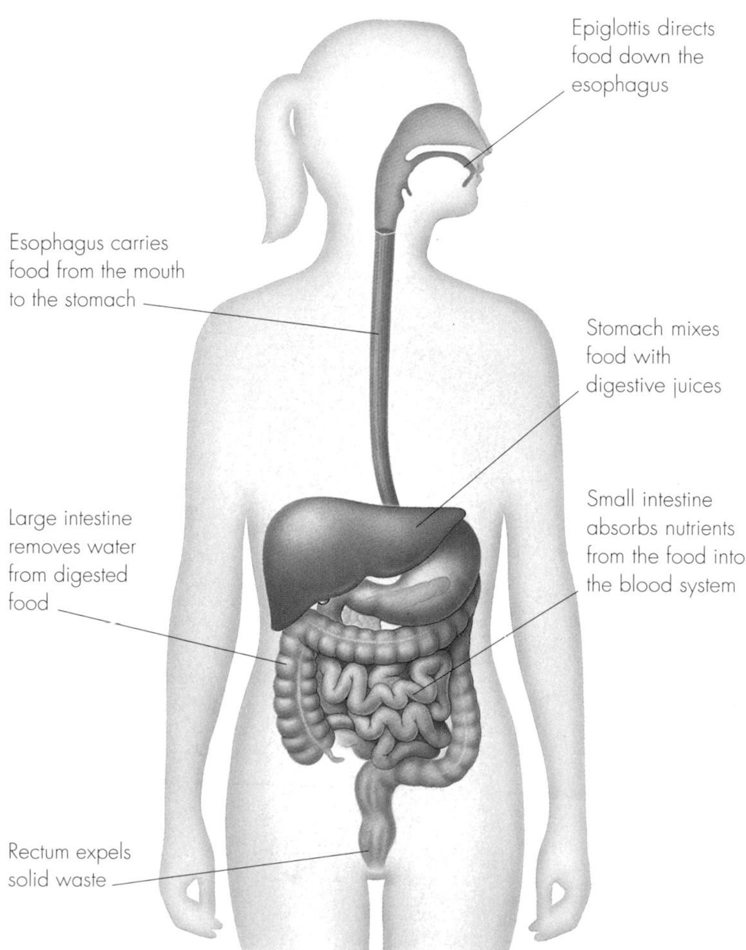

ABOVE *There are many natural remedies that can be used for digestive complaints, including homeopathic and herbal remedies.*

TREATMENT

AYURVEDA

• Crush fresh root ginger to extract the juice. Mix with the juice of a lime and a lemon, add a pinch of salt, and drink. *(See page 47.)*

CHINESE HERBALISM

• Treatment would address a weakness of the Spleen and Stomach. Rice and wheat sprouts would be used.

HERBALISM

• Try an infusion of peppermint or fennel tea after meals or when feeling full and windy. *(See pages 121 and 125.)*

• Improve the general tone of the digestive tract with bitter aperient herbs such as dandelion, gentian, and wormwood, taken 20 minutes before food. *(See page 133.)*

• A cold stomach can be warmed by eating 3 cardamom pods, or a pinch of ginger or cayenne. *(See pages 118 and 139.)*

• Fresh dill, added to boiling water and steeped, will reduce flatulence and gas pains.

TRADITIONAL HOME AND FOLK REMEDIES

• Eat a slice of fresh pineapple after meals to ease symptoms.

• Clove tea and cinnamon tea are both digestive and will soothe away the symptoms. *(See page 90.)*

• Fennel, eaten raw or cooked, or the bruised seeds infused and drunk, acts as a digestive.

• Peppermint leaves can be infused and drunk to relieve indigestion, and to soothe any gas pains. Peppermint oil can be rubbed into the abdomen for instant relief.

• Drink a little warmed vinegar and honey in a cup of hot water to ease digestive complaints. *(See pages 101 and 102.)*

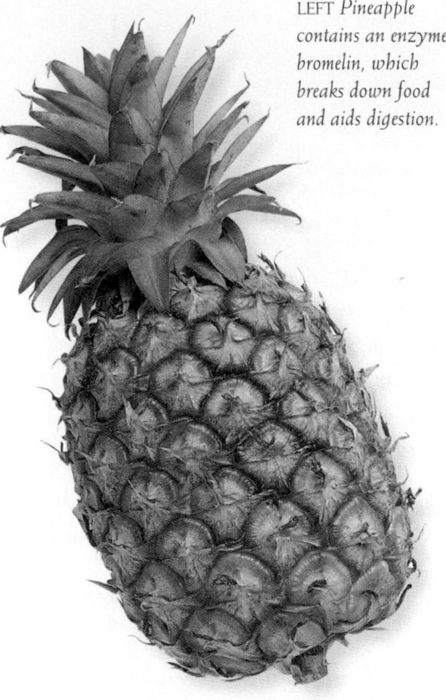

LEFT *Pineapple contains an enzyme, bromelin, which breaks down food and aids digestion.*

HOMEOPATHY

Chronic indigestion should be treated constitutionally, but the following remedies may be useful during an attack:

• Carb. veg., after rich foods, with gas and belching. *(See page 188.)*

• Nux vomica, after spicy food, and overindulgence in cigarettes and alcohol. *(See page 214.)*

• Arsenicum, when there is burning pain, particularly between midnight and 2A.M. *(See page 182.)*

• Pulsatilla, for an attack brought on by rich food, and accompanied by a bad taste in the mouth, nausea, and weepiness. *(See page 209.)*

• China, for windy stomach, and a bloated and sluggish feeling, and where stools have the appearance of chopped egg. *(See page 190.)*

• Lycopodium, for a bloated stomach with heartburn, and a full feeling even when hungry, especially where food causes instant discomfort. *(See page 203.)*

• Graphites, for burning pains which are relieved by food or milk, but followed by ingestion. *(See page 196.)*

• Bryonia, for a heaviness in the stomach, which is worse after food, with heartburn, nausea, and faintness; and which is made worse by movement but improved by lying down. *(See page 185.)*

Travel Sickness

Travel or motion sickness is a sensitivity to the constant passive movement of the body while in a car, boat, airplane, train, or bus. Some people may even experience it in lifts. Why only some people experience travel sickness is unclear. The syndrome appears to arise from sensory mismatch, when the information coming to the brain from various sensory inputs does not add up, as when the eyes report a steady horizon, but the balancing (vestibular) system reports a rocking motion. Travel sickness appears to be more common in women, and children under the age of two. Elderly people do not seem to be so troubled by the problem. Severe travel sickness can cause a complete lack of coordination.

Symptoms

• *progressive nausea* • *vomiting* • *pallor, faintness, and dizziness* • *abdominal discomfort* • *headache* • *sweaty palms and face* • *increased salivation*

TREATMENT

AYURVEDA
• Ginger, chewed fresh, may help symptoms. *(See page 47.)*
• Oral syrup of Vilwadi lehya will be useful.

CHINESE HERBALISM
• Sipping a warm drink with grated root ginger may be helpful.

HERBALISM
• Chew fresh angelica leaves, and hang them in the car while traveling. *(See page 115.)*
• Chew fresh or crystallized ginger to ease nausea. *(See page 139.)*
• Fennel or chamomile tea will ease the symptoms. *(See pages 119 and 121.)*
• Fresh peppermint leaves can be chewed, or drink an infusion to soothe and settle the stomach. *(See page 125.)*

HOMEOPATHY
Take the following remedies hourly when symptoms begin:
• Nux vomica, for a feeling of chilliness, which is improved by vomiting. *(See page 214.)*
• Arnica, when you are overtired and irritable. *(See page 182.)*
• Cocculus, for nausea with a metallic taste in the mouth.
• Sepia, when nausea is made worse by the smell of food and improved by eating. *(See page 212.)*
• Tabacum, for nausea with giddiness, and pale, cold sweat, with a band around the head.

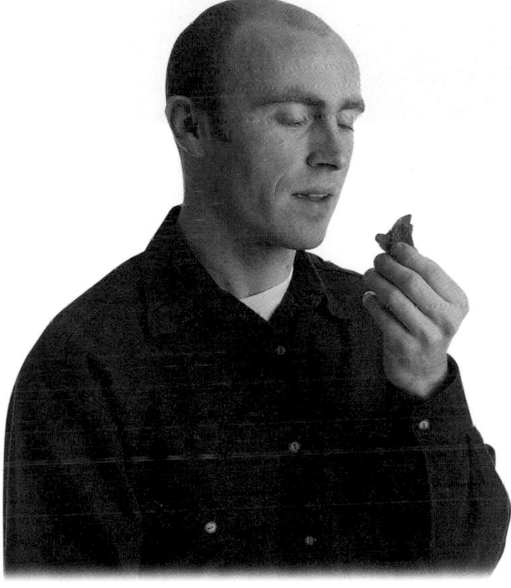

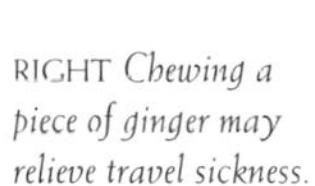

RIGHT *Chewing a piece of ginger may relieve travel sickness.*

Gallstones

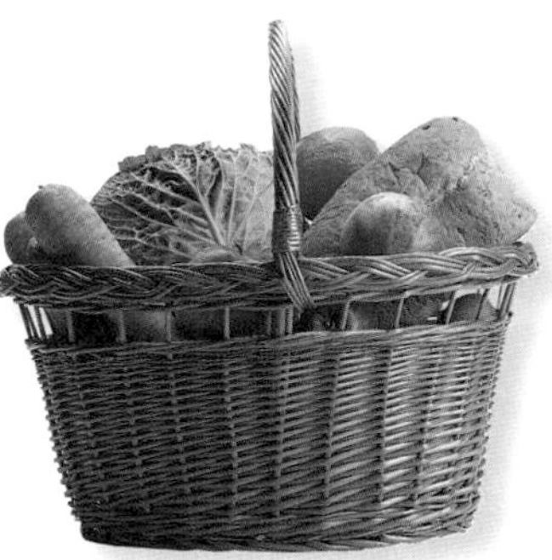

ABOVE *To minimize the risk of gallstones, increase your intake of dietary fiber.*

Gallstones are hard stone-like masses occurring in the gallbladder or in the bile duct. They are usually about the size of a pebble, and most are composed of cholesterol, calcium, or both. Abnormal composition of bile (too much cholesterol, for example), blockage of bile outflow, infection, or hereditary factors may all cause gallstones. Risk factors include obesity, advancing age, a high-fat diet, and food intolerance. Far more women than men are affected by gallstones. Gallstones occur in about 10 percent of the U.S. population, particularly in women. There may be from one to ten or more stones, ranging in size, about 1–25mm. across. Gallstones are rare in childhood, but become progressively more common with age. Autopsies show that 20 percent of all women have gallstones when they die. The use of oral contraceptives may cause gallstones to form earlier than they would have otherwise.

Symptoms

• *acute upper abdominal pain* • *possibly high fever* • *inflammation of the gall bladder (cholecystitis)* • *there may be some jaundice if the stones cause bile duct obstruction* • *severe pain if a stone passes from the bile duct into the duodenum (biliary colic)*

TREATMENT

AYURVEDA
• Kalanchoe can be used to treat gallstones.

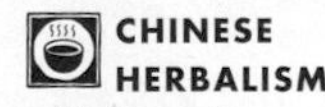

CHINESE HERBALISM
• Herbs such as lysimachia, pyrrosia leaf, and rhubarb may break up and dissolve small stones. *(See page 73.)*

HERBALISM
• The following herbs will dissolve the gallstones, but it will take several months. Blend infusions of balmony, dandelion leaves, stone root, and fringetree bark. Take 2 or 3 times a day. *(See page 133.)*

AROMATHERAPY
• Massage lavender and rosemary oils over the gallbladder area to relieve the pain. *(See page 161.)*

HOMEOPATHY
Treatment would always be constitutional, but the following remedies may help until you are able to seek advice:
• Berberis, for relief of normal symptoms.
• China, if berberis is not effective. *(See page 190.)*

VITAMINS AND MINERALS
• Reduce your intake of all fats, except olive oil, which has been proved to break up gallstones.
• Increase your intake of dietary fiber, and ensure that you drink plenty of water.

LEFT *Increasing your intake of water is crucial to prevent gallstones.*

Hepatitis

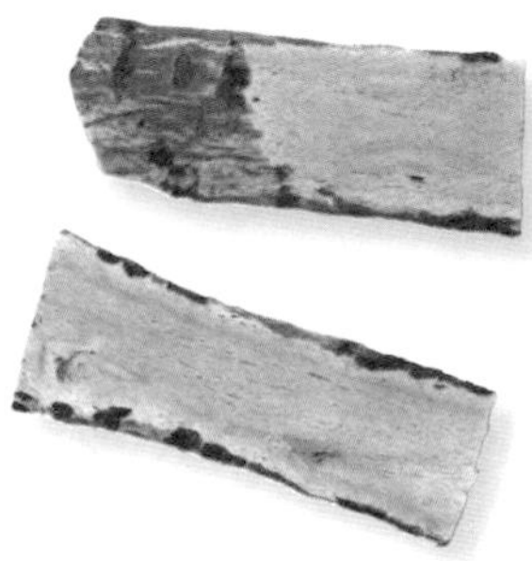

ABOVE *Astragalus is used by Chinese herbalists to strengthen the liver and treat deficient qi.*

Hepatitis is a disorder involving inflammation of the liver. Hepatitis A, once called infectious hepatitis, is the most common cause of acute hepatitis and is usually transmitted by food and water contaminated by human waste. Hepatitis B is spread mainly by blood or blood products, but can be transmitted from mother to fetus, and by intimate contact, including sexual intercourse. It often causes an initial episode of liver disease and occasionally leads to chronic hepatitis. Hepatitis C is the most common form of viral hepatitis. Type C is transmitted in blood and blood products (which are now screened for the virus), and it may be present in the body for many years before it damages the liver. Hepatitis C is a leading cause of chronic hepatitis and is considered a serious public health threat.

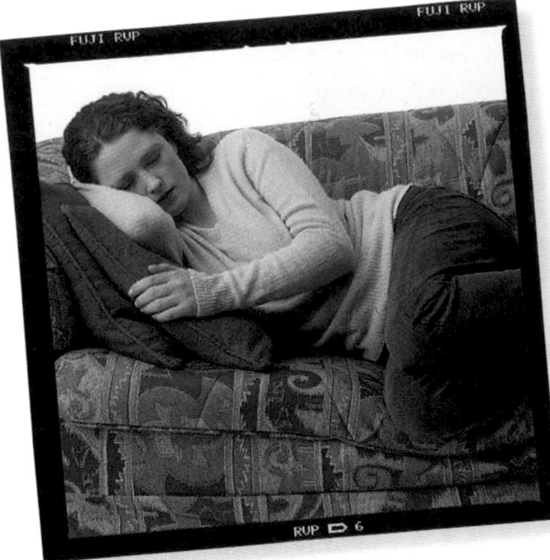

LEFT *Hepatitis leaves the sufferer feeling extremely weak and tired.*

Symptoms

• loss of appetite • dark urine • fatigue • sometimes fever • the liver may become enlarged • jaundice may occur, giving the skin a yellow tinge • hepatitis may be acute or chronic: the acute form can subside after about two months or, rarely, can result in liver failure

DATA FILE

- Hepatitis C accounts for 10–40 percent of all hepatitis, and 90–95 percent get the disease from blood transfusions.
- Another strain of hepatitis C is uncommon in Europe and the U.S., but common in Mexico, Africa, and Asia, and usually contracted from contaminated water.
- According to recent research, 25 percent of people in the U.S. who receive blood transfusions will develop hepatitis.
- Of those contracting chronic hepatitis, most are women under the age of 45.
- Chronic hepatitis leads to cirrhosis and liver damage.
- Acute hepatitis may arise secondary to various infections that involve the liver.

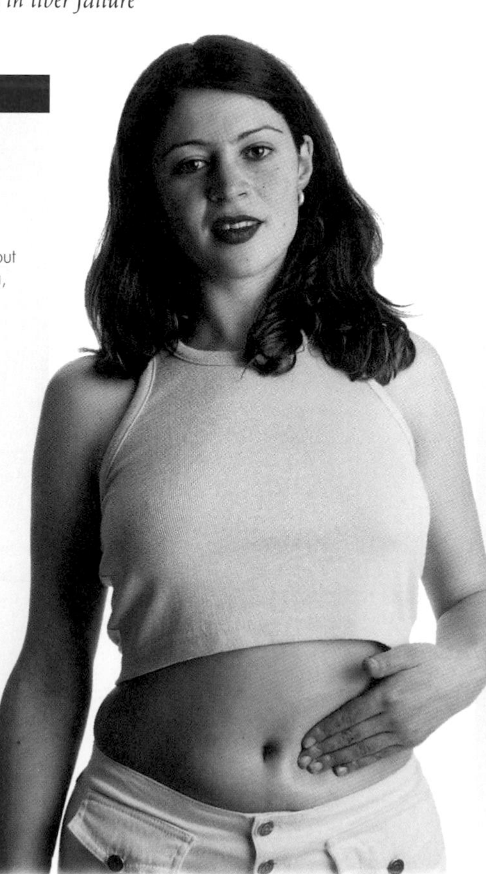

LEFT *Certain essential oils rubbed on the abdomen, act as tonics to the liver.*

TREATMENT

CHINESE HERBALISM

• Hepatitis A would require treatment for excess liver and gall bladder Damp Heat. Suitable herbal remedies include gardenia fruit and oriental wormwood.

• Hepatitis B would require treatment for deficient qi and a weakened liver. Suitable herbs include peony root, mulberry, ginseng, licorice, and astragalus. *(See pages 57, 64, 67, and 116.)*

HERBALISM

• Liver tonics may be taken daily to encourage healing and rejuvenation. Any of the following herbs can be used: golden seal, verbena, barberry, blue flag, dandelion, and wild yam. *(See pages 120 and 123.)*

TRADITIONAL HOME AND FOLK REMEDIES

• Drink barley or rice water as an overall tonic. *(See pages 92 and 96.)*

AROMATHERAPY

• Oils which act as tonics to the liver include juniper, grapefruit, chamomile, and cypress. Massage them, in a little carrier oil, into the abdominal area, or add a few drops to your bath. *(See pages 146–71.)*

HOMEOPATHY

Chronic hepatitis, which is rare, will be treated constitutionally. Cases of acute hepatitis may respond to the following:

• Bryonia, for symptoms that come on after exposure to cold, with sharp pain in the liver area. *(See page 185.)*

• Mercurius, for a yellow tongue and bad breath, with jaundice and sensitivity to cold and heat. *(See page 205.)*

• Hydrastis, for swollen, tender liver, and catarrh.

• Lachesis, when the liver feels tender and swollen, and the abdomen is distended and painful. *(See page 216.)*

VITAMINS AND MINERALS

• Plenty of fluids are necessary to cleanse the system.

• Extra vitamin C will help overcome the infection. *(See page 256.)*

Cirrhosis of the Liver

The liver is the second-largest organ in the human body, after the skin. It is a spongy, reddish brown gland that lies just below the diaphragm in the abdominal cavity, and it serves to metabolize carbohydrates and store them as glycogen; metabolize lipids (fats, including cholesterol and certain vitamins) and proteins; manufacture a digestive fluid, bile; filter impurities and toxic material from the blood; produce blood-clotting factors; and destroy old, worn-out red blood cells.

ABOVE *Taking a bath containing a few drops of the recommended essential oils, such as chamomile, relieves pain associated with liver damage.*

The liver is able to regenerate itself after being injured or diseased; if a disease progresses beyond the tissue's capacity to regenerate new cells, the body's entire metabolism is severely affected. Severely impaired livers are sometimes replaced, and in the early 1990s the one-year survival rate was 76 percent.

Cirrhosis of the liver is the replacement of normal tissue by nonfunctioning fibrous tissue, causing scarring (or fibrosis). Cirrhosis occurs as the last stage in a range of liver disorders which have been so damaging as to cause a breakdown in the liver's regeneration process. Normal liver function is prevented and any remaining healthy liver cells are cut off from the blood supply they need. Cirrhosis may be caused by hepatitis B, poisoning, and long-term alcohol abuse.

Symptoms

• appetite and weight loss • continuous indigestion • nausea and vomiting with general malaise • loss of muscle power • itching of the skin • bad breath • bleeding varicose veins (caused by the blood's attempt to use an alternative route from the liver back to the heart) • vomiting blood

TREATMENT

HERBALISM
• Good liver tonics include barberry, dandelion root, golden seal, vervain, wild yam, and yellow dock. Make an infusion of one or more and sip 2 or 3 times daily. *(See pages 120, 128, 134, and 138.)*

AROMATHERAPY
• Oils which work as a tonic to the liver and improve its function include chamomile, cypress, grapefruit, juniper, lemon, and orange. Mix a few drops in a warm carrier oil and massage into the abdomen, or add a few drops to your bath. *(See pages 146–71.)*

HOMEOPATHY
Constitutional treatment with an experienced homeopath will be necessary, but the following remedies will help until you have arranged treatment:
• Arsenicum, when there is fluid retention, and the patient feels chilly, restless, and worse between midnight and 2A.M. *(See page 182.)*
• Phosphorus, when there is jaundice, a craving for cold water (which makes symptoms worse), and a tendency to bleed easily. *(See page 208.)*
• China, when the liver is swollen and painful, and you feel chilly and full of wind. *(See page 190.)*

Pancreatitis

A long, thin organ, the pancreas has both digestive and endocrine functions, and for this reason contains two completely different types of cells. It measures about 5–6in. (12–15 cm.) in length and is situated within the curve of the duodenum.

Pancreatitis is an inflammation of the pancreas which can be either acute or chronic. Acute pancreatitis may be caused by interference (often from gallstones) with the outflow of digestive juices from the pancreas, as a result of which the pancreas begins to digest itself. Alcoholism is another cause, and is almost always responsible for cases of chronic pancreatitis. Chronic pancreatitis is more common in men than in women and is most commonly due to alcoholism. The dominant feature of chronic pancreatitis is upper abdominal and back pain. Diagnosis of pancreatitis can be difficult since it closely resembles peptic ulcer and acute appendicitis. Pancreatic cancer is the fourth leading cause of cancer death in the U.S.

Symptoms

• acute pancreatitis: – severe central abdominal pain, spreading to the back and shoulder, then the whole abdomen – nausea, vomiting, and shock • chronic pancreatitis: – constant pain, often in the back – weight loss • if bile duct obstruction occurs there will be jaundice

RIGHT *An infusion of yellow dock is recommended for an inflamed pancreas.*

TREATMENT

HERBALISM
• Soothing herbs include licorice and yellow dock, drunk as an infusion in an attack. *(See pages 122 and 128.)*
• Treatment would be individual, according to the cause of the illness.

HOMEOPATHY
• For acute pancreatitis, ring for emergency medical attention, and give Aconite, every 10 minutes, until help arrives. *(See page 178.)*
• For chronic pancreatitis, constitutional treatment is necessary, but the following remedies may help in an attack:
• Phosphorus, when there is jaundice and a craving for cold drinks, that are then vomited up. *(See page 208.)*
• Iris, for watery stools, a burning sensation in the bowels, and cutting pains in the abdomen.
• Mercurius, for stabbing pains in the abdomen, a chilly feeling, jaundice, and offensive sweat. *(See page 205.)*
• Arsenicum, for burning pains which are worse between midnight and 2A.M., feeling chilled and restless. *(See page 182.)*

Crohn's Disease

For sufferers of Crohn's disease, segments of the bowel become inflamed, ulcerated, and greatly thickened, while the sections in between remain normal. Any part of the bowel may be affected, but usually it is the last part of the small intestine, the terminal ileum, that is involved. It is a chronic disease whose cause is unknown, although there may be a genetic factor. Complications of Crohn's disease include arthritis, red swellings on the skin, mouth ulcers, eye inflammation, gallstones, urinary infections, and kidney stones. Crohn's most often affects young adults and people over sixty.

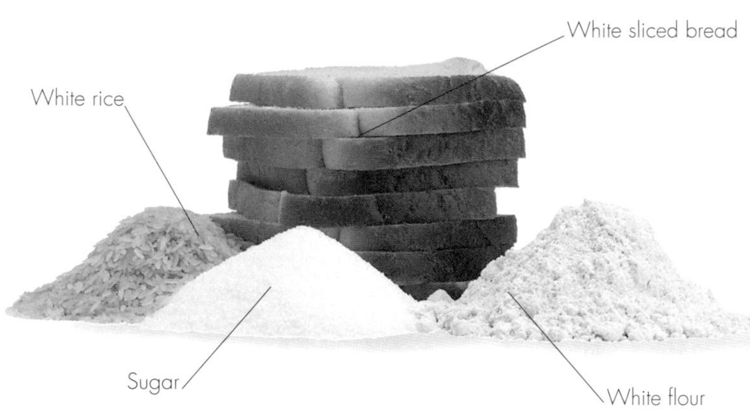

ABOVE *Diet may be a contributory factor to Crohn's disease. Avoid sugar and other refined carbohydrates and seek advice from a professional nutritionist as you may be allergic to some foods.*

Symptoms

• *spasms of lower abdominal pain* • *diarrhea* • *appetite and weight loss* • *anemia* • *rectal bleeding in older sufferers*

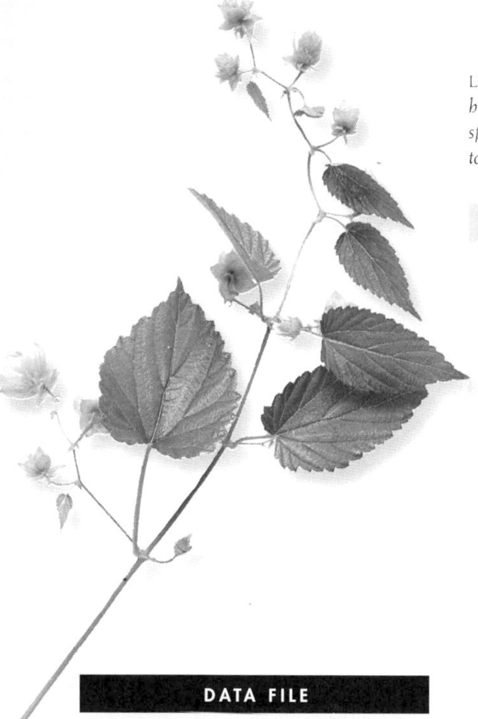

LEFT *Hops are used herbally to relieve abdominal spasms and as a general aid to the digestive system.*

DATA FILE

- Commonly occurs between the ages of 20 and 40.
- Four times more common in Caucasians and Jews than any other ethnic group.
- Crohn's may be hereditary, affecting multiple family members.
- Crohn's mainly affects the small intestine, but can occur anywhere along the digestive tract.
- Bowel obstruction and various other complications which arise may require surgical intervention.
- The cause of the potentially fatal disorder remains unknown.

TREATMENT

AYURVEDA
- Henbane can be used for bowel spasms and colic. It has sedative and antispasmodic actions.
- Coriander can help with diarrhea and the pain of Crohn's disease. It is an anti-inflammatory. *(See page 35.)*
- Hollyhock is often used to treat bowel irritation.

HERBALISM
- An infusion of peppermint can help protect the gut lining from irritation, and help to soothe the griping of the condition. The bitters stimulate and cleanse the bowels, and have an antiseptic and antibacterial action. *(See page 125.)*
- Hops have an antispasmodic action which reduces tension in the body, relieving colic and spasm in the gut. The bitters in hops also enhance the action of the digestive system.

AROMATHERAPY
- Lavender oil will help you to relax and to reduce the effects of stress. Add it to your bath water, or use in an overall body massage for best effect. *(See page 161.)*
- Roman chamomile oil, rubbed into the abdomen, may help to soothe the pain. *(See page 150.)*

HOMEOPATHY
Treatment would be constitutional, but some of the following remedies may be appropriate:
- Colocynthis, for diarrhea accompanied by griping pains, and also copious, thin, frothy stools. *(See page 191.)*
- Pulsatilla, for symptoms made worse by onions, rich food, and cold drinks, with diarrhea worse at night. *(See page 209.)*

RIGHT *Some herbs, such as peppermint, have a soothing effect on the digestive system and may be drunk as a tea.*

VITAMINS AND MINERALS
- You may need to take extra vitamin A, B, and D, and zinc supplement daily. *(See pages 252–5 and 256.)*
- You may be allergic to some foods, such as dairy produce or wheat – see a nutritional therapist for advice.
- Avoid sugar and other refined carbohydrates.

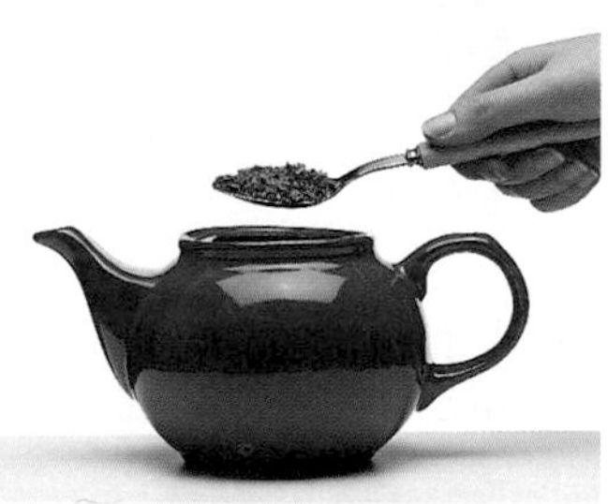

Place chopped peppermint leaves in a pot and pour boiling water over the herb. Cover with a lid.

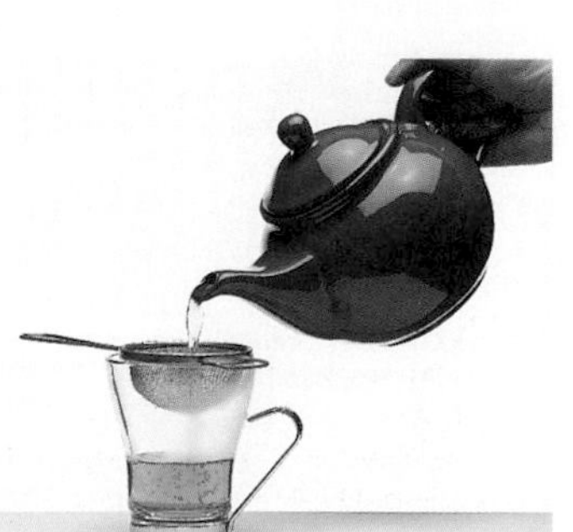

Allow the peppermint to infuse for approximately 4 minutes before pouring.

Constipation

Constipation refers to unduly infrequent or irregular bowel movements, with difficulty, discomfort, and sometimes pain on passing dry, hard feces. It is usually harmless but may be an indication of an underlying disorder, especially in adults over the age of 40. Constipation may result from: insufficient fiber in the diet, immobility, hemorrhoids *(see page 377)*, an anal fissure *(see page 376)*, iron tablets, hypothyroidism *(see pages 404–405)*, or hormonal changes, such as those in pregnancy. Dietary causes include inadequate fluid intake; a lack of vitamin B1, B5, B6, potassium, magnesium, and zinc; too much animal protein, too many dairy products; too much vinegar, pepper, salt, spices, and aluminum. If the diet is not at fault, the cause may be eating meals too fast, not taking enough exercise, tension, anxiety, depression, taking antibiotics, abusing laxatives, or abuse of certain over-the-counter drugs, such as cough mixtures.

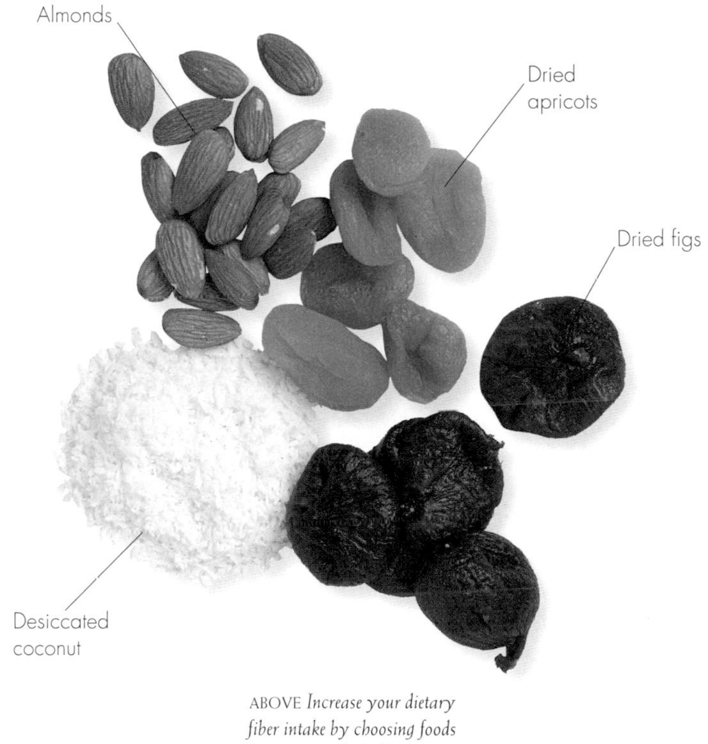

ABOVE *Increase your dietary fiber intake by choosing foods that contain a high fiber content.*

ABOVE *Senna leaves act as a stimulating laxative and will help with constipation.*

Symptoms

- *pain during bowel movements*
- *weight loss*
- *sufferers may experience headaches, furred tongue, loss of appetite, nausea, fatigue and depression, all arising largely from anxiety about constipation*

TREATMENT

CHINESE HERBALISM

Constipation is believed to be caused either by Heat, stagnation of qi, Deficiency (of qi, yang, Blood, or yin), or interior Cold. Some suitable pills include:

- Ma Ren Wan, for Heat (dry stools, thirst, dark urine).
- Run Chang Wan, for chronic constipation of any kind, especially in old age or after childbirth.
- Mu Xiang Shun Qi Wan, for qi stagnation.

HERBALISM

- Laxative herbs, which can be drunk as herbal infusions up to 3 times daily, include licorice, marshmallow root, rhubarb root, buck thorn, and senna leaves. *(See pages 114, 122, and 127.)*

AROMATHERAPY

- Massage a few drops of marjoram, rosemary, or fennel oil, diluted in grapeseed oil, into the abdomen, to relieve constipation. *(See pages 146–71.)*

HOMEOPATHY

Constipation is regarded as a constitutional problem, but the following remedies can help with occasional symptoms:

- Lycopodium, when there is flatulence but no need to open bowels for long periods of time; then stools are hard, and passed with pain. *(See page 203.)*
- Nux vomica, for constipation that alternates with diarrhea. *(See page 214.)*
- Sepia, when the belly feels full. *(See page 212.)*
- Opium, when there is no desire to pass stool. *(See page 207.)*
- Silicea, when there is a burning sensation after a bowel movement. *(See page 211.)*
- Causticum, for a stitch-like pain accompanying a bowel movement. *(See page 189.)*
- Bryonia, for large, hard, dry stools, with congestion in the abdomen causing distension, and a burning feeling in the rectum. *(See page 185.)*
- Alumina, when there is no desire to open bowels until the rectum is full; the stool may be covered in mucus.

VITAMINS AND MINERALS

- Increase your intake of dietary fiber, which will help to bulk out stools.
- Acidophilus will encourage the health of the intestines and make bowel movements more normal. *(See page 271.)*
- Chronic constipation may respond to an increased intake of B-complex vitamins, particularly if it follows a course of antibiotics. Vitamin B1 is most effective. *(See page 252.)*

BELOW *Rhubarb root contains a natural laxative. Drink an infusion 3 times a day to relieve constipation.*

Diarrhea

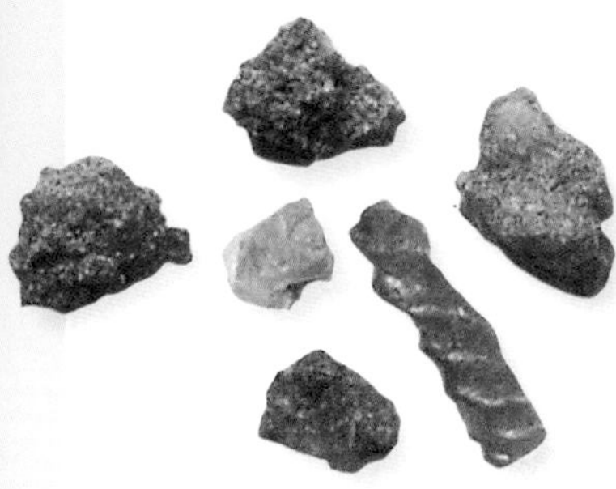

ABOVE *Myrrh is an old herbal remedy for diarrhea. Add a few drops of myrrh tincture to water to relieve symptoms.*

Diarrhea occurs when normal reabsorption of water from the stools has not taken place, so that stools are characteristically loose and runny. The two basic mechanisms involved in diarrhea, which may operate independently or together, are excessive accumulation of fluid in the intestinal tract and excessive propulsive action in the intestines. Excessive fluid in the intestines can result from conditions that decrease the absorption of water from the colon, or from conditions that cause water to be secreted into the intestines, as in cholera and other infections. The body secretes excess water in order to "flush" disease and toxins. Excessive propulsive action may be caused by nervous and chemical factors or by partial obstruction of the intestine.

Diarrhea is a feature of many conditions, including dysentery, food poisoning, cholera, typhoid, gastroenteritis, and parasitic infestation. It can also be brought on by stress or anxiety, and in babies it may be caused by lactose intolerance. Chronic diarrhea may be caused by Crohn's disease (see page 372), ulcerative colitis, or cancer of the colon.

CAUTION

CONSULT A PHYSICIAN REGARDING EPISODES OF DIARRHEA LASTING MORE THAN 48 HOURS, PARTICULARLY IF THERE IS FEVER AND/OR VOMITING.

Symptoms

- *Depending on the cause, associated symptoms may include:*
- *abdominal cramps*
- *vomiting*
- *wind*

RIGHT *Make sure that you drink enough fluids as you are at risk of dehydration with diarrhea. Restrict your food intake to soups as they are easily digestible.*

TREATMENT

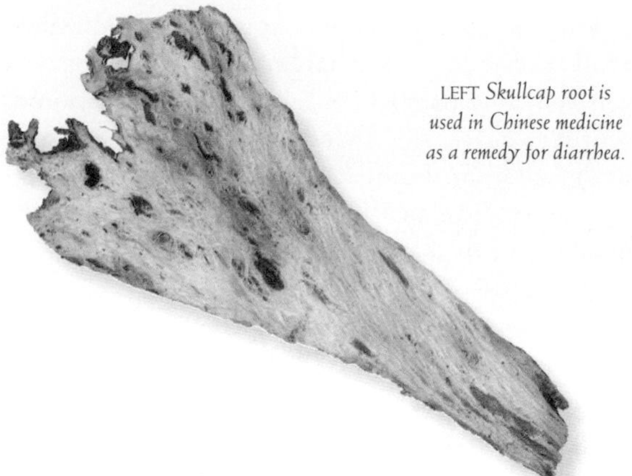

LEFT *Skullcap root is used in Chinese medicine as a remedy for diarrhea.*

AYURVEDA

- Cassia pods, henbane, and coriander can be used to treat diarrhea. *(See pages 32 and 35.)*

CHINESE HERBALISM

- The full condition is caused by Cold Damp or Damp Heat; the empty condition is due to a Spleen, Stomach, or Kidney yang deficiency. *(See page 48.)*
- Skullcap root may be suitable for acute diarrhea, as well as golden thread, kapok flowers, and dandelion root. *(See pages 61 and 74.)*
- For chronic diarrhea, a treatment of psoralea fruit, codonopsis root, and astragalus may be given. *(See pages 57 and 60.)*
- Huo Xiang Zheng Qi Wan/Agastache upright qi powder, for gastric flu. *(See page 54.)*
- Mu Xiang Shun Qi Wan and Shen Ling Bai Zhu Wan, 2 pills taken together for alternating diarrhea and constipation (Liver qi stagnation with Spleen qi deficiency). The latter can be taken for chronic loose stools with poor appetite, tiredness, etc. *(See page 57.)*
- Liu Jun Zi Pian, or Six Gentlemen Tablet, for loose stools, diarrhea, indigestion resulting from Spleen qi deficiency.
- Xiang Sha Liu Jun Zi Wan, for loose stools, diarrhea, and indigestion, accompanied by nausea.

TRADITIONAL HOME AND FOLK REMEDIES

- Carrot juice or soup is very helpful, especially for infants. *(See page 89.)*

HERBALISM

- For acute diarrhea take a gentle laxative such as dock to clear away the cause of the irritant.
- A few drops of myrrh tincture in water will clear many infections.
- For chronic and nervous diarrhea use chamomile or marigold mixed with a soothing, astringent herb such as raspberry leaf. *(See pages 117, 119, and 128.)*

HOMEOPATHY

Chronic diarrhea should be treated constitutionally, but acute attacks may be treated with one of the following remedies:

- Aconite, for diarrhea that comes on suddenly, where the patient has a distended abdomen. *(See page 178.)*
- Pulsatilla, for diarrhea which is worse at night and made worse by rich foods. *(See page 209.)*
- Colocynthis, for diarrhea accompanied by griping pains, with yellowish, thin, and copious stools. *(See page 191.)*
- Arg. nit., for diarrhea caused by anxiety, characterized by episodes of belching and cravings for sweet and salty food. *(See page 181.)*
- China, for stools accompanied by wind, and made worse by fruit. *(See page 190.)*
- Phosphoric acid, when stools contain undigested food and you feel better after passing them.

VITAMINS AND MINERALS

- Increase your intake of potassium, which is easily lost in diarrhea and vomiting. *(See page 262.)*
- Increase your intake of vitamins B1 and B3, which will address the digestive system. *(See pages 252 and 253.)*
- Drink plenty of water, to flush the system.
- Take a multivitamin and mineral supplement with food when you are able to eat properly again, to replace lost nutrients. *(See page 248.)*
- Take plenty of fresh acidophilus for at least a month after an attack, to ensure the health of the bowels. *(See page 271.)*

Irritable Bowel Syndrome (IBS)

Irritable bowel syndrome (or spastic colon) is a very common disorder with recurrent abdominal pain, intermittent diarrhea alternating with constipation. This may be caused by a disturbance in the muscle movement in the large intestine, triggered by anxiety, stress, or food intolerance. IBS affects far more women than men.

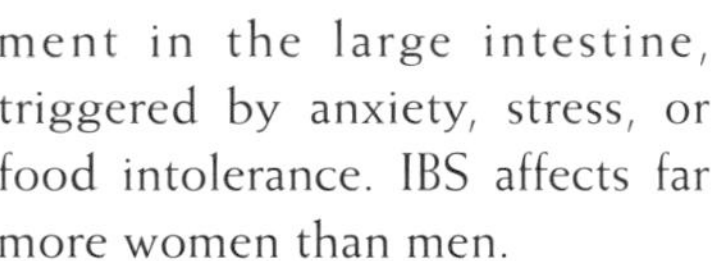

DATA FILE

- 10–20 percent of the population suffers or has suffered from IBS.
- Up to 50 percent of all health cases dealt with by gastroenterologists are caused by IBS.
- The vast majority of sufferers are women, and the young to middle-aged are particularly vulnerable.

Symptoms

• cramp-like abdominal pain, usually after eating, relieved by going to the toilet • swelling of the abdomen • excessive wind and abdominal rumblings • headache and back pain • general malaise • a sensation of fullness halfway through a meal • undue awareness of bowel action • anxiety

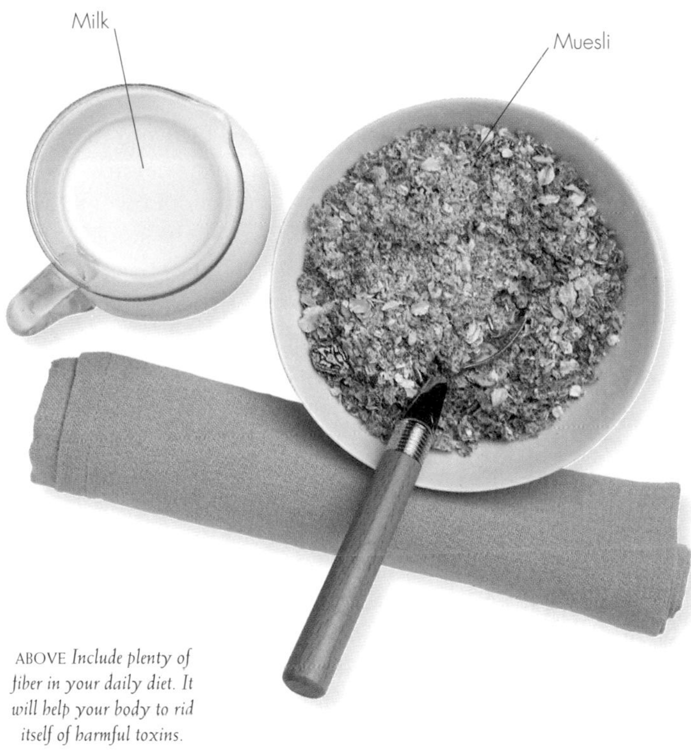

ABOVE *Include plenty of fiber in your daily diet. It will help your body to rid itself of harmful toxins.*

TREATMENT

AYURVEDA
- Coriander and hollyhock are suitable herbs to treat IBS. *(See page 35.)*

CHINESE HERBALISM
- Treatment would address weakness of the Kidneys and Spleen, excess Damp in the intestines, and stagnation of Liver qi. Some suitable herbs might include rhubarb, dandelion, magnolia, and angelica. *(See pages 65 and 73.)*

HERBALISM
- Slippery elm has a soothing action along the length of the gut. *(See page 136.)*
- Try calming herbal teas such as chamomile, peppermint, and balm, all of which have an antispasmodic action. *(See pages 119 and 125.)*
- Chew fresh ginger to help relieve spasms. *(See page 139.)*

AROMATHERAPY
- Massage the abdomen with lavender or chamomile oils, which have antispasmodic qualities. *(See pages 161 and 150.)*
- Detoxifying oils include juniper, garlic, fennel, and rose; add to your bath water or use in massage. *(See pages 146–71.)*

HOMEOPATHY
Treatment must be constitutional, but the following remedies may provide some relief:
- Arg. nit., when there is flatulence, constipation alternating with diarrhea, and mucus in the stools. *(See page 181.)*
- Cantharis, for burning pain in the abdomen, great thirst, nausea, and accompanying cystitis. *(See page 188.)*
- Colocynthis, for griping pains brought on by anger. *(See page 191.)*
- Colchicum, for water stools, and tearing pains and nausea made worse when food is smelt.

FLOWER ESSENCES
- Consider whether or not your condition is stress-related *(see Stress, page 284)* and choose a remedy that fits your emotional symptoms. *(See page 219.)*
- Rescue Remedy is useful during attacks, to calm. *(See page 244.)*
- Mimulus will help if you are frightened by the thought of eating or of experiencing another attack. *(See page 235.)*

VITAMINS AND MINERALS
- Vitamin A is necessary to keep the intestinal tract healthy. *(See page 252.)*
- Take acidophilus to encourage the growth of healthy bacteria. *(See page 271.)*
- A deficiency of zinc and vitamin B6 is indicated in many cases; ensure that your intake is adequate. *(See pages 265 and 254.)*
- Dietary fiber helps to detoxify.

LEFT *Stress and anxiety may act as triggers for irritable bowel syndrome. Take Bach's Rescue Remedy during attacks to calm you.*

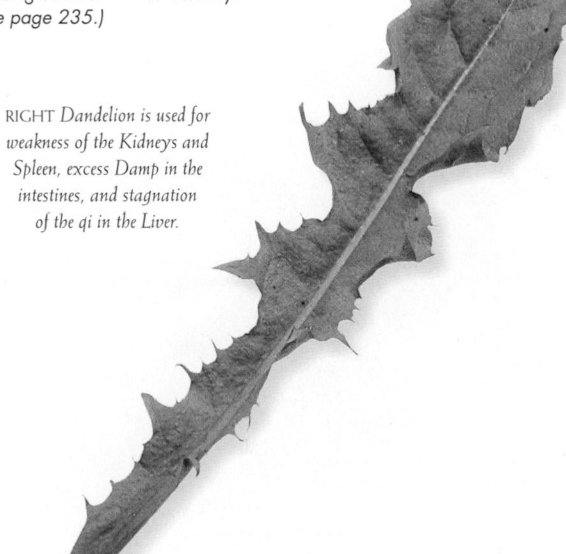
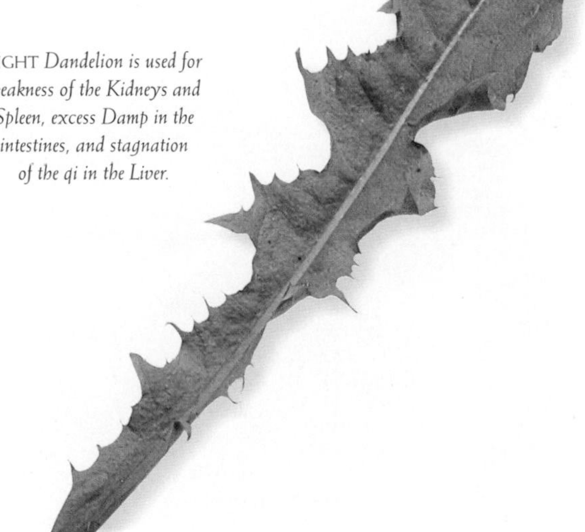

RIGHT *Dandelion is used for weakness of the Kidneys and Spleen, excess Damp in the intestines, and stagnation of the qi in the Liver.*

Anal Fissure

An anal fissure is a tear in the lower anal canal, close to the anal sphincter, and is often associated with internal hemorrhoids. The condition is fairly rare, but is most common in middle age, although it affects some children. When the stool is passed, the split is irritated, causing the sphincter muscles to go into painful spasm. Constipation is the root cause in most cases. Usually it heals quickly without complications but occasionally it may be chronic, spreading to the sphincter muscle and ending in infection. In some cases an anal fissure may be linked with other gut diseases.

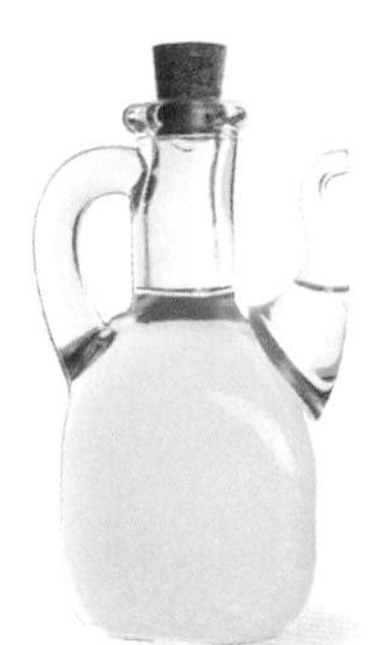

ABOVE *Relieve pain by dabbing olive oil onto the affected areas.*

Symptoms

- *pain during bowel movements*
- *minor bleeding*
- *irritation and discomfort*

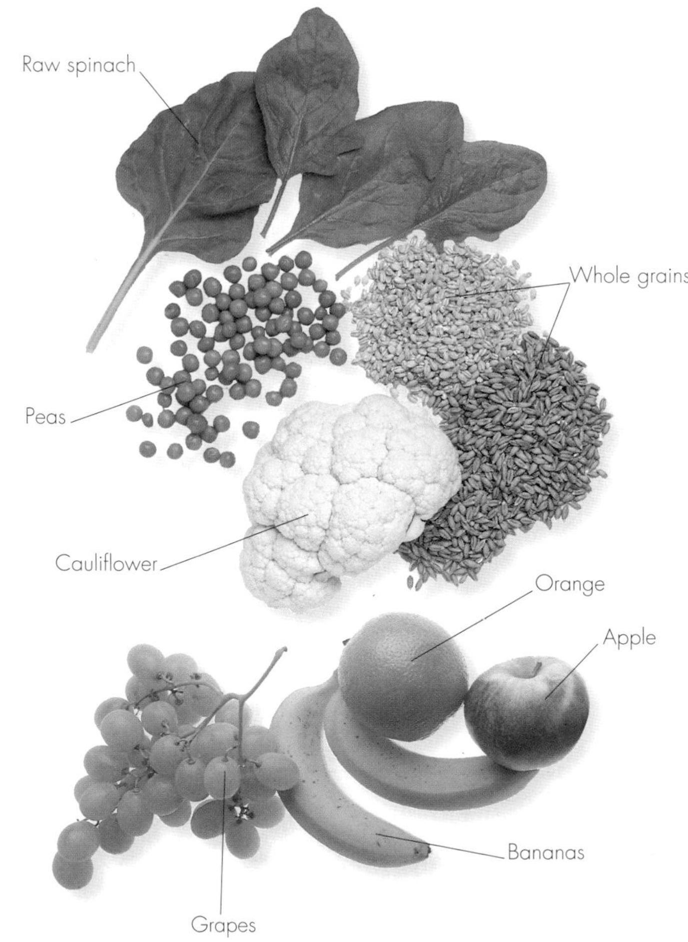

ABOVE *Eating fiber-rich foods will prevent constipation which is the major cause of anal fissures.*

TREATMENT

AYURVEDA

- The following preparations may be helpful if the fissure is caused by constipation: Abhayarishta (an oral tonic), Gin (oral pills), or Sukumara ghritha (oral ghee).

TRADITIONAL HOME AND FOLK REMEDIES

- Dab a little olive oil on to the fissure to encourage healing and relieve pain. *(See page 95.)*
- Fresh lemon juice, applied to the fissure, will prevent infection and dull the pain. *(See page 87.)*

HERBALISM

- Dandelion coffee is a mild laxative, and can be drunk, as required, on a daily basis. *(See page 134.)*
- Take a drink made of a cup of psyllium or flax seeds in a cup of water before bedtime to moisten stools and encourage regular bowel movements.
- Butternut, cascara, licorice, and yellow dock, decocted and mixed with a little honey, can help to stimulate bile, which will help produce normal bowel movements. *(See pages 122 and 128.)*
- Slippery elm and cinnamon will lubricate. *(See page 136.)*
- Comfrey root can help to heal the sore and inflamed tissues. *(See page 132.)*

AROMATHERAPY

- Apply a few drops of neat lavender or tea tree oil to the fissure to encourage healing and prevent infection. It may sting. *(See pages 161 and 162.)*

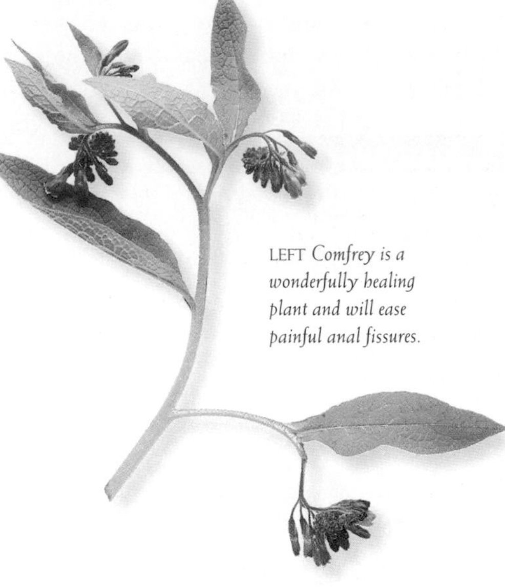

LEFT *Comfrey is a wonderfully healing plant and will ease painful anal fissures.*

HOMEOPATHY

- Constitutional treatment would be appropriate, particularly if you are prone to fissures, but the following remedies, taken four times daily, may help:
- Nitric acid, for sharp pains during the passing of stools, also afterwards; constipation, irritability.
- Ratanhia, for relieving a burning sensation in the rectum which worsens after a bowel movement (loose or constipated).
- Aesculus, for sore, burning pain in the fissure, and an aching lower back, with stools large and hard.

VITAMINS AND MINERALS

- Acidophilus encourages the health of the bowels, and so should be taken daily as required. *(See page 271.)*
- Eat plenty of foods that are high in dietary fibers, including whole grains, fresh, raw vegetables and fruits, and dried fruits.

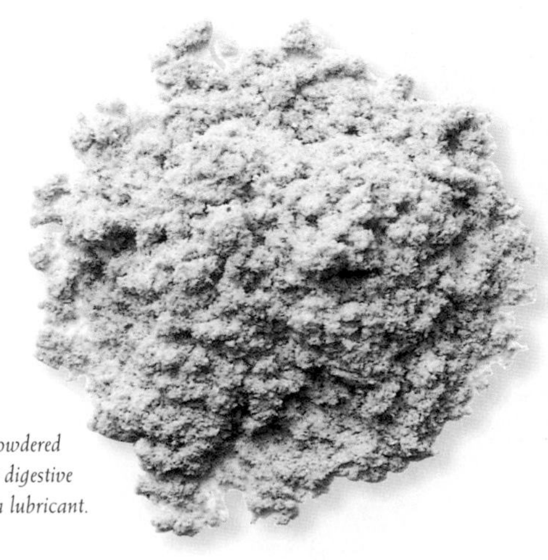

RIGHT *Use powdered slippery elm for digestive disorders and as a lubricant.*

Piles (Hemorrhoids)

Piles are swollen (or varicose) veins in the lining of the anus. The varicosity may be just above the anal canal, causing "internal" hemorrhoids, or at the lower end of the canal, causing "external" hemorrhoids. The latter may even protrude outside the anus ("prolapsed" hemorrhoids). Piles are caused by increased pressure on the veins of the anus, most commonly as a result of chronic constipation with straining, pregnancy, and childbirth. There may, however, be a congenital predisposition. Piles affect 50–75 percent of the U.S. population, and become more common with age.

ABOVE *As its common name suggests, pilewort is a good treatment for piles.*

Symptoms

- *pain and bleeding during bowel movements* • *soreness and itching around the anus* • *possibly a mucus discharge from prolapsed hemorrhoids*

TREATMENT

AYURVEDA
- There are several Ayurvedic preparations available from health food stores, including Abhayarishta, which is an oral tonic, and Dadimadi ghritha (oral ghee).

TRADITIONAL HOME AND FOLK REMEDIES
- Red potato can be cut into a slim cigar shape and inserted into the anus to relieve symptoms. *(See page 98.)*
- Sit on a cold bowl of water, or use a cold bidet, several times daily to reduce inflammation and swelling. *(See page 103.)*

HERBALISM
- Make a small witch hazel compress, and keep it on the affected area for as long as possible to reduce inflammation and encourage healing. *(See page 123.)*
- Pilewort ointment is useful, and should be applied 2 or 3 times daily.
- Bayberry and yellow dock are both astringent herbs, and can be added to cocoa butter, which can then be shaped into a suppository and placed in the anus. *(See page 128.)*
- Internally, a course of dandelion root, horse chestnut, stone root, or yarrow can be helpful. *(See pages 112 and 134.)*
- Externally, horse chestnut can be applied.
- Clear congestion in the area with a good diet and teas of bitter herbs such as dock or dandelion root. *(See page 134.)*

AROMATHERAPY
- Apply a local compress of astringent essential oils of cypress, frankincense, lavender, or myrrh. *(See pages 146–71.)*
- Add a little rosemary oil to a warm bath to improve the circulation. *(See page 168.)*

HOMEOPATHY
- Ratanhia, for pain that feels like splinters on the anus when passing a stool.
- Hamamelis, for a bruised, sore, and congested feeling.
- Sulfur, for hot, burning, and itching piles. *(See page 215.)*
- Sepia, for the sensation of having a ball in the rectum, along with a tendency to prolapse. *(See page 212.)*

Wind

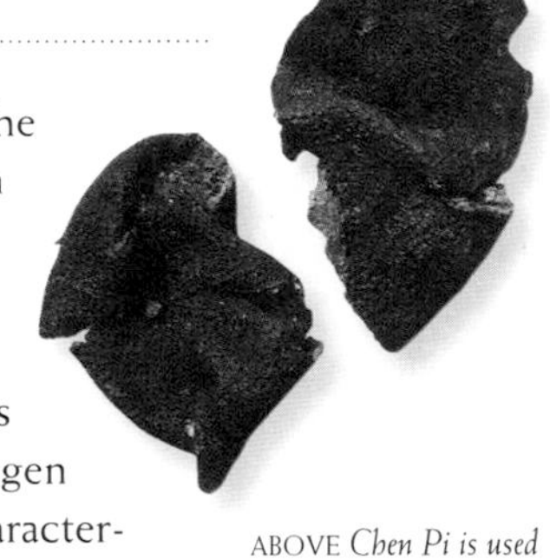

ABOVE *Chen Pi is used to treat Wind as it invigorates stagnant qi.*

Wind (or flatulence) refers to the expulsion from the body of an excessive amount of air or gas, via the anus (breaking wind) or the mouth (belching or burping). Gas discharged via the anus is called flatus and comprises a number of gases, including hydrogen sulfide, which is responsible for the characteristic unpleasant smell. Wind can be caused by excessive swallowing of air (aerophagy), which may be a response to stress, or a consequence of eating too quickly. It is also a feature of disorders such as indigestion and irritable bowel syndrome. Certain foods such as pulses and beans produce more flatus than others. Gas is formed in the large intestine as a result of the action of bacteria on carbohydrates and amino acids in digested food; the gas consists of hydrogen, carbon dioxide, and methane. Gas formed in the intestine is passed only through the anus.

CAUTION

EXCESSIVE FLATULENCE ACCOMPANIED BY WEIGHT LOSS, SEVERE ABDOMINAL PAIN, OR BLEEDING DURING BOWEL MOVEMENTS REQUIRES MEDICAL ATTENTION.

Symptoms

- *besides its characteristic sounds, flatulence can also often cause abdominal discomfort*

TREATMENT

AYURVEDA
- Ayurvedic preparations available include Digesic, which is an oral tablet, as well as Gasex and Ramabana.
- Henbane may also be useful.

CHINESE HERBALISM
- Treatment would be aimed at stagnant Stomach energy, and suitable herbs include magnolia bark, and orange or lemon peel.

TRADITIONAL HOME AND FOLK REMEDIES
- Charcoal is excellent for reducing gas in the stomach and intestines.
- Celery seeds can reduce flatulence. *(See page 83.)*

HERBALISM
- Fresh dill, added to boiling water and steeped, will reduce flatulence and gas pains.
- Try making an infusion of sweet flag, drinking half a cup before meals.

HOMEOPATHY
The following remedies can be taken in every 30 minutes, for up to 6 doses:
- Lycopodium, when gas feels stuck, is painful, and is made worse by onions, garlic, and fried foods. *(See page 203.)*
- Arsenicum, for a burning discomfort. *(See page 182.)*
- Arg. nit., for the feeling that the stomach is full of gas. *(See page 181.)*

BELOW *If you suffer from gas in the intestine, try taking charcoal or celery seeds.*

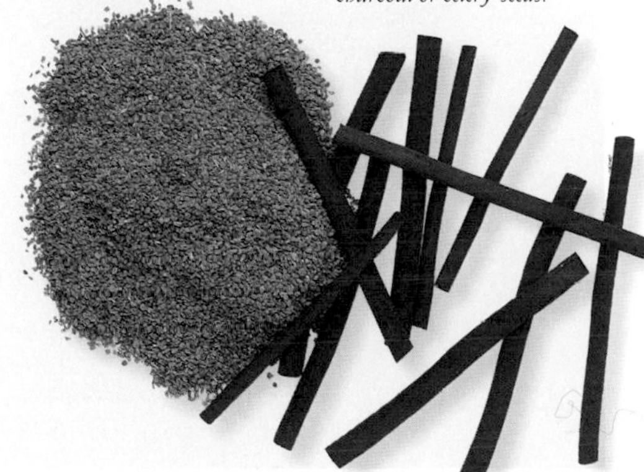

DISORDERS OF THE URINARY SYSTEM

Kidney Stones

Kidney stones (calculi) may occur anywhere in the kidneys or ureters and are the result of the crystallization of various substances in the urine, often when the body is dehydrated, causing the urine to be more concentrated. Dehydration alone, however, will not cause the formation of stones, and there is usually some other factor involved, such as kidney disease, infection, a bodily disturbance, or certain drugs. Most stones are combinations of calcium, magnesium, phosphorus, and oxalate. Collections of small kidney stones are known as "gravel," while much larger ones are called "staghorn" calculi.

ABOVE *Add a few drops of juniper essential oil to your bath, or massage into the bladder area, to relieve kidney stone pain.*

SYMPTOMS

• if a stone is lodged in the ureter it may cause agonizing pain – ureteric colic – through muscle contractions – the pain may spread to the lower abdomen and the groin • often there is blood in the urine • if stones cause blockage of the urinary tract, this can cause serious damage to kidney function

DATA FILE

- The most common types of stones contain various combinations of calcium, magnesium, phosphorus, or oxalate. Up to 80 percent of stones are formed mainly of calcium.
- Kidney stones affect approximately 1 in 1,000 Americans – an estimated 10 percent of U.S. men and 3 percent of U.S. women.
- Most common in the south-eastern U.S., known as the "stone belt."
- Less common types are due to inherited disorders characterized by excretion of abnormal amounts of cystine or xanthine.
- Recurrence of most stones can be prevented by therapy based on analysis of the stones, the urine, and the blood.
- Kidney stones range in size from less than 2/10in. (5mm.) to over 1in. (2.5cm.) in diameter.
- They tend to run in families, and four out of every five patients with kidney stones are male, usually between the ages of 20 and 30.
- Differences in dietary and fluid intake may put certain people at higher risk for kidney stones.

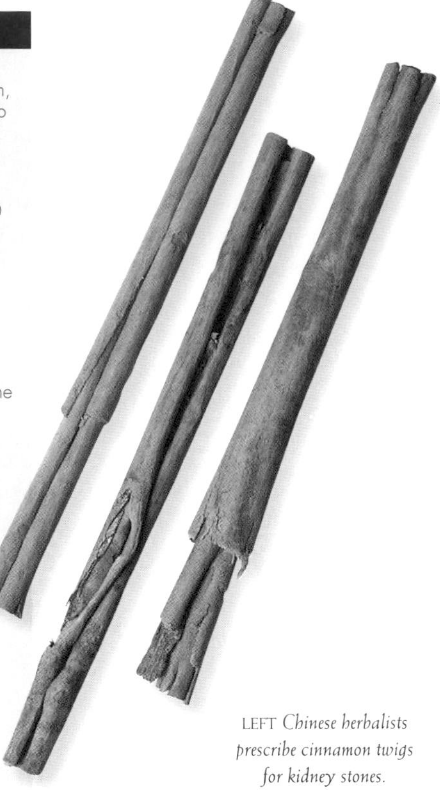

LEFT *Chinese herbalists prescribe cinnamon twigs for kidney stones.*

TREATMENT

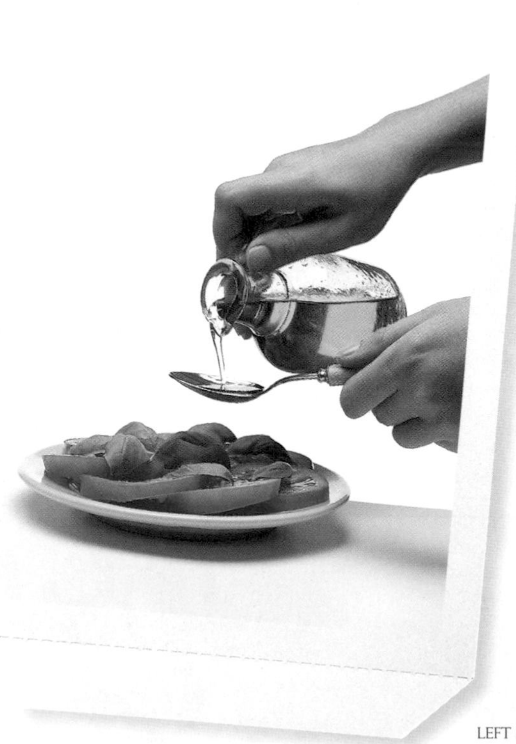

CHINESE HERBALISM

• Herbs which may help with correcting Kidney deficiency include ginseng, water plantain, poria, cinnamon twigs, and ephedra. *(See pages 59, 67, and 71.)*

TRADITIONAL HOME AND FOLK REMEDIES

• Include 2 tablespoons of extra virgin olive oil in your diet each day. *(See page 95.)*

• Fresh lemon juice, drunk in a little hot water every morning, will help to flush the kidneys and break down kidney stones. *(See page 87.)*

HERBALISM

• Herbs that can be used to dissolve the stones include celery seed, gravel root, parsley, and stone root. Sip a decoction 3 times daily.

• During an acute attack, try infusions of corn silk, coughgrass, or yarrow. *(See page 112.)*

AROMATHERAPY

• Oils used to treat kidney stones include fennel, geranium, juniper, and lemon. These can be added to a light carrier oil and massaged into the bladder area, or used in the bath. *(See pages 146–71.)*

HOMEOPATHY

Treatment would be constitutional, but the following remedies may be useful for up to 10 doses:

• Tabacum, for pains shooting to the urethra, causing nausea and cold sweat.

• Nux vomica, for right-sided pain, causing nausea and vomiting, or an urgent need to empty the bowels, accompanied by weak urine flow and irritability. *(See page 214.)*

• Berberis, for stitching pain in the lower ribs and hips when urinating, which worsens if moving about.

• Lycopodium, for pain in the right side which stops at the bladder, and which is worse between 4 and 8P.M. *(See page 203.)*

VITAMINS AND MINERALS

• Drink plenty of water (about 6pt. [3l.] a day) to flush the kidneys.

• Avoid long-term use of vitamin C, calcium, or vitamin D supplements. *(See pages 256 and 258.)*

• Extra magnesium and vitamin B6 will help. *(See pages 262 and 254.)*

LEFT *Include at least 2 tablespoons of olive oil in your daily diet. If you can afford it, choose extra virgin olive oil.*

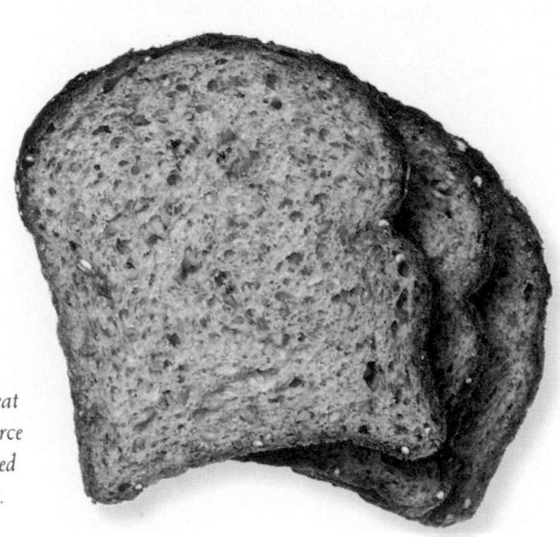

RIGHT *Whole wheat bread is a good source of magnesium needed for a healthy diet.*

Bladder Stones

Most bladder stones (calculi) are made up of crystals of calcium oxalate or uric acid. They are caused by the precipitation from solution of substances present in the urine. The stones may cause obstruction to urinary output, resulting in infection, although often they remain unrecognized. They occur with greater frequency in developing countries, and may be a result of a diet low or deficient in phosphate and protein. Bladder stones mainly affect men. Gout sufferers may experience bladder stones, and any disease which causes a high level of calcium in the blood and urine, such as hyperparathyroidism, may contribute to the formation of stones.

SYMPTOMS

• *difficulty in passing urine* • *stress incontinence* • *if infection develops there may also be: – burning pain on passing urine – small amounts of urine, cloudy in appearance and with an unpleasant smell – fever – a dull ache in the lower abdomen*

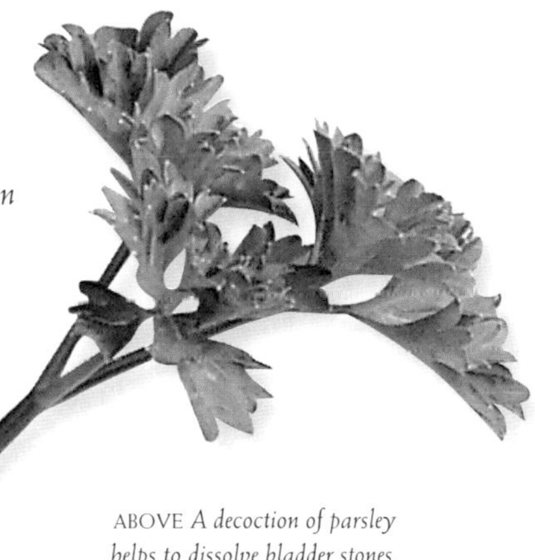

ABOVE *A decoction of parsley helps to dissolve bladder stones. Sip three times daily.*

TREATMENT

CHINESE HERBALISM
• Herbs which may help include ginseng, water plantain, poria, cinnamon twigs, and ephedra. *(See pages 59, 67, and 71.)*

TRADITIONAL HOME AND FOLK REMEDIES
• Fresh lemon juice, drunk in a little hot water every morning, will help to flush the bladder and break down bladder stones. *(See page 87.)*
• Barley or rice water will help to encourage the flow of urine and act as a tonic to the urinary system. *(See pages 92 and 96.)*

HERBALISM
• Herbs that can be used to dissolve the stones include celery seed, gravel root, parsley, and stone root. Sip a decoction 3 times daily.
• During an acute attack, try infusions of corn silk, coughgrass, or yarrow. *(See page 112.)*

AROMATHERAPY
• A number of essential oils work on the urinary tract, including tea tree, sandalwood, juniper, and eucalyptus. They should be applied in repeated hot compresses over the bladder area. *(See pages 146–71.)*

HOMEOPATHY
Treatment would be constitutional, but the following remedies may be useful for up to 10 doses:
• Lycopodium, for red sediment in the urine and a frequent urge to urinate, particularly at night. *(See page 203.)*
• Sarsaparilla, for slimy, sandy urine, with severe pain around the urethra when the flow stops.
• Uva ursi, when stones stop the flow of urine, which contains blood and mucus.

VITAMINS AND MINERALS
• Drink plenty of water (about 6pt. [3l.] a day) to flush the bladder.
• Extra vitamin C acts as a natural diuretic and will help to flush the urinary system. *(See page 256.)*

Cystitis

Cystitis is inflammation of the urinary bladder and/or urethra (the tube through which urine passes from the bladder out of the body). Inflammation usually occurs as a result of infection, bruising, or irritation. In the case of infection the bacteria involved are most often Escherichia coli, which will have traveled from the anus, via the urethra, to the bladder. Irritation and bruising can be caused by barrier contraceptives and sexual intercourse. Other causes of cystitis include chemical irritants (soap, bubble bath, bath oils), poor hygiene, insufficient drinking, food irritants, fruit juices, pregnancy, and the menopause. Cystitis is far more common in women than in men.

DATA FILE

• More frequent in women because of the close proximity of the urethra and the vagina to the anus.

• 50–80 percent of the bacteria in our bodies are resistant to allopathic (conventional) treatment.

• Prevalent in women during childbearing years, especially during pregnancy.

• Drugs such as methenamine mandelate, nitrofurantoin, and cyclophosphamide may also cause cystitis.

SYMPTOMS

• *burning pain on passing water* • *frequent and urgent need to pass water, although little if any is passed* • *dragging pain in lower abdomen and lower back* • *nausea and possibly vomiting* • *possibly unpleasant smelling urine, which may contain blood*

TREATMENT

AYURVEDA
• Hollyhock is a diuretic, and can treat cystitis.
• Boil 4 tablespoons of coriander seeds in 4 cups of water until the liquid is reduced to 2 cups. Strain and drink with a little honey. *(See page 35.)*

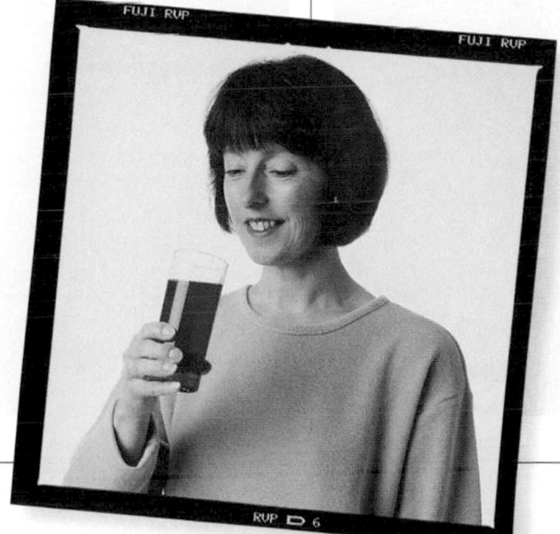

BELOW *Cranberry juice is an excellent remedy for cystitis. Drink as much as possible to flush the urinary system.*

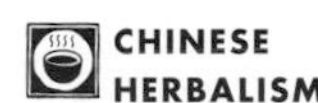

CHINESE HERBALISM
• Plantain seeds would be used to address Damp Heat.

TRADITIONAL HOME AND FOLK REMEDIES
• Eat live yogurt; use as a douche to ease symptoms and prevent recurrence. *(See page 93.)*
• Cranberry juice discourages bacteria from sticking to the walls of the bladder. *(See page 99.)*
• Garlic tincture added to food or warm drinks eases cystitis. *(See page 82.)*
• Drink barley water and lemon juice daily. *(See page 92.)*

HERBALISM
• Herbs used to treat cystitis include urinary antiseptics and diuretics. Drink infusions of buchu, corn silk, coughgrass, uva ursi, and yarrow. *(See pages 112 and 116.)*

AROMATHERAPY
• Add antiseptic bergamot, lavender, and sandalwood to the bath. *(See pages 146–71.)*

HOMEOPATHY
Chronic cystitis should be treated constitutionally, but take the following in an attack:
• Cantharis, for burning urine. *(See page 188.)*
• Staphisagria, for cystitis after intercourse.
• Mercurius, for violent pain with blood in the urine. *(See page 205.)*
• Apis, for stinging pain that is better for cold water. *(See page 180.)*
• Sarsaparilla, for burning after urinating.

VITAMINS AND MINERALS
• Drink plenty of water to flush the urinary system.
• Take 1g. of vitamin C daily, which acts as a natural diuretic and boosts the immune system. *(See page 256.)*

Urethritis

Urethritis is an inflammation of the urethra (the tube through which urine passes out of the body). In women it is usually caused by a bladder infection, while in men it may be a symptom of other diseases, including gonorrhea and Reiter's syndrome. It may also result from damage to the urethra, from a catheter for example. Nonspecific urethritis (NSU) is a milder form thought to be caused in most cases by chlamydia, although the cause may not be established. NSU may be caused by a large number of different types of micro-organisms, including bacteria and yeasts. Other possible causes include exposure to irritant chemicals, such as antiseptics and some spermicidal preparations. Urethritis may be followed by scarring and the formation of a urethral stricture (narrowing of a section of the urethra), which can make the passing of urine difficult.

CAUTION

ALL SUSPECTED CASES SHOULD BE INVESTIGATED BY A PHYSICIAN, IN CASE THE CAUSE IS CHLAMYDIA OR A SIMILAR INFECTION.

Symptoms

• *burning sensation and sometimes severe pain on passing urine* • *blood in urine and possibly a pus-filled yellow discharge* • *in NSU the symptoms are milder and the discharge in men is usually clear* • *in women there may be no symptoms, with occasionally increased discharge*

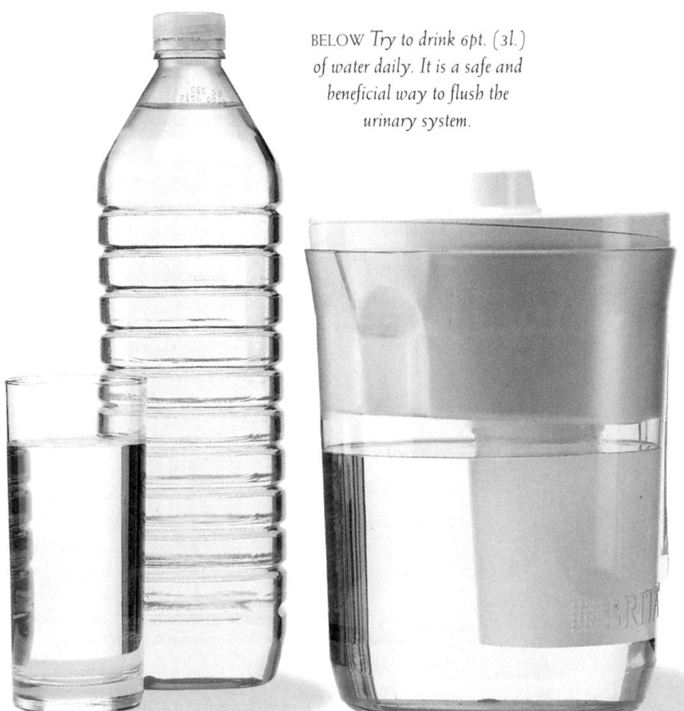

BELOW *Try to drink 6pt. (3l.) of water daily. It is a safe and beneficial way to flush the urinary system.*

TREATMENT

AYURVEDA
• Hollyhock is diuretic, and can be used to treat urethritis.
• Boil 4 tablespoons of coriander seeds in 4 cups or water until the liquid is reduced to 2 cups. Strain and drink with a little honey. *(See page 35.)*

TRADITIONAL HOME AND FOLK REMEDIES
• Eat live yogurt, and use as a douche to ease the symptoms of infection and inflammation, and prevent recurrence of the urethritis. *(See page 93.)*
• Cranberry juice, drunk daily, discourages bacteria from sticking to the urinary tract. It treats and prevents urethritis. *(See page 99.)*
• Garlic tincture, added to food or warm drinks, will ease inflammation and fight infection. *(See page 82.)*
• Drink barley water, several cups a day, with some lemon juice. *(See pages 87 and 92.)*

HERBALISM
• Herbs used to treat urethritis include urinary antiseptics and diuretics. You may drink infusions of any of the following herbs, alone or in combination: buchu, corn silk, coughgrass, uva ursi, and yarrow. *(See pages 112 and 116.)*
• Buchu will help to clear infection. Take as a tea, three times daily.

AROMATHERAPY
• Bergamot, lavender, and sandalwood are soothing and antiseptic. Add them to the bath water every evening. *(See pages 146–71.)*

HOMEOPATHY
For NSU, antibiotics should be taken, as prescribed, but the following may be helpful if it is not NSU:
• Cantharis, when the urine burns and is violently painful. *(See page 188.)*
• Staphisagria, for cystitis after intercourse.
• Mercurius, for violent pain with blood in the urine. *(See page 205.)*
• Apis, for stinging pain that is better for cold water. *(See page 180.)*
• Sarsaparilla, for burning pain which comes on after urinating.

VITAMINS AND MINERALS
• Drink plenty of water (6pt. [3l.] daily) to flush the urinary system.
• Take 1g. of vitamin C daily, which acts as a natural diuretic and boosts the immune system. *(See page 256.)*
• Vitamin C builds healthy mucous membranes. *(See page 256.)*
• Take acidophilus after a course of antibiotics. *(See page 271.)*

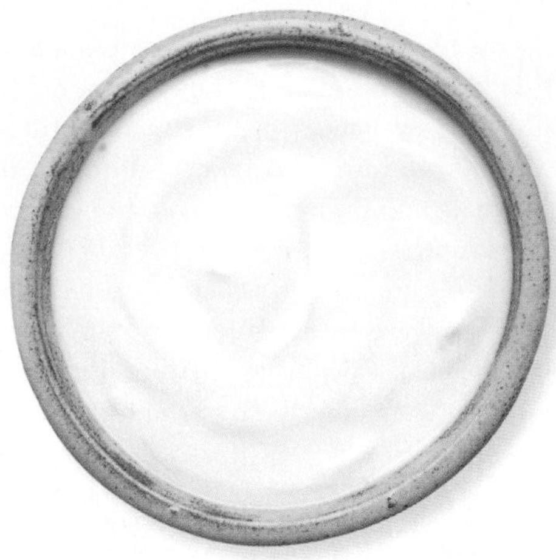

ABOVE *Antibiotics destroy good as well as bad bacteria in the intestinal tract. Eat plain live yogurt after taking antibiotics to restore the good bacteria.*

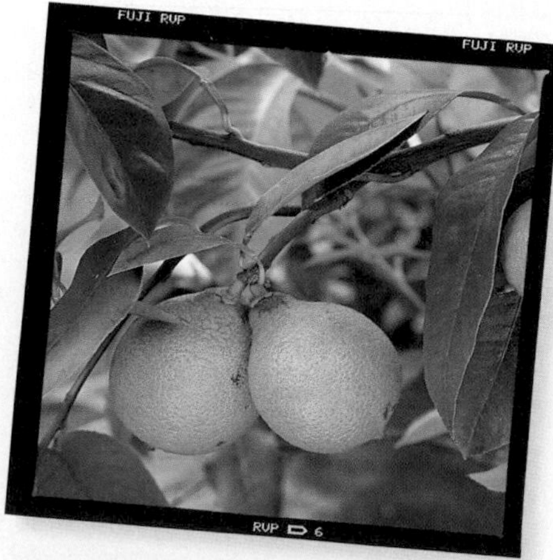

ABOVE *Vitamin C, contained in citrus fruits, will boost your immune system as well as building healthy mucous membranes.*

Incontinence

Incontinence is the inability to retain feces in the rectum, or an uncontrollable involuntary passing of urine. Incontinence, or involuntary urination, is extremely common. The most common form is stress incontinence, in which a small quantity of urine is "leaked" when there is increased pressure in the abdomen, as in laughing, sneezing, or coughing. Stress incontinence is often experienced after childbirth, as a result of injury or strain to the pelvic floor muscles, whose function it is to support the bladder and keep the urethra closed. Other causes include senile dementia, prostate enlargement, damage to nerve control as a result of stroke, multiple sclerosis, or local cancer, and bladder stones. Fecal incontinence (lack of normal control over passing feces) may occur in diarrhea, or if the controlling muscles have been damaged by disease or childbirth. Another cause is fecal impaction, which is often caused by long-standing constipation. *(See Constipation on page 373 and Diarrhea on page 374 for treatment of fecal incontinence.)*

ABOVE *Use a decoction or tincture of horsetail for incontinence of urine. It has toning properties that help strengthen the bladder.*

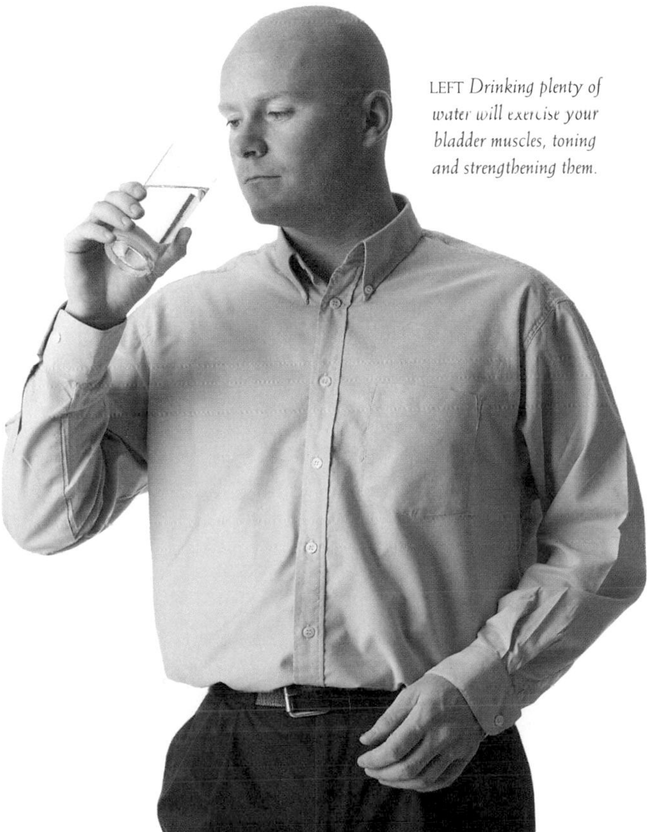

LEFT *Drinking plenty of water will exercise your bladder muscles, toning and strengthening them.*

TREATMENT

SWEET CHESTNUT

CHINESE HERBALISM

- Treatment would address Kidney Yang Deficiency with internal Cold, and the best herb to use is golden lock, taken as a tea. *(See page 61.)*
- If the condition accompanies prolapse, treatment will be given for Deficient qi, using central qi pills. This will help with the control of fecal and urinary incontinence.

HERBALISM

- The seeds of the ginkgo biloba plant act as a tonic to the kidneys and bladder, and have been used for incontinence and excessive urination. *(See page 122.)*
- Horsetail has toning and astringent properties, which make it useful both for incontinence and frequent urination. *(See page 120.)*

HOMEOPATHY

Treatment would be based on the cause of the incontinence, but some of the following might be useful:

- Causticum, for incontinence made worse by coughing or laughing. *(See page 189.)*
- Ferr. phos., for an inability to control the bladder, with pain and a frequent urge to urinate. *(See page 194.)*
- Nux vomica, for irritability and involuntary dribbles of urine. *(See page 214.)*
- Pulsatilla for stress incontinence which is made worse by sitting down. *(See page 209.)*
- Sepia, for incontinence related to weak pelvic floor muscles, accompanied by the feeling that the abdomen is falling out of the vagina. *(See page 212.)*

FLOWER ESSENCES

A number of the remedies will help with negative emotions and distress. Some to try are:

- Walnut, if incontinence is the result of change, such as pregnancy, a new baby, or menopause. *(See page 232.)*
- Sweet Chestnut, if you suffer from despair. *(See page 227.)*
- Agrimony, if you hide behind a cheerful face. *(See page 225.)*
- Crab Apple if you feel unclean. *(See page 234.)*

VITAMINS AND MINERALS

- Increase your intake of dietary fiber, which will prevent constipation and straining, a common cause of incontinence.
- Drink plenty of water to ensure regular use of the bladder muscles.

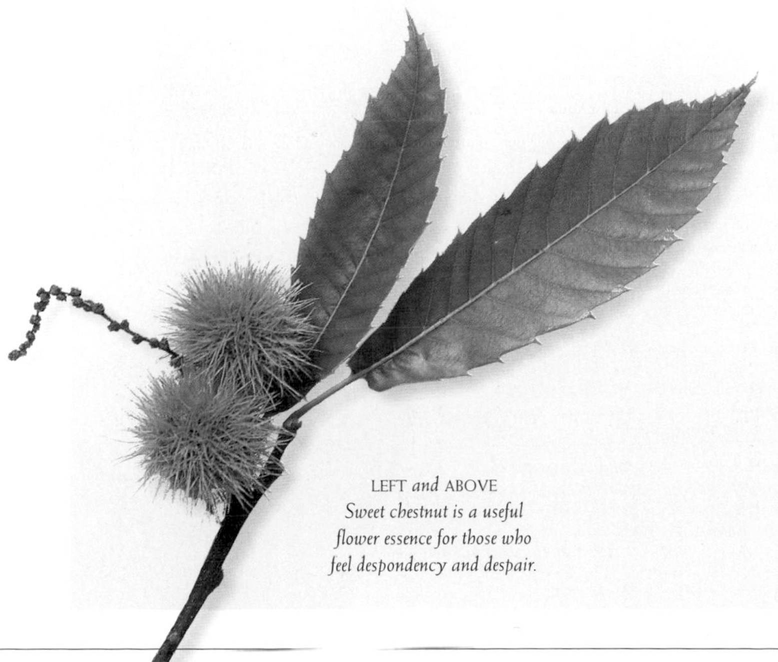

LEFT *and* ABOVE *Sweet chestnut is a useful flower essence for those who feel despondency and despair.*

DISORDERS OF THE REPRODUCTIVE SYSTEM: FEMALE

Breast Problems

The female breast consists mainly of a round mass of glandular tissue comprising about 15–20 lobes, each having a duct leading to an opening on the nipple; the duct system and glandular tissue develop fully with pregnancy. The amount of fat sheathing the glandular tissue determines the size of the breast. Connective tissues, or stroma, form the foundation or framework of the breast. The layer of ligaments directly beneath the breast sends strands into the breast itself, providing the firm consistency of the organ. The deep layer of connective tissue sends strands in the opposite direction into the covering of the chest muscles.

DATA FILE

Breast cancer is an important medical problem, with women of age 35 or older at increasing risk of developing some form of the disease. Physicians urge that women conduct monthly self-examinations of their breasts to detect potentially cancerous lumps, because the disease is more easily curable when found at an early stage. Another screening method is the X-ray process called mammography. Medical groups agree that women of 50 and older should have a yearly mammograph test. Some groups also advise an initial test for women between 35 and 40, and a test every one or two years for women between 40 and 50.

Some typical breast problems are:

- Tenderness, associated with pregnancy and PMS.
- Abscesses, which start as a bacterial infection in the breast tissue, producing swelling, redness, pain, and possibly fever. *(See also Breast-feeding Problems, page 383.)* They usually occur in women who are breast-feeding.
- Cysts, non-cancerous fluid-filled capsules in the ducts of the breast, appearing in groups or singly, occur mainly between the ages of 30 and 50, and in many women they cause one or more breasts to become lumpy and tender in the week or so before a menstrual period starts.
- Duct ectasia, blockage and inflammation of the milk ducts, is one of the most common causes of breast pain, particularly in women aged 40 to 50. It produces hot, red areas on the breast, a lump, and sometimes a watery discharge.
- Duct papillomas, which are benign, wart-like tumors in the ducts which, if not removed, may turn malignant. Their cause is uncertain, but may be hormonal.
- Fat necrosis, when fatty material released from the fat cells as a result of a blow to the breast forms into a hard lump of scar tissue, causing dimpling on the skin.
- Fibroadenoma, a benign breast tumor which is usually round, firm, and rubbery, causing no pain, can be moved around beneath the skin using the fingertips. These lumps are very common and most women will have one at some stage.

CAUTION

PREGNANT WOMEN SHOULD NOT TAKE CELERY SEED WITHOUT A PHYSICIAN'S APPROVAL.

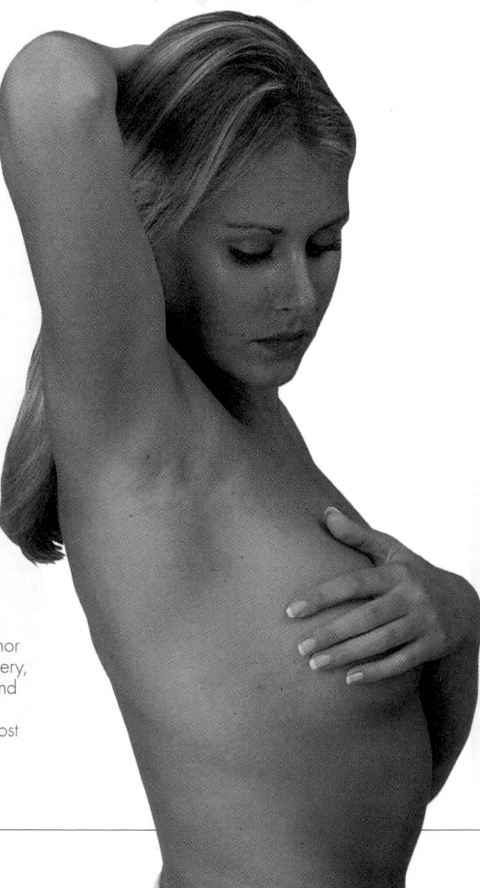

ABOVE *Celery seeds are used in Ayurvedic medicine to treat breast problems, particularly if they are swollen.*

LEFT *A change in diet may help some breast problems. Try cutting down on salty foods and caffeine and increase your intake of vitamin A.*

TREATMENT

AYURVEDA

- Barberry can be applied externally for its antibiotic and antifungal action. It also shrinks tumors (benign and cancerous), when it is taken internally. *(See page 29.)*
- Calamus oil will stimulate lymphatic drainage, and can be used for treating most breast problems. *(See page 24.)*
- Celery seed is diuretic, and can be useful when breast problems are related to swellings. *(See page 29.)*

CHINESE HERBALISM

- A poultice made from powdered dried rhubarb root can be applied to the breast to ease pain and swelling. *(See page 73.)*
- Madder root and dandelion may also be useful.

TRADITIONAL HOME AND FOLK REMEDIES

- Apply a bruised white cabbage leaf to the breast when there is infection, to heal and draw out the pus. *(See page 85.)*
- Apply continuous compresses of strong peach tea to the affected area for infection.
- Bruised parsley leaf poultices can be used for hard and lumpy breasts.

HERBALISM

- The herbs that are most useful for preventing and treating breast problems are those that encourage the action of the lymphatic system: cleavers, golden seal, marigold, marshmallow, nettles, and yellow dock. *(See pages 114, 117, 128, and 137.)*
- Consider taking the herb agnus castus for breast problems related to hormones (particularly premenstrually, and during the menopause). *(See page 139.)*

AROMATHERAPY

- Geranium oil can be used in the bath for relief of tenderness and edema, or massage it, blended into a little carrier oil, into the affected area. *(See page 165.)*
- Juniper, rosemary, lavender, and fennel oils will help to regulate hormone imbalance and relieve the symptoms of breast diseases. *(See pages 146–71.)*

HOMEOPATHY

For pain associated with PMS, try:

- Carb. an., for breast enlargement with shooting pains.
- Conium, for swelling, pain, and tenderness.
- Nat. mur., when the breasts are retaining water. *(See page 206.)*
- Calcarea, for heavy, pendulous breasts. *(See page 186.)*

Cysts should be dealt with constitutionally, but the following remedies may be useful in the short term:

- Pulsatilla, for sudden, inexplicable pains. *(See page 209.)*
- Conium, when the affected area is hard and painful.
- Phytolacca, for breasts that are more tender premenstrually, and when you are stressed.

For an abscess, try:

- Bryonia, for the early stages, with hardened breasts and pain. *(See page 185.)*
- Belladonna, for the early stages when there are red streaks. *(See page 183.)*
- Hep. sulf., for localized pain with irritability. *(See page 198.)*
- Silicea, for cracked, oozing nipples and feelings of exhaustion. *(See page 211.)*

For lumps, the following may be useful:

- Graphites, for hard, swollen, thickened breasts with blistered and sore nipples. *(See page 196.)*
- Belladonna, when the breasts are red, throbbing, and heavy. *(See page 183.)*
- Mercurius, for when the breasts are painful and full of milk at the time of menstruation. *(See page 205.)*

VITAMINS AND MINERALS

- Cut down on salty food to prevent water retention.
- Supplements of evening primrose oil and vitamin B6 may be useful. *(See pages 270 and 254.)*
- Cut down on caffeine, which can encourage the formation of cysts and lumps in the breast.
- Breast pain and lumps may be alleviated by increasing your daily intake of vitamin A. *(See page 252.)*
- Women with low levels of selenium may have a greater risk of suffering fibrocystic breast disease. *(See page 264.)*
- Apply vitamin E cream to heal cracked nipples. *(See page 257.)*

Breast-feeding Problems

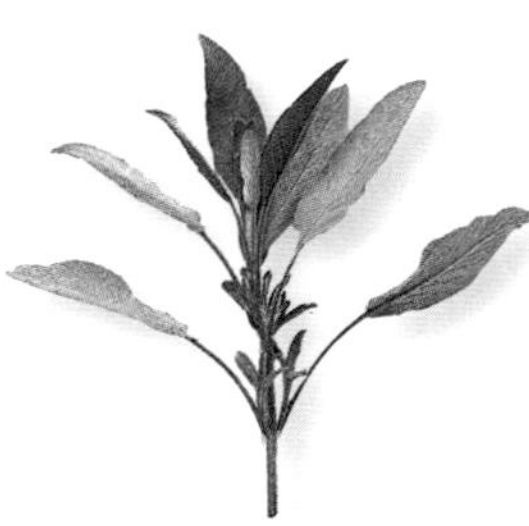

ABOVE *If you need to stop producing milk quickly try red sage as a safe alternative to drugs.*

After the birth of a child a mother's breast begins to produce milk, a natural process designed to provide complete nourishment for a baby for several months after its birth. Before milk is produced the mother's breast produces colostrum, a deep-yellow liquid containing high levels of protein and antibodies. A newborn baby who feeds on colostrum in the first few days of life is better able to resist the bacteria and viruses that cause illness. The mother's milk, which begins to flow a few days after childbirth when the mother's hormones change, is a blue-white color with a very thin consistency. If the mother is well nourished the milk provides the baby with the proper balance of nutrition. The fat contained in human milk, compared with cow's milk, is more digestible for infants and allows for greater absorption of fat-soluble vitamins into the bloodstream from the baby's intestine. Calcium and other important nutrients in human milk are also better utilized by infants. Antigens in cow's milk can cause allergic reactions in a newborn child, whereas such reactions to human milk are rare. Human milk also promotes growth, largely due to the presence of certain hormones and growth factors.

Breast-fed babies have a very low risk of developing meningitis or severe blood infections, and have a 500–600 percent lower risk of getting childhood lymphoma. Breast-fed babies also suffer 50 percent fewer middle ear infections.

DATA FILE

Typical breast-feeding problems are:

- Aching breasts, usually caused by engorgement either through increased blood pressure or overproduction of milk. Symptoms include fever, with hard, lumpy, and painful breasts.
- Blocked duct, a small red lump on the breast or a white lump on the nipple caused by rushed feeds, or by not emptying the breast properly.
- Cracked nipples, possibly caused by poor feeding position or by using damp breast pads.
- Mastitis, inflammation of the breast, usually caused either by a blocked duct or by infection. Symptoms include fever, redness and pain in the affected breast.
- Slow let-down reflex, that is to say a delay in the breast's milk-releasing response.
- Sore nipples, tenderness caused by prolonged suckling.
- Vaginal dryness caused by the suppression of estrogen production during lactation.

BELOW *A drink of dill tea can help prevent wind or colic in a baby, making it easier for the baby to suckle.*

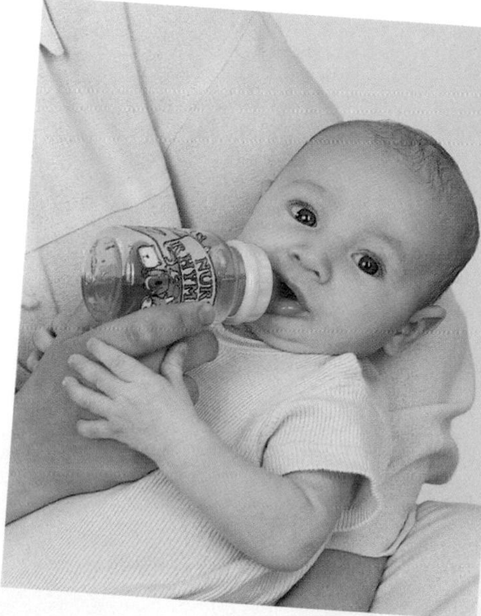

TREATMENT

AYURVEDA
- Cumin can increase milk production. *(See page 36.)*
- Fenugreek seeds will increase milk production. *(See page 45.)*

CHINESE HERBALISM
- Dandelion, peony bark, Chinese gentian, and madder root can be used for relieving mastitis. *(See page 67.)*

TRADITIONAL HOME AND FOLK REMEDIES
- Bruise parsley leaves, and apply them to hardened or knotty breasts during breast-feeding.
- Feed your baby a little diluted dill tea to prevent wind, which may be causing his or her breast-feeding problems.

HERBALISM
- Calendula cream will soothe and encourage the healing of sore and cracked nipples, and is safe for the baby to swallow. *(See page 117.)*
- Caraway, aniseed, dill, and fennel promote the flow of best milk, and can be taken in the form of teas or infusions. *(See page121.)*
- Compresses of marshmallow and slippery elm can often help with engorgement. *(See pages 114 and 136.)*
- Red sage will dry up breast milk almost instantly, if necessary. *(See page 129.)*
- Dilute tinctures of St. John's wort and marigold in boiled water and dab on to cracked nipples after each feed. *(See pages 117 and 124.)*
- Take echinacea for any infection. *(See page 120.)*

ABOVE *Ayurvedic practitioners give cumin to promote the flow of breast milk.*

AROMATHERAPY
- Lavender oil, in the bath or in a vaporizer, can encourage the let-down reflex. Better still, try massaging your baby with 1 drop in a little light carrier oil before a feed, to relax you both. *(See page 161.)*
- Caraway and verbena oils can be massaged into the breasts to stimulate the production of milk. *(See pages 146–71.)*
- Calendula and chamomile oils are anti-inflammatory, and can be applied to the breasts to ease inflammation and pain. Wash off before feeding. *(See pages 148–150.)*
- Peppermint oil, in cold compresses, can reduce the flow of milk when there is engorgement. *(See page 164.)*

HOMEOPATHY
- Chamomilla, Pulsatilla, Sulfur, and Graphites for sore and cracked nipples. *(See pages 204, 209, 215, and 196.)*
- Pulsatilla and Calcarea, for hard, engorged breasts. *(See page 209.)*
- Agnus will help with loss of breast milk.
- Calcarea, for poor-quality milk, when the mother is prone to chills. *(See page 186.)*
- Aconite, for sudden, excessive milk production, or, equally, sudden loss of milk caused by shock. *(See page 178.)*
- Bryonia, for hard and swollen breasts. *(See page 185.)*
- China, for exhaustion from breast-feeding. *(See page 190.)*
- Ignatia, for loss of milk due to grief or trauma. *(See page 200.)*

FLOWER ESSENCES
- Apply Rescue Remedy or Emergency Essence cream to the nipples when they are sore or cracked, to soothe and encourage healing. *(See page 244.)*
- Take either essence internally for distress caused by pain. *(See page 244.)*
- Olive is useful for overwhelming fatigue. *(See page 235.)*
- Walnut is useful for helping with change – in this case, the birth of your baby. *(See page 232.)*

VITAMINS AND MINERALS
- Breast-feeding mothers need plenty of protein, vitamins, and iron. *(See page 260.)*
- Drink plenty of fluids while breast-feeding.
- Apply vitamin E oil to sore and cracked nipples to help them heal. *(See page 257.)*

Menstrual Problems

The most common menstrual problems are dysmenorrhea (painful menstruation), menorrhagia (heavy menstrual bleeding), and amenorrhea (no menstrual bleeding). In primary dysmenorrhea there is either an increased level of or increased sensitivity to prostaglandin, the hormone-like substance that produces uterine contractions. Secondary dysmenorrhea (unusual menstrual cramps) begins at least three years after menstruation begins and may be caused by endometriosis, fibroids, a pelvic infection, stress, or a thyroid disorder. The symptoms for both include sharp pain or a dull ache in the lower abdomen and lower back, headaches, sweating, diarrhea. In severe cases there may be vomiting and fainting. Menorrhagia is best described as bleeding that is so heavy that it interferes with normal life. It may be caused by fibroids, polyps, pelvic infection, endometriosis, hypothyroidism, blood-clotting disorders, stress, or use of an IUD or injectable contraceptive. Primary amenorrhea refers to menstruation not starting by the age of 18. This is usually due to low body weight or heredity. Secondary amenorrhea occurs when menstruation stops for more than six months due to pregnancy, weight loss, starting oral contraceptives, severe shock, stress, anemia, thyroid disorder, or a fibroid.

ABOVE *Take bioflavonoids to regulate your menstrual cycle. They will also balance your hormone levels.*

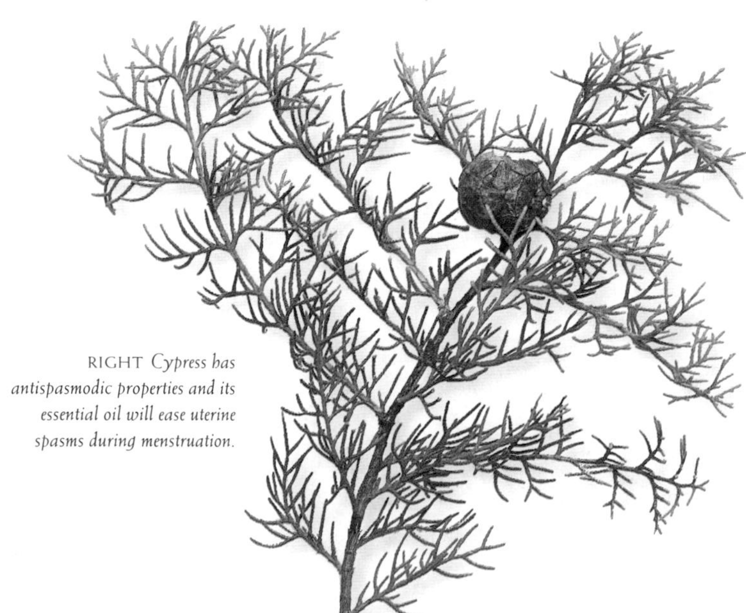

RIGHT *Cypress has antispasmodic properties and its essential oil will ease uterine spasms during menstruation.*

TREATMENT

AYURVEDA

- Aloe vera can induce menstruation. *(See page 27.)*
- Basil can be used to promote menstruation. *(See page 42.)*
- Caraway relaxes uterine tissue and is beneficial for menstrual cramps. *(See page 30.)*
- Cardamom will help digestive problems associated with menstruation. *(See page 38.)*
- Cedar stimulates the menstrual cycle, and celery seeds can treat irregular menstruation. *(See page 32.)*

CHINESE HERBALISM

- Excessive flow is considered to be caused by Heat in the Blood; scanty flow, late menstruation, and painful menstruation are due to Cold in the Blood.
- Warming herbs, such as ginger, ginseng, and cinnamon, may be used. *(See pages 59 and 67.)*
- Cornelian Asiatic cherry can be used in the treatment of heavy menstrual bleeding. *(See page 60.)*

TRADITIONAL HOME AND FOLK REMEDIES

- Dried carrot powder taken daily may help to regulate the menstrual cycle. *(See page 89.)*
- Cayenne pepper regulates bleeding. Add a few grains to any herbal tea.
- Cinnamon bark will help to control menstrual flow.
- Diluted lemon juice cleanses the system and helps to control bleeding. *(See page 87.)*
- Beets help to regulate menstrual problems.
- Strawberry leaves, taken over a long period, can help to regulate menstrual flow and ease pain.

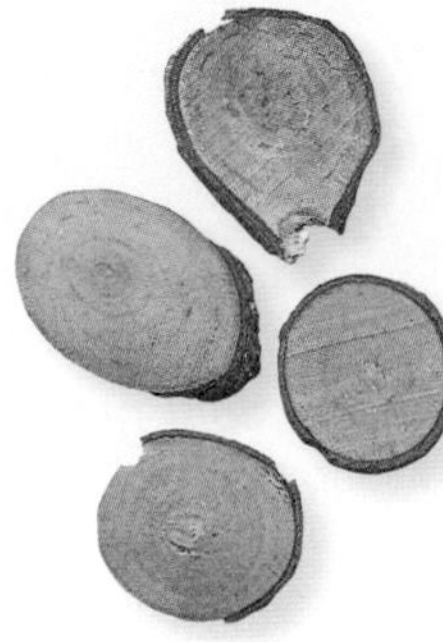

ABOVE *The Chinese use warming herbs, such as cinnamon, for menstrual problems.*

HERBALISM

- Cramp bark is helpful for menstrual cramps. *(See page 138.)*
- Lady's mantle is an astringent and is useful for heavy menstrual bleeding. Take 3 times daily, as required. *(See page 113.)*
- Yarrow will help to regulate menstruation. *(See page 112.)*
- Raspberry leaves can help to control an excessive flow of blood. *(See page 128.)*
- Thyme tea, drunk each morning and evening, can control excessive flow. *(See page 135.)*
- Angelica root can help to promote menstruation which is delayed. *(See page 115.)*
- Catnip tea, drunk each evening and morning during menstruation, will help to ease pain.
- Peppermint tea will ease any bloating and pain during menstruation. *(See page 125.)*

AROMATHERAPY

- Antispasmodic oils, such as clary sage, cypress, and lavender, will help to ease cramps. *(See pages 146–71.)*
- Clary sage and fennel oils, massaged into the lower back, can help to regulate hormone balance, and, through that, the menstrual cycle. *(See pages 146–71.)*
- Heavy menstrual bleeding can be treated with geranium, rose, or cypress essential oils. Add to the bath water or use in a local massage. *(See pages 146–71.)*

HOMEOPATHY

- China, for spasmodic bleeding with dark clots and cramps. *(See page 190.)*
- Belladonna, for pain, bright red blood, and nagging headache. *(See page 183.)*
- Ipecac., for heavy bleeding and bright red blood with nausea. *(See page 189.)*
- Sepia, for a bearing-down type pain. *(See page 212.)*
- Aconite, for menstruation that stops after an emotional shock. *(See page 178.)*
- Ignatia, for menstruation that stops after grief, trauma, or loss. *(See page 200.)*
- Colocynthis, for cramping pain which is improved by pressure. *(See page 191.)*
- Sabina, for pain and dark red blood with clots.
- Chamomilla, for pains that resemble labor pains. *(See page 204.)*

VITAMINS AND MINERALS

- Vitamin B6, taken twice daily, can help prevent menstrual cramps. *(See page 254.)*
- Iron and zinc will help in cases of heavy menstrual bleeding. *(See pages 260 and 265.)*
- Take vitamin A and B6 for heavy bleeding. *(See pages 252 and 254.)*
- Bioflavonoids can help to balance hormone levels and regulate the menstrual cycle. *(See page 272.)*
- Deficiencies of zinc and vitamin B6 can result from absence of menstruation. *(See pages 265 and 254.)*

Premenstrual Syndrome (PMS)

Premenstrual syndrome is the term used to describe a huge range of symptoms, at least some of which are experienced by most women (especially those over 30) every month between ovulation and menstruation. The symptoms may be physical, emotional, or behavioral in character and are thought to be caused either by hormonal imbalance (possibly due to recent childbirth or a gynecological disorder) or by marginal (sub-clinical) nutritional deficiencies which can affect the fine hormone balance in the body. Interestingly, women who regularly consume caffeine are more likely to suffer from severe PMS, and there is sometimes a connection with a thyroid condition.

Symptoms

• *physical: – breast enlargement and tenderness – bloated abdomen – headaches/migraines – pelvic discomfort – fluid retention and weight gain – constipation or diarrhea – greasy hair and skin – tiredness* • *emotional: – irritability and confusion – anxiety – disturbed sleep – depression and, in severe cases, suicidal thoughts* • *behavioral: – clumsiness and lack of coordination – poor concentration – violent or aggressive outbursts*

LEFT *Eating fresh apples, celery, and grapes will help to prevent bloating in the week before your menstrual period is due.*

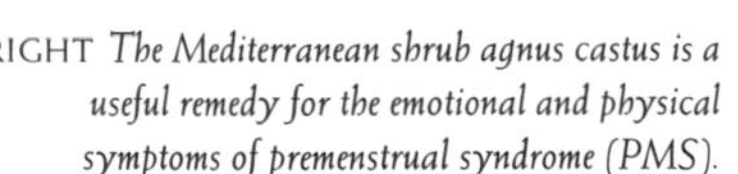

RIGHT *The Mediterranean shrub agnus castus is a useful remedy for the emotional and physical symptoms of premenstrual syndrome (PMS).*

TREATMENT

AYURVEDA

• Calamus root stimulates the adrenals, which will help PMS associated with stress. *(See page 24.)*
• Caraway is useful for digestive problems associated with PMS, and is a natural diuretic. *(See page 30.)*
• Myrrh is used for treating many conditions relating to menstruation. *(See page 34.)*
• Angelica is specific for PMS. *(See page 28.)*

CHINESE HERBALISM

• PMS is believed to be caused by an imbalance of Spleen, Kidneys, and Liver, and can be treated with angelica, peony, hoelen, and skullcap. *(See pages 56, 67, 71, and 74.)*

TRADITIONAL HOME AND FOLK REMEDIES

• Swelling can be prevented by eating plenty of fresh, crunchy apples in the week prior to menstruation. *(See page 94.)*
• Celery is also a good diuretic, and acts on the kidneys to encourage their action. *(See page 83.)*
• Eat fresh grapes to prevent bloating.
• Barley water, which is rich in B vitamins, can be drunk freely throughout your menstrual cycle to ease symptoms. *(See page 92.)*
• To ease irritability and other emotional symptoms, eat plenty of oats. *(See page 84.)*

HERBALISM

• Try an infusion (herbs steeped in boiling water) of agnus castus or false unicorn, which have a balancing effect on the hormones. *(See page 139.)*
• Herbs which help to reduce some of the symptoms of stress and anxiety include oats, vervain, and passiflora. *(See pages 117 and 138.)*
• Water retention can be eased with couchgrass or dandelion teas, drunk two or three times each day during the premenstrual phase. *(See page 133.)*
• Rosemary, oats, cinnamon, and lemon balm will help to lift the spirits. *(See pages 117 and 127.)*
• Skullcap, wood betony, and vervain are good for addressing tension, anxiety, and depression. *(See pages 131 and 138.)*
• Cornsilk and burdock are useful for symptoms associated with bloating. *(See page 115.)*
• Cleavers and poke root will help with monthly breast tenderness.
• Take valerian for extreme tension. *(See page 136.)*
• Chamomile, cinnamon, and peppermint will help with nausea and vomiting. *(See pages 119 and 125.)*
• Yellow dock and wormwood will balance the blood sugar levels. *(See page 128.)*

AROMATHERAPY

• Try essential oils of geranium and rosemary in your bath to relieve symptoms, including water retention and irritability. *(See pages 165 and 168.)*
• Clary sage and rose may help with depression. *(See pages 169 and 168.)*
• A light massage (whole body, or over the abdominal area) with lavender oil or clary sage will balance hormones and ease symptoms. *(See pages 161 and 169.)*

HOMEOPATHY

Treatment will be constitutional, but useful remedies include:
• Lachesis, for symptoms which are worse first thing in the morning; also good for painful breasts. *(See page 216.)*
• Nux vomica., for irritability and chilliness, constipation, frequent urination, and various food cravings. *(See page 214.)*
• Sepia, for irritability, weepiness, emotional flatness, feeling turned off by sex, and cravings for sweet or salty foods. *(See page 212.)*
• Kali carb., for tension, exhaustion, feeling overweight, and where the symptoms become worse around 3A.M.
• Pulsatilla, for suddenly bursting into tears, nausea, depression, irregular menstruation, and painful breasts. *(See page 209.)*
• Lycopodium, for bad temper, depression, and a craving for sweet things. *(See page 203.)*
• Sulfur, when the main symptom is a craving for sweets. *(See page 215.)*

FLOWER ESSENCES

• Mustard, for depression. *(See page 239.)*
• Scleranthus, for mood swings. *(See page 239.)*
• Olive, for fatigue. *(See page 235.)*
• Crab Apple, for feeling repulsive and unliked. *(See page 234.)*

VITAMINS AND MINERALS

• Evening primrose oil, with the following supplements: vitamins C, E, and B6, magnesium, zinc, iron, and chromium. These should be taken continuously for one month, and subsequently during the fortnight preceding menstruation. *(See pages 270, 256, 257, 254, 265, 260, and 259.)*

Infertility

The term infertility, or failure to reproduce, is generally applied when failure to conceive follows regular, unprotected sex over an 18-month period. Infertility indicates a fault in the reproductive system and is very often treatable.

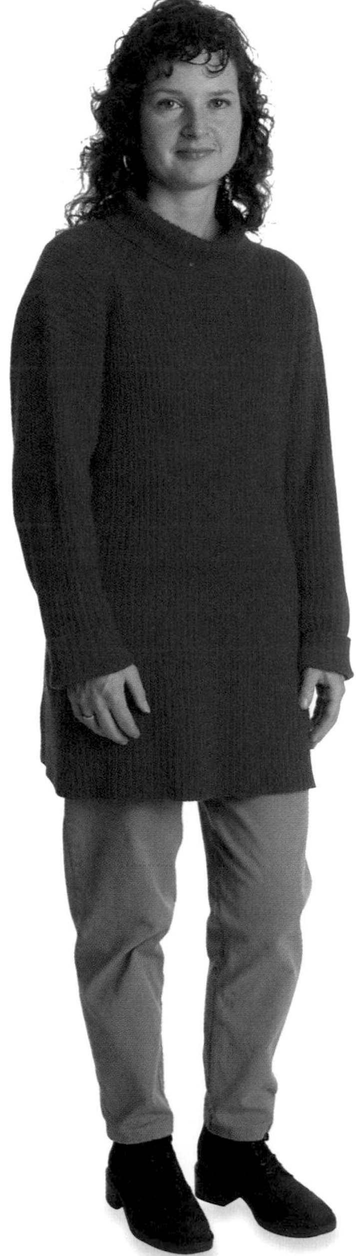

ABOVE *White Chestnut is an excellent flower essence to take if the problems of infertility are causing you great anxiety.*

TREATMENT

Evening primrose capsules
Nuts
Yogurt
Pumpkin seeds
Garlic perles
Kidney beans
Black-eyed peas

LEFT *Increasing your intake of essential fatty acids will help stimulate the production of your sex hormones.*

AYURVEDA

• Cloves can tone the uterus, and garlic has a rejuvenating effect on the reproductive system. *(See page 38.)*
• Saffron is aphrodisiac, and can help when infertility is associated with sexual problems. *(See page 36.)*

CHINESE HERBALISM

• Infertility is believed to be caused by Damp Heat and imbalance of yin and yang. Golden lock tea may be useful, but treatment is always individually prescribed, so see a practitioner.

TRADITIONAL HOME AND FOLK REMEDIES

• Oats are calming, and can help with the effects of stress, as well as toning the body. Eat as often as possible. *(See page 84.)*

HERBALISM

• Agnus castus is an excellent hormone regulator and will help if your menstruation is irregular, or you are not ovulating for hormonal reasons. It may also be useful if you are prone to early miscarriage. *(See page 139.)*
• False unicorn root helps to regulate the ovaries and strengthen the endometrium.
• Balm, passiflora, and skullcap will help to reduce the effects of stress, which may be causing the condition. *(See page 131.)*

AROMATHERAPY

• Rose oil is said to increase sperm count and quality, as well as acting as a mild aphrodisiac. Add a few drops to your partner's bath, or perhaps engage in a little gentle massage, with 2 or 3 drops of rose essential oil in a mild carrier oil such as sweet almond oil. *(See page 168.)*
• A few drops of geranium and melissa can be used neat in the bath, or diluted in a gentle carrier oil and massaged over the abdomen on a regular basis. *(See pages 165 and 163.)*
• Tea tree and lavender oils are anti-infective and anti-inflammatory, and can be useful in abdominal massage, for treating any pelvic infection or inflammation which may be preventing the woman conceiving. *(See pages 161 and 162.)*
• If infertility is causing the patient great anxiety, one of the relaxing oils, such as lavender, marjoram, or chamomile, can be used in the bath, or try it in a vaporizer. *(See pages 150, 161, and 165.)*
• When repeated attempts to get pregnant have failed and you need a little encouragement to continue with love-making, ylang ylang is a lovely, relaxing oil that acts as an aphrodisiac. Use as a massage oil or in the bath. *(See page 148.)*

HOMEOPATHY

Treatment would be constitutional, but the following remedies may be helpful:
• Conium, when breasts are tender, with areas of hard swelling, and sexual desire is suppressed.
• Saline, for previous miscarriages before 12 weeks.
• Sepia for irregular menstruation, and a feeling of chilliness, weeping, and irritability. *(See page 212.)*

FLOWER ESSENCES

• White Chestnut may be useful if you are extremely upset or tormented by the problem. *(See page 224.)*
• For despondency, try Gorse. *(See page 240.)*

VITAMINS AND MINERALS

• Cutting out alcohol, smoking, and drugs may be suggested for the period before conception.
• Eating plenty of whole foods rich in vitamins and minerals will not only ensure that sperm and egg are healthy, but that the woman's body is a welcoming home for the growing embryo. Good nutrition increases the chances of conception and gives the baby every chance of being healthy.
• Vitamin E and B6 may be supplemented, as low intake is often linked to a low sperm count. Vitamin E may regulate the production of cervical mucus in women. *(See pages 257 and 254.)*
• Increase intake of EFAs (essential fatty acids): in oily fish, fish liver oils, seeds, nuts, pulses, beans, evening primrose oil, unrefined vegetable oils), to stimulate sex hormone production.
• Zinc deficiency has been linked to infertility. *(See page 265.)*

DATA FILE

Causes of infertility include:

- Age. Fertility declines in women over the age of 35.
- Cervical mucus may be too thick and sticky, or contain hostile antibodies.
- Endometriosis, when pieces of the womb lining migrate to the Fallopian tubes or the ovaries, causing tube blockage or clogging of the area.
- Fibroids, benign growths of muscle.
- Narrowed or scarred cervix, which may have resulted from surgery in the cervical area.
- Ovulation problems due to congenital abnormality, damage to the ovaries, or hormonal problems.
- Pelvic infections. Scar tissue from infections can cause blockage of the Fallopian tubes.
- Polycystic ovaries, repeated or multiple ovarian cysts.
- Smoking, which can cause constriction of blood vessels supplying the reproductive organs, which then inhibits their action.
- Stress. There are possible links between stress and infertility.
- Womb problems such as adenomyosis, where scar tissue forms on the womb wall, an abnormal womb shape, and polyps.
- Approximately 10–15 percent of couples, or one in every seven marriages, in the United States is affected by infertility.
- In approximately 40 percent of cases, infertility is due to a female factor, 40 percent of cases are due to a male factor *(see page 398)*, and in the remaining instances no cause can be found despite thorough evaluation.
- In as many as 35 percent of couples, multiple conditions causing infertility can be identified.
- In female infertility, ovulatory dysfunction, including lack of ovulation and poor progesterone production, is responsible for approximately 15 percent of infertility cases.
- Fallopian tube obstruction and pelvic adhesions, which may result from pelvic inflammatory disease, endometriosis, and post-partum infections, account for 30 percent of infertility cases.
- Cervical factors, which may impede the passage of sperm into the uterus, are responsible for approximately 5 percent of infertility cases.
- Uterine factors, including polyps, adhesions, leiomyomata (fibroid tumors), and congenital anomalies, may interfere with implantation of the embryo. Approximately 5 percent of infertility cases are caused by these abnormalities.

Miscarriage

Spontaneous abortion, or miscarriage, occurs when the embryo fails to develop, when there is complete or incomplete expulsion of the embryo or fetus, and placenta, or when the fetus dies prior to 20 weeks. If fetal death occurs at 20 weeks or more after the last period, it is termed a late fetal death or a stillbirth.

Up to three-fourths of conceptions abort spontaneously. Most occur before the woman's pregnancy can be confirmed, prior to six weeks after her last period. These constitute about one-fifth of confirmed pregnancies and about one-tenth of all pregnancy hospitalizations in the United States.

In many cases the womb sheds an embryo because it is not developing normally. Often, however, there is no explanation for miscarriage at all, although the following may be at greater risk: women over 40, pregnancies resulting from fertility treatment, twin or multiple pregnancies, pregnancies where the placenta is faulty.

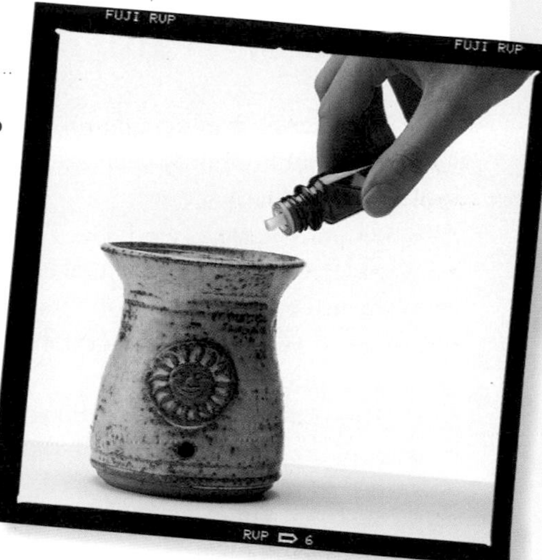

ABOVE *The therapeutic vapors of essential oils such as lavender can help you through the grieving period that follows the loss of a baby.*

CAUTION

SUDDEN, SEVERE ABDOMINAL PAIN BETWEEN THE FIFTH AND TENTH WEEKS OF PREGNANCY MAY INDICATE AN ECTOPIC PREGNANCY (ONE THAT DEVELOPS IN THE FALLOPIAN TUBE). THIS IS A LIFE-THREATENING CONDITION REQUIRING URGENT MEDICAL ATTENTION.

Symptoms

• of a threatened miscarriage: – bleeding, clots or a dark discharge from the vagina – mucus in the vaginal blood – abdominal pain, possibly cramp-like pain similar to menstrual cramps – back pain • of inevitable miscarriage: – opening of the cervix and continuous bleeding (inevitable abortion) – emptying of the uterus, after which the cervix closes and bleeding stops (complete abortion) – partial emptying of the uterus, after which the cervix remains open and bleeding continues (incomplete abortion)

TREATMENT

AYURVEDA

- Herbs to tone the uterus and improve circulation may be useful, but treatment must be undertaken by a registered practitioner. *(See page 20.)*

CHINESE HERBALISM

- Dodder seeds are used to prevent miscarriages. *(See page 62.)*

HERBALISM

- Herbs for threatened miscarriage include false unicorn root decoction, which should be sipped every few minutes.
- Cramp bark can help to relax the uterus and prevent miscarriage. *(See page 138.)*
- Black haw can be used to avert miscarriage and ensure relaxation.
- Tonic herbs to prevent miscarriage include red raspberry leaves mixed with a little vervain. *(See pages 128 and 138.)*
- Following miscarriage, you can use raspberry leaves to aid the healing of the uterus, and antiseptic herbs such as thyme or echinacea to help prevent infection. *(See pages 120, 128, and 135.)*
- Rosemary and wild oats will help to support the nervous system following the trauma of miscarriage. *(See pages 117 and 127.)*

LEFT *Raspberry is an excellent healing remedy for the uterus after a miscarriage.*

AROMATHERAPY

- Lavender is relaxing, and can be used daily in the bath to calm – particularly if you are concerned about miscarriage. Use only in a vaporizer if you have a history of miscarriage. It will be useful following a miscarriage to help your body get back to normal. *(See page 161.)*
- Rose has an affinity with the reproductive system, and can be used in a vaporizer (not applied) to help prevent miscarriage. *(See page 168.)*

HOMEOPATHY

- Arnica, where there is risk of miscarriage following an accident or injury. *(See page 182.)*
- Take Hypericum, following amniocentesis, to prevent miscarriage. *(See page 199.)*
- Ipecac., for threatened miscarriage, when the blood is bright red with abdominal cramps. *(See page 189.)*
- Sabina, if the blood is dark and clotting, usually at the end of the first trimester.

FLOWER ESSENCES

- Rock Rose, for helplessness and terror. *(See page 231.)*
- Mimulus, for gnawing fear of miscarriage. *(See page 235.)*
- Star of Bethlehem, for shock. *(See page 235.)*
- Gentian, for despondency following a very early miscarriage. *(See page 230.)*
- Walnut, to help you adjust to the new situation. *(See page 232.)*

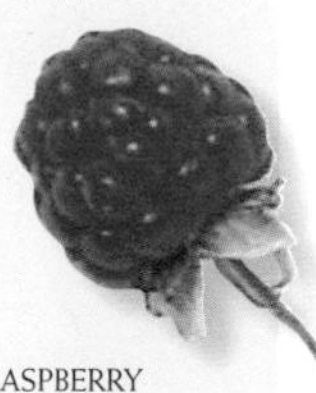

RASPBERRY

Pregnancy Problems

Women may experience problems during pregnancy, often as a result of hormonal changes. Some of the most common problems women experience are:

- ANEMIA (*see page* 357)
- BACKACHE, due either to postural changes made to accommodate the extra weight, or to the position in which the baby is lying
- BLEEDING GUMS, caused by hormonal changes which lead to a thickening and softening of the gums
- CONSTIPATION, when normal bowel action is slowed down by an increase of progesterone
- CRAMPS, which occur mainly in the feet, calves, and thighs due to inefficient circulation (as a result of increased progesterone), and possibly calcium deficiency
- FAINTING, caused by a shortage of blood to the brain due to lowered blood pressure and an increased demand for blood to the womb
- FLATULENCE, since digesting food is moved more slowly, which allows wind to build up
- FLUID RETENTION, when an upset in the balance of salt and potassium in the cells causes swelling in the hands, legs, and feet
- HEARTBURN, a burning sensation in the upper chest, and possibly a sour taste in the mouth, which are caused by acidic juices rising back up the esophagus
- INSOMNIA, caused by general inevitable bodily discomfort towards the end of pregnancy
- MORNING SICKNESS, nausea and/or vomiting usually in the first three months of pregnancy, but not necessarily confined to the morning
- PELVIC PAIN, pain in the groin or inside of the thighs when walking, caused by pressure on the pelvic nerves
- PILES (*see page* 377)
- STRETCH MARKS, fine red lines (which eventually turn silver) appearing on the breasts, abdomen, and thighs, and caused by stretching of the skin
- VARICOSE VEINS
- TIREDNESS, characterized by a desire to sleep a lot in the first three months
- INCREASED VAGINAL DISCHARGE, probably thickish and white

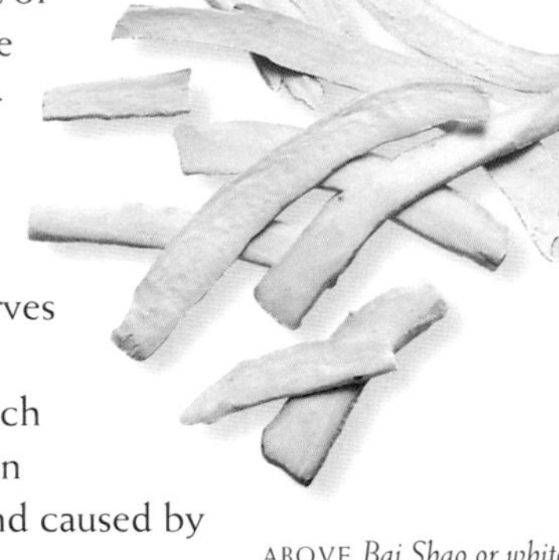

ABOVE *Bai Shao or white peony is considered one of the best women's tonics in Chinese medicine.*

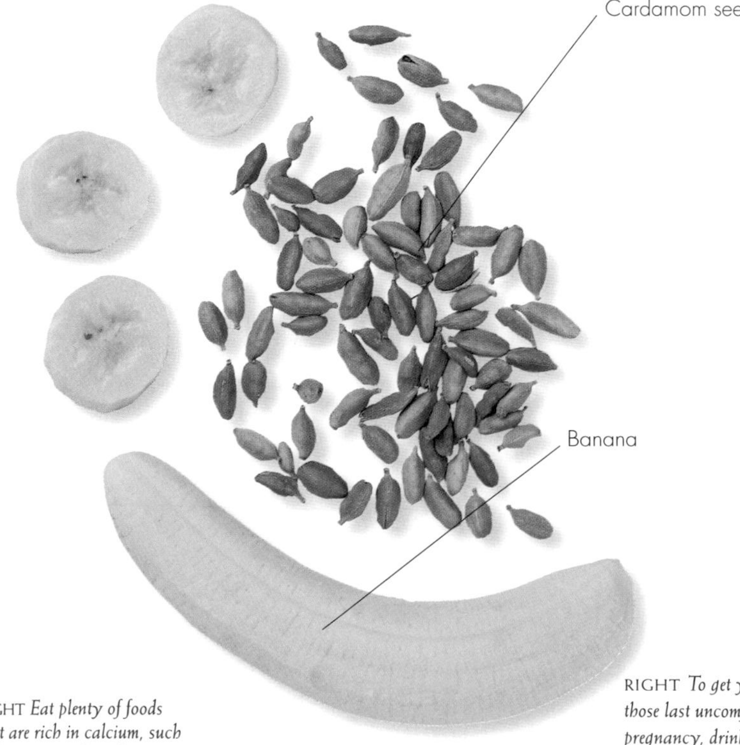

RIGHT *Eat plenty of foods that are rich in calcium, such as bananas and cardamom, to prevent cramps.*

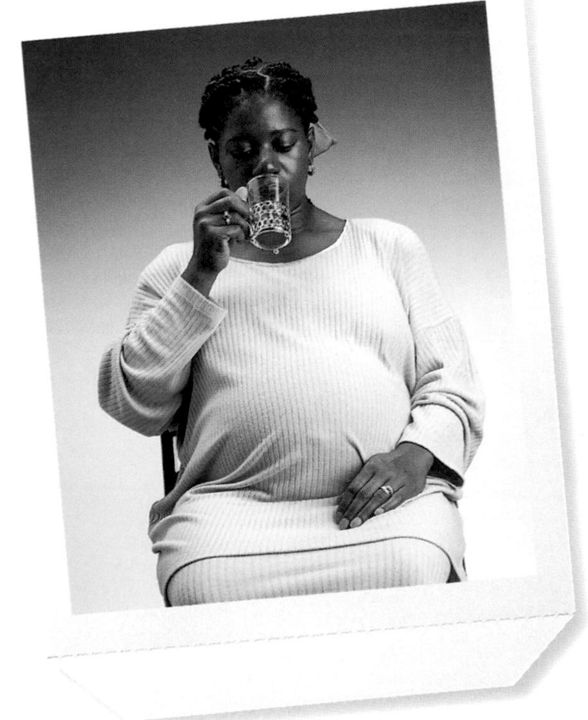

RIGHT *To get you to sleep during those last uncomfortable months of pregnancy, drink a glass of honey and apple cider vinegar in warm water before you retire.*

TREATMENT

AYURVEDA
• Aloe vera can be applied externally to prevent stretch marks. *(See page 27.)*
• Ginger, for recurrent nausea in pregnancy. *(See page 47.)*
• Eating caraway seeds deals with constipation and digestive problems. *(See page 30.)*
• Cardamom suppresses vomiting when eaten with a banana. *(See page 38.)*
• Cayenne, used externally, can ease muscle pain. *(See page 31.)*
• Clove tones muscles and expectant mothers are recommended to eat them in the last month of pregnancy to strengthen the uterus. *(See page 38.)*
• Licorice, for constipation, and digestive problems. *(See page 39.)*
• Long pepper, for muscle soreness, digestive problems, and constipation. *(See page 43.)*
• Mustard can help with muscle and joint pain, and acts as a laxative. *(See page 30.)*

CHINESE HERBALISM
• Teasel root, ginseng, and acanthopanax root, for persistent back pain. *(See page 54.)*
• Peony root and astragalus, for high blood pressure. *(See pages 57 and 67.)*
• Ginseng, licorice, and tangerine peel, for an acid stomach. *(See pages 59, 64, and 67.)*
• Gui Pi Wan, for anemia.
• Astragalus, for overwhelming exhaustion. *(See page 57.)*
• Wild jujube and fleece-flower stem, for insomnia. *(See pages 71 and 75.)*
• Dittany bark, for itching.
• Ginger, for morning sickness.
• Water plantain, poria, cinnamon twigs, and ephedra, for edema. *(See pages 59 and 71.)*
• Gentian and oriental wormwood, for thrush.

TRADITIONAL HOME AND FOLK REMEDIES
• Eating yogurt will cool the pain of heartburn. *(See page 93.)*
• Use a witch hazel compress on varicose veins – either in the legs or the vulva. *(See page 91.)*
• For relief of varicose veins in the legs or vulva, apply neat lemon juice. *(See page 87.)*
• Garlic helps the circulation, and can prevent cramping, varicose veins, and piles. *(See page 82.)*
• Apply a witch hazel compress to piles to reduce inflammation and encourage healing. *(See page 91.)*
• Drink a glass of honey and apple cider vinegar in warm water before bed to help you sleep peacefully. *(See pages 101 and 102.)*
• Celery juice can help you sleep when taken before bedtime. *(See page 83.)*
• Chamomile, fennel, and thyme have antifungal properties, and can be used as a compress and pressed against the vagina to ease and treat thrush.

HERBALISM
• Dandelion tea is a mild diuretic, and so will help with edema. *(See page 133.)*
• Chamomile or peppermint tea will ease heartburn. *(See pages 119 and 125.)*
• Dandelion leaves, nettles, chives, sorrel, and coriander leaves are rich in iron, which will prevent anemia. *(See pages 133 and 137.)*
• Chamomile, fennel, burdock, and ginger are gentle laxatives, safe for preventing constipation. *(See pages 115, 119, 121, and 139.)*
• Lavender, vervain, and lemon balm will soothe the nerves and relax muscles. *(See page 138.)*
• Nettles, meadowsweet, and celery seeds are rich in calcium, which can help to prevent cramping. *(See pages 121 and 137.)*
• Lemon balm and chamomile tea can help prevent nausea, as can ginger and fennel. Take as infusions as required. *(See pages 119, 121, and 139.)*
• Slippery elm helps to soothe the digestive tract, and can help morning sickness and weak digestion. *(See page 136.)*
• Hops can be used for treating severe vomiting.
• False unicorn root and agnus castus can balance the hormones, which will prevent many symptoms. *(See page 139.)*
• Calendula, marjoram, and comfrey are astringent and can be applied to the legs or vulva as required. *(See pages 117 and 132.)*
• Peppermint and cleavers can be drunk as an infusion to improve circulation and treat varicose veins. *(See page 125.)*
• Chamomile, catnip, and vervain can help with insomnia, when taken before bedtime or during the night. *(See pages 119 and 138.)*
• Chamomile, dandelion root, nettle, and licorice can be taken three times daily for piles. *(See pages 119, 122, 134, and 137.)*
• Calendula flowers can be infused, added to coconut oil, and rubbed into the skin to prevent stretch marks. *(See page 117.)*

AROMATHERAPY
• Lavender oil can be rubbed into the temples for headaches, and into the back for muscle pains. *(See page 161.)*
• Geranium, fennel, marjoram, and ylang ylang can be added to the bath to prevent constipation. *(See pages 146–71.)*
• Roman chamomile and marjoram are excellent in a full-body massage to ease the muscular pains of pregnancy. *(See pages 150 and 165.)*
• Thyme, cypress, lavender, and lemon oils can be added to the bath water to strengthen the veins and increase circulation. *(See pages 146–71.)*
• Essential oil of geranium can be added to the bath for piles. *(See page 165.)*
• A gentle massage with lavender, chamomile, or lemon balm can relax and help you sleep. *(See page146–71.)*
• Add a few drops of tea tree or cinnamon oil to a cup of cool water and apply to the vaginal area on a clean cloth to treat thrush. *(See pages 162 and 150.)*
• A light massage of lavender and neroli, in a carrier oil, can prevent stretch marks. *(See pages 162 and 152.)*
• Massage lavender, geranium, or ginger oils into the lower back to ease pain and reduce tension. *(See pages 146–71.)*

HOMEOPATHY
• Nat. mur., for help with water retention. *(See page 206.)*
• For anemia *(see page 357)*, try Kali carb., when the back feels weak and tired, and there are unpleasant dragging pains.
• Belladonna, when there is a hard tense feeling in the lower abdomen. *(See page 183.)*
• Nux vomica., for nausea that is worse in the morning, and when the vomit contains mucus. *(See page 214.)*
• Ipecac., for nonstop nausea and vomiting. *(See page 189.)*
• Pulsatilla, for nausea which comes on in the evening. *(See page 209.)*
• Ferr. phos., for nausea a few hours after eating. *(See page 194.)*
• Nat. mur., for nausea with an aversion to bread and fat, with a craving for salt and great thirst. *(See page 206.)*
• Capsicum, for heartburn with a burning sensation behind the breastbone.
• Phosphorus, for heartburn with a craving for cold drinks that are then vomited. *(See page 208.)*
• Sulfur, for heartburn that is worse around 11 A.M. *(See page 215.)*

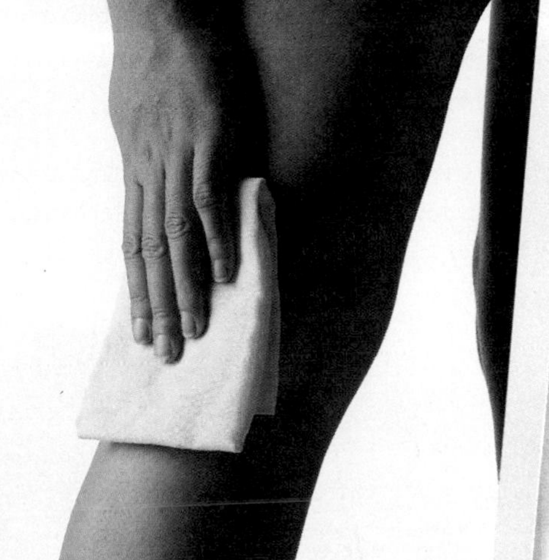

ABOVE *A witch hazel compress will help relieve painful varicose veins.*

FLOWER ESSENCES
• Olive is useful for dealing with general exhaustion. *(See page 235.)*
• Crab Apple may help with relief of nausea. *(See page 234.)*
• Rescue Remedy or Emergency Essence may be useful for vomiting. *(See page 244.)*

VITAMINS AND MINERALS
• Ensure you get plenty of iron, to prevent and treat anemia. Take vitamin C together with iron, in order to aid iron absorption. *(See pages 256 and 260.)*
• Folic acid is necessary during pregnancy for the healthy development of the fetus. *(See page 255.)*
• Dietary fiber will help to prevent constipation.
• Eat plenty of foods rich in calcium to prevent cramp. *(See page 258.)*
• Supplements of vitamin B6, zinc, and magnesium may help with nausea. *(See pages 254, 265, and 262.)*
• Vitamins C and E, and bioflavonoids, zinc, and brewer's yeast will help to heal damaged blood vessels which are the cause of varicose veins. *(See pages 256, 257, 265, and 272.)*
• Take acidophilus for thrush. *(See page 271.)*
• Ensure you have plenty of vitamins E, C, zinc, silica, and pantothenic acid, which can help to prevent stretch marks. *(See pages 257, 256, 263, 264, and 254.)*
• Vitamin E oil can be applied neat to areas that are likely to become stretched, including the perineum. *(See page 257.)*

Labor Pains

Labor pains are caused by womb contractions. In the first stage of labor the contractions slowly dilate the cervix until it is wide enough to allow the baby's head to pass through. During the second stage, more powerful and more frequent contractions push the baby into the lower part of the birth canal and into the world. In the third stage, continued contractions help to expel the placenta. The pain itself varies at different stages. At first it may be no more than a dull discomfort eased by moving around. Later it may be likened to severe menstrual cramps which reach a peak then die out as the contraction ends. Pain may be felt in the lower abdomen, lower back, and the legs. The pain experienced appears to be different between women, and is related to their "pain threshold." Most women describe severe, in many cases unbearable, pain.

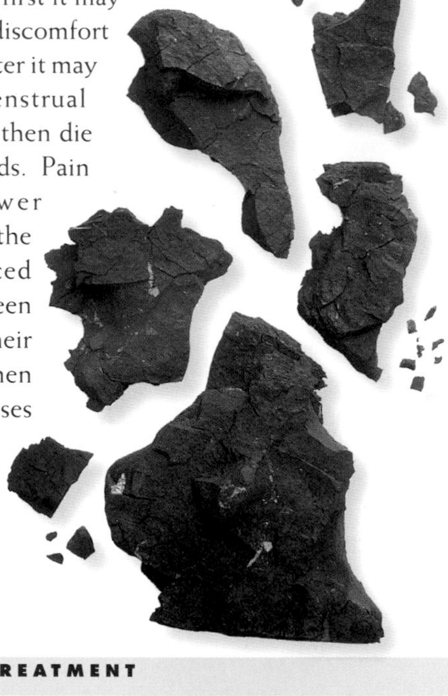

LEFT *Add a few drops of relaxing lavender essential oil to a birthing pool.*

RIGHT *Carb. veg. is the homeopathic remedy to try for exhaustion during the first stage of labor.*

TREATMENT

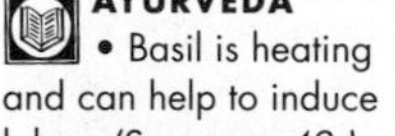

AYURVEDA

• Basil is heating and can help to induce labor. *(See page 42.)*

CHINESE HERBALISM

• Chinese angelica and peony root, for abdominal pains experienced during and after childbirth. *(See pages 56 and 67.)*

• Jing Jie may be useful as a painkiller, and will help to prevent hemorrhaging.

HERBALISM

• Blue cohosh can be taken throughout labor to tone the uterus and help keep contractions strong.

• Raspberry leaf, black cohosh, and motherwort can help during the second stage of labor. *(See page 128.)*

• Angelica root and raspberry leaf can help with the delivery of the placenta. *(See pages 115 and 128.)*

• Chamomile tea can be sipped to soothe and calm. *(See page 119.)*

• Ginger may be used to speed up a slow labor. *(See page 139.)*

AROMATHERAPY

• Clary sage, jasmine, and rose can be massaged into the lower back to relax the mother between contractions. *(See pages 146–71.)*

• Melissa oils can help to relieve the pain of childbirth, and should be used throughout the labor. *(See page 163.)*

• Rub lavender oil into the lower back, or add it to the water of a birthing pool to ease pain. *(See page 161.)*

HOMEOPATHY

• Coffea, for violent, unbearable pain when the mother cries out and is understandably nervous between contractions. *(See page 192.)*

• Belladonna, for violent contractions, with delirium and staring eyes. *(See page 183.)*

• Nux vomica., when the pains are accompanied by a need to pass water or a stool, and the mother is irritable. *(See page 214.)*

• Secale can speed a slow labor, when the uterus seems unable to contract any longer.

• Carb. veg. is useful when the mother becomes exhausted during labor. *(See page 188.)*

• Caulophyllum for weak, irregular contractions.

• Gelsemium, if the mother is anxious and trembles, and contractions are not productive. *(See page 195.)*

FLOWER ESSENCES

• Rescue Remedy can be sipped for anxiety and tension. *(See page 244.)*

• Olive, for overwhelming fatigue. *(See page 235.)*

• For overstraining, use Vervain. *(See page 241.)*

• Sweet Chestnut is good for utter despair, and for the feeling that the baby will never be born. *(See page 227.)*

• Impatiens, when things do not seem to be happening fast enough. *(See page 233.)*

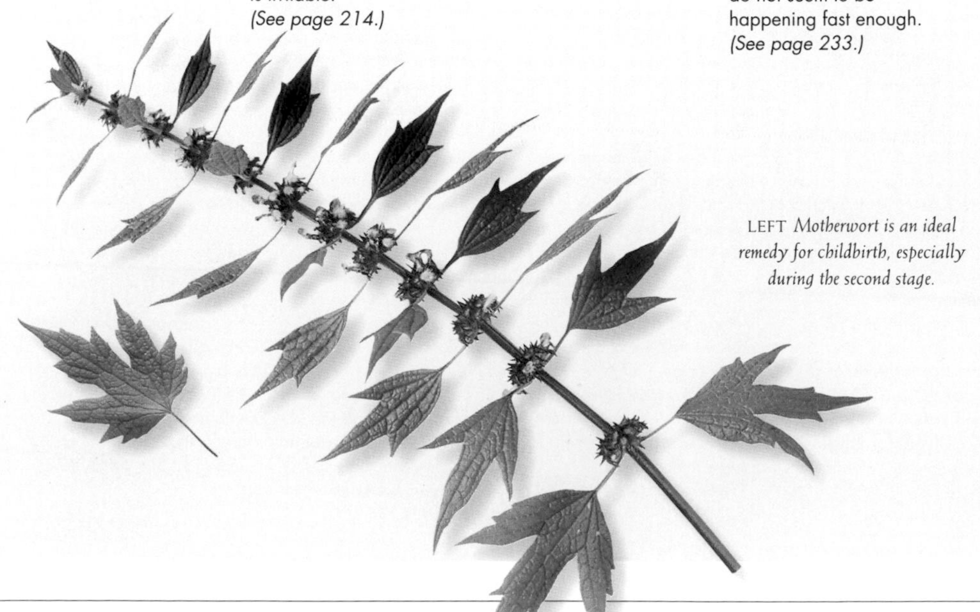

LEFT *Motherwort is an ideal remedy for childbirth, especially during the second stage.*

Post-delivery Problems

Almost all women suffer from problems of some kind following the trauma of childbirth, whether physical or emotional. These may include:

- ABDOMINAL SORENESS, usually resulting from a Cesarean section, from which it can take up to 12 weeks to recover
- ANEMIA caused by blood loss during delivery *(see page 357)*
- BACKACHE, which may very well relate to back strain during the birth process
- BREAST-FEEDING PROBLEMS *(see page 383)*
- EXHAUSTION as a result of the birth, coupled with sheer lack of sleep due to the needs of a crying baby
- HAIR LOSS caused by normal hormonal changes after the birth
- HEADACHE, which may be severe and last up to 48 hours after the delivery, for those who have an epidural injection
- PILES *(see page 377)*
- POST-NATAL DEPRESSION *(see page 392)*
- PROLAPSE *(see page 394)*
- SORENESS in the genital area, caused by stitches from a tear or episiotomy, which may last for some days

ABOVE *In Ayurveda, saffron is traditionally prescribed for post-natal problems.*

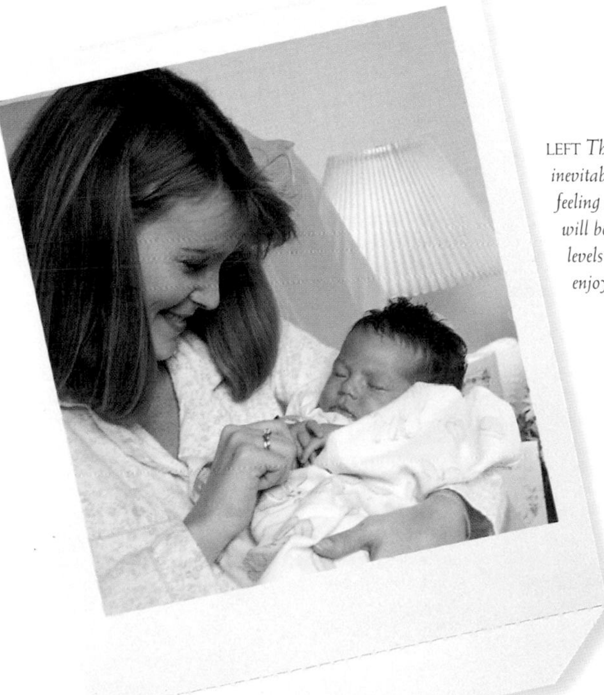

LEFT *The birth of a baby inevitably leaves you feeling exhausted. Ginseng will boost your energy levels and help you to enjoy motherhood.*

TREATMENT

AYURVEDA

- Aloe vera will encourage healing, and soothe spasm and inflammation. *(See page 27.)*
- Vetovert is excellent for exhaustion and depression. *(See page 46.)*
- Turmeric can be used for bruising. *(See page 37.)*
- Saffron is a good overall herb for post-natal problems. *(See page 36.)*

CHINESE HERBALISM

- San Qi will relive swelling, stop hemorrhaging, and disperse bruising. *(See page 68.)*
- Tian Ma (castrodia rhizome) will help relieve headaches which come on after childbirth. *(See page 62.)*
- Ginseng will help to restore, boost energy levels, prevent infection, and encourage healing. *(See page 67.)*

HERBALISM

- Good pain-relieving herbs include pulsatilla, black cohosh, lavender, and wild yam. *(See page 120.)*
- St. John's wort and calendula will help healing. *(See page 124.)*
- An infusion of calendula can be used to assist in healing the perineum. *(See page 117.)*
- Witch hazel can be applied to the perineum to encourage healing and soothe pain. *(See page 123.)*
- A comfrey compress can be applied to the perineum to speed healing. *(See page 132.)*
- Golden seal will help with bleeding, as will beth root and false unicorn root.
- Golden seal and myrrh are excellent for dispelling uterine infections.
- Cramp bark will help with uterine infections, pain, and cramping. *(See page 138.)*
- Black haw is useful for any afterpains suffered.
- Beth root and horsetail can be added to the bath for incontinence and weak pelvic floor muscles. *(See page 120.)*
- Nettles, chickweed, and coriander will act as tonics for fatigue. *(See page 137.)*

AROMATHERAPY

- Geranium, rose, and clary sage act as uterine tonics and help the pelvic tissues to regain their elasticity after the birth. *(See pages 146–71.)*
- Lavender is useful for relief of afterpains. *(See page 161.)*
- Chamomile, massaged into the abdomen, helps relieve pain and cramps. *(See page 150.)*
- Jasmine has a tonic action on the womb. *(See page 161.)*
- Apply lavender and chamomile, diluted in a little apricot kernel oil, to the affected area for sore stitches. *(See pages 161 and 150.)*

HOMEOPATHY

- Coffea, for sharp afterpains and exhaustion. *(See page 192.)*
- Nux vomica., for afterpains associated with an urgent need to pass water. *(See page 214.)*
- Pulsatilla, for pains if part of the placenta is retained. *(See page 209.)*
- China, for exhaustion following loss of blood. *(See page 190.)*
- Carb. veg., for exhaustion with sweating. *(See page 188.)*
- Sepia, for exhaustion with bearing-down pains. *(See page 212.)*
- Belladonna, for troublesome incontinence. *(See page 183.)*
- Pulsatilla, for piles. *(See page 209.)*
- Ferr. phos., for bleeding (the blood is bright red, clots easily), accompanied by a burning face. *(See page 194.)*
- Secale, for a post-partum hemorrhage.
- Pulsatilla, for continuing labor pains and dark red blood. *(See page 209.)*
- Arnica, to encourage healing and prevent bruising. *(See page 182.)*
- Hypericum or Arnica tincture, diluted in water, to cleanse the perineum and any stitches. *(See pages 199 and 182.)*
- Ledum, where stitching has been necessary. *(See page 202.)*

VITAMINS AND MINERALS

- Ensure that you are getting plenty of iron, which can help with fatigue. *(See page 260.)*
- Vitamin B and chromium stabilize energy levels. *(See pages 252–5 and 259.)*
- Vitamin E will encourage healing, and can be applied to stitches. *(See page 257.)*

RIGHT *Dab witch hazel on the perineum to encourage healing and relieve pain.*

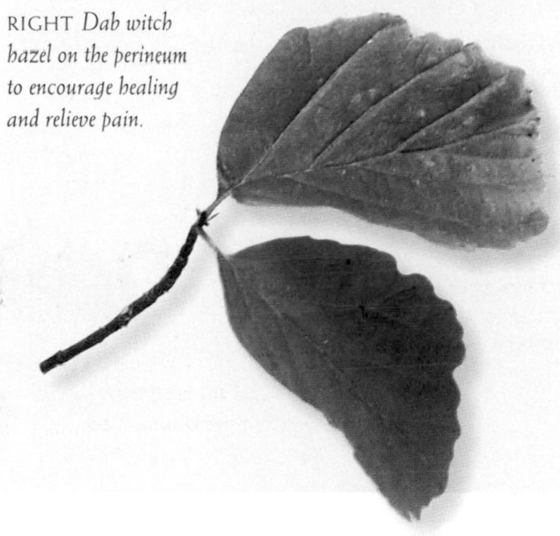

Post-natal Illness (PNI)

The term post-natal illness covers the varying degrees of anxiety, fearfulness, and depression experienced by women after the birth of a baby. Its cause is thought to be the massive drop in pregnancy hormones, aggravated by general exhaustion and discomfort in the days following delivery. Mild "baby blues" usually begin three to four days after delivery, and last only a few days. Some women experience symptoms for several weeks. Many women suffer from baby blues, but in a few women the symptoms, initially a natural response to a new situation, last for much longer than a few weeks and seriously undermine their ability to cope. Post-natal depression (PND) generally starts within weeks of the birth and may last for a year or more. In extreme cases there may be post-partum psychosis, characterized by virtual breakdown. Post-natal depression is most common in women with other stresses – marriage or relationship problems, anxiety about coping with a new baby, financial problems – as well as hormonal imbalances, blood sugar problems, and previous episodes of post-natal depression.

ABOVE *Known as the women's ginseng in China, angelica is a good tonic for PNI.*

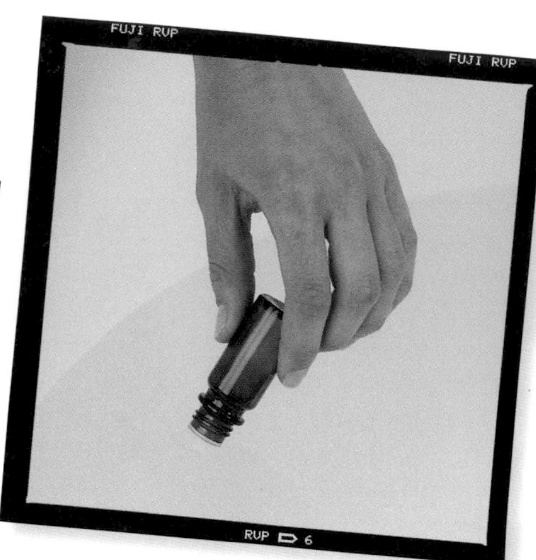

RIGHT *If you are suffering from PND relax in a warm bath with a few drops of ylang ylang or neroli oils.*

Symptoms

• *baby blues: – irritability – tearfulness and vulnerability – mild depression and anxiety – fears about responsibility* • *post-natal depression: – constant feeling of sadness – feeling unable to cope – feelings of guilt and inadequacy – loss of sex drive – excessive worrying* • *post-partum psychosis: – hyperactive, manic and euphoric – depressive, with panic attacks and insomnia – almost schizophrenic behavior – hallucinations*

RIGHT *Flower essence therapists recommend Olive for the sheer exhaustion that follows the birth of a baby.*

TREATMENT

AYURVEDA
• Camphor clears the mind and helps the nervous system. *(See page 33.)*
• Cumin may be useful. *(See page 36.)*
• Licorice strengthens the nerves. *(See page 39.)*
• Individual treatment will be necessary to lift the spirits and to address any hormonal problems. *(See page 22.)*

CHINESE HERBALISM
• Angelica, peony root, licorice, and thorowax root may be useful. *(See pages 56, 64, and 67.)*
• Ginseng will help to restore and to strengthen the whole person. *(See page 67.)*
• Chinese senega can reduce insomnia and bouts of depression. *(See page 70.)*
• Dodder seed may help to restore hormone imbalances to normal. *(See page 62.)*

HERBALISM
• Agnus castus can help to restore the hormone balance in the body. *(See page 139.)*
• St. John's wort and oats are nervine, and will help to reduce stress symptoms and anxiety. *(See page 124.)*
• Rosemary or lemon balm teas or tinctures will help the nervous system and lift depression. *(See page 127.)*
• False unicorn root balances the hormones and can be added to any herbal preparation.

AROMATHERAPY
• Clary sage has a balancing effect on hormones, and so can help to treat and prevent post-natal illness. *(See page 169.)*
• Jasmine and bergamot are overall tonics and relaxants, and can be used daily, either in the bath or in massage, to ease symptoms. *(See pages 161 and 153.)*
• Ylang ylang and neroli are specific to PND, and can be used in a long, enjoyable, warm bath in order to ease symptoms. *(See pages 148 and 152.)*

HOMEOPATHY
Treatment would be constitutional, but the following remedies may help:
• Pulsatilla, for curtailing episodes of weepiness. *(See page 209.)*
• Nat. mur., for coping with feelings of irritation, guilt, and withdrawal. *(See page 206.)*
• Sepia, for allaying exhaustion, lack of interest, and irritability. *(See page 212.)*

FLOWER ESSENCES
• Rescue remedy or Emergency Essence will help after the trauma of the birth. *(See page 244.)*
• Gorse is good for feelings of hopelessness. *(See page 240.)*
• Mustard, when you feel as if you are under a dark cloud for no apparent reason. *(See page 239.)*
• Olive will help to address exhaustion. *(See page 235)*
• Walnut will help you to deal with change. *(See page 232.)*
• Sweet Chestnut is for fits of utter despair. *(See page 227.)*

VITAMINS AND MINERALS
• Some experts believe that nutritional deficiencies are at the root of the problem; ensure you eat plenty of foods rich in vitamins C and B, calcium, iron, magnesium, and also potassium. *(See pages 256, 252–5, 258, 260, and 262.)*
• Tyrosine and tryptophan, amino acids, can help to ease post-natal depression. *(See page 269.)*

Menopause Symptoms

Menopause is the cessation of menstruation and a woman's reproductive capacity. It usually occurs around the age of 50, but may happen prematurely, or artificially after removal of the ovaries. Most symptoms that occur during menopause result directly from the estrogen deficiency produced by the failing ovaries. Interestingly, Japanese women suffer far fewer symptoms of the menopause because they eat more plant estrogens like tofu, soya, and miso.

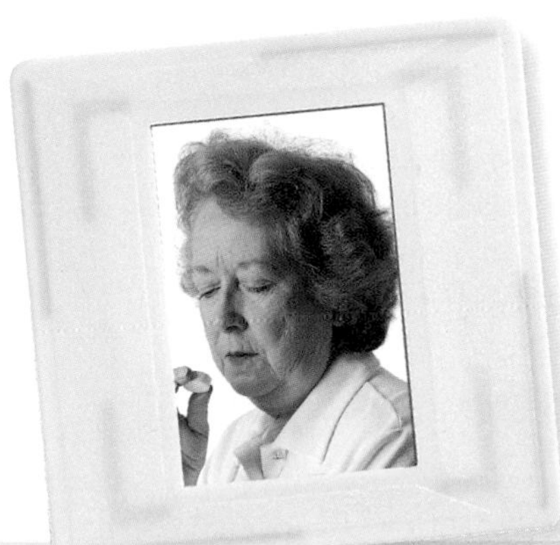

LEFT *Menopausal symptoms, including hot flushes, and depression, may be relieved with homeopathic remedies.*

Symptoms

• back pain • dry, thinning hair and dry skin • flooding (very heavy periods) • very light periods • hot flushes, mostly affecting the face and neck, and varying in frequency and duration • incontinence, one of the most common menopausal symptoms; through wear and tear, childbearing, and lack of estrogen • osteoporosis • psychological problems such as irritability, anxiety, insomnia, and poor memory • increased hair growth on the face, stomach, or chest, due either to an increase in the male hormone, androgen, or the drop in estrogen production • vaginal looseness, a feeling of slackness, or of something protruding into the vaginal passage – possibly a prolapsed uterus, or a section of the urethra, bladder or rectum dropping downward as a result of lost muscle tone • about 20–25 percent of menopausal women experience pain during intercourse, called dyspareunia. Mostly, this is due to thinning of the vaginal wall and a lack of lubrication, both caused by estrogen deficiency

TREATMENT

AYURVEDA

• Calamus root can be good for memory problems and mental stress. *(See page 24.)*
• Celery seeds and cedar are balancing, and may help with menstrual problems. *(See page 29.)*
• Cinnamon is especially powerful during menopause, and is particularly useful for low libido and edema. *(See page 34.)*
• Coriander is cooling, and acts as a diuretic and diaphoretic. It is also thought to be aphrodisiac. *(See page 35.)*
• Aloe vera cools and cleanses the liver when taken internally, helping with any "hot" symptoms of menopause, including flushes, sweats, and swelling. *(See page 27.)*

CHINESE HERBALISM

• Shan Zhu Yu can be used for flooding, with ginseng for heavy sweating and hot flushes. *(See pages 60 and 67.)*
• Chinese senega may be useful for irritability, insomnia, and depression. *(See page 70.)*
• Angelica, peony root, and thorowax root are the ideal herbs to treat the symptoms of menopause, which is believed to be a weakness of the Kidneys, deficient Blood, and an imbalance between Kidney and Liver. *(See pages 56 and 67.)*

HERBALISM

• Valerian will help with anxiety and tension, and combined with skullcap relaxes the nervous system. *(See pages 131 and 136.)*
• Ginseng will help with anxiety and irritability, and increases mental alertness. It will also boost vitality and prevent feelings of fatigue. *(See page 126.)*
• Herbal laxatives include butternut, blue flag, and senna.
• Shepherd's purse, lady's mantle, yarrow, golden seal, beth root, and periwinkle help with heavy bleeding. *(See pages 112 and 113.)*
• Dandelion cleanses the liver and helps the body to detoxify, which can reduce the risk of breast growths and other cell changes. *(See page 133.)*
• Milk thistle can be used to treat lumpy and painful breasts. *(See page 131.)*
• Agnus castus can be used for breast tenderness and any problems of the menopause, as it works to normalize the levels of female hormones. *(See page 139.)*
• Black cohosh can restore female hormonal balance and help to prevent night sweats and hot flushes. Other herbs to consider are licorice, alfalfa, and Dong Quai. *(See page 122.)*
• American ginseng can increase libido, as can agnus castus and black cohosh. *(See pages 126 and 139.)*
• Ginkgo biloba can help with memory and concentration problems. *(See page 122.)*
• Cramp bark is antispasmodic and will help with painful menstruation. *(See page 138.)*
• Burdock root helps with dry and scaly skin, and licorice or chamomile, applied directly to the skin, will soothe and soften. *(See pages 115, 119, and 122.)*
• Valerian can help improve the quality of sleep and treat insomnia. *(See page 136.)*
• Passiflora will help you to sleep.
• Motherwort can restore thickness and elasticity to the walls of the vagina, and dong quai can help with dryness. *(See page 124.)*
• Dandelion is a natural diuretic and will help with any swelling associated with water retention. *(See page 133.)*

AROMATHERAPY

• Clary sage will lift your mood and help to deal with fluctuating hormones. *(See page 169.)*
• Chamomile, diluted in a little carrier oil, is adaptogenic, and will balance hormone levels causing night sweats, hot flushes, and other symptoms. *(See page 150.)*
• Essential oils of damian, and geranium or ylang ylang are aphrodisiacs for low libido. *(See pages 146–71.)*
• Fennel can be massaged into the abdomen for water retention and symptoms of hormonal imbalance. *(See page 159.)*

HOMEOPATHY

• Sepia is enormously useful, and can treat hot flushes, headaches, irritability, and heavy menstrual bleeding. *(See page 212.)*
• Conium, for loss of libido.
• Graphites, for weight gain, hot flushes, and scanty menstrual bleeding. *(See page 196.)*
• Lachesis, for flooding, irritability, memory loss and concentration problems, hot flushes, and headaches. *(See page 216.)*
• Pulsatilla, for depression, weepiness and changeable moods. *(See page 209.)*
• Sanguinara, for tender breasts and flooding.

FLOWER ESSENCES

• Mustard, for depression with no identifiable cause. *(See page 239.)*
• Olive, for fatigue. *(See page 235.)*
• Mimulus, for fear of aging and death. *(See page 235.)*
• Walnut, for life changes. *(See page 232.)*

VITAMINS AND MINERALS

• Take magnesium and vitamin B-complex for anxiety and irritability. *(See pages 262 and 252–5.)*
• Vitamin E, linseed oil, acidophilus, and vitamin B-complex will help with tender and lumpy breasts. *(See pages 257, 271, 252–5.)*
• For constipation, try extra vitamin C. *(See page 256.)*
• Co-enzyme Q10 will help lack of energy and fatigue; check that you are not anemic.
• Quercetin can help with migraine and headaches associated with menopause, as can vitamin C and E. *(See pages 256 and 257.)*
• Vitamin C can help regulate heavy bleeding (flooding) when combined with bioflavonoids. *(See page 256.)*
• Vitamin A, zinc, iron, and vitamin B-complex can also help with heavy menstrual bleeding. *(See pages 252, 265, 260, and 252–5.)*
• Selenium may help to reduce hot flushes and night sweats, as will vitamin C, which is a more effective preventive than HRT. *(See pages 264 and 256.)*
• Zinc, vitamin C, vitamin E, and magnesium will help with painful menstruation. *(See pages 256, 265, 257, and 262.)*
• Linseed oil, evening primrose, vitamin B-complex and zinc can be taken for skin problems. *(See pages 270, 252–5, and 265.)*
• Magnesium is helpful for insomnia and sleep problems. *(See page 262.)*
• A vitamin E capsule can be placed inside the vagina for vaginal dryness. *(See page 257.)*

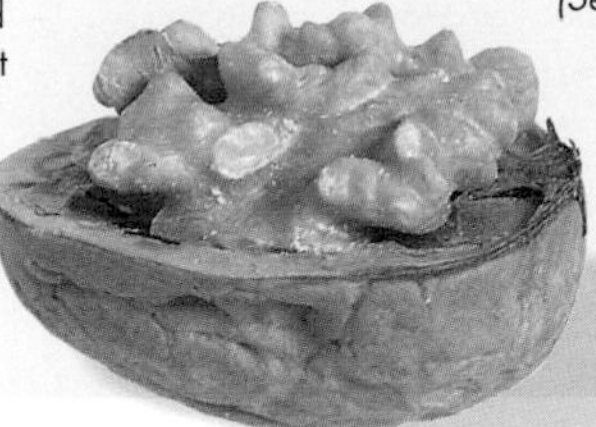

LEFT *Walnut is an excellent flower essence to take during the important life transitions.*

Prolapse

Prolapse occurs when the uterus and/or vagina slip downward due to a weakening or stretching of the structures that would normally keep them in place. It occurs when ligaments and muscles which hold the uterus and vagina in place become weak or slack with age, or as a result of childbirth, allowing the uterus to bulge into the vagina and press on the bladder or rectum. If prolapse is complete a large part of the vagina or uterus may actually protrude through the vaginal opening, causing soreness or ulceration, and encouraging infection. The risk of a prolapse may be heightened by a chronic cough, chronic constipation, or obesity. Neither prolapse is serious at first, but may become so if neglected. Surgery to tighten pelvic floor muscles may be necessary if exercises do not improve the muscle tone. A ring pessary, fitted behind the pubic bone, may be necessary in an elderly woman. Sixty-five percent of all women who prolapse do so before the age of 55. Women who have had several children, or a difficult labor, seem to be more prone to prolapse.

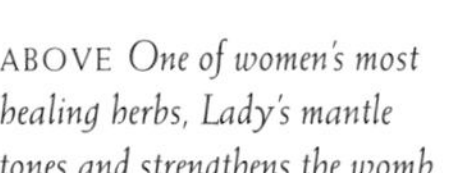

ABOVE *One of women's most healing herbs, Lady's mantle tones and strengthens the womb.*

Symptoms

• *a sensation of something dropping down* • *dragging feeling in lower abdomen* • *backache* • *fatigue* • *in addition to the above, prolapse of the vagina may involve: – frequent urge to pass water – stress incontinence – possibly urine infections*

TREATMENT

CHINESE HERBALISM
• Treatment would be aimed at Deficient qi, and Central qi pills would be useful. *(See page 49.)*

HERBALISM
• Motherwort, lady's mantle, and life root can help to restore the tone of the uterus and vagina. *(See pages 113 and 124.)*
• Use astringent herbs such as horsetail, shepherd's purse, false unicorn, and bayberry. These can be taken as teas, tisanes, decoctions, pills, etc. They can also be used as a poultice and applied to the abdomen. Barberry stimulates the uterus to contract: do not use in pregnancy. *(See page 119.)*
• For a prolapse after the menopause, try sage, calendula, ginseng, and wild yam: all estrogenic. *(See pages 117, 120, 126, and 129.)*
• Chickweed ointment or douche can soothe and heal soreness of the vagina or cervix.
• Pessaries with glycerin and golden seal can be helpful.

AROMATHERAPY
• Massage the lower abdomen and back with diluted oils of rosemary and lemon to improve the circulation and tighten tissues. *(See pages 168 and 154.)*

HOMEOPATHY
• Sepia, for a pressing feeling that something is coming out. *(See page 212.)*
• Aloe, for long-standing prolapse with a feeling of fullness and sometimes morning diarrhea.

VITAMINS AND MINERALS
• Uterus glandular tissues give support to your uterus.
• Vitamin E increases the elasticity of the tissues, and helps them respond to stress more effectively. *(See page 257.)*

Ovarian Cysts

A cyst is an abnormal sac or cavity that contains liquid or semi-solid material enclosed by a membrane. Ovarian cysts most commonly occur in women between the ages of 35 and 55. Usually they are benign, but they can sometimes cause problems because of their size. Ovarian cysts may be caused by slight ovulation disorders, or by swelling of the lining of the ovary through fluid collection. The most common ovarian cyst is a follicular cyst that contains watery fluid. Pseudomucinous cysts contain a thick mucous fluid and can lead to complications if they rupture or become infected.

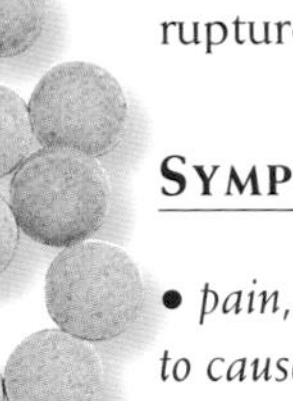

ABOVE *If you suffer from ovarian cysts, try taking vitamin E supplements.*

Symptoms

• *pain, once the cyst has grown large enough to cause problems* • *abdominal discomfort* • *possibly an increase in the size of the abdomen* • *breathlessness* • *may lead to varicose veins (see page 361) or piles (see page 377)* • *repeated or multiple cysts may affect fertility (see page 398)*

TREATMENT

CHINESE HERBALISM
• Dodder seeds can balance the reproductive system. *(See page 62.)*
• San qi, for general relief of pain. *(See page 68.)*
• Tree peony may be useful. *(See page 67.)*

HERBALISM
• False unicorn root or blue cohosh can help to restore the function of the reproductive system.
• Kelp can be added to ensure normal thyroid function. *(See page 122.)*
• Take dandelion root to help the liver metabolize estrogen. *(See page 134.)*
• Agnus castus acts to restore estrogen levels. *(See page 139.)*

AROMATHERAPY
• Basil, marjoram, and lavender can be massaged into the abdomen to ease pain and restore balance. *(See pages 146–71.)*
• Clary sage will help to balance hormones. *(See page 169.)*

HOMEOPATHY
Treatment should be constitutional, but the following remedies may be useful.
• Colocynthis, is for small round cysts which cause boring pain which is improved by pressure. *(See page 191.)*
• Apis, for stinging pains, particularly in the right ovary. *(See page 180.)*
• Lachesis, for local pain which is worse in the morning, and occurs mainly in the left ovary. *(See page 216.)*
• Ledum, for driving pain through the ovary and womb. *(See page 202.)*

FLOWER ESSENCES
• Take Rescue Remedy or Emergency Essence to restore a sense of calm during pain and discomfort. *(See page 244.)*

VITAMINS AND MINERALS
• Increase your intake of iodine, since thyroid problems may be at the root of the cysts. *(See page 261.)*
• Vitamin E is helpful for preventing and treating cysts. *(See page 257.)*
• The B-complex vitamins will help to re-establish hormone balance and the metabolism of estrogen by the liver. *(See pages 252–5.)*

BELOW *Kelp stimulates the thyroid gland and may be taken to ensure normal function.*

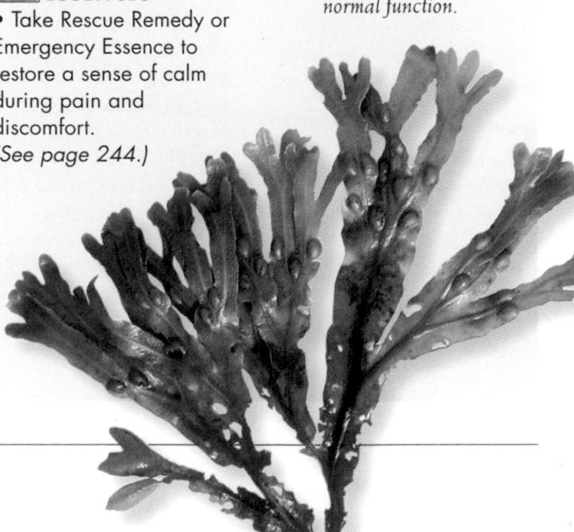

Pelvic Inflammatory Disease (PID)

ABOVE *Use myrrh in conjunction with unicorn root. Its anti-inflammatory properties will relieve PID.*

Pelvic inflammatory disease (PID) is an umbrella term for infections and inflammations that have penetrated the reproductive system, i.e. the ovaries (ovaritis), Fallopian tubes (salpingitis), and the uterus (endometritis). Left untreated, these infections can develop and recur for years. Possible causes of PID are gonorrhoea and chlamydia cystitis (*see page 379*), various viruses, or the natural flora of the vagina. Triggers include anything that allows a lurking infection to travel, such as childbirth, abortion, surgery on the reproductive system or in the pelvic area, or an IUD (intrauterine device, which prevents pregnancy).

Symptoms

- *acute: – fever with shaking – painful intercourse – unusual vaginal discharge – vaginal bleeding after sex or in mid-menstrual cycle – severe lower abdominal pain – back pain*
- *chronic: – weight loss – backache and lower abdominal pain – nausea – diarrhea – tiredness – pain on urination – reduced fertility (caused by scarring which blocks the Fallopian tubes)*

TREATMENT

AYURVEDA

- Aloe vera relieves inflammation, soothes muscle spasms, and purifies the blood. *(See page 27)*
- Angelica has antibacterial properties and can help with pain. *(See page 28.)*
- Gotu kola may be useful if the infection is linked to STDs. *(See page 33.)*

CHINESE HERBALISM

- Peony root can be used for abdominal pain. *(See page 67.)*
- Cinnamon treats pain and other symptoms. *(See page 59.)*
- Pseudoginseng root (San Qi) may be useful. *(See page 68.)*

TRADITIONAL HOME AND FOLK REMEDIES

- Peel a clove of garlic, wrap it in gauze, and tie a piece of string to one end. Place in the vagina and change daily. *(See page 82.)*

HERBALISM

- Fresh garlic, taken as often as possible throughout the day, can act to fight infection and boost the immune system. *(See page 113.)*
- Echinacea will help to boost immunity as well as addressing the infection. *(See page 120.)*
- Thyme and parsley will help to fight infection. *(See page 135.)*
- Blue cohosh has an affinity with the reproductive system. Take daily.
- False unicorn root and myrrh combine well.

AROMATHERAPY

- Add lavender, rosemary, or geranium oils to the bath water to relax and help to fight infection. *(See pages 146–71.)*

HOMEOPATHY

Treatment should be constitutional, but the following may help:

- Mercurius, for chills and sweat that is unpleasant, and where the condition is improved by rest. *(See page 205.)*
- Apis, for stinging, burning pains, mainly on the right side. *(See page 180.)*
- Aconite, for sudden onset, with mild fever and anxiety. *(See page 178.)*
- Belladonna, for sudden onset, with red face and burning. *(See page 183.)*
- Colocynthis, is for cramping pains relieved by pressure. *(See page 191.)*

VITAMINS AND MINERALS

- Include vitamin C, E, and zinc in your diet to boost the immune system. *(See pages 256, 257 and 265.)*
- Acidophilus encourages the growth of healthy bacteria, and is especially useful if you have taken a course of antibiotics. *(See page 271.)*

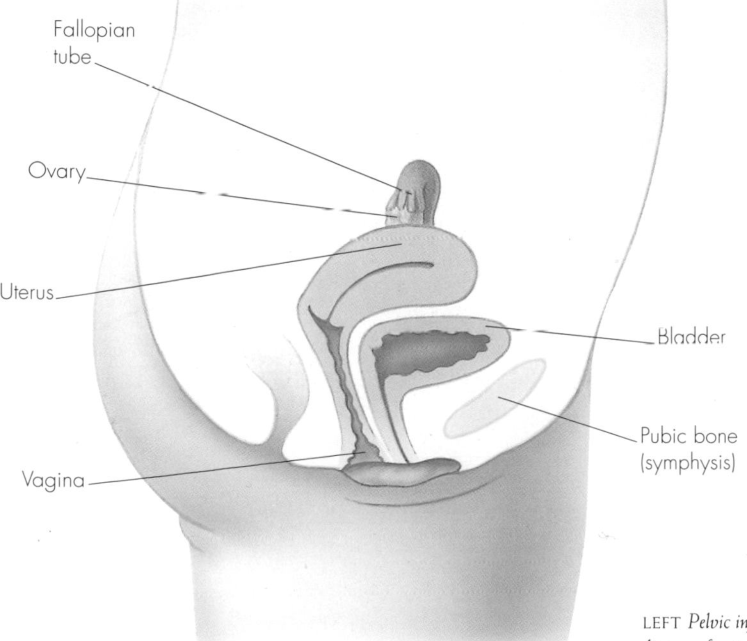

LEFT *Pelvic inflammatory disease refers to any infections of the reproductive system.*

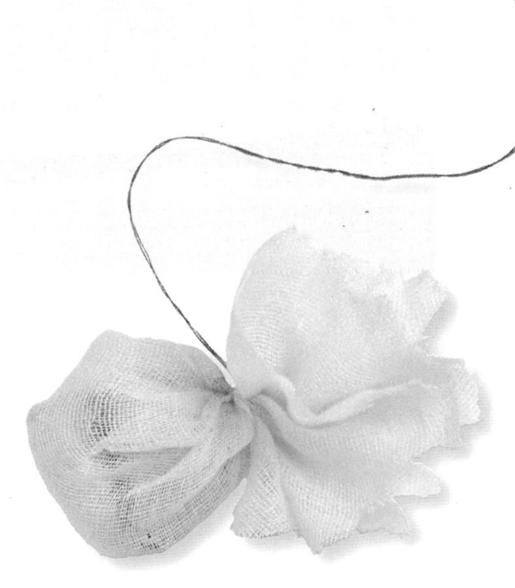

ABOVE *Place a piece of garlic wrapped in gauze inside the vagina. Its antibiotic and antiseptic actions may help to fight PID.*

Thrush

Thrush is caused by the yeast organism *Candida albicans*, which lives naturally in the vagina and also the mouth, bowel, and, to some extent, the skin. It only begins to cause problems when there is an overgrowth of it. Antibiotics, immuno-suppressive drugs, a compromised immune system, periods of hormonal change and stress can all encourage Candida growth, and thrush as a result. Other aggravating factors include a high sugar intake, tight clothing, poor personal hygiene, and scented bath oils. Women seem to suffer more frequently from thrush, or candidiasis, than men.

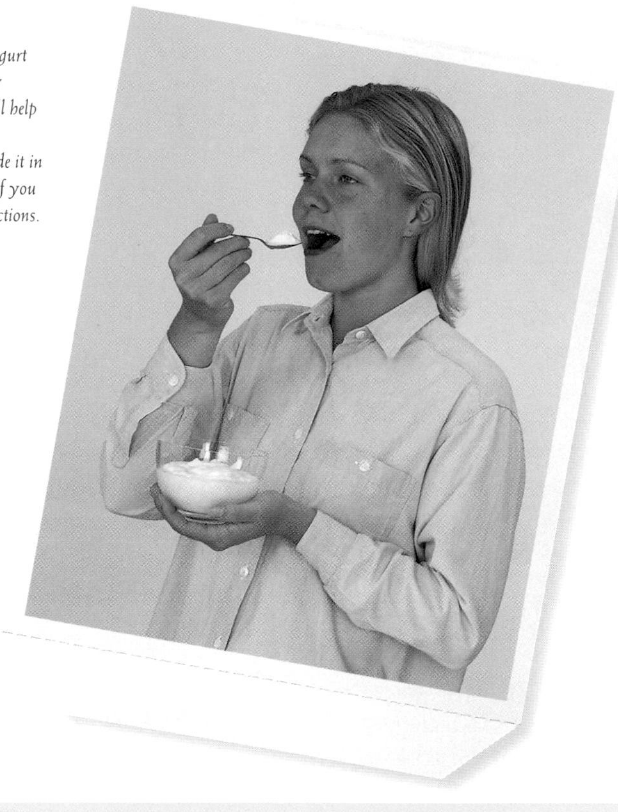

RIGHT *Live yogurt contains healthy bacteria that will help prevent fungal infections. Include it in your diet daily if you are prone to infections.*

Symptoms

- *an itchy, white vaginal discharge*
- *sore, red, dry, itchy vulva*
- *stinging pain on urination*
- *soreness and discomfort during intercourse* • *possibly a red rash extending down the thighs, or around to the anus*

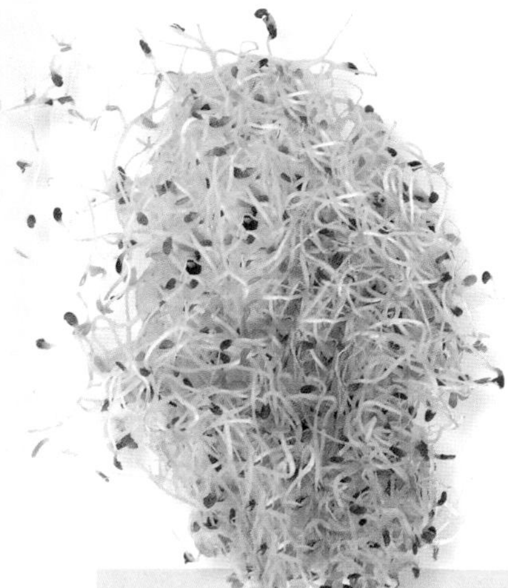

LEFT *Alfalfa has antifungal properties and is used in Ayurveda to treat thrush.*

TREATMENT

AYURVEDA

• Garlic is a useful anti-infective agent, and works against fungi. *(See page 26.)*

• The following herbs may be used in internal and external preparations, for their antifungal properties: barberry, alfalfa, basil, cinnamon, coriander, myrrh, and elecampane. *(See pages 29, 34, 35, 40, 41, and 42.)*

• Treatment would be individual, to balance the system.

CHINESE HERBALISM

• Treatment would address excess Damp and Damp Heat. Suitable herbs might include gentian and oriental wormwood.

• Dang Gui or ginger will be used when you feel generally depleted. *(See page 56.)*

TRADITIONAL HOME AND FOLK REMEDIES

• A live yogurt douche will encourage the growth of healthy bacteria (flora) which will prevent fungal infection. Use regularly if you are prone to thrush. Apply to patches of oral thrush, and include live yogurt in your daily diet. *(See page 93.)*

• Apple cider vinegar, added to a pint of warm water, can be used as a douche. *(See page 102.)*

• Sit in a bowl of water to which a little vinegar or lemon juice has been added, to correct pH imbalance and maintain an acid environment. *(See page 102.)*

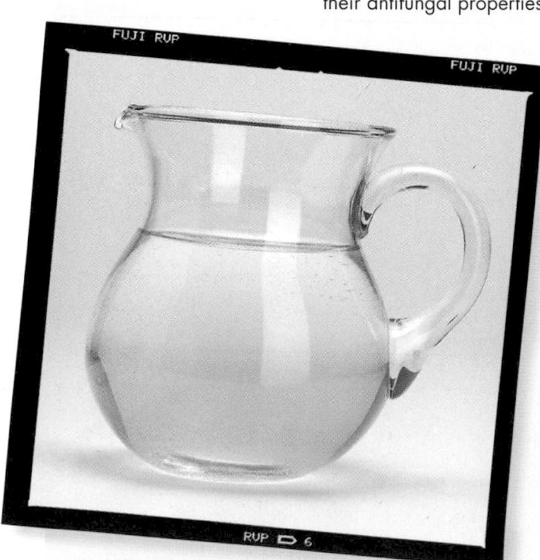

ABOVE *Use a douche of cider vinegar and warm water to treat vaginal thrush.*

HERBALISM

• Drink an infusion of echinacea or marigold to encourage healing, boost the immune system, and clear infection. *(See pages 117 and 120.)*

• A douche of marigold or lavender flowers will ease symptoms. *(See page 117.)*

• Take echinacea 3 times daily for chronic cases of thrush, and every 2 hours in acute attacks, to boost the immune system. *(See page 120.)*

• Useful antifungal herbs include calendula, cinnamon, and rosemary. *(See pages 117 and 127.)*

• Chamomile cream and chickweed ointment can be applied externally to soothe itching and irritation. *(See page 117.)*

• Soak a tampon in water with a few drops of golden seal tincture and insert; remove after one hour.

AROMATHERAPY

• A tiny drop of tea tree oil, added to 2pt. (1.2l) of warm, already boiled water, can be used as a douche. *(See page 162.)*

• Massage with lavender or tea tree oil can boost the immune system and prevent further infections. *(See pages 162 and 161.)*

HOMEOPATHY

• Pulsatilla, for cloudy or watery discharge which causes smarting and soreness. *(See page 209.)*

• Lachesis, for burning discharge, with weariness, bloating, and symptoms that are worse around menstruation. *(See page 216.)*

• Graphites, for a sore vagina with small ulcers appearing on the labia. *(See page 196.)*

• Calcarea, if there is vaginal itching, a yellow or milky discharge, and increased itchiness around the time of menstruation. *(See page 186.)*

• Aluminia, for frequent, straw-colored discharge which causes itching and stiffens underwear.

VITAMINS AND MINERALS

• Take acidophilus tablets to restore the healthy bacteria in the body, which will fight the infection. *(See page 271.)*

Painful Intercourse

Many women experience pain or discomfort during sexual intercourse (called dyspareunia) at different points in their lives, and it may be attributed to a number of causes:

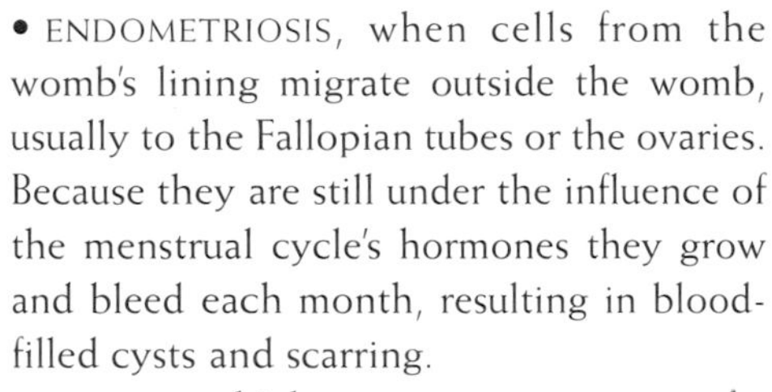

- ENDOMETRIOSIS, when cells from the womb's lining migrate outside the womb, usually to the Fallopian tubes or the ovaries. Because they are still under the influence of the menstrual cycle's hormones they grow and bleed each month, resulting in blood-filled cysts and scarring.

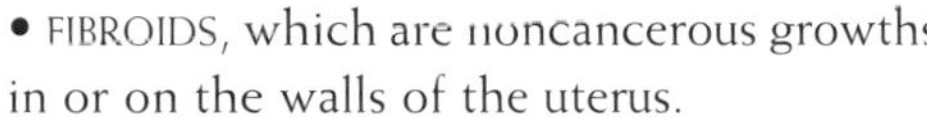

- FIBROIDS, which are noncancerous growths in or on the walls of the uterus.

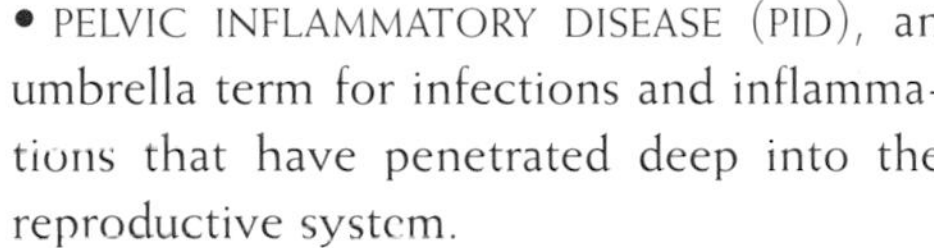

- PELVIC INFLAMMATORY DISEASE (PID), an umbrella term for infections and inflammations that have penetrated deep into the reproductive system.
- SEXUALLY TRANSMITTED DISEASES (STDs).
- THRUSH (*see page 439*).
- CHILDBIRTH. The labor and delivery process can cause soreness and discomfort for some weeks, particularly if the woman has had an episiotomy.
- Menopause (*see page 393*).

ABOVE *Marjoram is a warm, relaxing, and sedative herb. Use the essential oil in a massage or burn in a vaporizer.*

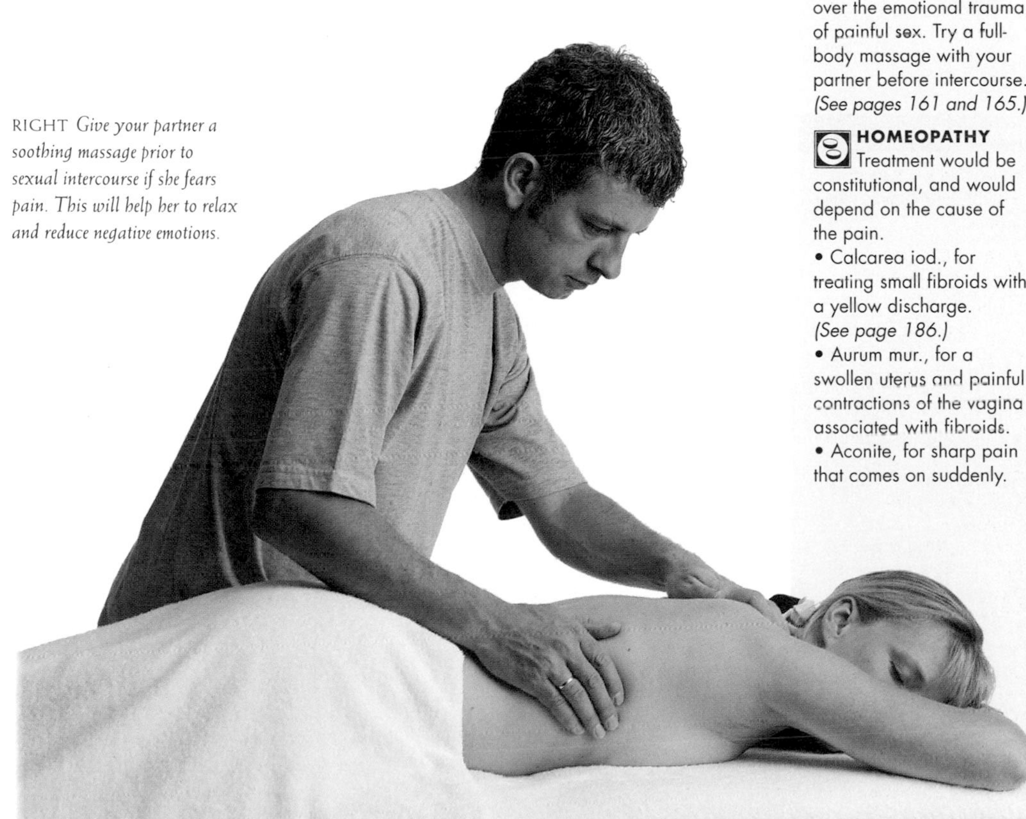

RIGHT *Give your partner a soothing massage prior to sexual intercourse if she fears pain. This will help her to relax and reduce negative emotions.*

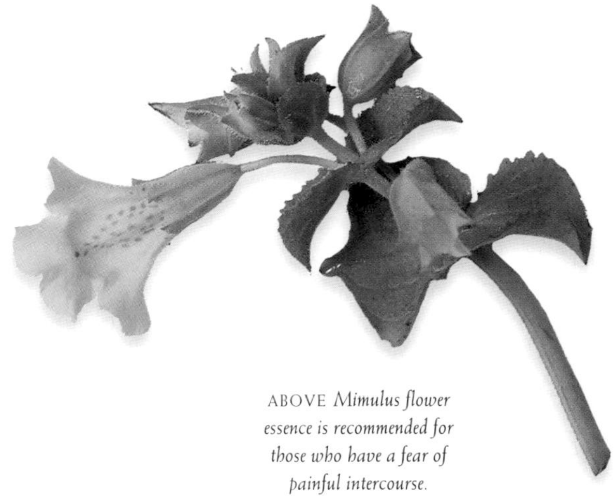

ABOVE *Mimulus flower essence is recommended for those who have a fear of painful intercourse.*

TREATMENT

(See treatment for Thrush on page 396, Menopause on page 393, Pregnancy Problems on page 388, and PID on page 395.)

AROMATHERAPY

- Lavender and marjoram are relaxing, and can help you to get over the emotional trauma of painful sex. Try a full-body massage with your partner before intercourse. *(See pages 161 and 165.)*

HOMEOPATHY

Treatment would be constitutional, and would depend on the cause of the pain.

- Calcarea iod., for treating small fibroids with a yellow discharge. *(See page 186.)*
- Aurum mur., for a swollen uterus and painful contractions of the vagina associated with fibroids.
- Aconite, for sharp pain that comes on suddenly.
- Sepia or Belladonna, when the problem is associated with prolapse. *(See pages 212 and 183.)*

FLOWER ESSENCES

- Mimulus, for fear of pain during sex. *(See page 235.)*
- Rescue Remedy or Emergency Essence, taken before making love, to calm and reduce feelings of panic and anxiety. *(See page 244.)*

VITAMINS AND MINERALS

- Take plenty of vitamin A and E, which will help restore the health of the reproductive system. *(See pages 252 and 257.)*
- Acidophilus will help to maintain the balance of healthy flora in the body. *(See page 271.)*
- Vitamin E capsules can be placed in the vagina to ease pain and dryness. *(See page 257.)*

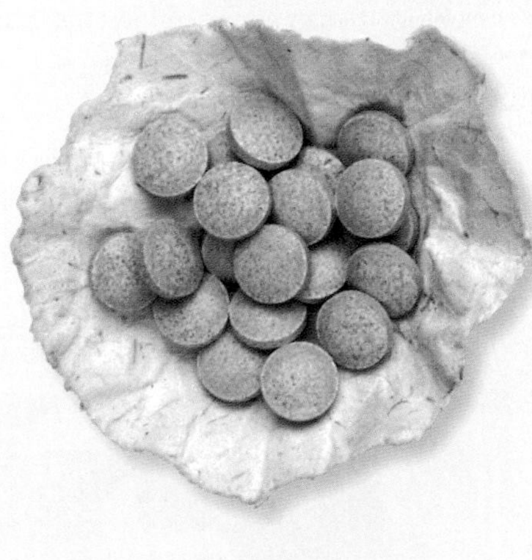

ABOVE *Supplement your diet with vitamins A and E to promote a healthy reproductive system.*

DISORDERS OF THE REPRODUCTIVE SYSTEM: MALE

Infertility

The term infertility is generally applied when failure to conceive follows an 18-month period of regular, unprotected sexual intercourse. It is usually a sign that something in the body is not working properly. The most common cause of infertility in men is a low sperm count (possibly due to environmental pollution). Poor sperm quality, inadequate mobility of sperm, no sperm at all, or an abnormality in the penis may also be responsible. In some cases the problem may be hormonal. Risk factors include smoking, excessive alcohol consumption, raised temperature around the testes (caused by tight trousers, or by varicose veins on the scrotum), certain prescription drugs, stress, or infection with mumps. A diet lacking in vitamins and minerals can also cause a man to be less fertile. One research study discovered that organic farmers had twice the sperm count of other men!

ABOVE *Low sperm counts, abnormal, or immobile sperm all contribute to male infertility.*

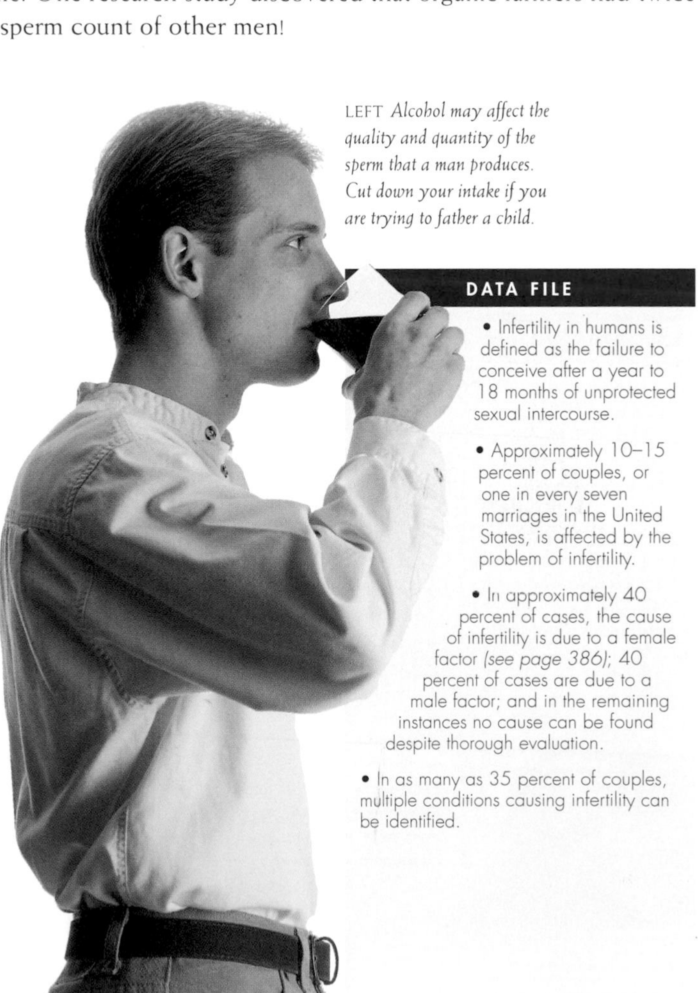

LEFT *Alcohol may affect the quality and quantity of the sperm that a man produces. Cut down your intake if you are trying to father a child.*

DATA FILE

- Infertility in humans is defined as the failure to conceive after a year to 18 months of unprotected sexual intercourse.
- Approximately 10–15 percent of couples, or one in every seven marriages in the United States, is affected by the problem of infertility.
- In approximately 40 percent of cases, the cause of infertility is due to a female factor *(see page 386)*; 40 percent of cases are due to a male factor; and in the remaining instances no cause can be found despite thorough evaluation.
- In as many as 35 percent of couples, multiple conditions causing infertility can be identified.

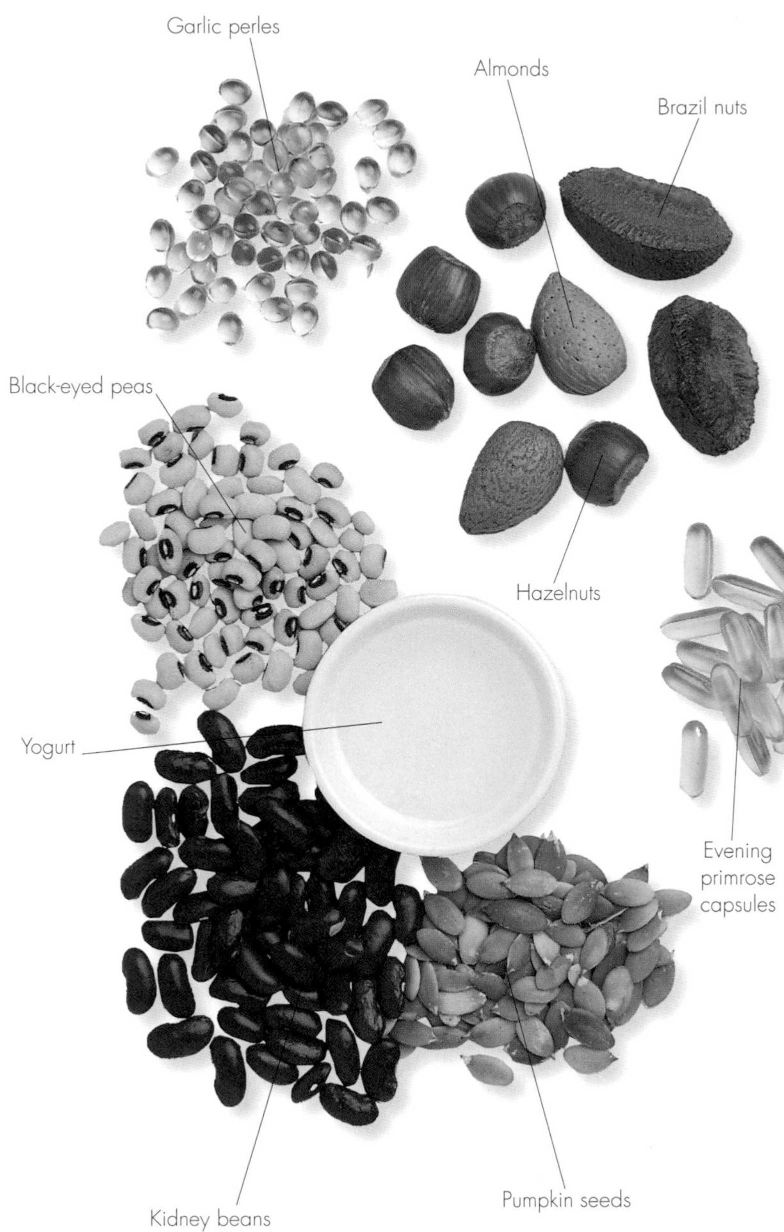

ABOVE *Foods that contain essential fatty acids, such as these, are believed to stimulate the production of sex hormones.*

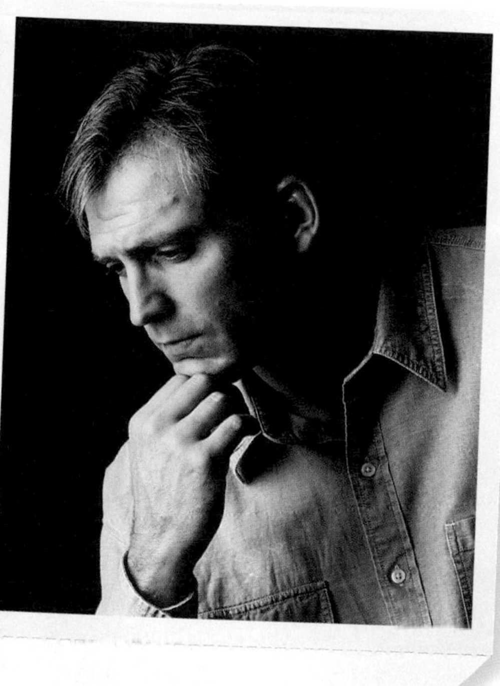

ABOVE *White Chestnut flower essence is useful to calm persistent worrying thoughts.*

TREATMENT

AYURVEDA

• Saffron is used for the treatment of infertility. *(See page 36.)*
• Sandalwood can help with impotence and acts as an aphrodisiac. *(See page 44.)*
• Clove, ginger, cardamom, cinnamon, vetiver, and coriander are aphrodisiac, which may help. *(See pages 34, 35, 38, 46, and 47.)*

CHINESE HERBALISM

• Infertility is believed to be caused by Damp Heat, and an imbalance of yin and yang; treatment will be according to the nature of your infertility. The following combinations may be useful: Yi Zhi Ren, He Shou Wu, Gou Qi Zi, Du Zhong, and Wu Wei Zi, for problems associated with sperm. *(See pages 63, 66, 70, and 74.)*

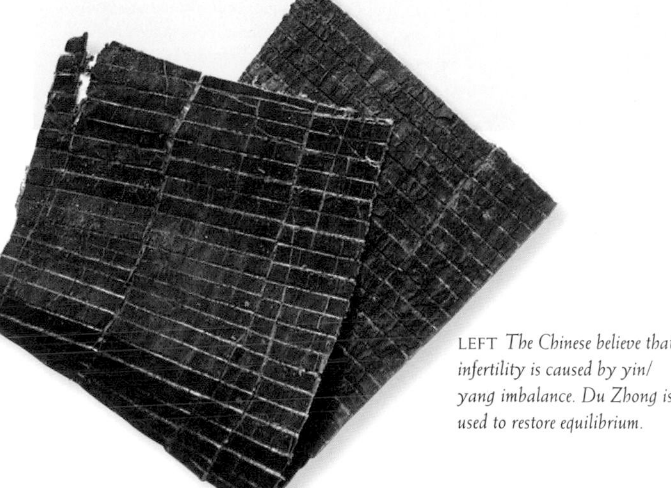

LEFT *The Chinese believe that infertility is caused by yin/yang imbalance. Du Zhong is used to restore equilibrium.*

HERBALISM

• Remedies such as damiana and saw palmetto have hormonal effects, stimulating the male reproductive system while also acting as useful nerve restoratives. *(See pages 131 and 135.)*

AROMATHERAPY

• Rose oil is said to increase sperm count and quality, as well as acting as a mild aphrodisiac. Add a few drops to your partner's bath, or perhaps engage in a little gentle massage, with 2 or 3 drops of rose essential oil in a mild carrier oil such as sweet almond oil. *(See page 168.)*
• If infertility is causing anxiety, any of the relaxing essential oils, such as lavender, marjoram, or chamomile, can be vaporized or used in a bath. *(See pages 146–71.)*
• When repeated attempts to get pregnant have failed and you need a little encouragement to continue with love-making, ylang ylang is a lovely, relaxing oil that will act as an aphrodisiac. *(See page 148.)*

HOMEOPATHY

Treatment would be constitutional, but the following remedies may be helpful:
• Conium, for inability to sustain an erection.
• Lycopodium, for an increased desire for sex, but where intercourse is spoiled by anticipation of failure. *(See page 203.)*
• Sepia, for a dragging sensation in the genitals, and no desire for sex. *(See page 212.)*

FLOWER ESSENCES

• Willow can be taken for resentment, bitterness, and self-pity about the problem. *(See page 239.)*
• White Chestnut, for worrying thoughts. *(See page 224.)*
• Pine, for guilty feelings. *(See page 236.)*
• Olive, for exhaustion and overwhelming fatigue. *(See page 235.)*

VITAMINS AND MINERALS

• There is a possibility that a zinc deficiency might cause problems with male fertility. Studies in the U.S. have shown that zinc is essential for sperm formation, and men who have zinc deficiencies may produce zero or reduced sperm counts. Zinc is also linked to a man's sex drive. *(See page 265.)*
• Cutting out alcohol, smoking, and drugs may be suggested for both couples for the period before conception.
• Vitamins E and B6 may be supplemented, as a deficiency is often linked to a low sperm count. *(See pages 257 and 254.)*
• An increased intake of EFAs (essential fatty acids, found in oily fish, fish liver oils, seeds, nuts, pulses, beans, evening primrose oil, and unrefined vegetable oils) stimulates sex hormone production.

BELOW *Rose essential oil has aphrodisiac qualities, well as relaxing the mind.*

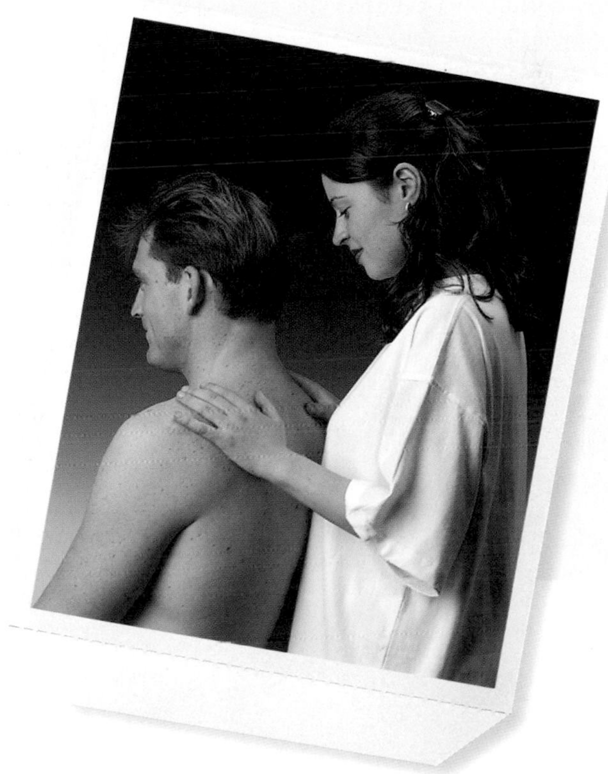

Prostate Problems

The prostate is a small sex gland which surrounds the urethra (urine tube) under the bladder. Its function is to produce the fluid which transports and nourishes sperm as it is ejaculated. Common prostate problems include:

• BENIGN PROSTATIC HYPERPLASIA (BPH), a slow, noncancerous enlargement of the prostate, progressively constricts the urethra, causing obstruction in the flow of urine. Incomplete emptying of the bladder as a result causes a frequent urge to urinate at night as well as during the day.

• PROSTATITIS, inflammation of the prostate gland, is common in younger men and may be chronic or acute. Symptoms include a frequent urge to urinate, burning pain, and difficulty in urinating, lower back pain, painful ejaculation, and inflamed testes.

• PROSTATE CANCER, the second most common form of cancer in men. The prostate is enlarged, as in BPH, but is felt to be hard on examination. As well as an urge to urinate more frequently, there may be blood in the urine and pain on urinating. If the cancer is advanced there may also be bone pain and weight loss.

• CANCER of the prostate occurs in 1 of 8 American men. Prostate cancer is more common after the age of 55; approximately 80 percent of all cases occur in men over 65; by the age of 80, 80 percent of all men have the cancer to some degree. Cancer of the prostate also becomes increasingly common in men over the age of 60; its development is stimulated by male hormones and retarded – to a variable extent – by female hormones. A male baby has a 13 percent chance of contracting prostate cancer, and a 3 percent chance of dying from it. For early detection of prostate cancer, the ACS (American Cancer Society) recommends that men over age 40 should have an annual digital rectal examination. After age 50, men should have an annual prostate-specific antigen blood test.

• BENIGN PROSTATIC HYPERTROPHY occurs in half of all men over the age of 50, and in three-quarters over the age of 70 – a total of about 10 million men.

Watercress has powerful antibiotic properties and will help fight urinary infections

Sesame seeds are believed to enhance sexual vigor

Pumpkin seeds act as a male sexual tonic and protect the prostate

LEFT *Certain foods, such as those shown here, may be of particular benefit to the prostate gland.*

TREATMENT

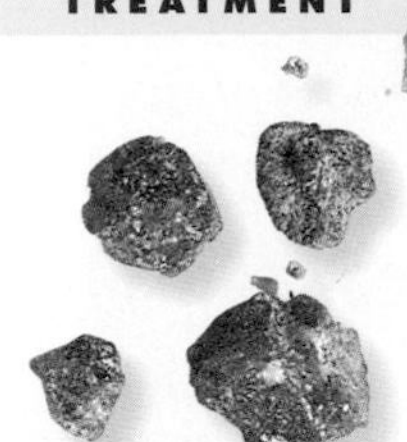

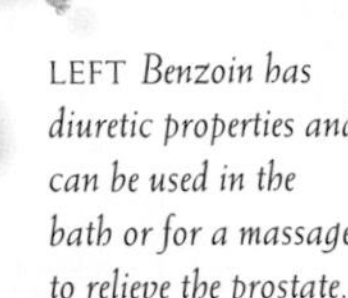

LEFT *Benzoin has diuretic properties and can be used in the bath or for a massage to relieve the prostate.*

AYURVEDA
• Gotu kola is cooling, rejuvenating, and diuretic. *(See page 33.)*
• Cedar and celery seed are natural diuretics and will encourage urination. *(See pages 29 and 32.)*
• Cinnamon is diuretic and analgesic, which will help ease the discomfort. *(See page 34.)*
• Coriander is diuretic and aphrodisiac, which will help address the low libido that is associated with this condition. *(See page 35.)*

CHINESE HERBALISM
• Prostate problems are believed to be caused by excess dampness and stagnant qi. The herbs cinnamon bark, cork tree bark, and water plantain will be useful treatments. *(See pages 59 and 68.)*
• Panax ginseng is recommended for an enlarged prostate. *(See page 67.)*

TRADITIONAL HOME AND FOLK REMEDIES
• Watercress leaves are tonic and should be eaten as often as possible to help alleviate the problem. *(See page 94.)*
• Sesame seeds have a beneficial effect in maintaining and enhancing sexual vigor.
• Pumpkin seeds are a male sexual tonic, and are used in the treatment of prostate problems.

HERBALISM
• Saw palmetto is able to reduce inflammation of the prostate. *(See page 131.)*
• Couchgrass and horsetail can be given to help encourage urination, and can be drunk freely throughout the day as a natural diuretic.

AROMATHERAPY
• Clary sage and geranium, which have estrogen-like oils, can be used in whole-body massage or in the bath to treat the condition. *(See pages 165 and 169.)*
• Bergamot, chamomile, and myrrh are anti-inflammatory, and will ease symptoms, particularly of prostatitis. *(See pages 146–71.)*
• Benzoin, sandalwood, frankincense, and cedarwood are all diuretic, and can be used both in the bath and for a full-body massage. *(See pages146–71.)*

HOMEOPATHY
Constitutional treatment would be required, but in the meantime the following remedies can be taken 4 times daily for 3 to 4 weeks:
• Arg. nit., for impotence because erection is lost on penetration, and for pain on intercourse and low libido. *(See page 181.)*
• Sabal, for difficult or painful urination, and spasms of pain. Also for enlarged prostate, and if intercourse is painful.
• Pulsatilla, for thick yellow discharge from the penis and an urgent desire to urinate. *(See page 209.)*
• Thuja, for burning at the neck of the bladder and a frequent need to urinate. *(See page 216.)*
• Baryta carb., for a frequent urge to urinate, a slow stream of urine, and premature ejaculation. *(See page 185.)*
• Iodum, for loss of potency, with shrunken testicles and hard prostate gland.

VITAMINS AND MINERALS
• Lecithin, calcium, and magnesium may help treat prostate disorders. *(See pages 271, 258, and 262.)*
• An increased intake of zinc can help to prevent and treat prostatitis. *(See page 265.)*
• Evening primrose has been successfully used for prostate problems. *(See page 270.)*
• Cold-pressed linseed oil can help if the condition is mild but recurrent.
• Flower pollen is widely used to treat problems of the prostate gland. *(See page 271.)*

Erection Problems

Failure to achieve an erection that is firm enough, or sustained for long enough, to allow normal sexual intercourse is generally known as impotence. Its cause may be physical (organic), psychological, or a combination of both. Organic impotence may be due to an imperfect blood supply to the penis, an age-related loss of male sex hormones, diabetes, medicinal drugs, or various neurological conditions. Psychological factors such as lack of desire, depression, or fear of failure may be responsible for impotence, and alcohol, while enhancing sexual desire, can actually impede performance.

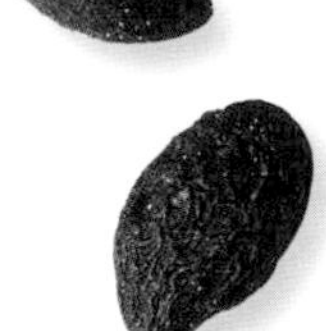

ABOVE *Saw palmetto is a strengthening tonic and will help the male reproductive system.*

DATA FILE

- Approximately 30 million men in the U.S. suffer from impotence.
- It is now believed that up to 85 percent of cases have a physical cause.
- The Association for Male Sexual Dysfunction recognizes over 200 drugs that may cause it, including alcohol, antihistamines, antidepressants, narcotics, diuretics, sedatives, nicotine.
- Primary impotence is the case in which the male has never maintained an erection of long enough duration to engage in sexual intercourse.
- Secondary impotence is when a previously potent male loses the ability to maintain an erection during intercourse.
- Fear of failure and performance anxiety are frequently underlying negative psychological sources of impotence.

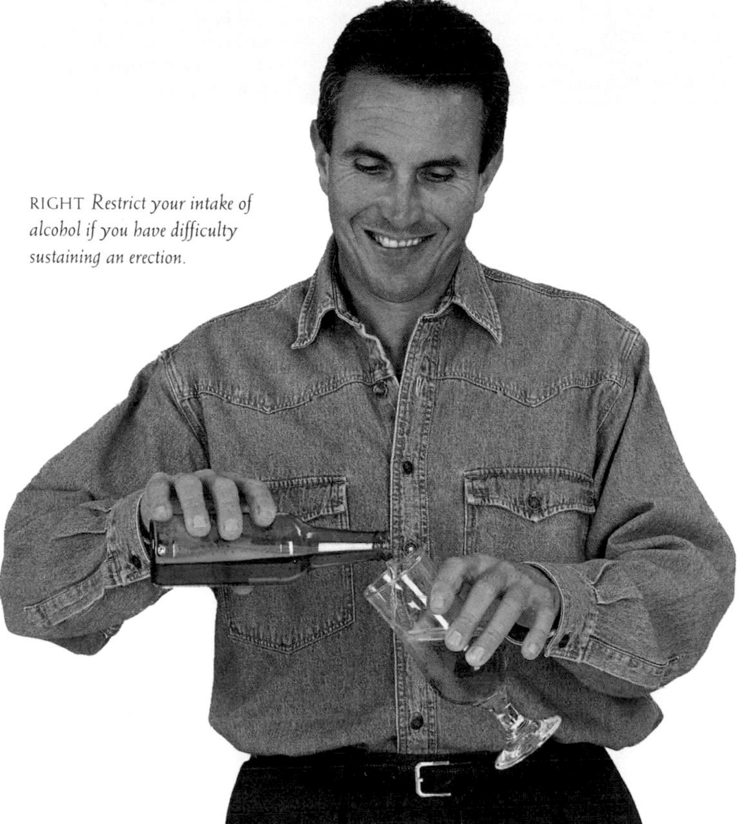

RIGHT *Restrict your intake of alcohol if you have difficulty sustaining an erection.*

TREATMENT

AYURVEDA

- Sandalwood is good for impotence, and accompanying anxiety and nervousness. *(See page 44.)*
- Cinnamon tones the muscles and is noted for treating impotence. *(See page 34.)*
- Ginger is warming and can help improve matters. *(See page 47.)*
- Saffron is used for impotence and anxiety. *(See page 36.)*
- Clove, ginger, cardamom, cinnamon, vetiver, and coriander are aphrodisiac, which may help. *(See pages 34, 35, 38, 46, and 47.)*

CHINESE HERBALISM

- Ginseng can improve vitality and help to reduce feelings of anxiety. *(See page 67.)*
- Impotence is believed to be caused by weakness of the Kidneys and Liver, with Liver qi stagnation, and cibot root may be useful.
- Chinese angelica, white peony root, and thorowax will help feelings of anxiety. *(See pages 56 and 67.)*

TRADITIONAL HOME AND FOLK REMEDIES

- Watercress leaves are tonic and should be eaten as often as possible to help alleviate the problem. *(See page 94.)*
- Sesame seeds have a beneficial effect in maintaining and enhancing sexual vigor.
- Pumpkin seeds are a male sexual tonic.
- Avocado pear is excellent if you suffer from sexual problems. *(See page 96.)*

HERBALISM

- Peppermint leaves stimulate and warm the body, and will help to reduce feelings of anxiety. *(See page 125.)*
- Anise is a powerful tonic: drink small amounts to treat impotence.
- Remedies like damiana and saw palmetto have dual hormonal effects, stimulating and toning the male reproductive system, and restoring nerves. *(See pages 131 and 135.)*

AROMATHERAPY

- Essential oils of clary sage, sandalwood, and ylang ylang are natural aphrodisiacs and will help you to relax. Try a full-body massage, or a few drops in the bath. *(See page 146–71.)*

HOMEOPATHY

- Lycopodium, when you feel surges of desire, but anticipate failure. *(See page 203.)*
- Agnus, for an erection that is not firm enough for successful penetration.
- Conium, for an erection which does not last.
- Caladium, for erections which occur during sleep, but disappear on waking, and a lack of erection even when sexually excited. *(See page 91.)*

FLOWER ESSENCES

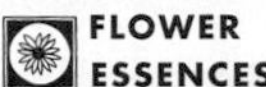

- Larch, for lack of sexual confidence and feelings of inadequacy. *(See page 233.)*
- Gentian, for a sense of failure. *(See page 230.)*
- Sweet Chestnut, for despair and hopelessness. *(See page 227.)*
- Crab Apple, for feeling unclean on any level. *(See page 234.)*

VITAMINS AND MINERALS

- Avoid alcohol, drugs, and caffeine, which constrict the blood vessels and inhibit the blood flow needed to achieve an erection.
- Molybdenum can prevent impotence and sexual difficulties. *(See page 263.)*
- Zinc is required for the healthy functioning of the reproductive organs, and should be included in a varied, healthy diet. *(See page 265.)*
- L-tryptophan may help to prevent feelings of anxiety from causing sexual difficulties. *(See page 269.)*

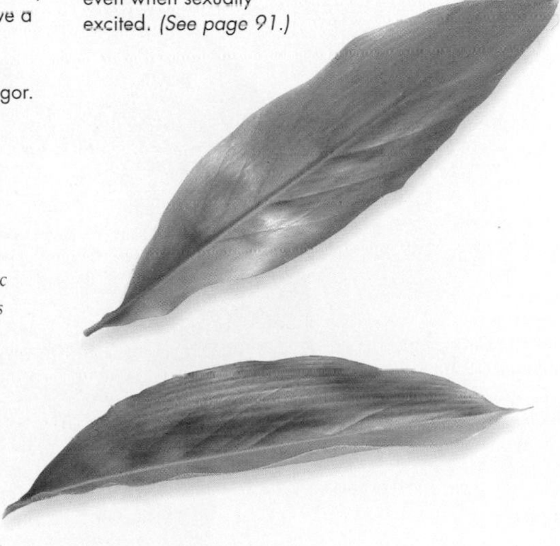

RIGHT *In Ayurvedic medicine cardamom is recommended as an aphrodisiac.*

Ejaculation Problems

For men, orgasm is usually accompanied by ejaculation. A single ejaculate contains about 300 million sperm in a fluid medium called semen. Ejaculation is a two-phased process. In the emission phase seminal fluid accumulates in the bulb of the prostate. In the expulsion phase the neck of the urinary bladder closes to ensure that no urine will mix with the semen, and the muscles at the base of the penis and of the penile urethra contract to force the semen out of the urethral opening. Some men experience a "retrograde," or dry, ejaculation as a result of genetics, illness, medication, surgery, or damage to the valves of the urethra that control the flow of semen.

In most cases ejaculation problems are psycho-sexual in origin, and not due to any physical abnormality, so that a man may experience sexual failure with one partner, but function quite normally with another. There are two main problems: premature ejaculation and absence of ejaculation. Premature ejaculation is very common indeed and refers to the occurrence of the male orgasm at the time of penetration, or very soon after. In extreme cases it may even take place before physical contact is made. Premature ejaculation is usually a feature of early sexual experience, or a sign of performance anxiety. The absence of ejaculation is very rare but can occur as a result of overindulgence, inadequate stimulation of the penis, or age-related loss of penile sensitivity.

ABOVE *Ginseng works as an aphrodisiac and is recommended for men who have sexual problems due to anxiety.*

RIGHT *Most ejaculation problems have a psychological origin. Eat oats, which have relaxing and therapeutic qualities.*

TREATMENT

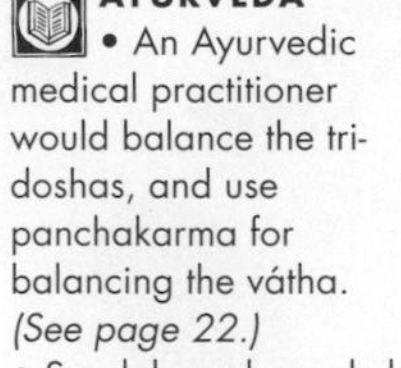

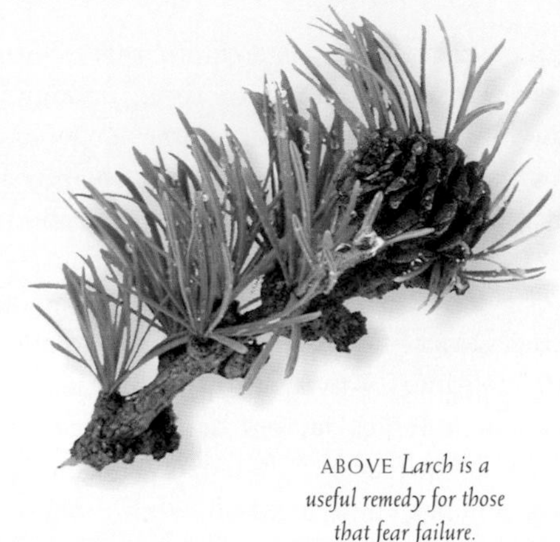

ABOVE *Larch is a useful remedy for those that fear failure.*

AYURVEDA

- An Ayurvedic medical practitioner would balance the tri-doshas, and use panchakarma for balancing the vátha. *(See page 22.)*
- Sandalwood may help to relieve anxiety, and has an anesthetic effect on the area which can reduce premature ejaculation. *(See page 44.)*
- Saffron may be helpful. *(See page 36.)*

CHINESE HERBALISM

- Treatment may address weakness of the Kidneys and Liver, and deal with Liver qi stagnation. Cibot root may work well.
- Problems causing or associated with anxiety may be treated with ginseng, Chinese angelica, white peony root, and thorowax root. *(See pages 56 and 67.)*

TRADITIONAL HOME AND FOLK REMEDIES

- Oats contain thiamine and pantothenic acid, which act as gentle tonics for the nerves and will relax and calm you. Take regularly. *(See page 84.)*

HERBALISM

- Herbal remedies would be used to calm the nervous system and to relax. *(See page 104.)*
- Skullcap and valerian are useful herbs, and should be blended together for best effect. Drink this as a tea three times daily to calm. *(See pages 131 and 136.)*
- Lady's slipper and lime blossom may also work to ease anxiety and tension associated with the condition.
- Remedies like damiana and saw palmetto have hormonal effects, stimulating and toning the male reproductive system and restoring nerves. *(See pages 131 and 135.)*

AROMATHERAPY

- A relaxing blend of essential oils of lavender, geranium, and bergamot in sweet almond oil or peach kernel oil may be used in the bath at times of great stress and anxiety. *(See pages 146–71.)*

HOMEOPATHY

Constitutional treatment will be necessary, but the following remedies may be of some use:

- Lycopodium, for an increased sexual desire; lack of self-confidence and expectation of failure with premature ejaculation. *(See page 203.)*
- Nux vomica., for impatience, craving excitement, short temper, and use of stimulating drugs. *(See page 214.)*
- Graphites, for loss of sex drive, premature or non-existent ejaculation. *(See page 196.)*
- Nitric acid, for irritability, self-criticism, and extreme sensitivity.
- Ignatia, for problems caused by grief or disappointment. *(See page 200.)*
- Mercurius, when thrush or urethritis causes the problem. *(See page 205.)* *(See also Prostate Problems, page 400).*

FLOWER ESSENCES

- Try Elm for anxiety accompanying a feeling of being unable to cope. *(See page 241.)*
- Larch may help with lack of self-confidence. *(See page 233.)*
- Gentian may be useful for a sense of failure. *(See page 230.)*
- Rescue Remedy or Emergency Essence, taken before intercourse, can help to calm and relax you. *(See page 244.)*

VITAMINS AND MINERALS

- Increase your intake of B vitamins, which work on the nervous system, and avoid caffeine or other stimulants in any form. *(See pages 252–5.)*

Priapism

Priapism is the name given to prolonged and painful erection in the absence of sexual interest. It is caused by failure of the blood to return from the penis to the circulation after a period of sexual activity. This may be because of a disturbance in the nervous system's control of blood flow, due to a disease of the spinal cord or brain. It may also be caused by clotting due to leukemia or sickle-cell anemia, inflammation of the prostate, bladder stones, or urethritis.

CAUTION

LONG-SUSTAINED ERECTION CAN BE DANGEROUS AS THERE IS A RISK OF THROMBOSIS, WHICH MAY CAUSE PERMANENT LOSS OF ERECTILE FUNCTION.

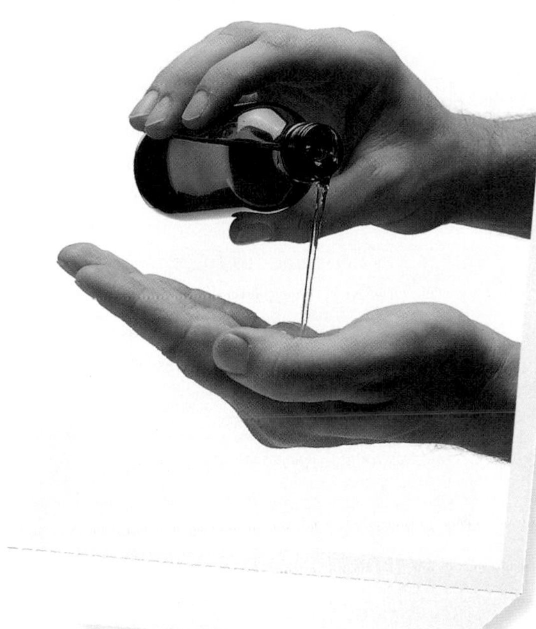

LEFT *Bergamot oil is recommended for priapism as it is anti-inflammatory. Massage the area or use the oil in a bath.*

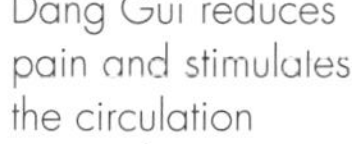

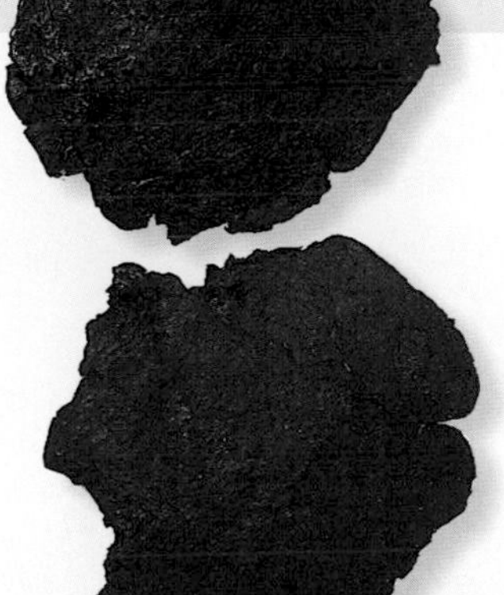

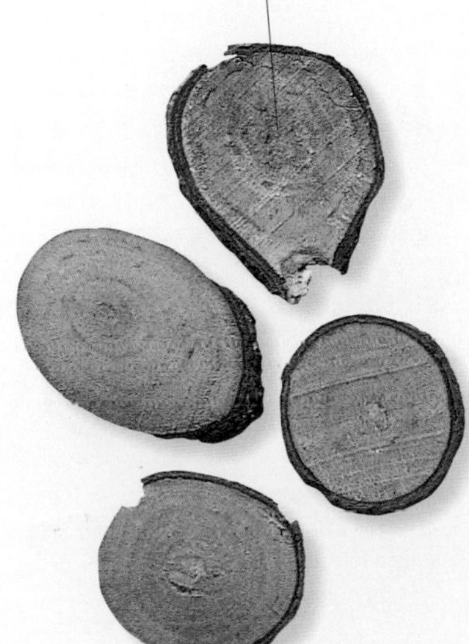

ABOVE *Chinese medicines that are used to treat priapism include Gui Zhi and Dang Gui.*

TREATMENT

AYURVEDA

- Angelica can improve circulation. *(See page 28.)*
- Black pepper increases blood circulation and feeds the nervous system. *(See page 44.)*
- Calamus oil massage will improve circulation in the area. *(See page 24.)*
- Cayenne pepper is analgesic and warming. *(See page 31.)*

CHINESE HERBALISM

- Gui Zhi may be useful when the yang qi has failed to move fluids through channels. *(See page 59.)*
- Dang Gui will reduce pain and invigorates blood circulation. *(See page 56.)*

HERBALISM

Herbs which encourage circulation include:

- Broom, which tones the arteries.
- Ginger, hawthorn tops, and rosemary, which are stimulating and work to encourage circulation. *(See pages 119, 127, and 139.)*
- Lavender and vervain, which are calming, and can be sipped during an attack to ease symptoms. *(See page 138.)*

See also the sections on Prostate problems, page 400; Urethritis, page 380; and Bladder Stones, page 379.

AROMATHERAPY

- Local massage with rosemary or peppermint is stimulating and will help normalize the blood flow in the area. *(See pages 164 and 168.)*
- Massage the area with diluted juniper, marjoram, myrrh, or tea tree, which will act as a tonic. *(See pages 146–71.)*
- Bergamot is anti-inflammatory, and may be used in local massage or in the bath to ease inflammatory conditions causing priapism. *(See page 153.)*

HOMEOPATHY

Treatment would be constitutional, but during an attack the following remedies may help:

- Carb. veg., for sluggish circulation, and possibly piles and varicose veins. *(See page 188.)*
- Kali brom., for the treatment of impotence.
- Cantharis, for a painful erection. *(See page 188.)*

VITAMINS AND MINERALS

- Vitamin E is suggested. *(See page 257.)*
- Vitamin C, which affects the health of the circulatory system, may be useful. *(See page 256.)*

DISORDERS OF THE ENDOCRINE SYSTEM

Thyroid Problems

The thyroid gland, found in the neck, is responsible for controlling the general level of activity of the body. An overactive gland (hyperthyroidism) causes a racing heart, increased digestion, and enormous physical energy. Untreated, this condition can lead to heart failure and extreme weight loss, among other things. An underactive gland (hypothyroidism) leads to apathy, overwhelming fatigue, heart problems, menstrual problems, and weight gain. Thyroid problems are very common and, fortunately, they can be diagnosed long before they become serious, and various remedies can then be applied. Occasionally thyroid disease forms part of a wider disease process, including diabetes and rheumatoid arthritis. Other causes of thyroid disease include iodine deficiency, which may exist from birth and features in mental retardation, enlargement of the thyroid gland (goiter), inflammation, and, rarely, cancer.

TREATMENT

AYURVEDA

• An Ayurvedic medical practitioner may suggest panchakarma Method for detoxification. *(See page 22.)*

CHINESE HERBALISM

• Hyperthyroidism is believed to be caused by Heat in the Liver, and marine plants and seaweed are prescribed.

HERBALISM

• Bugleweed is excellent, and should be drunk 3 times daily for hyperthyroidism.
• Bladderwrack helps to regulate the function of the thyroid gland. Take 3 times daily, in any form. *(See page 122.)*

AROMATHERAPY

• Geranium oil balances hormone production, and will help to ensure that the thyroid gland is working effectively. Use the oil in the bath, or in an overall massage for best effect. *(See page 165.)*

HOMEOPATHY

Treatment will be constitutional and aimed at controlling acute symptoms. Long-term control of the condition should be undertaken by a physician. However, specific remedies which may help control symptoms are:

Hyperthyroidism:
• Iodum, when the sufferer feels hot, cannot stop activity, is obsessive, and probably dark-haired and brown-eyed.
• Nat. mur., for symptoms accompanied by constipation, palpitations and earthy-colored complexion. *(See page 206.)*
• Belladonna, when symptoms include a flushed face and staring eyes. *(See page 183.)*
• Lycopus, when the heart is pounding and racing.

Hypothyroidism:
• Arsenicum can be taken for up to five days, twice daily, while constitutional treatment is being sought. *(See page 182.)*

VITAMINS AND MINERALS

• Nutritional deficiencies (for example, zinc, Vitamin A, selenium, and iron) and a toxic overload are thought to be the main factors involved in the onset of hypothyroidism. Ensure that you eat a good healthy diet, with plenty of fresh organic vegetables, seafood, and onions.
• Garlic and onions are both particularly valuable if the patient's thyroid gland is underactive.
• Supplement your diet with natural thyroid hormones created from iodine, and the amino acid tyrosine for hypothyroidism. *(See pages 261 and 269.)*
• Garlic is a rich source of iodine, which can help regulate thyroid function. *(See page 261.)*

Onions are beneficial if the thyroid is underactive
Curly Kale is a rich source of vitamin A and calcium
Vitamin A can be found in oily fish, such as mackerel
Shellfish contain zinc, necessary for a healthy thyroid gland
Garlic contains iodine, which helps regulate thyroid function

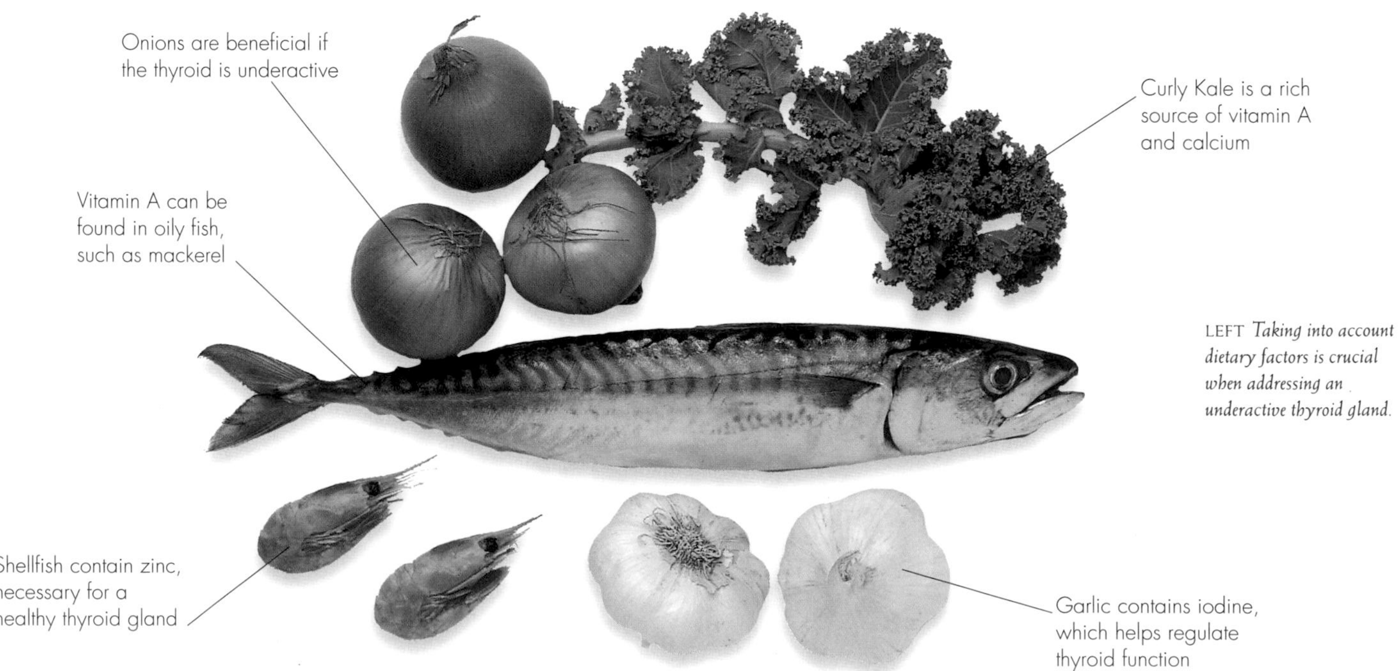

LEFT *Taking into account dietary factors is crucial when addressing an underactive thyroid gland.*

DATA FILE

Disorders of the thyroid include:

- Iodine deficiency. Iodine is an essential element in the thyroid hormone. Deficiency of iodine is rare, but can cause cretinism – physical and mental retardation featuring poor feeding, constipation, a characteristic cry, and a large tongue.
- Hypothyroidism, underaction of the thyroid. Features slowing of physical and mental processes, sensitivity to cold, obesity, no sweating, loss of hair, a puffy face, coronary artery disease. Untreated, hypothyroidism may lead to coma.
- Hyperthyroidism, overaction of the thyroid. Features weight loss, increased appetite, palpitations, anxiety, irritability, dislike of heat, sweating, and infrequent menstruation. Untreated it may lead to heart failure.
- Goiter *(see page 405)*.
- Cancer. Thyroid cancer is quite rare and is usually found as a single firm lump in the neck. It may spread to the lymph nodes in the neck and can involve the vocal cords, causing hoarseness or loss of the voice.
- Over 5 million people in the U.S. suffer from thyroid problems; 90 percent of them are women.
- In the U.K. researchers discovered that one in ten people suffering from Parkinson's also suffered from hyperthyroidism.
- Various conditions can cause goiter, an enlargement of the thyroid gland.
- Overproduction of hormones in the thyroid gland, which may follow emotional or physical stress, results in toxic diffuse goiter (Grave's disease) or toxic nodular goiter (Plummer's disease), both of which are characterized by nervousness, sweating, weight loss, and hyperactivity.
- If goiter is caused by a low dietary intake of iodine, it is termed endemic (colloid) goiter.

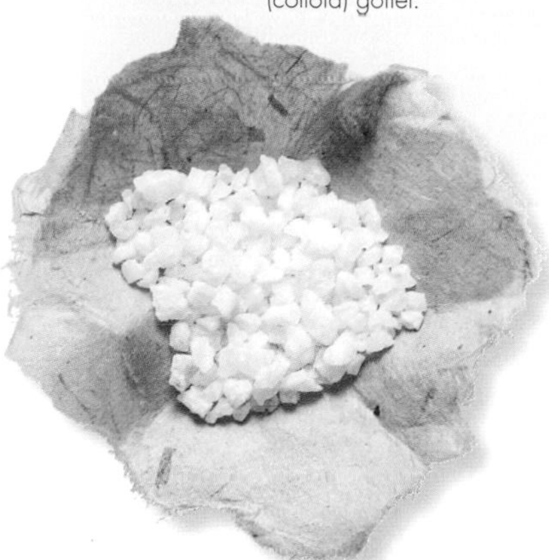

ABOVE *Nat. mur., made from rock salt, is a possible homeopathic remedy for thyroid problems.*

ABOVE *Clary sage oils helps to balance hormones, which may stimulate an underactive thyroid.*

Goiter

Goiter is an enlargement of the thyroid gland, visible as a swelling on the neck, and is fairly common. In order for the thyroid to produce hormones it requires iodine in the diet for their synthesis. If there is insufficient iodine in the diet the gland increases its activity and swells, resulting in a goiter. The nontoxic enlargement of the thyroid due to insufficient iodine is common and easily remedied by eating more fish and iodized salt, thereby increasing iodine intake. Conditions of which goiter is a feature are:

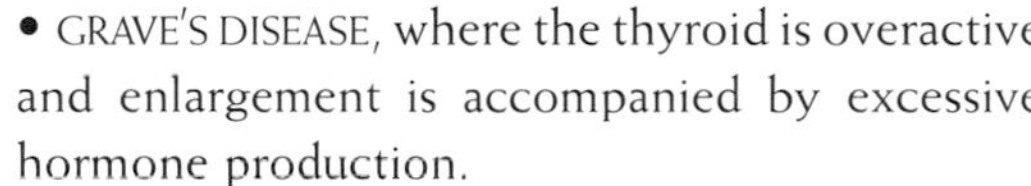

- GRAVE'S DISEASE, where the thyroid is overactive and enlargement is accompanied by excessive hormone production.
- HASHIMOTO'S THYROIDITIS, where the thyroid is underactive due to antibodies to thyroid hormone. Causes an ache in the neck and difficulty in swallowing.
- SUB-ACUTE THYROIDITIS, probably a viral infection which causes inflammation and pain.
- DYSHORMONOGENESIS, a genetic enzyme deficiency which interferes with normal hormone synthesis.
- TUMORS of the thyroid gland which may be benign or malignant.

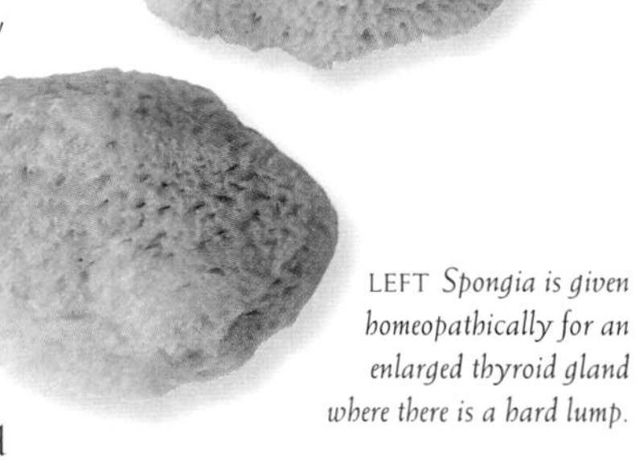

LEFT *Spongia is given homeopathically for an enlarged thyroid gland where there is a hard lump.*

Symptoms

- *swelling at the front of the neck, which may vary from a small lump to a very large mass* • *difficulty in swallowing or breathing in severe cases* • *hyperthyroidism (overactive thyroid):- weight loss – increased appetite – warm, dry skin – tremor – insomnia – bulging eyes –*
- *hypothyroidism (underactive thyroid):- tiredness – muscle weakness – weight gain – flaky skin – hair loss – deepening voice*

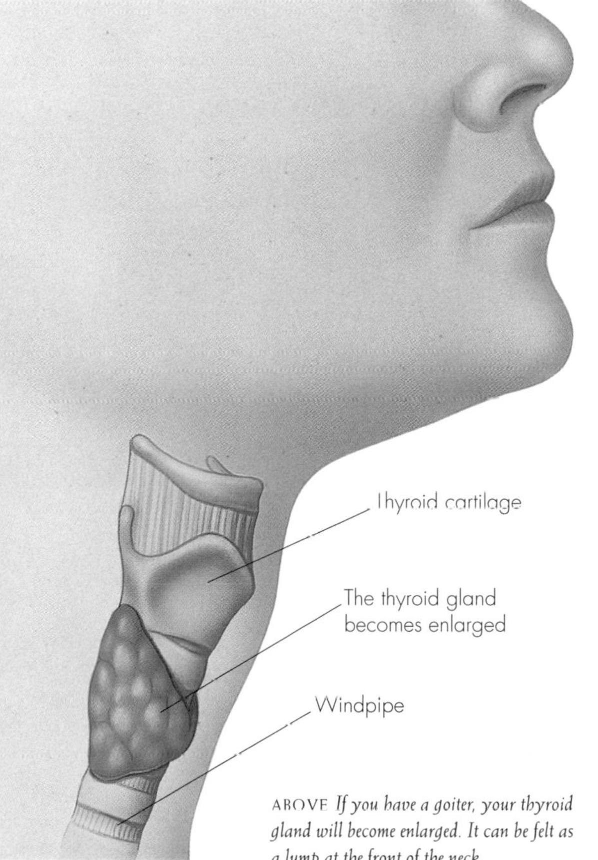

ABOVE *If you have a goiter, your thyroid gland will become enlarged. It can be felt as a lump at the front of the neck.*

TREATMENT

HERBALISM
- Bladderwrack, brown seaweed, can help goiter caused by an underactive thyroid. *(See page 122.)*
- Bugleweed is used to treat an overactive thyroid.

AROMATHERAPY
- Clary sage has a balancing effect on hormones, and since it is now believed that an underactive thyroid may be linked to an excess of female hormones, this may be a useful oil. *(See page 169.)*

HOMEOPATHY
The following remedies, taken twice daily for up to 2 weeks, should improve the condition:
- Iodum, for someone who is always in a hurry and feeling hot.
- Spongia, for a long-standing condition, where there is a hard lump. *(See page 213.)*
- Calcarea, for a pale, chilly, overweight person. *(See page 186.)*
- Fluoric acid, for elderly sufferers who are young-thinking, vigorous, and with varicose veins.

VITAMINS AND MINERALS
- Increase your intake of salt, fish, seafish, and kelp to ensure adequate iodine. *(See page 261.)*

Diabetes

The most common form of diabetes is diabetes mellitus. It is caused by a lack of, or insufficient, insulin (the hormone produced by the pancreas), as a result of which the body is unable to process glucose. This causes a high level of glucose in the blood, and low absorption of the vital energy-producing glucose by the tissues. In Type I (insulin-dependency) diabetes the sufferer produces little or no insulin and requires lifelong monitoring. Blood sugar levels can swing wildly between hypoglycemia (featuring strange feelings, abnormal behavior, and a risk of coma) and hyperglycemia (causing overproduction of ketones, and coma). Type I usually first appears in those who are under the age of 35, particularly adolescents, and develops rapidly. Type II, maturity-onset diabetes, is thought to be caused by the body's cells' lack of response to insulin. It usually affects people aged 40 and over, and there is an association with obesity and pregnancy. The onset of Type II is gradual and may go unnoticed for some time.

ABOVE *Scientific studies have shown that onions reduce blood sugar levels for longer periods than insulin, but more slowly.*

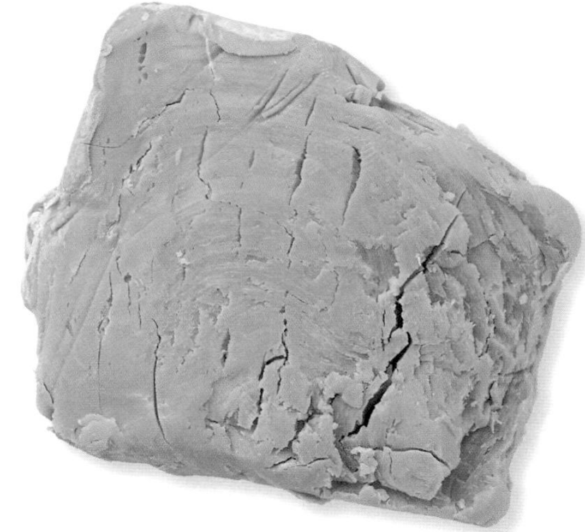

ABOVE *The chromium content of Brewer's yeast may help blood sugar levels to remain constant.*

SYMPTOMS

• excessive thirst • excessive urination • weight loss • fatigue, weakness, and apathy • hunger • bad breath • complications include: – nerve damage (causing damage to the eye muscles and double vision as a result) – damage to blood vessels affecting the eyes (sometimes causing blindness), kidneys, circulation in the legs – organic impotence – arterial disease and gangrene

DATA FILE

- Diabetes affects over 10 million people in the United States and causes about 300,000 deaths each year.
- An estimated 5 million adults have undetected Type II diabetes, and another 20 million have a glucose intolerance that could lead to diabetes.
- Complications due to diabetes are the third most frequent cause of death in the U.S.
- Damage to the retina from diabetes is the main cause of blindness in the U.S.
- Its prevalence increases with age, from about 0.2 percent in persons under 17 years of age to about 20 percent in persons aged 65 years and over, and is greater in females.
- Prevalence is inversely related to family income and varies markedly among ethnic groups, with occurrence about two times higher in non-Caucasians than in Caucasians.

TREATMENT

AYURVEDA
- An Ayurvedic practitioner would recommend oral preparations from herbs that act upon the levels of glucose in the blood. There have been good results from treatment, with some cases being resolved within as little as 2 months. *(See page 22.)*
- For non-insulin-dependent diabetes, boil and cut one karella into small pieces and eat with the seeds every morning and evening.

CHINESE HERBALISM
- Lilyturf root, grassy privet, lotus seed, and Chinese yam are suggested.
- Treatment aimed at nourishing the Spleen, Kidneys, and Stomach would use Chinese yam, lotus seed, and mulberry.

HERBALISM
- Onions and garlic lower blood sugar levels. Ensure that you have plenty in your diet; take garlic oil supplements if not. *(See page 113.)*
- Fenugreek seed works to control blood sugar levels. Drink daily.
- Alfalfa is recommended for diabetics, and it should be taken daily.

HOMEOPATHY
Constitutional treatment will be balancing and can be taken alongside conventional medication. In some cases the condition has been completely cured through homeopathy, but it must be undertaken by a registered practitioner.

VITAMINS AND MINERALS
- Brewer's yeast contains chromium, which helps to normalize blood sugar levels and metabolism. Take 2–3 tablespoons daily. *(See page 272.)*

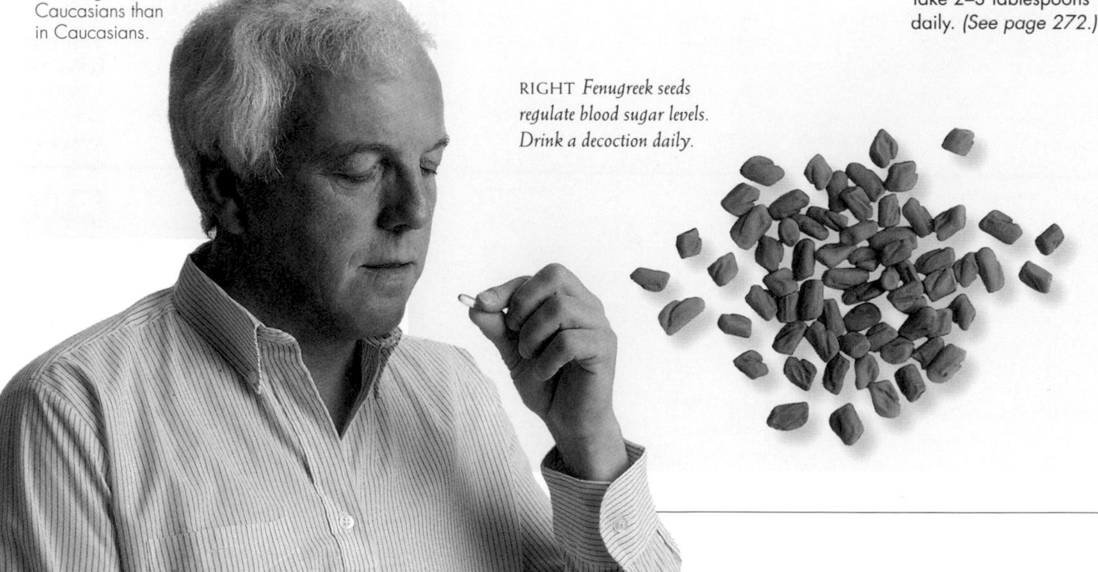

RIGHT *Fenugreek seeds regulate blood sugar levels. Drink a decoction daily.*

RIGHT *Try to ensure that you include garlic in your diet. If you do not like the taste, take garlic oil supplements.*

Addison's Disease

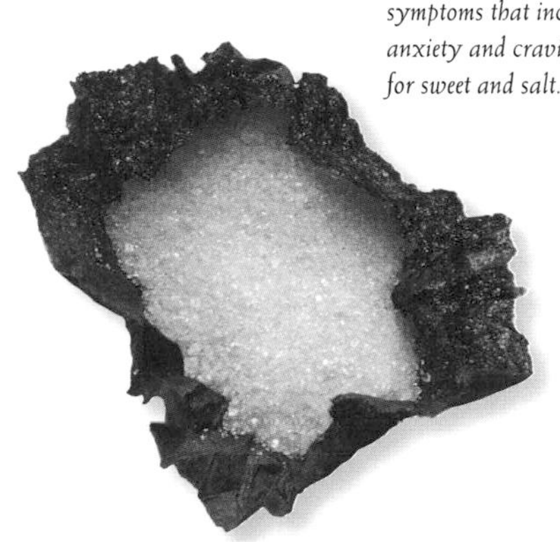

BELOW *Argentum nitricum is the homeopathic remedy for symptoms that include anxiety and cravings for sweet and salt.*

Addison's disease is a disorder of the adrenal glands which leads to insufficient output of cortisol and aldosterone – the steroid hormones which help the body to react to stress and control water balance, respectively. The disease is caused by an inflammation followed by atrophy of the outer layer (cortex) of the adrenal gland. This in turn is caused by abnormal action of the immune system in which it behaves towards the gland tissue as though it were foreign. Addison's is therefore known as an auto-immune disease. Addison's disease is usually due to damage by an auto-immune reaction, tuberculosis, or fungal infections. Addison's disease is rare, and generally has a slow onset and chronic course, with symptoms developing gradually over months or years. Acute episodes, called Addisonian crises, can be brought on by infection, injury, or other stresses, and they occur because the adrenal glands cannot increase their production of steroid hormones which normally help the body to deal with stress. The condition was invariably fatal before hormone treatment became available in the 1950s.

Symptoms

• weakness • fatigue • low blood pressure • excessive urination • dehydration • skin discoloration, as the pituitary gland attempts to compensate for insufficient adrenal output by overproducing another hormone which stimulates the pigment cells

TREATMENT

HERBALISM
• Treatment to stimulate the endocrine system; herbs to boost the immune system may also be appropriate. Treatment would be individual.

AROMATHERAPY
• Oils which strengthen the adrenal system include: rosemary, ginger, and lemongrass. *(See pages 146–71.)*

HOMEOPATHY
Treatment would be constitutional; however, the following treatments may help. If you don't feel any better after a week or so, see your doctor.
• Silicea, when your feet are sweaty and smelly, cold weather makes the symptoms worse, and you feel really exhausted. *(See page 211.)*
• Nat. mur., for when you have constipation, dry lips, a craving for salt, and symptoms which are made worse by sun. *(See page 206.)*
• Arg. nit., for apprehension, salt and sweet cravings, and tremors. *(See page 181.)*

LEFT *Lemongrass essential oil is used by aromatherapists to strengthen the adrenal system.*

Hypoglycemia

Hypoglycemia is a condition in which there is an abnormally low level of glucose in the blood. It is extremely dangerous because the brain is dependent on a constant supply of glucose. The most common cause of hypoglycemia is a relative insulin overdose by diabetics (i.e. the actual amount of insulin taken may be correct, but the intake of carbohydrate or the amount of exertion may have used up the supply too quickly). Excessive exercise and insufficient carbohydrate may, in fact, lead to hypoglycemia in non-diabetics.

DATA FILE

- The condition occurs in association with a number of diseases, most notably insulin overdose in diabetics.
- Repeated severe attacks can cause permanent brain damage.
- There are two main types of hypoglycemia: organic and functional.
- Any endocrine malfunction in the pancreas and adrenal glands, as well as the pituitary, thyroid, or sex glands, may result in organic hypoglycemia. Alcoholism, which impairs the liver's ability to produce glucose, can also lead to organic hypoglycemia, as can other disorders of the liver and tumors of the liver or pancreas.
- Functional hypoglycemia is a temporary condition of markedly lowered blood sugar, most commonly occurring 2–3 hours after a meal high in carbohydrates.
- 50 percent of sufferers over the age of 50 have a thyroid problem.

Symptoms

• headache and faintness • rapid pulse and palpitations • profuse sweating • mental confusion and loss of memory • irrational and disorderly behavior • slurred speech • numbness, temporary paralysis • fits and, eventually, potentially fatal coma

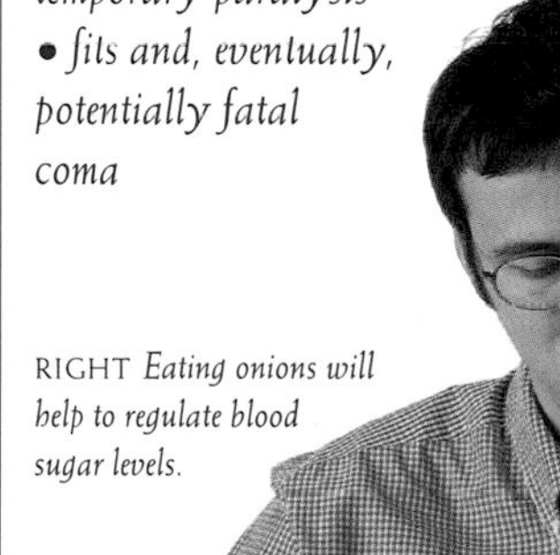

RIGHT *Eating onions will help to regulate blood sugar levels.*

TREATMENT

AYURVEDA
• Plants which act on blood sugar levels will be prescribed, as well as detoxification treatment to ensure that the system is working efficiently. *(See page 22.)*

TRADITIONAL HOME AND FOLK REMEDIES
• Onions and garlic will help to regulate blood sugar levels. Eat raw or cooked, as often as possible. *(See page 82.)*

CHINESE HERBALISM
• Chinese yam and lotus seed will help to normalize blood sugar levels.

HOMEOPATHY
• Homeopathic treatment would be constitutional, but well worth it, because in many cases the condition can be cured completely.

FLOWER ESSENCES
• Take Rescue Remedy if you feel an attack coming on. It will calm you and help to reduce the severity. *(See page 244.)*

VITAMINS AND MINERALS
• Take extra Vitamin C and B-complex tablets, chromium (to regulate blood sugar levels), magnesium, potassium, zinc, and manganese. *(See pages 256, 252–5, 259, 262, 265, and 263.)*

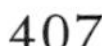

Obesity

Obesity is the excessive storage of energy in the form of fat, and applies to a body weight that is more than 20 percent over the recommended maximum for a person's height. The main cause of obesity is excessive calorie intake, but other factors include a low basal metabolic rate, genetic factors, emotional problems, metabolic disorders such as thyroid problems, taking steroids or insulin. Obesity can aggravate or trigger other conditions such as heart attack, gallstones, arthritis, hiatus hernia, varicose veins, kidney disorders, and fertility problems. In particular, the chances of suffering from high blood pressure, stroke, and maturity-onset diabetes are greatly increased by obesity. Obese women are more likely to be at risk from cancer of the ovaries, womb, and breast; obese men are at risk from cancer of the colon, rectum and prostate. The strain on the joints of the back, knees, and hips from the extra weight can cause problems.

ABOVE *Increase your intake of pungent foods, such as peppers, to encourage the body to eliminate waste more easily.*

THE BODY MASS INDEX

• The Body Mass Index (BMI) is reached by dividing your weight in kilograms by your height in meters squared. So, if you weigh 80kg. and are 2m. tall, your BMI is 80 divided by 2x2 – 80 divided by 4 – which is 20. The graphic below shows how the index works.

• If you have a BMI of 27 or more, you double the risk of high blood pressure, heart disease, and gallstones, and are 14 times more likely to contract diabetes.

• If it is over 30, you have 4 times the risk of heart disease, high blood pressure, and gallstones, and are 30–50 times more likely to contract diabetes. You are also 4 times more likely to get degenerative arthritis.

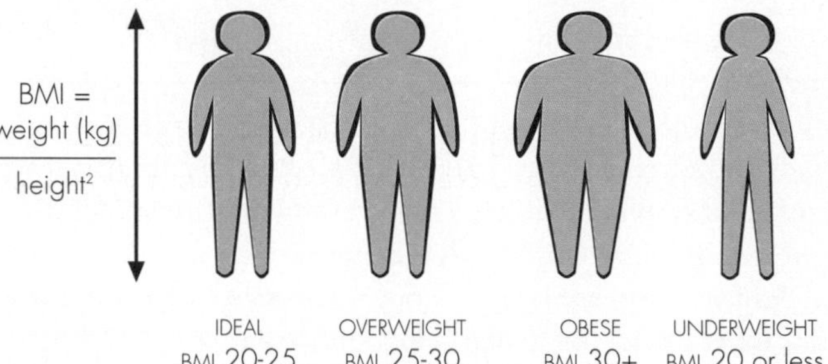

ABOVE *People are judged to be obese if they weigh more than 20 percent above their ideal body weight*

DATA FILE

• Affects approximately 20–30 percent of the U.S. population.

• Fat should account for up to 25 percent of body weight in a healthy woman, and 17 percent in a healthy man.

• At least one-third of Americans are 20 percent or more overweight.

• 25–50 percent of adult Americans are currently on a diet; $30 billion is spent on diet aids annually.

• One in every four U.S. teenagers carries enough weight to put them at risk of later health problems.

• Individuals who weigh more than 20 percent above their supposed "ideal body weight" according to the standard height and weight tables of the Metropolitan Life Insurance Company may be judged as obese.

• Obesity may be classified according to the age of onset, family history, degree of obesity, and adipose tissue cell size and distribution.

• Obesity significantly increases the risk of premature death, heart attack, diabetes mellitus, hypertension, atherosclerosis, gall bladder disease, osteoarthritis, and certain cancers.

• Obese individuals with an apple shape (fat in the upper body or abdomen) are at greater risk of medical diseases than those with a pear shape (fat confined to the lower body or hips).

TREATMENT

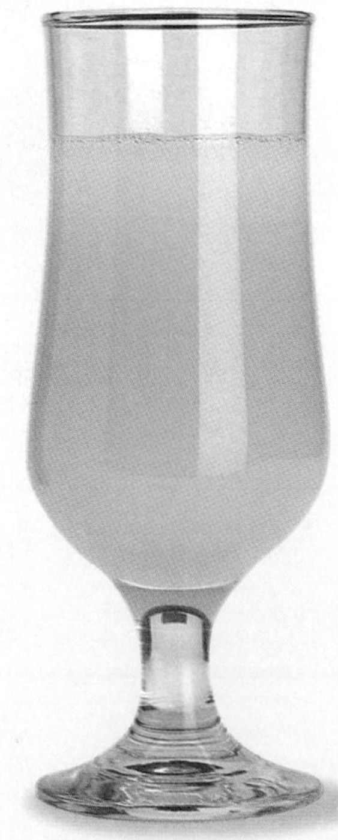

ABOVE *A daily glass of grapefruit juice will suppress the appetite and help break down fats.*

AYURVEDA

• Treatment would be aimed at addressing an addiction to food, accompanied by marma puncture and a diet modified to your dosha type. *(See page 22.)*

• A complete detoxification will encourage weight loss naturally.

CHINESE HERBALISM

• Increase your intake of foods that are bitter, pungent, astringent, and hot, which will encourage your body to eliminate waste more efficiently.

• Cut down on salty, sweet, and sour foods.

TRADITIONAL HOME AND FOLK REMEDIES

• Drink a glass of freshly squeezed grapefruit juice every morning to cleanse, help break down fats, and suppress appetite. *(See page 88.)*

HERBALISM

• Bladderwrack may help to encourage the metabolism. *(See page 122.)*

• Nettles are good diuretics and generally help the metabolism. Try drinking nettle tea before meals. *(See page 137.)*

HOMEOPATHY

Constitutional treatment is most appropriate, but some of the following remedies might be useful:

• Graphites, if you suffer from constipation and skin problems, and feel cold. *(See page 196.)*

• Kali carb., if you are clogged with catarrh, have backache, and feel cold.

• Ferr. phos., if you are oversensitive and flush easily. *(See page 194.)*

• Capsicum, if you are lazy, have a red face, and suffer from burning sensations in the digestive tract.

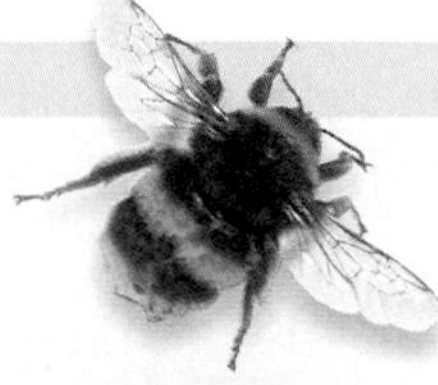

ABOVE *A teaspoon of bee pollen will stimulate the body's metabolism.*

• Calcarea, if you suffer from indigestion, and crave hot food and eggs. *(See page 186.)*

VITAMINS AND MINERALS

• Bee pollen stimulates the metabolism and helps to curb appetite. Take up to 1 teaspoon daily. *(See page 271.)*

• Brewer's yeast will help to reduce various cravings for food and drink. *(See page 272.)*

• Chromium supplements will help to ensure that your blood sugar levels are stable, and regulate appetite. *(See page 259.)*

• Phenylalanine, taken on an empty stomach before bed, encourages weight loss. *(See page 268.)*

Gout

Gout is an acute disease of the joints. It is caused by the deposition of chalky crystals around the joints, tendons, and other body tissues when there is an abnormally high level of uric acid in the body. Severe inflammation and tissue damage result, and possibly structural damage to the kidneys and stone formation. Gout affects more than 1 million Americans, mostly men between the ages of 40 and 50. Primary gout appears to involve a hereditary factor.

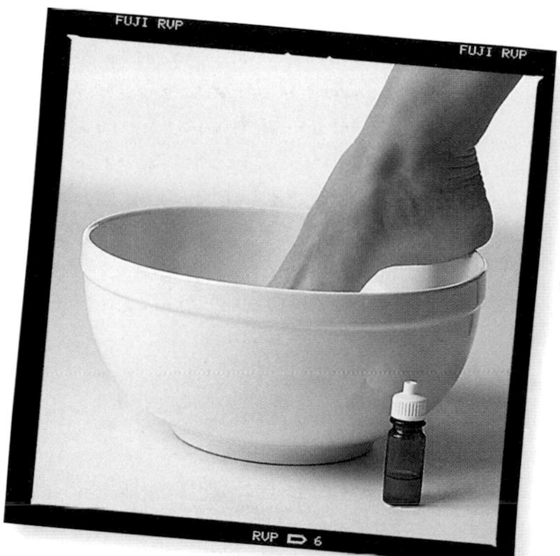

LEFT *Add a few drops of a recommended essential oil such as pine to a foot bath. This will increase the circulation and relieve the painful symptoms associated with gout.*

SYMPTOMS

The first sign of gout is usually excruciating pain and inflammation of the innermost joint of the big toe (or, less frequently, the ankle, knee joint, hand, wrist, or elbow). An attack can last for days or weeks, and then subsides, but usually there are recurrences, until eventually gout is a constant presence.

TREATMENT

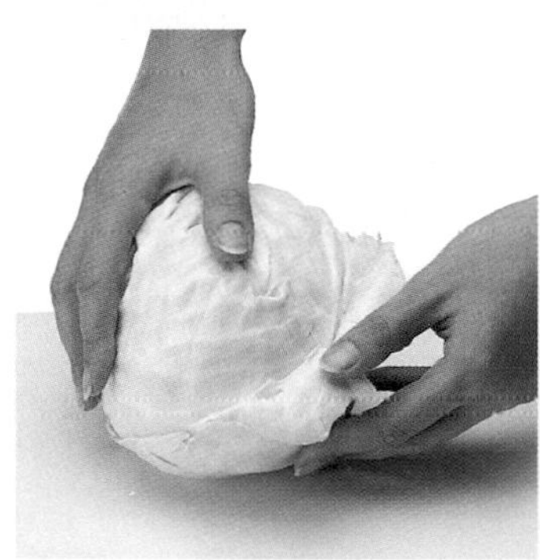

To make a soothing compress, take a few cabbage leaves.

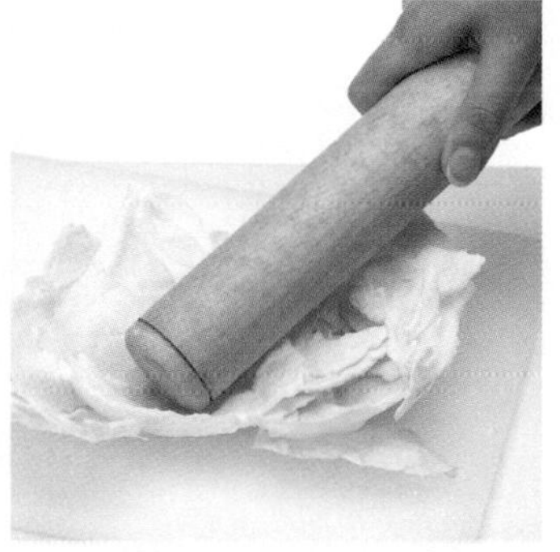

Crush the leaves with a rolling pin. Apply in a compress to the inflamed area.

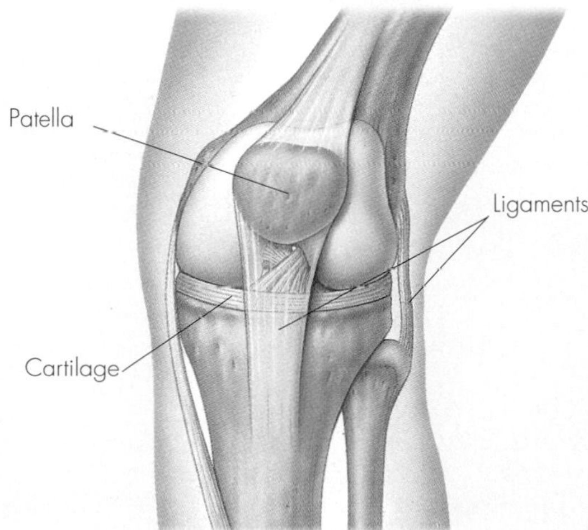

ABOVE *The symptoms of gout include acute pain in the affected joints as a result of uric acid deposits.*

CHINESE HERBALISM
• Painful joints are said to be caused by Wind Cold, and some of the most useful herbs to relieve Cold and Damp include cinnamon, aconite root, angelica root, and wild ginger.
(See pages 56 and 59.)

TRADITIONAL HOME AND FOLK REMEDIES
• Raw apple and cucumber juice will help to reduce the severity and incidence of attacks.
(See pages 89 and 94.)

HERBALISM
• Drink plenty of water and cleansing infusions such as celery seed tea.
• Bring down the acute inflammation with a compress made of crushed cabbage leaf.
• Nettle tea is helpful in preventing attacks.
(See page 137.)

AROMATHERAPY
• Rub a few drops of lavender and frankincense, mixed in a little grapeseed oil, into the affected joints.
(See pages 146–71.)
• Pine, rosemary, or juniper oils, which increase circulation, can be added to the bath or added to a foot-bath to ease the condition. Rub them neat into the affected joints.
(See pages 146–71.)

HOMEOPATHY
Homeopathic treatment would be constitutional, but in an attack one of the following remedies may be appropriate:
• Pulsatilla, for fleeting pains. *(See page 209.)*
• Lycopodium, for symptoms that are worse between 4–8P.M.
(See page 203.)
• Urtica, for joints that feel hot and itchy.
(See page 217.)
• Arnica, for painful joints which feel bruised.
(See page 182.)
• Ledum, for joints that are cold and swollen, and are improved by moving about. *(See page 202.)*

VITAMINS AND MINERALS
• A good diet is the key. Eat plenty of fresh, green vegetables and avoid high-protein foods such as red meat and sea- food.
• Eat food containing plenty of vitamin C (or take supplements of 1g. daily). *(See page 256.)*
• Avoid alcohol, which increases uric acid.
• Charcoal tablets may help to reduce the levels of uric acid in the body.
(See page 273.)

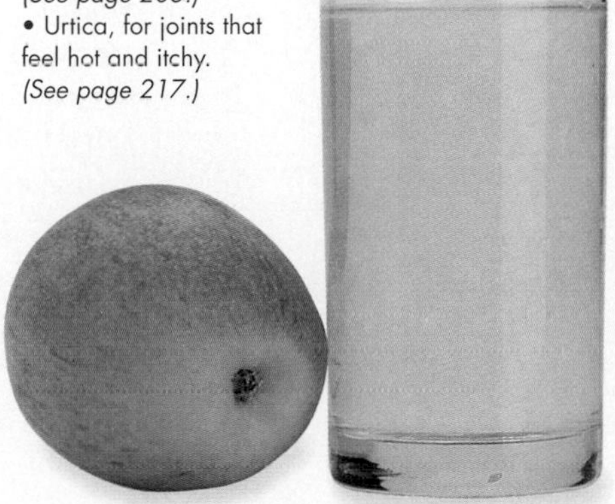

RIGHT *A change of diet will help symptoms of gout to subside. Include fresh fruit and plenty of water.*

DISORDERS OF THE IMMUNE SYSTEM

HIV and AIDS

HIV is the human immunodeficiency virus, which makes the immune system unable to fight off infections. HIV is believed to be responsible for AIDS (acquired immune deficiency syndrome). Once acquired, HIV remains in the body for life, although there may be no symptoms for years. HIV may be contracted from transfusion of contaminated blood; from infected blood passing through the skin barrier via a deep graze, needle puncture, or a wound; in the womb or at birth; by breast-feeding; or through unsafe sex. When the immune system reaches a particular stage of deterioration due to HIV, certain bacteria which are usually kept in check by healthy immune functioning are able to thrive (opportunistic infections). AIDS is diagnosed when one or more of these infections is present, but AIDS is not a disease in itself. Previously an AIDS diagnosis suggested that death would follow quickly, but improvement in drugs treatments may change the implications of an AIDS diagnosis.

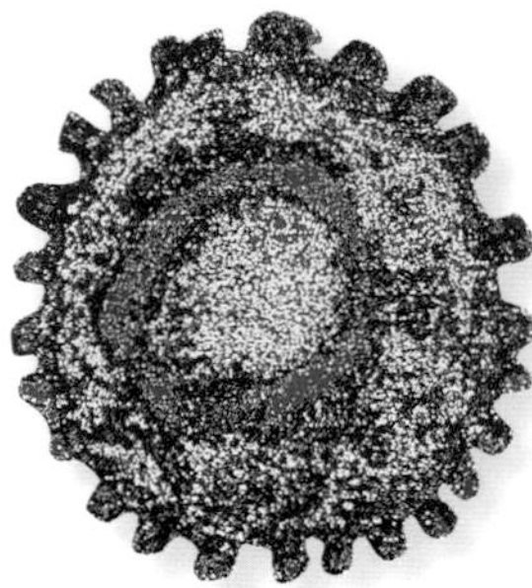

ABOVE *The HIV virus, which weakens the human immune system, leaving it open to infection.*

DATA FILE

- Since the first AIDS cases were reported in 1981, through mid-1995, more than 476,000 AIDS cases and more than 295,000 deaths have been reported in the U.S.
- Nearly 1 million Americans were infected with HIV through the mid-1990s but do not yet have clinical symptoms.
- AIDS cases have also been reported in almost every country in the world, with an estimated cumulative 19 million adults and children infected worldwide since the late 1970s.
- Many of those infected with HIV may not even be aware that they carry and can spread the virus.
- 90 percent of HIV-positive children under the age of 13 acquired HIV from their infected mothers; around one child in twelve born to infected women is HIV-positive. All babies born to infected mothers will test positive for HIV at birth, because the test is for antibodies to HIV and the baby has the mother's antibodies in its blood. Babies who test positive after 18 months (when the baby has developed its own antibodies) are actually infected with the virus.
- The period between initial infection and production of antibodies is three to six months.
- Estimates indicate that somewhere between 26–46 percent of the infected individuals will go on to develop AIDS within a little more than seven years following infection with HIV.
- Once AIDS is diagnosed, the clinical course generally follows a rapid decline; most people with AIDS die within three years. However, recent scientific advances in triple-drug therapy may extend life expectancy.

Symptoms

• flu-like symptoms when HIV first enters the system (seroconversion) • once the virus has begun to work on the immune system there will be: – night sweats and fevers – exhaustion – weight loss – diarrhea – thrush and herpes – mouth ulcers and bleeding gums • conditions associated with AIDS itself include: – neurological problems – fits and confusion – yellow skin and swollen painful joints – Kaposi's sarcoma, a rare form of skin cancer characterized by raised purple blotches – eye infections, particularly cytomegalovirus (CMV), which can lead to blindness – gut infections – pneumocystis carinii pneumonia (PCP)

TREATMENT

CHINESE HERBALISM

- Tonic herbs, such as astragalus, ganoderma, and ginseng will help your overall constitution. *(See page 57 and 67.)*
- Salvia, millettia, and peony will improve the Blood and help promote good circulation. *(See page 67.)*
- Chinese angelica can restore energy and stimulate white blood cells and antibody formation. *(See page 56.)*

HERBALISM

Treatment will always be tailored to the individual, but there are a number of herbs which can be used to boost immunity, including:

- Licorice, to enhance recovery, stimulating the formation and efficiency of white blood cells and antibodies. It is also useful in preventing stress. *(See page 122.)*
- Garlic, to prevent infections of all kinds, including those which have now become immune to antibiotics. *(See page 113.)*
- Echinacea, widely prescribed for treatment of chronic and acute infections – it cleanses the blood and lymphatic system, stimulating production of white blood cells and antibodies. *(See page 120.)*
- Ginseng, to boost immunity and encourage the body to deal efficiently with stress, as well as stimulating white blood cell production, and aiding recovery after illness. *(See page 126.)*

AROMATHERAPY

- Antiviral oils include tea tree, niaouli, eucalyptus, and thyme, and they can be used in any form – lymphatic massage is particularly recommended for its ability to stimulate the immune system. *(See pages 146–71.)*
- Lavender, tea tree, and bergamot stimulate production of white blood cells, and are active against one or more bacteria and viruses. *(See pages 146–71.)*
- Tea tree in particular has antiviral, antibacterial, and fungicidal properties, with a stimulating action on the immune system. *(See page 162.)*
- Mood-enhancing and uplifting oils, such as bergamot, lavender, geranium, rose, sandalwood, and ylang ylang, may be useful. *(See pages 146–71.)*

HOMEOPATHY

- Homeopathic remedies are designed to encourage the immune system to fight for itself, increasing the number of white blood cells in the body, and allowing you to reach a state of mental and emotional balance, which makes your body more responsive. Constitutional treatment is often aimed at the present ailment, as well as tendencies and symptoms which have not yet become proper ailments. Your homeopath will suggest improved nutrition, fresh air, exercise, and rest, which can restore the ability of the immune system to cope. Homeopathic remedies will be prescribed in conjunction with this advice.

VITAMINS AND MINERALS

- Include a variety of vegetables each day, with wholegrain cereals like brown rice and whole wheat bread, fruit, pulses (beans and lentils), and a few nuts and seeds for their oils.
- A daily multivitamin and multimineral preparation – especially one containing high amounts of the antioxidant nutrients – acts to boost immune activity. *(See page 251.)*
- Vitamin C stimulates immunity and is antiviral. *(See page 256.)*
- Acidophilus will encourage the healthy bacteria in your gut, which will help to fight off infections and infestations. *(See page 271.)*
- Zinc stimulates the immune system, and acts as an antiviral agent. *(See page 265.)*

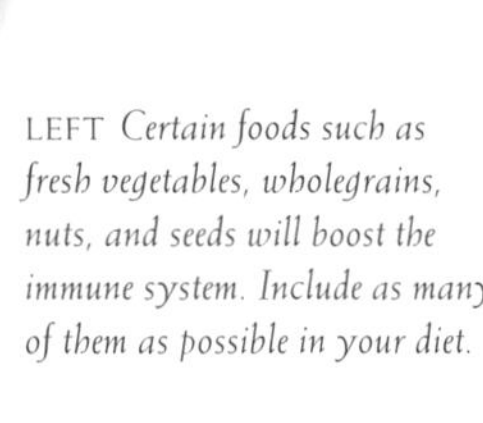

LEFT *Certain foods such as fresh vegetables, wholegrains, nuts, and seeds will boost the immune system. Include as many of them as possible in your diet.*

Glandular Fever

Glandular fever, or infectious mononucleosis as it is also known, is caused by the Epstein-Barr virus (a herpes virus). The virus multiplies in the white blood cells, eventually harming the immune system's efficiency. Glandular fever is usually transmitted via saliva, hence its nickname of the "kissing disease." While symptoms may last for only six weeks, recovery is slow and fatigue and low energy levels may linger for months. The disease occurs most commonly in adults 15–30 years old, and one attack confers immunity.

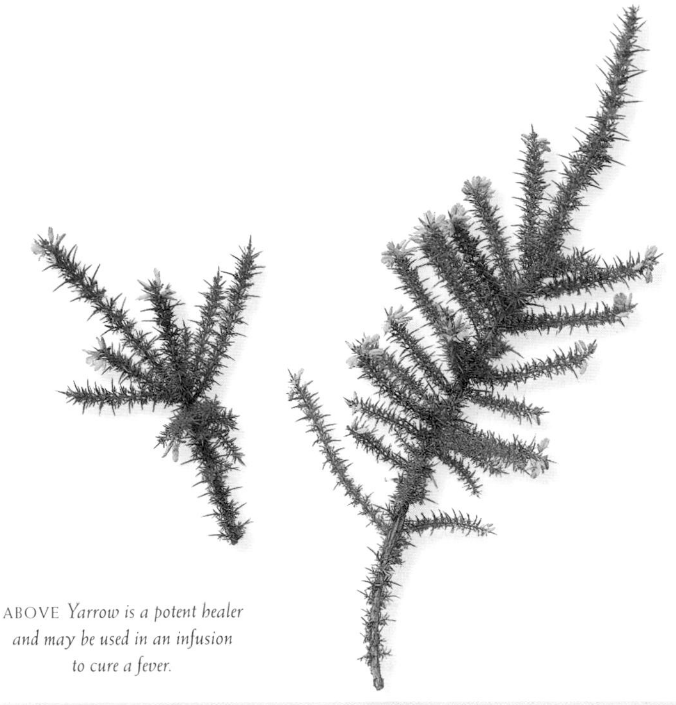

ABOVE *Yarrow is a potent healer and may be used in an infusion to cure a fever.*

Symptoms

• *flu-like symptoms, including fever, sore throat, headache* • *fatigue and lethargy* • *swollen lymph glands in the neck, armpits, and groin* • *a rash of small, slightly raised red spots* • *chest pain, with breathing difficulty and a cough* • *enlarged spleen and possibly damaged liver, causing jaundice*

BELOW *For an easy home remedy for glandular fever, try applying apple cider vinegar to the neck glands.*

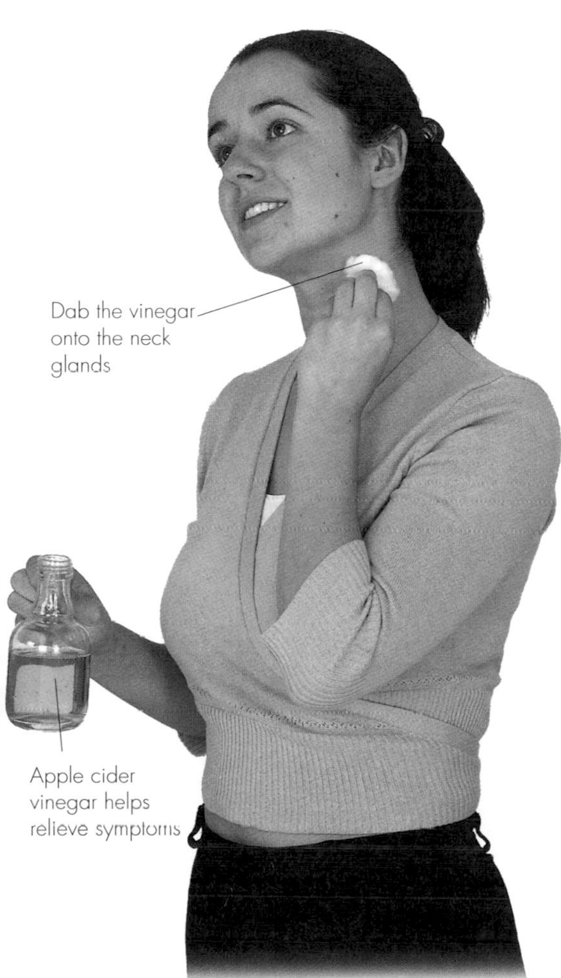

Dab the vinegar onto the neck glands

Apple cider vinegar helps relieve symptoms

Treatment

Chinese Herbalism

• Tonic herbs such as astragalus, ganoderma, and ginseng will help your overall constitution. *(See pages 57 and 67.)*

• Salvia, millettia, and peony will improve the Blood, and give the circulation a boost. *(See page 67.)*

• Chinese angelica can restore energy and stimulate white blood cells and antibody formation. *(See page 56.)*

Traditional Home and Folk Remedies

• Apply apple cider vinegar to the neck glands daily. Drink it in a cup of warm water to encourage healing. *(See page 102.)*

• Ginseng acts to balance the glands. Chew the fresh or dried root, or add the powder to hot herbal teas. It will prevent fatigue and stimulate you.

Herbalism

• Herbs to promote healing include cleavers, echinacea, and nettles, all of which stimulate immune activity as well as fighting infection. *(See pages 120 and 137.)*

• Balm, oats, and skullcap, if depression accompanies the fever. *(See pages 117 and 131.)*

• Infusions of yarrow and elderflower will help to control fever and also induce sweating. *(See pages 112 and 130.)*

Aromatherapy

• Essential oils can be used in the bath, or in massage, which also has therapeutic benefits. Oils to consider are eucalyptus, lavender, rosemary, and tea tree, which will encourage immune activity and fight the virus. *(See pages 146–71.)*

Homeopathy

Constitutional treatment is recommended, but the following remedies may be useful, taken up to six times daily, for two days.

• Belladonna, for sudden high fever, with a reddish face and agitation. *(See page 183.)*

• Mercurius, for tender glands and smelly sweat. *(See page 205.)*

• Calcarea, for chilliness, sweating, a sour taste in the mouth, and fatigue. *(See page 186.)*

• Cistus, for a chilly feeling, with painful neck and glands, exacerbated by cold air and mental exertion.

• Baryta carb., for swollen glands. This is particularly useful for children. *(See page 185.)*

Flower Essences

• Flower essences are often used by practitioners to help you cope with the physical and emotional effects of glandular fever.

• Olive will help if you feel exhausted on all levels. *(See page 235.)*

• Mustard controls feelings of depression that have no identifiable cause. *(See page 239.)*

• Gorse will help with feelings of hopelessness. *(See page 240.)*

Vitamins and Minerals

• Take extra vitamin C, B-complex, and zinc. *(See pages 256, 252–5, and 265.)*

• Evening primrose oil will help to encourage healing. *(See page 270.)*

• Royal jelly will help fight feelings of fatigue and depression, and stimulate the immune system. *(See page 276.)*

• Eat plenty of foods containing antioxidants. *(See page 251.)*

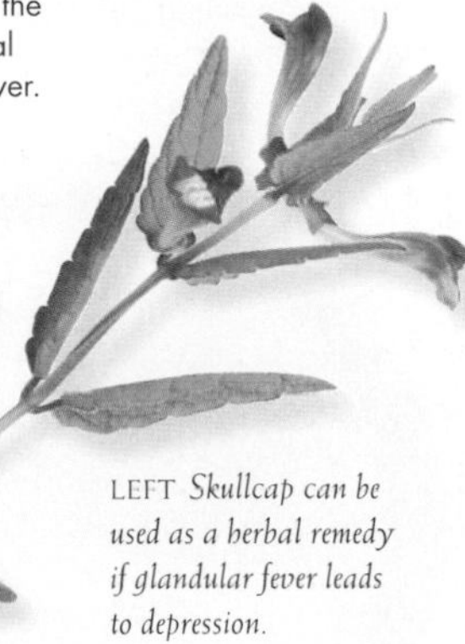

LEFT *Skullcap can be used as a herbal remedy if glandular fever leads to depression.*

Allergies

An allergy is the immune system's abnormal response to contact with a specific substance. The system overreacts when faced with foreign substances or organisms – allergens – and deals with them as if they were harmful, as it would with invading bacteria, for example. The result is an allergic reaction, also known as a histamine reaction (histamine being the substance produced in response to attack). Common allergens include certain foods, grass pollens, spores, fabrics, drugs, household chemicals, and stress. Some of the most common allergic responses are urticaria (*see page 303*), dermatitis (*see page 300*), asthma (*see page 344*) and hay fever/rhinitis (*see page 330*). An estimated 35 million people in the United States suffer from various allergies, some of which are mistaken for the common cold.

BELOW *Dermatitis is a common allergy. It is characterized by red, itchy patches on the skin.*

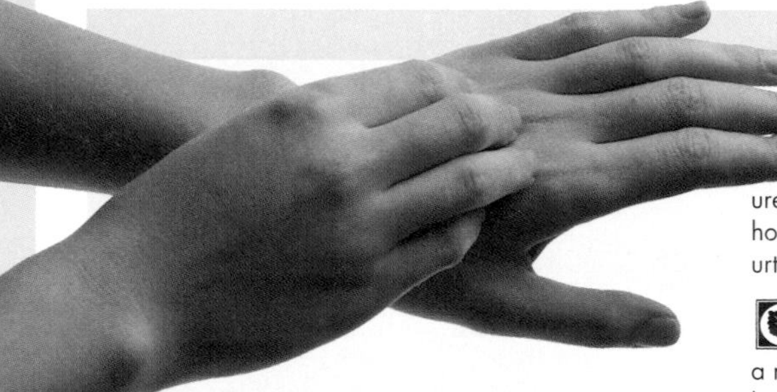

SYMPTOMS

RED CLOVER

• sneezing and runny nose • wheezing • excess catarrh • urticaria • anaphylactic shock (sometimes fatal), causing breathing difficulty, edema, constriction of air tubes, and heart failure

TREATMENT

AYURVEDA

• Cleansing and detoxification will be followed by a varied diet of organic foods.

• Herbal preparations to boost immunity may be appropriate, including Chebulic myrobalan (Harithaki), which helps in cases of eczema; bitter orange for asthma and other respiratory allergies; and stramonium. *(See page 22.)*

CHINESE HERBALISM

• Bi Yan Pian/Nose inflammation pills, for Wind Cold or Wind Heat to the face, indicated by sneezing, itchy eyes, facial congestion and sinus pain, acute and chronic rhinitis, and nasal allergies. Herbal prescriptions will be offered. *(See page 52.)*

• Yu Ping Feng San/Jade screen helps prevent hay fever and guards against allergies.

• Cang Er Zi Tang/ xanthium powder, for allergic rhinitis, with thick yellow catarrh or blocked nose.

TRADITIONAL HOME AND FOLK REMEDIES

• Eat the local honey if you suffer from hay fever. *(See page 101.)*

• Honey and apple cider can be drunk in a glass of warm water to restore and prevent allergies. *(See pages 101 and 102.)*

• Drink nettle tea to increase resistance.

• Apply nettle tea to skin, or use Urtica urens cream or homeopathic remedy for urticaria.

HERBALISM

• Echinacea acts as a natural antibiotic while building the immune system. Take three times daily, as an infusion, or a few drops of tincture in a glass of warm water, during attacks or when you are run down. *(See page 120.)*

• Other useful herbs include chamomile, elderflower, red clover, yarrow. *(See pages 112, 119, and 130.)*

• Add a small amount of ginseng powder to herbal drinks to overcome the tendency to allergic attacks, such as hay fever. *(See page 126.)*

• Eat the local honey in a cup of warm water with 2 tablespoons of apple cider vinegar to reduce the reaction to allergens. This is particularly useful during the hay fever season.

• Herbs to boost immunity include garlic, angelica, borage, wild yam. *(See pages 113, 115, and 120.)*

• Strengthen the weakened area with tonic teas, 2 cups taken over a period of time: the sinuses with elderflower tea; the stomach with chamomile, linden, and a warming digestive like cardamom; the skin with chamomile washes and rosemary in the bath. *(See pages 119, 127, and 134.)*

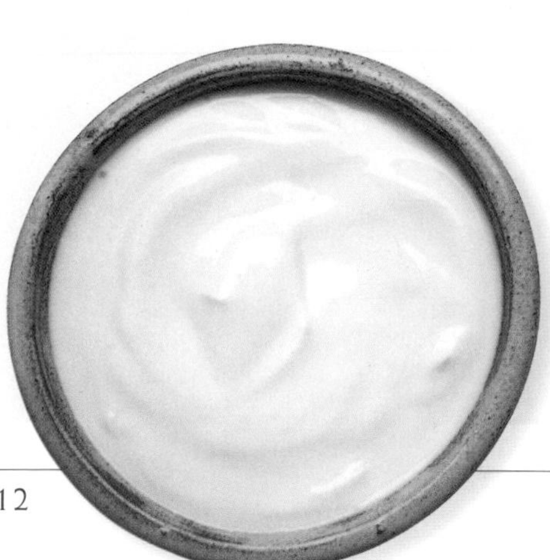

LEFT *Live natural yogurt will encourage the growth of beneficial bacteria in the gut.*

AROMATHERAPY

• Place a few drops of Roman chamomile in a vaporizer or on a light bulb to treat an allergic reaction, including asthma. *(See page 150.)*

• Melissa, in the bath or a vaporizer, soothes and reduces a reaction's severity. *(See page 163.)*

• Lavender essential oil, in a light carrier oil, can be massaged into the chest or other affected area to reduce spasm and generally boost immunity. *(See page 161.)*

HOMEOPATHY

Homeopathic treatment has proved to be very successful in the treatment of allergies. Remedies will be prescribed according to your individual case, so it is best to see a registered practitioner to ensure that prescription is exact.

• Urtica, for urticaria. *(See page 217.)*

• Pulsatilla or Arg. nit., for relief of conjunctivitis. *(See page 209.)*

• Apis, for bee stings. *(See page 180.)*

Anaphylactic shock is a medical emergency, and you must summon emergency medical care immediately. The following remedies can be given until help arrives:

• Aconite, when the patient is frightened and restless. *(See page 178.)*

• Veratrum, when the skin is cold and mottled, and the victim is in a cold sweat.

• Arnica, for shock brought on by injury. *(See page 182.)*

FLOWER ESSENCES

• If suffering a sudden allergic reaction, take Rescue Remedy or Emergency Essence. *(See page 244.)*

VITAMINS AND MINERALS

• Take steps to boost immunity, by increasing intake of magnesium (seafood, beans, and nuts), B vitamins (yeast extract, meat, or yeast), zinc (eggs, nuts, and seeds), vitamin A (fish and yellow and green vegetables), iron (liver, sesame seeds, and dried fruit) and vitamin C (fresh fruit and vegetables). *(See pages 262, 252–5, 265, 252, 260, and 256.)*

• A diet high in protein will help to build up immunity, while roughage from fruit, vegetables, nuts, seeds, and pulses will keep the digestive tract working and encourage the growth of beneficial bacteria in the gut (called flora), which helps the body to resist infection.

• Acidophilus, taken daily, will also work to encourage bowel health. *(See page 271.)*

• Evening primrose oil and blackcurrant seed oil are rich sources of essential fatty acids, which can prevent allergies in susceptible people. *(See page 270.)*

• Pollen supplements are useful for preventing allergies, in particular hay fever. *(See page 271.)*

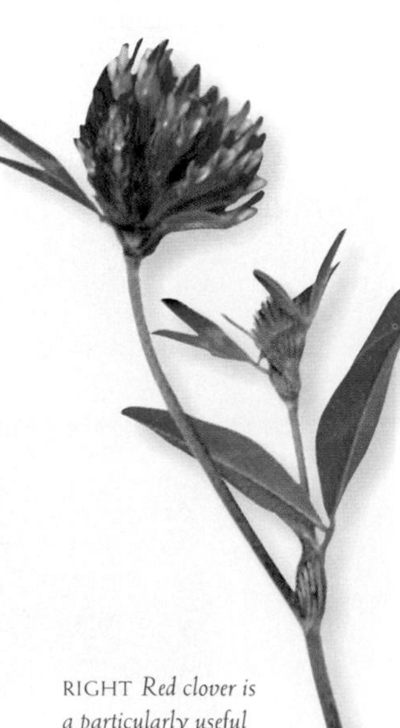

RIGHT *Red clover is a particularly useful remedy for skin allergies.*

Hodgkin's Disease

Hodgkin's disease (or Hodgkin's lymphoma) is a cancer that attacks the lymphatic tissue and the lymph nodes in particular. As the tissue becomes more and more damaged, relatively minor infections may become life-threatening. Late in the disease's development the bone marrow may also be affected. The cause of Hodgkin's is unknown, although it is thought that cancer-causing viruses are involved. In the United States, about 30 people out of every million have this ailment; it is more common in males between the ages of 20 and 40, although both sexes can suffer from the condition. Untreated, Hodgkin's disease is invariably fatal. *(See also Cancer, page 457)*

Symptoms

• *painless enlargement of lymph nodes, which acquire a rubbery feel* • *liver and spleen enlargement* • *anemia and fever* • *appetite and weight loss* • *night sweats* • *possible secondary effects caused by pressure on other structures from enlarged nodes: – neurological damage – obstruction to veins – difficulty in swallowing and breathing – jaundice*

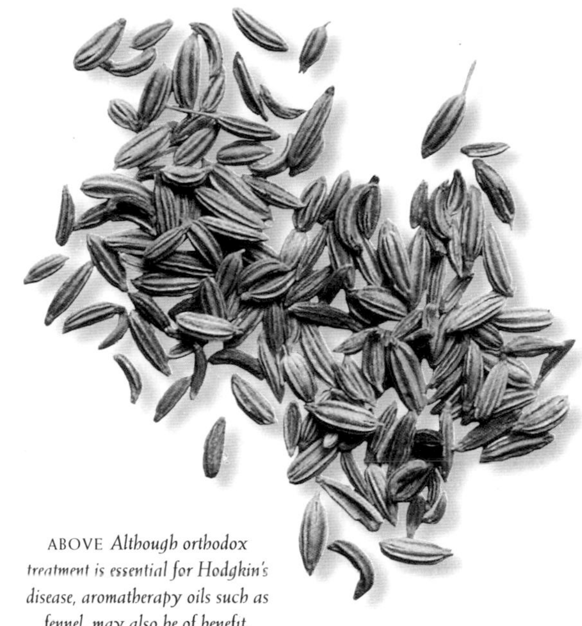

ABOVE *Although orthodox treatment is essential for Hodgkin's disease, aromatherapy oils such as fennel, may also be of benefit.*

TREATMENT

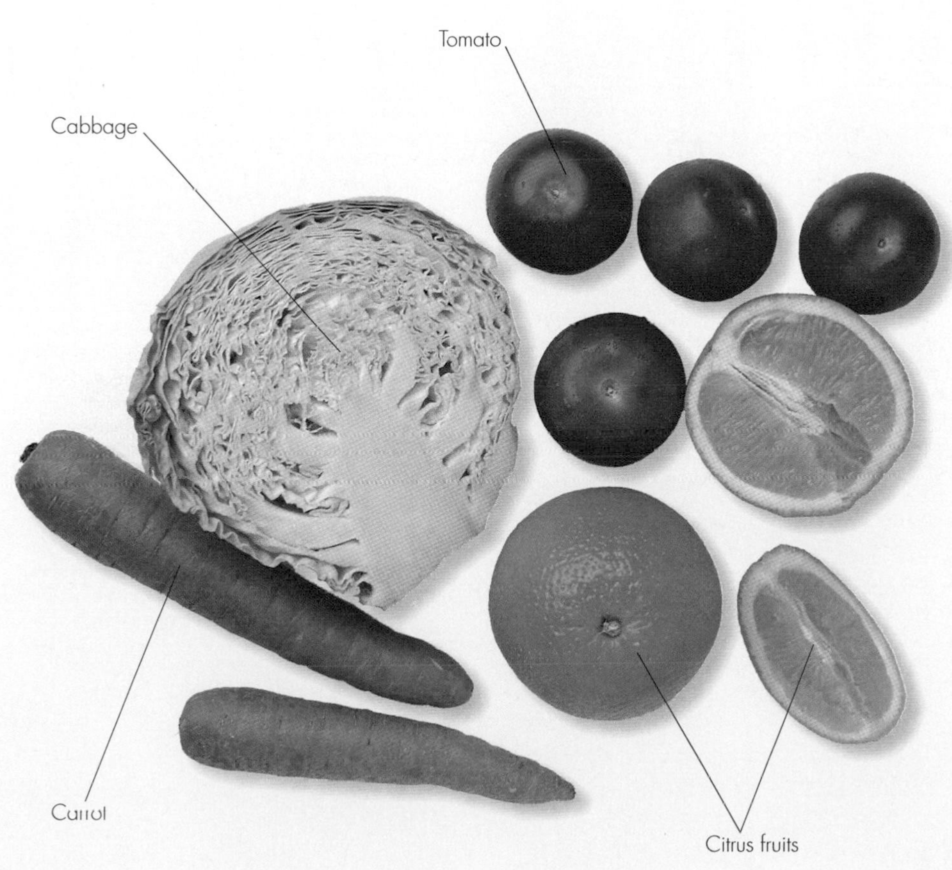

LEFT *Eat foods that contain antioxidants to strengthen your immune system.*

AROMATHERAPY

• Extra treatments to try are fennel, garlic, juniper, and rose, which can be used in the bath or in a vaporizer to detoxify the body. *(See pages 146–71.)*

• Tea tree and lavender essential oils strengthen the body's defenses. *(See pages 161 and 162.)*

• Oils which strengthen the action of the adrenals include geranium and rosemary, along with peppermint and thyme. *(See pages 146–71.)*

VITAMINS AND MINERALS

• Eat as much fresh fruit and vegetables as you can, paying particular attention to those containing antioxidants. *(See page 251.)*

• Reduce your intake of animal fats and avoid processed foods.

• A deficiency of vitamin C has been found in conjunction with certain tumors. Ensure you get plenty in your diet. *(See page 256.)*

• Vitamin A can protect against cancer in smokers to some degree. *(See page 252.)*

• Digestive enzymes may be offered to halt activities of trophoblastic cancer cells.

• Vitamin E is said to prevent a number of cancers. Ensure that you get plenty in your diet or take supplements. *(See page 257.)*

DISORDERS OF THE MUSCULOSKELETAL SYSTEM

Osteoporosis

In osteoporosis (meaning porous bones) the bones lose their density, becoming fragile and brittle. This is caused by alterations, with age, of the amounts of the various growth and sex hormones which control chemical changes in the bones, leading to progressive calcium and protein loss. Osteoporosis affects women more than men, and may be triggered or accelerated by a sedentary lifestyle, loss of activity, a low-calcium diet, smoking, heavy alcohol consumption, hereditary factors, or prolonged lack of estrogen. An overactive thyroid gland, chronic liver disease, and prolonged use of corticosteroids all predispose a person to osteoporosis.

DATA FILE

- Bone mass reaches a peak in women between the ages of 30 and 45; between the ages of 55 and 70, a woman will have lost 30–40 percent of her bone mass.
- Most common in white women after menopause.
- Affects more women than heart disease, stroke, diabetes, breast cancer, and arthritis.
- 50 percent of women between the ages of 45 and 75 suffer from some osteoporosis; 30 percent of these suffer from serious bone deterioration.
- Costs approximately $3.8 billion in treatment in the U.S. each year.
- Aggravated by a variety of factors, including smoking, excessive alcohol consumption, and a sedentary lifestyle.
- A dowager's hump is an abnormal curvature of the spine in the upper back. Typically affecting older women, the curvature is a result of collapse of the spinal column, caused by osteoporosis.

SYMPTOMS

- *loss of height from shrinkage of the spinal bones*
- *sudden breakage of a bone in the spine, with severe pain and disfigurement*
- *reduced ribcage movement, causing shortness of breath and pain*
- *wrist, forearm, neck, or hip fractures resulting from minor stumbles or falls*

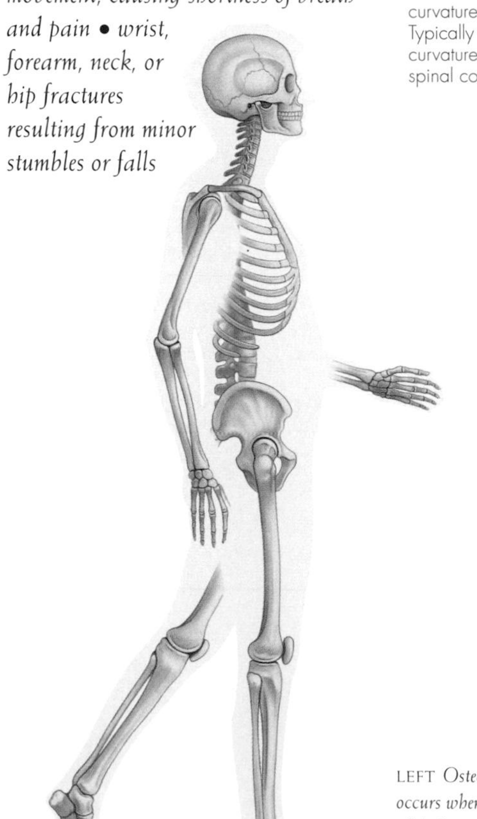

LEFT *Osteoporosis occurs when the density of the bones is reduced, causing them to become thin and weak.*

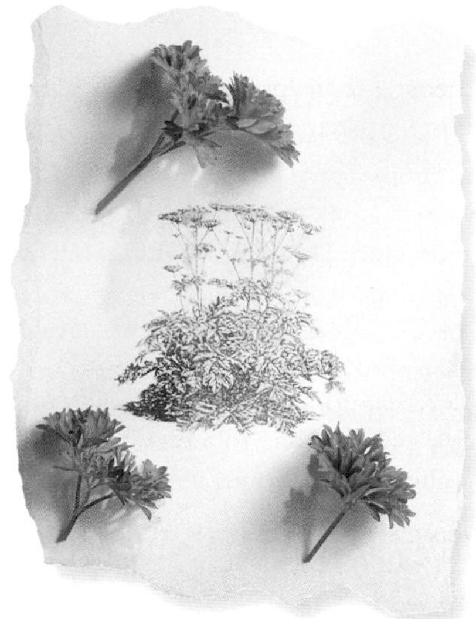

LEFT *Drink an infusion of parsley as a herbal remedy for osteoporosis. Its high calcium content will be of benefit.*

TREATMENT

CHINESE HERBALISM

- The condition is believed to be caused by Kidney Deficiency, and can be treated with cibot rhizome, drynaria tuber, and eucommia bark. *(See page 63.)*
- Cinnamon twigs will help to reduce pain. *(See page 59.)*

HERBALISM

- Drink a cup of comfrey leaf and bay leaf tea three times a day. *(See page 132.)*
- Many herbs, such as hops or sage, contain estrogen-like substances which can protect the bones against loss. *(See page 129.)*
- If you are in pain, use analgesic herbs such as white willow, meadowsweet, or wild yam. *(See pages 120, 121, and 129.)*
- Herbs that contain calcium include nettles, parsley, dandelion leaves, kelp, and horsetail, which can be drunk as often as possible. *(See pages 120, 122, 133, and 137.)*
- Take estrogenic herbs, which discourage the loss of calcium from the bones, including calendula, ginseng, false unicorn root, sage, hops, blue cohosh, wild yam, and licorice. *(See pages 120, 122, 126, and 129.)*
- Herbs which encourage the digestion and absorption of minerals from food include yellow dock root, rosemary, wormwood, and yarrow. *(See pages 112, 127, and 128.)*

HOMEOPATHY

Constitutional treatment will be necessary, but the following remedies may be useful to deal with bone pain:

- Ruta grav., for pain at the nape of the neck and in the lumbar region. *(See page 210.)*
- Aurum, for pains that are worse at night, mainly in the skull, nose, or palate. *(See page 184.)*
- Calcarea phos., for limbs that feel achy, numb, and chilly. *(See page 186.)*
- Fluoric ac., for stabbing pain.

VITAMINS AND MINERALS

- Recent evidence suggests that an increased intake of magnesium may help prevent the worst effects of osteoporosis. Magnesium sources include soybeans, nuts, and brewer's yeast. *(See page 262.)*
- Calcium can also be very helpful. Recommended doses are between 1,000mg. and 1,500mg. a day. *(See page 258.)*
- Vitamin D helps the body absorb calcium. *(See page 256.)*
- Increase your intake of foods containing boron, which reduces the body's excretion of calcium and magnesium, and increases the production of estrogen. *(See page 258.)*
- Fluoride may be useful for preventing and treating the condition because it stimulates new bone formation. *(See page 260.)*

Rheumatism

Rheumatism is a very general term applied to aches, pains, and stiffness in bones and muscles, occurring as a result of viral infection, food allergy, emotional stress, or an underlying joint disease. The following may all come under the umbrella term rheumatism:

- FIBROSITIS *(see page 423)*
- HYPERTHYROIDISM *(see page 405)*
- MYOSITIS, in which inflammation of muscles causes pain and weakness. It may develop from a bacterial or viral infection
- POLYMYALGIA RHEUMATICA, featuring pain and stiffness in the shoulders, neck, back, and arms, possibly due to a blood disorder
- VITAMIN D DEFICIENCY, which causes bone pain and muscle weakness

LEFT *The symptoms of rheumatism may be relieved by chewing horseradish leaves.*

DATA FILE

- Palindromic rheumatism is a disease that causes frequent and irregular attacks of joint pain, especially in the fingers, but leaves no permanent damage to the joints.
- Psychogenic rheumatism is common in women between the ages of 40 and 70, although men also contract this disease. Symptoms include complaints of pain in various parts of the musculoskeletal system that cannot be substantiated medically.
- One of the commonest forms of rheumatism is rheumatoid arthritis, affecting 1–3 percent of the population. Rheumatoid arthritis usually occurs between ages 35 and 40, but can occur at any age. It characteristically follows a course of spontaneous remissions and exacerbations, and in about 10–20 percent of patients remission is permanent.

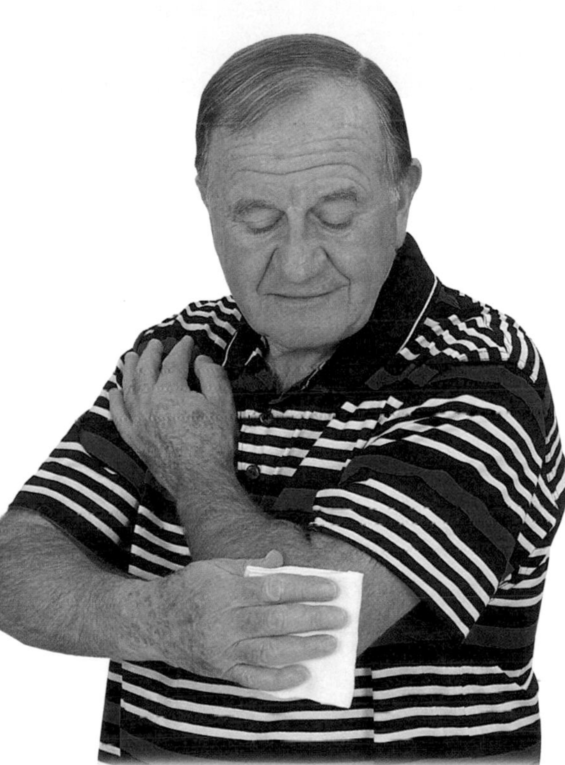

ABOVE *A poultice made from slippery elm may be applied to the part of the body affected by rheumatism.*

TREATMENT

AYURVEDA

- Ginger, coriander, and aloe vera (when there are hot pains) can be used to treat rheumatism. *(See pages 27, 35, and 47.)*
- Angelica is a good tonic and is warming for stiffness and discomfort. *(See page 28.)*
- Barberry, taken as a tea or applied as a compress, can be used to treat rheumatic ailments. *(See page 29.)*
- Basil relieves arthritis and rheumatism. *(See page 42.)*
- Rub calamus oil into the affected joints to improve circulation and drainage. *(See page 24.)*
- Camphor is indicated for arthritis, rheumatism, and many other musculoskeletal problems. *(See page 33.)*

CHINESE HERBALISM

- The condition is thought to be caused by qi stagnation, excess Wind, Damp, and Heat. Chinese herbalists use achyranthus root and cork tree bark. *(See page 68.)*

TRADITIONAL HOME AND FOLK REMEDIES

- Chew a tiny quantity of horseradish leaves, which is said to prevent attacks. *(See page 84.)*

HERBALISM

- Useful herbs, which may be taken internally or applied as a compress to the affected part of the body, include bogbean, feverfew, meadowsweet, and white willow. *(See pages 121, 129, and 133.)*
- Use a little cayenne pepper oil to warm the area and reduce pain and stiffness. *(See page 118.)*
- A poultice of slippery elm may be of benefit. *(See page 136.)*
- An infusion of celery seed may help reduce the level of acid in the blood, which is a contributory factor in rheumatism.

AROMATHERAPY

- Bergamot and myrrh reduce inflammation. Use in the bath, or massage the local area. *(See pages 135 and 153.)*
- There are many oils which can reduce swelling and inflammation and encourage the healing process. Try massage with pine, lemon, or juniper, in a suitable carrier oil. *(See pages 146–71.)*
- Massage with oil of black pepper or eucalyptus can stimulate the circulation and relieve stiffness. *(See pages 159 and 167.)*
- Lavender oil calms pain and helps to relieve stiffness. *(See page 161.)*

HOMEOPATHY

- Aconite, for sharp pains which tend to come on suddenly. *(See page 178.)*
- Bryonia, for pains that are worse in dry cold weather and on movement. *(See page 185)*
- Pulsatilla, for pains that move from joint to joint, and muscle to muscle. *(See page 209.)*
- Rhus tox., for stiffness that is worse in the morning or after rest. *(See page 210.)*
- Mercurius, for pain that is worse at night and for heat. *(See page 205.)*
- Calcarea hypophos., for sharp pains in the wrists and hands.
- Causticum, for pains in the jaw and neck, with spasm. *(See page 189.)*

FLOWER ESSENCES

- Rub a little Rescue Remedy, or the cream, into the affected area. *(See page 244)*

VITAMINS AND MINERALS

- Many cases of rheumatism respond to a dietary change, and it is suggested that the following foods are eaten as often as possible to reduce muscular and joint inflammation: cabbage, celery, turnip, lemon, dandelion, and oily fish.
- Drink plenty of water, which will flush the system and act as a detoxicant.
- Eliminate members of the "nightshade" family of plants from your diet, as these can cause joint problems. These include potatoes, peppers, eggplant (aubergine), and paprika.
- Evening primrose oil is a rich source of gamma-linolenic acid, which is necessary for the production of prostaglandins, which may have an anti-inflammatory effect. *(See page 270.)*

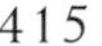

Fractures

A fracture is a break or crack in a bone. It may occur as a result of excessive force through injury (particularly in sport), an accident such as a car crash, or disease. A simple fracture is one where the soft tissue overlying the broken bone is still intact; a compound fracture is one where the skin is damaged so that the fractured bone is exposed and therefore vulnerable to infection. Fractures caused by disease (such as osteoporosis, or a tumor or cyst) are known as pathological fractures. In such cases there is a weakening of bones that predisposes them to break more easily. An estimated 200,000 hip fractures occur in people over the age of 65 each year. The tendency to fracture increases with age.

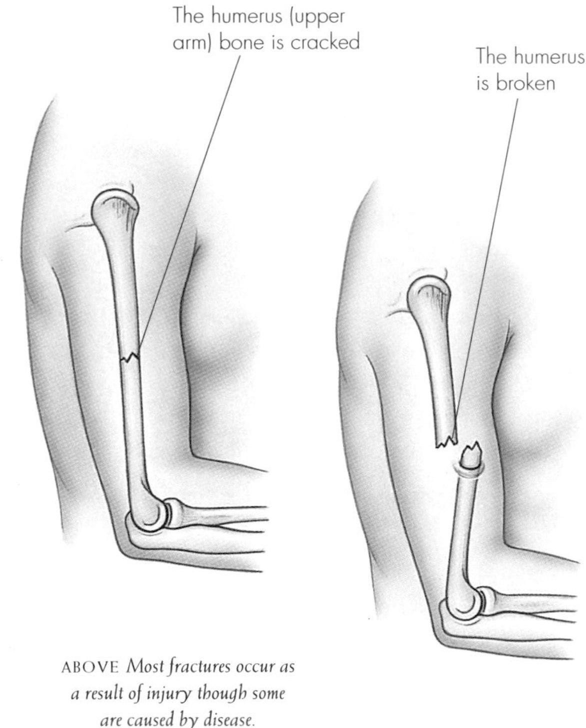

ABOVE *Most fractures occur as a result of injury though some are caused by disease.*

Symptoms

• swelling, pain, and tenderness • inability to move the affected part • possibly a protruding bone, deformity, and discoloration

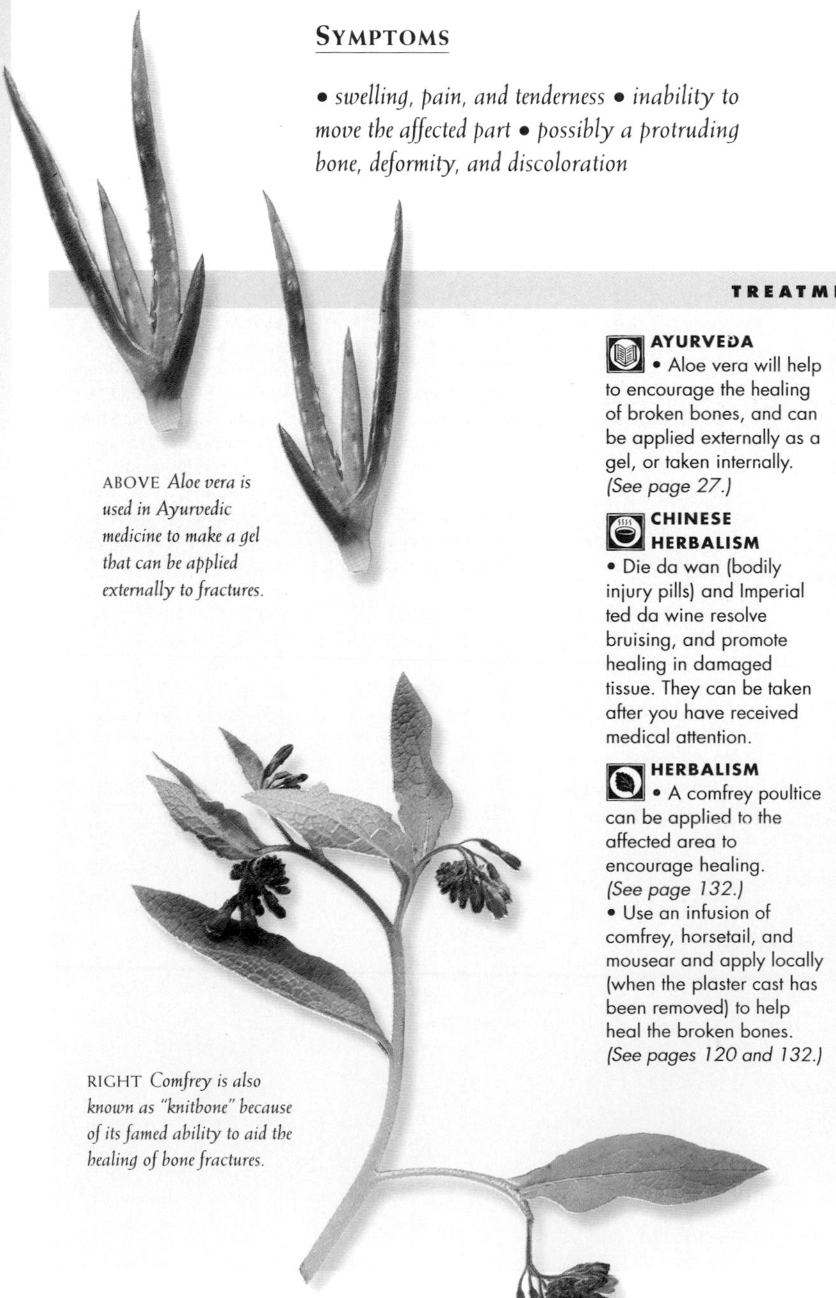

ABOVE *Aloe vera is used in Ayurvedic medicine to make a gel that can be applied externally to fractures.*

RIGHT *Comfrey is also known as "knitbone" because of its famed ability to aid the healing of bone fractures.*

TREATMENT

AYURVEDA

• Aloe vera will help to encourage the healing of broken bones, and can be applied externally as a gel, or taken internally. *(See page 27.)*

CHINESE HERBALISM

• Die da wan (bodily injury pills) and Imperial ted da wine resolve bruising, and promote healing in damaged tissue. They can be taken after you have received medical attention.

HERBALISM

• A comfrey poultice can be applied to the affected area to encourage healing. *(See page 132.)*

• Use an infusion of comfrey, horsetail, and mousear and apply locally (when the plaster cast has been removed) to help heal the broken bones. *(See pages 120 and 132.)*

• Comfrey root can be taken internally (in small amounts) to set the bone and encourage healing. *(See page 132.)*

AROMATHERAPY

• Elemi oil can help to encourage the circulation after a plaster cast has been removed.

• Lavender in a vaporizer will help to relax and calm. *(See page 161.)*

• Thyme, rosemary, and marjoram can be diluted and massaged into the area, or applied as a compress, to soothe pain and promote healing. *(See pages 146–71.)*

HOMEOPATHY

• Arnica, every 10 minutes after the injury, then every 8 or 10 hours thereafter, as necessary. *(See page 182.)*

• Symphytum (bone knit) can be used for up to 3 weeks to promote healing. Do not take this unless you are sure the bone is aligned, for the healing is profound.

FLOWER ESSENCES

• Rescue Remedy or Emergency Essence can be given at the time of the injury, and taken as required to calm and to treat any shock. *(See page 244.)*

VITAMINS AND MINERALS

• Increase your calcium, magnesium, and phosphorus intake. *(See pages 258, 262, and 263.)*

• Increase your intake of vitamin A. Foods such as carrots are a good source. *(See page 252.)*

BELOW *An infusion of comfrey, horsetail (shown here), and mouse ear may be applied externally to the fracture to encourage bones to mend.*

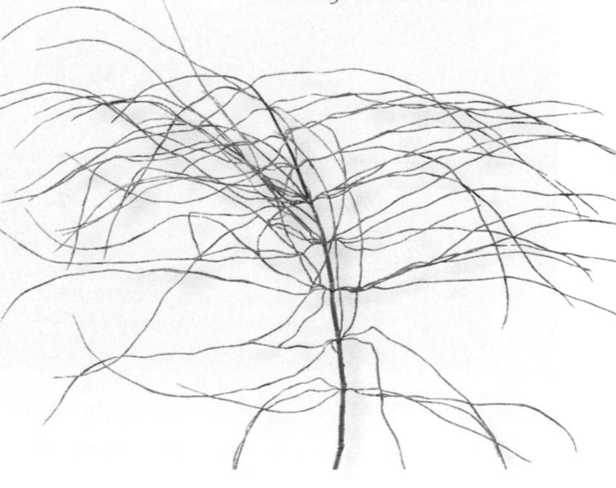

Sprains and Strains

A sprain is the result of an overstretching or tearing of the ligaments which bind the joints together, caused by a sudden pull. Severe sprains may lead to dislocation of the affected joint (particularly common in the case of the shoulder), and repeated injury of this nature can cause a loss of the ligaments' elasticity. The most commonly strained or sprained joint is the ankle, which is usually sprained as a result of going over on the outside of the foot so that the complete weight of the body is placed on the ankle. The back, fingers, knees, and wrists are also commonly sprained.

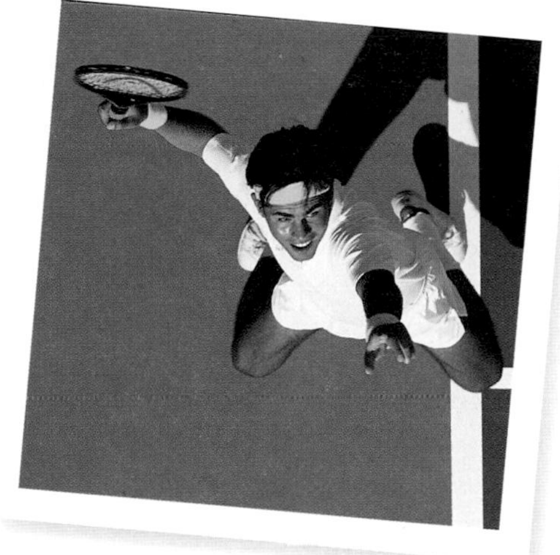

LEFT *Sprains and strains often occur during sports activities. Make sure you warm up muscles properly beforehand to minimize the chance of injury.*

SYMPTOMS

• *swelling in the affected area* • *pain in the affected joint, sometimes severe*

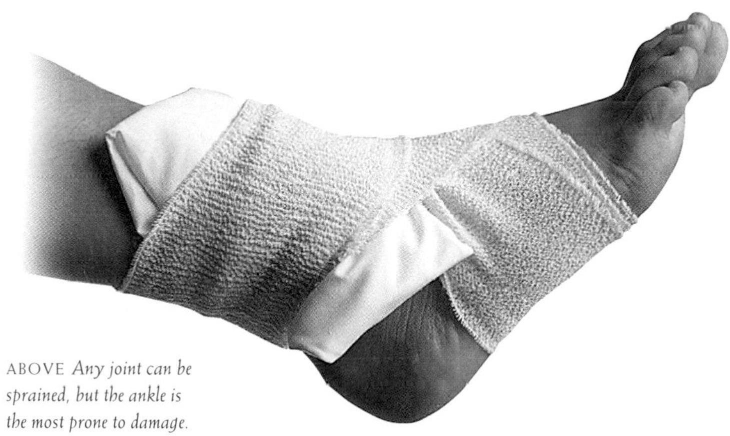

ABOVE *Any joint can be sprained, but the ankle is the most prone to damage.*

TREATMENT

CHINESE HERBALISM

• San Qi is useful after injury, for swelling and pain. *(See page 68.)*
• Die Da Wan will help with injuries to the soft tissues, inflammation, and bruising.

TRADITIONAL HOME AND FOLK REMEDIES

• Cider vinegar can be used as a compress in order to relieve pain and swelling. *(See page 102.)*
• Apply a poultice of raw onions to the sprain. *(See page 82.)*
• Raise the affected limb and apply a cold compress as soon as possible. Strains should be bandaged with an elastic bandage to provide support, but take care not to bind too tightly and cut off circulation. Keep the limb elevated until the swelling goes down and some normal movement is possible.

HERBALISM

• Burdock can be taken internally in the form of a tea, or applied as a poultice to the affected area. *(See page 115.)*
• Ginger can be added to bath water or a foot bath, or applied as a compress to encourage healing. *(See page 139.)*
• Chamomile can be taken internally to calm and reduce pain. *(See page 119.)*

AROMATHERAPY

• Use a little lavender oil in a foot bath, or on a cold compress applied to the area. Avoid massaging the area, which will increase inflammation. *(See page 161.)*
• A compress with essential oils of sweet marjoram and rosemary can be used to heal and to reduce inflammation. *(See pages 165 and 168.)*

HOMEOPATHY

• Arnica should be taken internally until the injury has healed. *(See page 182.)*
• Ruta grav. can be taken the day after the injury occurs. *(See page 210.)*
• A cold compress with Arnica tincture should be applied hourly for the first 8 hours to reduce swelling. *(See page 182.)*

FLOWER ESSENCES

• Rescue Remedy can be taken internally to reduce shock and to calm. A few drops on a cold compress, applied to the injury, can help to reduce pain. When the swelling has gone down, a little Rescue Remedy cream can be massaged into the joint area. *(See page 244.)*

VITAMINS AND MINERALS

• The following nutrients help to encourage healing in the body: vitamin C, beta carotene, zinc, selenium, and vitamin E. *(See pages 256, 265, 264, and 257.)*

CAUTION

IF YOU SUSPECT A FRACTURE, SEE YOUR PHYSICIAN IMMEDIATELY.

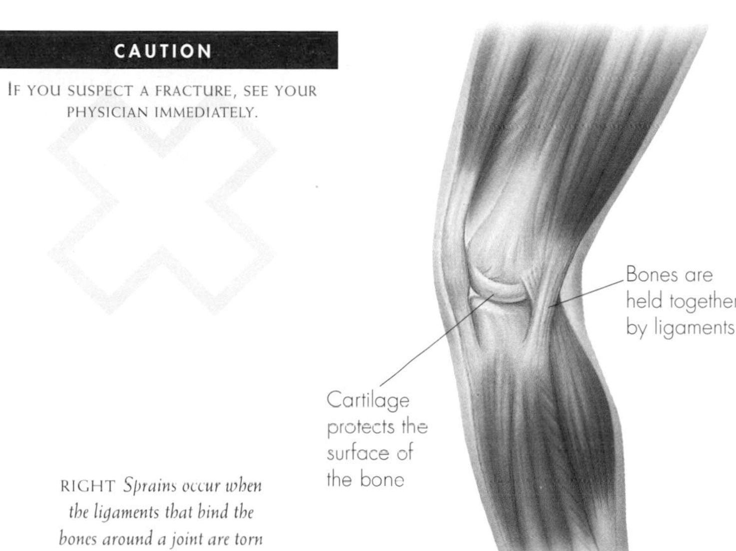

RIGHT *Sprains occur when the ligaments that bind the bones around a joint are torn due to excessive demands made on the joint.*

Neck Problems

Constant movement of the neck, along with its position and the number of structures within it, makes it particularly vulnerable to problems, which include:

- CERVICAL OSTEOARTHRITIS – the cartilage of the vertebrae of the neck wear away, most commonly in middle age, causing pain, stiffness, and sometimes tenderness to touch.
- CERVICAL RIB – this is an abnormal floating rib or pair of ribs attached to the lowest vertebra of the neck, which can cause compression of various nerves and arteries.
- CERVICAL SPONDYLOSIS – neurological damage is caused in the neck region as a result of compression of the spinal cord or nerve roots by an outgrowth of bone. Sufferers develop a walking disorder (spastic gait) and weakness in the arm muscles. Cervical spondylosis can begin from the age of 25 onward.
- LOCKED NECK – overstrain of ligaments or muscle spasms caused by an awkward or sudden movement, often occurring during sleep.
- NECK RIGIDITY – stiffness and pain on movement caused by neck muscle spasms. A classic symptom of meningitis.
- NECK SWELLING – swelling of any of the structures in the neck may be caused by tumors, allergy, bleeding, or inflammation. It can be extremely dangerous, seriously interfering with breathing. It may also affect swallowing.

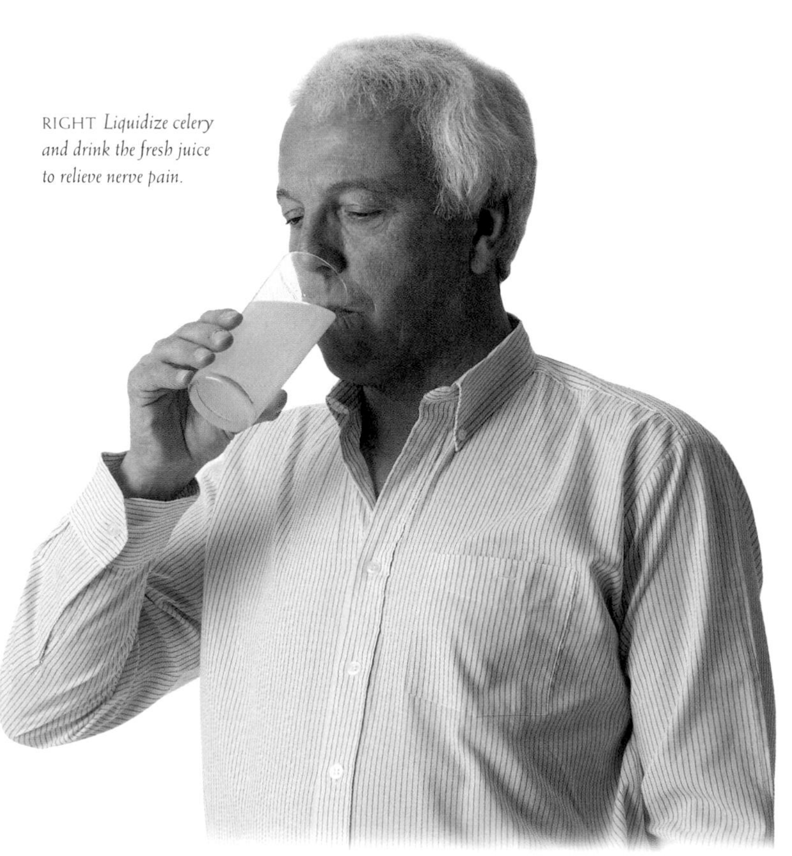

RIGHT *Liquidize celery and drink the fresh juice to relieve nerve pain.*

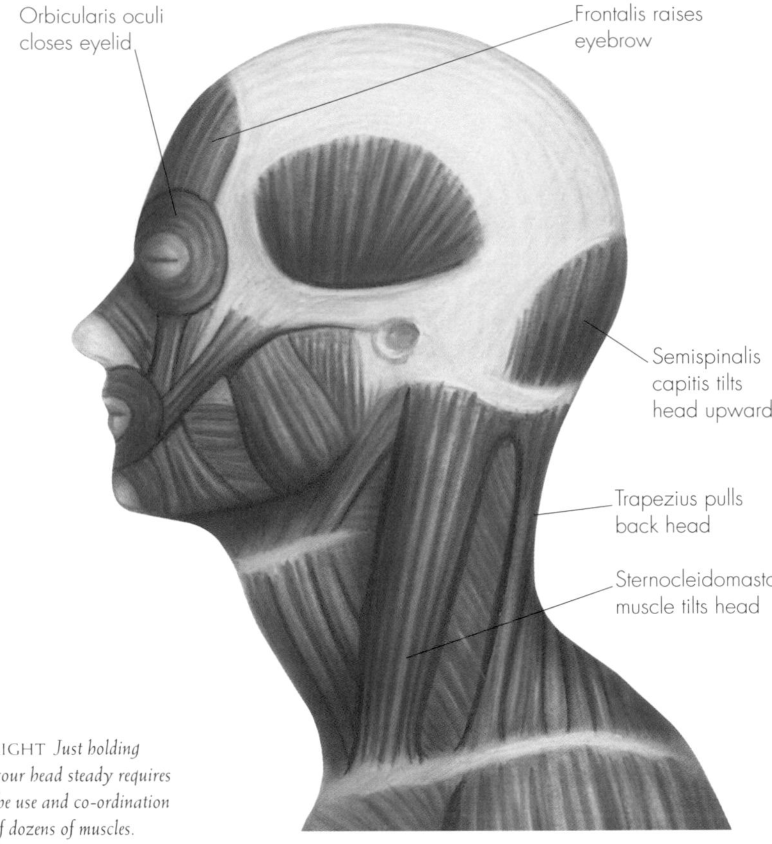

RIGHT *Just holding your head steady requires the use and co-ordination of dozens of muscles.*

- TORTICOLLIS (WRY NECK) – an abnormality in the head's position caused by permanent twisting of the neck, due possibly to muscle damage sustained at birth, a whiplash injury, a visual problem, or shortening of the skin of the neck through scarring.
- WHIPLASH INJURY – a sudden force (such as a car collision) causes a violent bending of the neck in one direction, followed by reflex muscle contraction which throws the neck in the opposite direction. The ligaments connecting the vertebrae are stretched or torn, causing prolonged pain and disability.

BELOW *Barberry has anti-inflammatory properties and is used internally for pain in the Ayurvedic tradition.*

CAUTION

A STIFF NECK ACCOMPANIED BY HEADACHE, NAUSEA, VOMITING, AND ABNORMAL SLEEPINESS MAY INDICATE MENINGITIS, AND IMMEDIATE MEDICAL ATTENTION IS REQUIRED.

TREATMENT

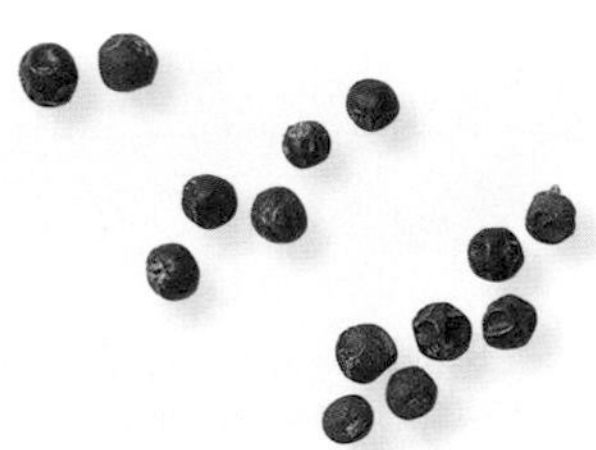

ABOVE *Use crushed juniper berries externally to relieve pain.*

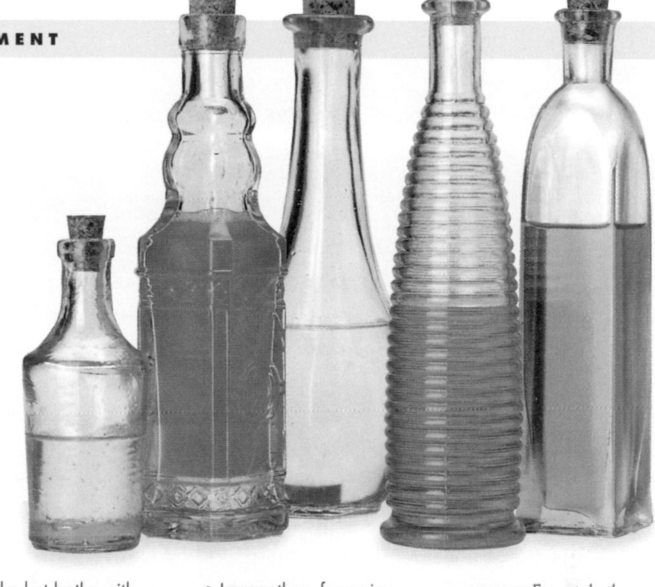

ABOVE *Essential oils, such as juniper or rosemary, can be added to a carrier oil and massaged into the painful area.*

AYURVEDA

• Barberry can be taken internally for pain. *(See page 29.)*
• Mustard oil relieves muscular pains and stiffness. *(See page 30.)*
• Turmeric and St. John's wort are also excellent for relieving stiffness, pain, and inflammation. *(See pages 37 and 40.)*

CHINESE HERBALISM

• The cause of stiffness and "freezing" may be caused by weak yang qi, external Cold and Damp. Useful treatments include cinnamon twigs and turmeric. *(See page 59.)*

TRADITIONAL HOME AND FOLK REMEDIES

• Drink celery juice to ease nerve pain. *(See page 83.)*
• Apply fresh horseradish to the affected area (do not leave on for long, or it will numb and burn). *(See page 84.)*
• Apply bruised juniper berries to muscular swellings for effective relief.
• Local heat will help to relax tense muscles.

HERBALISM

• St. John's wort has sedative, painkilling properties. It can be drunk as an infusion or applied to the affected area in an oil. *(See page 124.)*
• Valerian can reduce tension and help you to sleep. *(See page 136.)*
• The following herbs reduce inflammation and relieve pain: Jamaican dogwood, St. John's wort, vervain, and white willow. *(See pages 124, 129, and 138.)*

AROMATHERAPY

• A drop of juniper, mustard, or pepper oils, diluted in some carrier oil, can be massaged into the affected area. Wrap warmly afterwards. *(See pages 146–71.)*
• Wintergreen oil is good for muscular pains: massage into the affected area.
• Rosemary is stimulating and analgesic, and can be massaged into the area to relieve pain and stiffness. *(See page 168.)*
• Take hot baths with lavender, juniper, pine, or nutmeg to warm, reduce pain, and encourage the healing process. *(See pages 146–71.)*

HOMEOPATHY

• Cimicifuga, for a stiff neck, with the chin fixed in a raised position. *(See page 190)*
• Causticum, for dull pain at the nape of the neck, together with stiffness between the shoulders. *(See page 189.)*
• Bryonia, for pain made worse by the slightest touch. *(See page 185.)*
• Dulcamara, for pain at the top of the nape of the neck, as if from lying in an awkward position. *(See page 213.)*
• Lacnanthes, for pain down the right side of the neck, and in the upper arm and elbow.

FLOWER ESSENCES

• Rub Rescue Remedy cream into the affected area. *(See page 244.)*
• Star of Bethlehem can be taken internally after an injury to reduce the effects of shock and trauma. *(See page 235.)*
• Olive, if you feel exhausted and drained of spirit. *(See page 235.)*

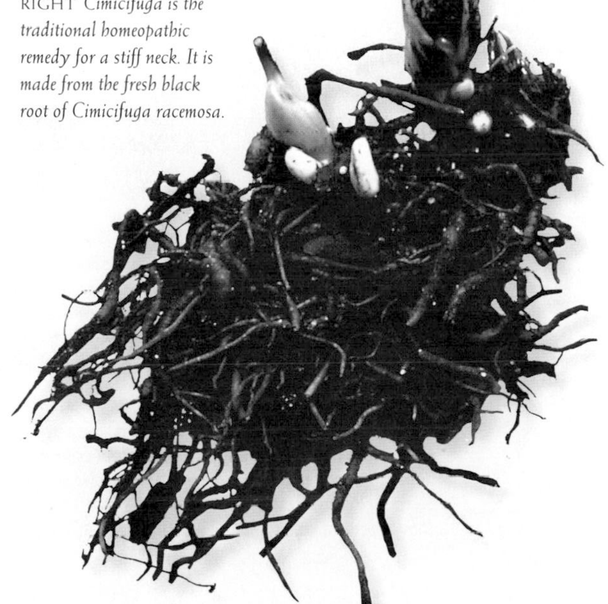

RIGHT *Cimicifuga is the traditional homeopathic remedy for a stiff neck. It is made from the fresh black root of Cimicifuga racemosa.*

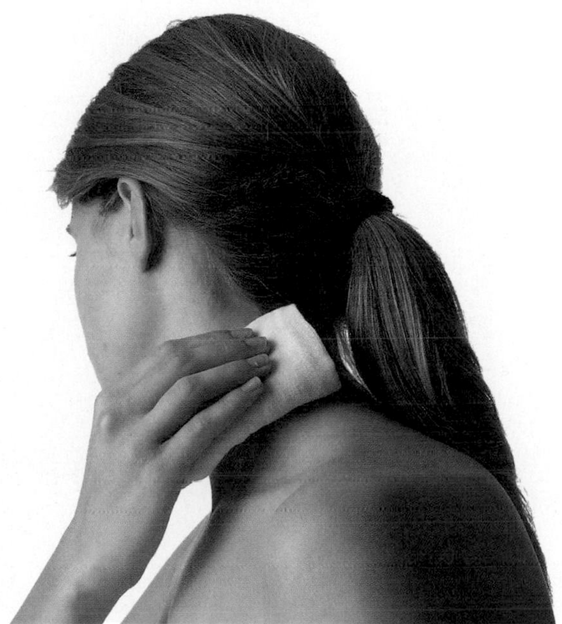

RIGHT *Healing herbs, such as vervain or valerian, may be made into a compress and applied to the affected area of the neck.*

Back Problems

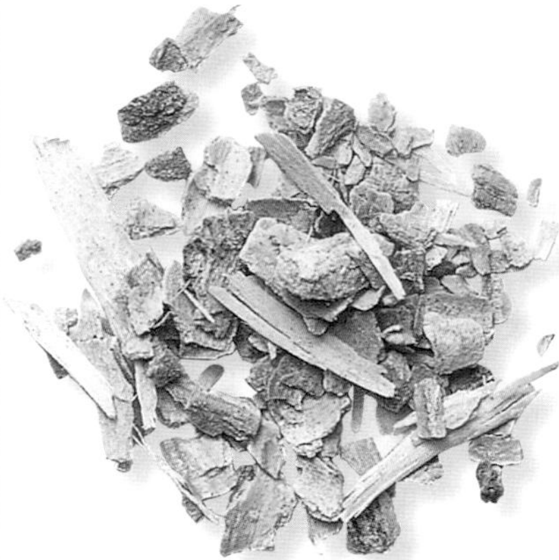

ABOVE *Cramp bark relaxes muscular spasms. It can be made into a cream, decoction, tincture, or capsules.*

Aches or pains in the back are due to mechanical disorders, which may cause or arise from damage to ligaments, muscles, vertebral joints, or discs. These may occur as a result of poor posture, lack of exercise, obesity, unaccustomed lifting or maneuvers, pregnancy, stress, or depression. A slipped disc is one of the most common causes of back pain, and this in turn may cause sciatica. Types of back pain vary according to the underlying cause.

DATA FILE

- A slipped disc does not, in fact, slip, but it herniates when the outer layer of the disc degenerates and the soft interior material extrudes into the spinal column, causing pain and sciatica.
- Most back pain is caused by a muscle strain. Injuries are the second most common cause of pain.
- Nearly 80 percent of all adults suffer from back pain at some time.
- The U.S. National Center for Health Statistics reports that back pain is the sixth most common reason for visits to the emergency room, and accounts for 13 million visits to general physicians' offices each year.
- In the U.K., the Back Pain Association estimates that every year over 3 million Britons consult a family physician because of back trouble.
- In the U.S., around 60 million working days are lost each year through back pain, and that figure is rising. Those days cost the economy around $5.2 billion (£3 billion) each year.

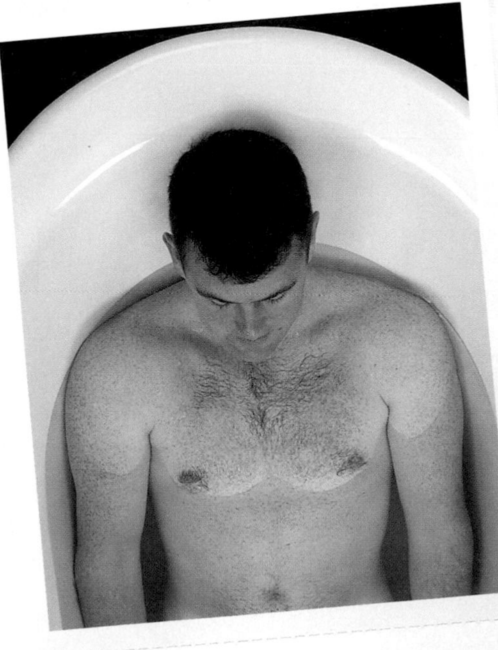

RIGHT *A relaxing bath with lavender oil can be extremely beneficial. It is one of the key oils for muscular pain.*

SYMPTOMS

• muscle spasms • lower back pain, ranging from mild to excruciating • stiffness • referred pain or pins and needles in other areas

TREATMENT

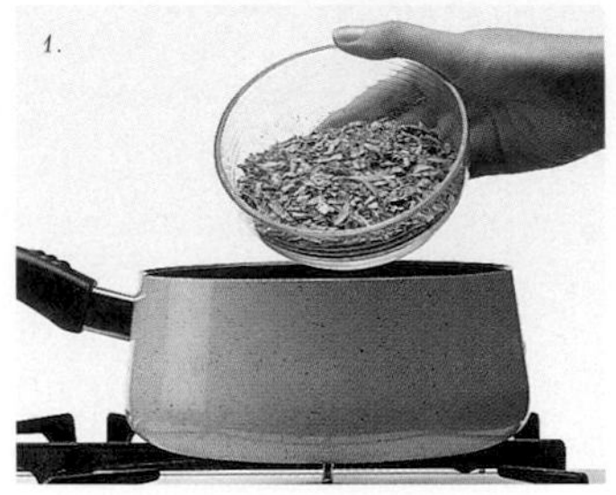

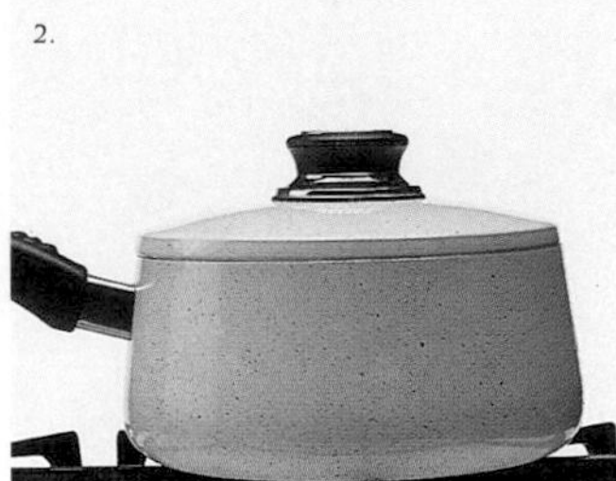

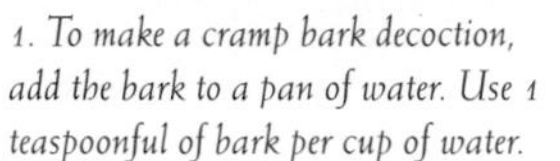

1. To make a cramp bark decoction, add the bark to a pan of water. Use 1 teaspoonful of bark per cup of water.

2. Cover the pan, bring the mixture to the boil, and simmer for about 10 to 15 minutes.

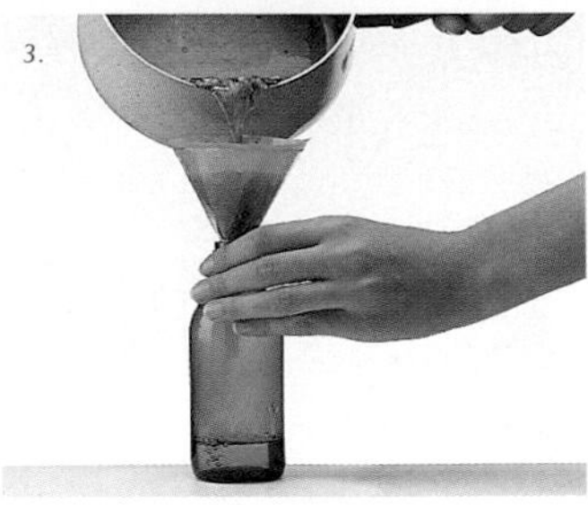

3. Pour the decoction through a strainer and store it in a dark glass bottle if you are not using it immediately.

AYURVEDA

- Aloe vera can be taken for inflammation, and applied externally for pain and inflammation. *(See page 27.)*
- Massage the painful area with mustard oil to reduce pain and aching. *(See page 30.)*
- Use cayenne externally for muscle soreness and stiffness. *(See page 31.)*

CHINESE HERBALISM

- Teasel root, ginseng, and acanthopanax can be used to relieve pain. *(See pages 54 and 67.)*
- Jing Jie can be used to stop swelling and to kill pain.
- Pseudoginseng root can be used to relieve swellings and for general relief of pain. *(See page 68.)*

TRADITIONAL HOME AND FOLK REMEDIES

- It may be helpful to chew a small quantity of horseradish leaves every day to ease pain. *(See page 84.)*
- A mustard poultice, applied to the area, will ease pain and reduce any congestion in the area. *(See page 98.)*

HERBALISM

- Massage cramp bark cream into the back. Or take cramp bark decoction, tincture, or capsules. *(See page 138.)*
- Rub macerated comfrey or St. John's wort into the back to relieve pain. *(See page 124.)*
- The following herbs reduce inflammation and relieve pain: Jamaican dogwood, St. John's wort, vervain, and white willow. *(See pages 124, 129, and 138.)*

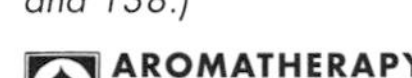

AROMATHERAPY

- Relaxing in a warm bath to which lavender oil has been added can be very soothing. *(See page 161.)*
- Pain due to fatigue or tension can be treated with a massage of ginger, juniper, marjoram, or rosemary; the same oils can be added to the bath. *(See page 146–71.)*
- Massage with ginger or black pepper can be used when there is acute pain. *(See pages 167 and 171.)*
- Marjoram can help to treat the muscular problem in the longer term, as well as reducing pain. *(See page 165.)*
- Bergamot and myrrh are anti-inflammatory, useful for massage or in the bath. *(See pages 153 and 155.)*

HOMEOPATHY

Treatment would be constitutional, but the following remedies may be useful:

- Calc. fluor., for backache that is worse when starting to move but eases if you continue to move.
- Arnica, for bruising and pain resulting from an injury. *(See page 182.)*
- Ruta grav. helps relieve pain at the nape of the neck and in the lumbar region. *(See page 210.)*
- Aconite, for sharp pain made worse by exposure to cold or dry weather. *(See page 178.)*
- Rhus tox., when the lower back feels stiff and bruised, especially after resting and in damp weather. *(See page 210.)*
- Sulfur, for violent sharp pain on stooping. *(See page 215.)*
- Bryonia, for pain that comes on in cold dry weather and is made worse by movement. *(See page 185.)*

Lumbago

Lumbago is the term used to describe any persistent or recurrent lower back pain. It is muscular in origin and usually concerns the large group of muscles surrounding the spine. Lumbago may vary in severity from a dull ache to severe pain; often it is experienced as a sudden excruciating pain on bending, on standing up from sitting, on twisting round, or on lifting heavy objects. It is generally brought on or exacerbated by cold, damp weather conditions, muscle strain, poor posture, obesity, and pregnancy. Lumbago is one of the most commonly reported symptoms and it generally becomes more frequent with age.

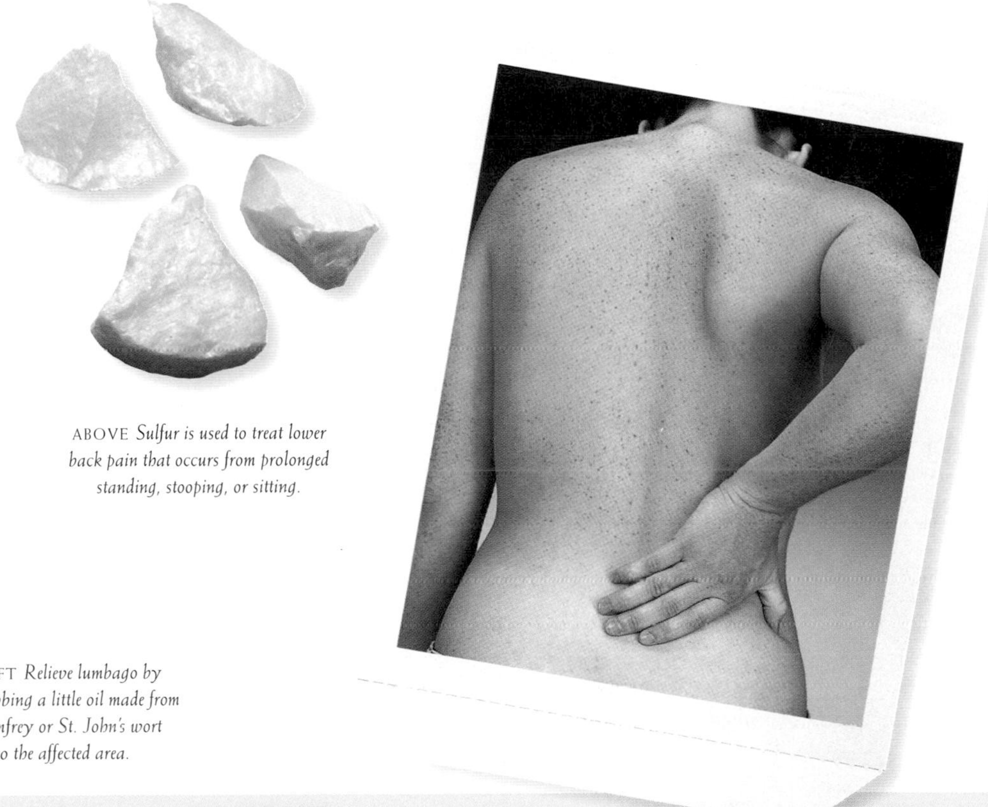

ABOVE *Sulfur is used to treat lower back pain that occurs from prolonged standing, stooping, or sitting.*

ABOVE *Lumbago pain is centred in the small of the back and may be quite severe.*

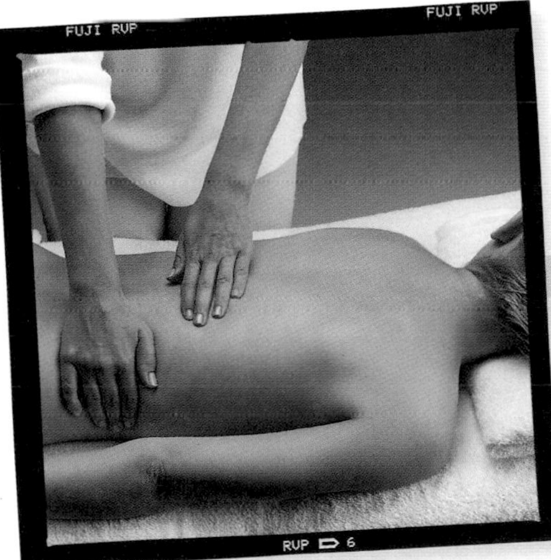

LEFT *Relieve lumbago by rubbing a little oil made from comfrey or St. John's wort onto the affected area.*

TREATMENT

AYURVEDA

• Saffron is anodyne and has antispasmodic properties. *(See page 36.)*

CHINESE HERBALISM

• Apart from physical injury, the cause may be excess internal Cold. Treatment would include tincture of achyranthes root and acanthopanax bark.

HERBALISM

• Rub a little oil made from comfrey or St. John's wort into the affected area, to relieve the pain. *(See pages 124 and 132.)*

• The following herbs reduce inflammation and relieve pain: Jamaican dogwood, St. John's wort, vervain, and white willow. *(See pages 124, 129, and 138.)*

AROMATHERAPY

• Add a little mustard, rosemary, and thyme oils to the bath to relieve pain. Hot baths are most effective. *(See pages 146–71.)*

• Juniper, oregano, pine, and rosemary poultices ease inflammation and pain. *(See pages 146–71.)*

HOMEOPATHY

• Aconite can be taken when the pain comes on suddenly and is made worse by cold dry weather. *(See page 178.)*

• Arnica, for pain that comes on after injury. *(See page 182.)*

• Rhus tox., for a painful lower back that feels bruised and stiff, and that improves with movement. *(See page 210.)*

• Sulfur, for violent sharp pain on stooping. *(See page 215.)*

• Bryonia, for pain that comes on in cold dry weather and is made worse by movement. *(See page 185.)*

• Ant. tart., for continuous pain with nausea and vomiting. *(See page 179.)*

• Dulcamara, for pain which is aggravated by stooping and exertion. *(See page 213.)*

FLOWER ESSENCES

• Agrimony is useful for those who make light of the pain and do not let it show in front of others. *(See page 225.)*

• Hornbeam, for weariness at the prospect of doing daily tasks that cause pain. *(See page 227.)*

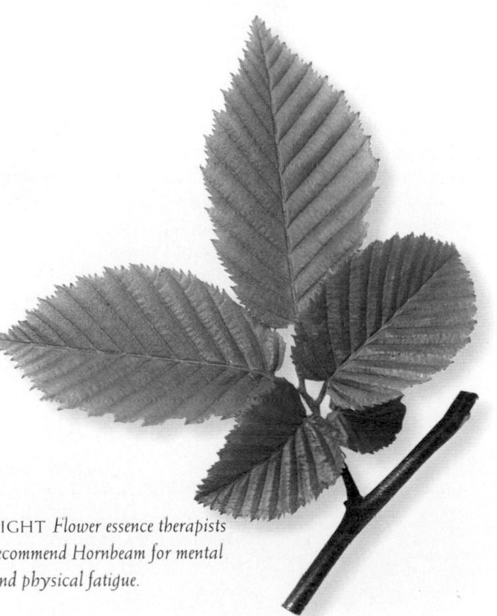

RIGHT *Flower essence therapists recommend Hornbeam for mental and physical fatigue.*

Sciatica

Sciatica is the name given to the aching or pain along the route of the sciatic nerve. This is the largest nerve in the body, running from the spinal cord, through the buttock and the back of each leg. Sciatica is usually caused by pressure on the roots of the sciatic nerve, most commonly from a prolapsed disc (*see page 420*), but other possible causes include pregnancy and childbirth, heavy lifting, stress, or a tumor. The type of pain varies from mild to more severe and "shooting" in nature. There may also be associated symptoms. Sciatica and other back pains may be eased by lying on the floor for fifteen minutes. Prop the head up on a small pile of paperback books and keep the knees bent. Repeat daily.

CAUTION

SEE YOUR PHYSICIAN IF YOU HAVE PROLONGED SCIATICA.

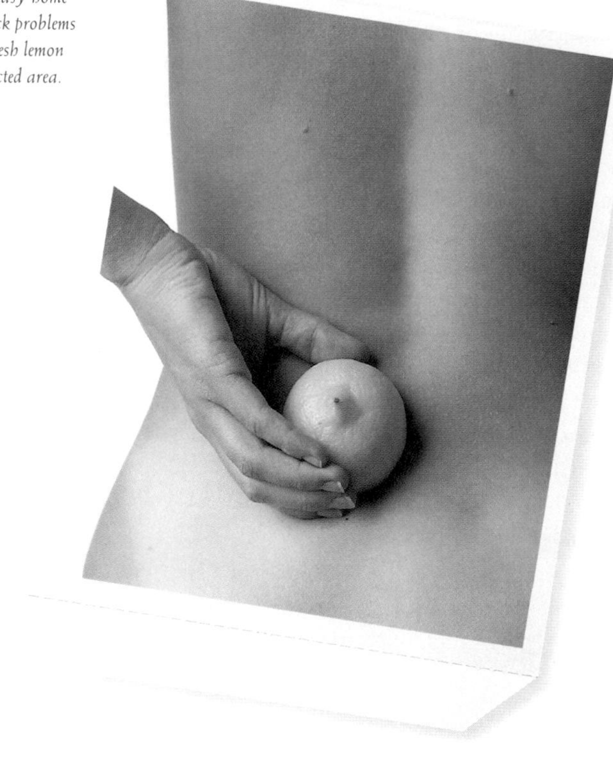

RIGHT *An easy home remedy for back problems is to rub a fresh lemon over the affected area.*

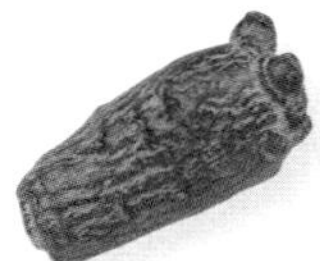

ABOVE *Gou Teng is recommended by Chinese herbalists as a remedy for sciatica.*

Symptoms

• a burning sensation and muscle weakness • numbness or pins and needles in the leg, foot, or toes • muscle spasms in buttock or leg • diminished reflexes in knees and ankles

TREATMENT

AYURVEDA

• Saffron is used for neuralgia and is warming. *(See page 36.)*

• Mustard oil can be rubbed into the affected area to warm it. *(See page 30.)*

CHINESE HERBALISM

• Sciatica is believed to be caused by Heat stagnation in the Liver. Gou Teng may be useful, and San Qi can help with the general relief of pain. A practitioner will select herbs specific to your symptoms and the cause of the condition. *(See page 68.)*

TRADITIONAL HOME AND FOLK REMEDIES

• Take a warm bath to which nettles have been added to help relieve the pain.

• Celery juice or tea can alleviate some forms of sciatica. *(See page 83.)*

• Rub fresh lemon over the affected area – it works! *(See page 87.)*

HERBALISM

• Apply bruised juniper berries to the affected area for pain relief

• Coltsfoot leaf or tincture can be used in a soothing compress (hot) and applied on the affected area.

• Elderberry wine is a traditional remedy for sciatica. *(See page 130.)*

• For pain relief, try cajeput cream or ointment rubbed on the affected area.

AROMATHERAPY

• Lavender oil is antispasmodic and anti-inflammatory. Use in the bath or in local massage. *(See page 161.)*

• Chamomile compresses or massage will reduce the irritation and lessen the pain. *(See page 150.)*

• Mix a few drops of juniper, mustard, or pepper essential oil in a little carrier oil and rub into the affected area. Cover with warm clothing. *(See pages 146–71.)*

• Oregano and thyme can be added to the bath to relieve the symptoms. *(See page 170.)*

HOMEOPATHY

• Colocynthis, is for shooting pains down the right leg to the foot, causing numbness. *(See page 191.)*

• Rhus tox., for tearing pain which is better for heat and movement. *(See page 210.)*

• Arsenicum, for sciatic pain in an elderly person. *(See page 182.)*

• Lycopodium, for pain in the right leg, and which is worse between 4 and 8P.M. *(See page 203.)*

• Carbon sulf., for pain in the left leg, which is worse for heat and cold.

• Gelsemium, for burning pains which are worse at night. *(See page 195.)*

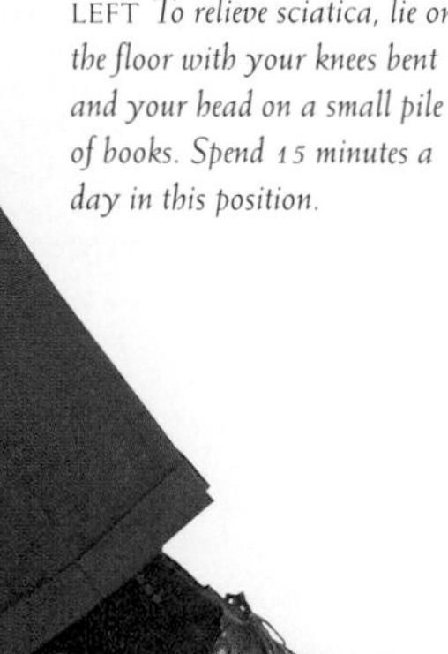

LEFT *To relieve sciatica, lie on the floor with your knees bent and your head on a small pile of books. Spend 15 minutes a day in this position.*

Fibrositis

Fibrositis (or fibromyalgia) is a chronic stress- or occupation-induced condition in which a series of muscular spasms causes intermittent aches and pain, usually in the back and trunk. It seems to be triggered by cold weather conditions or emotional upset. Fibrositis is most common in middle-aged and elderly people, and may occur more often in anxious people, and in those who spend time sitting in a cramped position. Tender areas (there are nine specific spots) are felt on the affected muscles. Pain and stiffness may be felt in the neck, shoulders, chest, buttocks, knees, and back. In some cases the attacks are accompanied by exhaustion and disturbed sleep. Fibrositis is not considered to be a medical term, and some doctors refuse to recognize the condition because investigation usually fails to reveal any detectable reason for the symptoms.

ABOVE *Basil is known as tulsi in Ayurvedic medicine and is used for pain relief.*

Symptoms

• aches and pain in muscles or tendons • tenderness in particular spots on the affected muscles • possibly stiffness

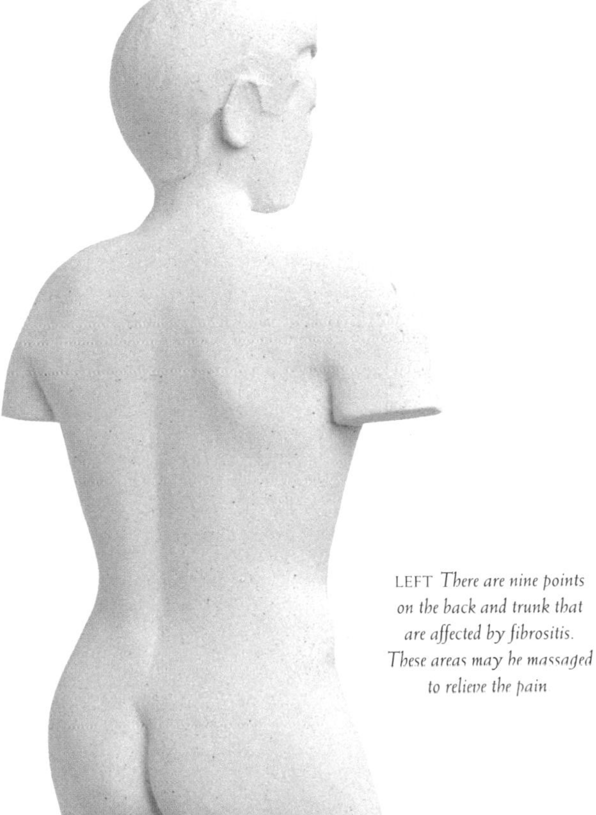

LEFT *There are nine points on the back and trunk that are affected by fibrositis. These areas may be massaged to relieve the pain*

TREATMENT

AYURVEDA

• Barberry, taken as a tea or applied as a compress, treats fibrositis. *(See page 29.)*

• Basil can provide pain relief. *(See page 42.)*

• Rub calamus oil into the affected joints to improve circulation and drainage. *(See page 24.)*

• Camphor can be rubbed into the affected area to warm and encourage healing. *(See page 33.)*

CHINESE HERBALISM

• Gan Caeo is good for spasm in the legs. *(See page 64.)*

• Bai Shao helps spasm in the feet and hands. *(See page 67.)*

• Ginseng will be useful as an overall tonic. *(See page 67.)*

TRADITIONAL HOME AND FOLK REMEDIES

• Apply compresses of apple cider vinegar to the affected area; use several cups of vinegar in bath water. *(See page 102.)*

• Make a honey and vinegar drink, with 1 tablespoon of each in a cup of hot water, and drink. *(See pages 101 and 102.)*

HERBALISM

• A decoction of cramp bark taken 4 or 5 times a day should bring relief. Cramp bark can also be taken as a tincture or in capsule form. The ointment is useful for massaging into the affected area. *(See page 138.)*

• Make a fresh peppermint poultice and apply to the area of spasm. *(See page 125.)*

AROMATHERAPY

• Essential oil of lavender relieves pain and reduces inflammation. Use in the bath or in a gentle massage of the affected area. *(See page 161.)*

• Chamomile, lavender, and rosemary are anti-inflammatory and pain-relieving, and are good for local massage or using in compresses. *(See page 146–71.)*

• Black pepper, eucalyptus, marjoram, and benzoin will improve the circulation in the area and reduce stiffness. *(See page 146–71.)*

HOMEOPATHY

• Aconite, for pain that starts suddenly and worsens with movement. *(See page 178.)*

• Arnica, for muscles that feel bruised and are made worse by movement. *(See page 182.)*

• Bryonia, for fibrositis in the back, neck, and limbs, which worsens with movement. *(See page 185.)*

• Chamomilla, for pain, stiffness, and bad temper. *(See page 204.)*

• Ledum, for a cold feeling in the muscles, with pain and stiffness alleviated by cold. *(See page 202.)*

• Nux vomica., for pain and stiffness which are worse in damp weather and improved by pressure. *(See page 214.)*

• Rhus tox., for muscles stiff from overuse, which are better for movement. *(See page 210.)*

• Causticum, for tearing pains in the muscles, with stiffness, and which are made worse by cold. *(See page 189.)*

FLOWER ESSENCES

• Rub a little Rescue Remedy cream into the affected area to encourage healing and provide pain relief. *(See page 244.)*

• Take Rescue Remedy or Emergency Essence during an attack to calm and restore. *(See page 244.)*

VITAMINS AND MINERALS

• Royal jelly may help to relieve symptoms. *(See page 276.)*

• Take extra calcium, magnesium, and vitamin C to encourage the health of the muscles and joints. *(See pages 258, 262, and 256.)*

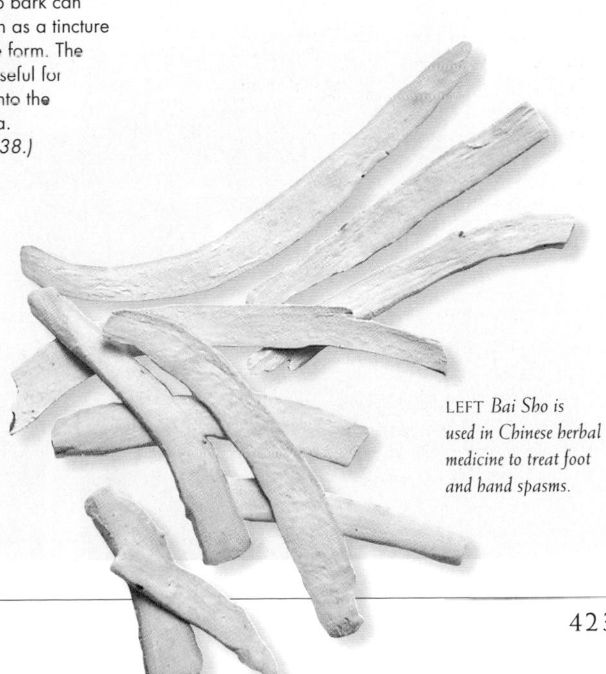

LEFT *Bai Sho is used in Chinese herbal medicine to treat foot and hand spasms.*

Arthritis

Arthritis is an inflammation of the tissues of one or more joints, usually with pain, swelling, and redness. The two most common forms of arthritis are osteoarthritis and rheumatoid arthritis. Other disease processes and infections which cause arthritis include gout, psoriasis, tuberculosis, rubella, and gonorrhea.

Osteoarthritis is a degenerative disorder in which the cartilage between the joints wears away. The body attempts to repair this damage by producing bony outgrowths at the margins of affected joints, but these, in fact, cause pain and stiffness. It is usually age-related and affects the hips, knees, spine, and shoulders in particular. Obesity is an aggravating factor.

DATA FILE

- Over 50 million Americans suffer from some form of arthritis.
- Rheumatoid arthritis affects 1–3 percent of the American population (about 2.1 million people).
- The usual age of onset for arthritis is between 30 and 40, but the disease may start at any age and may even strike children (juvenile rheumatoid arthritis or Still's disease).
- Juvenile rheumatoid arthritis affects 71,000 young Americans each year, 6 times as many girls as boys, and figures are increasing.
- Women are affected by rheumatoid arthritis three times as often as men, and about 16 percent of the female population over 65 have the disease.
- Osteoarthritis rarely attacks before the age of 40, but most people over the age of 60 have it.

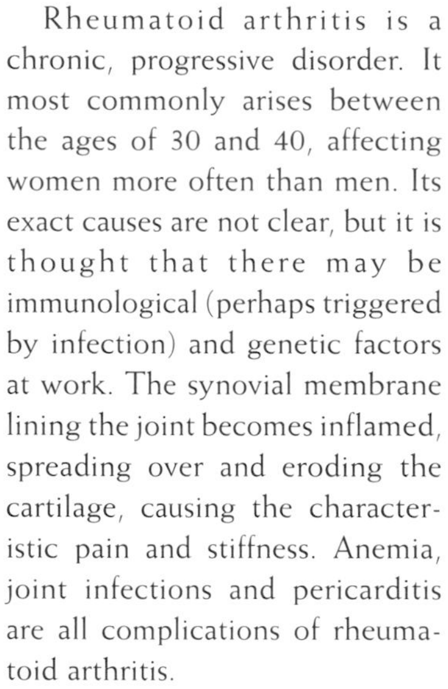

Rheumatoid arthritis is a chronic, progressive disorder. It most commonly arises between the ages of 30 and 40, affecting women more often than men. Its exact causes are not clear, but it is thought that there may be immunological (perhaps triggered by infection) and genetic factors at work. The synovial membrane lining the joint becomes inflamed, spreading over and eroding the cartilage, causing the characteristic pain and stiffness. Anemia, joint infections and pericarditis are all complications of rheumatoid arthritis.

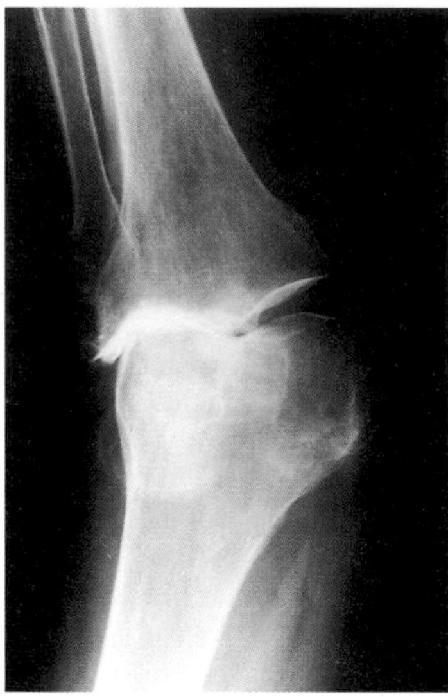

ABOVE *Arthritis is characterized by painful, swollen, and inflamed joints. As the disease progresses, the joints often become deformed.*

Symptoms

• osteoarthritis – intermittent pain in affected joints, gradually becoming more frequent – progressive movement limitation – audible creaking in affected joints – swelling and redness • rheumatoid arthritis – morning stiffness, taking up to an hour for the joints to loosen – weakness and inflammation of the ligaments, tendons, and muscles – eventually there may be deformity of joints (typically the fingers/hands), causing pain and debility – eye inflammation – bursitis – general feelings of being unwell include lethargy, appetite and weight loss, muscle pain

CAUTION

BLADDERWRACK SHOULD BE AVOIDED BY ANYONE SUFFERING FROM AN OVERACTIVE THYROID. DEVIL'S CLAW SHOULD NOT BE USED DURING PREGNANCY; IT IS BEST AVOIDED IF YOU SUFFER FROM STOMACH ACIDITY OR ULCERS. DO NOT USE SIBERIAN GINSENG DURING PREGNANCY UNLESS ADVISED TO DO SO BY A QUALIFIED HERBALIST.

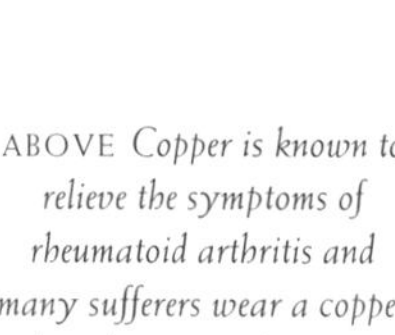

ABOVE *Copper is known to relieve the symptoms of rheumatoid arthritis and many sufferers wear a copper bracelet to ease the pain.*

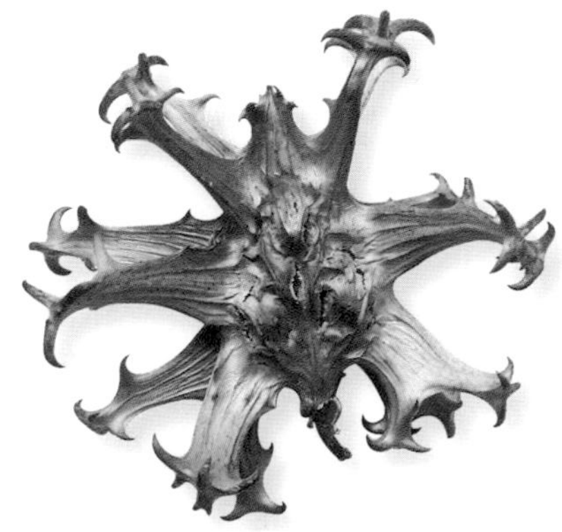

ABOVE *A tincture made from the Devil's claw tuber is used to treat all kinds of arthritis.*

TREATMENT

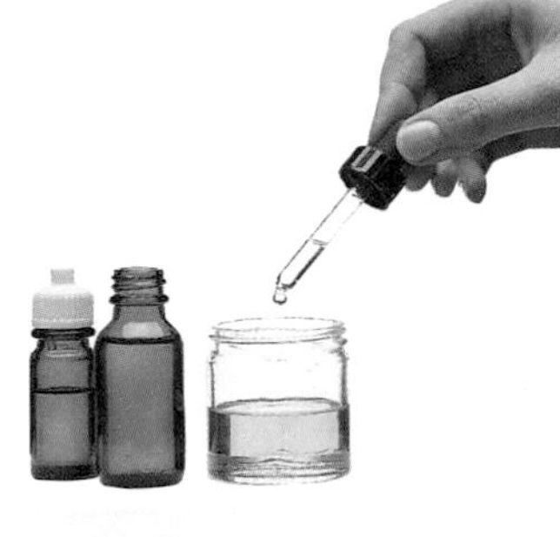

Make a liniment with comfrey tincture and black pepper oil. Pour some olive oil into a small jar.

Add a few drops each of comfrey tincture and black pepper oil. Leave the liniment to mature.

AYURVEDA

- Ginger, coriander, and aloe vera can be used to treat arthritis. (See pages 27, 35, and 47.)
- Angelica is a good tonic and is warming. (See page 28.)
- Barberry, taken as a tea or applied as a compress, can be used to treat arthritis. (See page 29.)
- Basil can provide relief from the pain of arthritis and rheumatism. (See page 42.)
- Rub calamus oil into the affected joints to improve circulation and drainage. (See page 24.)
- Camphor is indicated for the treatment of arthritis and rheumatism, and many other musculoskeletal problems. (See page 33.)

CHINESE HERBALISM

- The source of the problem is considered to be Wind Damp. Painful joints are caused by Wind Cold. Arthritis with hot, swollen, but not painful, joints is considered to be caused by Wind Heat.
- Treatment would include cinnamon twigs to release qi; aconite root, angelica root, and wild ginger to relieve Cold and Damp. (See pages 56 and 59.)
- Gentian and cork bark tree can be used for Wind Heat. (See page 68.)
- Pupleuri root, licorice, and Chinese skullcap are recommended for their powerful anti-inflammatory effects. (See pages 64 and 74.)
- Osteoarthritis is thought to be a weakness in the Kidneys, and Blood stagnation. Use cinnamon twigs, tinospora stem, angelica, and ledebouriella root. (See pages 56 and 59.)

TRADITIONAL HOME AND FOLK REMEDIES

- Eating nettles or drinking nettle tea is an old remedy for arthritis. The "stings" in stinging nettles contain histamine, which is anti-inflammatory.
- Vinegar and honey is another old remedy. (See pages 101 and 102.)
- Apple cider baths or ginger root baths can help to reduce symptoms and encourage healing. (See page 102.)
- Apples are good detoxifiers. Eat them daily to improve symptoms and cure the condition. (See page 94.)

HERBALISM

- Apply a poultice of slippery elm and cayenne to the affected joints. (See pages 118 and 136.)
- Herbs that work to heal arthritis include feverfew, meadowsweet, celery seed, and white willow. They can be taken internally, or used externally, as required. (See pages 121, 129, and 133.)
- Bladderwrack capsules, tablets, or powder used regularly may prevent the progress of the disease. (See page 122.)
- For aching joints, try a liniment made with tincture of comfrey and a few drops of black pepper essential oil. (See page 132.)
- Dandelion root and horsetail tea or tincture is recommended for degenerative arthritis. (See pages 120 and 134.)
- For inflamed hand joints, take a decoction or tincture of devil's claw. (See page 123.)
- Siberian ginseng is beneficial for rheumatoid arthritis. (See page 126.)

AROMATHERAPY

- Use juniper oil in the bath or in a massage oil blend. It is stimulating and anti-rheumatic. (See page 160.)
- Massage petitgrain into the limbs for osteoarthritis. (See page 152.)
- Lemon and cypress oils are detoxifying, and can be used in the bath and in massage to help the body eliminate poisons. (See pages 154 and 156.)
- Chamomile, lavender, and rosemary are anti-inflammatory and pain-relieving; use in local massage or compresses. (See pages 146–71.)
- Black pepper, eucalyptus, marjoram, and benzoin will improve the circulation in the area and reduce stiffness. (See pages 146–71.)

HOMEOPATHY

- Bryonia is useful for arthritis where stitching pains occur in swollen pale or red joints. (See page 185.)
- Colchicum, when it is worse in warm weather, with inflamed joints, irritability, and sensitivity to touch.
- Rhododendron, when it is worse in stormy weather.
- Rhus tox., when the arthritis symptoms include pain and stiffness, and are made worse after rest and in cold damp weather, as well as improving with movement. (See page 210.)
- Pulsatilla, when pain moves from one joint to another. (See page 209.)
- Apis, for hot, stinging pain. (See page 180.)

VITAMINS AND MINERALS

- There is some evidence to show that the antioxidants – Vitamins A, C, and E, plus selenium – may have beneficial effects on arthritis. (See pages 252, 256 and 257.)
- Magnesium is required to form the synovial fluid which surrounds the joints, and an adequate intake will ensure health. (See page 262.)
- Cod liver oil and evening primrose oil capsules are reported to help rheumatoid arthritis. (See pages 269 and 270.)
- Copper may help relieve the symptoms of rheumatoid arthritis, and many sufferers use copper bracelets as a result. (See page 259.)

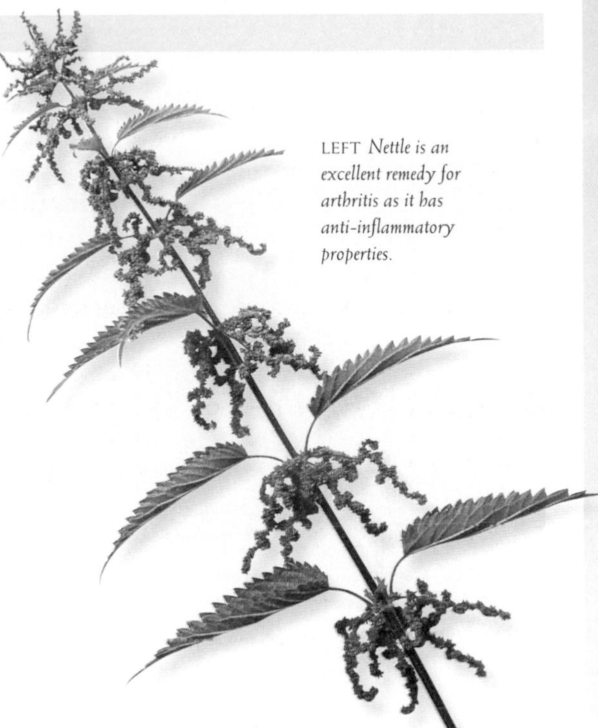

LEFT *Nettle is an excellent remedy for arthritis as it has anti-inflammatory properties.*

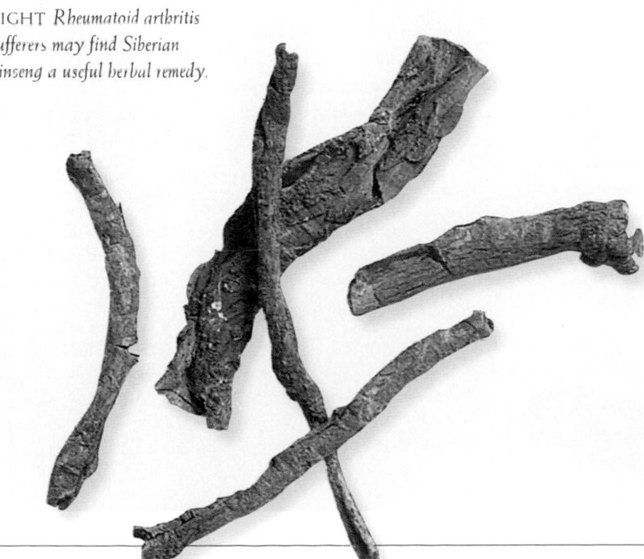

RIGHT *Rheumatoid arthritis sufferers may find Siberian ginseng a useful herbal remedy.*

Cramp

Cramp is a painful muscular spasm which occurs most frequently in the feet and legs, but can also affect the abdomen, arms, and hands (writer's cramp). Excess salt loss through sweating is the most common cause, and pregnancy, prolonged sitting or standing, strenuous or unaccustomed exercise, or lying in an unusual position may all be triggers. The muscle contraction is usually short-lived, lasting minutes only, but in some cases it may be prolonged, and repeated. Many old people suffer from night cramps. Some research indicates that a vitamin E deficiency may be partly to blame, and there may also be an imbalance of magnesium and calcium in the body.

ABOVE *One traditional remedy for cramp that works well is to take lemon with a pinch of salt. If taken before bed, it will help to prevent night cramps.*

CAUTION

SEEK MEDICAL ADVICE IF CRAMP IN THE CHEST OCCURS DURING OR AFTER EXERCISE, AS THIS MAY BE ANGINA.

Symptoms

- *twitching, followed by severe pain and a sensation of contortion in the affected muscle*

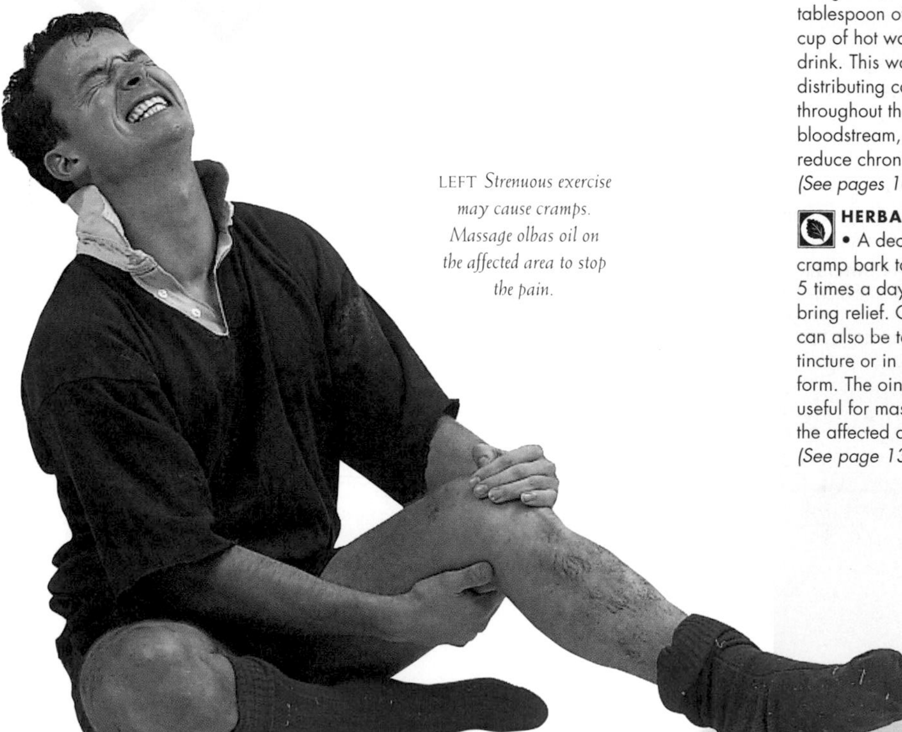

LEFT *Strenuous exercise may cause cramps. Massage olbas oil on the affected area to stop the pain.*

TREATMENT

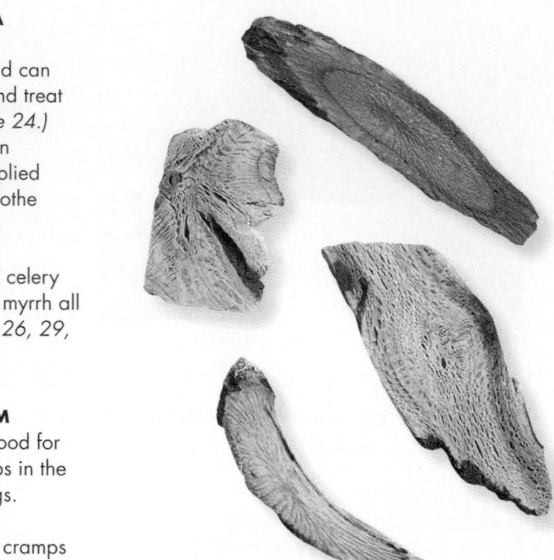

ABOVE *Gan Caeso is used in Chinese medicine to stop spasms and relieve pain.*

AYURVEDA

- Yarrow is antispasmodic and can help to prevent and treat cramp. *(See page 24.)*
- Aloe vera, taken internally and applied externally, can soothe muscular spasm. *(See page 27.)*
- Basil, caraway, celery seed, garlic, and myrrh all help. *(See pages 26, 29, 30, 34, and 42.)*

CHINESE HERBALISM

- Gan Caeo is good for spasm and cramps in the abdomen and legs. *(See page 64.)*
- Bai Shao helps cramps in the feet and hands. *(See page 67.)*

TRADITIONAL HOME AND FOLK REMEDIES

- Apply compresses of apple cider vinegar to the affected area, and use several cups of vinegar in the bath. *(See page 102.)*
- A pinch of salt and a sip of lemon juice before bed may prevent night cramps. *(See page 87.)*
- Make a honey and vinegar drink, with 1 tablespoon of each in a cup of hot water, and drink. This works by distributing calcium throughout the bloodstream, which can reduce chronic cramp. *(See pages 101 and 102.)*

HERBALISM

- A decoction of cramp bark taken four or 5 times a day should bring relief. Cramp bark can also be taken as a tincture or in capsule form. The ointment is useful for massaging into the affected area. *(See page 138.)*
- Make a fresh peppermint poultice and apply directly to the area affected by the spasm. *(See page 125.)*
- Olbas oil is effective for sports-induced muscle cramps and spasm.

AROMATHERAPY

- Lavender is antispasmodic and can be usefully employed for cramp as a massage oil. *(See page 161.)*
- Rub the affected area with geranium essential oil. *(See page 165.)*
- Use melissa and chamomile oils for abdominal cramps, diluted in a light carrier oil. *(See pages 150 and 163.)*

HOMEOPATHY

- Take Mag. phos. (6c) every five minutes when cramp occurs. It is especially useful for writer's cramp and cramp that occurs after excessive exercise. *(See page 204.)*
- For menstrual cramp, take Mag. phos. every 30 minutes. *(See page 204.)*
- Cuprum metallicum, for the spasm and subsequent pain. *(See page 192.)*
- Arnica, for cramps caused by muscle fatigue following prolonged exercise. *(See page 182.)*

FLOWER ESSENCES

- Rub a little Rescue Remedy cream into the affected area to encourage healing and provide pain relief. *(See page 244.)*
- Take Rescue Remedy or Emergency Essence during an attack to calm and restore. *(See page 244.)*

VITAMINS AND MINERALS

- Increase your intake of calcium if you are susceptible to cramp. *(See page 258.)*
- Vitamin D is essential for the absorption of calcium. *(See page 256.)*
- Vitamin E supplements have been proved to help prevent night cramps. *(See page 257.)*
- Increase your intake of salt and magnesium. *(See page 262.)*
- Calcium tablets taken with vitamin C are said to prevent night cramps. *(See page 258.)*

Restless Legs

Restless legs is the term used to describe a condition associated with insomnia in which the legs ache and are constantly moved about in order to achieve comfort. It is thought to be due either to problems in the nervous system, or to hereditary factors. It is more common in older people and smokers, and it may be triggered by cold, damp weather conditions or overexertion of muscles. There is also an association with diabetes, vitamin B and iron deficiency, excess caffeine intake, and withdrawal from drugs.

ABOVE *Add a few drops of ylang ylang essential oil to a vaporizer in your bedroom to help you sleep.*

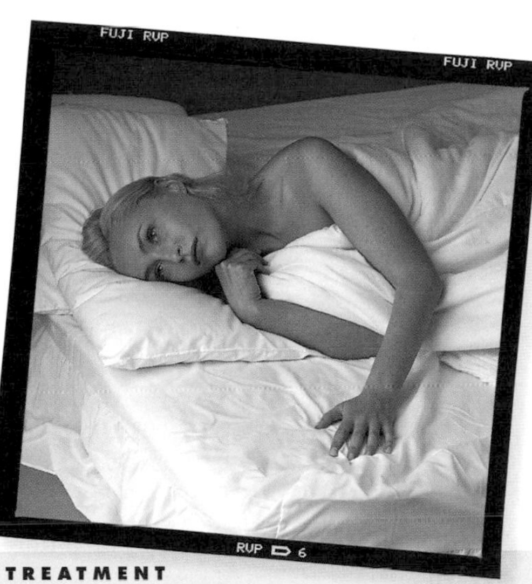

RIGHT *If you have trouble sleeping, try using sedative oils such as chamomile or ylang ylang. They may be inhaled safely from a vaporizer as you sleep.*

Symptoms

• tickling sensation under the skin • burning or prickling sensation • aching, twitching, and jerking • restlessness relieved by movement

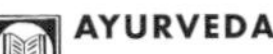

TREATMENT

AYURVEDA

- Warming herbs such as mustard (seeds and oil) and turmeric may be recommended. *(See pages 30 and 37.)*
- Black pepper stimulates circulation and the nervous system. *(See page 44)*
- Camphor stimulates the nervous system and body tissues. *(See page 33.)*
- Cumin is useful for nervous conditions and is generally warming. *(See page 36.)*

CHINESE HERBALISM

- Restlessness is thought to be caused by yin or Blood Deficiency, and possible treatments are lotus seed sprouts and felskrone root tea.

HERBALISM

- A chamomile infusion or compress can help dispel the condition. *(See page 119.)*
- Valerian root works on the nervous system and can help to calm. *(See page 136.)*
- Bruised cloves can be added to any tea to relieve nervous conditions.

AROMATHERAPY

- Benzoin, bergamot, and frankincense have a calming action on the nervous system and can be used in the bath, in a vaporizer, or in local massage to ease. *(See pages 146–71.)*
- If you have trouble sleeping, try using a few drops of chamomile, lavender, marjoram, and ylang ylang, which are hypnotic. *(See pages 146–71.)*

HOMEOPATHY

- Arsenicum, for general restlessness and feelings of chilliness. *(See page 182.)*
- Sepia, for twitching which is worse during the day, and better for taking exercise. *(See page 212.)*
- Belladonna, for legs that jerk into spasm, and for feeling hot, with cold extremities. *(See page 183.)*
- Ignatia, when the problem comes on after grief or a broken love affair. *(See page 200.)*

FLOWER ESSENCES

- Rescue Remedy cream can be rubbed into the muscles of the legs, as required, to calm. *(See page 244.)*

VITAMINS AND MINERALS

- Vitamin E will help to control the condition. *(See page 257.)*
- Iron or vitamin B deficiency may be at the root of the condition, so ensure that you include plenty in your diet. *(See pages 260 and 252–5.)*
- Cut consumption of stimulants, such as caffeine, alcohol, and tobacco.
- Keep the affected muscles warm, and take plenty of hot baths.
- Zinc, for trembling, twitching feet, and restless legs, even while sleeping.

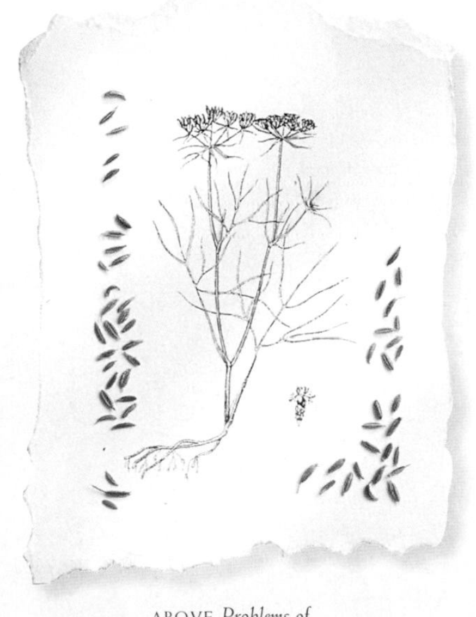

ABOVE *Problems of the nervous system are treated with cumin in Ayurvedic medicine.*

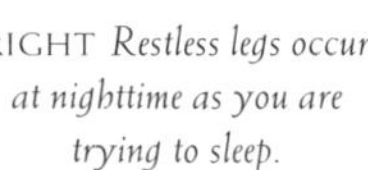

RIGHT *Restless legs occur at nighttime as you are trying to sleep.*

Bursitis

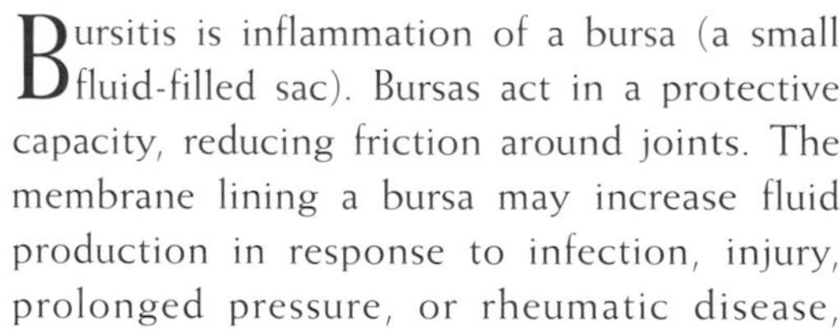

Bursitis is inflammation of a bursa (a small fluid-filled sac). Bursas act in a protective capacity, reducing friction around joints. The membrane lining a bursa may increase fluid production in response to infection, injury, prolonged pressure, or rheumatic disease, causing the bursa to swell. This may occur in any of the large joints of the body, such as the ankle or shoulder, and is commonly associated with bunions at the joint between the big toe and the foot. The build-up of calcium deposits on tendons associated with a joint is a frequent precipitating cause. The calcium deposits trigger an inflammatory reaction that can spread to a nearby bursa and even rupture it. Constant kneeling is a trigger for bursitis, causing a condition known as "housemaid's knee."

ABOVE *A compress of feverfew will relieve painful and hot joints.*

Symptoms

- *restricted movement in the affected joint, caused by swelling*
- *pain and tenderness in the affected area*

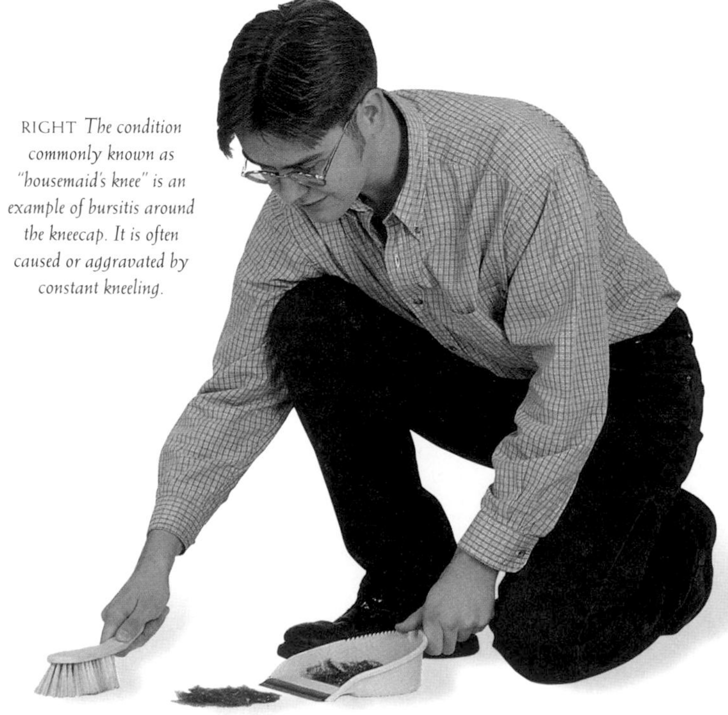

RIGHT *The condition commonly known as "housemaid's knee" is an example of bursitis around the kneecap. It is often caused or aggravated by constant kneeling.*

TREATMENT

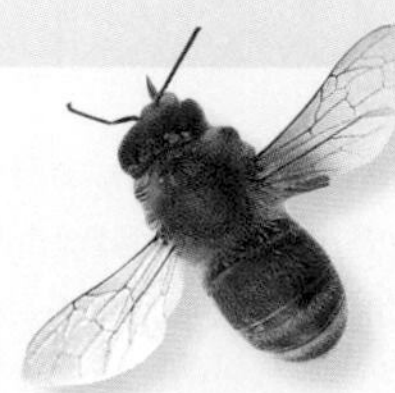

ABOVE *The honey bee, the source of the Apis homeopathic remedy.*

AYURVEDA

- Ginger, coriander, and aloe vera can be used to treat bursitis. *(See pages 27, 35, and 47.)*
- Angelica is a good tonic and is warming. *(See page 28.)*
- Barberry, taken as a tea or applied as a compress, can be used to treat pain and inflammation. *(See page 29.)*
- Rub calamus oil into the affected joints to improve circulation and drainage. *(See page 24.)*

CHINESE HERBALISM

- Pupleuri root, licorice and Chinese skullcap are recommended for their powerful anti-inflammatory effects. *(See pages 64 and 74.)*
- Cinnamon twigs, tinospora stem, angelica, and ledebouriella root may also be helpful. *(See pages 56 and 59.)*

TRADITIONAL HOME AND FOLK REMEDIES

- Eating nettles, or drinking nettle tea, is a traditional remedy for pain and inflammation. The "stings" in stinging nettles contain histamine, which is anti-inflammatory.
- Apple cider foot baths or ginger root baths can help to reduce symptoms and encourage healing. *(See page 102.)*
- Hot or cold compresses on the area will help to disperse swelling. *(See page 80.)*

HERBALISM

- Apply a poultice of slippery elm and cayenne to the affected joints. *(See pages 118 and 136.)*
- Herbs that work to heal bursitis include feverfew, meadowsweet, celery seed, and white willow. They can be taken internally, or used externally, as required. *(See pages 121, 129, and 133.)*
- For relief of aches and pains, try a liniment made with tincture of comfrey and a few drops of black pepper essential oil. *(See page 132.)*
- For improving inflamed joints, take a decoction or tincture of devil's claw. *(See page 123.)*
- Siberian ginseng is a beneficial herb. *(See page 126.)*

AROMATHERAPY

- Use juniper oil in the bath or as part of a massage oil blend. It has stimulating and anti-rheumatic qualities. *(See page 160.)*
- Chamomile, lavender, and rosemary are anti-inflammatory and relieve pain. Use on a compress or for local massage. *(See page 146–71.)*
- Black pepper, eucalyptus, marjoram, and benzoin will improve the circulation in the area and reduce stiffness. *(See pages 146–71.)*

HOMEOPATHY

- Belladonna, for pain which is made worse by the slightest movement, with red hot joints that are swollen and throbbing. *(See page 183.)*
- Kali iod., for pains that are worse at night.
- Rhus tox., for tearing pains with stiff, swollen joints, and which are made worse by heat and cold. *(See page 210.)*
- Pulsatilla, for dragging pain and tightness over the bursa, with chilliness. *(See page 209.)*
- Apis, for burning, stinging pain made worse by heat. *(See page 180.)*
- Sticta, for shooting pains.
- Bryonia, for pain made worse by movement or heat. *(See page 185.)*

FLOWER ESSENCES

- Rub a little Rescue Remedy cream into the affected area to encourage healing and provide pain relief. *(See page 244.)*
- Take Rescue Remedy or Emergency Essence during an attack to calm and restore. *(See page 244.)*

BELOW *Chinese herbalists use licorice to treat complaints where there is inflammation.*

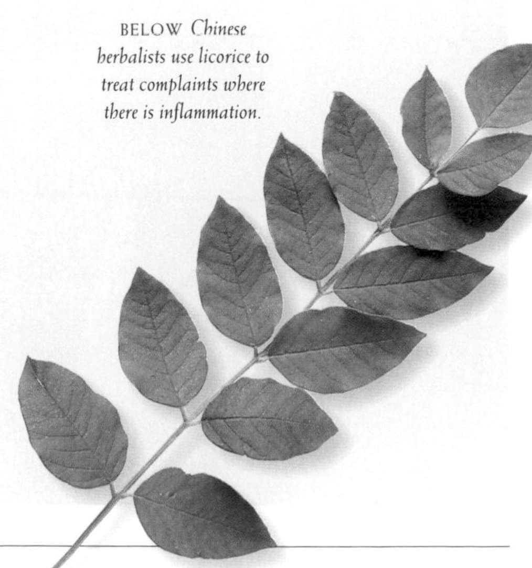

Tendinitis

Tendinitis is an inflammation and thickening of the tendons, usually caused by an injury or overuse of the muscles. There is some association with bursitis *(see page 428)*, and indeed the diagnosis is often difficult to make. Bursitis is characterized by a dull pain, whereas the pain of tendinitis is sharp.

Symptoms

• *sharp pain and limited movement in the affected area* • *swelling* • *pins and needles and numbness*

LEFT *Turmeric has anti-inflammatory properties and may be used to treat tendinitis.*

TREATMENT

AYURVEDA • Turmeric is anti-inflammatory, can be used externally, as an infused oil, or taken internally, 3 times daily, between meals. *(See page 37.)*

TRADITIONAL HOME AND FOLK REMEDIES
• Apply a vinegar compress to reduce areas of inflammation. *(See page 102.)*
• Wrap a bruised wet plantain leaf around the affected area to reduce swelling and stiffness, and to encourage healing.

HERBALISM • Apply a poultice of slippery elm and cayenne to the affected joints. *(See pages 118 and 136.)*
• Herbs that work to heal arthritis include feverfew, meadowsweet, celery seed, and white willow. They can be taken internally or used externally, as required. *(See pages 121, 129, and 133.)*
• For aching joints, try a liniment of tincture of comfrey and a few drops of black pepper essential oil. *(See page 132.)*
• For inflamed joints in the hand, take a devil's claw decoction or tincture. *(See page 123.)*

AROMATHERAPY • Chamomile, lavender, and rosemary are anti-inflammatory and pain-relieving. Use in local massage or compresses. *(See pages 146–71.)*
• Black pepper, eucalyptus, marjoram, and benzoin improve the circulation in the area and reduce stiffness. Use as cold or warm compresses. *(See pages 146–71.)*

HOMEOPATHY • Ruta grav., for tearing pains and lameness. *(See page 210.)*
• Rhus tox., for tearing pains made worse by rest, damp, and movement. *(See page 210.)*

VITAMINS AND MINERALS
• The following nutrients in the diet help encourage healing of the soft tissues: vitamin C, beta carotene, zinc, selenium, vitamin E. *(See pages 256, 264, and 257.)*
• Bromelain, a digestive enzyme, is an anti-inflammatory agent.

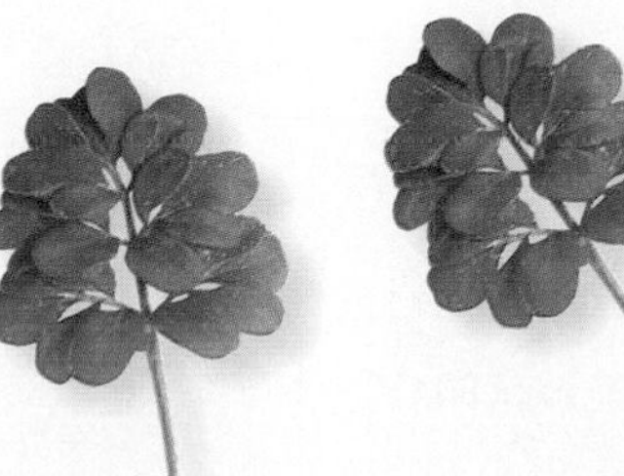

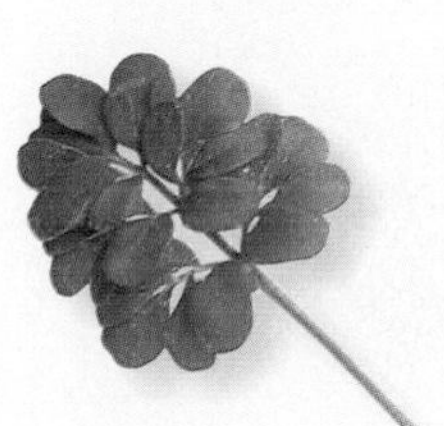

ABOVE *Ruta grav. is used homeopathically to treat bruised, aching, and inflamed tendons.*

Bunions

A bunion (or hallux valgus) is an inflammation of the soft tissue at the base of the big toe due either to ill-fitting shoes or an inherited weakness. Women are more prone to bunions than men, and there is also an association with flat feet. A bunion pushes the big toe outward at the base and in towards the other toes at the top. In some cases a bunion is so large it may distort the sufferer's shoe. Bunions are known as bursitis *(see page 428)*.

Ensure that shoes fit properly and are designed to suit the foot, not the fashion. High-heeled shoes and shoes with narrow toes are especially bad for the feet. Go barefoot as often as is practical, walking on a variety of surfaces to exercise the small bones in the feet. Practice picking up small objects, such as marbles, with the toes.

Symptoms

• *pain and discomfort in the affected foot* • *the bunion is aggravated by continuous and prolonged pressure*

TREATMENT

Make a warming mustard foot bath to reduce pain and inflammation. Crush some mustard seeds in a pestle and mortar and add to a bowl of warm water (as hot as is comfortable).

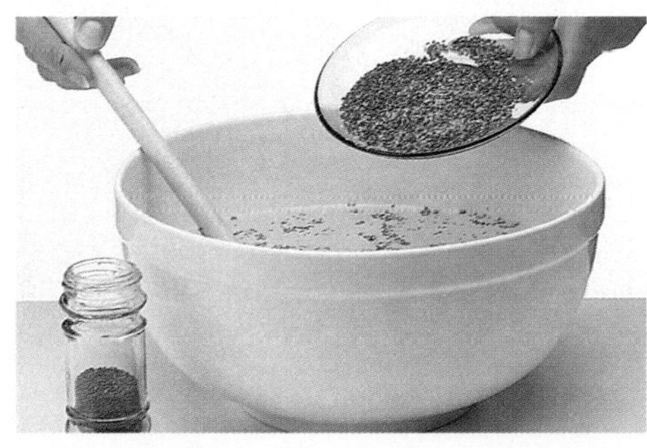

AYURVEDA • Cedarwood can be used as a rub for sore joints and pain. *(See page 32.)*
• Camphor can be used externally to ease the pain caused by bunions. *(See page 33.)*
• St. John's wort can be taken internally and also used externally in the treatment of bunions. *(See page 40.)*
• Mustard, used in a foot-bath, will reduce pain and inflammation, and encourage healing. *(See page 30.)*

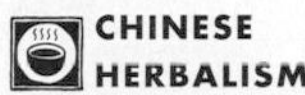

CHINESE HERBALISM
• Ginger is a useful anti-inflammatory agent.
• Other herbs to try, for external use, include: San Qi, for general relief of pain and swelling, and Jing Jie for inflammation, stiffness, and pain. *(See page 68.)*

HERBALISM • Treatment to ease inflammation and swelling includes compresses of marshmallow, linseed, comfrey, and slippery elm. *(See pages 114, 132, and 136.)*
• Chamomile infusions, taken internally, will help. *(See page 119.)*

AROMATHERAPY • For inflamed bunions, add a drop of melissa or chamomile essential oil to the massage oil and rub in gently. *(See pages 150 and 163.)*
• Lavender or marjoram oil will relieve pain. *(See pages 161 and 165.)*

HOMEOPATHY • Antimonium is the most effective remedy. *(See page 179.)*
• Apis, for burning, stinging pain made worse by heat. *(See page 180.)*
• Sticta, for shooting pains.
• Kali iod., for pain which is much worse at night.
• Ruta grav., when the bunion feels bruised and painful. *(See page 210.)*
• Rhus tox., when the skin is itchy, red, swollen, and burning and the joints are stiff, but pain decreases with moving about. *(See page 210.)*

Sleep Problems

All babies and children need different amounts of sleep, and most of them experience some difficulty sleeping at some point. Common causes of sleep problems in babies are diaper rash, teething, colic, illness, being too hot or cold, or simply being wakeful. Older children may be worried about something at school, or a stressful event in the family home. Illness usually disrupts sleep patterns in some way. Some children experience night terrors, which may cause the child to waken suddenly, screaming.

BELOW *Babies will enjoy a gentle massage to help them drift off to sleep.*

CAUTION

IF YOU ARE CONCERNED ABOUT THE CAUSE OF YOUR CHILD'S SLEEP PROBLEMS, SEE YOUR PHYSICIAN.

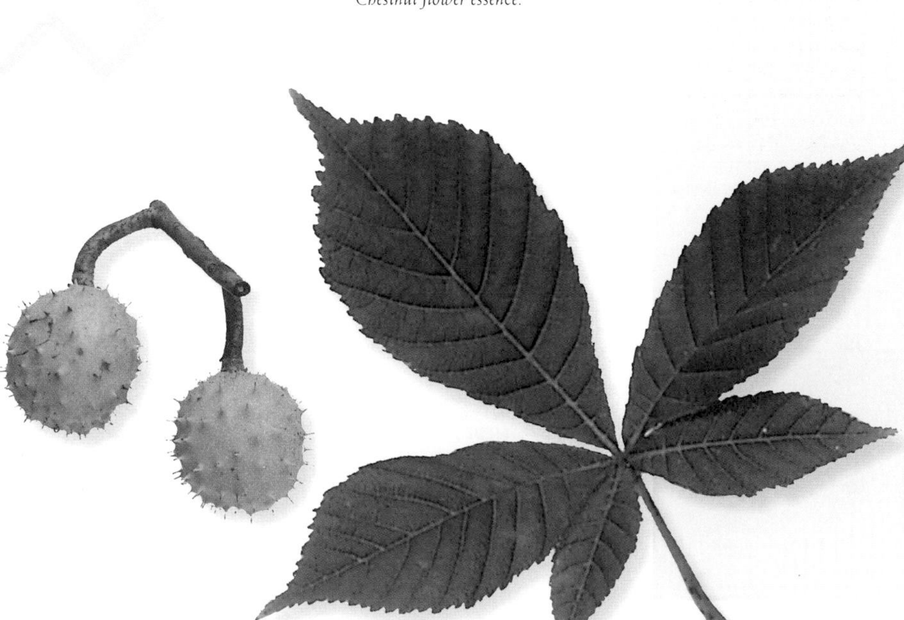

BELOW *If your child is kept awake by worries about the next day, try White Chestnut flower essence.*

TREATMENT

TRADITIONAL HOME AND FOLK REMEDIES

- A little brewer's yeast, mixed with honey and warm milk, makes a soothing bedtime drink for children from the age of four upwards. *(See page 101.)*

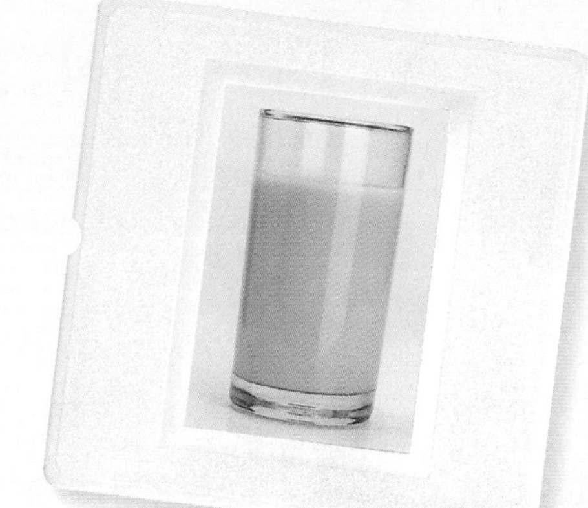

ABOVE *The traditional bedtime drink of warm milk gets extra power from the addition of yeast and honey.*

HERBALISM

- Vervain is a gentle sedative, and can help children fall asleep – particularly if they are fighting against it. *(See page 138.)*
- Limeflowers will be useful for calming nervous, sensitive children. *(See page 134.)*
- Motherwort can be useful for calming a frightened child or baby. *(See page 124.)*
- A crying baby may be soothed with an infusion of chamomile, offered an hour or so before bedtime or upon waking. *(See page 119.)*
- A strong infusion of chamomile, hops, lavender, or limeflower can be added to a warm bath to soothe and calm a baby or child. *(See pages 119 and 134.)*
- Tincture of catmint, added to a little honey, can be given to a distressed child as and when required.

AROMATHERAPY

- A few drops of chamomile, geranium, rose, or lavender can be added to the bath water. *(See pages 141–71.)*
- Lavender oil, on a handkerchief tied near the cot or bed, will help your baby or child to sleep. *(See page 161.)*
- Lavender or chamomile can be used in a vaporizer in your child's room. *(See pages 150 and 161.)*
- A gentle massage before bedtime, with a little lavender or chamomile blended with a light carrier oil, may ease any tension or distress. *(See pages 150 and 161.)*

HOMEOPATHY

- Ant. tart. for night terrors. *(See pages 186 and 179.)*
- For constant crying use Colocynthis or Bryonia. *(See pages 191 and 185.)*
- Phosphorus, for thirst, and alternating anger and affection. *(See page 208.)*
- Pulsatilla, for a weepy and clingy child. *(See page 209.)*
- Chamomilla, if sleep is being disturbed by teething. *(See page 204.)*
- Nux vomica, for irritability, and after a busy, stressful day. *(See page 214.)*

FLOWER ESSENCES

- White Chestnut will be helpful for children with overactive minds. *(See page 224.)*
- A distressed child or baby can be given Rescue Remedy, which will calm him or her. *(See page 244.)*
- Rock Rose, for night terrors. *(See page 231.)*
- Aspen, for anxiety for no identifiable cause. *(See page 236.)*
- Walnut will be useful for change – a new baby, school, or house. *(See page 232.)*
- A few drops of Mimulus will soothe a child who is afraid of the dark. *(See page 235.)*

VITAMINS AND MINERALS

- Avoid cold-energy foods such as bananas and cucumbers, which can cause colic and digestive problems.
- A warm glass of goat's milk will encourage sleep without causing any digestive disturbance.
- Older children may suck a zinc lozenge before bedtime to help them to go to sleep. *(See page 265.)*

Hyperactivity

Hyperactivity is a behavioral disorder which appears to be becoming more common. A hyperactive child has an excessively high energy level, being restless, inattentive, and easily frustrated. There are often prolonged and regular tantrums, and fidgeting. Intelligence is common among hyperactive children, but there is such a short attention span that they often do not do well at school. Psychiatrists have labeled the problem attention-deficit hyperactivity disorder, or ADHD. (Some children display attention-deficit disorder, or ADD, without hyperactivity.) ADHD appears in children before the age of four, but its signs are often missed until the child attends school.

There is a widespread belief that food additives, such as preservatives, are at the root of the problem, but this has not been conclusively proved. Others believe that minor brain damage may be the cause of hyperactivity.

ABOVE *Sandalwood essential oil calms the nervous system and soothes a restless child.*

ABOVE *Tantrums may be caused by food additives – try to eliminate them from your child's diet.*

SYMPTOMS

- *restlessness* • *inattentiveness*
- *tantrums* • *fidgeting*

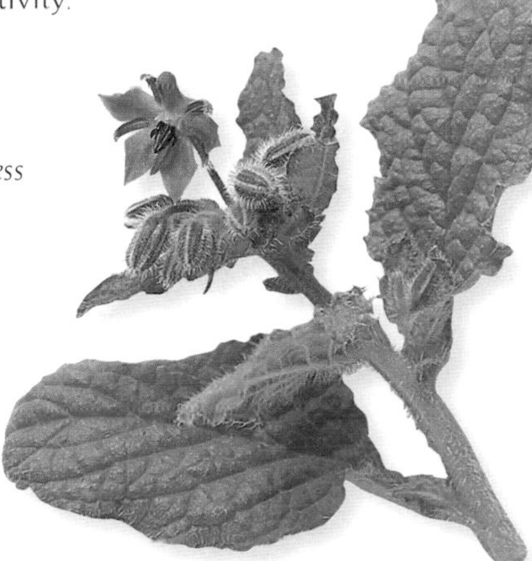

RIGHT *The adrenal gland is overworked by stress: borage helps redress the balance.*

DATA FILE

- Up to 3 percent of all children manifest significant symptoms of ADHD, with boys greatly outnumbering girls.
- A low frustration threshold predisposes such children to uncontrollable tantrums.
- There are many causes of ADHD, only some of which are known. In addition to genetic influences, various factors affecting the pregnant mother have been implicated, including the use of prescription or illicit drugs and the use of alcohol and nicotine.
- There is mounting evidence that the overprocessing of foods – including artificial colorings, flavorings, preservatives, and other additives – may be a factor, coupled with the depletion of various vitamins and minerals from the processed foods.
- Allergy-like intolerance of certain foods, especially milk, wheat, and corn, produces ADHD in some children.
- Pollutants such as lead, mercury, cadmium, insecticides, and herbicides may also be causative.

TREATMENT

HERBALISM

- Black root and fringe tree may be useful herbs if poor digestion is causing hyperactivity.
- Herbs to support a stressed nervous system include vervain and skullcap. *(See pages 131 and 138.)*
- Oats act as a tonic to the nervous system. *(See page 117.)*
- Chamomile, limeflowers, and skullcap, for tense and anxious children. *(See pages 119, 131, and 134.)*
- Borage and licorice will work to address an overworked adrenal gland. *(See page 122.)*

AROMATHERAPY

- Massage may calm hyperactivity in children. If the child can be persuaded to lie quietly for a few minutes, both mother and child may benefit from the feeling of peace and calm created during the massage. Use a little lavender or Roman chamomile oil to calm. *(See pages 150 and 161.)*
- Neroli, rose, and sandalwood essential oils have a calming action on the nervous system. *(See pages 146–71.)*
- Add a few drops of Roman chamomile to the bath water to soothe and encourage sleep. *(See page 150.)*

HOMEOPATHY

- Constitutional treatment is recommended, but China may be appropriate if food allergies or digestive problems are at the root. *(See page 190.)*
- Chamomilla will calm an overexcited, demanding child. *(See page 204.)*

FLOWER ESSENCES

- Vervain, for an over-enthusiastic child. *(See page 241.)*
- Impatiens, for a child who is talkative, quick thinking, and impatient. *(See page 233.)*
- Cherry Plum, for loss of control. *(See page 236.)*

VITAMINS AND MINERALS

- Include plenty of vitamin B-complex, vitamin C, zinc, and essential fatty acids in the diet, which help behavioral problems. *(See pages 252–5, 256 and 265.)*
- It will probably be necessary to take a good multivitamin and mineral tablet each day.

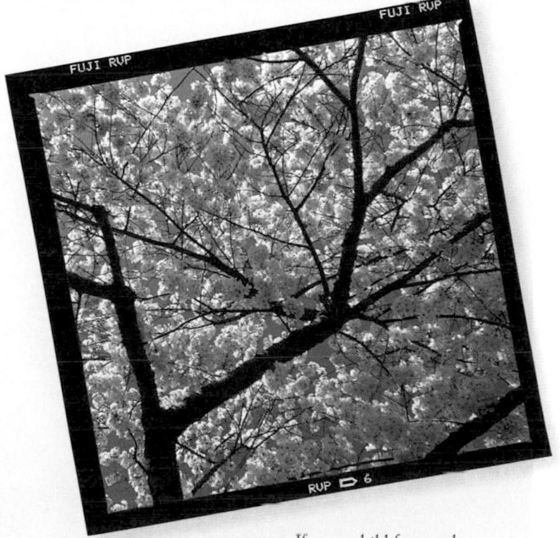

ABOVE *If your child frequently loses self-control, the flower essence Cherry Plum may help.*

Bedwetting

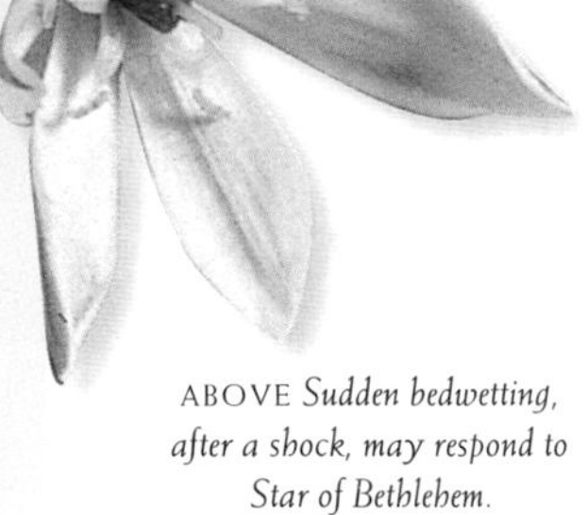

ABOVE *Sudden bedwetting, after a shock, may respond to Star of Bethlehem.*

Bedwetting is not considered to be a problem until your child is at least five years old. Many children, boys in particular, are slow in getting the message that they should get up to use the toilet at night, but that is no reflection on the state of their health – mental or otherwise. If a child sleeps heavily it may take longer for night dryness, but many children manage it by two or three years of age. Bedwetting in children who have already established a pattern of dry nights is usually caused by stress of some sort, like moving house, changing schools, family fighting. Children who have never been dry at night may suffer from immature nerves and muscles controlling bladder function. Other medical causes include diabetes, urinary infection, a structural abnormality, nutritional deficiencies, and food allergies.

TREATMENT

HERBALISM
• Offer St. John's wort and horsetail teas throughout the day, sweetened with honey, to soothe an irritable bladder and encourage control of the bladder. *(See page 124.)*
• If the bedwetting stems from an emotional upset or disturbance, vervain and lemon balm relax and soothe. *(See page 138.)*

AROMATHERAPY
• Massage oil of chamomile into the lower back and tummy while settling your child down to sleep. *(See page 150.)*

HOMEOPATHY
• Equisetum, when the wetting occurs during dreams.
• Belladonna, when it occurs early in the night. *(See page 183.)*
• Kreosotum, when wetting occurs during dreams early in the night and during deep sleep.
• Causticum, for wetting in first sleep, and when the problem is worse in clear weather or when your child has a cough. *(See page 189.)*
• Plantago, when all else fails.

FLOWER ESSENCES
• Try Wild Rose if your child drifts through life. *(See page 238.)*
• Walnut will help if the bedwetting is brought on by change, such as a new house, school, or baby. *(See page 232.)*
• Chestnut Bud, if the child does not seem to learn from the experience. *(See page 224.)*
• Star of Bethlehem, if bedwetting is related to a trauma or shock. *(See page 235.)*
• Mimulus, when the problem is linked to fear. *(See page 235.)*

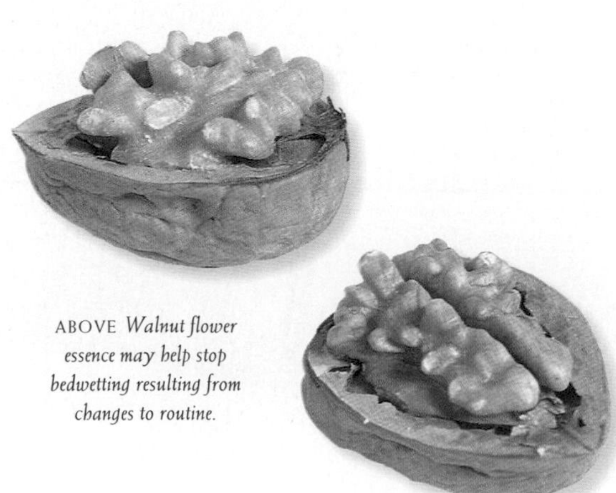

ABOVE *Walnut flower essence may help stop bedwetting resulting from changes to routine.*

Cradle Cap

Cradle cap (seborrheic eczema) is common during the first three months of life and is characterized by a thick encrusted layer of skin on the baby's scalp. Nearly 90 percent of all babies will suffer from cradle cap at some point during the first few months. There will be yellow scales, which form in patches, especially on the top of the head. In severe cases, cradle cap can last for up to three years. Like dandruff, cradle cap is a condition in which the seborrheic glands are overactive, and it is often associated with seborrheic dermatitis, a skin condition in which there are red, scaly areas on the forehead and eyebrows, among other places.

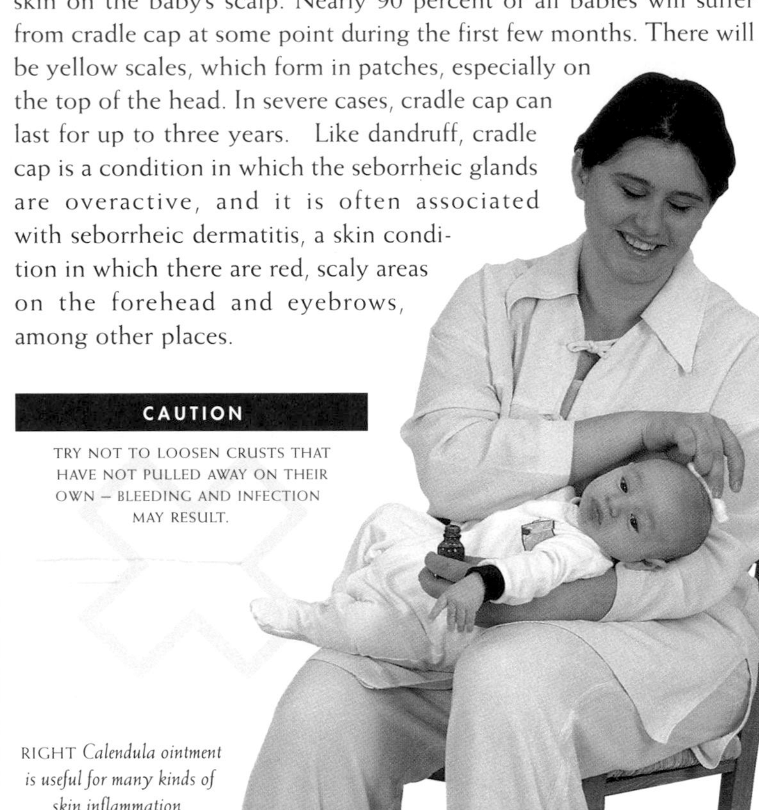

CAUTION

TRY NOT TO LOOSEN CRUSTS THAT HAVE NOT PULLED AWAY ON THEIR OWN – BLEEDING AND INFECTION MAY RESULT.

RIGHT *Calendula ointment is useful for many kinds of skin inflammation.*

TREATMENT

TRADITIONAL HOME AND FOLK REMEDIES
• Massage olive oil into the scalp each evening, and then gently shampoo away in the morning. *(See page 95.)*
• Mash an avocado, apply to the scalp, and then gently rinse. Rub the skin of the avocado across the head to moisten and heal. *(See page 96.)*
• Over-washing will make the condition much worse. Gently brush away loosened crusts with a soft brush.

HERBALISM
• Rinse the scalp after washing with an infusion of meadowsweet, which acts as an anti-inflammatory and will reduce any itching. *(See page 121.)*
• Burdock may also be used to rinse the scalp after washing your baby's hair. *(See page 115.)*
• Butternut can be taken internally (1 drop, 3 times daily, mixed in water) to encourage healing.

AROMATHERAPY
• Massage a few drops of lavender or lemon oil, mixed in a light carrier oil, into the scalp before bedtime. Rinse gently each morning. *(See pages 154 and 161.)*

HOMEOPATHY
• Massage the scalp with Calendula ointment. *(See page 187.)*
• Lycopodium, taken internally, is useful if the skin is dry but uninfected. *(See page 203.)*

FLOWER ESSENCES
• Rock Rose is useful if the itching causes distress. Rescue Remedy cream may be massaged into the scalp to reduce symptoms. *(See page 231.)*
• Add 2 drops of Rescue Remedy to the rinse water, and use after a shampoo. *(See page 244.)*

Impetigo

(*See under Skin and Hair, page 311*).

ABOVE *Distilled witch hazel is an old standby. Dilute with water and apply to the eyelid.*

Sticky Eye

Sticky eye is a mild infection of the eyes which causes a yellowish discharge and crusting. It is most common in the first week of life, and is usually the result of a foreign object entering the eye during birth, or from the blood or amniotic fluid. This condition is not serious and usually rights itself without treatment. In an older child, sticky eyes are usually a sign of conjunctivitis, which is a condition in which the conjunctiva of the eye becomes infected (*see page 318*). It may indicate a blocked tear duct.

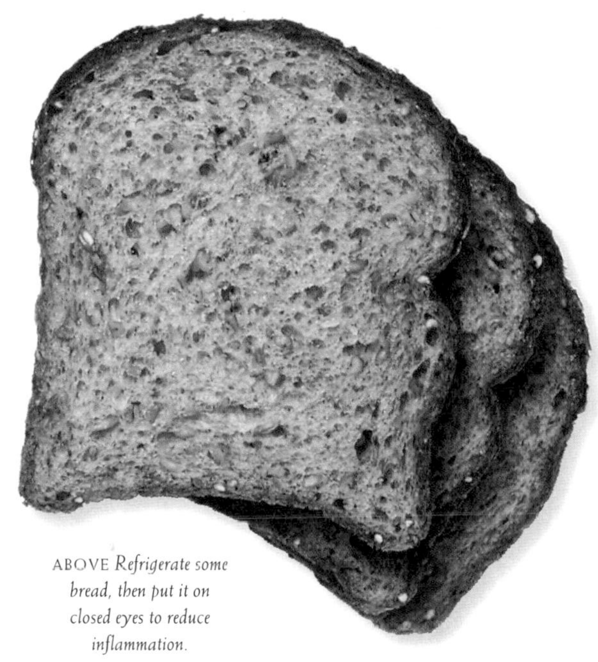

ABOVE *Refrigerate some bread, then put it on closed eyes to reduce inflammation.*

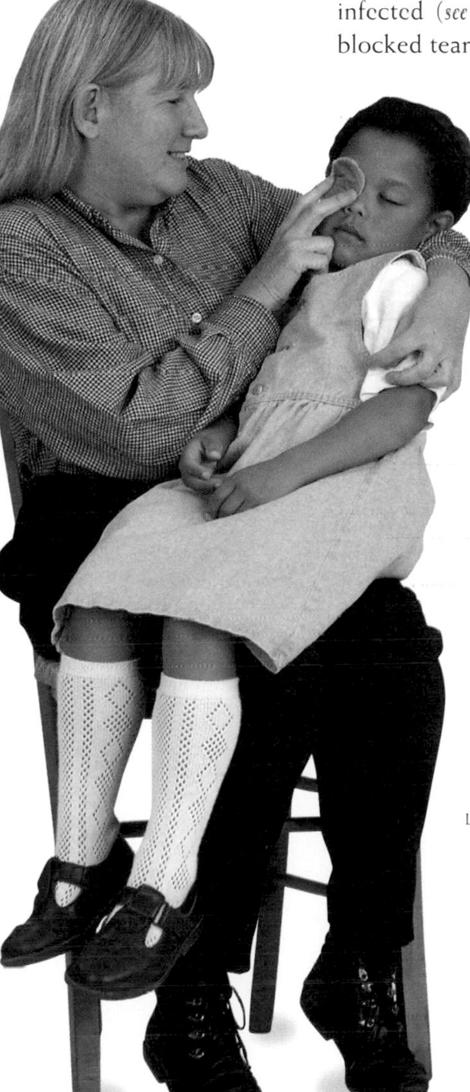

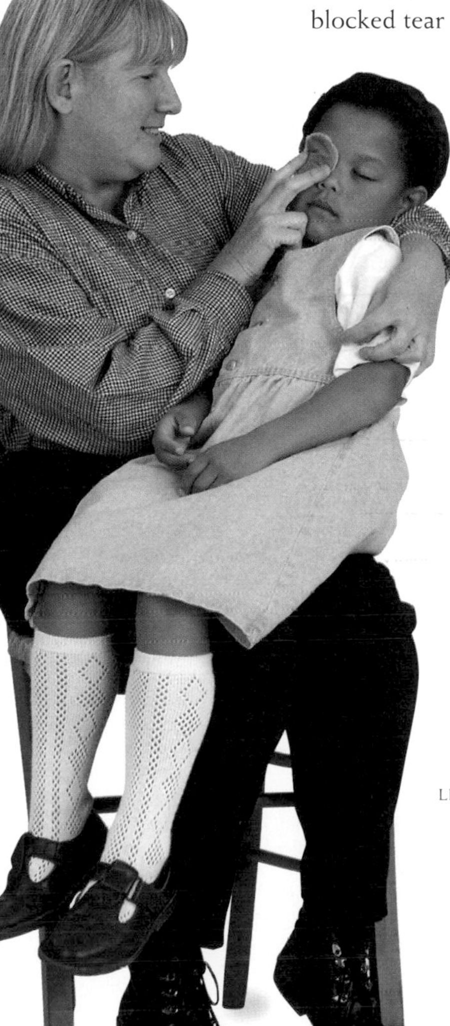

CAUTION

ALWAYS USE VERY WEAK HERBAL INFUSIONS FOR BABIES AND TODDLERS – ONE-FIFTH OF THE DOSE FOR ADULTS. CHILDREN SHOULD HAVE HALF DOSES BETWEEN THE AGES OF SIX AND TWELVE.

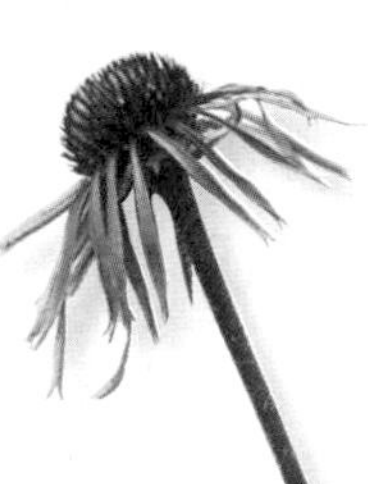

LEFT *A soaked chamomile tea bag will clean and soothe the eye.*

TREATMENT

TRADITIONAL HOME AND FOLK REMEDIES

- Apply cold bread to closed eyes to reduce the inflammation and soothe itching. *(See page 101.)*
- Boil fennel seeds to make an eyewash for conjunctivitis and sore and inflamed eyes.
- Honey water can be used to cleanse the eye; it acts to destroy any infection, soothe, and encourage healing. *(See page 101.)*

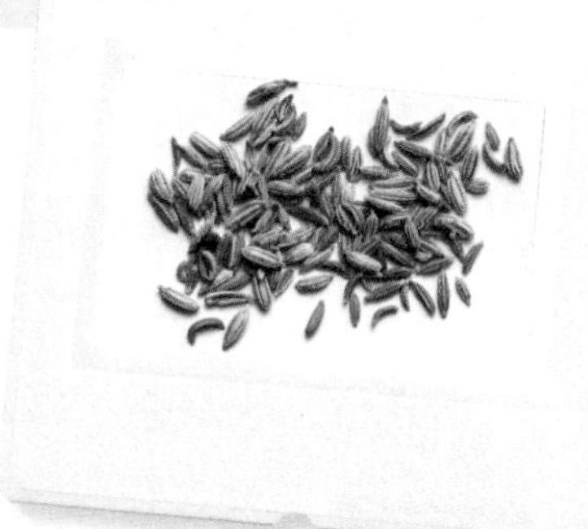

ABOVE *An eyewash made from fennel seeds reduces inflammation.*

HERBALISM

- Infusions of the following herbs can be taken internally to ease the condition: echinacea (which boosts the immune system and acts as a natural antibiotic), eyebright, and golden seal. *(See page 120.)*
- Infusions of chamomile, elderflower, eyebright, and golden seal can be applied externally. Some of these herbs can also be bought as a tincture and then used to make a soothing eyewash. *(See pages 119, 120 and 130.)*
- Soak a chamomile tea bag and hold to the eyelids to soothe. Use it to gently clean the eyes (a new bag for each eye). *(See page 119.)*
- Distilled rosewater or witch hazel can help. *(See page 123.)*

LEFT *Drinking echinacea infusion brings antibiotic benefits.*

HOMEOPATHY

- Euphrasia, for burning, itching eyes. *(See page 194.)*
- 1 or 2 drops of Euphrasia tincture can also be used to bathe the eyes. *(See page 194.)*
- Pulsatilla can be used when there is mucus collecting in the corner of the eyes. *(See page 209.)*
- Hep. sulf. will be useful to draw out infection. *(See page 198.)*

Earache and Middle Ear Infections

Earache may be caused by inflammation of the lymph nodes in the neck, or by another illness like mumps. There may be an ear infection in the inner, middle, or outer parts of the ear. Occasionally a boil can crop up in the outer ear, which can be very painful. The most common ear infections in children are middle ear infections. These are usually caused by the transmission of infection from the nose or throat by the Eustachian tube. Because this tube is short and small in babies and young children, it is easily blocked, and infection does not have far to travel to the middle ear itself. Ear infections can cause a great deal of pain, and the pressure may burst the eardrum, causing a discharge. Earache is also occasionally a sign of dental problems.

Symptoms

pain • possibly a discharge • possibly fever and a sore throat • malaise

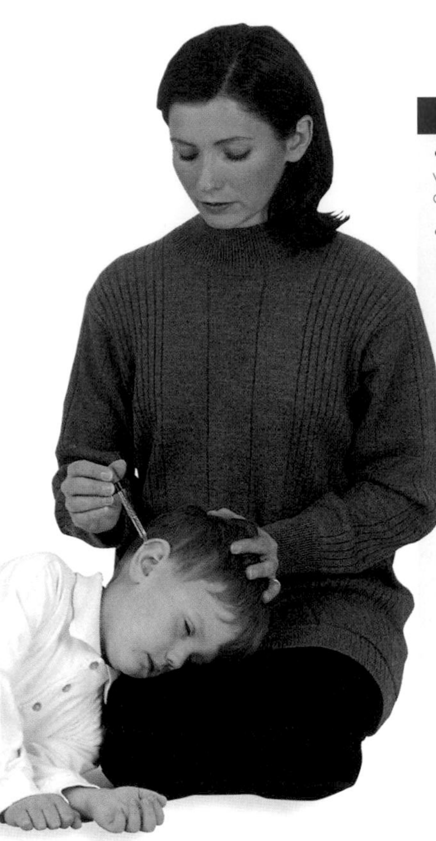

DATA FILE

- As many as 95 percent of all children will have at least one ear infection by the age of six.
- If untreated, ear infections may become chronic.
- Chronic infections may also be associated with allergies, tuberculosis, measles, and other diseases.
- Up to 30 percent of children under the age of six suffer from chronic ear infections.
- Young children, who have shorter and straighter Eustachian tubes than adults, are especially prone to middle ear infections.
- The tendency to ear infections is now believed to be inherited.
- Researchers have also linked recurrent middle ear infections in young children to food allergies.

LEFT *Use a dropper to administer witch hazel and St. John's wort to relieve pain and inflammation.*

TREATMENT

CAUTION

UNTREATED EAR INFECTION MAY SCAR THE EARDRUM AND CAUSE PERMANENT HEARING DAMAGE. INFECTION CAN ALSO SPREAD FROM THE EAR TO OTHER PARTS OF THE HEAD, WHICH MAY BE LIFE-THREATENING.

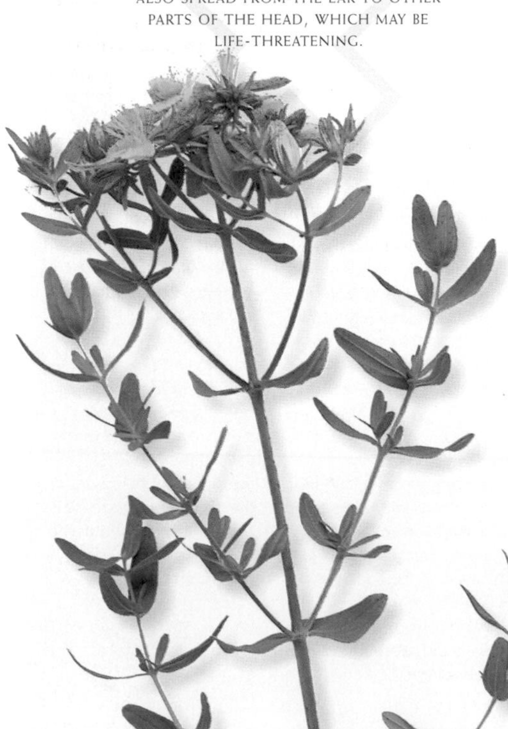

LEFT *A hot St. John's wort compress is anti-inflammatory and comforting.*

TRADITIONAL HOME AND FOLK REMEDIES

- Witch hazel can be added to a teaspoon of oil of St. John's wort and dropped into the ear. This will take away the pain and inflammation. *(See page 91.)*
- Crush fresh garlic and mix with a little honey to encourage the body to fight off the infection. *(See page 82.)*
- Drink honey and lemon, or a little cider vinegar in some warm water to help rid the body of catarrh and strengthen immunity. *(See pages 87, 101, and 102.)*
- Blackcurrant tea will help to boost the immune system and to reduce catarrh.

HERBALISM

- Passiflora will help if there is panic.
- Echinacea can be taken to boost the immune system and clear the pus. *(See page 120.)*
- Apply a hot compress or poultice to the neck and ears using mullein or St. John's wort, which are anti-inflammatory. *(See pages 124 and 137.)*
- Give chamomile tea to drink, to soothe pain and distress. *(See page 119.)*
- For an acute attack, use black root and hops to lower fever and reduce the inflammation present.
- A few drops of tincture of myrrh or golden seal can be added to a light oil, warmed, and dropped into the ear canal.
- Soak a cotton ball with a few drops of warmed garlic oil and press gently into the ear canal. *(See page 113.)*

AROMATHERAPY

- A few drops of neat lavender oil can be placed in the ear on a cotton ball, or gently eased in with a Q-tip. *(See page 161.)*
- Gently massage the neck and head around the ear with oil of mullein or lavender in a light carrier oil. *(See page 161.)*
- Tea tree or lavender oil can be used in a vaporizer for their antiseptic properties. *(See pages 161 and 162.)*
- Use a few drops of lavender oil on a handkerchief by the bed to help your child to stay calm and to sleep. *(See page 161.)*

HOMEOPATHY

- Hep. sulf. is useful for acute attacks, with an earache accompanying a sore throat; and where the child feels chilly. *(See page 198.)*
- Aconite can be used in the early stages, particularly when the symptoms set in suddenly. *(See page 178.)*
- Belladonna, when the affected ear is red and hot, and the child is feverish and perhaps delirious. *(See page 183.)*
- Chamomilla when the child is inconsolable and the pain is made worse if the child is in a draft. *(See page 204.)*

FLOWER ESSENCES

- Rub a little Rescue Remedy (stock or cream) into the painful parts just below the ears to stop the child panicking and reduce inflammation. *(See page 244.)*
- Rescue Remedy or Rock Rose will ease panic. *(See pages 244 and 231.)*
- Olive can be used during recuperation. *(See page 235.)*

VITAMINS AND MINERALS

- Make sure your child's diet is rich in foods containing vitamin C and zinc, which boost the immune system and help to treat infection. *(See pages 256 and 265.)*

Glue Ear

Glue ear is a chronic condition affecting a large number of children. It is characterized by a thick, often smelly, mucus which builds up in the middle ear, due to Eustachian tube obstruction, impairing hearing, and causing the eardrum to perforate to allow the mucus to be discharged. Glue ear is common in children who have frequent colds or other infections, which block the Eustachian tube (*see Middle Ear Infection on page 323 and Outer Ear Infection on page 324*). There is some indication that overuse of antibiotics may encourage the condition, and many children have excess or chronic catarrh (*see page 329*) which may be linked to food allergies or intolerance. Usually both ears are affected, and it is often accompanied by enlarged adenoids and frequently occurs with viral upper respiratory infections, such as the common cold. The first and often the only sign of glue ear is some degree of deafness.

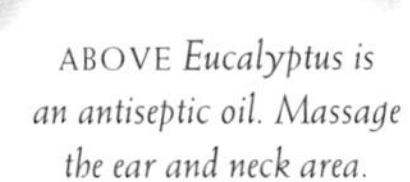

ABOVE *Eucalyptus is an antiseptic oil. Massage the ear and neck area.*

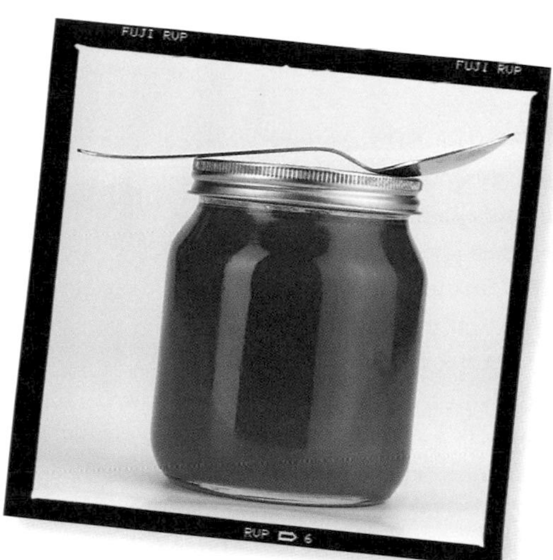

RIGHT *Make garlic-infused honey. It is an expectorant.*

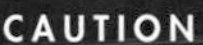

CAUTION

SEVERE INATTENTION AMONG CHILDREN UNDER TWO YEARS COULD WELL BE DUE TO PARTIAL DEAFNESS CAUSED BY GLUE EAR. IT IS ESSENTIAL THAT THIS IS INVESTIGATED IN ORDER TO AVOID LONG-TERM SPEECH, COMPREHENSION, AND INTELLECTUAL IMPAIRMENT.

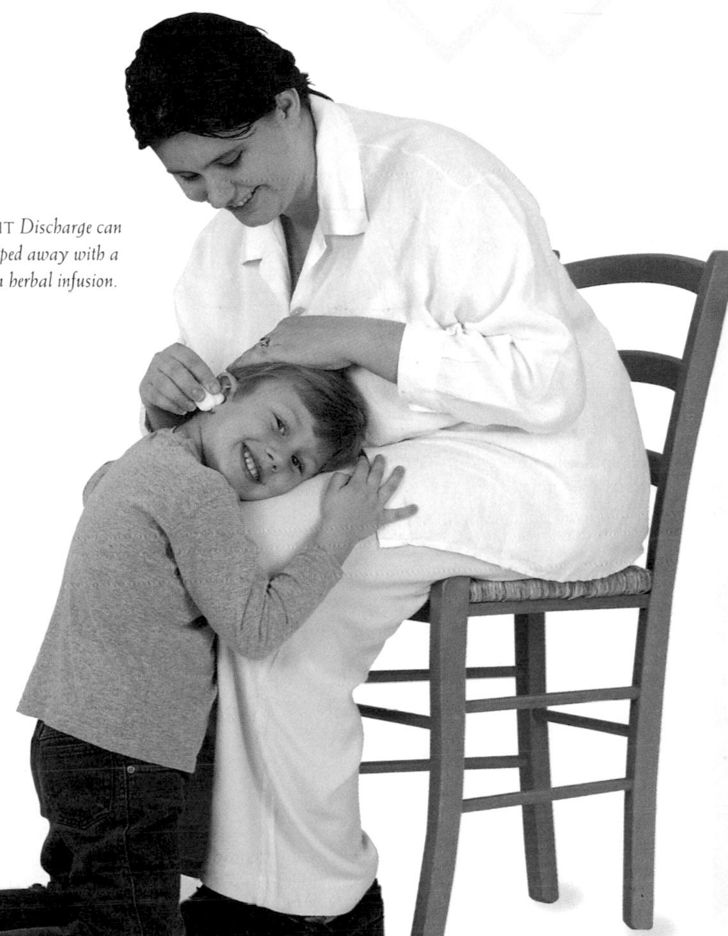

RIGHT *Discharge can be wiped away with a warm herbal infusion.*

TREATMENT

CHINESE HERBALISM

- Herbs to reduce inflammation and Mucus (Phlegm) would be Sheng di Huang or Chinese senega root/Polygala. *(See pages 70 and 72.)*

TRADITIONAL HOME AND FOLK REMEDIES

- Drink lemon and honey or cider vinegar to clear the mucus and to strengthen the immune system. *(See pages 87, 101, and 102.)*
- Garlic is excellent at shifting catarrh and cleansing the blood. Offer as garlic perles, or chop fresh garlic and serve with a teaspoon of honey. *(See page 82.)*
- Blackcurrant tea is excellent for catarrh and will encourage healing of the ear.

HERBALISM

- Chamomile and echinacea are antiseptic, and can be taken internally or added to a foot or hand bath to reduce subsequent infection and to relieve unpleasant symptoms. *(See pages 119 and 120.)*
- Clean away discharge with a warm infusion of antiseptic herbs, such as chamomile or golden seal. *(See page 119.)*
- Herbal remedies to boost the immune system include chamomile, echinacea, peppermint, and wild indigo. *(See pages 119, 120, and 125.)*
- Herbs to help clear the catarrh include elderflowers, euphrasia, golden rod, and hyssop. *(See page 130.)*
- Herbs which work to reduce catarrh include golden rod, ground ivy, and elderflower. *(See page 130.)*

AROMATHERAPY

- Dilute essential oils of lavender, chamomile, eucalyptus, or rosewood in a light carrier oil, warm, and massage around the ear and neck. *(See pages 146–71.)*
- Massage the ear area with a few drops of essential oil of lavender blended in a light carrier oil. *(See page 161.)*
- A steam inhalation of eucalyptus, chamomile, or lavender can help to reduce catarrh and ease accompanying symptoms. *(See pages 146–71.)*
- Apply a hot compress to the nose, ears, and throat made using diluted essential oils of lavender, rosewood, or chamomile *(See pages 146–71.)*

HOMEOPATHY

- Kali mur., when there are cracking sounds in the affected ear, accompanied by swollen glands in the neck.
- Lycopodium, when there is deafness and a roaring sound in the affected ear. *(See page 203.)*
- Pulsatilla, for a full feeling in the ear, and a feeling of weepiness. *(See page 209.)*
- Mercurius, when there is thick, smelly discharge. *(See page 205.)*

VITAMINS AND MINERALS

- Chronic infection can be caused by a build-up of catarrh (see page 329). Reduce consumption of dairy produce and any other possible allergens, including wheat.
- Take cod liver oil and vitamin C to boost the immune system. *(See page 269.)*

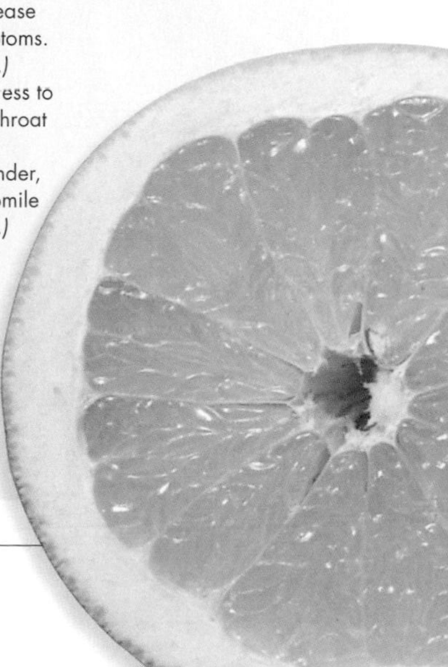

RIGHT *Citrus fruits are high in vitamin C to help fight off infection.*

Colds

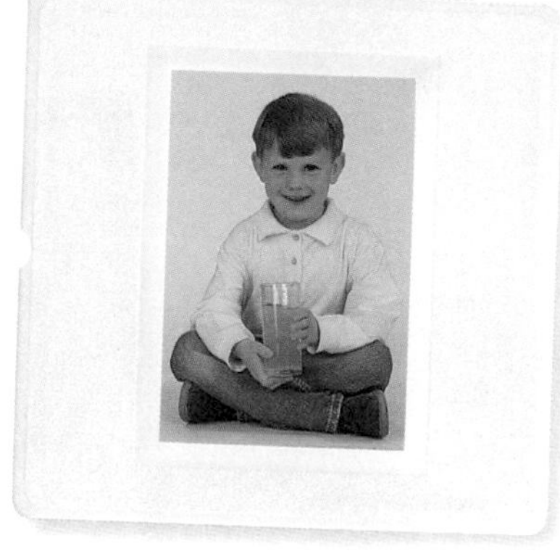

ABOVE *Hot lemon and honey is a tried and tested cold cure.*

Small children are more susceptible than adults to the viruses causing colds and flu because their immune systems are immature. Do not be surprised if your child seems to contract every cold he or she comes into contact with. Symptoms of a cold include a running nose, headache, and sometimes a cough. There may be a mild fever and a feeling of general malaise. Most colds run their course within 7–10 days. Some colds may be symptoms of allergy (particularly when the mucus remains clear) or common childhood illnesses and fevers, or part of a pattern of symptoms associated with asthma or cystic fibrosis. Recurrent colds (almost constantly suffering) may indicate a lowered immune capacity, which can be treated by complementary remedies. (*See Colds, page 352.*)

ABOVE *Include garlic in food for its antibiotic, immune-enhancing properties.*

Symptoms

• *running nose* • *headache* • *sometimes a cough* • *possibly a mild fever and a feeling of general malaise*

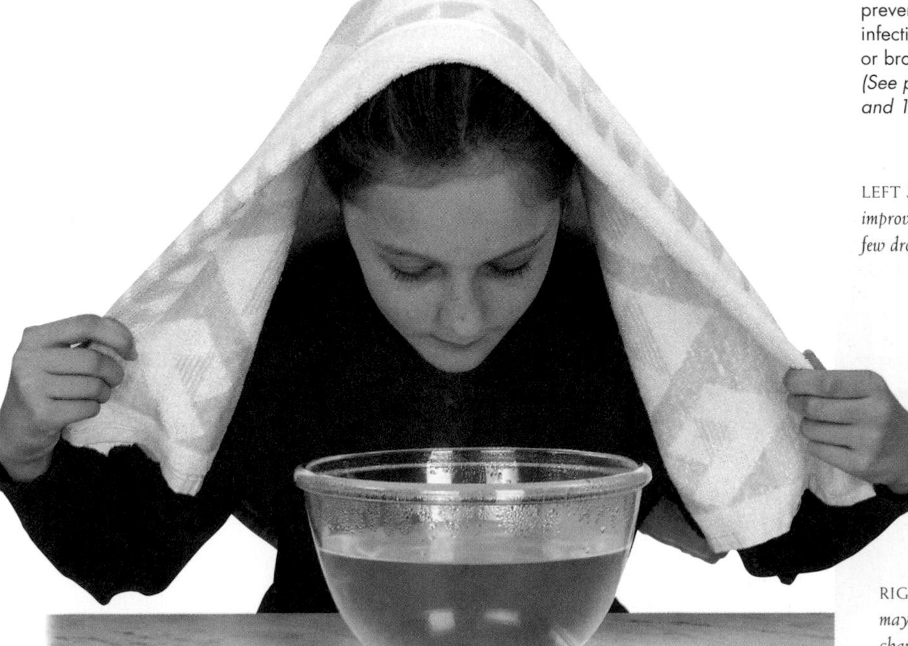

LEFT *Steam inhalation improves congestion. Use a few drops of cinnamon oil.*

TREATMENT

TRADITIONAL HOME AND FOLK REMEDIES

• Blackcurrant tea is excellent for catarrh and infections.

• Eat plenty of fresh garlic and onions to reduce catarrh and cleanse the blood. Garlic is also antibiotic and boosts the immune system. *(See page 82.)*

• Hot lemon and honey will help to clear catarrh, prevent a secondary infection (such as tonsillitis or bronchitis), and soothe discomfort. *(See pages 87 and 101.)*

HERBALISM

• Blue flag or poke root, for swollen glands.

• Golden seal and elecampane, for chronic colds, to clear mucus from the lungs and nasal passages.

• Elderflowers, drunk as an infusion, will reduce catarrh and help to decongest. *(See page 130.)*

• Peppermint is another decongestant and will also work to reduce a fever. *(See page 125.)*

• Eucalyptus, rosemary, and thyme will help to clear congestion and work as antiseptics, which may help to prevent a secondary infection of the tonsils or bronchi (bronchitis). *(See pages 127 and 135.)*

• Chamomile will soothe an irritable child and help him or her to sleep. Chamomile also has antiseptic action, which will help to rid the body of infection, and it works to reduce fever and feverish symptoms. *(See page 119.)*

• Try adding a strong infusion of chamomile or yarrow to the bath. *(See pages 112 and 119.)*

• Mullein or comfrey can be drunk or used as a compress around the neck to soothe a sore throat. *(See pages 132 and 137.)*

• Herbs to strengthen the immune system, including echinacea, can be taken throughout a cold. *(See page 120.)*

AROMATHERAPY

• Place your child's head over a steaming bowl of water with a few drops of essential oil of cinnamon. Place a towel over her head to make a tent, and let her sit there for 4 or 5 minutes to ease congestion. *(See page 150.)*

• Massage a few drops of pine or eucalyptus, blended in a light carrier oil, into the chest area. *(See pages 159 and 166.)*

• Try a few drops of lavender or tea tree oil in a warm bath to encourage healing and open up the airways. *(See pages 161 and 162.)*

• Use chamomile, cloves, lavender, pine, lemon, and thyme together or separately in a room vaporizer to help ease symptoms and promote healing. *(See pages 146–71.)*

HOMEOPATHY

• Nat. mur., for dealing with watery colds. *(See page 206.)*

• Kali mur., for colds with catarrh.

• Ferr. phos., for hot colds. *(See page 194.)*

• Arsenicum, for watery colds, particularly if your child is prone to frequent colds. *(See page 182.)*

• Euphrasia, for colds affecting the eyes. *(See page 194.)*

• Pulsatilla is useful if your child is clingy and irritable, and when there is thick yellow discharge. *(See page 209.)*

• Bryonia, for an irritable child who is thirsty and wants to be left alone. *(See page 185.)*

• Mercurius, for a child with earache and swollen lymph nodes in the neck. *(See page 205.)*

FLOWER ESSENCES

• Rescue Remedy will soothe any distress. *(See page 244.)*

• Olive will help with fatigue. *(See page 235.)*

• Willow, if the child feels sorry for him or herself. *(See page 239.)*

VITAMINS AND MINERALS

• Eat plenty of foods with vitamin C and zinc, which will help discourage a cold and reduce its duration. *(See pages 256 and 265.)*

RIGHT *Feverish coughs may be improved by sipping chamomile infusion.*

BELOW *Lavender oil, sprinkled on the pillow, promotes sleep.*

Coughs

Coughing expels foreign bodies and irritating mucus from the trachea and airways of the lungs. The membranes lining the whole respiratory tract are very sensitive and react to inhaled particles or infection by producing mucus, which is then coughed up. The color of the mucus or phlegm indicates the nature or the degree of irritation or infection. There are many types of coughs, some of which accompany a cold. Others are caused by chemicals, other infections, like ear and tonsil infections, excess catarrh, inflammation of the airways, and many other things. A chronic cough is one that lasts for more than 10 days, or one that recurs frequently.

CAUTION

IF A COUGH IS ACCOMPANIED BY A HIGH FEVER AND YOUR CHILD HAS DIFFICULTY BREATHING, SEE YOUR PHYSICIAN IMMEDIATELY. IF A COUGH DOES NOT IMPROVE WITHIN A FEW DAYS, SEE YOUR PHYSICIAN.

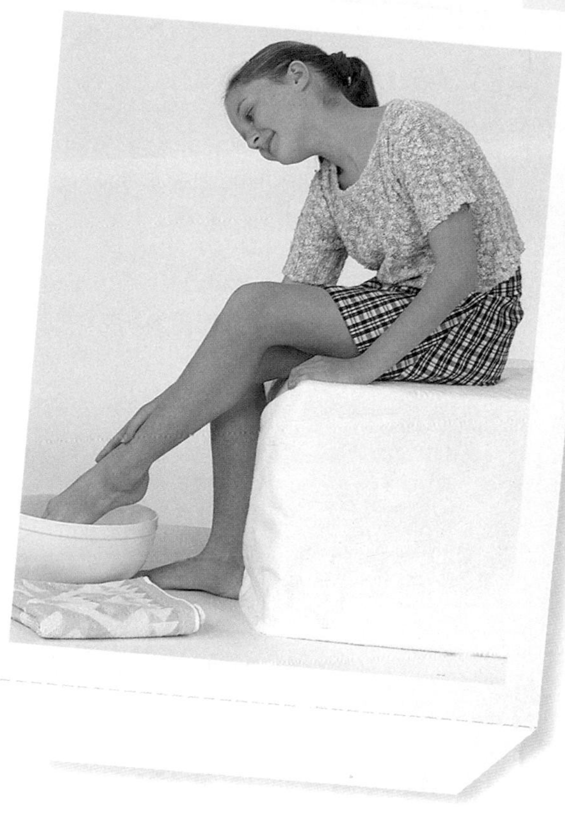

RIGHT *A thyme oil foot bath helps shift stubborn catarrh.*

TREATMENT

TRADITIONAL HOME AND FOLK REMEDIES

- Fresh garlic should be eaten as often as possible to cleanse the blood, improve the immune response, and encourage healing. *(See page 82.)*
- Give your child lots of honey, which has antibacterial action and will also soothe a sore throat. *(See page 101.)*
- Blackcurrant tea will ease the pain of a sore throat and help to reduce catarrh.
- Ginger, added to meals, will help to get rid of any lingering catarrh.
- Pineapples are traditionally used for expelling excess catarrh.
- Lemon and honey will soothe a sore throat and ease a tickly cough. *(See pages 87 and 101.)*

HERBALISM

- Aniseed and fennel will warm the system and help to shift a cough. *(See page 121.)*
- Cayenne pepper can be added to food (a few grains) to stimulate the body's immune defenses and clear the wet secretions from the lungs. *(See page 118.)*
- Pasque flower and lobelia will clear fever and reduce inflammation.
- For fever, try infusions of chamomile, catmint, hyssop, and yarrow. *(See pages 112 and 119.)*
- Comfrey and coltsfoot help expel mucus from the lungs and airways. Mix 10 drops of each tincture with warmed honey. Serve by the teaspoonful. *(See page 132.)*
- Elecampane and thyme can be infused and used to treat a wet cough. *(See page 135.)*
- When the mucus is tough to shift, try strong infusions of ginger and fennel or thyme. *(See pages 121, 135, and 139.)*
- Elecampane root tea, sweetened with honey and ginger, will help to reduce inflammation and reduce mucus.

AROMATHERAPY

- Use lavender, myrrh, eucalyptus, or thyme in a vaporizer. *(See pages 146–71.)*
- A few drops of oil of thyme, pine, cinnamon, clove, or eucalyptus can be used in combination or on their own in a foot bath to ease congestion. *(See pages 146–71.)*
- Add a few drops of eucalyptus and sandalwood to a carrier oil or some petroleum jelly, and rub into the chest and upper back. *(See pages 159 and 169.)*
- Myrrh can be massaged into the body in the same way, to reduce mucus. Or put a few drops on a handkerchief and tie it to the bed. *(See page 155.)*
- Lavender oil on a handkerchief or pillow will encourage sleep and aid the healing process. *(See page 161.)*

HOMEOPATHY

- Belladonna can be taken when the cough is accompanied by a fever, and the child has bright red cheeks and neck. *(See page 183.)*
- Pulsatilla may be useful if there is a thick yellow discharge and your child is clingy and tearful. *(See page 209.)*
- Ant. tart., for a cough that causes the chest to rattle and makes breathing painful. *(See page 179.)*
- Bryonia, for a painful, dry cough which is made worse by movement. *(See page 185.)*
- Spongia is excellent for croup *(see page 438)* and for a loud, crowing cough. *(See page 213.)*
- Drosera, for a tickling cough which is worse when lying down. *(See page 193.)*
- Try aconite if the symptoms come on suddenly. *(See page 178.)*
- Chamomilla will soothe an inconsolable child, who is better for being held. *(See page 204.)*

FLOWER ESSENCES

- Use Rescue Remedy when your child experiences distress, or panics because breathing is difficult. Rescue Remedy may also help your child to sleep. A few drops can be taken internally or applied to pulse points. *(See page 244.)*
- Olive is good for a child who is overwhelmed by fatigue. *(See page 235.)*

VITAMINS AND MINERALS

- Plenty of fluids and bed rest will make it easier for your child to shift a cough. Offer fluids only for the first couple of days, and then just light meals. Avoid dairy produce altogether until the catarrh has shifted.

RIGHT *If your child is worn out by coughing, try Olive flower essence.*

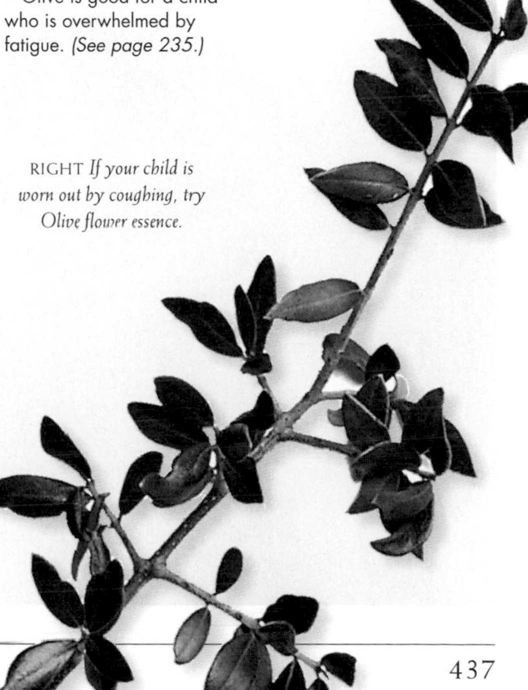

Croup

Croup is an acute inflammation and narrowing of the air passages, especially the larynx, in young children. The disorder is caused by various viruses, particularly the para-influenza virus, or by bacteria. The primary symptoms are coughing, hoarseness, and noisy, difficult breathing, which can sometimes be alleviated with steam inhalations. The characteristic cough of croup is a definite loud bark or whistle, caused by inflammation of the vocal cords. Infectious croup occurs mainly in the winter, when the larynx (voice box) or trachea (windpipe) become inflamed and swollen after what seems to be simply a cold. Other causes include allergy or the inhalation of a foreign body. Because the larynx swells and blocks the passage of air, breathing can be very difficult, which can panic a child.

CAUTION

IF YOUR CHILD TURNS BLUE, CALL A PHYSICIAN IMMEDIATELY.

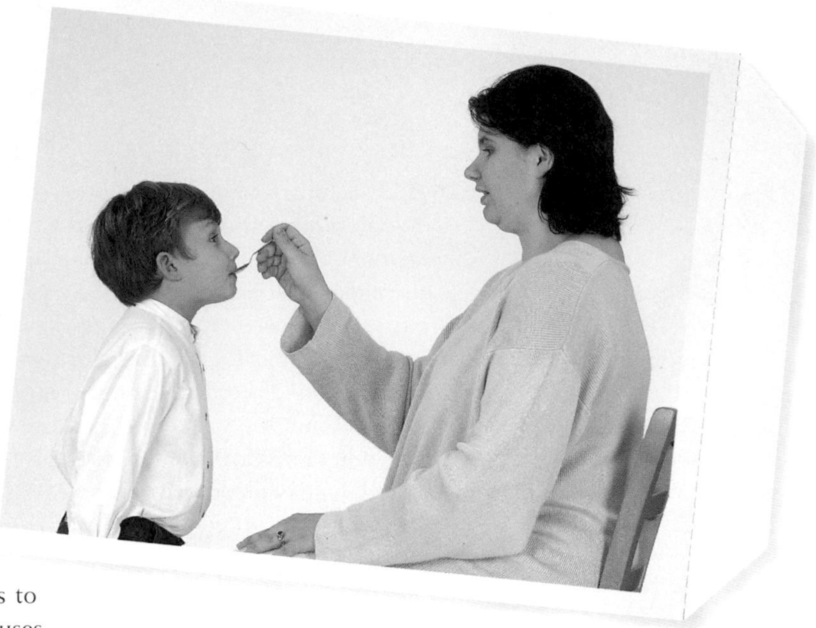

ABOVE *Give wild cherry syrup to calm painful spasms.*

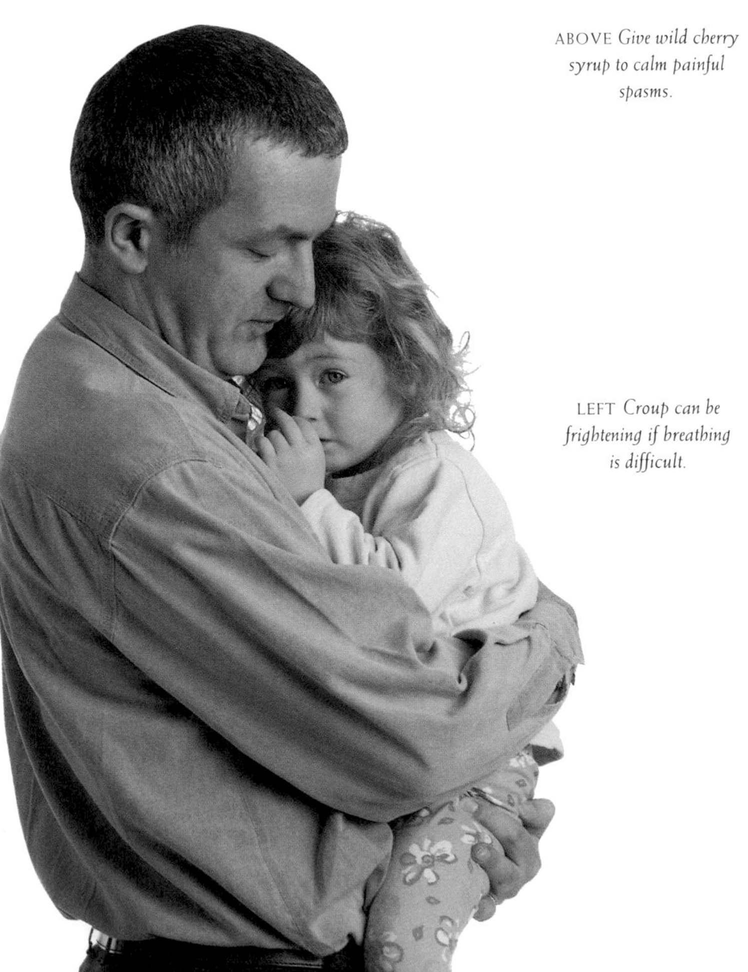

LEFT *Croup can be frightening if breathing is difficult.*

TREATMENT

TRADITIONAL HOME AND FOLK REMEDIES

- Offer a hot honey and lemon drink to ease the symptoms. Honey has strong antibacterial properties and will be useful if the cause of the croup is bacterial infection. *(See pages 87 and 101.)*
- A little cider vinegar mixed with a mug of warm water can be sipped to ease symptoms. *(See page 102.)*
- Blackcurrant tea is helpful and restorative.
- Put your child in a bathroom with the door shut and the hot taps running, or fill a bowl with boiling water and gently place your child's head over it, covered by a towel. Steam will open the airways and reduce symptoms. Raise the upper end of the cot or bed so that breathing is easier. *(See page 103.)*

HERBALISM

- Lobelia and black cohosh will reduce spasm, soften the phlegm, and clear the lungs.
- Wild cherry syrup can reduce spasm and help deal with phlegm.
- Try infusing lavender flowers or chamomile in a bowl of hot water, then ask your child to lean over it, to help breathing. *(See page 119.)*
- Infuse some chamomile, catmint, or wild cherry, and give your child small sips before bedtime and during an attack. *(See page 119.)*
- Mix catmint, horehound, and wild cherry together with a little honey or licorice and give by the teaspoonful as necessary.
- A foot bath with some thyme or eucalyptus oil added should help. *(See page 135.)*

AROMATHERAPY

- Essential oils of eucalyptus, lavender, pine, chamomile, thyme and cinnamon can be added, together or individually, to a vaporizer or a foot-bath. *(See pages 146–71.)*
- A few drops of eucalyptus or lavender can be placed on a handkerchief by the child's cot or bed to ease breathing and encourage the child to relax. *(See pages 159 and 161.)*
- Rub a few drops of lavender oil mixed with petroleum jelly into your child's chest and upper back. *(See page 161.)*

HOMEOPATHY

- Spongia is the traditional treatment for croup, and can be taken every 20 minutes during an attack. *(See page 213.)*
- Aconite can be taken alongside Spongia. *(See page 178.)*
- Phosphorus may be useful when there is a thirst for cold drinks (which may be vomited up). *(See page 208.)*
- Drosera, for a deep hoarse-sounding cough, with gasping and retching. *(See page 193.)*

FLOWER ESSENCES

- Rescue Remedy will help to calm the child, which will make breathing easier. *(See page 244.)*
- Rock Rose will help if your child is frightened. *(See page 231.)*
- Olive can be taken following an attack, if the child is exhausted. *(See page 235.)*

Thrush

Thrush, or candidiasis, is a fungal, or yeast infection of the Candida albicans fungus, which is very common in those with immature immune systems, or those with immune systems that are compromised or very stressed. Thrush takes many forms, the most common of which are oral and that which develops in the diaper area.

The immune system can be impaired by poor diet, pollution, the overuse of drugs – which suppress it and upset the balance of the intestinal flora, causing Candida, or thrush, to flourish – injury, or surgery, among others. In babies, it usually occurs in conjunction with diaper rash. Oral thrush is characterized by sore, white, raised patches in the mouth. In the diaper area or skin folds it takes the form of an itchy red rash with a white top.

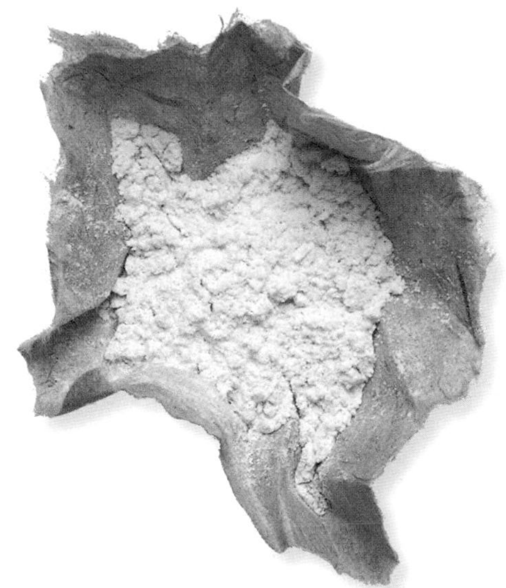

LEFT *Arsenicum is useful for sores on the mouth, especially if brought on by exhaustion.*

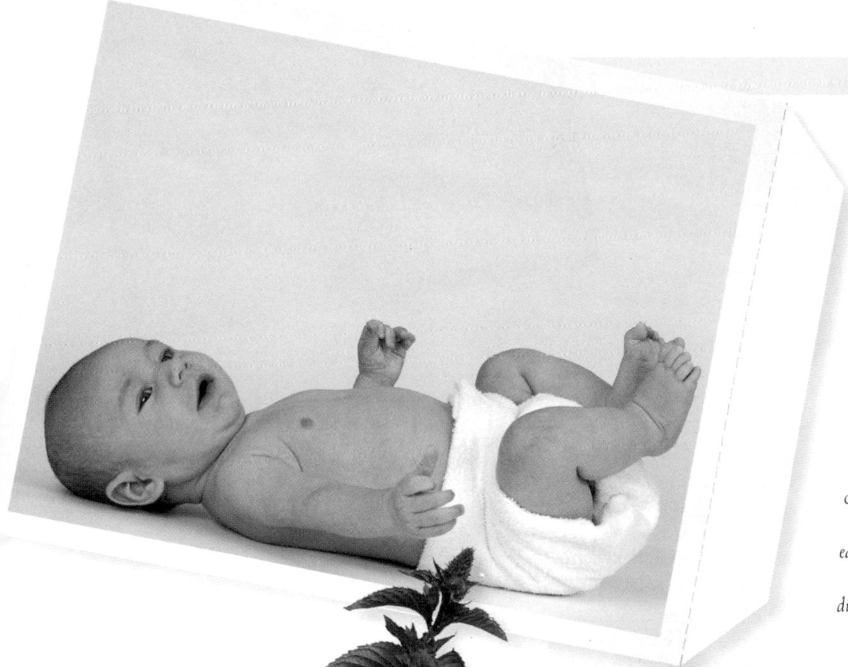

LEFT *Diaper rash is a common fungal infection in young babies and is easy to treat, particularly with the use of a very diluted blend of tea tree oil.*

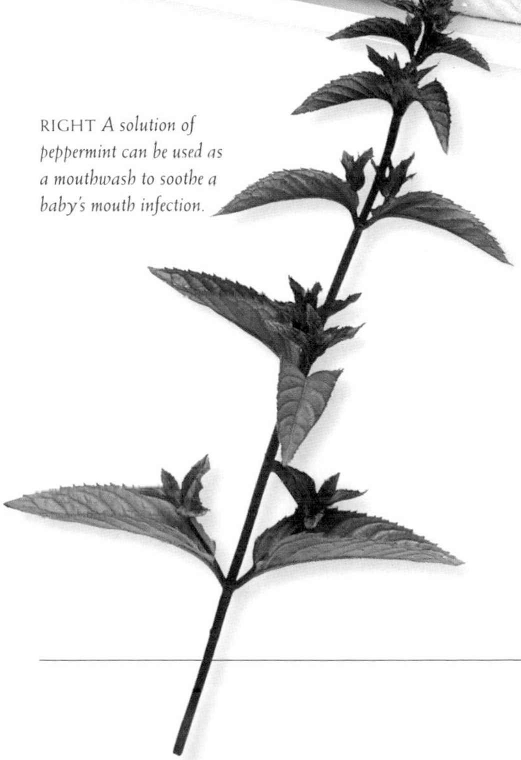

RIGHT *A solution of peppermint can be used as a mouthwash to soothe a baby's mouth infection.*

TREATMENT

HERBALISM

- Echinacea, to boost the immune system, will help to prevent chronic thrush and help the body to fight infection. *(See page 120.)*
- Oral thrush may be helped by preparing a mouthwash solution with lavender, lemon, or peppermint in spring water. Rinse the baby's mouth, or dab a few drops on the affected areas. *(See page 125.)*

AROMATHERAPY

- Use tea tree oil in a vaporizer in your child's room, to boost the immune system and act as an antifungal agent. *(See page 162.)*
- Extremely dilute lavender oil or tea tree oil can be dabbed on to patches in the mouth and on the bottom. Avoid the genitals. *(See pages 161 and 162.)*

HOMEOPATHY

Treatment will be constitutional, but the following remedies may be useful:

- Borax, at the first sign of an outbreak.
- Mercurius, when there is more saliva than usual and the tongue trembles. *(See page 205.)*
- Capsicum, for sore, hot patches.
- Arsenicum, for burning pains, mouth ulcers, and feeling worn out. *(See page 182.)*

FLOWER ESSENCES

- Apply a little Rescue Remedy cream to the affected area (externally) and a few drops of diluted stock remedy to sores in the mouth. *(See page 244.)*
- Olive can be useful if outbreaks are linked to exhaustion. *(See page 235.)*

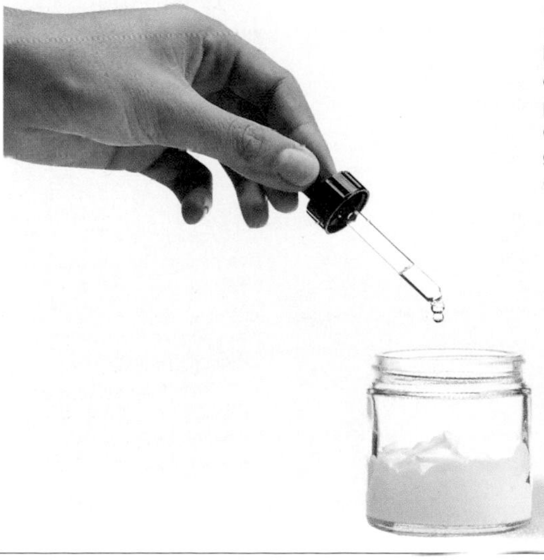

LEFT *Rescue Remedy applied in a cream is a useful external application.*

Teething Problems

Your baby's first teeth will probably appear at about six months of age, and there may be problems with teeth coming through until the age of two or three. Most babies experience some discomfort, which can range from quite mild, which may make them clingy and fractious, to severe, accompanied by dribbling, loosened stools, and sleeping problems. A classic symptom is a red patch on one cheek.

ABOVE *A little honey, rubbed into the gums, lessens the discomfort of teething.*

CAUTION

VOMITING IS NOT A SYMPTOM OF TEETHING. SEE YOUR PHYSICIAN IF YOUR BABY SEEMS UNWELL.

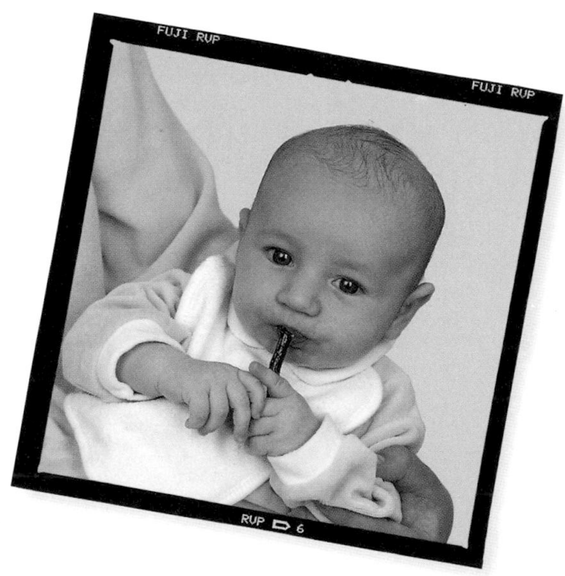

RIGHT *Try a piece of licorice root as a teether for your baby.*

TREATMENT

TRADITIONAL HOME AND FOLK REMEDIES

- Rub a little honey into the gums for relief. Make sure it is pasteurized. *(See page 101.)*
- Give your baby a cold licorice root to gnaw on. *(See page 91.)*
- Cold raw carrots are useful teethers, but watch your baby carefully to make sure he or she doesn't bite off a piece and choke on it. *(See page 89.)*

LEFT *Rock Rose is a component of Rescue Remedy which will soothe a child who seems inconsolable.*

HERBALISM

- Syrup made from the marshmallow root will soothe inflamed gums. Add a few teaspoons to your baby's normal meals. *(See page 114.)*
- Offer infusions of chamomile or fennel to calm and to soothe. *(See pages 119 and 121.)*

AROMATHERAPY

- Put a few drops of lavender oil on the bedclothes to help your baby to sleep. Essential oils of chamomile and lavender can be added to the bath water to calm a distressed baby. *(See pages 150 and 161.)*
- Rub the gums with a little chamomile oil mixed with a teaspoon of honey. Clove oil also acts as a local anesthetic, and a minute amount can be diluted and rubbed into the gums. *(See page 150.)*

HOMEOPATHY

- Chamomilla is the standard remedy for teething, and can be taken up to 6 times daily. *(See page 204.)*
- Calc. phos. may also be useful. *(See page 186.)*

FLOWER ESSENCES

- Rub a little diluted Rescue Remedy directly into the gums, or apply to pulse points if your baby is crying inconsolably. A few drops at nighttime will keep your baby calm, enabling him or her to sleep. *(See page 244.)*
- Walnut will help the child through the transition. *(See page 232.)*

BELOW *Make an infusion by pouring boiling water on lightly crushed fennel seeds. Leave for ten minutes.*

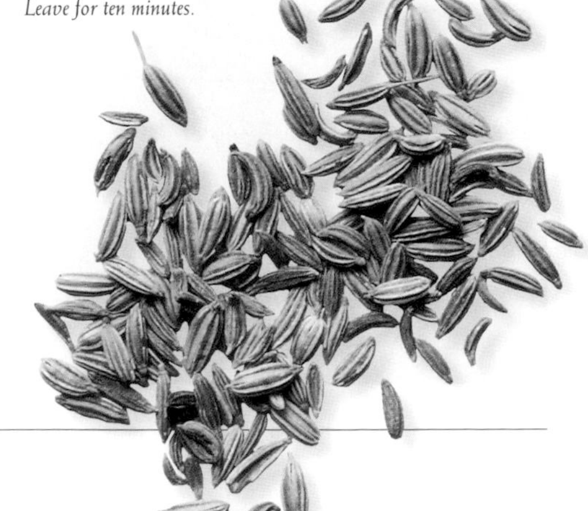

Colic

Colic is characterized by apparently unending frantic crying, usually at around the same time of day or night. The legs are drawn up to the abdomen, and the baby appears to be in severe pain. Excessive crying causes the baby to swallow air, which can exacerbate the problem and lead to abdominal bloating. The cause is unknown, but colic may be caused by contractions of the colon, an allergy to something in the formula (if bottle-fed) or the mother's diet (if breast-fed), or simply excessive air which is gulped in through repeated bouts of crying. The most common form of colic is three-month colic, typically coming on in the evening and lasting anything from a few minutes to several hours. Burping or laying the baby over the knee or shoulder usually has little effect.

CAUTION

VOMITING OR DIARRHEA ARE NOT SYMPTOMS OF COLIC AND TREATMENT MUST BE SOUGHT IMMEDIATELY.

LEFT *Try adding lemon balm infusion to your baby's bath.*

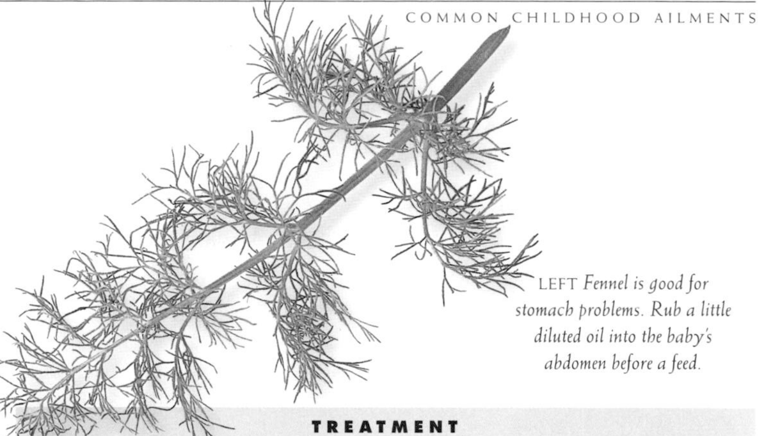

LEFT *Fennel is good for stomach problems. Rub a little diluted oil into the baby's abdomen before a feed.*

TREATMENT

TRADITIONAL HOME AND FOLK REMEDIES

- Caraway water can be diluted and given to even a very young baby in a sterilized bottle. Offer a few sips just before a feed.

HERBALISM

- Because colic is exacerbated by tension, relaxing herbs are often suggested – used in the bath, or infused, cooled slightly and taken by bottle. Chamomile, lemon balm, and limeflowers are the most effective. *(See pages 119 and 134.)*
- A warm bath with an infusion of dill, fennel, marshmallow, or lemon balm will soothe a colicky baby. *(See pages 114 and 121.)*
- Catmint, infused and diluted, can be added to your baby's bath water to relax any abdominal spasm.

AROMATHERAPY

- Rub a little very dilute fennel oil into the abdomen before feeds to prevent colic. *(See page 159.)*
- A gentle massage of the abdominal area with one or a blend of essential oils of chamomile, dill, lavender, or rose will help to ease symptoms and calm a distressed baby. *(See pages 146–71.)*
- If your baby is wakened by discomfort, place a handkerchief with a few drops of lavender oil by the bed. *(See page 161.)*
- Try a few drops of lavender or chamomile oil in a warm bath, just before evening feeds. *(See pages 150 and 161.)*

HOMEOPATHY

- Chamomilla is useful for babies who seem better when they are held. *(See page 204.)*
- Pulsatilla is used for babies who are better in the fresh air and when they are rocked. *(See page 209.)*
- Cuprum met. is used when the tummy rumbles, and the child curls fingers and toes in discomfort. *(See page 192.)*

FLOWER ESSENCES

- Rock Rose is excellent for extreme fright. *(See page 231.)*
- Rescue Remedy can be used to calm and should therefore help to reduce any spasm. *(See page 244.)*

VITAMINS AND MINERALS

- If you are breast-feeding, avoid dairy produce for a few days to see if this helps.
- Other foods which should be avoided are very spicy foods, citrus foods, gassy foods (beans, onions, cabbage, etc.), and sugar.

BELOW *Breastfeeding mothers should avoid dairy foods, which may cause colic in babies.*

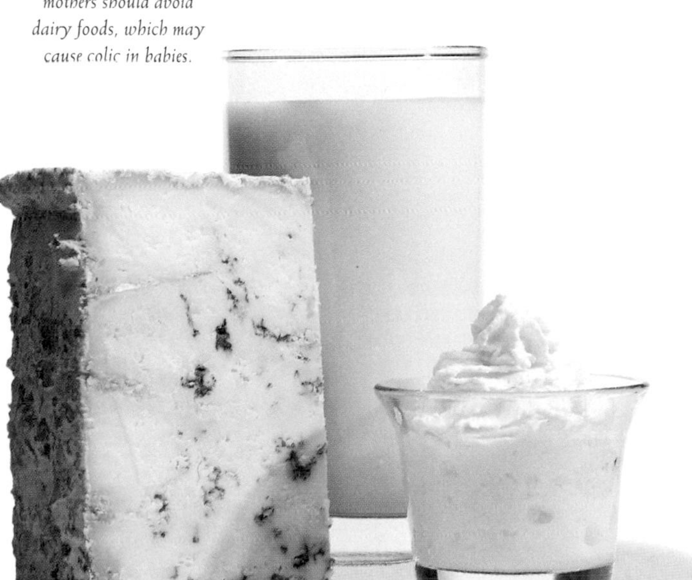

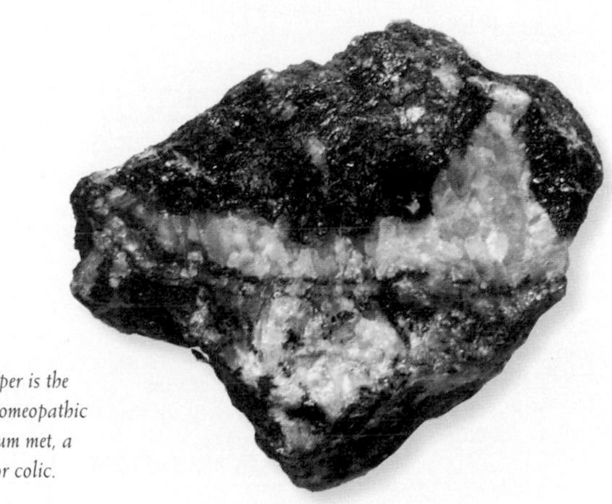

RIGHT *Copper is the source for the homeopathic remedy Cuprum met, a treatment for colic.*

Vomiting and Diarrhea

There are many causes of vomiting and diarrhea in children including infections such as gastroenteritis, eating rich or fatty foods (or, indeed, overeating), emotional upsets, food poisoning, and many others. These conditions are not usually serious, unless they recur.

Gastroenteritis is usually present if there is fever of 38°C (100°F), vomiting, lack of enthusiasm for feeds, and torpor. Occasionally diarrhea is due to too early reintroduction of milk after an attack of gastroenteritis. Remember that babies and children can dehydrate quickly, and you must ensure that they drink plenty of liquids.

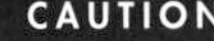

CAUTION

BABIES AND CHILDREN CAN VERY EASILY BECOME DEHYDRATED BY VOMITING OR DIARRHEA, AND IT IS IMPORTANT THAT YOU SEEK MEDICAL TREATMENT URGENTLY. SEE YOUR PHYSICIAN IF THERE IS BLOOD IN THE VOMIT OR FECES.

LEFT *Very ripe bananas help restore beneficial intestinal bacteria.*

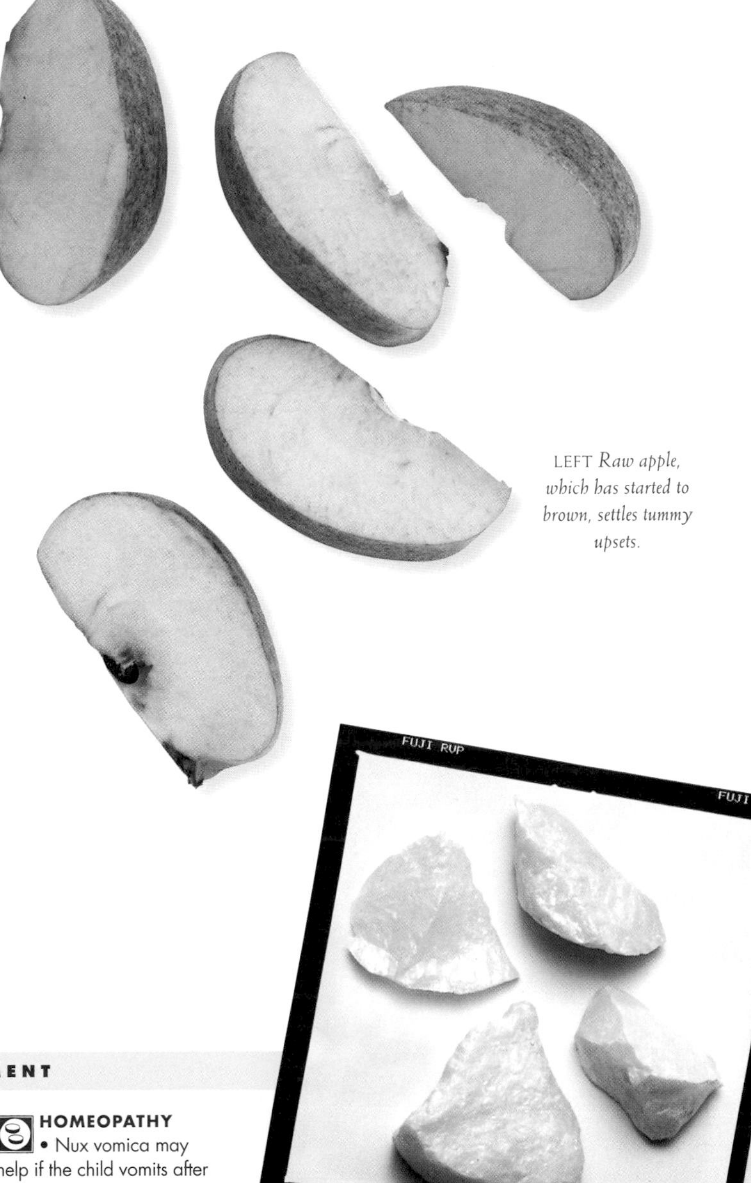

LEFT *Raw apple, which has started to brown, settles tummy upsets.*

ABOVE *Sulfur, prepared as a homeopathic remedy, helps to drive toxins out of the body.*

TREATMENT

TRADITIONAL HOME AND FOLK REMEDIES

- Milk and honey are excellent for treating an attack of food poisoning. *(See page 101.)*
- Mustard is a natural emetic and can be taken internally, mixed with a few teaspoons of warm water. *(See page 98.)*
- Garlic is excellent to fight infection, boost immunities, and cleanse the blood. It is also a natural antibiotic, so is excellent in cases of bacterial infection. *(See page 82.)*
- Drink fresh lemon juice, warmed and mixed with a little honey, to cleanse the gut. *(See pages 87 and 101.)*
- Drink blackcurrant juice, as a gut astringent.
- Raw apple which has gone brown is useful for settling an upset stomach. Offer in small quantities. *(See page 94.)*

HERBALISM

- Chamomile or melissa tea will help to settle and calm an excited child. *(See page 119.)*
- Meadowsweet or marshmallow syrup can help with vomiting. *(See pages 114 and 121.)*
- Gentian and barberry can be added to water and sipped frequently.
- Chamomile and vervain can be taken internally to soothe a child whose illness is exacerbated or caused by emotional upset, or who is distressed by the vomiting. *(See pages 119 and 138.)*
- Try ginger, crushed or decocted, to ease nausea. *(See page 139.)*
- Chamomile, echinacea, peppermint, and thyme can be drunk as infusions or added to a foot-bath when infection causes the illness. *(See pages 119, 120, 125, and 135.)*

AROMATHERAPY

- Massage the tummy and chest with a few drops of lavender or chamomile essential oil in a light carrier oil. *(See pages 150 and 161.)*
- Use essential oil of thyme or tea tree in a vaporizer for their antiseptic properties. *(See pages 162 and 170.)*
- A few drops of lavender essential oil in the bath or by the bedside will calm. *(See page 161.)*

HOMEOPATHY

- Nux vomica may help if the child vomits after eating too much, or too quickly. *(See page 214.)*
- China, for diarrhea with wind, particularly when the child is very irritable. *(See page 190.)*
- Colocynthis, if diarrhea is copious, thin, and yellow, accompanied by episodic pain. *(See page 191.)*
- Arsenicum, when there is burning and the child is restless, anxious, and cold. *(See page 182.)*
- Veratrum alb., when there is vomiting and diarrhea with cold sweats.
- Pulsatilla, after a rich, fatty meal, when there is no thirst. *(See page 209.)*
- Sulfur, for red orifices, smelly burps, and cravings for sweets. *(See page 215.)*

FLOWER ESSENCES

- Rescue Remedy will relieve the distress caused by vomiting and diarrhea. *(See page 244.)*
- Olive flower essence is useful for recuperation. *(See page 235.)*
- If the vomiting is caused by emotional problems select a remedy that will help with those problems.

VITAMINS AND MINERALS

- Following an attack of vomiting or diarrhea, offer lots of live yogurt and very ripe bananas to restore the proper bacterial balance of the gut.
- An acidophilus tablet can be taken for the same purpose. These are available in vanilla flavor. *(See page 271.)*

Diaper Rash

Diaper rash is caused by contact with urine or feces, which cause the skin to produce less protective oil and therefore provide a less effective barrier to further irritation. It can also be caused by irritating chemicals in feces, not thoroughly rinsing soap or detergent out of diapers, and the chemicals contained in disposable diapers. The baby's buttocks, thighs, and genitals become sore, red, spotty, and weepy in areas touched by diapers. In boys, the foreskin may become inflamed, making urination painful. The rash may become secondarily infected with the Candida fungus if the baby has been given antibiotics or if breast milk has antibiotics in it, or if the mother has oral or genital thrush.

CAUTION

ANY DIAPER RASH WHICH DOES NOT HEAL WITHIN A WEEK OR SO SHOULD BE SEEN BY A PHYSICIAN.

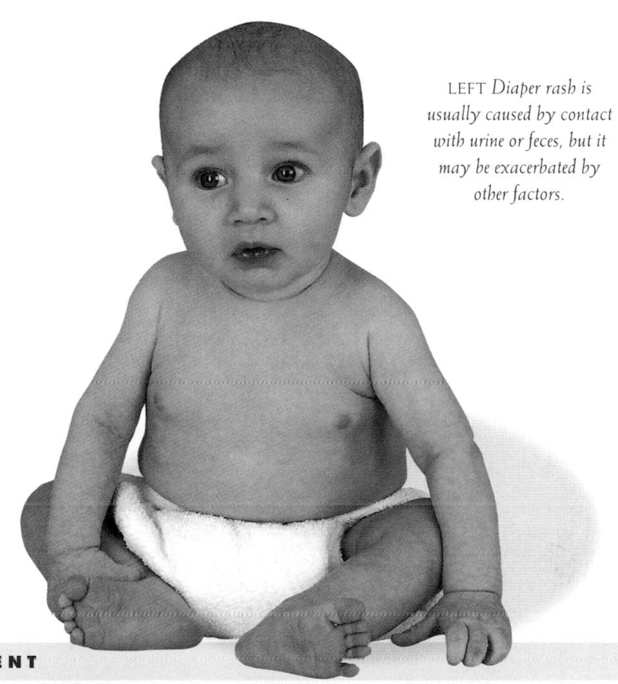

LEFT *Diaper rash is usually caused by contact with urine or feces, but it may be exacerbated by other factors.*

TREATMENT

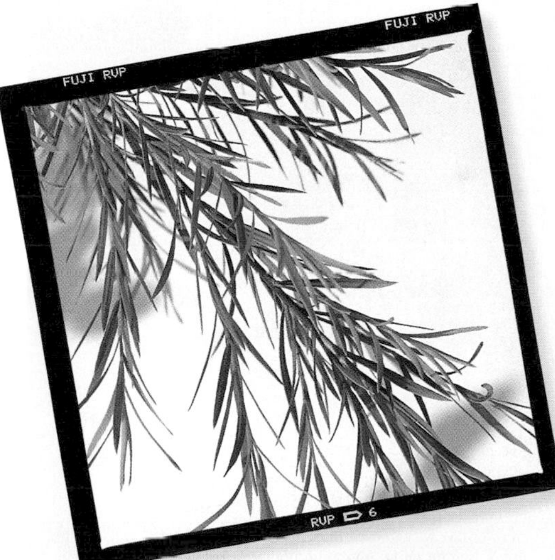

ABOVE *A natural disinfectant, tea tree oil can be added to rinsewater to get diapers extra clean.*

TRADITIONAL HOME AND FOLK REMEDIES

- Rub the skin of an avocado on the rash to encourage healing. *(See page 96.)*
- Wash the bottom with a little diluted cider vinegar and allow it to dry before putting on the diaper. *(See page 102.)*
- Live yogurt can be spread on the diaper area to soothe, and to prevent thrush from occurring in the folds of the skin. *(See page 93.)*
- Egg white can be painted on the sore bottom and allowed to dry before putting on a diaper. This will encourage the skin to heal and prevent further irritation.
- Avoid using soap or other detergents on the diaper area. Rinse carefully with clean water at each diaper change. Frequent diaper changes are suggested, and using a disposable diaper liner may help to reduce irritation. Allow your baby to go for as long as possible with a bare bottom, to allow it to dry and heal. Give plenty to drink.

HERBALISM

- Buchu will reduce the acidity of the urine.
- Marigold ointment can be rubbed on to the diaper area to soothe and to reduce inflammation. *(See page 117.)*
- Wash the diaper area with infusions of marigold, rosemary, or elderflower. *(See pages 117, 127, and 130.)*
- Powdered golden seal can be applied to a clean diaper area before putting on the new diaper.
- Give your baby lots of soothing drinks, such as diluted chamomile tea, to reduce the acidity of the urine. *(See page 119.)*

AROMATHERAPY

- Add a few drops of tea tree to the rinse cycle of your machine when using cloth diapers to disinfect. Cloth diapers are much kinder to your baby's delicate skin. *(See page 162.)*
- A few drops of lavender or rose oil in a peach kernel carrier oil can be gently rubbed into the diaper area. Use this blend to protect against diaper rash as well. *(See pages 161 and 168.)*
- A drop of oregano or thyme oil, in a light carrier oil, can be used to discourage thrush. *(See page 170.)*

HOMEOPATHY

- Calendula ointment can be applied to the diaper area. *(See page 187.)*
- Internally, you can try giving Rhus tox. for an itchy, blistered rash. *(See page 210.)*
- Sulfur may be appropriate if the skin is dry and scaled. *(See page 215.)*
- Merc. sol. can help to reduce the acidity of the urine. *(See page 205.)*
- Cantharis, when the urine is scalding and the skin is red and raw. *(See page 188.)*
- Rhus tox., when the rash appears as mounds or pimples. *(See page 210.)*

FLOWER ESSENCES

- Rescue Remedy cream may be gently massaged into the affected area to reduce inflammation and ease pain or itching. A few drops of Rescue Remedy on pulse points will calm a distressed baby. *(See page 244.)*

BELOW *Live yogurt cools the sore area and prevents the rash spreading.*

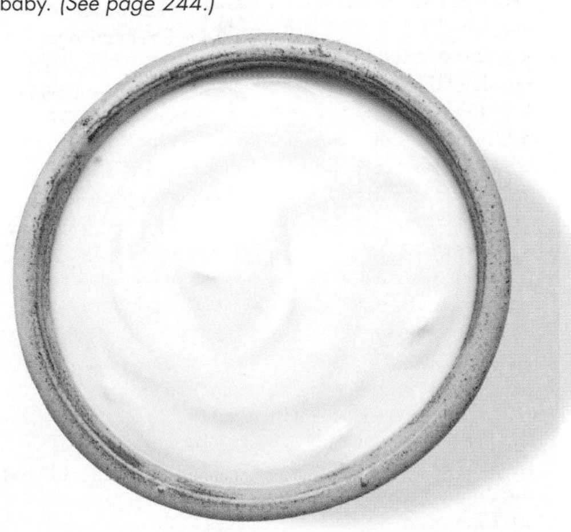

Worms

An infestation of worms in the digestive system is quite common, particularly in young children, who usually contract them at school. Worms can sometimes be seen around the anus, or in the feces, and they inflame the area of the bowel or rectum where they attach themselves. Several types of worms can exist as parasites in humans, ranging in size from microscopic to many meters in length. Most infestations are uncommon in the U.K. and the U.S., apart from threadworms. Threadworms, which are tiny, white threadlike worms which infest the rectum, are not dangerous, although they do tend to disturb sleep. They cause itching around the anus, and sometimes mild, colicky abdominal pain. Worms may be acquired by eating undercooked, infected meat, by contact with soil or water contaminated by worm larvae, or by accidental ingestion of worm eggs (from the fingers or from food) from soil contaminated by infected feces.

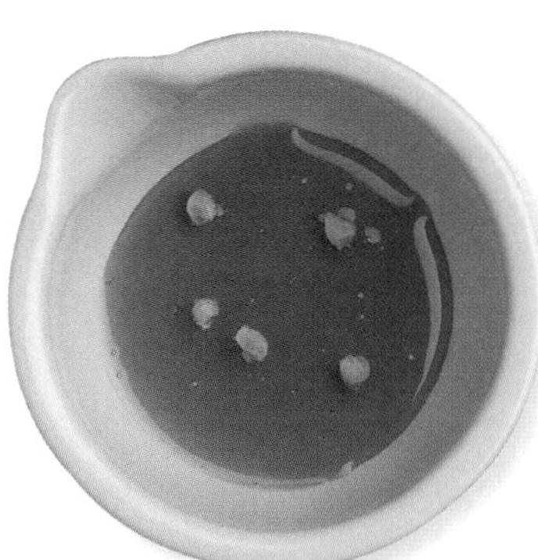

ABOVE *Grind lemon pips with honey for worm treatment.*

CAUTION

WHATEVER TREATMENT YOU GIVE, REPEAT IT AFTER TWO WEEKS TO EXPEL THE WORMS THAT WERE EMBRYOS AT THE FIRST TREATMENT.

TREATMENT

TRADITIONAL HOME AND FOLK REMEDIES
- Raw garlic, which is toxic to worms and parasites, can be eaten, or a small piece, wrapped in some gauze, can be inserted into the anus. *(See page 82.)*
- Give 5 lemon pips, ground and mixed with honey, daily for 5 days. *(See pages 87 and 101.)*

HERBALISM
- Cayenne pepper and senna can be combined; the former stuns the worms and the latter encourages them to be expelled. Mix in a little live yogurt, to avoid irritating the digestive tract. *(See page 118.)*
- Wormwood tea will stun worms.

AROMATHERAPY
- Rub a little black pepper oil, very diluted in grapeseed oil, into the abdominal area. *(See page 167.)*

HOMEOPATHY
- China may alter the balance of the body so that the child expels threadworms naturally. *(See page 190.)*
- Teucrium, for an itchy bottom and nose, which are worse in the evening and accompanied by restless sleep patterns.
- Santoninum, when all else fails.

FLOWER ESSENCES
- Rescue Remedy for distress caused by discomfort. *(See page 244.)*
- Crab Apple, if your child feels unclean or polluted. *(See page 234.)*

VITAMINS AND MINERALS
- Acidophilus tablets should be taken for several weeks to improve the health of the bowel. *(See page 271.)*

Whooping Cough (Pertussis)

CAUTION

THERE IS A RISK OF SECONDARY INFECTION, IN PARTICULAR PNEUMONIA AND BRONCHITIS. ALL CASES OF WHOOPING COUGH SHOULD BE SEEN BY A PHYSICIAN. IF THE COUGH IS ACCOMPANIED BY VOMITING, MAKE SURE THERE IS ADEQUATE INTAKE OF FLUID TO PREVENT DEHYDRATION. CALL YOUR PHYSICIAN IMMEDIATELY IF YOUR CHILD BECOMES BLUE AROUND THE LIPS.

Whooping cough is an acute, highly infectious, and quite serious illness which occurs mostly in children under the age of five. The incubation period of whooping cough is seven to ten days, and the condition can last for about six weeks – sometimes longer. Pertussis, as it is known, usually begins with a normal cold, which develops into a cough. The infection is bacterial and irritates the airways, causing them to become swollen and lined with thick, infected mucus. The coughing becomes severe, with long bouts that have a characteristic "whoop" sound to them. Vomiting often accompanies the coughing. Whooping cough is more dangerous in infants, who can suffer anxiety from being unable to breathe normally. Children should be kept away from others.

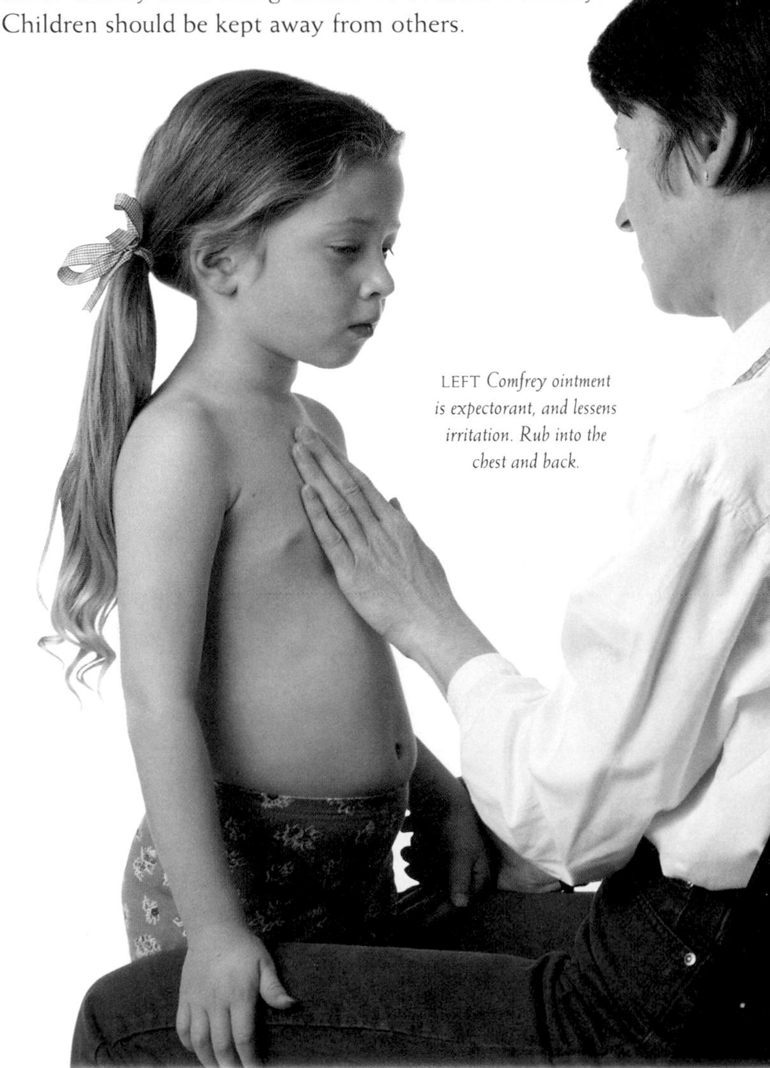

LEFT *Comfrey ointment is expectorant, and lessens irritation. Rub into the chest and back.*

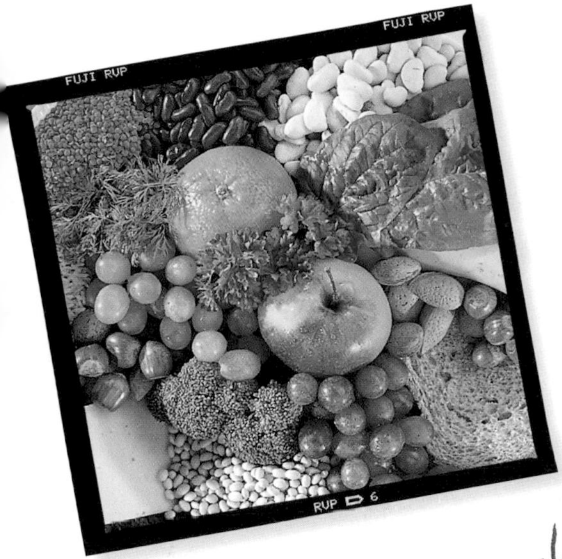

ABOVE *Make sure your child eats a good, balanced diet to cope with what can be a long illness.*

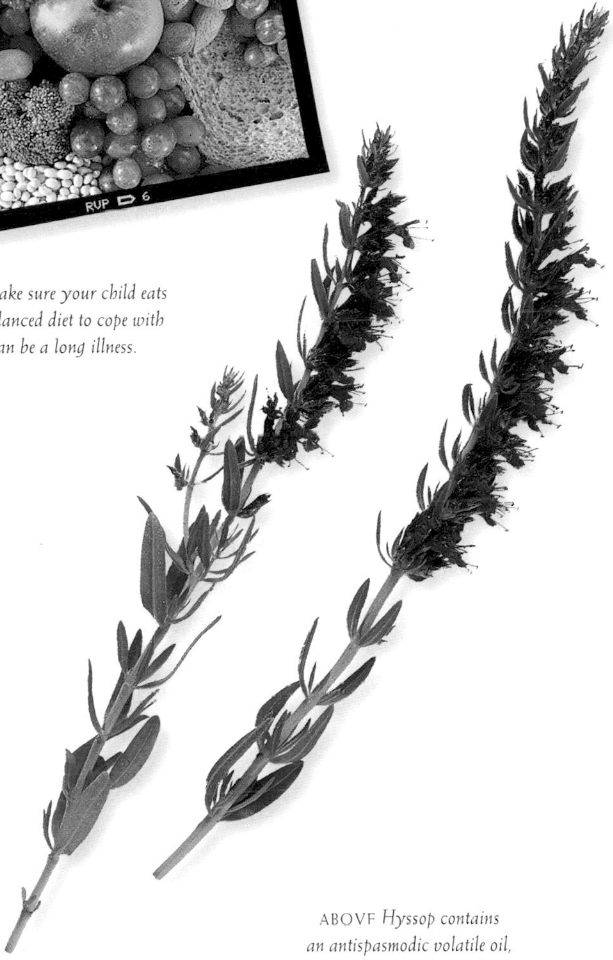

ABOVE *Hyssop contains an antispasmodic volatile oil, to ease a painful cough.*

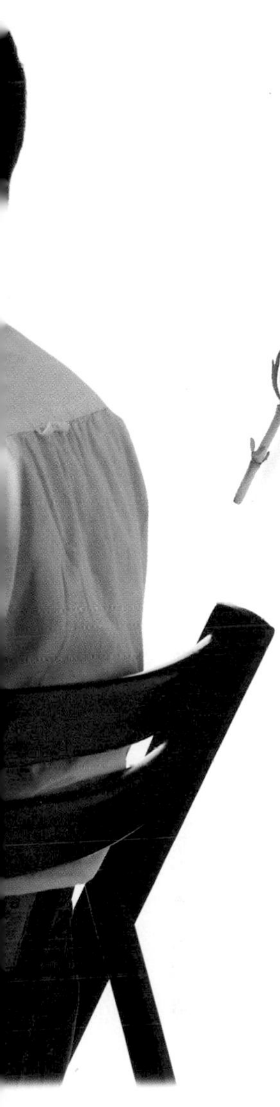

DATA FILE

- Whooping cough is caused by a bacteria, Bordetella pertussis.
- Because of mass vaccination of children, whooping cough is now relatively rare, affecting only a small proportion of the population.
- After an incubation period of about a week, symptoms at first resemble those of the common cold; after 7–10 days, coughing increases and takes on the distinctive attributes of whooping cough.
- The younger the patient, the greater the risk of serious illness; most deaths from whooping cough occur in the first six months of life.

TREATMENT

TRADITIONAL HOME AND FOLK REMEDIES

- Honey and licorice can be mixed with a little hot water to make a drink to relieve the cough. *(See pages 91 and 101.)*
- A garlic poultice, placed on the chest and back area, is recommended to help expel the phlegm. Do not leave the poultice on for too long, because it can cause blistering. *(See page 82.)*

HERBALISM

- A combination of coltsfoot and elecampane can prevent the infection by strengthening the body and clearing phlegm.
- Sundew is very successful in treating a number of bacterial infections, and also works to relax the muscles of the breathing tubes. It should be made into an infusion and taken by the teaspoonful, as necessary.
- Hyssop and lobelia should be used to help allay the spasmodic cough.
- Coltsfoot can be used to loosen the cough and help to expel the mucus.
- The bark of the wild cherry has a profound effect on the cough reflex.
- Red clover will help to reduce any spasm of the bronchi.
- A few drops of tincture of thyme should be taken to loosen and expel the mucus. Thyme also works as an antiseptic. *(See page 135.)*
- Massage comfrey ointment into the chest and back to relax the lungs. *(See page 132.)*
- Lemon balm tea will soothe anxiety.
- Elecampane is commonly used for children's coughs, and can be purchased in easy-to-use syrup form.
- Offer a little black root if there is vomiting.
- After the bath, massage a little comfrey ointment into the chest and back to relax and expand the lungs. *(See page 132.)*

AROMATHERAPY

- Mix a few drops of lavender and chamomile oils in a light carrier oil, and massage into the chest and back area to calm, and to relax tensed muscles. *(See pages 150 and 161.)*
- Tea tree, lavender, chamomile, and eucalyptus can be used in a vaporizer to help open up the lungs and reduce spasm. *(See pages 146–71.)*
- A few drops of oil of thyme, in the bath, will soothe and reduce the severity of the cough. *(See page 170.)*

HOMEOPATHY

- Pertussin may be given in one dose towards the end of the disease to prevent an "echo" effect.
- Aconite can be taken during an attack or at the beginning of the illness. *(See page 178.)*
- Ant. tart., when there is a rattling cough with gasping. *(See page 179.)*
- Sanguinaria, for a harsh, dry cough.
- Arnica, when there is bleeding, or the child is distressed before the coughing starts. *(See page 182.)*
- Drosera is useful when the cough is made worse by lying down and there are pains below the ribs. *(See page 193.)*
- Bryonia, when there is a dry, painful cough and vomiting. *(See page 185.)*

FLOWER ESSENCES

- Rescue Remedy is excellent for calming a child who has difficulty drawing breath, and who is frightened by the condition. A few drops on pulse points, or sipped in a glass of cool water, will help. *(See page 244.)*
- Cherry Plum will help if there is any serious spasmodic coughing. *(See page 236.)*
- Mimulus and olive are good during the later stages of the condition. *(See page 235.)*

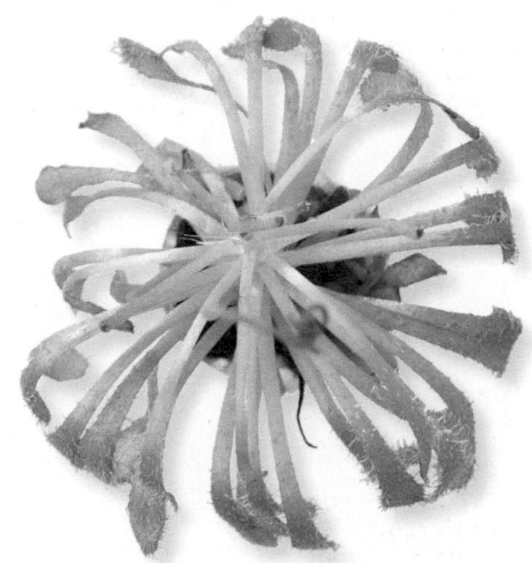

RIGHT *Drosera contains plumbagin, which fights streptococcus, pneumococcus, and staphylococcus bacteria.*

German Measles (Rubella)

Rubella, also called German measles, is a viral infection that begins with symptoms of a cold and loss of appetite, occasionally accompanied by a sore throat and swelling of the lymph nodes in the neck. The rash will appear about a day later and consists of tiny pink spots that may be so concentrated that the overall area appears red and inflamed. There may be mild fever. German measles is very infectious, with an incubation period of two or three weeks. The illness itself only lasts three to five days.

CAUTION

THE SYMPTOMS IN SMALL CHILDREN MAY BE MILD, BUT IF A PREGNANT WOMAN COMES INTO CONTACT WITH THE CONDITION THERE IS A SERIOUS RISK OF MISCARRIAGE AND BIRTH DEFECTS. SUFFERERS ARE INFECTIOUS FROM ONE WEEK BEFORE THE RASH APPEARS TO THREE WEEKS AFTERWARD.

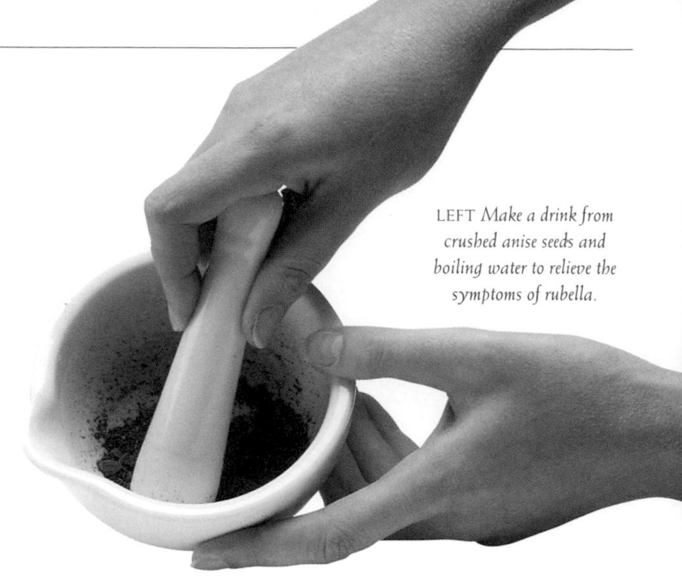

LEFT *Make a drink from crushed anise seeds and boiling water to relieve the symptoms of rubella.*

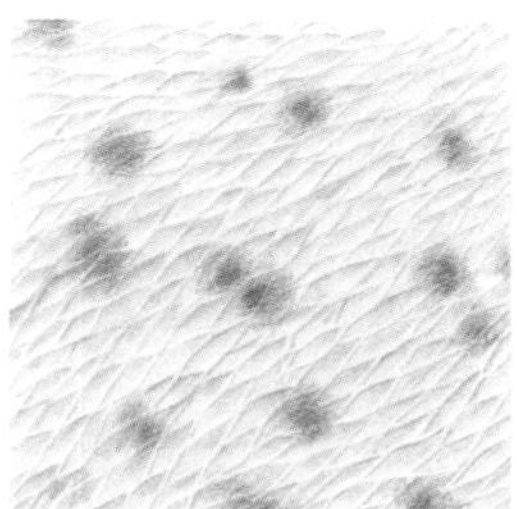

RIGHT *German measles produces a rash of pale pink, possibly itchy, spots that spread from the face.*

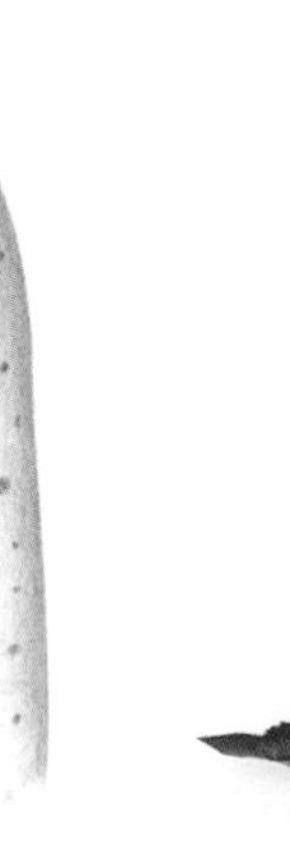

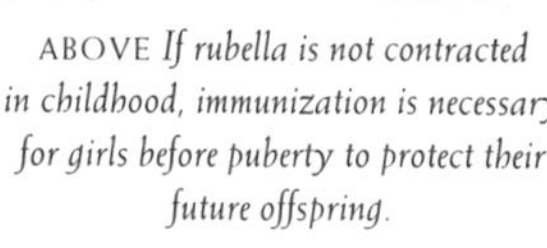

ABOVE *If rubella is not contracted in childhood, immunization is necessary for girls before puberty to protect their future offspring.*

TREATMENT

CHINESE HERBALISM

- Rubella is believed to be caused by external Wind and Heat. Use mulberry, honeysuckle, and chrysanthemum. *(See page 65.)*

TRADITIONAL HOME AND FOLK REMEDIES

Pound some anise seeds, allow them to steep in boiling water for about 30 minutes, and then offer the drink by the teaspoonful to relieve symptoms.

- Honey and lemon in a little hot water can be drunk to reduce discomfort of the cold-like symptoms. *(See pages 87 and 101.)*
- Frequent, cool baths will relieve any itchiness and bring down a fever. *(See page 103.)*

HERBALISM

- Borage stimulates the kidneys and can help when fever is present.
- Yarrow tea, cooled and drunk several times daily, will relieve symptoms. *(See page 112.)*
- An infusion of elderflower, combined with peppermint, will cool a fever and calm your child. *(See pages 125 and 130.)*
- Very high fever can be treated with an infusion of catmint, taken as required.

AROMATHERAPY

- A few drops of lavender oil on the bedclothes, or on a handkerchief near the bed, will help ease symptoms and calm the child. *(See page 161.)*
- If there is a build-up of phlegm, use a few drops of tea tree or eucalyptus essential oil in a vaporizer to assist easier breathing. *(See pages 159 and 162.)*

HOMEOPATHY

- Pulsatilla, when there is thick, yellow discharge and hot, red eyes. *(See page 209.)*
- Belladonna, for fever, a bright red rash, and a hot face. *(See page 183.)*
- Phytolacca, for painful ears and swollen glands which are improved by taking cool drinks.
- Aconite, if there is a high fever and not too much mucus present. *(See page 178.)*
- Merc. sol., where there is yellow discharge and a fever. *(See page 205.)*

FLOWER ESSENCES

- Rescue Remedy will ease distress and calm the child. *(See page 244.)*

VITAMINS AND MINERALS

- Eat a good amount of raw fruits and vegetables to cleanse the system.
- Increase the intake of foods containing vitamin C and zinc to aid the action of the immune system. *(See pages 256 and 265.)*
- Vitamin E oil can be applied to the spots to prevent scarring. Take vitamin E supplements for the same reason. *(See page 257.)*
- Acidophilus should be taken after any illness to encourage the production of healthy bacteria in the gut. *(See page 271.)*

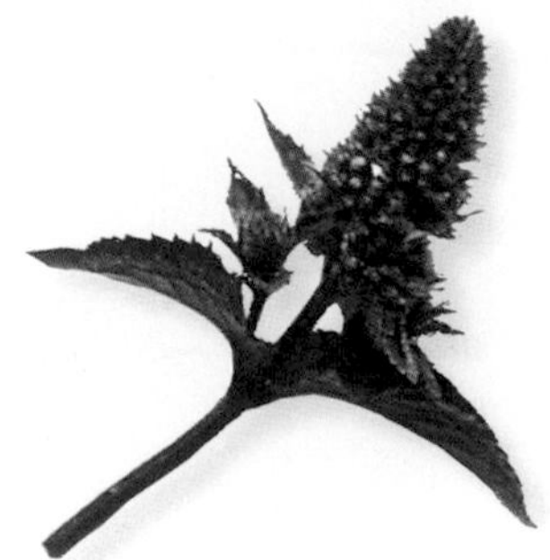

LEFT *Peppermint can be infused with elderflower to promote sweating and bring down a fever.*

DATA FILE

- German measles is highly contagious but mild.
- Symptoms usually disappear without complication in about a week.
- Many people may have had German measles without knowing it, because a skin rash is not always present.
- Natural infection apparently produces lifelong immunity.
- Pregnant women who become infected with rubella have a high risk of giving birth to a baby with serious defects, including blindness, cardiovascular disorders, deafness, or mental retardation.

Measles

Measles is a highly infectious disease caused by a virus which is normally inhaled. The incubation period is about fourteen days, and just before the rash appears spots can be seen in the mouth. It begins like a cold, with runny nose or cough, then a fever, and occasionally conjunctivitis occurs. Fever tends to become high as the rash comes out. The rash is characterized by flat, brown-red spots, which usually begin behind the ears and on the face. The lymph nodes will become swollen and there will be little or no appetite, perhaps vomiting and diarrhea. Measles spots are not itchy, but your child will feel profoundly unwell. Complications of measles are common, and they include pneumonia, middle ear infections, and bronchitis. Encephalitis may also occur.

DATA FILE

- Measles usually affects children, but the disease can occur at any age in susceptible people.
- The early symptoms – fever, malaise, sore muscles, headache, eye irritation, and sensitivity to light – occur about 11 days after infection.
- Nasal discharge, sneezing, and coughing develop rapidly.
- Measles reduces normal resistance, making a patient susceptible to more serious secondary bacterial infections.
- In rare cases, the virus enters the brain to cause a form of encephalitis.
- Measles was once common throughout the world, but in 1963 the measles vaccine was introduced, which greatly reduced the incidence.
- The 1980s saw a marked increase in measles cases in the U.S., which may have been due to the failure to vaccinate many infants at the age of 15 months.
- About 5 percent of vaccinated adults are not adequately protected by a single dose of vaccine.
- Infection confers lifelong immunity.

CAUTION

IF FEVER RECURS SEVERAL DAYS AFTER THE SPOTS HAVE BEGUN TO HEAL, SEE YOUR PHYSICIAN.

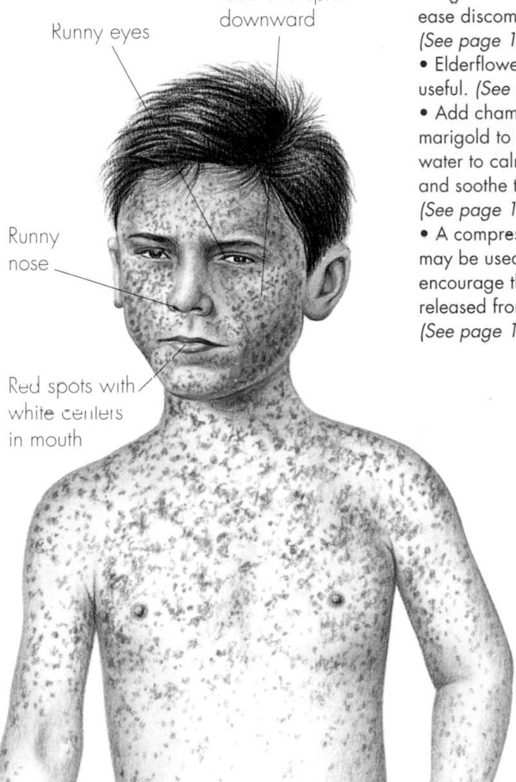

LEFT *Measles is a potentially dangerous illness, as it weakens the immune system. The blotchy reddish-brown rash spreads from the face.*

TREATMENT

CHINESE HERBALISM

- The source of the illness is believed to be excess Heat in the Blood and Stomach. Peppermint, safflower, and honeysuckle may be used to treat measles. *(See pages 58 and 65.)*

TRADITIONAL HOME AND FOLK REMEDIES

- Garlic will encourage the spots to "come out," which means that the body is expelling toxins. *(See page 82.)*
- Ginger can be used as a compress directly on the spots.
- Hot honey and lemon drinks are soothing and will encourage healing. *(See pages 87 and 101.)*

HERBALISM

- Garlic and echinacea can be taken to improve the action of the immune system. *(See pages 113 and 120.)*
- Catmint and yarrow teas can be sipped to bring down fever and ease discomfort. *(See page 112.)*
- Elderflower is also useful. *(See page 130.)*
- Add chamomile or marigold to the bath water to calm your child and soothe the symptoms. *(See page 117 and 119.)*
- A compress of ginger may be used to help encourage the toxins to be released from the body. *(See page 139.)*

AROMATHERAPY

- A few drops of Roman chamomile in the bath will ease symptoms and help encourage sleep. *(See page 150.)*
- Lavender oil can be dropped on the bedclothes or on a handkerchief by the bed to calm. It can also be applied neat to spots to encourage healing. *(See page 161.)*
- When there is a build-up of phlegm and other symptoms of a cold, a gentle chest massage with a few drops of tea tree oil in a light carrier oil base will help. *(See page 162.)*
- Use essential oil of eucalyptus, tea tree, or chamomile in a vaporizer. *(See pages 146–71.)*

HOMEOPATHY

- Aconite and Belladonna can be taken for a high fever. *(See pages 178 and 183.)*
- Pulsatilla, when there is diarrhea, yellow discharge, and a cough. *(See page 209.)*
- Bryonia, when there is a hard, painful cough, and a high temperature, accompanied by thirst. *(See page 185.)*
- Stramonium, when there is a high fever, a red face, and convulsions.
- Morbillinum can be taken for 3 days if your child has been in contact with a sufferer. This will help reduce the severity of the symptoms.

FLOWER ESSENCES

- Rescue Remedy eases distress and discomfort. *(See page 244.)*
- Cherry Plum, Hornbeam, and Chicory are suggested for all childhood illnesses. *(See pages 236, 227, and 228.)*

VITAMINS AND MINERALS

- Eat plenty of raw fruits and vegetables every day to cleanse the system.
- Increase the intake of foods containing vitamin C and zinc to aid the action of the immune system. *(See pages 256 and 265.)*
- Vitamin E oil can be applied to the spots to prevent scarring. Take vitamin E supplements for the same reason. *(See page 257.)*
- Acidophilus should be taken after any illness to encourage production of the healthy bacteria in the gut. *(See page 271.)*

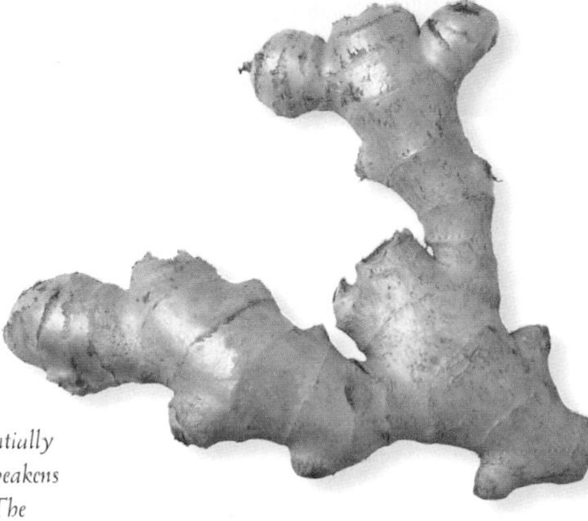

ABOVE *A ginger compress helps to relieve the rash of spots.*

Chickenpox

Chickenpox is an extremely contagious viral infection, which features headache, fever and general malaise, with spots starting usually on the trunk and spreading to most parts of the body, including the mouth, anus, vagina, and ears. They appear as pimples, which soon fill with fluid to become little blisters. Eventually the spots dry up and form a scab, which may cause scars. These spots are very itchy and it is important that the child does not scratch, for scarring and bacterial infection can result. The incubation period is ten to fourteen days, and sufferers are contagious from just before the spots appear.

ABOVE *Make a witch hazel compress to help soothe the itchiness of the spots and to stop the child scratching.*

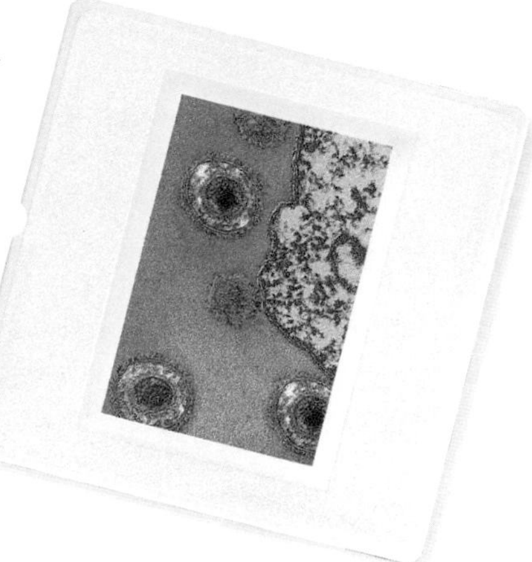

ABOVE *The chickenpox virus can cause shingles in adults.*

DATA FILE

- Chickenpox is usually contracted before the age of nine.
- The chickenpox virus, varicella zoster, usually lies dormant in the body. When immune activity is low, it can resurface as shingles.
- The rash develops into itching blisters that break in a few days and are covered by scabs, which leave no scars unless they become infected by bacteria from scratching.
- Chickenpox can be life-threatening to children with depressed immune systems.
- A mother with chickenpox may transmit the virus to her baby during the last days of her pregnancy.
- In 1995 a vaccine called Varivax was approved for use in children over the age of one. The vaccine is 70–90 percent effective in preventing chickenpox over the short term.

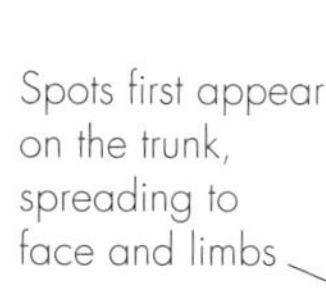

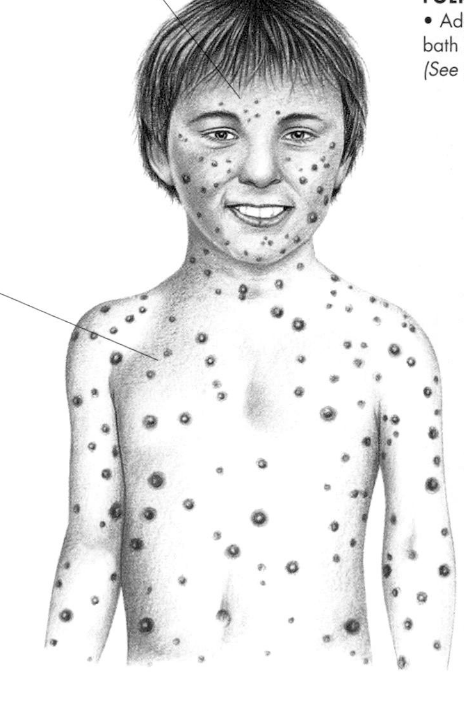

LEFT *Chickenpox rash is characterized by small, raised spots which develop into inflamed blisters. They become very itchy before drying to a scab.*

CAUTION

WHEN FEVER LASTS FOR MORE THAN A COUPLE OF DAYS, OR THERE IS AN OBVIOUS CHEST INFECTION ACCOMPANYING THE RASH, SEE YOUR PHYSICIAN. VERY RARELY, CHICKENPOX PNEUMONIA CAN OCCUR AS A SECONDARY INFECTION.

TREATMENT

CHINESE HERBALISM

- The illness is believed to be caused by Wind and Heat invasion. Safflower, cimicifuga, and honeysuckle may be used in the treatment. *(See pages 58 and 65.)*

TRADITIONAL HOME AND FOLK REMEDIES

- Add baking soda to the bath to ease itching. *(See page 100.)*

HERBALISM

- A witch hazel compress can be applied directly to the spots, or a little added to the bath, to ease discomfort.
- Tincture of comfrey or elderflower can be applied directly to the spots to encourage healing and to relieve the itching. *(See pages 130 and 132.)*
- Add burdock infusion to your child's bath. *(See page 115.)*
- Crushed peppermint leaves, applied to the spots, relieve symptoms. *(See page 125.)*

AROMATHERAPY

- A few drops of Roman chamomile can be used in the bath to soothe. *(See page 150.)*
- Essential oil of lavender can be dabbed directly on spots to ease the itching and encourage healing. Lavender also has an antibacterial action, which will help prevent a secondary infection. *(See page 161.)*

HOMEOPATHY

- Variolinum can be taken once before your child acquires the illness, during an epidemic of chickenpox, and symptoms should be less severe.
- Rhus tox. can be taken for a few days after contact with an infected child, and then again as soon as the first spots appear. *(See page 210.)*
- Aconite, in the early stages of the illness. *(See page 178.)*
- Belladonna, for fever. *(See page 183.)*

FLOWER ESSENCES

- If the child is unreasonably demanding of attention, Chicory may be helpful. *(See page 228.)*
- Impatiens can ease fractious behavior. *(See page 233.)*
- Crab Apple may be diluted and applied directly to the spots to encourage healing. *(See page 234.)*
- Olive will be useful for the convalescence period. *(See page 235.)*

CAUTION

THERE ARE COMPLICATIONS WHICH CAN DEVELOP IN TEENAGE BOYS WHO CONTRACT MUMPS: INFLAMMATION OF THE TESTICLES CAN LEAD TO STERILITY. IF THE ILLNESS IS FOLLOWED BY SEVERE HEADACHE, STIFFNESS, OR FEVER, SEE YOUR PHYSICIAN IMMEDIATELY.

Mumps

Mumps is a viral infection which usually affects children, causing fever and swelling of the main salivary glands, the parotids. This swelling furnishes the sufferer with the characteristic chipmunk appearance. The condition rarely occurs in children under two or three years of age, and takes about two or three weeks to incubate. It is infectious from a day before the glands begin to swell until about a week after they have gone down. The virus is spread by coughing and sneezing.

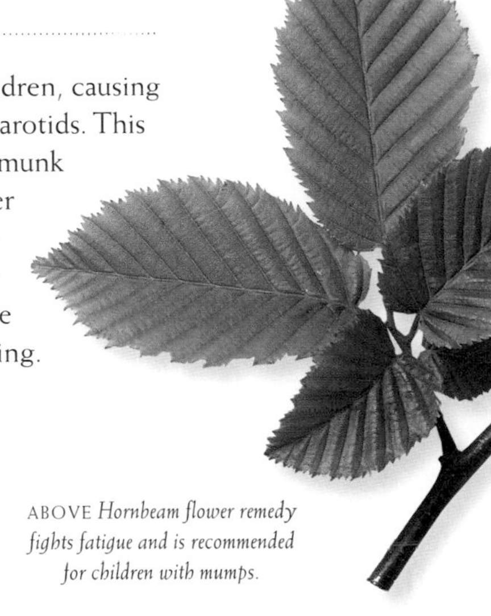
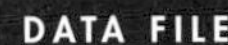

ABOVE *Hornbeam flower remedy fights fatigue and is recommended for children with mumps.*

Symptoms

• *general malaise* • *fever* • *headache* • *pains around the neck* • *swallowing will be painful*

DATA FILE

• Because mumps is a systemic infection, other parts of the body may also be affected, including salivary glands, the testicles, the ovaries, the pancreas, and the central nervous system.

• Mumps is communicable, though less so than measles, and occurs with great frequency in heavily populated areas.

• While the disease can occur at any age, it is children aged 5–15 who are primarily affected.

• Once a person has had mumps, this ensures permanent immunity.

• In adult males, inflammation and swelling may first occur in the testicles. Testicular inflammation, orchitis, occurs in about 20 percent of adult males who have mumps; it can be very painful and occasionally causes sterility.

• An infection involving the ovaries, oophoritis, occurs occasionally in women. Oophoritis causes high fever, chills, and lower back pain.

• A condition called aseptic meningitis sometimes occurs when the virus enters the central nervous system.

• Involvement of the pancreas occurs in less than 10 percent of cases.

LEFT *A gentle neck massage with a chamomile oil blend will ease pain.*

TREATMENT

CHINESE HERBALISM

• The source of mumps is considered to be Wind and Damp Heat, and dandelion, honeysuckle, skullcap, and rhubarb may be suggested. *(See pages 65, 73, and 74.)*

TRADITIONAL HOME AND FOLK REMEDIES

• Chop fresh ginger and apply as a compress directly to the swollen glands to provide relief.
• Cayenne powder, mixed with vinegar, can be warmed and applied to the affected area. *(See pages 86 and 102.)*

HERBALISM

• Catmint, marigold, or chamomile infusions can be sipped to reduce fever, or added to a bath of cool water. *(See pages 117 and 119.)*
• Garlic, peppermint, and echinacea can be taken internally to boost immunity and encourage healing. *(See pages 113 and 120, and 125.)*
• Red clover and cleavers can help to reduce the inflammation and swelling. Drink both as a lukewarm infusion.
• A warm compress with poke root or marigold can be applied to the swelling. *(See page 117.)*

AROMATHERAPY

• Eucalyptus and thyme can be used for steam inhalations and in the bath (use sparingly). *(See pages 159 and 170.)*
• Massage the neck area with chamomile or lavender oil, diluted in a little grapeseed oil. Take care to do so gently. *(See pages 150 and 161.)*

HOMEOPATHY

• If your child has not had mumps, Phytolacca or Parotidium can be taken during an epidemic to reduce the severity of symptoms.
• Rhus tox., when the left glands are more severely affected than the right. *(See page 210.)*
• Belladonna, when there is high fever, shooting pains, and a bright red face and throat. *(See page 183.)*
• Merc. sol., when the patient sweats heavily and has a coated tongue. *(See page 205.)*
• Pulsatilla may help to prevent orchitis, and is useful if fever continues. *(See page 209.)*

FLOWER ESSENCES

• Rescue Remedy can be used to ease distress caused by discomfort. *(See page 244.)*
• Willow may be helpful if the child resents the fact that brothers and sisters are still well. *(See page 239.)*

VITAMINS AND MINERALS

• Eat a good selection of raw fruits and vegetables to cleanse the system.
• Increase the intake of foods containing vitamin C and zinc to aid the action of the immune system. *(See pages 256 and 265.)*
• Acidophilus should be taken after any illness to encourage production of the healthy bacteria in the gut. *(See page 271.)*

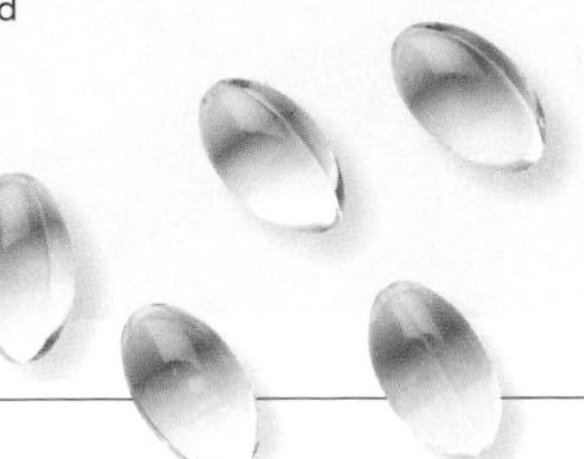

LEFT *Garlic oil capsules help revitalize a flagging immune system.*

COMMON AILMENTS IN THE ELDERLY

Depression

Many elderly people feel a sense of worthlessness as they age; they feel that they no longer matter to others, that their dependency is problematic, and that they have lost any sense of purpose or usefulness. Often this is exacerbated by the refusal of others to allow an elderly person to participate in daily chores, inadequate social intercourse, and lack of mental stimulation. A feeling of isolation develops, and withdrawal and depression are common responses to the dependency and loss of control that old age often brings. (*See also under Mind and Emotions, page* 283.)

BELOW *Sage has stimulant qualities. Add fresh sage to food.*

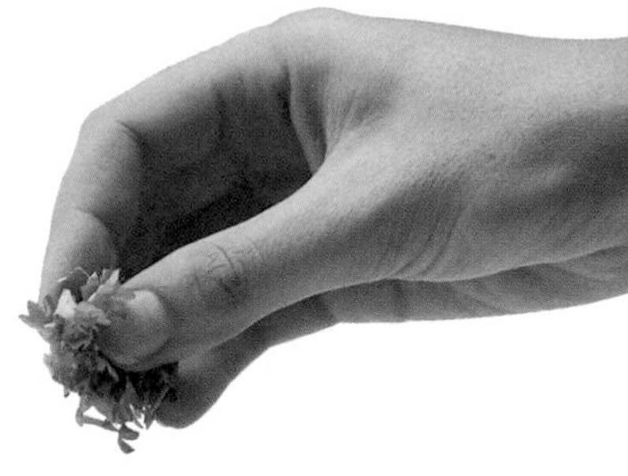

SYMPTOMS

- *irritability or aggression*
- *bewilderment and disorientation*
- *fecal incontinence can be a feature of depression in the elderly*

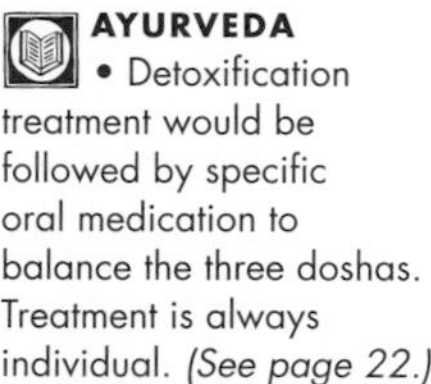

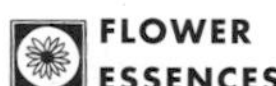

LEFT *The value of human touch, received through massage, is great.*

TREATMENT

AYURVEDA
• Detoxification treatment would be followed by specific oral medication to balance the three doshas. Treatment is always individual. *(See page 22.)*

CHINESE HERBALISM
• Depression is believed to be caused by stagnation of the Liver qi, and may be treated with angelica, peony root, licorice, and thorowax root. *(See pages 56, 64, and 67.)*

TRADITIONAL FOLK AND HOME REMEDIES
• Clove tea, or bruised cloves added to herbal teas such as chamomile or peppermint, are able to lift mild depression. *(See page 90.)*
• Drink sage tea, and add fresh sage to food, to fight depression.

HERBALISM
• The best antidepressant and nervine (with specific action for nerves) herbs include: balm, borage, limeflower, oats, rosemary, and vervain. These can be taken as herbal teas, added to the bath, or taken as tablets, or in tincture form (herbs suspended in alcohol). *(See pages 117, 127, 134, and 136.)*
• Ginseng is an antidepressant herb and will help with other problems accompanying old age, such as confusion, memory problems, and a weakening system. *(See page 126.)*

AROMATHERAPY
• Antidepressant oils include: bergamot, chamomile, clary sage, jasmine, geranium, lavender, melissa, neroli, orange, rose, sandalwood, and ylang ylang. These may be blended or used singly in massage (which will also be very therapeutic), or in the bath or a vaporizer. *(See pages 146–71.)*
• Basil, chamomile, juniper, marjoram, and tea tree will act as a general tonic, and can be used in any of the same ways. *(See pages 146–71.)*

HOMEOPATHY
Treatment should be constitutional, but some of the following remedies may help:
• Ignatia, for a depression which results from a trauma or a bereavement. *(See page 200.)*
• Arsenicum, for restlessness, chilliness, exhaustion, and obsessive tidiness. *(See page 182.)*
• Cadmium phos. for depression after illness, with exhaustion.
• Pulsatilla, for bursting into tears for no reason. *(See page 209.)*

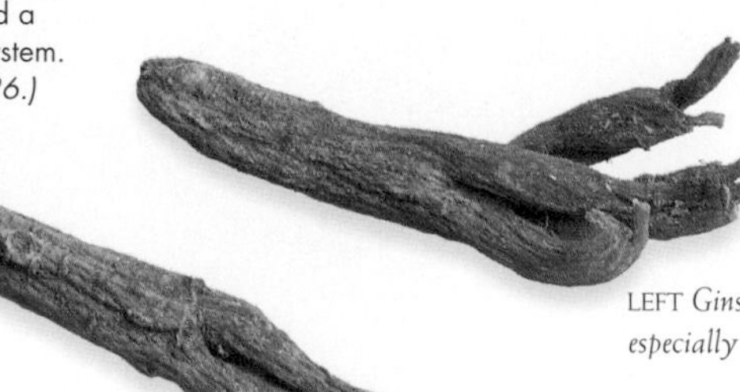

LEFT *Ginseng fights depression, especially when due to debility.*

FLOWER ESSENCES
• Cherry Plum, for "fear of the mind being overstrained, of doing dreaded things," and of doing violence to oneself or others. *(See page 236.)*
• Agrimony, for deeply held emotional tensions which are hidden from others. *(See page 225.)*
• Gorse, for feelings of great hopelessness. *(See page 240.)*
• Gentian, for relief of feelings of despondency or a mild depression. *(See page 230.)*
• Mustard, for blacker and deeper feelings that seem to have no identifiable cause. *(See page 239.)*
• Sweet Chestnut should be taken if the person is anguished and stretched beyond endurance. *(See page 227.)*

VITAMINS AND MINERALS
• Do not include an excessive amount of vitamin D, zinc, copper, or lead in the diet. *(See pages 256, 265, and 259.)*
• Ensure you have an adequate intake of vitamin C and the B vitamins, which help the health of the mind and nervous system. *(See pages 256 and 252–5.)*
• Calcium, potassium, and magnesium may also need to be supplemented. *(See pages 258 and 262.)*
• Take plenty of the antioxidant nutrients, which help to delay some of the effects of aging. *(See page 251.)*
• Some therapists may recommend using the amino acid tryptophan. *(See page 269.)*

Confusion

One of the most common problems among elderly people is confusion. This may be a symptom of dementia (*see page 452*), hypothermia (very common among old people, who tend to economize on fuel and heating), or acute brain syndrome (caused by pneumonia, circulatory problems, or drug side-effects). Most often, however, it is a consequence of being cut off from the mainstream of life. Without visitors and possibly with no access to daily news, one day seems very much like another.

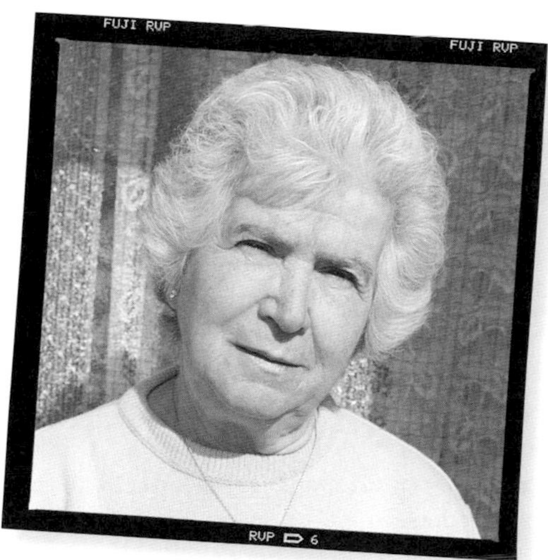

ABOVE *Ginseng powder helps improve powers of memory. Add it to herbal tea.*

Symptoms

• self-neglect can be a natural consequence of confusion, with less attention paid to personal appearance and diet than previously • forgetfulness, sometimes with serious consequences • a lack of orientation, particularly in terms of time • bewilderment and agitation • depression and its associated symptoms (see page 450) • hallucinations (in acute brain syndrome)

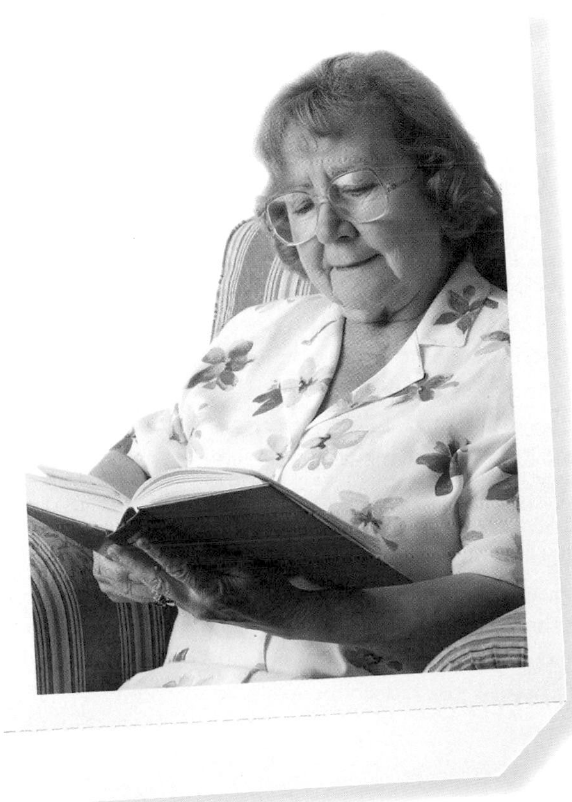

ABOVE *Keeping up interest in a subject or reading a novel will help to keep the mind sharp.*

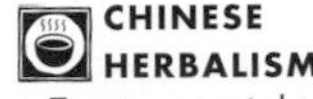

TREATMENT

AYURVEDA
• Henbane may be suggested, as well as lemon or lime juice.

CHINESE HERBALISM
• Treatment might address deficient Kidney essence, and useful herbs include dodder seeds, mulberry, and black ginger seed. *(See page 62.)*

TRADITIONAL FOLK AND HOME REMEDIES
• Ginseng powder, added to herbal teas, will improve memory and help with symptoms of confusion and agitation.
• Gotu kola can revive memory and focus the mind. Add a small amount to your tea for a few days running, but discontinue use occasionally.

HERBALISM
• Rosemary is a tonic, particularly for the elderly, as it stimulates and nourishes the nervous system. It improves memory and concentration. Use fresh in food, or drink an infusion. *(See page 127.)*
• Orange blossom, particularly in the form of neroli oil, works on the nervous system and effectively counteracts nervous exhaustion, confusion, and depression.

AROMATHERAPY
• Geranium oil regulates the nervous system, and helps fight confusion, panic, and anxiety. *(See page 165.)*

HOMEOPATHY
• Acute confusion can be treated with Belladonna, particularly if accompanied by a red face and fever. Consult a physician if symptoms do not get any better after a day. *(See page 183.)*
Chronic confusion can be treated with one of the following:
• Baryta carb., for confusion due to senile dementia. *(See page 185.)*
• Cannabis ind., for confusion, delusions.
• Alumina, for confusion, irritability, and obstinacy.

FLOWER ESSENCES
Flower essences have a tremendous effect on the mind and emotions. Some to try include:
• White Chestnut, a mind plagued by repetitive thoughts. *(See page 224.)*
• Wild Rose, if you drift through life resigned to accept any eventuality. *(See page 238.)*
• Gentian, for any feelings of despondency. *(See page 230.)*
• Scleranthus, if you suffer from indecision and cannot make up your mind. *(See page 239.)*

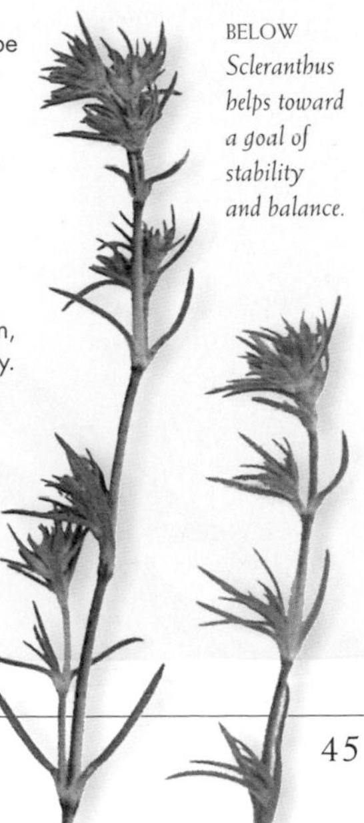

BELOW *Scleranthus helps toward a goal of stability and balance.*

Senile Dementia

Senile dementia is a form of chronic organic brain disease in which there is progressive loss of intellectual power due to shrinkage (atrophy) and deterioration of the brain in old age. The onset is subtle and is sometimes only identified retrospectively by slight personality changes. The risk of dementia increases with age, but not all older people will get dementia. Most dementias are not reversible, but people with dementia can function better with treatment of other medical or sensory problems, and optimal social and environmental support. Stimulation and activity can help people with dementia.

ABOVE *Basil oil's pungent fragrance helps concentration.*

SYMPTOMS

• *in the early stages: – insomnia – restlessness – loss of interest in work or hobbies – forgetfulness, particularly of recent events – impaired judgment and reasoning* • *later: – progressive memory loss, until only events in the distant past may be remembered – mood swings to the point of character change – failure to follow even the most simple instructions – simplified vocabulary and repetitive conversation – delusions – apathy and indifference – sufferers fail to feed and warm themselves, which leads to total dependency – incontinence*

RIGHT *Rosemary is uplifting, and is a tonic for the nervous system.*

TREATMENT

CHINESE HERBALISM
• Dementia may be treated with herbs such as Chinese wolfberry or black ginger seed. *(See page 66.)*
• Treatment might be aimed at deficient kidney essence, and herbs to address this include mulberry and dodder seeds. *(See page 62.)*

AROMATHERAPY
• Basil and rosemary oils can be used in the bath, or in a massage, diluted in a little carrier oil, to clear the mind and stimulate mental activity. *(See pages 164 and 168.)*
• Chamomile, melissa, rosemary, marjoram, and lavender strengthen the nervous system, and can be used in any way. *(See pages 146–71.)*
• Tea tree acts as a general tonic, to help overall health and well-being. *(See page 162.)*

HOMEOPATHY
Treatment would be constitutional, but the following remedies may help:
• Phosphorus, for apprehension, cravings for salt, and accompanied by arteriosclerosis. *(See page 208.)*
• Baryta carb., for weakness, tiredness, when symptoms are worse in cold, and for degeneration of the blood vessels. *(See page 185.)*
• Ignatia, for symptoms stemming from a trauma or bereavement. *(See page 200.)*
• Lycopodium, for lack of self-confidence, use of the wrong words, particularly in a person who was once sharp and ambitious. *(See page 203.)*
• Aurum iod., when there is partial paralysis.

FLOWER ESSENCES
• The flower essences work on the mind and emotions specifically, and there are a variety to choose from, according to your specific feelings. *(See page 219 for a full list.)*

VITAMINS AND MINERALS
• Ensure that your diet contains plenty of vitamins B and C, as well as zinc and magnesium. *(See pages 252–5, 256, 265, and 262.)*
• Taking lecithin, which contains phosphatidyl choline, improves memory when taken daily. *(See page 271.)*
• Take supplements which contain all 22 amino acids to improve brain function.

TREATMENT

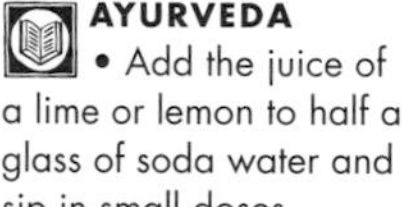

AYURVEDA
• Add the juice of a lime or lemon to half a glass of soda water and sip in small doses.

CHINESE HERBALISM
• Fresh ginger, cinnamon twigs, and peppermint may be useful. *(See page 59.)*
• Mulberry will be used to nourish the blood.

HERBALISM
• Small sips of fresh ginger tea, made with root ginger, will help to ease the symptoms. *(See page 139.)*
• Teas of rock rose flowers or wild rose flowers, with a little honey, will be helpful.

HOMEOPATHY
Treatment will be constitutional, particularly if dizziness is a chronic problem, but some of the following may help:
• Causticum, when dizziness is worse in cold water and coughing causes urine to leak. *(See page 189.)*
• Silicea, for poor circulation, and when symptoms are worse when lying on the left side. *(See page 211.)*
• Arnica, when dizziness follows injury and occurs when standing suddenly. *(See page 182.)*
• Lycopodium, when it accompanies senile dementia, with an inability to concentrate, and when symptoms are worse between 4 and 8P.M. *(See page 203.)*

FLOWER ESSENCES
• If dizziness is associated with panic, stress, or anxiety, Rescue Remedy will be calming and restorative. Take as required. *(See page 244.)*

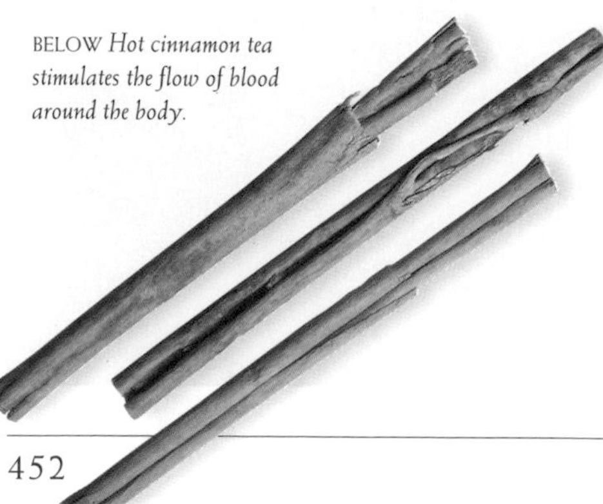

BELOW *Hot cinnamon tea stimulates the flow of blood around the body.*

Dizziness

CAUTION

CHRONIC, UNDIAGNOSED DIZZINESS SHOULD BE INVESTIGATED BY A PHYSICIAN.

One of the most common features of aging is dizziness, often a cause of stumbles and falls. It may stem from age-related loss of orientation, side-effects of drugs, a failure in the balancing mechanism of the inner ear, or from neurological disturbances. (*See also page 299.*) It can also be a symptom of hypothermia, which is common among the elderly, partly because many tend to economize on fuel and heating, and partly because the brain's control of heat regulation is less efficient than that of younger people. Dizziness can be both frightening and debilitating, particularly for those elderly people who live alone.

SYMPTOMS

• *a spinning sensation* • *nausea and vomiting* • *headache* • *pallor and sweating*

LEFT *Squeeze the juice of a lemon into soda water to sip.*

Falls and Accidents

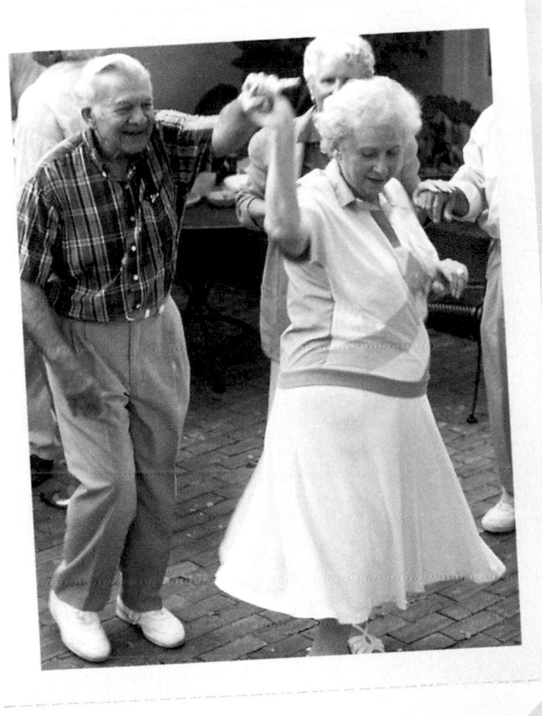

ABOVE *Finding hobbies which keep you active is one of the best ways of retaining mobility.*

Failing vision, unsteadiness, slower reflexes, dizziness, stiffness, and muscle weakness all contribute to the vulnerability of elderly people, making them more prone to falls and accidents. Often a stumble that would be little more than an inconvenience to a younger person is a serious hazard to the elderly, causing physical disability and, often, emotional complications. This may be partly explained by problems in the Data File alongside. *(See also First Aid, page 458.)*

DATA FILE

- Cataracts (*see page 317*).
- Osteoporosis (*see page 414*). Old people, and old women in particular, are susceptible to fractures even from minor accidents. The resultant immobility can trigger other problems, such as chest and urinary infections, and depression.
- Delicate skin. An older person's skin is more delicate and bruises or tears much more easily than previously.
- Slower healing processes. Muscular injuries are slow to heal among the elderly, causing long periods of disability and dependency. This in turn can lead to depression (*see page 450*).

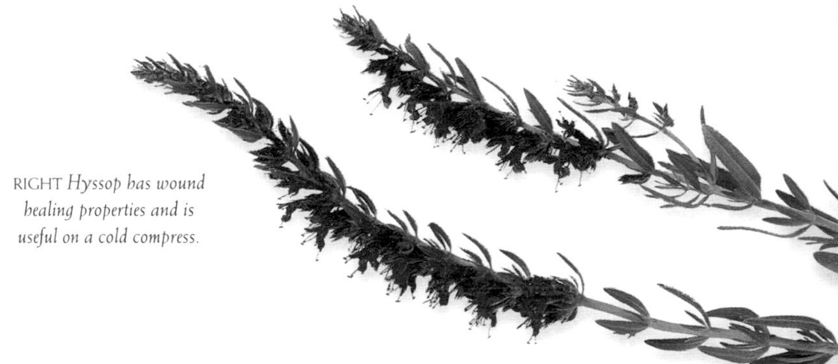

RIGHT *Hyssop has wound healing properties and is useful on a cold compress.*

TREATMENT

AYURVEDA
- Harithaki can help for conditions related to impaired vision, which can help to prevent accidents.

HERBALISM
- Use witch hazel on a cold compress for bruises. *(See page 123.)*
- Calendula cream will help healing of sprains, cuts, and bruises. *(See page 117.)*
- Compresses of herbs like hyssop, lavender, or fennel will reduce swelling and bruising. As it heals, essential oil of rosemary can be applied as a compress to encourage the circulation and, through that, the healing process. *(See page 121.)*
- Rosemary is a tonic, particularly for the elderly, as it stimulates and nourishes the nervous system and will help keep you alert. *(See page 127.)*
- Orange blossom, particularly in the form of neroli oil, is an effective nervine tonic (for the nervous system), which can help prevent accidents that are caused by a lack of concentration, and general confusion.

AROMATHERAPY
- Oils that refresh and invigorate will help focus the mind, which prevents accidents. Use one or more of the following in the bath: rosemary, peppermint, geranium, eucalyptus. *(See page 146–71.)*
- Basil oil also clears the mind and stimulates mental activity. *(See page 164)*
- Bergamot, chamomile, lavender, marjoram, and rosemary will help to ease pain in the event of an accident. Do not apply to broken skin, but use in a vaporizer or in massage, avoiding the affected areas. *(See page 146–71.)*

HOMEOPATHY
- Arnica aids healing in someone who is constantly falling or having accidents. *(See page 182.)*
- Arnica followed by Symphytum, for fractures, to promote healing. *(See page 182.)*
- Aconite, for shock. *(See page 178.)*
- Veratrum, for shock, with cold pale skin and a cold sweat.
- Calendula will help heal deep and painful wounds. *(See page 187.)*
- Hypericum, for wounds that are characterized by shooting nerve pains. *(See page 199.)*

FLOWER ESSENCES
- Rescue Remedy or Emergency Essence can be used after an accident and in cases of shock. *(See page 244.)*

VITAMINS AND MINERALS
- Keeping physically and mentally active will help to prevent accidents. Ensure that you have a good intake of vitamin C and zinc, and B vitamins, which feed the nervous system. *(See pages 256, 265, and 252–5.)*
- Vitamin E will help healing. *(See page 257.)*

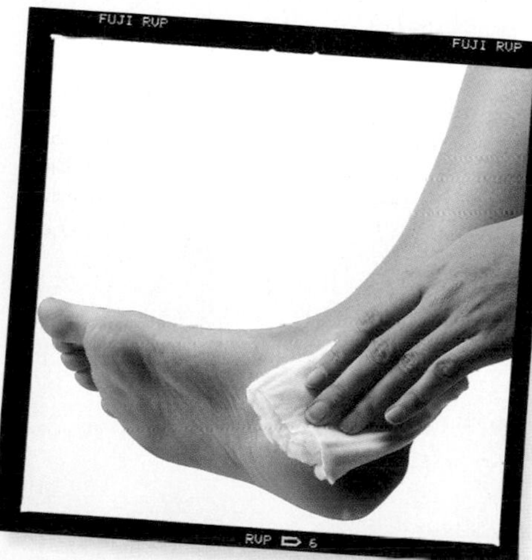

ABOVE *Distilled witch hazel, on a cold compress, treats a bruise.*

Trigeminal Neuralgia

Trigeminal neuralgia is a condition in which sudden nerve impulse discharges occur in the sensory nerve of the face on one side. These discharges cause severe pain and may be triggered by chewing, swallowing, or sometimes speaking. Usually there are repeated attacks over a period of some weeks, and the periods in between tend to become shorter. The cause of trigeminal neuralgia is unclear. Trigeminal neuralgia is unusual under the age of 50. When the condition occurs in young people it may be associated with MS.

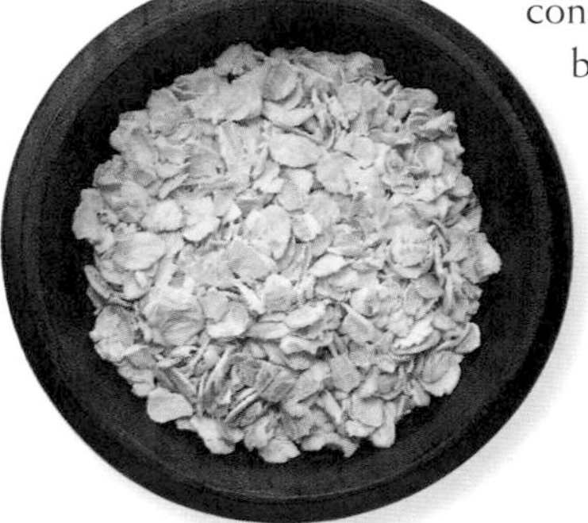

ABOVE *Cereals such as oats contain magnesium phosphate, itself the source of a homeopathic remedy.*

Symptoms

• excruciating pain lasting from a few seconds to one or two minutes • a feeling of being on edge in constant anticipation of the next attack • a tic caused by the wincing of the facial muscles (hence trigeminal neuralgia is also known as tic douloureux)

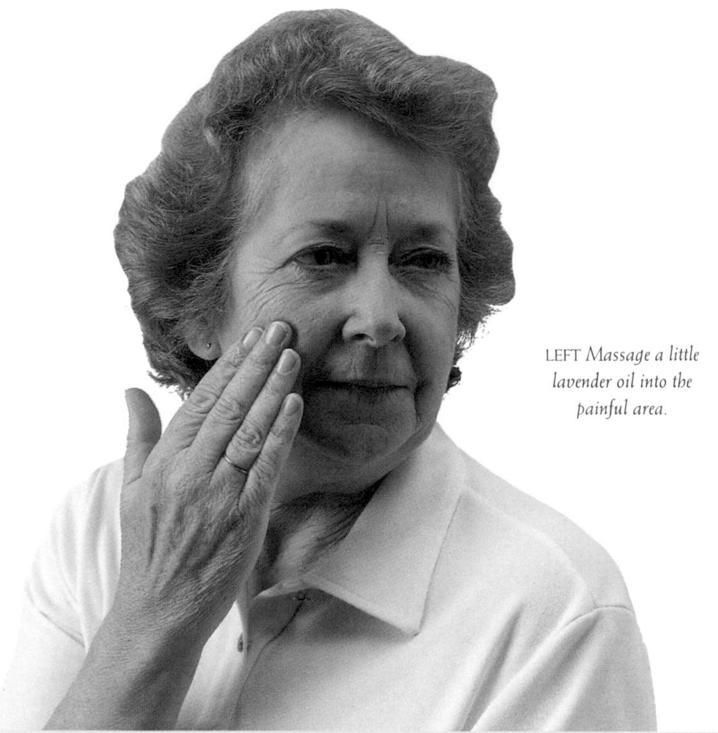

LEFT *Massage a little lavender oil into the painful area.*

TREATMENT

CHINESE HERBALISM

• Treatment would be aimed at addressing Wind, Damp, and Heat which have entered the meridians. Gentian and oriental wormwood may be useful.

TRADITIONAL HOME AND FOLK REMEDIES

• Celery juice or celery tea will help to ease the pain of neuralgia. *(See page 83.)*
• Rub lemons on the affected area for relief. *(See page 87.)*
• Rub peppermint oil into the affected area.
• Clove oil can be used where pain is experienced inside the mouth. *(See page 90.)*
• A compress of warm cider vinegar can bring relief. *(See page 102.)*

HERBALISM

• Ask a dentist to check your teeth, your bite, and jaw alignment.
• Drink rosemary and lavender infusions to relieve the pain. *(See page 127.)*
• Rub in cayenne-infused oil for neuralgia. *(See page 118.)*
• Warm chamomile compresses, applied to the affected area, will ease inflammation and pain. *(See page 119.)*

AROMATHERAPY

• Massage essential oil of eucalyptus, lavender, or chamomile into the affected area, or add the infused herbs to the bath. *(See pages 146–71.)*
• A compress of rosemary essential oil will invite the circulation to the area, which will encourage healing. *(See page 168.)*
• Blend 1 drop each of mustard and pepper oils in some grapeseed oil, and massage into the affected area. *(See pages 146–71.)*

HOMEOPATHY

Treatment should be constitutional, supervised by an experienced homeopath. Some of the following remedies may be helpful:
• Arsenicum, for an attack brought on by dry cold. You feel chilly, tired, restless, with burning pains. *(See page 182.)*
• Lachesis, for pain that is worse after sleep. *(See page 216.)*
• Mag phos., for pain that is relieved by heat and pressure. *(See page 204.)*
• Aconite, when symptoms come on suddenly, particularly after exposure to cold; the body feels congested and numb. *(See page 178.)*
• Colocynthis, for an attack brought on by cold or damp, and which is improved by heat. *(See page 191.)*

VITAMINS AND MINERALS

• Vitamins B1, B2, and biotin help nerve health. *(See pages 252, 253, and 257.)*
• Take extra vitamin E and chromium. *(See pages 257 and 259.)*

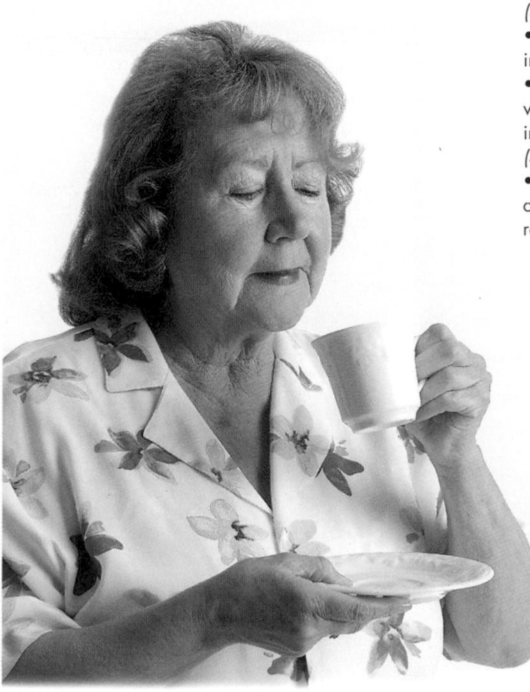

LEFT *Brew up some celery seed tea by infusing 1-2 teaspoonsful of seeds in boiling water.*

Incontinence

Incontinence, or involuntary urination, is extremely common among the elderly and usually has a physical cause. In men this may be prostate disease, and in women a prolapse of the bladder. Urinary infections or damage to the nervous system, such as acute or chronic brain disease, may also be responsible. Fecal incontinence is less common. It may be caused by constipation (if watery feces escape around the obstruction) or depression. Both types of incontinence are very distressing. (*See also page 381.*)

LEFT *Walnut flower essence helps with a change in life.*

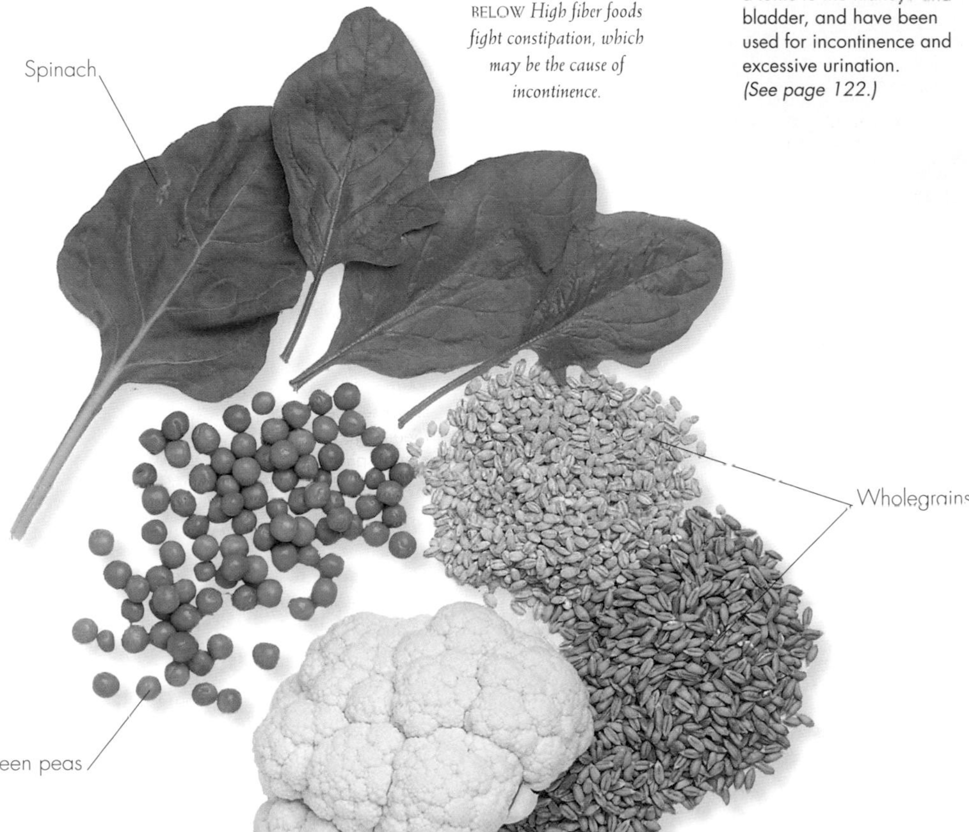

BELOW *High fiber foods fight constipation, which may be the cause of incontinence.*

TREATMENT

Fecal incontinence should be treated according to the cause (see constipation, senile dementia, depression, and gastroenteritis). Urinary incontinence can be treated in a variety of ways.

CHINESE HERBALISM

- Treatment would address Kidney Yang Deficiency with internal cold, and the best herb to use is golden lock, taken as a tea.
- If the condition accompanies prolapse, treatment will be given for deficient qi, using central qi pills. These will help with the control of fecal and urinary incontinence.

HERBALISM

- The seeds of the ginkgo biloba plant act as a tonic to the kidneys and bladder, and have been used for incontinence and excessive urination. *(See page 122.)*
- Horsetail has toning and astringent properties, making it useful for treating incontinence and frequent urination. *(See page 120.)*

HOMEOPATHY

Treatment would be based on the cause of the incontinence, but some of the following might be useful:

- Causticum, for incontinence made worse by coughing or laughing. *(See page 189.)*
- Ferr. phos., for an inability to control the bladder, with pain and a frequent urge to urinate. *(See page 194.)*
- Nux vomica, for irritability and involuntary dribbles of urine. *(See page 214.)*
- Pulsatilla, for stress incontinence which is made worse by sitting down. *(See page 209.)*
- Sepia, for incontinence related to weak pelvic floor muscles, with a feeling as if the abdomen is falling out of the vagina. *(See page 212.)*

FLOWER ESSENCES

A number of the remedies will help with negative emotions and distress. Some to try are:

- Sweet Chestnut, for feelings of despair. *(See page 227.)*
- Agrimony, if you hide behind a cheerful face. *(See page 225.)*
- Crab Apple, if you feel unclean. *(See page 234.)*

VITAMINS AND MINERALS

- Increase your intake of dietary fiber, which will prevent constipation and straining – a common cause of incontinence.
- Drink plenty of water to ensure regular use of the bladder muscles.

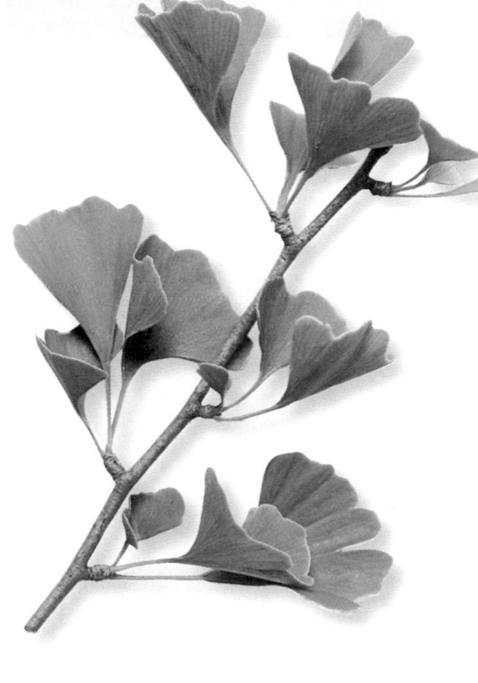

ABOVE *Gingko biloba seeds help to treat incontinence. The plant comes from China.*

CHRONIC ILLNESSES

Chronic Fatigue Syndrome (CFS)

Chronic fatigue syndrome (CFS) is also known as post-viral fatigue syndrome and myalgic encephalitis (ME), and its cause is the subject of controversy: it is thought by some to be caused by a viral infection (possibly herpes, polio, or Epstein-Barr), while others hold that it may be a psychological or neurological disorder, and others still that it is the result of damage to the immune system. There are recurrent acute attacks and rarely a full return to health in between. Symptoms may persist for years, aggravated by periods of stress or exertion.

SYMPTOMS

• *profound fatigue* • *fever* • *headache*
• *nausea and dizziness* • *muscle pain*
• *weight fluctuation* • *sleep disturbance*
• *depression* • *memory loss*

DATA FILE

- At one time CFS was known as the "yuppie flu," because it was initially identified most commonly among young professional people.
- Most common in women between the ages of 18 and 35.
- First reports of CFS appeared in the mid-1980s.
- Recent research has confirmed variations in basic bodily functions of people with CFS.
- The Epstein-Barr or herpes virus is often present in persons with these symptoms, but researchers have ruled out this virus as the cause, which remains unknown.

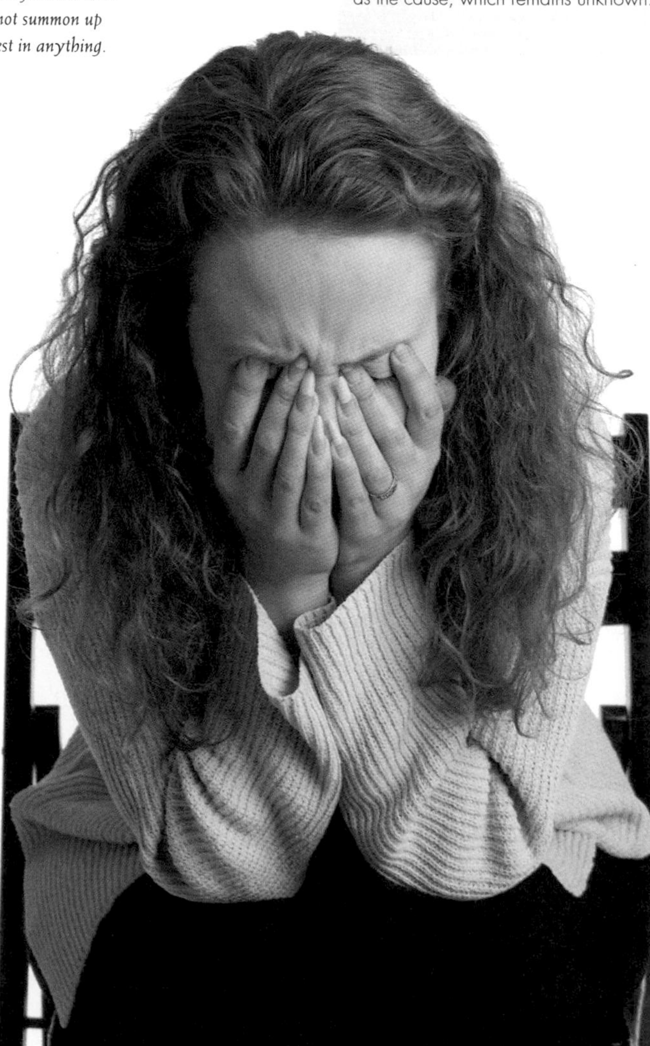

RIGHT *Olive flower essence is for those who cannot summon up interest in anything.*

TREATMENT

AYURVEDA
• Complete detoxification will help, along with oral preparations to strengthen the immune system and balance the doshas. Cluster fig and ginger may be useful to stimulate. *(See page 22.)*

CHINESE HERBALISM
• ME is believed to be caused by weakness of qi, Deficient Blood, and Damp Heat, and herbal treatment would be given accordingly, probably in conjunction with acupuncture. Chinese angelica can restore energy and stimulate white blood cells and antibody formation. *(See page 56.)*

HERBALISM
• Herbs that address the immune system, such as echinacea, will be most useful. *(See page 120.)*
• Ginseng and gingko biloba will encourage energy. *(See pages 122 and 126.)*
• Rosemary and sage wines act as an excellent tonic when you are run down and tired. *(See pages 127 and 129.)*
• Licorice can enhance recovery and stimulate the formation of white blood cells. *(See page 122.)*
• Astragalus can increase energy levels and resistance to disease. *(See page 116.)*

BELOW *Add some deliciously fragrant rose oil to your bath: a treat for the senses.*

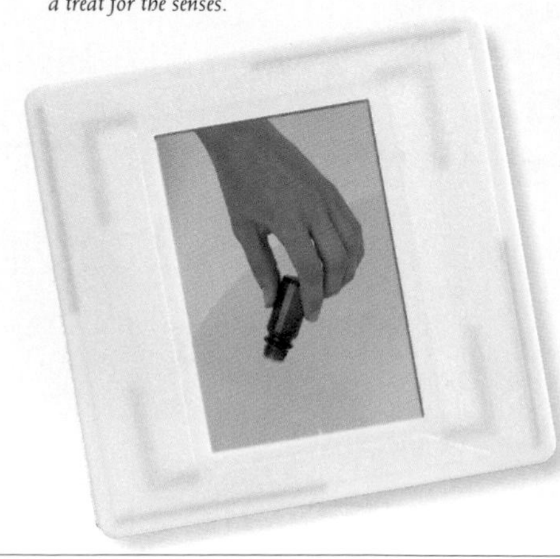

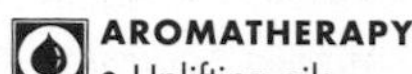

AROMATHERAPY
• Uplifting oils, such as bergamot, rose, and neroli, will help with flagging spirits. Use them in a massage or in the bath. *(See pages 146–71.)*
• Tea tree and niaouli will strengthen the immune system. Use these in a massage or in the bath. *(See pages 162 and 163.)*
• Rosemary is stimulating, and can be added to the bath, used in massage, or put in a vaporizer while you are working. *(See page 168.)*

HOMEOPATHY
• Homeopathic treatment would be constitutional, based on individual needs, but many promising studies have been done into its effects.
• China may be taken every 12 hours, for a few days, while waiting for constitutional treatment. *(See page 190.)*

ABOVE *Astragalus root decoction fights chronic fatigue.*

FLOWER ESSENCES
• Mustard, for depression, when you feel gloomy for no known reason. *(See page 239.)*
• Olive, when you are exhausted on all levels. *(See page 235.)*
• Rock Rose, for feelings of terror at the thought that you will never get better. *(See page 231.)*
• Crab Apple, if you feel unclean or impure on any level. *(See page 234.)*
• Hornbeam for exhaustion at the thought of doing anything. *(See page 227.)*

VITAMINS AND MINERALS
• A good B-complex vitamin tablet will help to ensure the health of the nervous system and give you more energy. *(See pages 252–5.)*
• Some sufferers have food allergies that may exacerbate or even cause the condition. Try an elimination diet to see if you are allergic to anything – in particular, dairy produce and wheat.
• Chronic yeast infection may be at the root of the condition. Taking an acidophilus supplement, or eating plenty of live yogurt will help fight the infection. *(See page 271.)*
• Evening primrose oil, taken over three months, has proved to be a useful treatment for ME. *(See page 270.)*

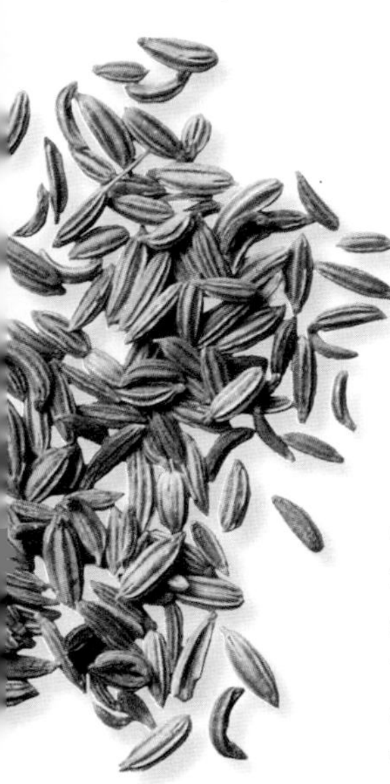

ABOVE *Use fennel essential oil for the nausea of chemotherapy.*

HIV/AIDS

(See under Immune System, page 410.)

Cancer

Cancer is a chronic disease that may occur anywhere in the body, beginning with a malignant tumor which may be either a carcinoma or a sarcoma. Carcinomas arise in the lining of the skin and internal organs. Sarcomas arise from solid tissues such as muscle, bone, lymph glands, blood vessels, and other connective tissues. Both are invasive – a cell becomes cancerous, divides, and forms an abnormal mass which grows until the healthy cells are outnumbered. The mass then spreads into adjacent tissues and structures, often destroying them. Secondary cancers occur if an invading cancer grows through the wall of a blood vessel so that the blood then carries cancerous cells to other parts of the body.

A tumor of low malignancy may take months or years to cause problems, whereas a high-malignancy tumor may have spread widely before the sufferer is aware of it.

ABOVE *A healthy diet, high in antioxidants, helps the immune system*

Symptoms

• It is impossible to enumerate all the symptoms of all cancers here, but awareness of signs that a change has occurred is important. They may have a harmless explanation, but include:
• unusual bleeding or discharge, especially from the vagina or rectum
• a lump or thickening in the breast or elsewhere
• a wound that does not heal • persistent change in bowel habits
• persistent hoarseness or coughing • persistent indigestion or difficulty in swallowing • change in the size or shape of a wart or mole
• persistent unexplained weight loss • nagging pain in the chest

TREATMENT

CHINESE HERBALISM

• Treatment will be aimed at supporting the immune system and reducing the harmful effects of chemotherapy and radiotherapy.
• Ginseng protects the immune system and helps to restore vitality. *(See page 67.)*
• Dang Gui will protect the Liver. *(See page 56.)*
• Huang Qi will act as a tonic, support the nervous system, and invigorate the immune system, as will ginger and ginseng. *(See pages 57 and 67.)*
• Chinese angelica can restore energy, and stimulate white blood cells and antibody formation. *(See page 56.)*

HERBALISM

• Herbs that calm the nervous system will be useful. Try chamomile, valerian, and limeflowers. *(See pages 119, 134, and 136.)*
• Echinacea can be used to promote healing. *(See page 120.)*
• Sweet violet, cleavers, red clover, and burdock will help to boost the immune system. *(See page 115.)*
• St. John's wort is a mild antidepressant which acts as a restorative and helps treat depression. *(See page 124.)*
• There are several herbs which have been found to have anticancer properties, and which can be used in conjunction with conventional medical treatment. These include yellow dock, garlic, nettle, myrrh, cleavers, thyme, calendula, poke root, and plantain. *(See pages 113, 116, 117, 128, 135, and 137.)*

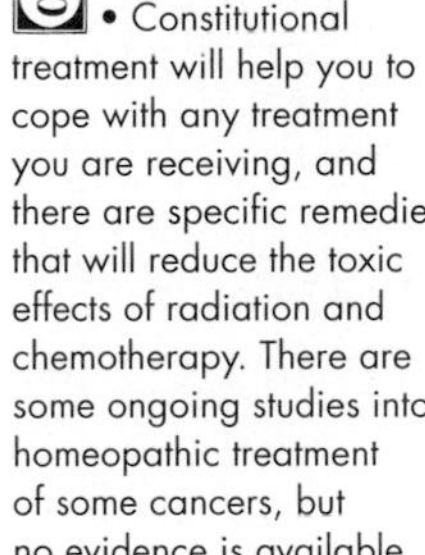

AROMATHERAPY

• An aromatherapy massage will restore the body's equilibrium.
• Geranium and rose, for lifting depression. *(See pages 165 and 168.)*
• Rosemary, bergamot, and sandalwood, for fatigue. *(See pages 146–71.)*
• Fennel, for nausea. *(See page 159.)*
• Do not massage the body immediately prior to or just after chemotherapy because it can encourage the spread of cancer cells throughout the body. In the early stages of cancer, use aromatherapy oils in the bath or in a vaporizer only. *(See page 144.)*

HOMEOPATHY

• Constitutional treatment will help you to cope with any treatment you are receiving, and there are specific remedies that will reduce the toxic effects of radiation and chemotherapy. There are some ongoing studies into homeopathic treatment of some cancers, but no evidence is available at the current time.

FLOWER ESSENCES

• Flower Essences are often used by practitioners to help you cope with the physical and emotional effects of cancer. *(See page 219 for a list of those that might be the most suitable.)*
• Mimulus is particularly good for feelings of fear. *(See page 235.)*
• Rock Rose is good if you feel helpless and experience terror or panic. *(See page 231.)*
• Olive will help if you feel exhausted on all levels. *(See page 235.)*
• Sweet chestnut will help if you feel there is no way out. *(See page 227.)*
• Gorse will help with feelings of hopelessness. *(See page 240.)*

VITAMINS AND MINERALS

• Eat as much fresh fruit and vegetables as you can, particularly those containing antioxidants. *(See page 251.)*
• Reduce animal fats and avoid processed foods.
• A deficiency of vitamin C has been found in conjunction with certain tumors. Ensure you get plenty in your diet. *(See page 256.)*
• Vitamin A can protect against cancer in smokers to some degree. *(See page 252.)*
• Digestive enzymes may be offered as a treatment to halt the activities of trophoblastic cancer cells.
• Vitamin E is said to prevent a number of cancers. Ensure that you get plenty in your diet or take supplements. *(See page 257.)*

DATA FILE

• In the 1990s nearly 6 million new cancer cases and more than 4 million deaths from cancer were being reported worldwide each year.

• The leading fatal cancer in the world today is lung cancer, which has risen rapidly because of the spread of cigarette smoking in developing countries.

• Stomach cancer, prevalent in Asia, is the second most fatal form of cancer in men, after lung cancer.

• Also on the increase is the leading killer of women, breast cancer, particularly in China and Japan.

• The fourth on the list is cancer of the colon or rectum, a disease that mainly strikes the elderly.

• In the U.S. in the early 1990s more than one-fifth of all deaths were caused by cancer; only cardiovascular diseases accounted for a higher percentage of deaths.

• In 1993 the American Cancer Society predicted that about 33 percent of Americans will eventually develop some form of cancer.

• Skin cancer is the most prevalent cancer in both men and women, followed by prostate cancer in men and breast cancer in women.

• Lung cancer, however, causes the most deaths in both men and women.

• Leukemia, cancer of the blood, is the most common type seen in children.

• An increasing incidence of cancer has been observed over the past few decades, due to improved cancer screening programs, to the increasing age of the population, and also to the large number of tobacco smokers.

• Researchers have estimated that if Americans stopped smoking, lung-cancer deaths could virtually be eliminated within 20 years.

	AYURVEDA	CHINESE HERBALISM	TRADITIONAL HOME AND FOLK REMEDIES
## Bites and stings Insect bites and stings are common, and may cause discomfort, but unless you suffer from an allergic reaction, the best course of treatment is to soothe the pain and reduce swelling. The stinging insects inject a toxin through a stinger at the tail end of the abdomen. The reaction is usually local, but if the sting occurs in the mouth or throat, swelling can cut off the air supply and cause death by asphyxiation. Death can occur in individuals who are hypersensitive to bee venom. Animal bites should always be cleaned carefully and seen by a doctor. Dogs and other animals can transmit the infectious disease rabies through bites. Symptoms include fever and convulsions. **Bruises** *See page 363*	• Aloe vera can be applied to the bite or sting to soothe; it also has anti-inflammatory and antiseptic properties. *(See page 27.)* • Bitter orange is anti-inflammatory and bactericidal. • Rub ghee on the affected area. *(See page 464.)* • Place a slice of raw onion on the bite or sting for natural relief. *(See page 25.)*	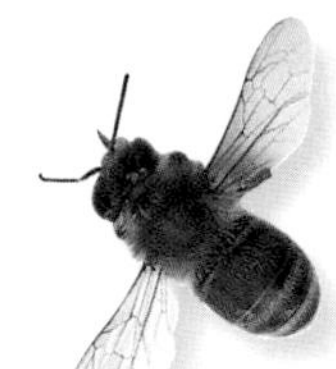 ABOVE *The homeopathic remedy Apis is made from bees and their venom.*	• The juice of a spring onion or a cucumber can be applied to stings to soothe and reduce inflammation. *(See page 82.)* • The juice of daikon radish is useful for spider bites. • Bathe stings in a bowl of water with several teaspoons of baking soda. *(See page 100.)* • A slice of raw onion placed on an animal bite will discourage infection and draw out poison. *(See page 82.)* • Apply garlic and onion to ant bites, and cucumber juice to ease the discomfort. *(See page 82.)* • Make a compress from a pad of cotton wadding soaked in lemon juice or cider vinegar and apply to a wasp sting. *(See pages 87 and 102.)* • Granulated sugar can be used to prevent a bite wound from scarring. Apply a poultice of sugar to the wound, after it has been cleaned, and bandage it with gauze.
## Blisters A blister occurs when a small area of the skin becomes raised and swollen by an accumulation of blood serum beneath it. If a blister is punctured the flesh beneath it becomes open to infection. It is therefore essential that it is kept clean and dry in order to heal effectively. Blisters can be caused by a number of things, including injuries – such as burns, scalds, or chafing (in new or ill-fitting shoes, for example) – insect bites, or infections. Some diseases will produce blisters, including chickenpox, herpes, eczema, and impetigo, and the disease can be transmitted by the virus particles inside the blisters.	• Aloe vera juice can be applied to the blister to encourage healing. *(See page 27.)* • Barberry can be used for an infected blister. *(See page 29.)* • Apply a basil oil poultice to the area. *(See page 42.)* • Cedar is a natural insect repellent. Spray around the room in an atomizer half full of water. *(See page 32.)*		• Boiled and mashed carrots can be applied to blisters to help to heal the area, and this is particularly good for infection. *(See page 89.)* • Use roasted onions, applied as a poultice to blisters, particularly those which have become infected. *(See page 82.)* • Peach pit tea is recommended to heal blisters. *(See page 103.)* • Ice will also reduce inflammation and any itching or pain. *(See page 103.)* • Bathe the blister with cold, salty water, which will discourage infection and help the blister to dry out. *(See page 103.)* • You can also apply surgical spirit, and then petroleum jelly to areas which may be susceptible to blisters caused by chafing. • Cover blisters in the daytime to prevent damage and infection. Remove bandages at night to allow them to dry out.

HERBALISM	AROMATHERAPY	HOMEOPATHY	FLOWER ESSENCES	CAUTION
• *Marigold petals are useful on a bee sting. (See page 117.)* • *Calendula cream will reduce swelling. (See page 117.)* • *The leaves of wormwood, sage, or rue can be macerated and applied to spider, scorpion, or jellyfish stings. (See page 129.)* • *Cover bites and stings with a wet, macerated plantain leaf. When it dries, replace with a wet leaf. (See page 126.)* • *Witch hazel is useful on mosquito bites. (See page 123.)*	• Use neat lavender oil on stings to reduce swelling and discomfort. *(See page 161.)* • 1 drop of tea tree oil can be rubbed into an insect bite or sting. *(See page 162.)* • A few drops of geranium oil, applied to water, can be used to clean a bite wound and encourage it to heal. *(See page 165.)* • Prevent insect bites by diluting essential oils of eucalyptus or citronella in half a mug of water, and then gently applying to exposed areas, avoiding the eyes and mouth. Use cider vinegar in the same way. *(See pages 158 and 159.)*	• *Ledum is useful for animal bites. (See page 202.)* • *Clean stings and animal bites with pure tincture of Hypericum. (See page 199.)* • *Aconite, for shock. (See page 178.)* • *Arnica, for bruising. (See page 182.)* • *Apis can be used for bee stings, after you have removed the sting with a pair of tweezers. (See page 180.)*	• Rescue Remedy or Emergency Essence, diluted in a few ounces of cool water, or the cream, can be applied to the sting or bite. Take orally for shock, pain, or distress, or apply to pulse points. *(See page 244.)*	
• *Aloe vera can be applied to the blister to help it heal. (See page 114.)* • *Marigold (calendula) can be applied to a blister to promote healing. (See page 117.)* • *Witch hazel, applied neat to a blister, will quickly relieve pain and swelling, and encourage healing. (See page 123.)*	• Neat lavender oil can be applied to blisters. *(See page 161.)* • Benzoin, applied to areas which are susceptible to blisters, can prevent as well as heal them. *(See page 170.)* • Roman chamomile has antiseptic properties. Use a few drops in half a mug of water to cleanse punctured blisters and the area around them. *(See page 150.)*	• *Urtica urens ointment can be applied to blisters caused by infection or burns. (See page 217.)* • *Hypericum ointment will encourage the healing of blisters. (See page 199.)* • *Cantharis, for itching, burning blisters. (See page 188.)* • *Rhus tox., for red and itchy blisters, particularly those caused by the chickenpox virus. (See page 210.)* • *Punctured blisters can be cleansed with a few drops of tincture of calendula in clean water. (See page 187.)*	• Rescue Remedy or Emergency Essence can be diluted in water and applied directly to the blister. *(See page 244.)*	**CAUTION** TRY NOT TO BURST A BLISTER, WHICH WILL LEAVE THE SKIN OPEN TO INFECTION. THE TOP LAYERS OF THE SKIN ARE USUALLY AFFECTED BY BLISTERS. SEE YOUR PHYSICIAN IF BLISTERS BECOME VERY PAINFUL AND INFLAMED, OR IF BLISTERS APPEAR FOR NO REASON.

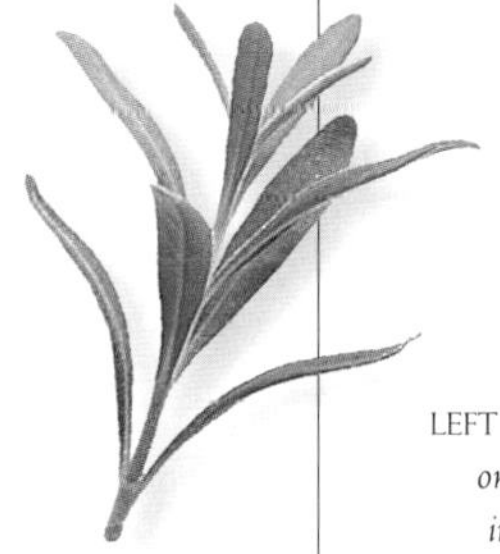

LEFT *Dab neat lavender oil on a sting. It has an insecticidal action.*

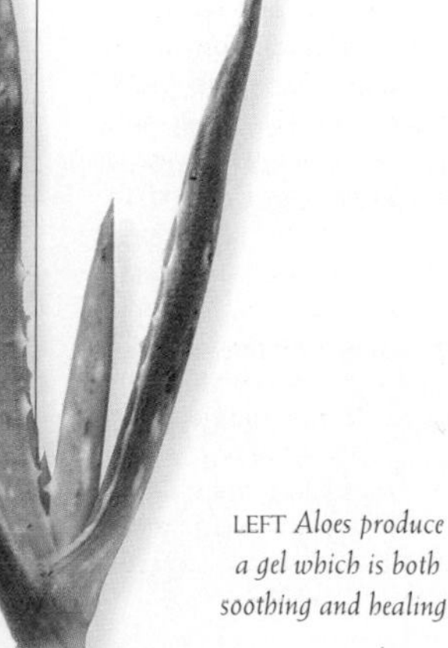

LEFT *Aloes produce a gel which is both soothing and healing.*

Mild shock

Injury or severe emotional trauma can lead to a potentially dangerous condition called shock, in which the blood fails to circulate properly. In serious cases of shock, the brain and other organs can be deprived of oxygen. Causes of shock include extreme pain, severe vomiting or diarrhea, blood infection, or violent allergy.

Toothache *See page 333*

AYURVEDA

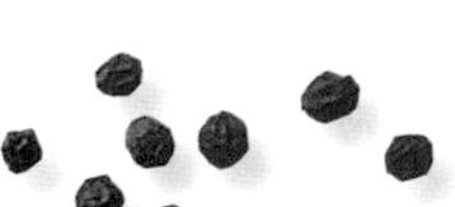

ABOVE Black pepper corns contain piperine, which helps to relieve pain.

CHINESE HERBALISM

- *Ginger and black pepper are warming and will help to restore circulation in cases of mild shock.*

Cuts and Abrasions

Minor cuts and abrasions should be cleaned with a mild antiseptic or cooled, previously boiled water to ensure that they do not become infected. More serious cuts, with damage to the skin and the structures below, should be seen by a physician.

Sprains *See page 417*
Travel Sickness *See page 369*
Nosebleed *See page 331*

AYURVEDA

- Aloe vera can be applied directly to cuts and grazes to encourage healing, reduce any inflammation, and prevent infection. *(See page 27.)*
- Yarrow improves blood clotting and may be useful for deeper wounds. *(See page 24.)*
- Myrrh can be used to clean the wound. *(See page 34.)*

CHINESE HERBALISM

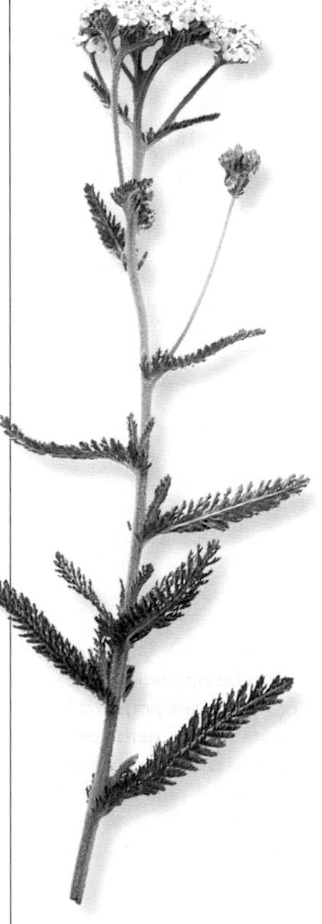

TRADITIONAL FOLK AND HOME REMEDIES

- Lemon juice is an excellent styptic, and can be diluted and applied directly to a clean wound. *(See page 87.)*
- A compress made of peach pit tea can be used on infected wounds.
- Sugar is said to prevent scar tissue. Press a few teaspoons of granulated sugar into a clean wound and dress with gauze. Rinse the wound carefully and dress again. Repeat up to five times daily, but take care not to disturb the clotting action.
- Direct pressure should be applied to the bleeding area, and maintained until the flow of blood ceases.

Burns and Scalds

A burn is an injury to the tissue of the body caused by heat, chemicals, electricity, or radiation. Serious burns must always be seen by a physician, as an emergency, but minor burns and scalds can be safely treated at home. Always cool a burn by letting cool water run over it until the pain has stopped. Try to avoid applying anything to the burn until it is cooled and you can see the extent of the damage. "Wet" burns should be dressed with a fabric, like gauze, which will "breathe." Change the dressing regularly.

Sunburn *See page 305*

AYURVEDA

- Aloe vera cools and prevents infection. *(See page 27.)*
- Onions may be used directly on the skin for instant relief. *(See page 25.)*
- St. John's wort can be used directly on the burn to cool and soothe. *(See page 40.)*

CHINESE HERBALISM

ABOVE *Yarrow helps to stop bleeding. The whole plant is used.*

TRADITIONAL FOLK AND HOME REMEDIES

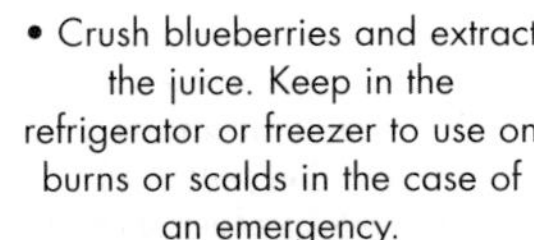

- Crush blueberries and extract the juice. Keep in the refrigerator or freezer to use on burns or scalds in the case of an emergency.
- Honey can be applied directly to a burn to facilitate healing and to help prevent infection. *(See page 101.)*
- Raw potatoes can be placed on a burn to provide instant relief. *(See page 98.)*
- Immerse the area in cool (not freezing water) for at least 10 minutes. Then apply hypericum lotion (about 10 drops of mother tincture, in a cup of water).

HERBALISM	AROMATHERAPY	HOMEOPATHY	FLOWER ESSENCES	CAUTION
• *Sip chamomile tea to calm. (See page 119.)* • *Add a little powdered ginseng to warm water with honey and lemon to restore. (See page 126.)*	• Lavender, melissa, or peppermint can be dropped on a handkerchief and held under the nose until help arrives or the condition stabilizes. *(See pages 146–71.)*	• *Aconite, for shock. Take every five minutes until it has subsided or help arrives. (See page 178.)* • *Arnica, for any bruising, injury, or trauma. (See page 182.)* • *Ignatia, for shock from an emotional upset or trauma. (See page 200.)*	• Four drops of Rescue Remedy or Emergency Essence can be taken internally or applied to the temples and pulse points, to reduce the effects of shock and ease a feeling of panic. *(See page 244.)* • Rock Rose is suitable if you are experiencing terror or panic. *(See page 231.)* • Try Mimulus for fear. *(See page 235.)*	**CAUTION** ONLY MILD SHOCK SHOULD BE TREATED WITH NATURAL REMEDIES.
• *Cayenne pepper is a very useful styptic, and a minute quantity can be applied directly to a clean wound to stop any bleeding. (See page 118.)* • *A few drops of marigold tincture in fresh, warm water can be used to clean the wound. This will help to prevent infection and encourage healing. (See page 117.)* • *Echinacea can be diluted and used directly on the wound to prevent infection. (See page 120.)* • *Comfrey ointment can be used on wounds which have become inflamed. (See page 132.)* • *Use a witch hazel compress on wounds and swellings. (See page 123.)* • *Tincture of myrrh is an excellent antiseptic. Apply a few drops to bandages before dressing a wound.*	• Lavender oil, applied directly to the nostrils or massaged in a light carrier oil into the temples, will provide relief from any accompanying shock or pain. *(See page 161.)* • A few drops of tea tree oil, in clear, warm water, can be used to clean a wound and act as an antiseptic. *(See page 162.)* • Geranium oil can be dropped on to a dressing to encourage healing. *(See page 165.)*	• *Ledum, for puncture wounds. This is particularly good if there is a risk of tetanus. (See page 202.)* • *Hypericum, for injuries that affect the nerve endings, such as the toes and fingers. (See page 199.)* • *Clean with calendula or hypericum tinctures. (See pages 187 and 199.)* • *Arnica should be used in the case of all injuries, to encourage healing and reduce the risk of bruising. (See page 182.)*	• Rescue Remedy or Emergency Essence can be applied neat to a graze to encourage healing and reduce pain, or applied to the temples and pulse points to calm. Use diluted in water on cuts, as the brandy may sting. *(See Shock, page 460.)* *(See page 244.)*	**CAUTION** IF YOU ARE UNABLE TO STOP THE BLEEDING, SEEK EMERGENCY MEDICAL ATTENTION. DO NOT OFFER FOOD OR DRINK.
• *Aloe can be applied directly to a burn in order to soothe and seal it from infection. It will also encourage healing. (See page 114.)* • *A few drops of echinacea tincture in a liter of water, poured over the burn, will help to prevent infection. (See page 120.)* • *Marigold tincture, applied sparingly to a dressing, is a useful healing agent. (See page 117.)*	• Lavender oil is ideal for burns and can be applied neat (use sparingly). *(See page 161.)* • A few drops of geranium oil in a liter of cooled boiled water can be poured over a burn or scald to encourage healing. *(See page 165.)*	• *Arnica can be taken to promote healing. (See page 182.)* • *Cantharis can help to relieve pain when taken immediately after the accident. (See page 188.)* • *Urtica can be used if the burn continues to be painful. (See page 217.)* • *Hypericum is useful for burns affecting the ends of fingers or toes, when there are sharp, stabbing pains. (See page 199.)* • *Aconite should be taken for shock. (See page 178.)* • *Urtica urens ointment may help to soothe a burn. (See page 217.)* • *Use hypericum ointment or calendula to prevent infection and encourage the burn to heal. (See page 199.)*	• Rescue Remedy or Emergency Essence will help to calm. A little bit of diluted tincture can be applied directly to a minor burn. *(See page 244.)*	**CAUTION** DO NOT PUNCTURE BLISTERS CAUSED BY BURNS, WHICH CAN CAUSE INFECTION. BURNS CAUSED BY CORROSIVE SUBSTANCES MUST BE WASHED OVER AND OVER AGAIN.

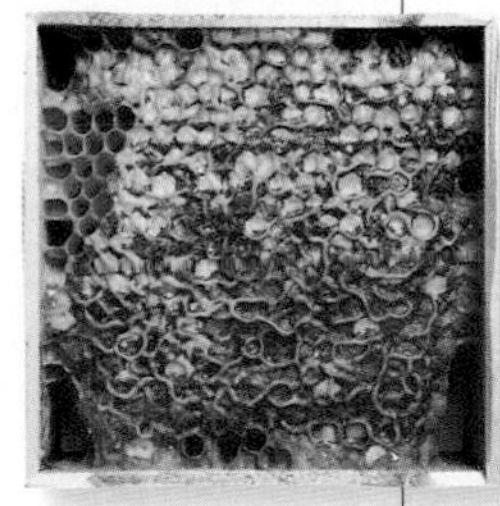

LEFT *Smear honey on burns, cuts or bruises, to help healing.*

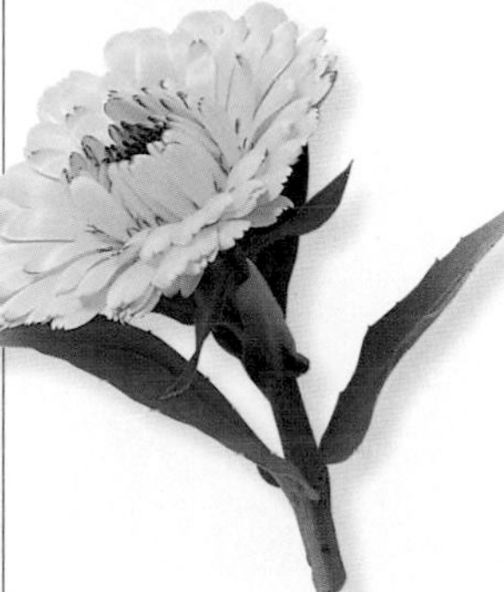

RIGHT *Calendula is antiseptic and promotes healing of any skin damage.*

Sunstroke

Sunstroke is a type of heat exhaustion, with symptoms that include headache, vomiting, fever, dizziness, and physical collapse. Heat exhaustion or sunstroke is usually caused by the excessive loss of water from the body that is the result of intensive heat. It is a mild form of shock. Sunstroke is also due to the body's inability to regulate internal heat. Heatstroke is a disorder that occurs when body-temperature regulating mechanisms are overwhelmed by excessive heat or fail in otherwise tolerable heat. Early nonspecific symptoms are faintness, dizziness, staggering, headache, dry skin, thirst, and nausea, which may be specifically related to heatstroke. In the latter stages of the condition, sweating ceases. Heatstroke is a medical emergency. The body temperature may be 40.5°C (105°F) or higher. Heatstroke differs from heat exhaustion, which lacks elevated body temperature and is characterized by persistent and heavy sweating.

AYURVEDA

- Add the juice of a lime or lemon to half a glass of soda water and sip in small doses.

CHINESE HERBALISM

- *Fresh ginger, cinnamon twigs, and peppermint may be useful. (See page 59.)*

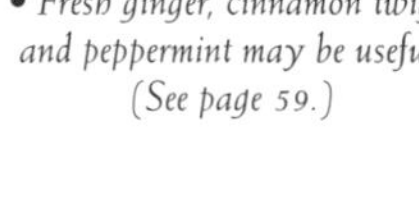

TRADITIONAL HOME AND FOLK REMEDIES

- Sip a little fresh cucumber juice to cool. *(See page 89.)*

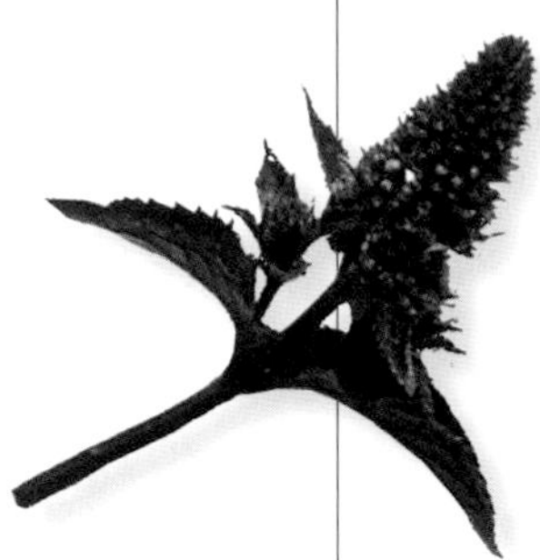

ABOVE *Peppermint soothes an upset stomach. Drink the tea as often as you like.*

Food Poisoning

Food poisoning is usually caused by eating food or drinking water that has been contaminated with bacteria, usually the salmonella strain. Symptoms of this kind of poisoning include diarrhea, fever, vomiting, and possibly pain in the abdomen. Gastroenteritis, an inflammation of the digestive system, can also result.

AYURVEDA

- Fresh lemon juice will help to cleanse, and fight infection.
- Strong spices like cayenne, curry, and turmeric have preventive properties against food poisoning.
- Combine 1 teaspoon of black pepper, 2 cloves of garlic, 1 tablespoon of cumin seeds, and a little salt in 4 cups of water. Boil until the liquid has reduced to 2 cups, and drink three times daily to cleanse and treat diarrhea.

CHINESE HERBALISM

- *Fresh ginger root will help to ease the nausea.*
- *Ping Wei Pian or Ren Dan may be useful.*

TRADITIONAL HOME AND FOLK REMEDIES

- Drink warm water with a little lemon juice to cleanse the system. *(See page 87.)*
- Add plenty of honey to a cup of warm water and sip for its antibacterial and immune-enhancing properties. *(See page 101.)*
- Chew ginger root to help ease the nausea.
- Cider vinegar, drunk with some warm water, will encourage vomiting to expel the poisons. *(See page 102.)*
- Drink plenty of cool fresh water, and avoid any food for at least twenty-four hours. *(See page 103.)*
- When the vomiting has ceased, ripe bananas can be eaten to help restore the bacterial balance in the gut. Live yogurt will have a similar effect. *(See page 93.)*

HERBALISM	AROMATHERAPY	HOMEOPATHY	FLOWER ESSENCES	CAUTION
• *Small sips of fresh ginger tea, made with root ginger, will help to ease the symptoms. (See page 139.)* • *Teas of rock rose flowers or wild rose flowers, with a little honey, will be helpful.*	BELOW *Chinese herbalists use ginger to restore yang in the body.* 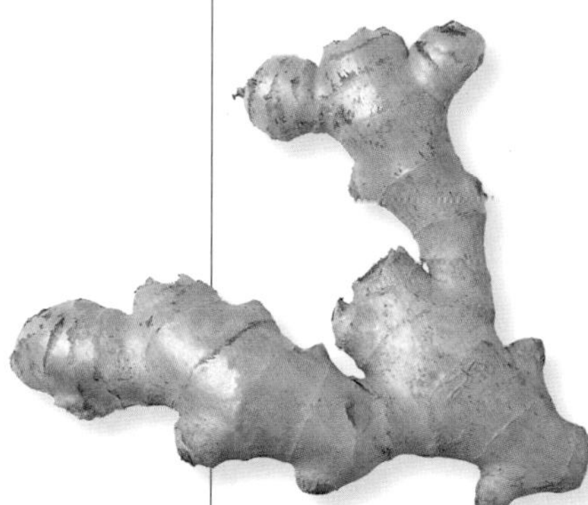 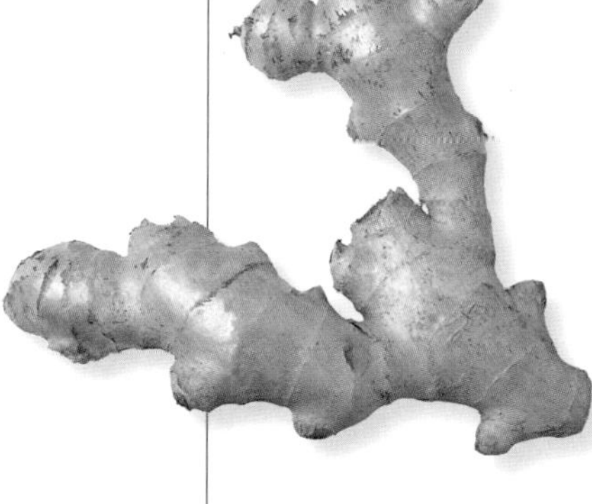	• *Take aconite initially, for symptoms of shock. (See page 178.) The following remedies will help in the aftermath:* • *Gelsemium, when there is accompanying trembling. (See page 195.)* • *Nux, when symptoms are made worse by flickering lights. (See page 214.)* • *Calcarea, when symptoms are worse on looking up. (See page 186.)* • *Borax, for symptoms made worse by downward motion.* • *Conium, when you feel worse lying down.*	• Rescue Remedy or Emergency Essence should be offered as soon as possible to treat shock. *(See page 244.)* • Olive will help in the aftermath. *(See page 235.)*	**CAUTION** FLUID MUST BE REPLACED AS SOON AS POSSIBLE, AND, IN SEVERE CASES, INTRAVENOUSLY. FIND A COOL PLACE AND SIT DOWN UNTIL ANY DIZZINESS SUBSIDES. IF YOU SUFFER FROM DIZZINESS THAT LASTS FOR MORE THAN AN HOUR OR VOMITING, SEE YOUR PHYSICIAN.
• *Make a tea of comfrey root and meadowsweet to treat infection and relieve symptoms. (See pages 121 and 132.)* • *Arrowroot or slippery elm tea can be sipped during the worst symptoms to soothe the digestive tract, and afterwards to help restore bowel health. (See page 136.)* • *Golden seal and meadowsweet can also be drunk as tisanes. (See page 121.)* • *Licorice tea will help to flush out the toxins. (See page 122.)* • *Fresh garlic, or garlic capsules, should be taken to reduce infection. (See page 113.)* • *Chamomile, drunk as a tea, will help to ease digestion and reduce inflammation. (See page 119.)*	• Chamomile oil, sprayed in the air or rubbed into the temples, will help to calm and ease symptoms. *(See page 150.)* • Tea tree, garlic, eucalyptus, and juniper all work to kill bacteria, and can be added to a cool bath or placed on a burner to help fight infection. *(See pages 146–71.)* • Rub a little diluted lavender oil into the abdomen to reduce any spasm and to help encourage healing. *(See page 161.)* • Bergamot will help to reduce any fever. Place on a cold compress on the head. *(See page 153.)*	• *Aconite, for symptoms that come on swiftly, causing some distress and shock. (See page 178.)* • *Baptisia, for salmonella infections. (See page 184.)* • *Pulsatilla, when the symptoms are worse at night and the sufferer feels tearful. (See page 209.)* • *Phosphorus, when there is diarrhea with a burning sensation, vomiting, and a craving for cold drinks. (See page 208.)* • *Arsenicum is excellent for many cases, particularly when there are burning pains and diarrhea. (See page 182.)* • *Nux vomica will help when the pain improves upon passing stools and there is a feeling of chilliness. (See page 214.)*	• Take Rescue Remedy or Emergency Essence initially. *(See page 244.)* • Olive will be useful as symptoms improve, to ease overwhelming exhaustion. *(See page 235.)*	**CAUTION** ANY CASE OF FOOD POISONING WHICH LASTS LONGER THAN 48 HOURS SHOULD BE SEEN BY A PHYSICIAN. ALL CASES OF SALMONELLA SHOULD BE REPORTED TO THE MEDICAL AUTHORITIES.

THE HOME HEALING REMEDY CHEST

The best way to learn about natural medicines is to try them out on yourself, your family, and friends. Assemble a stock of home medicines. Keep them in a box or cupboard along with a thermometer, scissors, an eye bath, cotton balls, and a selection of bandages, plasters, and sterile dressings. Use them for first aid and to treat minor ailments. The more you use, them the easier it becomes.

The list below includes remedies that most people will find useful. Check through the rest of the book and add remedies that are more specific to your family's needs. What are the most common medical conditions that arise in your family? Make or assemble suitable remedies so that they are always available. Try to treat illnesses as soon as the first symptoms appear. Do not wait for a runny nose to turn into sinusitis or bronchitis. Try to develop a general awareness of health. The aim of giving treatment at home should always be to prevent minor illnesses from turning into major ones – so avoiding visits to your practitioner.

ABOVE *Remember to keep a record of treatments, to refer to.*

Keep a notebook with the remedies to record your successes for future reference.

A short guide to indications and uses is given by each remedy below. Use this as a guide and consult the body of the book for more detailed information. The various remedies described can be used alone or in combination, but decide which is to be your main internal remedy for a specific situation, and use other suggestions as support. For example, use homeopathic Drosera for coughing attacks in children, and back this up with a drink of chamomile tea before bed, and eucalyptus essential oil in a vaporizer in the bedroom.

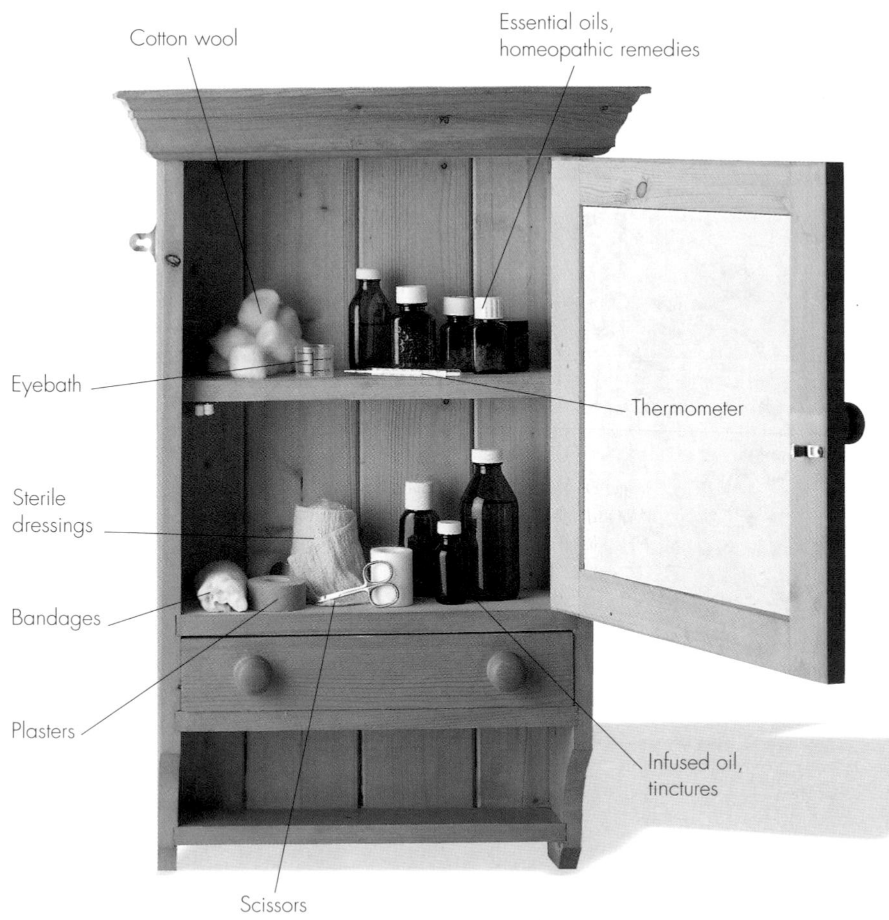

ABOVE *Be prepared! Keep a good stock of remedies and equipment at hand.*

Ayurveda

Coriander	USES	*Colds, flu, cystitis, sinus problems, and headaches.*
Mustard oil and seeds	USES	*Headaches, fever, rheumatism, sore feet, cold hands and feet.*
Curry leaves	USES	*Menstrual cramps.*
Garlic	USES	*Infections, chest pain, toothache.*
Ginger	USES	*Coughs and sore throats, indigestion, fungal infections.*
Black pepper	USES	*Diarrhea.*
Ghee	USES	*Bee and wasp stings, burning feet and hands.*
Karella	USES	*Tonic, calming.*
Lemon and lime juice	USES	*Dizziness.*
Aloe vera	ACTIONS	*Antiseptic, antibiotic, antiviral, anti-inflammatory and immune-enhancing.*
	USES	*Colds, colic, Candida, constipation, dermatitis, diabetes, water retention, ME, fungal infections, herpes, high blood pressure, inflammation, insomnia, indigestion, infections, menstrual cramps and irregularity, nausea, parasites, peptic ulcers, psoriasis, sprains, tinnitus.*

Chinese Herbalism

Patent Chinese herbal remedies for minor ailments are recommended for short-term use only. If you do not see an improvement within a week, stop using them and see a practitioner.

	REMEDY	PROPERTIES
Burns	Jing Wan Hung ointment	*Stops pain, resolves inflammation, clears Heat, promotes healing. Excellent for all types of burns. Can also be helpful for bedsores.*
Colds and Flu	Yin Qiao Jie Du Pian (honeysuckle and forsythia febrifugal pills)	*Expels Wind Heat. Best for colds and flu where you feel hot, have a sore throat, sneezing, and thick catarrh. Best in the first few days of illness. Not for when you are feeling chilled and achy, with watery catarrh. Not so useful once a cold has settled on your chest.*
	Tong Xuan Li Fei Wan	*Expels Cold and Wind. Best for colds and flu where you feel chilled and achy, and there is sneezing, maybe with watery catarrh. Best in the first few days of a cold or flu. Not for when you are feeling hot or have a sore throat. Not so useful once the cold has gone on to your chest.*
Coughs and Bronchitis	Qing Qi Hua Tan Wan (clear breathing and transform phlegm pills)	*Clears Phlegm and Heat from the lungs, stops coughing. Take for chest congestion and tightness in the chest, a cough, and coughing up thick yellow phlegm. The symptoms may be acute or chronic and may be accompanied by fever. It should produce an improvement in a couple of days, if it does not, seek professional help. Stop taking if you become thirsty. Not suitable for a dry, unproductive cough.*
	Chuan Bei Pi Pa Lu (fritillaria and loquat extract, cough syrup)	*Clears Phlegm and Heat from the Lungs, stops coughing. Use for an acute and chronic cough which produces thick phlegm, maybe yellow mucus. Not so good for dry coughs.*
Digestive Disturbances	Huo Xiang Zheng Qi Wan (herba agastachis pills)	*Regulates digestive system qi, clears Cold and Damp. For acute attacks of nausea, vomiting, and diarrhea with abdominal pain, especially when there are chills. Useful for gastric flu and for vomiting caused by food poisoning. If there is no improvement within a day, seek professional advice.*
Muscular Injuries	Die Da Wan (bodily injury pills) and Imperial Ted Da Wine	*Moves Blood and qi, resolves bruising, promotes healing in damaged tissue. The remedy is taken internally for bruises and sprains. Also useful for fractures after you have received medical attention. Not to be taken during pregnancy or if there is copious bleeding.*
Menstrual Problems	Dang Gui Pian (angelica tea), Shi Chuan Da Bu Wan (ten flavor tea), Wu Ji Rai Feng Wan (white phoenix pills)	*Supplements qi and Blood. There may be many causes of menstrual problems. For persistent problems it is wise to consult a practitioner. Dang Gui Pian is good for pain, but is not for excessive bleeding. Do not use Shi Chuan Da Bu Wan if you feel too hot.*

RIGHT *Sprinkle cayenne pepper in herbal tea for relief of indigestion.*

LEFT *Patent Chinese medicines are classic formulae developed over centuries.*

Traditional Home and Folk Remedies

Barley water (with lemon)	USES	*Digestive upsets, sore throats, cystitis.*
Black pepper	USES	*Congested head colds.*
Cabbage leaves	USES	*Mastitis, infections, hot swollen joints (crush and wrap around hot swollen joints).*
Cinnamon sticks	USES	*Colds, indigestion, circulatory problems.*
Celery	USES	*Neuralgia, headaches, muscle problems, spasm, kidney problems.*
Cloves	USES	*Neuralgia, indigestion, toothaches.*
Carrot juice	USES	*Stomach pains, children's diarrhea.*
Garlic	USES	*Internal and external infections and infestations.*
Honey	USES	*Weeping eczema, infected cuts, sore throats, flu, colds.*
Mustard	USES	*Colds, headaches, rheumatic pains, coughs.*

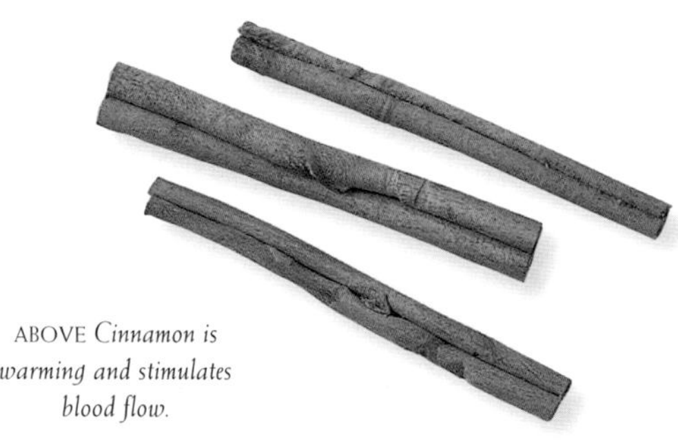

ABOVE *Cinnamon is warming and stimulates blood flow.*

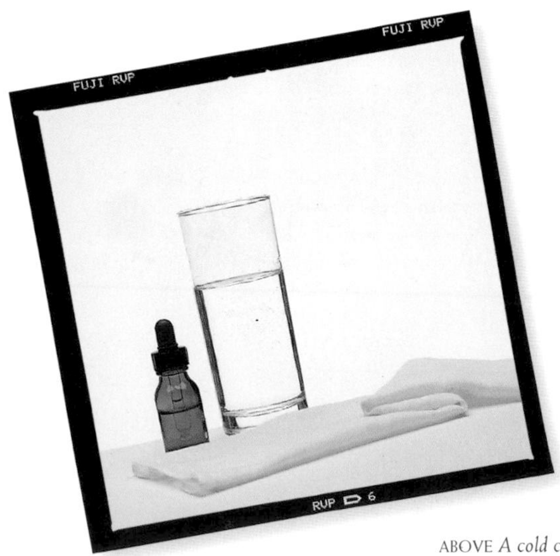

ABOVE *A cold compress, made with herbal tincture, has various uses.*

Aromatherapy

Keep essential oils in their original bottles. They last well but remember to screw the tops back on properly or they will slowly evaporate. If you buy them with the eyedropper attached, remember to keep them upright or the oil will eat away at the rubber top and leak. The home aromatherapist needs only a basic kit for minor ailments and first aid purposes. These ten oils are suitable for most people's needs.

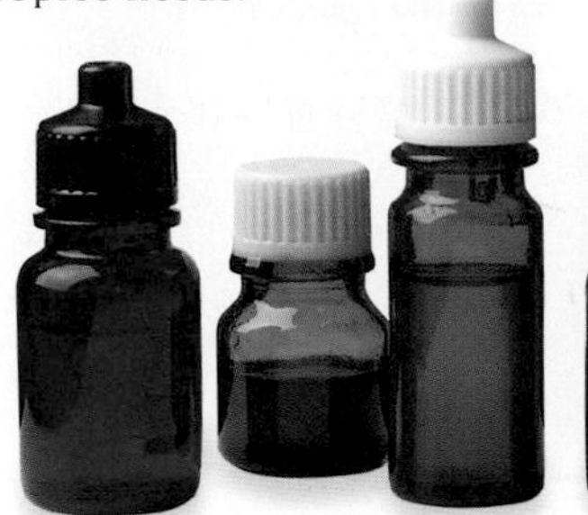

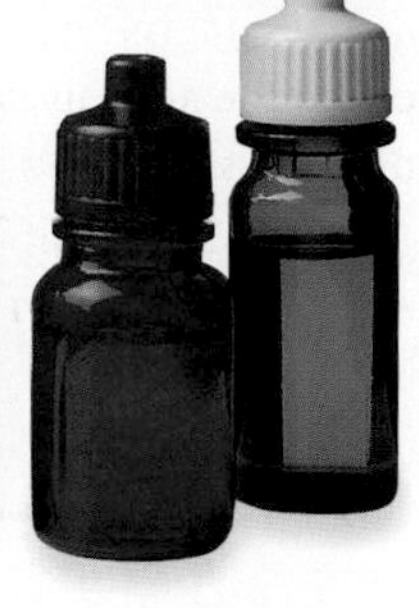

LEFT *Essential oils are usually diluted before skin application.*

Lavender	ACTIONS USES	*Relaxing, antiseptic, generally therapeutic.* *Dry skin, cuts, wounds, burns, bruises, insomnia, stress, indigestion, cystitis, headache.*
Chamomile	ACTIONS USES	*Calming, antiseptic, analgesic.* *Pain, indigestion, acne, eczema, sensitive skin, diaper rash, hay fever, toothache.*
Tea tree	ACTIONS USES	*Antifungal, antiseptic.* *Dandruff, mouthwash, cuts, insect bites, cystitis, thrush, colds, catarrh, infections.*
Geranium	ACTIONS USES	*Refreshing, relaxing, antidepressant, astringent.* *PMS, menopause, apathy, anxiety, cuts, fungal infections, eczema, bruises.*
Eucalyptus	ACTIONS USES	*Antiseptic, decongestant, anti-viral.* *Colds, chest infections, aches and pains.*
Rose	ACTIONS USES	*Soothing, tonic, antiseptic, antidepressant.* *Painful or irregular menstruation, menopause, insomnia, sensitive skin, sore throat, sinus congestion, depression.*
Rosemary	ACTIONS USES	*Stimulating, refreshing.* *Muscle fatigue, colds, poor circulation, aches and pains, mental fatigue.*
Peppermint	ACTIONS USES	*Digestive, refreshing.* *Bad breath, muscle fatigue, toothache, bronchitis, indigestion, travel sickness, sinus congestion.*
Lemon	ACTIONS USES	*Refreshing, antiseptic, stimulating.* *Cold sores, cuts, depression, acne, indigestion.*
Clary sage	ACTIONS USES	*Warming, soothing.* *Menstrual problems, depression, anxiety, high blood pressure.*

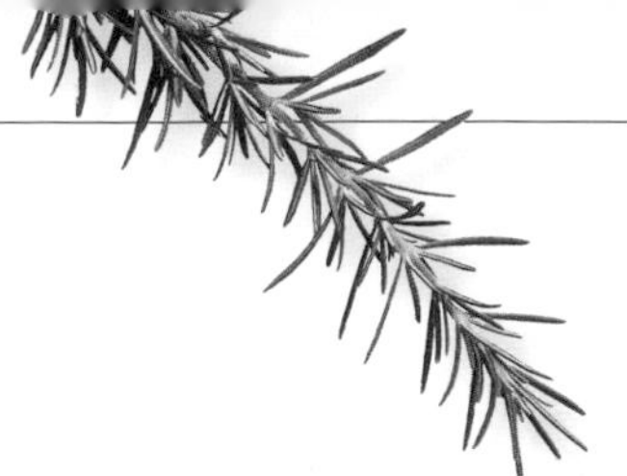

Herbalism

For most purposes keep either the dried herbs or their tinctures. Tinctures will keep, in dark-glass bottles in a cool place, for two or three years. Keep dried herbs in clean screw-top jars and replace them every year. Be sure to label all bottles and jars with the date and contents. Pills can be substituted where available and appropriate. They are especially useful for traveling and for unpleasant-tasting medicines. The creams and lotions can be bought or made at home. See the appropriate entry in the remedies section for methods of use (*pages 112–139*).

Angelica	USES	*Coughs, rheumatic pain, travel sickness, fever, pleurisy, nervousness.*
Basil	USES	*Insect bites, vomiting, constipation, nervous complaints.*
Bay	USES	*Rheumatism, fever, bruises, sprains.*
Calendula	USES	*Cuts, bruises, grazes, minor skin problems.*
Chamomile	USES	*Fever, nervous conditions, swelling, sores, fatigue, digestive complaints.*
Comfrey	USES	*Diarrhea, stomach ulcers, bleeding gums, menstrual problems, bruises, bites, sores, lung problems, whooping cough, broken bones.*
Echinacea	USES	*Fighting infection and warding off colds, flu and sore throats; boosts the immune system while acting as a natural antibiotic.*
Elder	USES	*Measles, bronchial problems, scarlet fever, colds, skin complaints.*
Garlic	USES	*Coughs and colds, thrush, wounds, bites, stings, infections, catarrh, cholesterol, high blood pressure.*
Ginger	USES	*Indigestion and wind, circulatory disorders, arthritis, morning sickness, travel sickness.*
Lavender	USES	*Relieves stress and promotes relaxation; treats stress and related disorders, insomnia, headaches, infection.*

BELOW *Chamomile is very versatile: antiseptic, nervine, sedative, and anti-inflammatory.*

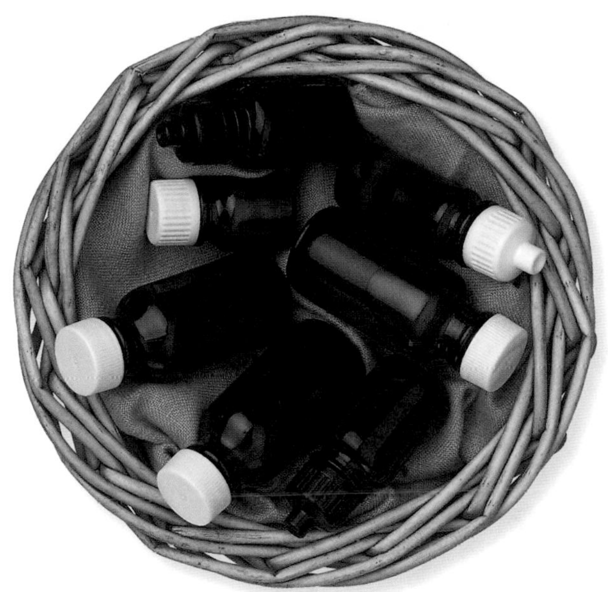

ABOVE *Herbal tinctures must be kept in dark glass bottles to preserve their medicinal actions.*

Limeflowers	USES	*Tension headaches and the effects of stress, including insomnia.*
Marjoram	USES	*Diarrhea, flatulence, coughs, cramps, colic, sprains, rheumatism, inflammation, sore throats, bruises.*
Meadowsweet	USES	*Pain relief, acid indigestion.*
Mint	USES	*Headaches, insomnia, nervousness, coughs, migraine, flatulence, abdominal aches.*
Parsley	USES	*Rheumatism, cystitis, insect bites, asthma, stings, urinary ailments, coughs.*
Peppermint	USES	*Indigestion, flatulence, headaches, colds.*
Rosemary	USES	*Circulatory disorders, stomachache, bruises, headaches, migraine, exhaustion.*
Sage	USES	*Gastritis, diarrhea, throat problems, nervousness.*
Thyme	USES	*Coughs and colds, sore throat, catarrh, headaches, whooping cough, diarrhea, rheumatism, bruises.*
Valerian	USES	*Flatulence, nervous headache, insomnia, stress, tension.*

RIGHT *Calendula is a very useful first aid remedy.*

Homeopathy

Although it is better to receive treatment from a qualified homeopath, homeopathy can be very useful in treating minor injuries at home. Bites, stings, bruises, cuts, travel sickness, and so on can be alleviated with the right remedy. But if you are in any doubt, seek professional help. For acute first aid problems in adults, children, and babies, use 30c. For less acute conditions, use 6c. Take every 2 hours up to 6 doses, then three times a day. Do not take more than 30c during pregnancy. Keep remedies in the original bottles. Keep away from essential oils. Replace before the "sell by" date. Homeopathic remedies work best when they fit the full symptom picture. Try to find the remedies that especially suit the individual.

Arnica	USES	*Cuts, grazes, broken skin, bruising, burns, scalds, nosebleeds, stings, sprains, dislocated joints, fractures, eye injuries, and shock.*
Apis	USES	*Stings, hives, water retention, cystitis, allergies affecting the throat, mouth, and eyes, bites, puncture wounds.*
Bryonia	USES	*Fractures, sprains, strains, mastitis, swollen joints, heat exhaustion, colds, flu, bursting headache with nausea.*
Calendula	USES	*Burns, cuts, grazes (more often used as a cream or tincture).*
Cantharis	USES	*Blisters, burns, scalds, burning diarrhea, cystitis, any stinging or burning sensation.*
Euphrasia	USES	*Conjunctivitis, bruising of the eye, sore eyes, eyestrain, constipation, bursting headaches.*
Hypericum	USES	*Cuts, grazes, bruising, crushed parts such as fingers, lacerations, puncture wounds, cut lip, diarrhea, and indigestion.*
Ledum	USES	*Cuts, bruises, insect stings, black eye, sore eye, bites, sprains and strains, particularly when they feel numb.*
Nux vomica	USES	*Travel sickness, digestive problems, hangovers, morning sickness, cystitis, nausea with headache.*
Phosphorus	USES	*Electrical burns or shock, nosebleeds.*
Rhus tox.	USES	*Red, swollen, itchy blisters, diaper rash, torn muscles, swollen joints, dislocated joints, cramp, muscle stiffness, arthritic or rheumatic pain which is helped by movement.*
Silicea	USES	*Splinters, recurrent colds and infection, migraine, spots.*

Flower Essences

Essence		
Rescue Remedy	USES	*Shock, trauma, injury, panic, anxiety.*
Star of Bethlehem	USES	*Shocks of all kind, accidents, bad news, sudden startling noise, trauma.*
Walnut	USES	*Change of any sort, including menopause, adolescence, divorce, a new school.*
Olive	USES	*Exhaustion and fatigue on all levels.*
Rock Rose	USES	*Helplessness, terror, panic.*

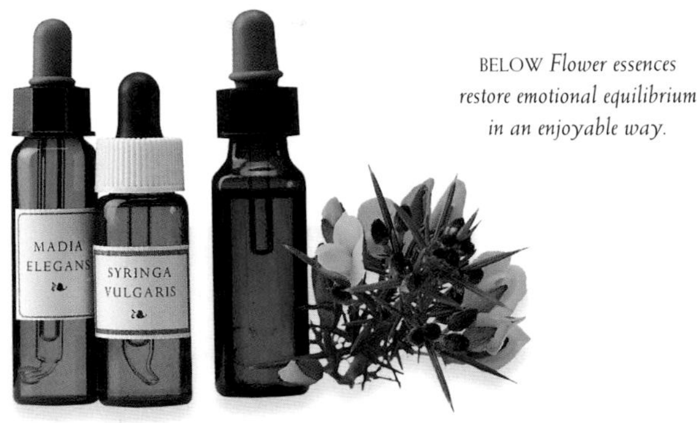

BELOW *Flower essences restore emotional equilibrium in an enjoyable way.*

Vitamins and Minerals

Supplement		
Royal jelly	USES	*Tonic, infections, allergies, stress.*
Ginseng	USES	*Stress, infections, colds, coughs, fatigue, circulatory problems.*
Vitamin C	USES	*Colds, infections (bacterial and viral), skin problems, circulatory problems, wounds, gum problems.*
Zinc	USES	*Colds, arthritis, fatigue, wounds.*
Chromium	USES	*Blood sugar swings, infections.*
Co-enzyme Q10	USES	*Colds, infection, heart problems, nervous problems, poor memory.*
Calcium	USES	*Insomnia, palpitations, arthritis, leg cramps, weak bones and teeth.*
Acidophilus	USES	*After antibiotics, constipation, diarrhea, infections, digestive problems, respiratory problems.*
Charcoal	USES	*Digestive problems, flatulence, indigestion.*

RIGHT *Charcoal has a long tradition of use for flatulence and indigestion.*

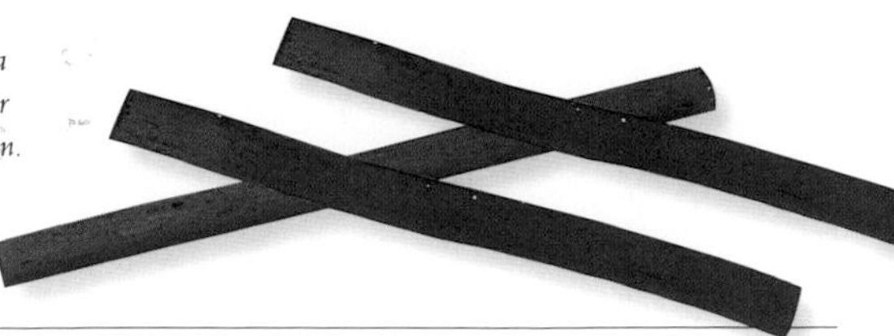

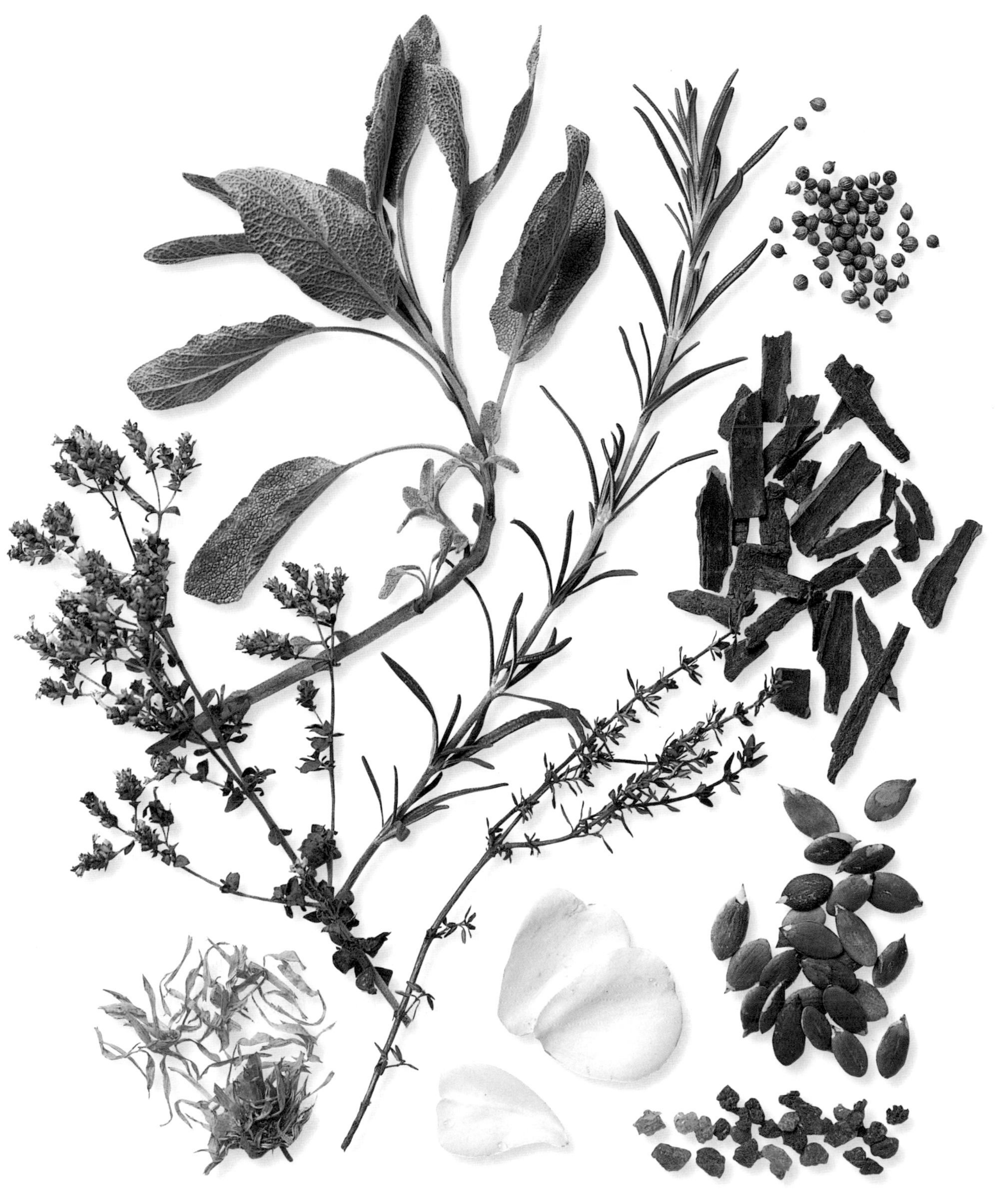

ABOVE *For regular and recurring health problems in the household, it is helpful to make up specific herb combinations. With time you will figure out particular mixtures that are beneficial to you and your family.*

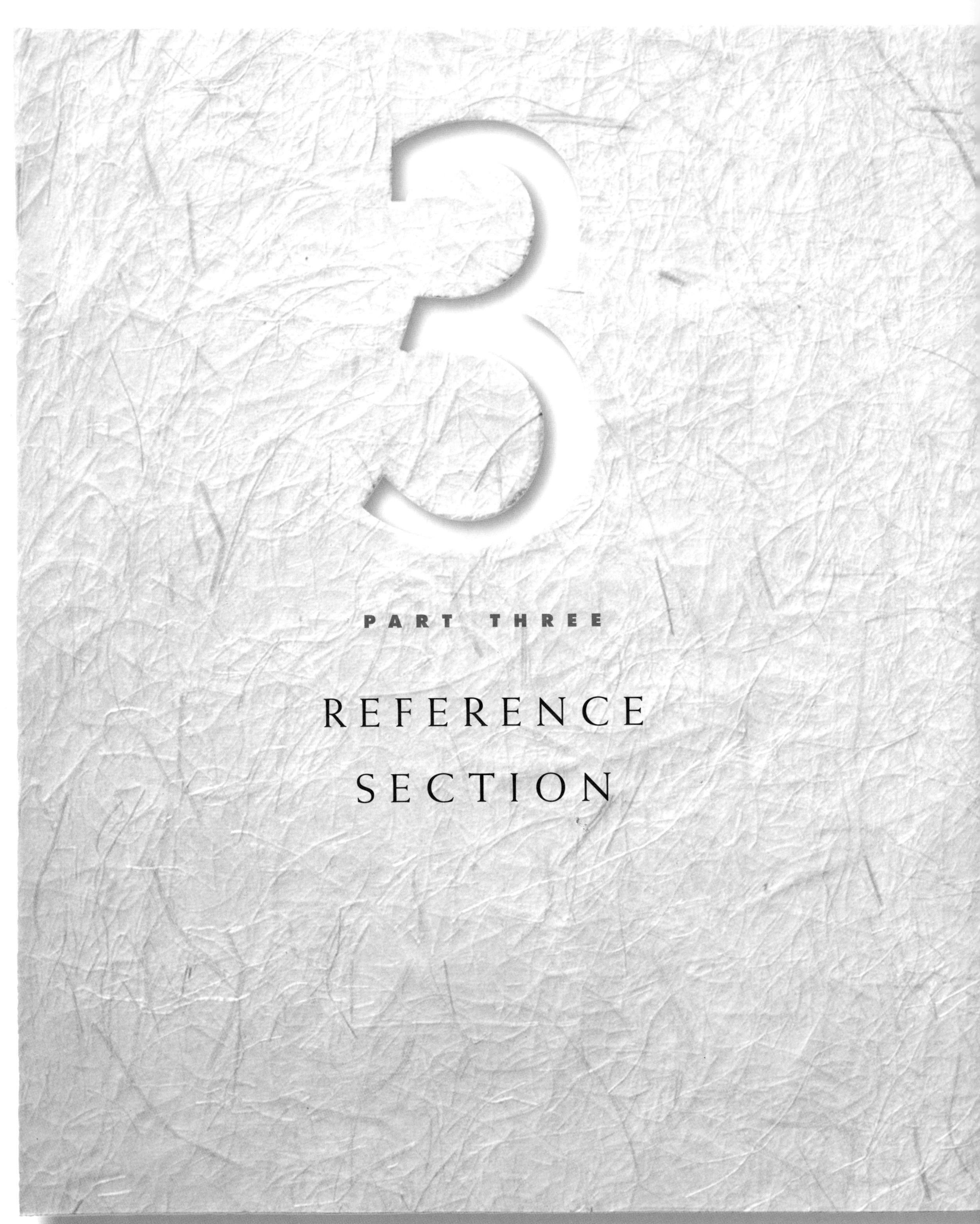

PART THREE

REFERENCE SECTION

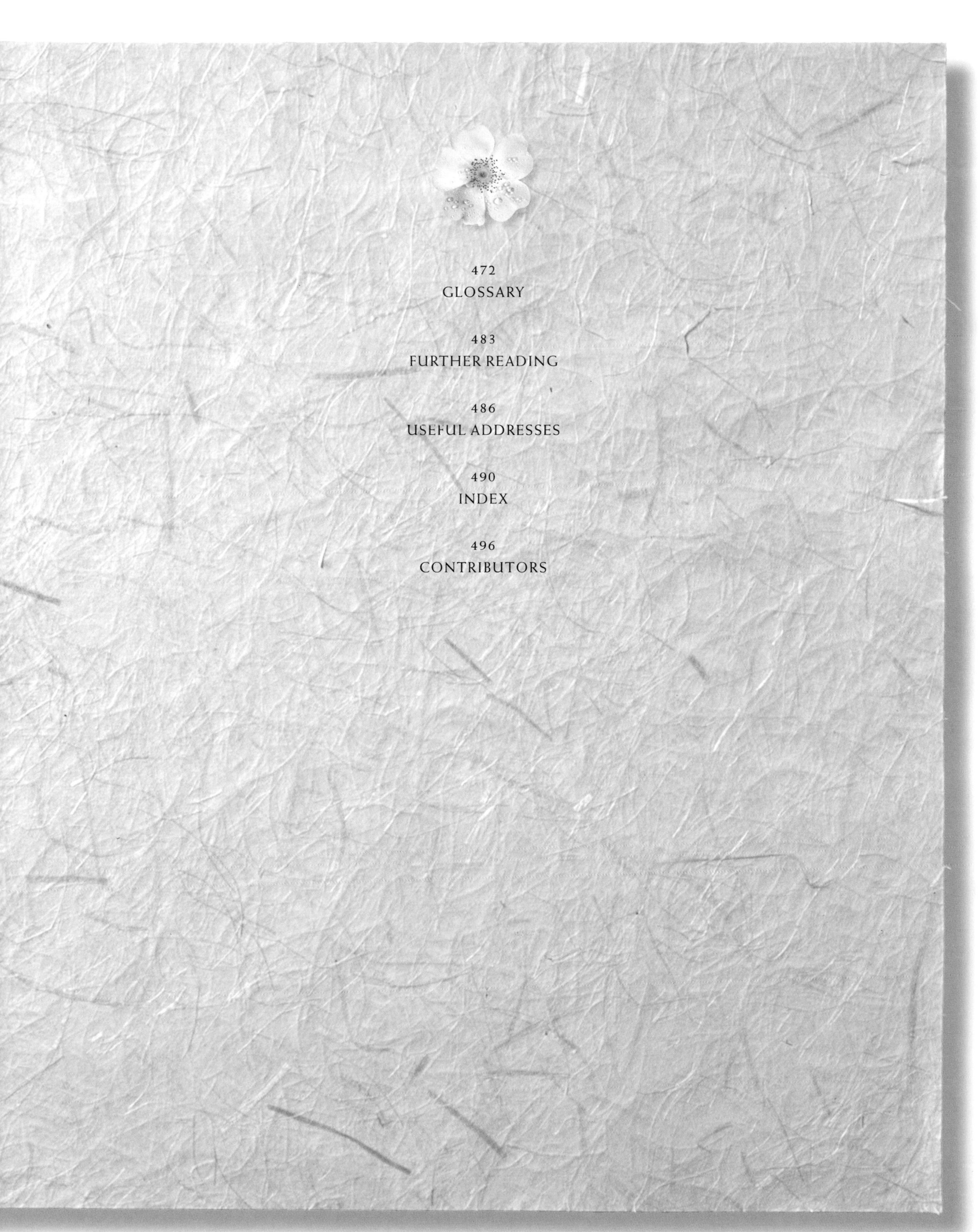

GLOSSARY

abortifacient
an agent that causes the early expulsion of a fetus

abscess
a self-contained pocket of pus that results from a bacterial infection, and causes inflammation of the local area

absolute
a highly concentrated viscous, semi-solid, or solid perfume, usually obtained by alcohol extraction from the concrete

acute
of sudden onset and brief duration

adaptogen
an agent that modulates hormones

adaptogenic
an agent that adapts itself to respond to the body's needs; for example, lavender is adaptogenic and will relax you if you need to be relaxed, or invigorate you if you are tired

adenoids
lymphatic tissue at the back of the nose

adrenal
the adrenal glands are a pair of endocrine glands, each located on the top of one of the kidneys, which secrete hormones that regulate the functions of other organs and systems into the bloodstream

adrenalin
a substance secreted by part of the adrenal gland that increases the heart rate in response to stress

aerophagia
excessive swallowing of air, which may be a response to stress or a consequence of eating too quickly

aggravation
the exacerbation of symptoms that can occur when taking some natural remedies, particularly in the case of chronic ailments

agni
meaning "fire," or the forces which break down substances consumed; in Indian medicine, considered to be metabolism

agoraphobia
fear of open or crowded places

alcohols
a group of chemical compounds with antiseptic, antiviral, and uplifting properties

aldehydes
chemicals that have a sedative and sometimes anti-inflammatory effect

aldosterone
the steroid hormone which helps the body to control water balance

-algia (suffix)
meaning "pain in"; for example, arthralgia, pain in the joints

allergen
a substance that causes an allergic reaction

allergy
an abnormal response by the body to a food or foreign substance

allopathic
Western medicinal treatment, based on treating symptoms rather than the underlying condition

alopecia
hereditary hair loss

alterative
corrects disordered body functions; works according to the needs of the body. Often used in the same way as "adaptogenic"

ama
in Ayurveda, a toxic substance believed to gather in the weak parts of the body and cause disease. Ama occurs when the metabolism is impaired due to an imbalance of agni

amenorrhea
absence of menses (menstrual periods)

analgesic
pain-relieving

anaphrodisiac
reduces sexual desire

anaphylaxis
an extreme allergic reaction to a foreign substance. Subsequent exposure can produce an overwhelming body reaction called anaphylactic shock

anemia
deficiency in either quality or quantity of red corpuscles in the blood

anodyne
pain-killing

anorexia nervosa
psychological problem causing extreme loss of appetite, drastic weight loss, and, sometimes, death

anosmia
loss of the sense of smell. It can be either temporary or permanent

antacid
a remedy or medicine that reduces stomach acidity

anthelmintic
a vermifuge, destroying or expelling intestinal worms

anthraquinone
a powerful laxative which can cause diarrhea and intestinal cramps

antiallergic
an agent that reduces allergic reactions

antiarthritic
an agent that combats arthritis

antibacterial
acts against bacteria; an agent that prevents bacteria forming, e.g. penicillin

antibilious
an agent that helps remove excess bile from the body

antibiotic
an agent that prevents the growth of, or destroys, bacteria

antibody
a chemical produced by the body's immune system to attack what it considers to be an invader, e.g. a bacterium, virus, or allergen

anticarcinogenic
an agent that acts to prevent or treat the development or spread of cancer

anticatarrhal
an agent that helps remove excess catarrh from the body

anticonvulsant
an agent that helps arrest or prevent convulsions

antidepressant
an agent that relieves depression

antidiarrheal
an agent that prevents or treats diarrhea

antidote
the term used to describe other remedies or substances that cancel or nullify the effect of a prescribed remedy

anti-emetic
an agent that reduces the incidence and severity of nausea or vomiting

antifungal
an agent that works to prevent the spread and incidence of fungal conditions

antihistamine
an agent that prevents or treats a histamine reaction (*see Allergy, page 412*)

antihypertensive
an agent that works to lower blood pressure

anti-infective
any agent that works to prevent or halt the spread of infection

anti-inflammatory
reducing inflammation

antimicrobial
acts against infection, particularly bacterial infection

antioxidant
a substance that prevents cell degeneration and decay

antiseborrheic
helps to control the production of sebum from sweat glands

antiseptic
helps to counter infection, by fighting bacteria

antispasmodic
prevents contractions of the muscles, or alleviates spasms and cramp

antiviral
inhibits the spread of viruses

aperitif
a stimulant to the appetite

aphrodisiac
increases or stimulates sexual desire; sexual stimulant, increases vitality and builds organs

aromatherapy
the therapeutic use of essential oils

aromatic
a substance with a strong aroma or smell

arteriosclerosis
hardening of the arteries

articulation
range of movement of the joints

asthma
spasm of the bronchi in the lungs, narrowing the airways

astringent
constricts the blood vessels or membranes in order to reduce irritation, inflammation, and swelling; has a binding and contracting effect, usually on the mucous membrane, to give it a protective coating against irritants or infective organisms; also one of the six tastes in Ayurveda; found in potatoes, beans, and witch hazel

athma
in Indian medicine, the unique, individual spirit which occupies the body and which is transferred to another body after death

atopic
persons with allergies are often called atopic. The common atopies include hay fever; asthma; infantile eczema, which is an itchy skin lesion; contact dermatitis, which is a skin inflammation caused by poison ivy or a variety of chemicals that may contact the skin; and perhaps some food or drug allergies

aura
every person, animal, and plant is said to have a visible aura, or magnetic field. These are said to indicate the state of health, emotions, mind, and spirit

autogenic discharge
sensations or muscle movements that accompany the release of stored tensions

autoimmune disorder
occurs when the body creates antibodies against itself and attacks healthy cells

B

bactericidal
an agent that destroys bacteria (a type of microbe or organism)

balsam
a resinous semi-solid mass or viscous liquid exuded from a plant, which can be either a pathological or a physiological product. A "true" balsam is characterized by its high content of benzoic acid, benzoates, cinnamic acid, or cinnamates

balsamic
a soothing medicine or application having the qualities of a balsam

benign
of a tumor, not cancerous or dangerous

bile
thick, oily fluid excreted by the liver; bile helps the body digest fats

biliousness
disorder of bile production (to excess)

bioflavonoids
also called vitamin P, bioflavonoids are widely found in food plants, where they impart color to flowers, leaves, and stems. There are at least 500 naturally occurring varieties, and they are said to strengthen or preserve the integrity of the veins, among other things

biopsy
removal of fluid or tissue from the body for examination

bitter
a tonic component that stimulates the appetite and promotes the secretion of saliva and gastric juices by exciting the taste buds; one of the six Ayurvedic tastes; found in barks, tannins, and resins

blepharospasm
a twitch or tic in which there is spasmodic closure of one or both eyes

Blood
in Chinese medicine, "Blood" has a specialized meaning

bronchio-dilator
a substance which dilates the bronchi, the tubes of the lungs

bursa
a small fluid-filled sac

C

calmative
a sedative agent

calcul
a kidney stone

Candida
Candida albicans, a fungus affecting the mucous membranes and skin; causes thrush

carbuncle
a bacterial infection of the skin, an interconnected group of boils that have many perforations, through which pus drains

carcinogenic
an agent that can cause cancer; cancer-causing

carcinoma
a cancerous tumor

cardiac
pertaining to the heart

cardioactive
an agent that stimulates heart activity

cardiotonic
having a stimulating effect on the heart

carminative
settles the digestive system and relieves flatulence

cathartic
an agent that purges the body, usually the intestine, and cleanses the system

cautery
burning tissue in the body

centesimal scale (c)
in homeopathy, the scale that measures the potency of remedies in hundredths. One drop of mother tincture is mixed with 99 drops of water or alcohol to make a remedy of 1c potency. This remedy is then diluted with a further 99 drops of water or alcohol to make a remedy of 2c potency. The sequence is repeated: 200c is usually the highest dose. The more the remedy is diluted, the more powerful it becomes

cephalic
remedy for problems relating to the head

cerebrovascular accident (CVA)
another term for stroke

chakras
in Eastern medicine, circles which are thought to be found along the mid-line of the body, in line with the spinal column

channels
invisible pathways in which qi (or chi) travels; also called meridians. They appear in and on the body

chelated
of mineral supplements, means that the mineral is combined with amino acids to make assimilation more efficient

chi (or qi)
the life force of the body, which circulates through its meridians or channels

chlamydia
a sexually transmitted disease caused by parasitic bacteria

cholagogue
an agent that stimulates the secretion and flow of bile into the duodenum

cholesterol
a steroid alcohol found in nervous tissue, red blood cells, animal fat, and bile. Excess can lead to gallstones

chronic
persisting for a long time; a state showing no change or very slow change

cicatrizant
an agent that promotes healing by the formation of scar tissue

coagulate
an agent that acts to clot or thicken the blood

complementary
the term used to describe alternative forms of medical treatment – emphasizing the fact that they support rather than replace orthodox medicine

compress
a lint or pad that is soaked in hot or cold substances and applied to the body for relief of swelling and pain, or to produce localized pressure

concomitant
in homeopathy, a symptom coming at the same time, but not directly related to, the main complaint

concrete
a concentrated, waxy, solid, or semi-solid perfume material prepared from previously live plant matter, usually a hydrocarbon type of solvent

congestion
abnormal accumulation of blood

constitutional
homeopathic term relating to the physical and mental constitution of a person, including hereditary factors and underlying health issues

contraindication
any factor in a patient's condition that indicates that treatment would involve a greater than normal risk and is therefore not recommended

cordial
a stimulant and tonic

corticosteroids
adrenal cortico hormones. There are two classes of corticosteroids. The glucocorticoids such as cortisone primarily affect carbohydrate and protein metabolism. They have limited use in the treatment of many immunologic and allergic diseases, such as arthritis. The mineralocorticoids such as aldosterone principally regulate salt and water balance. Synthetic steroids include anti-inflammatory drugs, oral contraceptives, and a synthetic adrenal steroid used to treat Addison's disease

cortisol
the steroid hormone which helps the body to react to stress

coryza
profuse discharge from the mucous membranes of the nose – "common cold"

counter-irritant
an application to the skin that relieves deep-seated pain, usually applied in the form of heat; see also rubefacient

dan tien
energy centers in the body. In Chinese medicine there are considered to be three: an upper (between the eyebrows); a middle (in the centre of the trunk); and a lower (the lower abdomen). Qi is stored here

decimal scale (x)
in homeopathy, the scale that measures the potency of remedies in tenths. One drop of mother tincture is mixed with nine drops of water or alcohol to make a remedy of 1x potency. This remedy is then diluted with a further nine drops of water or alcohol to make a remedy of 2x potency. The sequence is repeated. The more the remedy is diluted, the more powerful it becomes

decoction
a herbal preparation, where the plant material (usually hard or woody) is boiled in water and reduced to make a concentrated extract

decongestant
an agent for the relief or reduction of congestion, e.g. of the mucous membranes

decongestive
relieves or reduces mucus congestion

deficient
condition in Chinese medicine; any disorder that is caused by the body's inability to maintain balance, through improper function of the zangfu

degenerative
a condition in which there is irreversible and progressive decomposition

demulcent
an agent that protects mucous membranes and allays irritation

depurgative
cleanses the blood

detoxificant/detoxifier
an agent that acts to detoxify, or remove toxins from the body

detoxification
external and internal cleaning of the body; the removal of toxins from the body

dhatus
in Indian medicine, seven essential tissues which make up the body

dialogue
discussion on how habitual ideas and emotions can affect your mind, body, and spirit

diaphoretic
an agent that causes sweating

digestive
an agent that promotes or aids the digestion of food

digoxin
a glycoside isolated from the dried leaves of the foxglove plant. It is prescribed to millions of patients suffering from cardiac problems such as rapid atrial fibrillation or heart failure

dina chariya
a daily program recommended by Ayurveda for healthy living

discharge
an excretion or substance evacuated from the body

diuretic
an agent that aids production of urine, promotes urination, or increases flow, reducing the fluid level of the body

DNA
deoxyribonucleic acid, a chemical which makes up our chromosomes

doshas
the three basic constitutional types in Indian medicine – vátha, pitta, and kapha – which are known as the "tri-doshas"

douche
a substance used internally to cleanse or treat the vagina

drawing
draws poisons out from boils and abscesses etc.

dysfunction
abnormal functioning of a system or organ within the body

dysmenorrhea
severe pains accompanying the menstrual period

dyspepsia
difficulty with digestion associated with pain, flatulence, heartburn, and nausea

dyspnea
labored or difficult breathing

ectomorpe
one of three basic body types, characterized by thinness and weakness

ectopic
a pregnancy that occurs at a site other than inside the uterus, such as in the Fallopian tube, on the ovary, or at sites outside the abdomen, is termed ectopic

edema
a painless swelling caused by fluid retention beneath the skin's surface

EFAs
essential fatty acids

effleurage
slow, rhythmic massage

eight principal patterns
in Chinese medicine, the system of organizing diagnostic information according to the principles of yin, yang, interior, exterior, cold, hot, excess, and deficiency

emetic
an agent that induces vomiting

emmenagogue
an agent that induces or assists menstruation

emollient
an agent that softens and soothes the skin

Empty Heat
Internal Heat in the body resulting from a yin deficiency

endocrine
the endocrine system consists of specialized glands located in different parts of the body These glands secrete chemical substances called hormones, which transfer information from one set of cells to another

endometriosis
a common disease in women of reproductive age. It involves tissues of the endometrium, the inner lining of the uterus. During the menstrual cycle, built-up endometrial tissues normally are shed if pregnancy does not occur. In many women some endometrial cells escape from the womb into the pelvic cavity, where they attach themselves and continue their hormone-stimulated growth cycle. They may also migrate to remote parts of the body

endomorph
one of the three basic body types, characterized by roundness, fatness, and heaviness

endorphins
a group of chemicals manufactured in the brain that influence the body's response to pain

engorgement
congestion of a part of the tissues, or fullness (as in the breasts)

enuresis
bed-wetting

enzyme
complex proteins that are produced by the living cells and catalyze specific biochemical reactions

epidural
epidural anesthesia involves depositing anesthetic into the epidural space of the vertebral canal

epigastric
above the navel

epigastrium
the area above the navel

episiotomy
an incision made in the perineum (the area between the anus and the vagina) to prevent tearing while delivering a baby

esophagitis
inflammation of the lining of the esophagus

essence
the pure energy extracted from food that is transformed into qi by the body. Also the integral part of a plant, its life force, as used in flower remedies, herbalism, and aromatherapy

essential oil
a volatile and aromatic liquid (sometimes semi-solid) which generally constitutes the odorous principles of a plant. It is obtained by a process of expression or distillation from a single botanical form or species. A pure, concentrated essence taken from the plant; said to be its life force

esters
chemical compounds that are fungicidal and sedative

estrogen
a hormone produced by the ovary and necessary for the development of female secondary sexual characteristics

etiology
the science of the cause of illness and disease

excess condition
a condition in which qi, blood, or body fluids are imbalanced, accumulating in parts of the body

expectorant
promotes the removal of mucus from the respiratory system

expectoration
coughing up

external
in Chinese medicine, any factors influencing the body from the outside

exudative
a substance or agent that causes something to exude; for example, a warm compress would cause infection or pus to exude from a boil or wound

fast
abstention from all or most foods for a given period

febrifuge
an agent that combats fever

febrile
feverish

feces
excrement, stools

fever
elevation of body temperature above normal (36.8°C/98.4°F)

five elements
the system in Chinese medicine based on observations of the natural world. Built around the elements of fire, water, wood, metal, and earth

fixative
a material that slows down the rate of evaporation of the more volatile components in the composition of a perfume

fixed oil
the name given to a vegetable oil obtained from plants that, in contradistinction to essential oils, is fatty, dense, and nonvolatile, such as olive or sweet almond oil

flavonoids
antioxidants which act on the immune system

fomentation
a hot compress

four levels
the system of diagnosis in Chinese medicine

friction
small circular movements used in massage

fu
hollow yang organs in the body

fungicidal
an agent that prevents and combats fungal infection

fungicide
attacks fungal infestations

galactagogue
an agent that increases the secretion of milk

gan
sweet, used to assign taste to Chinese herbs

ganglion
swelling within a tendon or joint; also a group of nerves

gas exchange
the exchange of water carbon dioxide in the blood for fresh oxygen; it takes place in the alveoli of the lungs

generals
in homeopathy, symptoms relating to the whole person that can be expressed "I am . . . "; compare particulars

germicidal
destroys germs or micro-organisms such as bacteria

ghee
milk or butter fat, clarified by boiling and used in Indian cooking

giardiasis
an infectious parasite that attacks the gastrointestinal tract

giennial
a plant that completes its life-cycle in two years, without flowering in the first year

gliadin
a protein from wheat and rye cereals

gluten
a protein from wheat and other cereals

gum
"true" gum is little used in perfumery, being virtually odorless. However, the term "gum" is often applied to "resins," especially with relation to turpentines, as in the Australian "gum tree." Strictly speaking, gums are natural or synthetic water-soluble materials, such as gum arabic

gunas
in Indian medicine, characteristics which can be attributed to all matter, organic and inorganic, and to thoughts and ideas

halitosis
bad breath

hallucinogenic
causes visions or delusions

harmonize
to balance, or encourage something, such as the body, to work in harmony, with all systems at optimum level

hematoma
a collection of blood

hemorrhage
loss of blood

hemorrhoids
piles, anal varicose veins

hemostatic
stops the flow of blood; a type of astringent that stops internal bleeding or hemorrhaging

hepatic
relating to the liver; an agent that tones the liver and aids its function

herniate
to rupture, or burst out; a slipped disk herniates

holistic
aiming to treat the individual as an entity, incorporating body, mind, and spirit, from the Greek word holos, meaning whole

homeopathy
medical therapy devised by the 19th-century German doctor Samuel Hahnemann, based on the premise that like cures like; sick people are given minute doses of a remedy that will cause the symptoms of their disease, which helps the body to cure itself

homeostasis
the tendency of the internal environment of the body to remain constant in spite of varying external conditions

hormone
a product of living cells that produces a specific effect on the activity cells remote from its point of origin

humors
the four body fluids (blood, phlegm, choler, and melancholy) which are believed to determine emotional and physical disposition, in Chinese medicine

hybrid
a plant originating by fertilization of one species or subspecies by another

hypercalcemia
calcium deposits in the kidneys

hyperglycemia
a condition characterized by an abnormally high level of glucose (sugar) in the bloodstream

hyperhidrosis
excessive sweating caused by overactive sweat glands

hypermetropia
long-sightedness

hyperparathyroidism
secretion of parathyroid hormone resulting from a tumor, enlargement, or cancer of the thyroid glands

hypertension
raised blood pressure

hypertensive
raises blood pressure

hypnotic
causing sleep

hypoglycemia
a condition characterized by an abnormally low level of glucose (sugar) in the bloodstream

hypotension
low blood pressure, or a fall in blood pressure below the normal range

hypotensive
lowers blood pressure

I

immunodeficiency
a deficiency of immune activity

immuno-stimulant
an agent that stimulates immune activity, and the immune system

immunosuppressive
an agent or condition that suppresses the immune system, and normal or excessive immune activity

incontinence
partial or complete loss of control of urination

infection
multiplication of pathogenic (disease-producing) micro-organisms within the body

inflammation
protective tissue response to injury or destruction of body cells characterized by heat, swelling, redness, and usually pain

infusion
immersion of herbs in boiling water; also the liquid obtained from steeping a herb in hot or cold water

inhalant
a remedy or drug that is breathed in through the nose or mouth

insecticidal
an agent that repels or kills insects

insomnia
inability to sleep

internal
refers to aspects of disharmonies that arise within the body, in Chinese medicine

-itis
(*suffix*) "inflammation of"; for example, arthritis, inflammation of the joints

jin ye
body fluids – jin refers to the lighter fluids, and ye refers to the denser ones

Jing
the essence of all life in the body – the energy that governs our development

jingluo
Chinese term for the channels, or meridians, which run invisibly through the body, carrying the qi, or life force

kapha
the moon force, which is a basic life force or element in Ayurvedic medicine

ketogenic diet
a diet which is high in fat and very low in carbohydrates

ketones
chemical compounds that ease congestion and aid the flow of mucus

ku
bitter; a term used to describe the taste of Chinese herbs

kundalini
an energy which is believed to travel upwards through the chakras, promoting spiritual knowledge

lactagogue
a substance which encourages the production of milk in the breasts

laxative
a substance that provokes evacuation of the bowels

legume
a fruit or vegetable consisting of one carpel, opening on one side, such as a pea. Also called a "pulse"

lesion
a term used to describe an abnormality in or damage to the body

leucocyte
white blood cells responsible for fighting disease

leukorrhea
vaginal discharge

liniment
a warming rub, often made by mixing tinctures with herbal infused oils

lithotrophic
dispels stones

liverishness
a term used to describe inadequate liver function

lymph
a colorless fluid which contains mainly white blood cells, which are collected from the tissues of the body and transported through the lymphatic system

lymphatic
pertaining to the lymphatic system. A lymphatic remedy would encourage the flow of lymph

macerate
soak or pound until soft

mahabbutas
a Sanskrit term for the elements

malas
in Indian medicine, waste products of the body, including feces, urine, and sweat

malignant
cancerous and possibly life-threatening

MAOI
a type of antidepressant drug known as monoamine oxidase inhibitors

mammograph
an X-ray technique used to aid in the diagnosis of breast cancer in women

mantra
a syllable, word, or phrase which may be spoken aloud and repeated as an aid to meditation

marma puncture
in Indian medicine, the technique of inserting a needle into the marma points for certain treatments

marmas
in Indian medicine, energy points in the body where two or more important functions meet

marrow
in Chinese medicine, the substance that makes up the brain and spinal column

materia medica
a branch of science dealing with the origins and properties of remedies; a complete description of remedies suggested in therapies such as homeopathy and herbalism

medicated oil
2produced by steeping herbs or flowers for one or more months, then straining

meditation
exercising the mind in contemplation

meninges
the membranes that cover the brain and spinal cord

menopause
the normal cessation of menstruation, a life change for women

menorrhagia
an excess loss of blood occurring during menstruation

mentals
in homeopathy, symptoms relating to the mental state, mood, and ideas

meridians
channels that run through the body, beneath the skin, in which the life force, or qi, is carried. There are 14 main meridians running to and from the hands and feet to the body and head

mesomorph
one of the three basic body types, characterized by a muscular and prominent bone structure

metabolism
the complex process that is the fundamental chemical expression of life itself, and the means by which food is converted to energy to maintain the body

metrorrhagia
bleeding that occurs in the middle of the menstrual cycle

microbe
a minute living organism, especially pathogenic bacteria, viruses, etc.

micronutrients
vitamins, minerals, and other health-giving components of our food, such as amino acids, fiber, enzymes, and lipids

micturation
involuntary leakage of urine during coughing, laughing, or muscular effort

modality
in homeopathy, the factor that makes symptoms better or worse

mother tincture
in homeopathy or flower remedies, the source remedy, which is diluted to make the therapeutic dosages prescribed by practitioners

moxa
dried mugwort, which is burned on the end of needles or rolled into a stick, and then heated in moxabustion. It is said to warm the qi in the body in order to increase its flow

moxabustion
see moxa

moxides
a group of chemical compounds with expectorant properties

mucilage
a substance containing gelatinous constituents that are demulcent

mucilaginous
a substance that encourages the body to create more mucus

mucolytic
a substance that thins mucus

mucous membranes
surface linings of the body, which secrete mucus

musculoskeletal
anything pertaining to the muscles and bones (skeletal system) of the body

myopia
short-sightedness

N

narcotic
an agent that induces sleep; intoxicating or poisonous in large doses

nasya
in Ayurveda, inhalation of oils

naturopathy
treatment based on using natural agents and forces to bring about a cure. The naturopath tends to rely on natural products such as herbs and vitamins, rather than on synthetic drugs and surgery, and may also employ manipulation (such as osteopathy) and electrical treatments

nervine
strengthening and toning to the nerves and nervous system

noradrenaline
a hormone secreted by the adrenal gland

nosode
in homeopathy, a remedy made from a diseased source; for example, tuberculinum, made from tissue infected with tuberculosis

nutritive
a substance that promotes nutrition

nystagmus
abnormal, jerky movements of the eyes

oja
in Indian medicine, the ultimate vital energy that runs through the system

oleo gum resin
a natural exudation from trees and plants that consists mainly of essential oil, gum, and resin

oleoresin
a natural resinous exudation from plants, or an aromatic liquid preparation extracted from botanical matter using solvents. It consists almost entirely of a mixture of essential oil and resin

onycholysis
detachment of the nail from its bed

oophorectomy
removal of the ovaries

opacification
becoming opaque

orchitis
inflammation of the testes

orthodox
a term used to describe conventional medicine

overbreathing
breathing too quickly and too shallowly

palindromic
something which can be read the same when taken in reverse order

palpation
examination with the hands

panacea
a cure-all

panchakarma
in Ayurveda, internal cleansing, which consists of five forms of therapy, including vomiting, purging, two types of enema, and nasal inhalation. It is said to prevent disease and to rebalance vitality

parainfluenza
a type of cold virus

parasiticide
prevents and destroys parasites; a parasite killer

paronychia
an infection of the soft tissue around the nail, usually as a result of repeated minor injury, causing pain, swelling and inflammation. Pus may sometimes appear at the edge of the nail

particulars
in homeopathy, symptoms relating to a part of the person that can be expressed "My…"; compare generals

parturient
encouraging the onset of labor

pasteurized
heat treated to destroy harmful microorganisms

pathogenic
referring to any disease-causing agent

peculiars
in homeopathy, strange, rare, and peculiar symptoms which relate to the individual and are not common in illness

peptic
a term applied to gastric secretions and areas affected by them

percussion
vigorous drumming massage

pericarditis
inflammation of the pericardium of the heart

perineal
pertaining to the perineum, the area between the anus and the genital organs

periodontitis
loosening of a tooth, often caused by gingivitis

peristalsis
rhythmic movement of the gut to push food along the intestinal tract

pessary
a treatment that is inserted into the vagina or anus

petrissage
kneading massage movement

pharmacopeia
an official publication of drugs in common use in a given country

phenols
a group of chemical compounds with bactericidal and stimulating properties; they can be irritants

Phlegm
in Chinese medicine a disharmony of the body fluids produces either external (or visible) phlegm or internal (or invisible) phlegm; thick, shiny mucus produced in the respiratory passage

photosensitivity
a sensitivity to light

phototoxic
a substance that becomes poisonous on exposure to light

phthalides
chemicals which have a sedative effect and can ease insomnia

phytotherapy
the treatment of disease by plants; herbal medicine

pitta
in Ayurvedic medicine, the sun force, or one of the three basic life forces or elements controlling all physical and mental processes

plasma
the clear, yellowish fluid part of blood or lymph in which cells are suspended

polyphenols
antioxidants which have beneficial effects on the circulatory system

post-partum
following delivery of a baby; after pregnancy

potencized
diluted to homeopathic prescription

potency
the dilution of a homeopathic remedy; the higher the number, the higher the strength, and the greater the dilution

potentiate
in homeopathy, to shake a remedy to increase its potency

poultice
the therapeutic application of a soft moist mass (such as fresh herbs) to the skin to encourage local circulation and to relieve pain

prakruti
in Indian medicine, a person's individual constitution, determined by their "dosha" type

prana
the vital energy that runs through our bodies; in Indian medicine, also known as our life force

pranayama
the breathing exercises associated with yoga

priapism
prolonged penile erection, usually without sexually desire

progesterone
a female sex hormone that prepares the uterus for the fertilized ovum and maintains pregnancy

prolapse
the sinking or falling-down of an organ – usually refers to the vagina or uterus

prophylactic
preventive of disease or infection

prostaglandins
hormone-like substances that occur in tissues and organs of the human body. They affect several body systems, including the central nervous, cardiovascular, gastrointestinal, urinary, and endocrine systems

prostatitis
inflammation of the prostate gland

proving
the process used in homeopathy for testing a remedy; it can occur when the wrong remedy is prescribed and taken over a period of time, and the symptoms of the condition it is aimed at manifest themselves

psychogenic
symptoms or conditions of mental rather than physical origin

psychosomatic illness
the manifestation of physical symptoms resulting from a mental state

purgative
an agent stimulating evacuation of the bowels

purines
nitrogenous compounds in nucleic acids found in many foods including caffeine, anchovies, sardines, fish roe, sweetbreads and other organ meats. Some people who have difficulty metabolizing purines may be prone to gout

purulent
containing pus

purvakarma
in Ayurveda, a cleansing process involving oil and steam bath therapy

pustular
referring to elevated area of skin containing pus

pyorrhea
any condition characterized by discharge of pus

qi (chi)
the essential energy of the universe which is fundamental to all elements of life. It runs through the whole body in channels or meridians

Qi Ni
rebellious qi, which moves in the wrong direction

Qi Xian
sinking qi, which is too deficient to perform its holding function

Qi Zhi
stagnant qi that is sluggish and not moving efficiently

rajasic
in Ayurveda, energy-producing

rasayana
the branch of Ayurveda which involves rejuvenation

RDA
recommended daily allowance

RDI
recommended daily intake

rectification
the process of redistillation applied to essential oils to rid them of certain constituents

referred pain
pain that is felt in a different part of the body from the area that is actually affected

regulator
an agent that helps balance and regulates the functions of the body

rejuvenative
to invigorate, bring back to life or to the optimum level of functioning; to give new youth or restore vitality

relaxant
a substance that promotes relaxation (either muscular or psychological)

remedy picture
in homeopathy, the collection of symptoms that characterize a remedy

remission
a period in which the symptoms of a disease abate or lessen

Ren
the Chinese meridian that runs down the front of the body, from the lower lip to behind the genitalia

resin
a natural or prepared product, either solid or semi-solid in nature. Natural resins are exudations from trees, such as mastic; prepared resins are oleoresins from which essential oil has been removed

resolvent
an agent that disperses swelling or effects absorption of a new growth

restorative
an agent that helps strengthen and revive the body systems; strengthens and promotes well-being after illness

rhinitis
inflammation (often chronic) of the mucous membranes lining the nasal passage

rhizome
an underground plant stem lasting more than one season

Rishis
wise and holy men of ancient India who meditated and acquired the knowledge that was codified as Ayurveda

RNA
ribonucleic acid, or RNA, is needed in all organisms in order for protein synthesis to occur. It is also the genetic material of some viruses, which are referred to as RNA viruses

rubefacient
a mild irritant which causes redness of the skin

salpingitis
infection of the Fallopian tubes

salty
one of the six Ayurvedic tastes; found in rock salt, seaweed, sea salt, and vegetables

salve
a mixture of beeswax with vegetable oil used to preserve herbs and spices

samagni
in Indian medicine, a balanced appetite, when digestion, absorption, and metabolism function efficiently

san jiao
the triple warmer/heat/burner which is a process organ in the Chinese zangfu system

Sanskrit
ancient Indian language, sacred to Hinduism. Ayurveda was written in Sanskrit

saponins
chemicals which may affect red blood cells

sclerosis
hardening of tissue due to inflammation

seborrheic
involving the sebaceous glands, which secrete sebum into the hair follicles and on to most of the body surface

sebum
an oily, lubricating and protective substance

sedative
an agent that reduces functional activity; calming

self-limiting
a condition that lasts a set length of time and usually clears of its own accord

septic
putrefying due to the presence of pathogenic (disease-producing) bacteria

serotonin
a neurotransmitter in the brain which regulates and induces sleep, and is also said to reduce sensitivity to pain

shad rasa
the six basic food tastes identified by Ayurveda – sweet, acidic, salty, pungent, bitter, and astringent

shen
in Chinese medicine, an important aspect of mind or spirit; the spirit of the person

shiatsu
a type of massage that works on pressure points of the body

shock
sudden and disturbing mental or physical impression; also a state of collapse characterized by pale, cold, sweaty skin, rapid, weak, thready pulse, faintness, dizziness, and nausea

sialogogue
an agent that stimulates the secretion of saliva

six stage patterns
a Chinese diagnostic system

soft tissues
tissues of the body, including muscles, tendons, ligaments, and organs

soporific
an agent that induces sleep; sleep-inducing

sour
one of the six Ayurvedic tastes; found in fats, amino acids, fermented products, fruits, and vegetables

spasm
sudden, violent, involuntary muscular contraction

specific
remedy effective for a particular ailment

spermatorrhea
leaking of sperm

spermicidal
an agent or substance which acts to kill sperm

splenomegaly
abnormal enlargement of the spleen

spondylosis
progressive disease of the spine

sputum
spit

stagnant
when the flow of chi, or qi, is blocked in the meridians

STD
sexually transmitted disease

steroids
fat-soluble organic compounds that occur naturally throughout the plant and animal kingdoms and play many important functional roles

stimulant
increases activity in specific organs or systems of the body, warms and increases energy

stomachic
an agent that stimulates the functioning of the stomach

stroma
connective tissue that forms the foundation of the breast

sty
an infection of the follicle of an eyelash or of a sebaceous gland of an eyelid

styptic
an astringent agent that stops or reduces external bleeding

suan
sour; a description of taste for Chinese herbs

subclinical symptoms
symptoms which are not gross enough to be considered precursors to or evidence of clinically diagnosed disease

subfertility
below-normal fertility

succussion
the shaking method used in preparing homeopathic remedies

sweet
one of the six Ayurvedic tastes, found in sugar, carbohydrates, and dairy products

symptom picture
homeopathic term for the overall pattern of symptoms characterizing each individual patient

symptomatology
the study and interpretation of symptoms

symptoms
perceived changes in, or impaired function of, body or mind indicating the presence of disease or injury

synovial
referring to the fluid that bathes the joints

synthesization
to become synthesized, or amalgamated

T

tachycardia
an unduly rapid heartbeat

TCM
Traditional Chinese Medicine

tenesmus
a spasm of the rectum where one feels the need to defecate without being able to

terpenes
chemical constituents with anti-inflammatory and bactericidal properties

tincture
a herbal remedy prepared in an alcohol base

tisane
a type of herbal infusion, usually drunk as a tea

tissue salt
an inorganic compound essential to the growth and function of the body's cells

tonic
restores tone to the systems, balances, nourishes, and promotes well-being; strengthens and enlivens the whole or specific parts of the body

tonification
a process in Chinese medicine that involves strengthening and supporting the Blood and qi

tonify
to tone or balance; in Chinese medicine, to strengthen and support

topical
local application of cream, ointment, tincture, or other medicine

topical irritant
a substance that irritates the skin

torticollis
wry neck

toxin
a substance that is poisonous to the body

trauma
a physical injury or wound; also an unpleasant and disturbing experience causing psychological upset

trigeminal nerve
a nerve that divides into three and supplies the mandibular (jaw), maxillary (cheek), ophthalmic (eye), and forehead areas

tuber
a swollen part of an underground plant stem of one year's duration, capable of new growth

type
a term used by Bach and other flower remedy therapists to describe a person's general personality and approach to life. Also used by homeopaths to refer to a constitutional picture which relates to a particular remedy

ulcer
slow-healing sore occurring internally or externally

ureteric
referring to the ureter, the tube that carries urine from the kidney to the bladder

urethral
referring to the urethra, the canal that carries urine from the bladder out of the body

uterine tonic
a substance that has a toning effect on the whole reproductive system, in particular the uterus

váthá
the wind force in Ayurvedic medicine – one of the three basic life forces or elements that must be in balance for physical and mental processes to be balanced

vaginitis
inflammation or infection of the vagina

vasoconstrictor
an agent that causes narrowing of the blood vessels

vasodilator
an agent that dilates the blood vessels and so improves circulation

Vedic
relating to the Vedas, the ancient, sacred literature of Hinduism

vermifuge
an anthelmintic remedy that kills worms and intestinal parasites

verruca
a plantar wart

vesicant
causing blistering to the skin; a counter-irritant

vibrational medicine
any medicine which treats the body on a vibrational or "energy" level, such as homeopathy and flower essence therapy, based on the theory that we are all dense bodies of energy, and by taking substances that adjust that energy, or the rate at which our energy fields vibrate, we can effect a cure

virulent
extremely infective, or with a violent effect

volatile
unstable, evaporates easily, as in "volatile oil"; see essential oil

vulnerary
an agent that helps heal wounds and sores by external application; assists in the healing of wounds by protecting against infection and stimulating cell growth

vulval
relating to the vulva

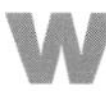

warming
any agent or substance which warms the body, usually by increasing circulation or the flow of qi

Wei Qi
defensive qi, which protects the body from invasion by external pathogenic factors. It flows just beneath the skin

xian
salty; a description of taste for Chinese herbs

xin
acrid; a description of taste for Chinese herbs

xu
deficiency; a common disharmony in Chinese medicine

yang
one aspect of the complementary aspects in Chinese philosophy; reflects the active, moving, and warmer aspects

yin
one aspect of the complementary aspects in Chinese philosophy; reflects the passive, still, reflective aspects

yin/yang
Chinese philosophy that explains the interdependence of all elements of nature. These contrasting aspects of the body and mind must be balanced before health and well-being can be achieved. Yin is the female force, and yang is the male

Ying Qi
nutritive aspects of qi that nourish the body

Yuan Qi
original or source qi; this aspect of qi is passed on from our parents

Zanfu Zhi Qi
qi of the organs; the qi that nourishes the organs of the body

zangfu
the complete yin and yang organs of the body; in Chinese medicine, the term for internal organs (different from those of Western medical science)

Zheng Qi
normal or upright qi; qi that circulates through the channels and the organs of the body

Zong Qi
gathering qi; the qi that gathers in the chest area through the coming together of Gu Qi and Kong Qi

FURTHER READING

Ayurveda

Ayurveda • Scott Gerson
ELEMENT BOOKS, 1993

The Complete Illustrated Guide to Ayurveda • Gopi Warrier and Dr. Deepika Gunawant
ELEMENT BOOKS, 1997

The Handbook of Ayurveda • Dr. Shantha Godagama
KYLE CATHIE, 1997

Quantum Healing • Dr. Deepak Chopra
BANTAM BOOKS, 1989

Return of the Rishi • Dr. Deepak Chopra
HOUGHTON MIFFLIN CO., 1988

The Seven Pillars of Ancient Wisdom • Dr. Douglas Baker
DOUGLAS BAKER PUBLISHING, 1982

Chinese Herbalism

Chinese Herbal Medicine • Richard Craze and Stephen Tang
PIATKUS, 1995

Chinese Herbal Medicine, Ancient Art and Modern Science • Richard Hyatt
WILDWOOD HOUSE LIMITED, 1978

Chinese Herbal Patent Remedies: A Practical Guide • Jake Fratkin
INSTITUTE FOR TRADITIONAL MEDICINE, 1986

In a Nutshell: Chinese Herbalism • Eve Rogans
ELEMENT BOOKS, 1997

Chinese Medicine • Tom Williams
ELEMENT BOOKS, 1995

The Chinese Way to Health • Dr. Stephen Gascoigne
HODDER HEADLINE, 1997

The Complete Family Guide to Chinese Medicine • Tom Williams
ELEMENT BOOKS, 1997

The Web That Has No Weaver • Ted J. Kaptchuk
CONGDON & WEED, 1983

Traditional Home and Folk Remedies

In a Nutshell: Aromatherapy • Sheila Lavery
ELEMENT BOOKS, 1997

The Complete Family Guide to Natural Home Remedies • Karen Sullivan
ELEMENT BOOKS, 1996

The Encyclopedia of Herbs and Herbalism • Malcolm Stuart
ORBIS PUBLISHING, 1979

The Golden Age of Herbs and Herbalists • Rosetta E. Clarkson
DOVER PUBLICATIONS, 1972

Healing Nutrients • Patrick Quillen
PENGUIN, 1989

Herbal Medicine • Anne McIntyre
OPTIMA, 1987

The Holistic Herbal • David Hoffman
FINDHORN, 1983

In a Nutshell: Natural Home Remedies • Karen Hurrell
ELEMENT BOOKS, 1996

Neal's Yard Natural Remedies • Susan Curtis, Romy Frasher, and Irene Kohler
ARKANA, 1988

The Power of Plants • Brendan Lehane
JOHN MURRAY, 1977

Traditional Home and Herbal Remedies • Jan De Vries
MAINSTREAM PUBLISHING, 1986

The Doctors Book of Home Remedies • The Editors of *Prevention* Magazine Health Books
RODALE BOOKS, 1990

The Doctors Book of Home Remedies for Children • The Editors of *Prevention* Magazine Health Books
RODALE BOOKS, 1994

The Doctors Book of Home Remedies for Women • The Editors of *Prevention* Magazine Health Books
RODALE BOOKS, 1997

Herbalism

The Complete Illustrated Holistic Herbal • David Hoffman
ELEMENT BOOKS, 1996

The New Holistic Herbal • David Hoffman
ELEMENT BOOKS, 1983

The Complete New Herbal • edited by Richard Mabey
PENGUIN BOOKS, 1991

The Family Medical Herbal • Kitty Campion
DORLING KINDERSLEY, 1988

The Herb Society's Complete Medicinal Herbal • Penelope Ody
DORLING KINDERSLEY, 1993

The Herbal for Mother and Child, • Anne McIntyre
ELEMENT BOOKS, 1992

Herbal Medicine: The Use of Herbs for Health and Healing • Vicki Pitman
ELEMENT BOOKS, 1994

Herbal Remedies: A Practical Beginner's Guide to Making Effective Remedies in the Kitchen • Christopher Hedley and Non Shaw
PARAGON, 1996

In a Nutshell: Herbalism • Non Shaw
ELEMENT BOOKS, 1998

Herbs for Common Ailments, • Anne McIntyre
GAIA BOOKS, 1992

The Home Herbal • Barbara Griggs
PAN BOOKS, 1995

Natural Medicine for Women • Julian and Susan Scott
GAIA BOOKS, 1991

Aromatherapy

The Complete Illustrated Guide to Aromatherapy • Julia Lawless
ELEMENT BOOKS, 1997

Aromatherapy • Christine Wildwood
ELEMENT BOOKS, 1991

Aromatherapy: An A–Z • Patricia Davis
C. W. DANIEL, 1988

Aromatherapy Blends and Remedies, • Franzesca Watson
THORSONS, 1996

The Aromatherapy Book • Jeanne Rose
NORTH ATLANTIC BOOKS, 1994

Aromatherapy for Pregnancy and Childbirth • Margaret Fawcett
ELEMENT BOOKS, 1993

In a Nutshell: Aromatherapy • Sheila Lavery
ELEMENT BOOKS, 1997

Aromatherapy: Massage with Essential Oils • Christine Wildwood
ELEMENT BOOKS, 1991

The Illustrated Encyclopedia of Essential Oils • Julia Lawless
ELEMENT BOOKS, 1992

The Fragrant Mind • Valerie Anne Worwood
DOUBLEDAY, 1996

The Fragrant Pharmacy • Valerie Anne Worwood
BANTAM BOOKS, 1995

Homeopathy

The Challenge of Homeopathy • Margery Blackie
UNWIN HYMAN, 1981

The Complete Family Guide to Homeopathy • Dr. Christopher Hammond
ELEMENT BOOKS, 1996

The Complete Homeopathy Handbook • Miranda Castro
PAN BOOKS, 1990

Emotional Healing with Homeopathy: A Self-help Manual • Peter Chappell
ELEMENT BOOKS, 1994

The Family Guide to Homeopathy • Andrew Lockie
HAMISH HAMILTON, 1990

Homeopathic Drug Pictures • Margaret Tyler
HEALTH SCIENCE PRESS, 1970

Homeopathy for Mother and Baby • Miranda Castro
PAN BOOKS, 1995

In a Nutshell: Homeopathy • Cassandra Marks
ELEMENT, 1997

Homeopathy: Medicine of the New Man • George Vithoulkas
THORSONS, 1985

The New Concise Guide to Homeopathy • Nigel and Susan Garion-Hutchings
ELEMENT BOOKS, 1993

The Woman's Guide to Homeopathy • Andrew Lockie and Nicola Geddes
HAMISH HAMILTON, 1992

Homeopathy for Children
• Henrietta Wells
ELEMENT BOOKS, 1993

Flower Remedies

In a Nutshell: Bach Flower Remedies
• Non Shaw
ELEMENT BOOKS, 1998

The Bach Flower Remedies: Illustrations and Preparations
• Victor Bullen and Nora Weeks
C. W. DANIEL, 1964

The Collected Writings of Edward Bach
• edited by Julian Barnard
FLOWER REMEDY PROGRAM, 1987

Flower Remedies: Natural Healing with Flower Essences • Christine Wildwood
ELEMENT BOOKS, 1991

A Guide to Bach Flower Remedies
• Julian Barnard
C. W. DANIEL, 1987

Heal Thyself • Dr. Edward Bach
C. W. DANIEL, 1931

The Original Writings of Edward Bach
• edited by Judy Howard and John Ramsell
C. W. DANIEL, 1990

The Twelve Healers and Other Remedies
• Dr. Edward Bach
C. W. DANIEL, 1936

Vitamins and Minerals

The Amino Revolution
• Robert Erdmann and Meirion Jones
CENTURY, 1987

The Complete Book of Minerals for Health • J. I. Rodale
RODALE BOOKS, 1976

The Complete Home Guide to All the Vitamins • Ruth Adams
LARCHMONT BOOKS, 1972

Doctor's Book of Vitamin Therapy: Megavitamins for Health
• Harold Rosenberg and A. N. Feldzaman
PUTNAM'S, 1974

The Doctors' Vitamin and Mineral Encyclopedia
• Sheldon Saul Hendler, M.D., Ph.D.
SIMON & SCHUSTER, 1995

Food and Health
• Elizabeth Morse, John Rivers, and Anne Heughan
BARRIE & JENKINS, 1990

Food: Your Miracle Medicine
• Jean Carper
SIMON & SCHUSTER, 1993

Nutritional Medicine
• Stephen Davis and Alan Stewart
PAN BOOKS, 1987

Raw Energy
• Leslie and Susannah Kenton
ARROW BOOKS, 1991

Superfoods • Michael Van Straten and Barbara Griggs
DORLING KINDERSLEY, 1992

Thorsons Complete Guide to Vitamins and Minerals • Leonard Mervyn
THORSONS, 1995

The Vitamin Bible • Earl Mindell
ARROW, 1993

Health Essentials: Vitamin Guide
• Hasnain Walji
ELEMENT BOOKS, 1992

In a Nutshell: Vitamins and Minerals
• Karen Sullivan
ELEMENT BOOKS, 1997

Which Vitamins Do You Need?
• Martin Ebon
BANTAM BOOKS, 1974

The Zinc Solution
• Derek Bryce-Smith and Liz Hodgkinson
ARROW BOOKS, 1987

USEFUL ADDRESSES

Ayurveda

AFRICA

Maharishi Ayurveda Health Centre
P.O. Box 5155
Halfway House
1685 South Africa

South African Ayurvedic Medicine
Association
85 Harvey Road
Morningside
Durban
4001 South Africa

AUSTRALASIA

Maharishi Ayurveda Health Centres
P.O. Box 81
Bundoora, Victoria 3083
Australia

EUROPE

Ayurvedic Company of Great Britain
50 Penywern Road
London SW5 9XS
U.K.

Ayurvedic Living
P.O. Box 188
Exeter EX4 5AB
U.K.

Ayurvedic Medical Association U.K.
The Hale Clinic
7 Park Crescent
London W1N 3HE
U.K.

Eastern Clinic
1079 Garrat Lane
Tooting, London SW17 0LN
U.K.

NORTH AMERICA

The Ayurveda Institute
P.O. Box 282
Fairfield, Iowa 52556
U.S.A.

The Ayurveda Institute
11311 Menaul N.E.,Suite A
Albuquerque, New Mexico 87112
U.S.A.

Mapi, Inc.
Garden of the Gods Business Park
1115 Elkton Drive, Suite 401
Colorado Springs, Colorado 80907
U.S.A.

Chinese Herbalism

AFRICA

The Herb Society of South Africa
P.O. Box 37721
Overport
South Africa

Western Cape Su Jok Acupuncture Institute
3 Periwinkle Close
Kommetjie
7975 South Africa

AUSTRALASIA

Australian College of Alternative Medicine
11 Howard Avenue
Mount Waverley, Victoria 3149
Australia

Australian College of Oriental Medicine
24 Price Road
Lalorama, Victoria 3766
Australia

Chinese and Herbal Centre
1st Floor, 2392–2394 Sussex Street
Sydney, New South Wales 2000
Australia

Holistic Health Centre
C.P.O. Box 2273
Auckland
New Zealand

EUROPE

British Acupuncture Council (BAC)
Park House, 206–208 Latimer Road
London W10 6RE
U.K.

British Herbal Medicine Association
P.O. Box 304
Bournemouth BH7 6JZ
U.K.

London School of Acupuncture and Traditional Chinese Medicine
60 Bunhill Row
London EC1Y 8QD
U.K.

Register of Chinese Herbal Medicine
21 Warbreck Road
London W10 8NS
U.K.

Register of Chinese Herbal Medicine (RCHM)
P.O. Box 400
Wembley
Middlesex HA9 9NZ
U.K.

NORTH AMERICA

American Association of Acupuncture and Oriental Medicine
1424 16th Street N.W., Suite 501
Washington, DC 20036
U.S.A.

American Herb Association
P.O. Box 1673
Nevada City, California 95959
U.S.A.

American Holistic Nurses Association
P.O. Box 2130
2133 E Lakin Drive, Suite 2
Flagstaff
Arizona 86003–2130
U.S.A.

American Holistic Medical Association
6728 Old McLean Village Drive
McLean, Virginia 22101
U.S.A.

Acupuncture Foundation of Canada
7321 Victoria Park Avenue, Unit 18
Markham, Ontario
Canada L3R 2ZB

Canadian Holistic Medical Association
42 Redpath Avenue
Toronto, Ontario
Canada M4S 2J6

Ontario Herbalists Association
1565 Carling Avenue, Suite 400
Ottawa, Ontario
Canada K1Z 8R1

Herbalism

AFRICA

South African Naturopaths and Herbalists Association
P.O. Box 18663
Wynberg
7824 South Africa

AUSTRALASIA

National Herbalists Association of Australia
Suite 305, BST House
3 Smail Street
Broadway, New South Wales 2007
Australia

EUROPE

The General Council and Register of Consultant Herbalists
18 Sussex Square
Brighton
East Sussex BN2 5AA
U.K.

The Herb Society
77 Great Peter Street
London SW1
U.K.

National Institute of Medical Herbalists
56 Longbrooke Street
Exeter EX4 8HA
U.K.

School of Herbal Medicine/Phytotherapy
Bucksteep Manor
Bodle Street Green
Near Hailsham
Sussex BN27 4RJ
U.K.

NORTH AMERICA

American Herbalists Guild
P.O. Box 1683
Sequel, California 95073
U.S.A.

Canadian Natural Health Association
439 Wellington Street
Toronto, Ontario
Canada M5V 2H7

Aromatherapy

AFRICA

Association of Aromatherapists South Africa
P.O. Box 23924
Claremont
7735 South Africa

EUROPE

Aromatherapy Organisations Council
3 Latymer Close
Braybrooke
Market Harborough
Leicester LE16 8LN
U.K.

International Federation of Aromatherapists
Stamford House
2–4 Chiswick High Road
London W4 1TH
U.K.

International Society of Professional Aromatherapists
Hinckley and District
Hospital and Health Centre
The Annexe
Mount Road
Hinckley
Leicestershire LE10 1AG
U.K.

NORTH AMERICA

The Aromatherapy Institute and Research
P.O. Box 1222
Fair Oaks, California 95628
U.S.A.

American Alliance of Aroma Therapy
P.O. Box 750428
Petaluma, California 94975–0428
U.S.A.

American Aromatherapy Association
P.O. Box 3679
South Pasadena, California 91031
U.S.A.

Nature's Apothecary
6350 Gunpark Drive 500
Boulder, Colorado 80301
U.S.A.

National Association of Holistic Aromatherapy
P.O. Box 17622
Boulder, Colorado 80308–0622
U.S.A.

The Pacific Institute of Aromatherapy
P.O. Box 6842
San Raphael, California 94903
U.S.A.

Homeopathy

AUSTRALASIA

Australian Federation of Homeopaths
238 Ballarat Road
Footscray, Victoria 3011
Australia

Australian Institute of Homeopathy
7 Hampden Road
Artermon
Sydney, New South Wales 2064
Australia

Institute of Classical Homeopathy
24 West Haven Drive
Tawa
Wellington
New Zealand

New Zealand Homeopathic Society
BOX 2929
Auckland
New Zealand

EUROPE

The British Homeopathic Association
27A Devonshire Street
London WC1N 1RJ
U.K.

The Faculty of Homeopathy
The Royal London Homeopathic Hospital
Great Ormond Street
London WC1N 3HR
U.K.

The Hahnemann Society
Humane Education Centre
Avenue Lodge
Bounds Green Road
London N22 4EU
U.K.

Homeopathic Development Foundation
19A Cavendish Square
London W1M 9AD
U.K.

Society of Homeopaths
2 Artizan Road
Northampton NN1 4HU
U.K.

NORTH AMERICA

American Foundation for Homeopathy
1508 Glencoe Street, Suite 44
Denver, Colorado 80220–1338
U.S.A.

Homeopathic Educational Services
2124 Kitteridge Street
Berkeley, California 94704
U.S.A.

International Foundation for Homeopathy
2366 East Lake Avenue, East Suite 301
Seattle, Washington
U.S.A.

National Center for Homeopathy
801 North Fairfax Street
Alexandria, Virginia 22314
U.S.A.

Canadian Society of Homeopathy
87 Meadowlands Drive West
Nepean, Ontario
Canada K2G 2R9

Flower Essences

AUSTRALASIA

Martin and Pleasance Wholesale Pty. Ltd.
P.O. Box 4
Collingwood
Victoria, New South Wales 3066
Australia

EUROPE

Bach Flower Remedies
The Bach Centre
Mount Vernon
Sotwell
Wallingford
Oxfordshire OX10 9PZ
U.K.

Flower Essence Fellowship
Laura Farm Clinic
17 Carlincott
Peasedown St. John
Bath BA2 8AN
U.K.

Healing Herbs
P.O. Box 65
Hereford HR2 OUW
U.K.

NORTH AMERICA

Dr. Edward Bach Healing Society
644 Merrick Road
Lynbrook, New York 11563
U.S.A.

Ellon (Bach U.S.A.), Inc.
P.O. Box 32
Woodmere, New York 11598
U.S.A.

Vitamins and Minerals

AUSTRALASIA

Australian College of Nutritional and Environmental Medicine
13 Hilton Road
Beamaris, Victoria 3193
Australia

EUROPE

The Council for Nutrition Education of Therapy (CNEAT)
1 The Close
Halton
Aylesbury
Buckinghamshire HP22 5NJ
U.K.

Health Education Authority
Hamilton House
Mabledon Place
London WC1H 9TX
U.K.

Institute of Optimum Nutrition
5 Jerdan Place
London SW6 1BE
U.K.

Society for the Promotion of Nutritional Therapy
P.O. Box 47
Heathfield
East Sussex TN21 8ZX
U.K.

NORTH AMERICA

American College of Advancement in Medicine
P.O. Box 3427
Laguna Hills, California 92654
U.S.A.

Canadian College of Naturopathic Medicine
60 Berl Avenue
Etobicoke, Ontario
Canada M8Y 3C7

National Institute of Nutrition
2565 Carling Avenue, Suite 400
Ottawa, Ontario
Canada K1Z 8RI

INDEX

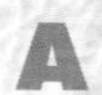

D

E

T

U

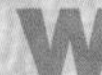

CONTRIBUTORS

KAREN SULLIVAN

is the author of numerous books on alternative health and nutrition including In a Nutshell: Vitamins and Minerals *(Element, 1996). She has also acted as general editor on* The Complete Illustrated Guide to Natural Home Remedies *(Element, 1996), and is health editor of a woman's magazine. She lectures widely on women's health and general health issues. Canadian by birth, she now lives in London with her two sons.*

MARY CLARK

has been a practitioner of healing and esoteric arts for over 20 years. She has studied Ayurveda, nutrition, herbalism, aromatherapy and stress management. Her skills also lie in the area of astrology and consulting the I Ching *with a focus on medical diagnosis. She provides a unique combination of approaches in her work for various corporations in the U.S., including Forbes, Sony, Barnes and Noble, and the Hebrew Hospital System in New York.*

EVE ROGANS

began studying Traditional Chinese Medicine in 1981, starting with acupuncture and moving onto herbalism. She has undergone clinical training in China on two occasions. As well as working in a private practice, where she specializes in pediatric acupuncture, she is also currently working in the field of drug abuse. Eve Rogans is the author of In a Nutshell: Chinese Medicine *(Element, 1997). She lives in London and is married with three children.*

NON SHAW

is a professional herbalist working from a private practice in North London. Trained in the Western herbal tradition, she also has a wide knowledge of other traditions and natural therapies. She teaches herbalism, massage, and Bach Flower Remedies and her written work has included the herbalism and Bach Flower Remedy sections of a range of Element health reference books. She writes for a number of health and women's magazines and is co-founder of a publication for independent herb users.

SHEILA LAVERY

writes widely on healthcare for several prestigious magazines and newspapers in the U.K. Her work, which often focuses on children's health issues, has also been included in various encyclopedias of alternative health. Along with herbalism, aromatherapy is one of her specialties and she is the author of In a Nutshell: Aromatherapy *(Element, 1996).*

PIPPA DUNCAN

is former editor of one of the U.K.'s leading health magazines and now works from home for a variety of monthly publications, including a number devoted to children's health. She has contributed to several reference books on family healthcare including The Complete Family Guide to Alternative Medicine *published by Element. She lives in Richmond with her husband and two children.*